NINTH EDITION

Caffey's Pediatric X-Ray Diagnosis

Volume 1

Walter E. Berdon, M.D.
Professor of Radiology
Columbia University College of Physicians and Surgeons
Director of Pediatric Radiology,
Columbia-Presbyterian Medical Center
Director of Radiology
Babies Hospital
New York, New York

Virgil R. Condon, M.D.
Associate Professor of Radiology and Pediatrics
University of Utah School of Medicine
Chairman, Pediatric Medical Imaging Department
Primary Children's Medical Center
Salt Lake City, Utah

Guido Currarino, M.D.
Professor of Radiology and Pediatrics
University of Texas Southwestern Medical School at Dallas
Radiologist, Children's Hospital Medical Center
Dallas, Texas

Charles R. Fitz, M.D.
Professor of Radiology and Pediatrics
George Washington University
Head, Division of Neuroradiology
Department of Radiology
Children's National Medical Center
Washington, D.C.

John C. Leonidas, M.D.
Professor of Radiology
Albert Einstein College of Medicine
New York, New York
Chief, Pediatric Radiology
Schneider Children's Hospital
New Hyde Park, New York

Bruce R. Parker, M.D.
Professor of Radiology and Pediatrics
Stanford University Medical Center
Stanford, California

Thomas L. Slovis, M.D.
Professor of Radiology
Wayne State University Medical School
Chief, Pediatric Radiology
Children's Hospital of Michigan
Detroit, Michigan

Beverly P. Wood, M.D.
Professor of Radiology and Pediatrics
University of Southern California School of Medicine
Radiologist-in-Chief
Children's Hospital of Los Angeles
Los Angeles, California

NINTH EDITION

Caffey's Pediatric X-Ray Diagnosis: An Integrated Imaging Approach
Volume 1

FREDERIC N. SILVERMAN, M.D.
Professor Emeritus
Diagnostic Radiology and Pediatrics
Stanford University
Stanford, California

JERALD P. KUHN, M.D.
Professor of Radiology
State University of New York at Buffalo
Director, Department of Radiology
Children's Hospital of Buffalo
Buffalo, New York

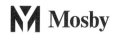 Mosby

St. Louis Baltimore Boston Chicago London Philadelphia Sydney Toronto

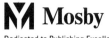

Sponsoring Editor: Anne S. Patterson
Developmental Editor: Elaine Steinborn
Assistant Managing Editor, Text and Reference:
   George Mary Gardner
Production Supervisor: Carol A. Reynolds
Proofroom Manager: Barbara M. Kelly

1 2 3 4 5 6 7 8 9 0 CL MV 97 96 95 94 93

Library of Congress Cataloging-in-Publication Data
Caffey's pediatric X-ray diagnosis: an integrated imaging approach.
   —9th ed. / [edited by] Frederic N. Silverman.
      p.   cm.
   Includes bibliographical references and index.
   ISBN 0-8151-1462-1
   1. Pediatric radiography.   I. Silverman, Frederic N. (Frederic Noah), 1914-   .   II. Caffey, John, 1895-1978.   Pediatric X-ray diagnosis.
   [DNLM: 1. Radiography—in infancy & childhood.   WN 240 C1291]
RJ51.R3C3   1992   92-18838
618.92'007572—dc20   CIP
DNLM/DLC
for Library of Congress

Sharon E. Byrd, M.D.
Associate Professor
Department of Radiology
Northwestern University Medical School
Head, Division of Neuroimaging
Department of Radiology
Children's Memorial Hospital
Chicago, Illinois

Richard B. Jaffe, M.D.
Associate Professor of Radiology and Pediatrics
Pediatric Medical Imaging
Primary Children's Medical Center
Salt Lake City, Utah

Lawrence R. Kuhns, M.D.
Professor of Radiology
Wayne State University Medical School
Pediatric Radiologist
Children's Hospital of Michigan
Detroit, Michigan

Massoud Majd, M.D.
Director, Section of Nuclear Medicine
Diagnostic Imaging and Radiology
Children's National Medical Center
Washington, D.C.

In this ninth edition of *Caffey's Pediatric X-ray Diagnosis* the editors and contributors continue the tradition of a broad-based work that provides both general and specific information necessary for the practice of diagnostic pediatric imaging. The term "x-ray" still is used, because this form of energy remains an important component of the relatively simple as well as the complex equipment and techniques used, and the concept of examination of structures within the body using primarily the sense of sight remains valid, notwithstanding the extensive use of nonionizing energy and computer-generated images. Much of the recent literature in diagnostic imaging has been directed to application of newly developed techniques of examination to specific anatomic, pathologic, and morbid features of disease entities. This is a necessary activity for their evaluation, which in the course of its pursuit also has provided important information on the nature of healthy human variability as demonstrated in images previously unavailable to physicians. Currently, numerous specialized publications are devoted to these types of examination, most of which continue to be developed to augment their already proved effectiveness. As in other medical fields, experience and availability determine selection of the appropriate tool in a given patient. Conventional radiography, however, still is the most widely available and used imaging method and often the first to be used as a diagnostic tool.

The authors have attempted to combine contributions of the imaging revolution with the continuing development of conventional radiographic methods in their applications to both health and disease in a specific age group: infants and children. Continuing as a general reference text, *Caffey's Pediatric X-ray Diagnosis* provides information relating to body systems that may assist in diagnosis in systems other than that being evaluated. Emphasis, as in previous editions, is on clinical correlations. Dr. Caffey used to make the point that, from the standpoint of patient care, images without a clinical history are comparable to findings on percussion by a blindfolded examiner: one method of physical examination used to the exclusion of the others. This concept applies to all the methods now subsumed under the term "body imaging." The strengths of imaging and clinical history are reciprocal, and rest on the clarification each can bring to the other. As always, attention is given to normal findings and to anatomic variations simulating disease. With the aggressive use of investigational tools available today and a litigious environment stimulating defensive practice, it is as important to not suggest erroneously the presence of disease as to miss its recognition.

Many new illustrations reflect the significance of ultrasound, computed tomography, magnetic resonance imaging, and other methods of examination increasingly used. Contributions from colleagues are indicated in the legends; to all we are exceedingly grateful. References have been revised and updated, with care to supplement statements made in the text. In many instances the specific author may not be cited in the text, but the appropriate reference should be recognized easily by the titles listed. We urge the use of listed references because they are informative in greater detail than what could be entered in the text and at times are stimulatingly provocative. They are placed at the end of each section of text in groups corresponding to the sequence of conditions discussed. Conditions noted briefly in one part of the text often are described in detail in another; the carefully developed index addresses these necessary cross referrals.

Several new contributors have been added to our list of authors. Dr. Sharon Byrd has joined Dr. Charles Fitz in a complete revision of the chapter on the brain and spinal cord; Dr. Thomas Slovis has joined Dr. Silverman in revision of the chapters on the neck and upper airway and on the thoracic walls, and also has collaborated with Dr. Kuhn in the chapters on the respiratory system; Dr. Richard Jaffe has prepared the chapters on the heart and great vessels with Dr. Virgil Condon; Dr. Bruce Parker has assumed responsibility for the chapters on the abdomen and gastrointestinal tract; and Drs. Beverly Wood and Massoud Majd have assisted Dr. Guido Currarino in the chapters on the genitourinary tract.

Since the eighth edition of this work and the one-volume *Essentials of Caffey's Pediatric X-ray Diagnosis*, Year Book Medical Publishers, Inc., who published these and all previous editions, has merged with The C.V. Mosby Company to form Mosby–Year Book, Inc., combining the strengths of both organizations. The editors and contributing authors of this edition have enjoyed the same willing support of the new publishing house as of the original. Mr. James D. Ryan of Year Book started us on this project, then turned it over to the able leadership of Mrs. Anne S. Patterson, Executive Editor, and Mrs. Elaine Steinborn, Developmental Editor, of Mosby–Year Book. Their enthusiastic response to our efforts and their professional expertise have helped direct us and have assisted in the preparation of this edition. To the many others of the professional staff of the combined organization who contributed to the production of this book we extend our sincere thanks. And to our friends, co-workers, and especially our families, who have supported our preoccupations and their consequences in relation to ordinary living activities, we are more than grateful.

Frederic N. Silverman, M.D.

Shadows are but dark holes in radiant streams, twisted rifts beyond the substance, meaningless in themselves.

He who would comprehend Röntgen's pallid shades needs always to know well the solid matrix whence they spring. The physician needs to know intimately each living patient through whom the racing black light darts, and flashing the hidden depths reveals them in a glowing mirage of thin images, each cast delicately in its own halo, but all veiled and blended endlessly.

Man—warm, lively, fleshy man—and his story are both root and key to his shadows; shadows cold, silent and empty.—(John Caffey.)

Within a few weeks after Röntgen announced his now renowned discovery to the world in December, 1895, the x-ray method of examination was applied to infants and children. The Vienna letter of February 29 (M. Rec. 49:312, 1896) contained a roentgen print of the arm of an infant made by Kreidl in Vienna: this is the second reproduction of a roentgen image in the American literature. Credit for the first recorded roentgen examination of an infant in the United States undoubtedly belongs to Dr. E. P. Davis of New York City, who described the roentgen shadows cast by the trunk of a living infant and the skull of a dead fetus in March, 1896. In his remarkable article (The study of the infant body and the pregnant womb by the roentgen ray, Am. J. M. Sc. 111:263, 1896) Dr. Davis also included three drawings of shadows visualized by means of a skiascope—shadows of the feet, elbows and orbit of a living infant. Feilchenfeld's discussion of spina ventosa in May, 1896, is probably the first roentgen description of morbid anatomy in children (Berlin. Klin. Wchnschr. 33:403, 1896). There were only two roentgen pediatric publications in 1896; the number increased to 14 in 1897.

In 1898, Escherich of Graz had had sufficient experience with pediatric roentgen examinations to write a general exposition on the merits and weaknesses of the method (La valeur diagnostique de la radiographie chez les enfants, Rev. d. mal. de l'enf. 16:233, May, 1898). This is a highly interesting and illuminating discussion in which Escherich points out that roentgen examination was already not being used as commonly in young patients as in adults. He states that a roentgen laboratory was established especially for children at Graz in 1897, and it seems probable that this was the first of its kind. A single film is reproduced—a print of an infantile hand and forearm which shows rachitic changes. The uncertainties of the mediastinal shadows, which still bedevil us, were fully appreciated by Escherich, and he was quite unhappy about this baffling structure "in which so many important infantile lesions lie concealed." He was enthusiastic in regard to the possible estimation of the state of hydration of soft tissues in infantile diarrhea from their roentgen densities.

Reyher's German monograph in 1908 is the earliest review of the world literature on pediatric roentgenology which I have found (Reyher, P.: Die roentgenologische Diagnostik in der Kinderheilkunde, Ergebn. d. inn. Med. u. Kinderh. 2:613, 1908). In it there are 276 references to articles published during the first 12 years following Röntgen's discovery, and these furnish a good key for the study of the early writings in this field. The appendix contains 40 small but clear roentgen prints.

Rotch's *The Roentgen Ray in Pediatrics* appeared in 1910—the first book in any language devoted exclusively to pediatric x-ray diagnosis and still, I believe, the only one in English. Dr. Thomas Morgan Rotch was Professor of Pediatrics, Harvard University, and an outstanding pediatrist of his time.* In this pioneer treatise he stresses the importance of mastering the shadows of normal structure before attempting

---

*Jacobi, A.: In memoriam Thomas Morgan Rotch, Am. J. Dis. Child. 8:245, 1914.

the recognition and interpretation of the abnormal, and he carefully correlates the clinical findings with the roentgen findings in the cases illustrated; 42 of 264 figures depict the "normal living anatomy of infants and children." This material was taken largely from the files of the Boston Children's Hospital, and the author's statement that more than 2,300 cases were available for study demonstrates that roentgen examination had long been a commonplace in his clinic. Dr. Rotch's early fostering of roentgen examination of infants and children, his appreciation of the special problems in applying this method to the young, his careful anatomicroroentgen studies and his text, monumental for this time, all mark him as the father of pediatric roentgenology in America.

Two years later—1912—the first German book, Reyher's *Das Roentgenverfahren in der Kinderheilkunde*, was published. Later and more familiar texts are Gralka's *Roentgendiagnostik im Kindesalter* (1927), Becker's *Roentgendiagnostik und Strahlentherapie in der Kinderheilkunde* (1931) and the *Handbuch der Roentgendiagnostik und Therapie im Kindesalter* by Engel and Schall (1933). As far as I have been able to determine, no book on pediatric roentgen diagnosis has been published in English during the 35 years which have passed since Rotch's unique publication in 1910. The absence of pediatric roentgenology in the flood of medical texts which has streamed from the American and English presses during the last three decades constitutes a dereliction unmatched in other equally important fields of medical diagnosis—a literary developmental hypoplasia which it is hoped *Pediatric X-Ray Diagnosis* will remedy.

This book stems from the roentgen conferences held semimonthly at the Babies Hospital during the last 20 years. The films reproduced herein were all selected from our own roentgen files save those for which credit to others is indicated in the legends. The purpose of the author is two-fold: description of shadows cast by normal and morbid tissues, and clinical appraisal of roentgen findings in pediatric diagnosis. Roentgen physics, technic and therapy have been omitted intentionally. As references and acknowledgments testify, the writer has borrowed freely from the literature and is indebted to many contributors for subject matter and illustrations. To all of them I am sincerely grateful. In the broad and deep field of pediatric diagnosis, selection of the most appropriate material has posed many dilemmas. In the main, data have been chosen which have proved the most useful and instructive in solving the common and important diagnostic problems which have arisen during two decades in a large and busy pediatric hospital and out-patient clinic.

The limitations of space do not permit adequate recognition here of all those to whom credit is due for the making of this book. The roentgen examinations which are its foundation could not have been made without the cooperation of thousands of patients—many weak and painweary; to all of these I am profoundly thankful. Intimate clinical contacts have been maintained and essential collateral examinations have been made possible through the sustained collaboration of my colleagues—attending physicians and surgeons, resident physicians and nurses. I am under deep and solid obligation to Dr. Rustin McIntosh who read the entire manuscript; his discerning criticism and valuable suggestions are responsible for numerous corrections and improvements in the text. The sympathetic reception given to our early endeavors by Dr. Ross Golden will always be remembered gratefully, as well as his continuing wise and friendly counsel. We have benefited much and often from the discipline of the necropsy table—from the instructive dissections of Dr. Martha Wollstein, Dr. Beryl Paige and Dr. Dorothy Andersen.

To none, however, do I owe more than to my loyal coworkers in the roentgen department of the Babies Hospital—Edgar Watts, Cecelia Peck, Moira Shannon, Mary Fennell and Mary Jean Cadman—for their gentle handling of patients, unfailing industry and superlative technical skill. Mrs. Cadman typed the manuscript; I am grateful to her for the speedy completion of a thorny chore. The drawings are the work of Alfred Feinberg, and they reflect his rich experience in medical illustration.

The final phase in the preparation of the manuscript was saddened by the death of Mr. H. A. Simons, President of the Year Book Publishers. His stimulating enthusiasm and generosity were indispensable to the completion of the book during these unsettled war years. His passing was a grievous loss. The task of publication has fallen to the capable and patient hands of Mr. Paul Perles and Mrs. Anabel Ireland Janssen.

John Caffey
Babies Hospital
New York 32
June 10, 1945

CONTENTS

Volume 1

CONTENTS

Volume 2

PART I

The Skull, Spine, and Central Nervous System

FREDERIC N. SILVERMAN

SHARON E. BYRD

CHARLES R. FITZ

1

The Skull

SECTION 1

Introduction to the Skull

The skull includes the skeletal head and mandible; the cranium is the skeletal head minus the mandible. The skull is divided into three interconnected portions: the neurocranium, the facial area, and the base. The neurocranium includes the calvaria, which is made up of the membranous portions of the occipital, parietal, frontal, and temporal bones, and is bounded inferiorly by the base of the skull, which is made up of the cartilaginous portions of these bones plus the sphenoid and ethmoid bones. The facial area is the portion of the skull between the forehead and the chin including the internal area below and in front of the brain case. The base of the skull is that part which separates the facial area from the calvaria. The neurocranium reflects the growth of the endocranial contents and follows the neural growth curve, whereas the facial area follows the somatic growth curve. The base also follows the somatic curve but does reflect changes secondary to neural growth.

The skull is still examined most commonly by conventional radiography. Computed tomography (CT) is extremely valuable in many circumstances, including closed head trauma with neurologic signs or signs of basilar injury, penetrating and open head trauma, craniofacial malformations, and neoplasms involving bone, among others. Insofar as osseous structures are concerned, nuclear medicine is less frequently used and magnetic resonance imaging (MRI) and ultrasound (US) have little to offer, although MRI is the procedure of choice for intracranial diagnosis. The several modalities may be complementary in special situations.

NEONATAL AND INFANT SKULL

Size and Shape

The neurocranium is larger relative to the face than at any other time during normal growth. Ratios of its respective areas in lateral projection are roughly 3:1 to 4:1 at birth and decrease to 2 to 2.5:1 by the age of 6 years. The bones of the calvaria lie in their incompletely mineralized membranous capsule, separated by broad strips of connective tissue which

form the sutures, and by patches of connective tissue, the fontanelles. The six constant or major fontanelles are located at the four corners of the parietal bones—two in the midline of the skull and two pairs on the sides (Fig 1–1). Accessory fontanelles may occur in several parts of the cranium but are usually located in the sagittal suture. The sutures and the synchondroses in the base are prominent in the newborn, diminishing in width during the first 2 to 3 months. Obliteration of the sutures does not begin until the second to third decades. The several sutures, fontanelles, and synchondroses are illustrated in Figures 1–1 to 1–4. The sphenoid bone at birth consists of three separate components: a single central mass made up of the body and the lesser wings, and two symmetric lateral osseous masses, each of which is made up of a greater wing and a pterygoid process. The pituitary fossa in the body of the sphenoid tends to be round with smooth margins; the dorsum sellae is short and blunt, and the clinoid processes are rudimentary. The angle between the body of the neonatal mandible and the ascending ramus in lateral projection is about 160 degrees; the relatively large bodies are separated in the midline by a prominent cartilaginous symphysis menti (see Fig 1–3). Natal teeth are occasionally present in normal children. Components of the individual bones, ununited in infancy, may lead to confusion in films unless correctly recognized. The frontal bone often is divided into two lateral halves by the metopic suture (see Figs 1–1 and 1–3); apparent discontinuity of the sphenoid bone with the frontal bone superiorly and the occipital bone posteriorly indicates the sites of its synchondroses with these two bones (see Fig 1–2). The four major components of the occipital bone (Figs 1–2 and 1–5) likewise may simulate discontinuities of structure.

Growth and Development

Most of the postnatal growth and differentiation of the skull occur during the first 2 years of life, so that after the 24th month, most of the features of the adult skull are present. During childhood, growth continues at a greatly reduced velocity, but does

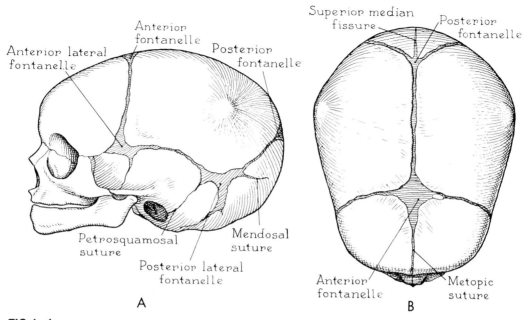

FIG 1–1.
The cranium at birth shows the greater and lesser fontanelles. Lateral **(A)** and superior **(B)** views.

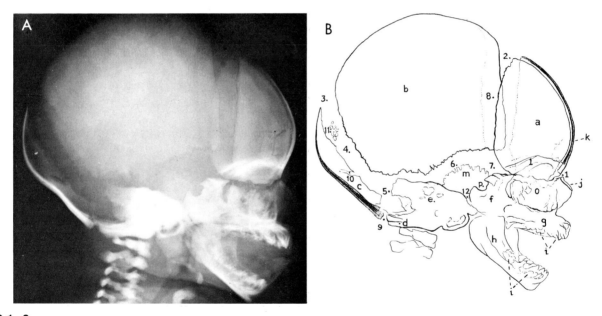

FIG 1–2.
A, roentgenogram of the normal neonatal skull, lateral projection. **B,** tracing of **A.**

a, frontal bone.
b, parietal bone.
c, squamous portion of the occipital bone.
d, exoccipital portion of the occipital bone.
e, superimposed petrous pyramids of the temporal bone.
f, body of the sphenoid.
g, upper maxilla.
h, mandible.
i, partially mineralized deciduous teeth and dental crypts.
j, nasal bone.
k, squamosa of the frontal bone.
l, horizontal plates of the frontal bone.
m, squamosa of the temporal bone.
o, orbit.
p, pituitary fossa.

1, frontonasal suture.
2, anterior fontanelle.
3, posterior fontanelle.
4, lambdoidal suture.
5, posterolateral fontanelle.
6, squamosal suture.
7, anterolateral fontanelle.
8, coronal suture.
9, synchondrosis between exoccipitals and supraoccipital portions of the occipital bone.
10, mendosal suture.
11, multiple ossification centers (wormian bones) in the lambdoidal suture.
12, occipitosphenoid synchondrosis.

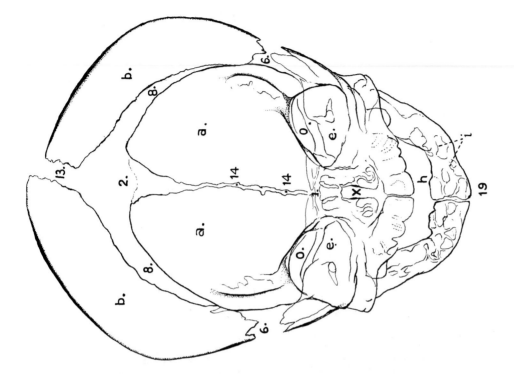

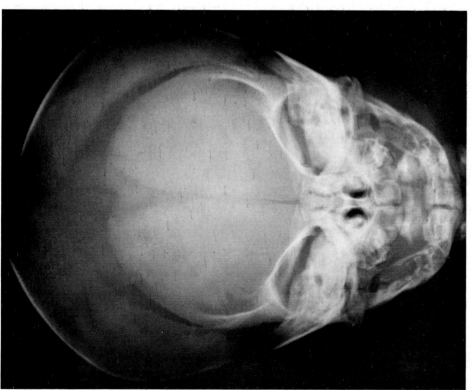

FIG 1–3.
A, roentgenogram of the normal neonatal skull, PA projection. **B,** tracing of **A.**

a, frontal bone.
b, parietal bone.
e, superimposed petrous pyramids of the temporal bone.
h, mandible.
i, partially mineralized deciduous teeth and dental crypts.
o, orbit.
x, nasal septum.

2, anterior fontanelle.
6, squamosal suture.
8, coronal suture.
13, sagittal suture.
14, metopic suture dividing the frontal bone.
19, symphysis of the mandible.

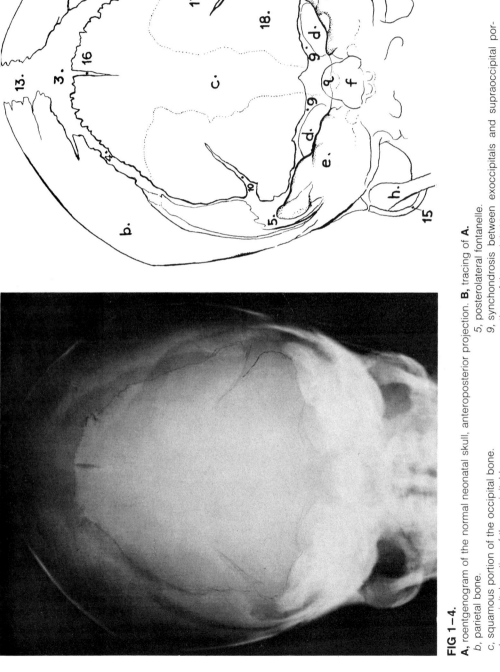

FIG 1–4.

A, roentgenogram of the normal neonatal skull, anteroposterior projection. **B,** tracing of **A.**

b, parietal bone.

c, squamous portion of the occipital bone.

d, exoccipital portion of the occipital bone.

e, superimposed petrous pyramids of the temporal bone.

f, body of the sphenoid.

h, mandible.

g, basioccipital portion of the occipital bone.

3, posterior fontanelle.

4, lambdoidal suture.

5, posterolateral fontanelle.

9, synchondrosis between exoccipitals and supraoccipital portions of the occipital bone.

10, mendosal suture.

13, sagittal suture.

15, zygomatic arch.

16, superior median fissure of the occipital bone.

17, interparietal portion of the occipital bone.

18, supraoccipital portion of the occipital bone.

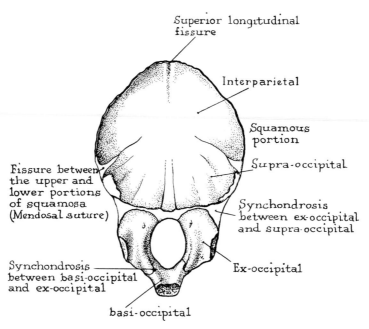

FIG 1–5.
The occipital bone at birth; internal surface.

demonstrate a slight postpubertal spurt. The thickness of the bones increases concomitantly. At about the 20th year, the skull attains its definitive size. The inner and outer tables, the diploic space, vascular markings, and grooves for the dural sinuses on the internal surface of the calvaria all make their appearance by the end of the second year.

With increasing age, the fontanelles and sutures become smaller and narrower. The anterior fontanelle usually is reduced to fingertip size during the first half of the second year; the posterior fontanelle may be closed at birth. No significant differences in size and age at closure were observed by Duc and Largo between term and preterm infants or between

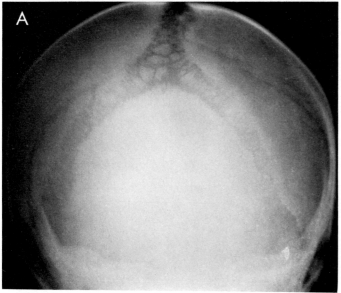

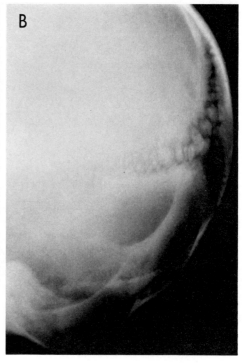

FIG 1–6.
Numerous large and small accessory ossification centers in, **A,** the sagittal and lambdoidal sutures (wormian bones) and, **B,** the posterior fontanelle (intrasutural bones) of a healthy boy 2 weeks of age.

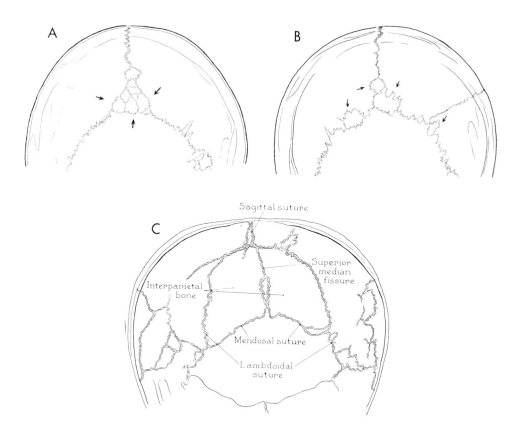

FIG 1–7.
A, multiple wormian bones *(arrows)* in the sagittal suture. **B,** multiple wormian bones *(arrows)* in the sagittal and lambdoidal sutures. **C,** interparietal bone bounded by the lambdoidal and persistent mendosal sutures. The superior median fissure is also still present and divides the interparietal bone into right and left halves. (Tracings of films.)

sexes. The age at closure was not significantly related to any growth parameter or to bone age. Closure of the fontanelles occurs clinically before it does radiographically. The great sutures of the vault do not begin to close anatomically until the middle of the third decade. The metopic suture is usually obliterated during the third year but persists throughout life in about 10% of cases. In the occipital bone, the mendosal suture (see Figs 1–4 and 1–5) usually disappears during the first 2 years, but it too can persist; the synchondrosis between the supraoccipital and exoccipital (supracondylar) portions usually disappears during the second or third year. The spheno-occipital synchondrosis begins to close near the time of puberty; it may persist until the 20th year. The variation and irregularity in disappearance times of suture lines make them unreliable criteria for estimation of the developmental age of the skull.

Variations of Normal

Variations of normal are common and are observed in both newborns and older infants and children. Intrasutural, or wormian, bones occur most frequently along the lambdoidal sutures (Figs 1–6 and 1–7).

They occur much less frequently in the fontanelles (Fig 1–8). The interparietal, or Inca, bone (Figs 1–9 and 1–10) results from division of the supraoccipital portion of the occipital bone into two parts by the mendosal suture, the superior part arising from

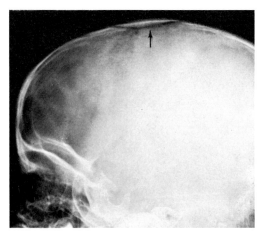

FIG 1–8.
Large independent bone *(arrow)* in the membrane of the anterior fontanelle of a normal girl 2½ years of age. Normal variants of this type must be kept in mind when evaluating films made after cephalic injuries. **(Courtesy of Dr. B.R. Girdany, Pittsburgh.)**

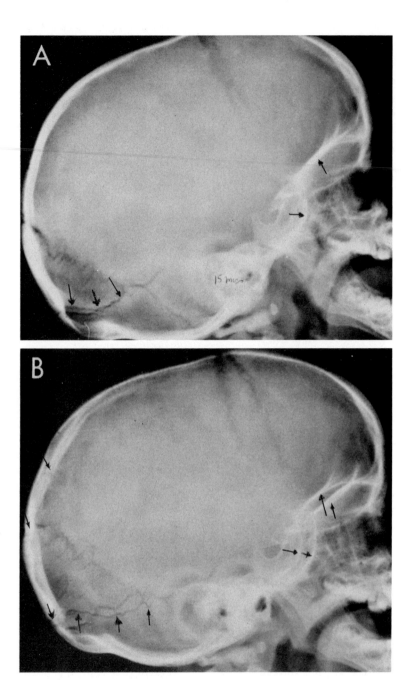

FIG 1–9.

A, direct lateral projection of the normal head of a boy 15 months of age; **B,** lateral projection of the same head with slight rotation on the vertical axis. In **A,** the *anterior arrows* point to the nearly exact overlays of the right and left horizontal plates of the frontal bone and of the right and left greater wings of the sphenoid bone; the *posterior arrows* indicate the right and left mendosal sutures in the occipital squama. The portion above the mendosal sutures is the interparietal (or Inca) bone. In **B,** the *anterior arrows* indicate the separation of the two structures previously superimposed as a result of the rotation. In addition, the overlap of the right and left arms of the mendosal suture has produced a series of small images that suggest four false fracture fragments or four false intrasutural (wormian) bones. The point of continuity of the right and left mendosal sutures is indicated by the *lowest arrow* posteriorly that is directed downward. The *middle posterior arrow* points to the lambda (which can be seen somewhat better in **A**). The *upper arrow* points to a convolutional marking exaggerated by the slight change in projection.

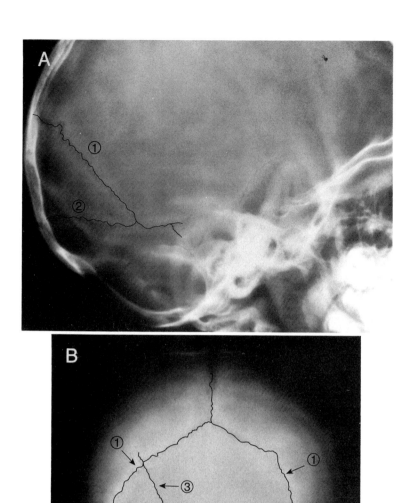

FIG 1–10.
Interparietal or Inca bone. **A,** lateral projection; **B,** AP Towne projection. *1,* right and left lambdoidal sutures; *2,* mendosal suture; *3,* accessory suture in interparietal bone. (Courtesy of Dr. J.P. Dorst, Baltimore, Md.)

membrane bone, and the inferior, from cartilage continuous with that of the supracondylar portions and the basiocciput. Beluffi described radiographic variations of the interparietal bone in a sample of 3,000 to 4,000 children from Italy, comparing them with a similar study in Bulgaria. Parker, in his comprehensive monograph, limits the term *interparietal bone* to that portion between the two limbs of the lambdoidal suture and a suture joining the right and left mendosal sutures that runs horizontally "scarcely 1½ cm above the inion." According to Grob, the term *mendosal* signifies something false or deceitful (viz. mendacious), as the suture is not a true one extending through the outer and inner tables. A rare synchondrosis/suture line runs vertically through the squamous portion of the occipital bone (Fig 1–11); persisting superior and inferior portions of the line are known as the superior longitudinal fissure or bi-interparietal suture, and the cerebellar synchondrosis or median cerebellar suture, respectively. Where the supraoccipital portion of the occipital bone forms the posterior border of the foramen magnum, accessory supraoccipital bones are occasionally found (Figs 1–12 and 1–13). The configuration caused by an outward bulge of the occipital squamosa just above the torcular Herophili in the

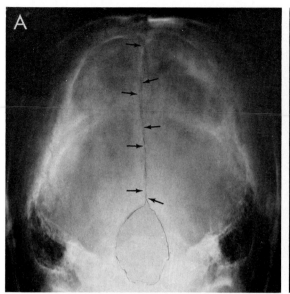
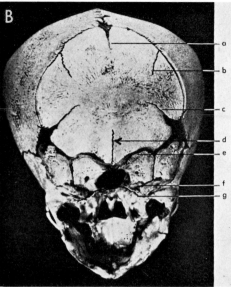

FIG 1–11.

A, Towne projection showing radiolucent midline longitudinal or cerebellar synchondrosis in the occipital squamosa of a girl 11 years of age, which resulted from failure of fusion mediad of its lateral paired ossification centers. This radiolucent strip can be mistaken for a fracture line. (Sutures retouched with pencil.) **B,** persistent longitudinal or cerebellar synchondrosis *(arrow d)* in the oc-

cipital squamosa of a skull of a newborn; only the caudal segment of the synchondrosis is still open in this case. (From Koehler A, Zimmer EA: *Borderlands of the Normal and Early Pathologic in Skeletal Roentgenology,* ed 3. Translated from 11th German ed by Wilk SP. Philadelphia, Grune & Stratton, 1968, p 209.)

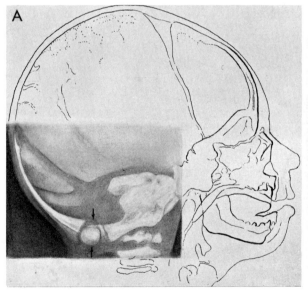
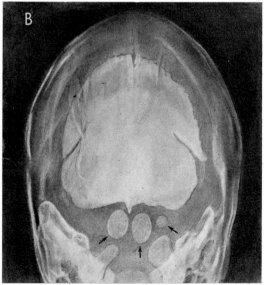

FIG 1–12.

Accessory bones of the supraoccipital bone. **A,** a lateral projection on the second day of life shows separate bony images *(arrows)* in the innominate synchondrosis. **B,** Towne projection of the same skull on the 20th day of life. There are three ossicles *(arrows)* in the

cartilage above the foramen magnum and a midline bony process on the underedge of the supraoccipital that is similar to the fetal process in this same site described by Kerckring (*Spicilegium Anatomicum.* Amsterdam, 1670).

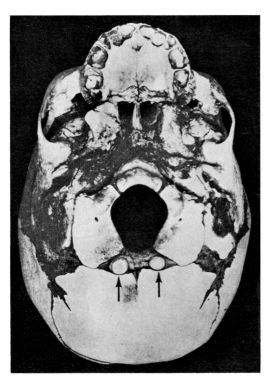

FIG 1–13.
Symmetric occipital ossicles above the foramen magnum in the photograph of a neonatal skull. (From Schulz AH: Anat Rec 1917; 12:357.)

newborn (Fig 1–14) is called *bathrocephaly;* it is believed by some to represent postural deformity resulting from a breech position. Rare anomalies seen in the basiocciput include unilateral or bilateral transverse clefts (Fig 1–15), and a posterior axial cleft that enlarges the foramen magnum anteriorly in the so-called keyhole defect. These are believed to represent remnants of the segmented embryonic spondylocranium that ultimately becomes the occipital bone. In some of the cases of the former type, cranial and cerebral abnormalities have been associated, so that its presence warrants consideration of other craniovertebral abnormalities even though most instances of both types are usually observations incidental to examination for unrelated indications. Associated abnormalities reported are choanal atresia and craniosynostosis. The increasing use of cranial CT may disclose more examples of both types.

Rarely, a horizontal interparietal suture divides the parietal bones into superior and inferior moieties (Fig 1–16). Compression of the fetal skull and its molding during passage through the maternal pelvis produce significant roentgen findings that persist several days after birth (Fig 1–17). During the first weeks and months of life, widths of sutures are so variable that caution is required in their evaluation for the diagnosis of increased intracranial pressure, particularly as positioning is difficult and partial superimposition of bilateral sutures can produce spurious widening (Fig 1–18).

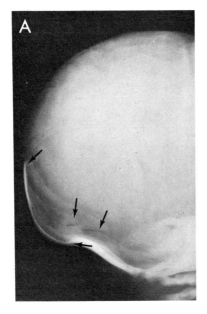

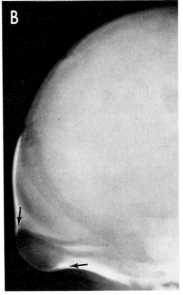

FIG 1–14.
Bathrocephaly in a newborn. **A,** the external bulge *(arrows)* extends from the lambda downward to the level of the mendosal suture of a normal infant 3 days of age. **B,** the bulge *(arrows)* in this normal infant of 5 days of age begins below the mendosal suture.

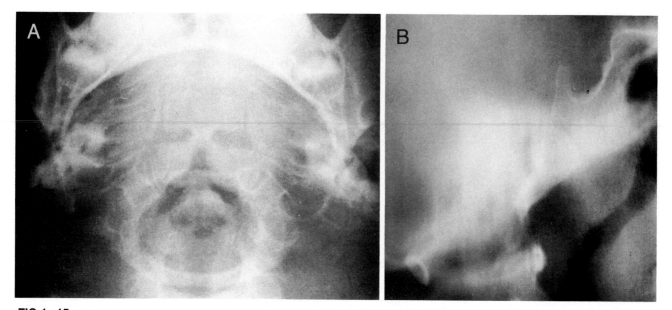

FIG 1–15.
Bilateral transverse clefts in the basiocciput in a 5-year-old, asymptomatic boy. **A,** basilar projection. In addition to the transverse clefts, there is an axial cleft extending toward the isthmus of the anterior and posterior portions of the basioccipital bone (keyhole defect). The axial defect filled in by age 15 but the transverse ones were unchanged. **B,** lateral tomogram at age 5 demonstrating the defect in the basiocciput between the spheno-occipital synchondrosis and the anterior margin of the foramen magnum. (Courtesy of Dr. G. Frank Johnson, Dayton, Ohio.)

In children older than 2 years the sutures extend through both tables and the diploic space. The outer table portion of the suture may be deeply serrated when the inner table portion is practically a straight line (Fig 1–19) and be erroneously interpreted as a "fracture through a suture." Persistence of the metopic suture may simulate a vertical fracture in the occipital bone in anteroposterior (AP), caudally angulated exposures, if extension of the superimposed radiolucent line into the area of the foramen magnum is not visible or if the inferior portion of the suture has been obliterated. The frontal crest on the internal surface of the frontal squamosa in the midsaggital plane may be sufficiently prominent to simulate calcification of the falx cerebri that attaches to it (Fig 1–20).

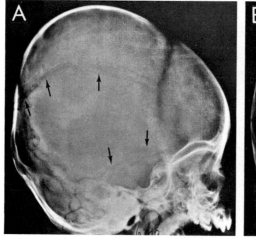
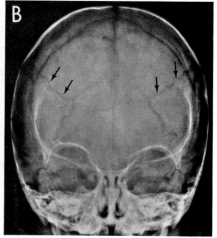

FIG 1–16.
Bilateral bifid parietal bones, each of which is divided into an upper and lower segment by an extra horizontal suture. The flattening of the occipital squamosa is postural in origin. The infant was 6 months of age and had not suffered a head injury. **A,** lateral, and **B,** frontal projections. The *upper arrows* point to the anomalous horizontal intraparietal sutures and the *lower arrows* to the normal squamosal (parietotemporal) sutures. (Courtesy of Dr. B.R. Girdany, Pittsburgh.)

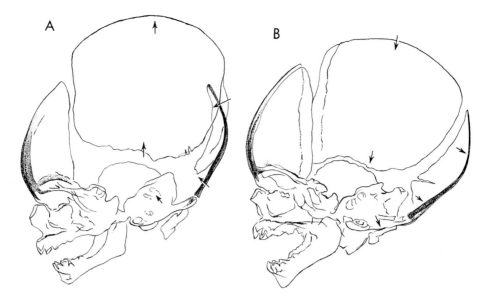

FIG 1–17.
A, tracing of a roentgenogram of the neonatal skull on the first day of life, demonstrating molding of the bones of the calvaria with overlapping of their edges and narrowing of the sutures caused by compression during passage of the head through the birth canal. The parietals are displaced upward, and the temporals and occip-ital are rotated counterclockwise. **B,** tracing of a roentgenogram on the third day of life, showing reexpansion of the cranium and wid-ening of the sutures and fontanelles, as compared with **A,** after the parietal, occipital, and temporal bones have returned to normal po-sitions. (Courtesy of Dr. H.C. Moloy.)

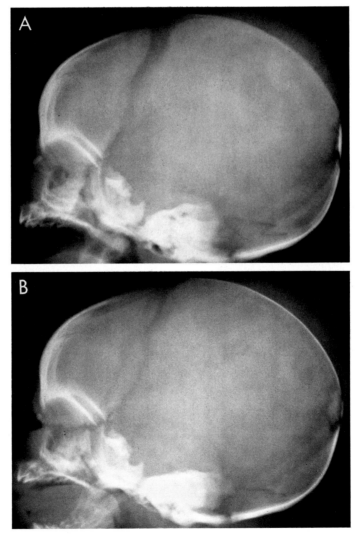

FIG 1–18.
Factitious widening of the coronal suture; **A,** a slightly oblique pro-jection in which the right and left limbs of the coronal suture over-lap; **B,** a little more oblique than **A,** in which the individual narrower right and left limbs are seen.

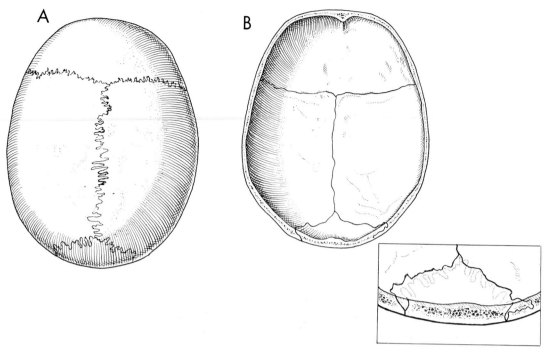

FIG 1–19.
Relation of the outer and inner tables and diploic space of the calvaria to the great sutures. **A,** the external aspect of the calvaria shows deep serrations in sutures of the outer table. **B,** the internal aspect shows the straight nonserrated sutures of the inner table. The inset depicts the lambdoidal suture near the lambda; the differences in position and course of the sutures of the outer and inner tables are shown. In the diploic space, the suture runs in a plane at approximately right angles to the course of the sutures in the tables (drawings of anatomical specimens).

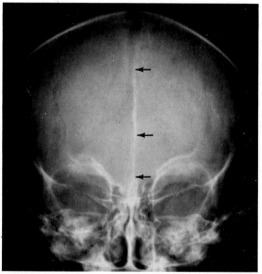

FIG 1–20.
Long, dense, and conspicuous—but normal—frontal crest on the internal surface of the frontal squamosa in its midsagittal plane. In lateral projection, there was no evidence that the falx cerebri behind the frontal crest was prematurely calcified. This boy, 5 years of age, was healthy.

JUVENILE SKULL: ROENTGENOGRAPHIC APPEARANCE

After the child is 2 years of age, the roentgenographic appearance of the skull is similar in most respects to that of the skull during adult life (Fig 1–21). With advancing age, the skull gradually grows and differentiates until late in childhood, when all of the essential characteristics of the adult skull have developed (Figs 1–22 and 1–23).

Normal Variations

The outstanding characteristic of the juvenile skull is its remarkable variability—in size, in shape, in thickness and mineral content, in depth of the grooves for the dural sinuses, in the pattern of the diploic structure and convolutional and vascular markings, in the degree of pneumatization of the temporal and paranasal bones, and in the size and shape of the pituitary fossa—in healthy persons. These normal variants are so marked that it is frequently difficult to distinguish normal variations from early pathologic changes.

A rarely observed anatomical variant of the base is the paracondylar process of the occipital bone (Fig 1–24). This was reported by Brocher in a 39-year-old

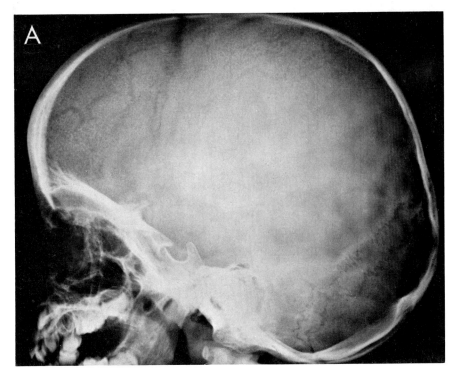

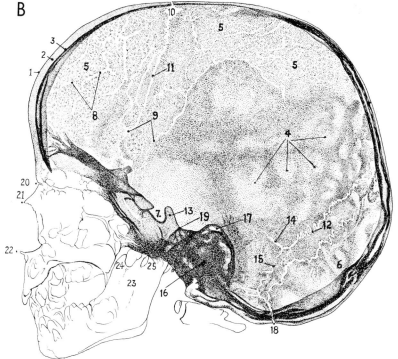

FIG 1–21.
A, roentgenogram of the normal skull at 2 years; lateral projection. **B,** tracing of **A.**

1, outer table.
2, diploic space.
3, inner table.
4, convolutional markings.
5, fine honeycomb of diploic structure.
6, internal occipital protuberance.
7, pituitary fossa.
8, diploic veins.
9, vascular grooves.
10, anterior fontanelle.
11, coronal suture.
12, lambdoidal suture.
13, dorsum sellae.

14, parietomastoid suture.
15, occipitomastoid suture.
16, petrous pyramids.
17, small temporal pneumatic cell.
18, synchondrosis between exoccipital and supraoccipital.
19, spheno-occipital synchondrosis.
20, nasofrontal suture.
21, nasal bone.
22, anterior nasal spine.
23, mandible.
24, coronoid process of the mandible.
25, condyloid process of the mandible.

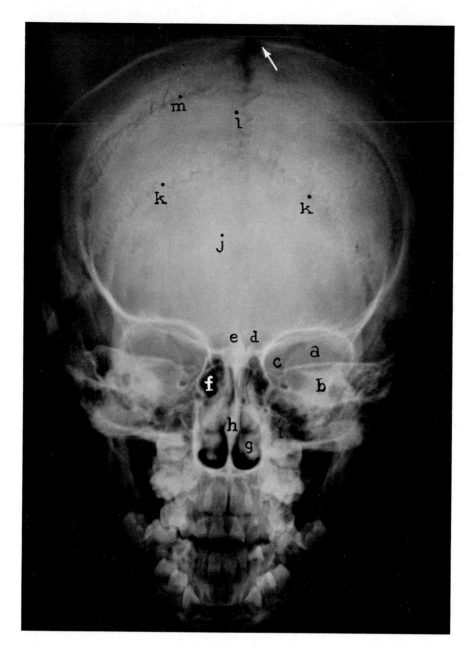

FIG 1–22.
Some roentgen features of the normal skull at 6 years; PA projection.
a, orbit.
b, petrous pyramid.
c, superior orbital fissure.
d, frontal sinus.
e, crista galli.
f, ethmoid cells.
g, inferior turbinate.

h, nasal septum.
i, maxillary sinus.
j, frontal bone.
k, lambdoidal suture.
l, sagittal suture.
m, coronal suture.

man with hemifacial microsomia and multiple segmentation deformities of the spine. The process arises from the lateral aspect of the condyloid process as a mass of bone that may be pneumatized and that extends toward the transverse process of the atlas, with which it may articulate or even fuse. In such cases, pain or torticollis may result. According to anthropologists, the process occurs in 7% to 8% of humans but is seldom reported by radiologists because it is not visible ordinarily by conventional radiography. The process is said to be common in ungulates and rodents but lacking in lower primates.

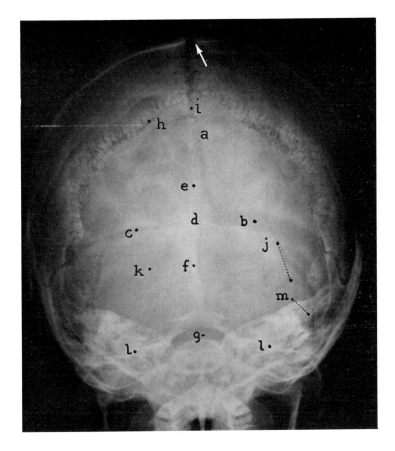

FIG 1–23.
Some important roentgen features of the normal skull at 3 years; AP projection.

a, groove for superior sagittal sinus.
b, groove for right transverse sinus.
c, groove for left transverse sinus.
d, torcular Herophili and superimposed external and internal occipital protuberances.
e, superior half of cruciate ridge.
f, inferior half of cruciate ridge.

g, foramen magnum.
h, lambdoidal suture.
i, lambda.
j, superimposed vascular markings in frontal bone.
k, posterior fossa.
l, petrous pyramid.
m, mastoid pneumatic cells.

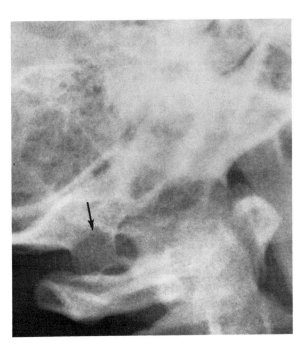

FIG 1–24.
Paracondylar process *(arrow)* in a girl 11 years of age. (Courtesy of Dr. Marie Capitanio, Philadelphia, Pa.)

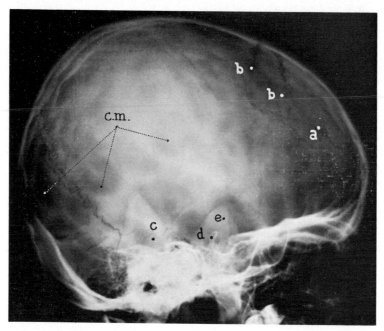

FIG 1–25.
Prominent convolutional markings in an asymptomatic girl 6 years of age: *c.m.*, convolutional markings; *a*, diploic veins; *b*, coronal suture; *c*, squamoparietal suture; *d*, dorsum sellae; *e*, shadow of external ear.

Convolutional (Digital) Markings

These are areas of diminished density in the calvaria that are separated by strips of normal density (Fig 1–25). Vignaud-Pasquier et al. demonstrated very clearly that they correspond very closely to the location and configuration of cerebral convolutions. They are probably formed by localized pressure of the pulsating brain on the inner table of the neurocranium.

Diploic and Vascular Markings

The diploic space between the external and inner tables of the calvaria is filled with a cancellous bony structure that is variable both in volume and pattern and is responsible for the fine, honeycomb texture of the cranial vault. The diploic veins of Breschet lie in large, irregular channels that appear in roentgenograms as irregular strips of diminished density extending through the bones of the vault in all direc-

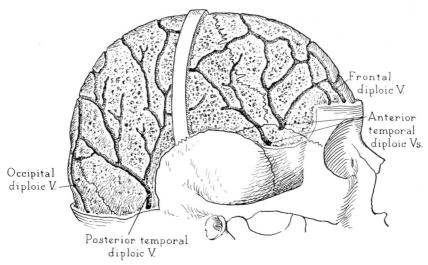

FIG 1–26.
The veins of the diploic space.

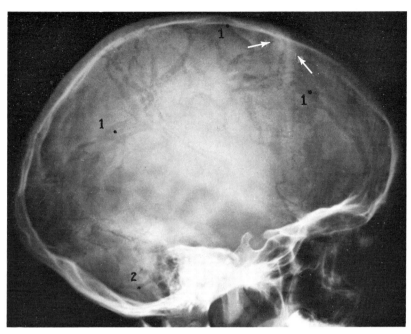

FIG 1–27.
Conspicuous large diploic veins in the frontal and parietal bones in a girl 8 years of age. The veins appear as wide strips of diminished density coursing through the frontal and parietal bones. *Arrows* are directed at the physiologic hyperostotic ridges on either side of the coronal suture. *1,* diploic venous lake; *2,* groove for the emissary vein of the mastoid.

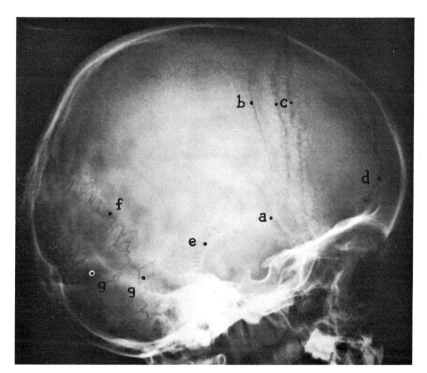

FIG 1–28.
Vascular markings: *a,* grooves for the middle meningeal artery; *b,* parietal diploic vein; *c,* coronal suture; *d,* frontal diploic veins; *e,* squamoparietal suture; *f,* lambdoidal suture; *g,* large groove for the transverse dural sinus.

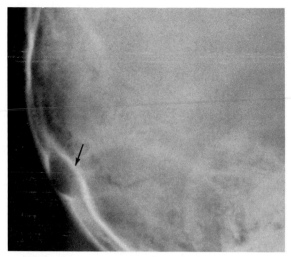

FIG 1–29.
Radiolucent patch in the occipital squamosa cast by an unusually deep sinus confluens (torcular Herophili) and transverse sinus of a healthy boy 11 years of age.

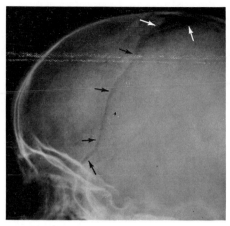

FIG 1–31.
Grooves of the bregmatic veins in a healthy girl, 11 years of age, near the ventral edge of the left parietal bone. This groove may be unilateral or bilateral. (From Lindblom K: *Acta Radiol Suppl (Stockh)* 1936; 30.)

tions (Figs 1–26 and 1–27). They are extremely variable in size, course, and visibility.

The grooves on the internal aspect of the calvaria for the arteries and veins appear in roentgenograms as strips of diminished density (Fig 1–28). Arterial grooves tend to taper more than the venous. The most constant of these channels is that of the middle meningeal artery, which courses upward and backward from the region of the pterion, where it may be surrounded by bone of the inner table. The largest and heaviest vascular markings on the internal surface of the calvaria are the bony thin-

nings over the venous sinuses of the dura mater. The superior sagittal sinus lies in a shallow groove on the internal surface at the median plane of the vault near the attachment of the falx cerebri. At the torcular Herophili, the channels for the superior longitudinal and transverse sinuses meet; one transverse sinus may be appreciably larger and deeper than the other (see Fig 1–23). The torcular Herophili in lateral projections may simulate an abnormal defect when it is unusually deep (Fig 1–29). At the bend where the transverse sinus turns caudad, near the mastoid process, superimposition of the lateral end of the sulcus of the transverse sinus and the sulcus of the sigmoid sinus may produce a rounded, ra-

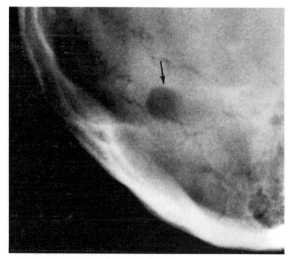

FIG 1–30.
Radiolucent patch *(arrow)* due to the superimposition of the sulci of an unusually deep transverse sinus and lateral sinus at their junction where the transverse sinus turns caudad. The patient was a healthy boy, 10 years old.

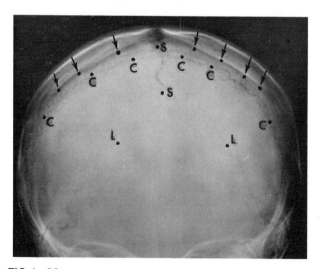

FIG 1–32.
Radiolucent grooves *(arrows)* for the left and right bregmatic veins in a healthy boy 2½ years of age. *L,* lambdoidal suture; *S,* sagittal suture; *C,* coronal suture.

diolucent patch when these sulci are unusually deep (Fig 1–30). Often, the groove for the bregmatic vein is seen as a conspicuous strip of diminished density on one or both lateral walls of the calvaria (Figs 1–31 and 1–32); this groove has also been called the sphenoparietal sinus, which is a misnomer here as the true sinus runs underneath the lesser wing of the sphenoid bone and does not always communicate with the bregmatic vein.

REFERENCES

Beluffi G: Os incae (l'osso dell' Inca). *Radiol Med* 1981; 67:135–140.

Bergerhoff W: *Atlas of Normal Radiographs of the Skull.* Berlin, Springer-Verlag. 1961.

Brocher JEW: Le processus paracondyleus s. apophyse paramastoïde (dans un cas de dysostose mandibulo-faciale unilatérale) *Radiol Clin* 1947; 16:392–396.

Caffey J: On the accessory ossicles of the supraoccipital bone: Some newly recognized roentgen features of the normal infantile skull. *Am J Roentgenol* 1953; 70:401–412.

Chasler CN: *Atlas of Roentgen Anatomy of the Newborn and Infant Skull.* St Louis, Warren H Green, 1972.

Duc G, Largo RH: Anterior fontanel size and closure in term and preterm infants. *Pediatrics* 1986; 78:904–908.

Etter LE: *Atlas of Roentgen Anatomy of the Skull.* Springfield, Ill, Charles C Thomas 1955.

Girdany BR, Blank E: Anterior fontanelle bones. *Am J Roentgenol* 1965; 95:148–153.

Grob M: Über die roentgenologischen Nahtverhältnisse der hintern Schädelgrube beim Kinde mit spezieller Berück-sichtigung der Sutura mendosa. *Fortschr Roentgenstr* 1938; 57:265–275.

Haberkern CM, Smith DW, Jones KL: The "breech head" and its relevance. *Am J Dis Child* 1979; 133:154–156.

Jacobson RI: Abnormalities of the skull in children. *Neurol Clin* 1985; 3:117–145.

Johnson GF, Israels H: Basioccipital clefts. *Radiology* 1979; 133:101–103.

Köhler A, Zimmer EA: *Borderlands of the Normal and Early Pathologic in Skeletal Roentgenology,* ed 10. Philadelphia, Grune & Stratton, 1956.

Kruyff E: Transverse cleft in the basiocciput. *Acta Radiol* 1967; 6:41–48.

Moloy HC: Studies on head molding during labor. *Am J Obstet Gynecol* 1942; 44:962–982.

Parker CA: *Wormian Bones.* Chicago, Roberts Press, 1905.

Pierce RH, Mainen MW, Bosma JF: *The Cranium of the Newborn Infant. An Atlas of Tomography and Anatomical Sections.* Bethesda, Md, US Department of Health, Education, and Welfare, 1978.

Popich GA, Smith DA: Fontanels, range of normal size. *J Pediatr* 1972; 80:749–752.

Silverman, FN: Some features of developmental changes observed clinically in the sphenoid and basicranium, in Bosma JF (ed): *Symposium on Development of the Basicranium.* DHEW Publication No (NIH) 76–989, 1976.

Vignaud-Pasquier J, Lichtenbert R, Laval-Jeantet M, et al: Les impressions digitales de la naissance à neuf ans. *Biol Neonate* 1964; 6:250–276.

Woon K-C, Kokich VG, Clarren SK, et al: Craniosynostosis with associated cranial base anomalies: A morphologic and histologic study of affected like-sexed twins. *Teratology* 1980; 22:23–35.

SECTION 2

Congenital Dysplasias

Involvement of the skull in generalized skeletal dysplasias is discussed in Part 4 in relation to the specific disorders. Eteson and Stewart have described craniofacial disorders associated with several dysplasias and offer insights into possible pathogenetic mechanisms.

CRANIOSCHISIS OR CRANIUM BIFIDUM

Cranioschisis, or cranium bifidum, usually occurs in the median sagittal plane, anteriorly or posteriorly (Fig 1–33). Both sites are characterized by bony defects and may accompany meningocele or meningo-

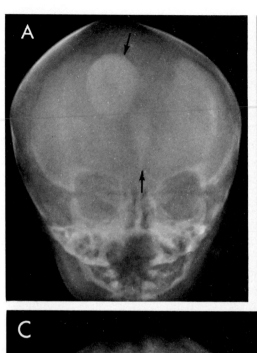

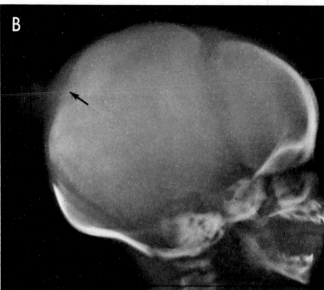

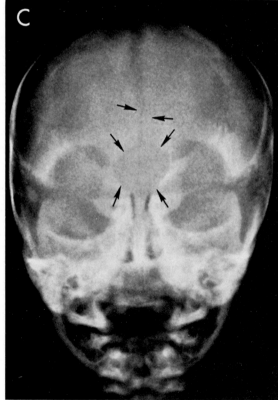

FIG 1–33.
Intrafrontal and interparietal cranium bifidum in the metopic suture and in the sagittal suture, with protrusion of a soft tissue sac (meningoencephalocele) at both anterior and posterior sites. **A,** frontal, and **B,** lateral projections. This girl was 2 days of age. The metopic suture is also widely open, and a smaller mass of soft tissue bulges externally between the two sides of the frontal squamosa. In **A,** the larger·superior patch of increased density *(upper arrow)* represents the interparietal protrusion and the lower small patch *(lower arrow)* represents the smaller and shallower intrafrontal protrusion. **C,** large circular bone defect (cranium bifidum) at the glabella in a widely open metopic suture. A lump of soft tissue bulged externally at this site. The patient was 11 days of age.

encephalocele. In meningoceles, a hernial sac (Fig 1–34) is covered with skin and contains only meninges and cerebrospinal fluid. As the name implies, meningoencephaloceles also contain brain (Fig 1–35). Rarely, cranioschisis or cranium bifidum may be associated with a scalp nodule only, with or without intracranial communication. Occasionally, small cranial defects are encountered through which there

is no herniation—cranium bifidum occultum (Fig 1–36). CT and MRI are most effective for evaluation.

Cranium bifidum with encephalocele often occurs in the sphenoid bone or in the cribriform plate of the ethmoid. In such cases, the protruding mass of brain and covering meninges may extend into the nasal cavity, nasopharynx, sphenoid sinus, posterior portion of one orbit, or into one of the pterygoid fos-

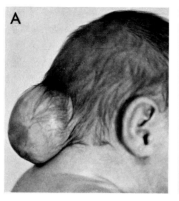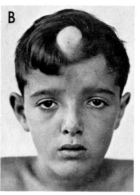

FIG 1–34.
Photographs of meningoceles. **A,** occipital meningocele in an infant 1 week of age. **B,** frontal meningocele in a boy 9 years of age.

sae. Important clinical signs include facial deformity (ocular hypertelorism) and broadened base of the nose. These conditions are discussed in more detail in Chapter 3.

LACUNAR SKULL OF NEWBORN (LÜCKENSCHÄDEL, CRANIOLACUNIA)

Lacunar skull develops during fetal life and is present at birth. It has been identified in films of the pregnant uterus, late in the gestational period. It is practically always associated with myelocele or encephalocele with associated meningocele, and with the Arnold-Chiari (Chiari II) malformation. The cause is not known but it is probably a dysplasia of the calvaria and its internal periosteum (i.e., the dura). It is not caused by fetal increased intracranial pressure, as it is found in heads that are normal or small in size without evidence of hydrocephalus. The characteristic "soap-bubble" rarefactions in the

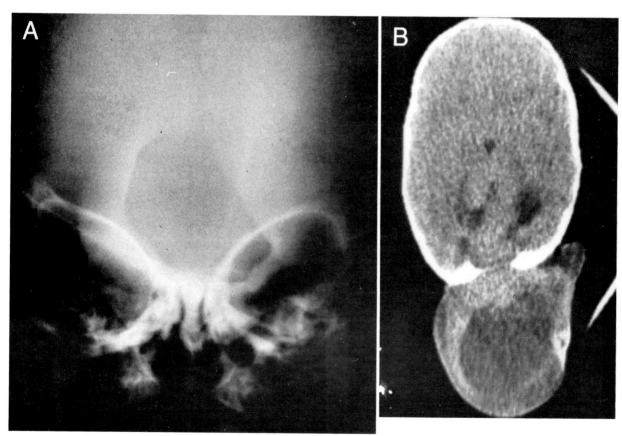

FIG 1–35.
Cranium bifidum in association with occipital cephalocele in an infant who also had macrocrania. **A,** the osseous defect was in continuity with the foramen magnum. A Dandy-Walker cyst protruded through the bony defect. **B,** CT of a 2-day-old boy with an encephalocele that was both supratentorial and infratentorial. The hernial sac contained occipital lobes and part of the cerebellar hemispheres as well as a large central cyst. (From Diebler C, Dulac O: *Pediatric Neurology and Neuroradiology.* New York, Springer-Verlag, 1987, pp 51–67. Used by permission.)

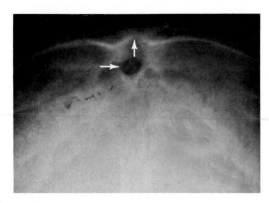

FIG 1–36.
Small round bony defect at the posterior end of the sagittal suture *(horizontal arrow)* in a patient 7 years of age, without protrusion of a hernial sac (cranium bifidum occultum). The *vertical arrow* points to the groove for the sagittal sinus.

upper part of the calvaria are easily recognized (Fig 1–37). These begin to fade after birth and usually disappear by the fourth or fifth month, notwithstanding progressive hydrocephalus in some instances. The normal convolutional rarefactions differ from the lacunar rarefactions in that they are not obvious until the end of the first year and tend to appear first in the posterior and lower lateral portions of the calvaria. The irregular, marked thinning of the bone in craniolacunia is clearly demonstrated in CT scans.

SYMMETRIC PARIETAL FORAMINA

About 60% of skulls show small defects in the superior posterior angles of the parietal bones through which emissary veins penetrate the calvaria. The veins generally communicate with the sagittal sinus internally and tributaries to the occipital veins externally. These small openings are the parietal foramina. Occasionally, large bone defects are present in these regions of the parietal bones, and these have been called enlarged parietal foramina. They are occasionally palpable on each side of the midline and, less frequently, are united to form a large, single defect (Fig 1–38). The defects result from a failure of mineralization of the membranous bone in this region and, in this sense, the term *enlarged parietal foramina* is a misnomer. They are usually not associated with other skeletal anomalies and have no clinical significance except in differential diagnosis of cranial defects such as those associated with meningocele, infection, certain types of histiocytosis, and such. Nevertheless, they have been reported in one case in which meningoceles protruded through them and, in an autosomal dominant familial form, were associated with hypoplasia of the lateral portions of the clavicles and acromial absence as well as other cranial dysmorphic features. Large parietal foramina have been recognized as an inherited trait ever since Goldsmith found them in 56 members of the Catlin family, giving rise to the term "Catlin mark." Lesions may persist throughout life, although they generally tend to become smaller and may be completely obliterated. Focal sclerotic residuals may remain in the areas where foramina have become obliterated. Nashold and Netsky classify radiologic defects in the area as due to parietal emissary foramina, parietal fenestrae, or parietal thinning. Somewhat similar, vascular-like defects have been

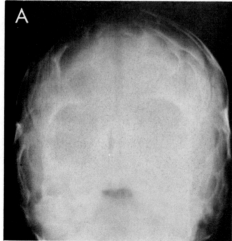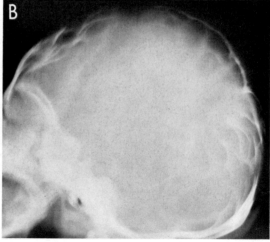

FIG 1–37.
Lacunar skull on the second day of life, associated with occipital meningocele. **A,** frontal, and **B,** lateral projections. All bones in the calvaria show checkered rarefaction separated by bands of heavier density. The shadow pattern resembles the mottling of beaten copper or silver.

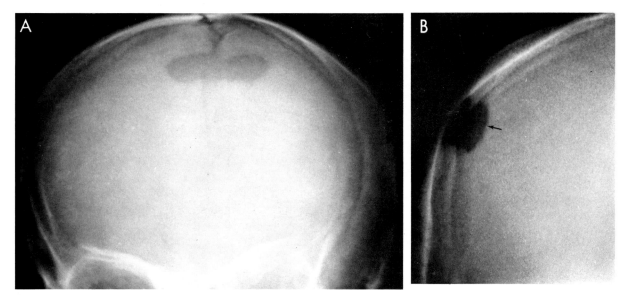

FIG 1–38.
Persistent interparietal fontanelle (parietal foramen) *(arrow)* in an otherwise healthy boy 5 years of age. **A,** frontal, and **B,** lateral projections.

described in the supracondylar portion of the occipital bone in a father and son. Currarino has reviewed the major, and some uncommon, normal variants and congenital anomalies in this region of the skull.

SINUS PERICRANII

This term is given to a soft, fluctuant mass, often of a red to blue color, observed in the scalp over the region of the sagittal or transverse sinuses. It responds in size to maneuvers that tend to increase intracranial pressure and may be associated with an underlying bony defect of the calvaria. It results from an abnormal communication between the intracranial and extracranial venous systems and its significance is only cosmetic. Confusion with lesions of more serious import warrants awareness of the condition that must be differentiated from arteriovenous malformations, angiomas and hemangiomas, sebaceous or dermoid cysts, meningocele, encephalocele, and abscess.

PREMATURE CRANIOSYNOSTOSIS

The basic clinical and radiologic features of this condition result from premature fusion of contiguous portions of calvarial bones across the membranous sutures between them. The sutures permit growth of the skull in a direction perpendicular to their long axis; consequently, with normal endocranial stimulus to growth, cessation in one suture is compensated by increased growth in others, resulting in de-

formity. Specific deformities follow premature synostosis of individual sutures and even combinations of sutures when their involvement is temporally related (Figs 1–39 to 1–41). Because the sagittal suture permits growth in width of the skull, its premature obliteration leads to a neurocranium that is high, long, and narrow (dolichocephaly) (Figs 1–42 and 1–43). Involvement of both limbs of the coronal suture results in a cranium that is high, wide, and decreased in length (brachycephaly) (Fig 1–44). Premature synostosis of one limb of the coronal suture results in an asymmetric pattern (plagiocephaly) (Fig

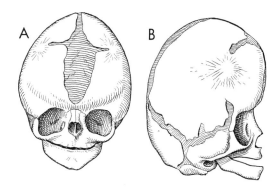

FIG 1–39.
Premature synostosis of the coronal suture; schematic representation. The suture is obliterated save for short, open terminal segments and open segments near the sagittal suture and anterior fontanelle. Radially striated ossification centers obliterate the rest of the coronal suture. The metopic, sagittal, lambdoidal, and temporoparietal sutures are all widely open. The calvaria is shortened ventrodorsally and elongated in the other axes. **A,** frontal aspect; **B,** lateral aspect.

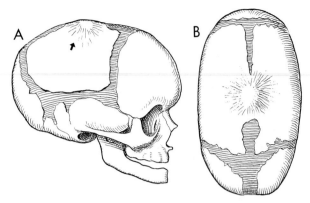

FIG 1–40.
Schematic drawings of premature synostosis of the sagittal suture, the central segment of which is filled with a radially striated ectopic ossification center. **A,** lateral aspect; **B,** superior aspect.

1–45); and a small, peaked anterior portion of the neurocranium with a relatively large posterior portion (oxycephaly) indicates premature synostosis of the sagittal and coronal sutures (Fig 1–46). Trigonocephaly is associated with premature synostosis of

the metopic suture that usually occurs before birth. It is also associated with ethmoid hypoplasia and, consequently, orbital hypotelorism (see Figs 1–50 and 1–51). It is of significance only in the rare occasion when there is, in addition, cerebral abnormality belonging to the holoprosencephalic group of malformations. The triangular-shaped forehead tends to become less obvious with age, and surgical intervention is neither necessary nor desirable. The lambdoidal suture may be synostosed alone (Fig 1–47) or on one or both sides in combination with other synostoses. If all the calvarial sutures are prematurely synostosed, a small neurocranium (microcrania) results (Fig 1–48). When bony union across individual sutures takes place at different times, bizarre cranial configurations may result that defy simple analysis. In many instances, deformities occur in the basilar and facial structures as associated or secondary phenomena. Currarino reported simulation of unilateral coronal synostosis by premature closure of the frontozygomatic suture together with possible involvement of the zygomaticosphenoidal and frontosphe-

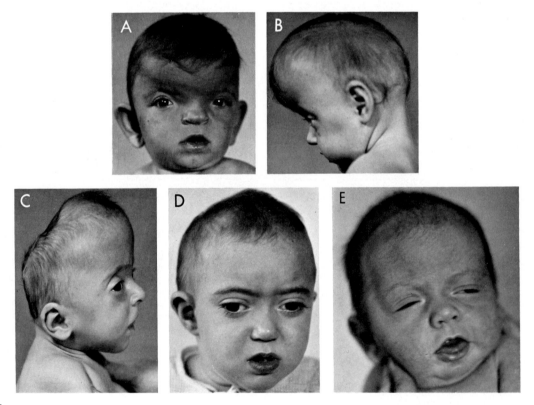

FIG 1–41.
The head and face in craniostenosis. **A,** the high, wide cranium of the brachycephalic type in a patient 8 months of age. Ocular hypertelorism is also present; there is a striking increase in width of the interorbital space. **B,** the long, narrow cranium of the dolichocephalic type in an infant 9 months of age with associated unilateral syndactylism. **C,** the high, pointed cranium of the oxycephalic type in an infant 3 months of age. **D,** the generally small cranium of

the microcephalic type in a patient 3 years of age who had severe optic atrophy and increased intracranial pressure. **E,** the asymmetric cranium of the plagiocephalic type in an infant 1 month of age. The ridge of bone along the margin of the open right half of the coronal suture is visible; the base of the left side of the coronal suture is prematurely closed.

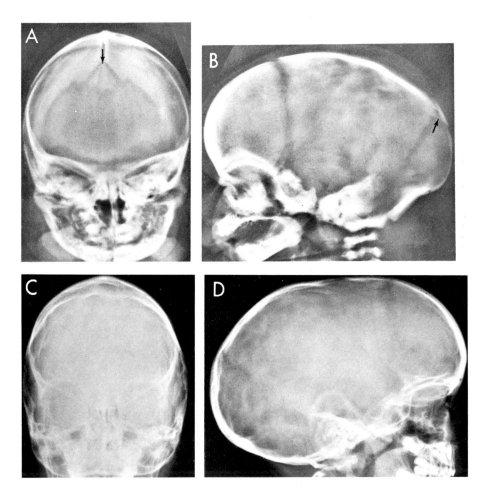

FIG 1–42.

Premature synostosis of the sagittal suture with elongation of the calvaria ventrodorsally, a decrease in the transverse axis of the calvaria, and relative (to length) decrease in vertical height. The sagittal suture is ridged externally. A sutural bone is present in the region of the posterior fontanelle (*arrows,* **A** and **B**). This infant was 2 days old. The coronal suture is widened, and the lambdoidal and squamosal sutures are normally wide, as is the squamocondyloid synchondrosis at the base of the occipital squamosa. **A,** frontal, and **B,** lateral projections. Similar changes are evident in the more mature skull of a girl 11 months of age. **C,** frontal, and **D,** lateral projections.

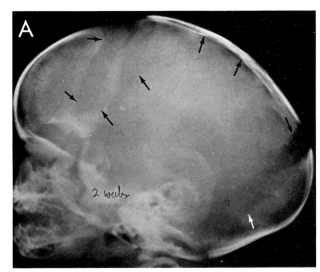

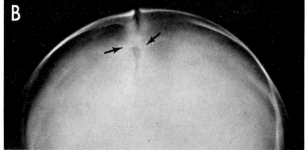

FIG 1–43.

Severe craniostenosis of the scaphocephalic type due to premature synostosis of only a short segment of the sagittal suture of an infant 2 weeks of age. In **A,** lateral projection, deformity due to the craniostenosis is clearly seen, but the sagittal suture itself is invisible. Coronal and lambdoidal sutures are widened, which suggests actively increased intracranial pressure. In **B,** frontal projection, the sagittal suture is visible in its entirety and is open save for a short segment only a few millimeters long.

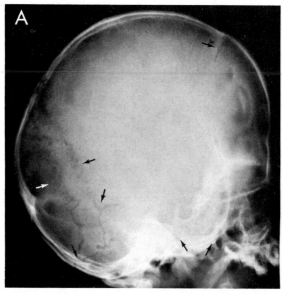

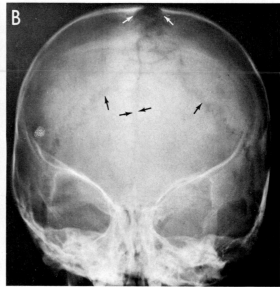

FIG 1–44.
Roentgenographic findings in the brachycephalic type of cranio-stenosis in a patient 13 months of age. **A,** lateral projection; **B,** frontal projection. The coronal suture is obliterated except for a short segment near the vertex. The AP diameter of the skull is shortened, and the vertical and lateral diameters are elongated.

There is no roentgenographic evidence of increased intracranial pressure. The sagittal, lambdoidal, and metopic sutures are open, as is the spheno-occipital synchondrosis at the base *(arrows)*. The orbital roofs and the greater wings of the sphenoid are elevated laterad.

noidal sutures. The ipsilateral coronal suture was not affected. Bertelsen first noted that the coronal, frontosphenoidal, and frontoethmoidal sutures form a continuous ring so that premature synostosis in any part of it can inhibit growth in the remainder.

Seeger and Gabrielsen stressed the role of fron-tosphenoidal synostosis in the radiologic evaluation of coronal synostosis.

Premature synostosis may be primary or second-ary. It is now generally accepted that abnormalities

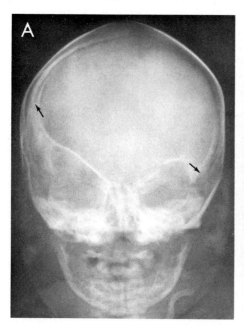

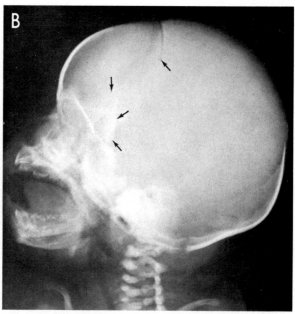

FIG 1–45.
Premature synostosis of the caudal segment of the right limb of the coronal suture in an infant 3 weeks of age. In **A,** frontal projection, the *arrows* are directed at the caudal ends of the right and left limbs of the coronal suture. The roof of the right orbit is lifted into a

more oblique position, as is the right wing of the sphenoid. In **B,** lateral projection, the right limb of the coronal suture stops abruptly a few centimeters below the anterior fontanelle. The lifting of the right orbital roof is also well seen *(two lower arrows)*.

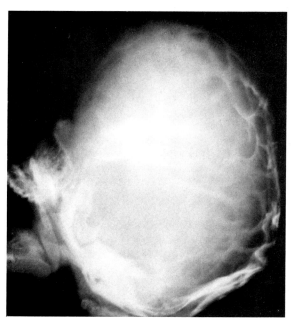

FIG 1–46.
Roentgenographic findings in the oxycephalic type of craniostenosis in a patient 3 months of age; lateral projection. The cranium is small and has a remarkably long vertical diameter. The deep convolutional markings indicate long-standing, severely increased intracranial pressure. The anterior fontanelle is widely open and bulging, and the margins flare outward. The synchondroses at the base are open.

toses occurs in association with other malformations and as components of syndromes, suggesting a widespread mesenchymal defect (Park and Powers). Syndromic craniostenosis is frequently combined with hydrocephalus as an associated rather than a derivative malformation. Secondary premature synostosis has resulted from rapid decompression of hydrocephalus through shunting procedures. Other instances of secondary synostosis are observed in rickets, particularly vitamin D–resistant rickets, hypophosphatasia, hypercalcemia, and primary hyperthyroidism or that secondary to overtreatment of hypothyroidism. The suggestion has been offered that hypersensitivity to, or intoxication with, vitamin D_3 is responsible for the craniosynostosis, at least in vitamin D–resistant rickets. Intrauterine constraint of the fetal head has been suggested as a cause of most instances of sporadic craniosynostosis (Graham et al.). The most common cause of secondary generalized craniosynostosis is cerebral maldevelopment.

in the base of the skull and the dural reflections are responsible for primary premature union of the calvarial bones (Moss; Smith and Töndury). However, corrective changes of the cranial base after correction of unicoronal synostosis (Marsh et al.) may indicate instances in which the basilar sutures are not involved. Another group of primary premature synos-

Cranial deformities mimicking premature synostosis may result from static forces such as prolonged recumbency that may be associated with occipital flattening (Fig 1–49). This may reflect either delayed motor development or mechanical restraints such as orthotic devices. The flattening is exaggerated in the soft heads of children with rickets or osteogenesis imperfecta. Plagiocephaly occurs as a result of postural stresses in torticollis. In contradistinction to that due to premature synostosis of one limb of the coronal suture, in which facial deformity is not present early, plagiocephaly due to torticollis does result in facial asymmetry. In the former, the ears are opposite each other when viewed from above, whereas they differ in size and position in the latter.

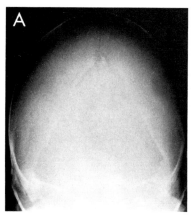
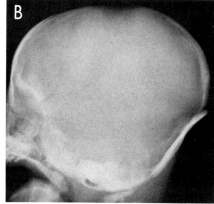

FIG 1–47.
Premature closure and ridging of the caudal two thirds of the lambdoidal suture and flattening of the occipital squamosa in an infant 1 month old. The uppermost segment of the lambdoidal suture is still open, and a small sutural bone is visible at the lambda itself.

The sides of the occipital squamosa are straight rather than convex, and the squamosa is narrower than is normal. **A,** AP, and **B,** left lateral projections.

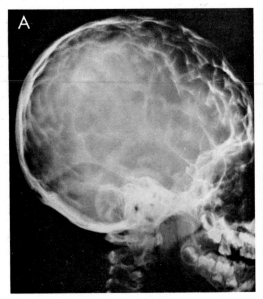 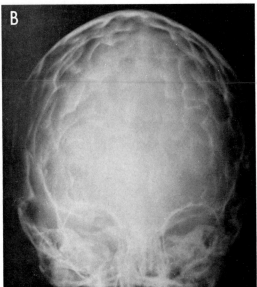

FIG 1–48.
Roentgenographic findings in the microcephalic type of craniostenosis in a patient 7 years of age. **A,** lateral, and **B,** frontal projections. All sutures of the cranium are obliterated and the skull is shortened in all its diameters. The long-standing increased intracranial pressure is indicated by the heavy convolutional markings.

Postural plagiocephaly can also result from persistent prone or supine positions in early life and may respond to positional changes or other mechanical forces. In postural plagiocephaly, three-dimensional reformatted CT images show fairly straight alignment of the metopic and sagittal sutures; with unicoronal synostosis, the metopic suture deviates toward the affected side.

The radiographic findings reflect the deformities of the cranium observed clinically. Obliteration of affected sutures may be observed. Basilar projections may demonstrate a decreased sphenopetrosal angle when frontosphenoidal synostosis complicates coronal synostosis. Closure of only a short segment of a suture is as effective in preventing separation of the opposing bones as is total obliteration (see Fig 1–43); identification of the actual site of synostosis in some cases may require special tangentially oriented projections or CT. Failure of growth at a suture may precede actual bony continuity across it. Often, sclerosis along one or both borders of a suture can be observed in instances of impending bony union. Increased convolutional markings are common, particularly when cranial expansion is limited and multiple sutures are involved. Increased intracranial pressure has been documented in many instances; hydrocephalus is somewhat less frequent. The most severe manifestations of increased intracranial pressure occur in primary synostosis of all the sutures (see Fig 1–48). The extreme degree of convolutional markings in such cases clearly differentiates them from those in which the condition is secondary to cerebral underdevelopment in which the inner table usually is smooth. Disturbances of cerebrospinal fluid circulation have been demonstrated with radionuclide scans with human serum albumin tagged with [131]I. Scans with ^{99m}Tc methylene diphospho-

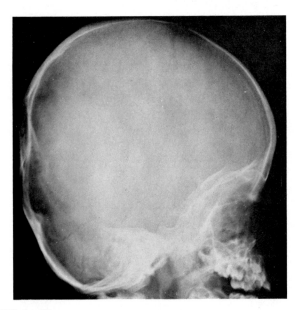

FIG 1–49.
Postural occipital flattening of the skull, in an infant 22 months of age, that resembles coronal suture premature synostosis (see Fig 1–44) in general contour. In this skull, however, the coronal sutures are open, the anterior fossa is deep, and the posterior fossa is shallow.

nate (MDP) have also been used to identify abnormal bone formation in cranial sutures. Correlation with radiographs and surgical findings indicated that the scan was not helpful when the radiograph was normal but was of value when the radiograph was abnormal to confirm fusion and detect other abnormal sutures.

Most of the radiographic features described above are better demonstrated with CT than by conventional radiography, but the former, especially three-dimensional CT, can be limited to cases in which findings are not clearly positive or negative, or to cases of complex, syndromic, craniofacial anomalies. The improved anatomical detail of three-dimensional CT facilitates the planning for surgical correction. The majority of patients treated surgically for sagittal synostosis demonstrate complete reossification within the first postoperative year. In the case of the other sutures, the process takes longer.

Trigonocephaly is the term applied to a triangular-shaped cranium, as viewed from above, that may be so narrow anteriorly that it results in a keel-shaped vertical ridge in the narrow forehead (Figs 1–50 and 1–51). The condition is probably always associated with premature closure of the metopic suture. Radiographic attempts to demonstrate the continuity of bone across the suture are probably not warranted, as surgical correction is not necessary and associated radiographic features in the width of the ethmoid bone, as seen in frontal projections, support the usually obvious clinical diagnosis. A decreased width of the ethmoid bone, resulting in orbital hypotelorism, is always present in trigonocephaly, but it may be present without trigonocephaly and even in the presence of an open metopic suture. The approximation of the orbits is expressed clinically by epicanthic folds and mild to moderate mongoloid slope to the palpebral fissures. Because of the orbital hypotelorism, trigonocephaly has been erroneously considered to be related to the group of holoprosencephalic cerebral malformations in which the orbits

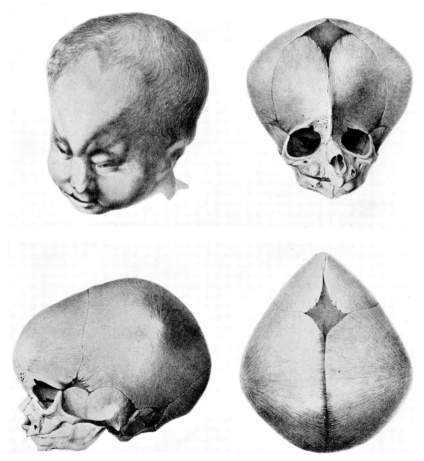

FIG 1–50.
Trigonocephaly in a newly born infant. Photograph of the head and face and three views of the skull—frontal, lateral, and superior.

(From Welcker H: *Untersuchungen über Wachstum und Bau des menschlichen Schädels.* Leipzig, W Engelmann, 1862.)

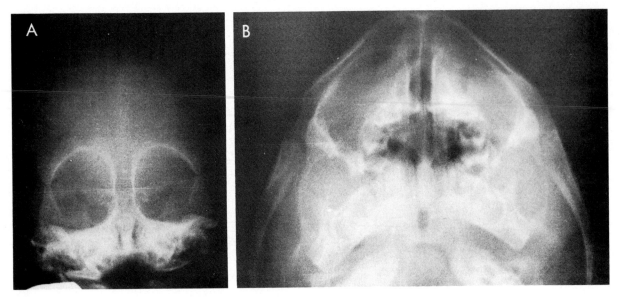

FIG 1–51.
Trigonocephaly. Frontal and basilar projections demonstrate the characteristic orbital hypotelorism and narrowing of the forehead. The metopic suture is invariably closed.

are characteristically approximated. In simple trigonocephaly, there is no increased incidence of neurologic or intellectual deficit. When there are these clinical findings, the specific group of brain malformations discussed in greater detail in Chapter 3 must be considered. Antley et al. called attention to a trigonocephaly syndrome in which there are also limb abnormalities, visceral defects, and abnormalities of the ear, mandible, and skin. With short ribs and, occasionally, pelvic dysplasia, the features of Jeune syndrome are simulated. The syndrome is currently designated the "Opitz C (trigonocephaly) syndrome."

Associated Abnormalities

Cohen reported that limb defects were the most common associated feature of syndromes associated with craniosynostosis, occurring in 84%. Syndactyly and polysyndactyly constituted 30% of the the limb defects, and deficiencies made up 22%. Several types of acrocephalosyndactyly and acrocephalopolysyndactyly have been described. Some are clearly defined; others are less certain and will probably undergo reclassification as further information becomes available. The best known is Apert syndrome (acrocephalosyndactyly type I) in which oxycephaly is associated with syndactyly of at least the second, third, and fourth manual and pedal digits, resulting in the so-called mitten-hand and sockfoot appearance (Fig 1–52). Mental retardation is variably present. Evaluation of craniofacial deformi-

ties in these patients can be assisted by CT (Fig 1–53).

Acrocephalosyndactyly types II, III, and IV are known, respectively, as Apert-Crouzon disease, Saethre-Chotzen syndrome, and Waardenburg syndrome; they involve varying degrees of facial abnormality and pedal and manual syndactylies in patterns generally repetitive for each type (Cohen). The last two are thought to represent the same condition. The next best-known form is acrocephalosyndactyly type V, or Pfeiffer syndrome. In this condition, there is only soft tissue syndactyly, which is not marked, but the thumbs and great toes are deformed and broad, and intelligence usually is not affected. All forms are transmitted by dominant inheritance.

The best known of three recognized types of acrocephalopolysyndactyly is Carpenter syndrome, which is characterized by a high incidence of mental retardation and the presence of preaxial polydactyly of the feet. These conditions, too, are genetically transmitted; Carpenter syndrome is autosomal recessive and the others (Noack and Sakati syndromes) are autosomal dominant.

In Crouzon's "hereditary cranifacial dysostosis," the cardinal elements originally included: (1) dolichocephalic and trigonocephalic deformities of the calvaria; (2) facial dysostosis with a hooked parrot nose, small maxilla, and a relatively larger mandible with overbite; (3) bilateral exophthalmos; and (4) genetic transmission and familial incidence (Fig 1–54). In some cases, fusions of the bones of the feet are

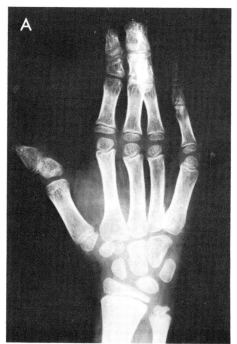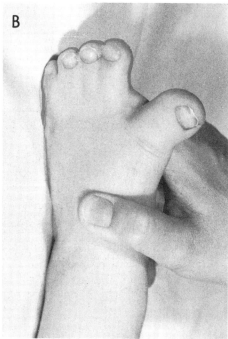

FIG 1–52.
Acrocephalosyndactyly, type I (Apert syndrome). **A,** the middle three digits of the hand are affected by bony and soft-tissue syndactyly. (From Kozlowski K, Maroteaux P, Silverman F, et al: *Ann* *Radiol* 1969; 12:965–1007. Used by permission.) **B,** typical appearance of a "sock-foot" deformity.

associated with the cranial changes. The serious complications are progressive exophthalmos, progressive loss of vision, progressive increase in intracranial pressure, and mental retardation; these are indications for surgical therapy, and early relief from these hazards should be urged by the pediatrician. In addition, the maxillary hypoplasia compromises the nasopharyngeal air space to such a degree that some affected children who appear retarded are only affected by hypercapnea secondary to this obstruc-

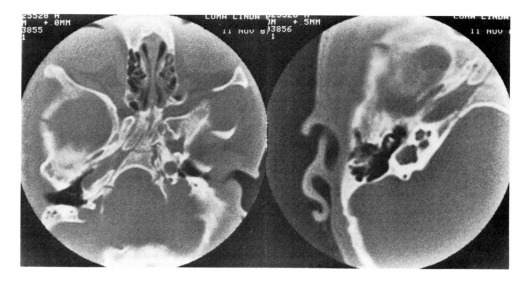

FIG 1–53.
Axial CT demonstrating bizarre deformity of the skull base caused by asymmetric craniosynostosis in a patient with Apert syndrome. In the figure on the left, the exposure is made through the lower portion of the body of the sphenoid, the spheno-occipital synchondrosis, and the basiocciput. The base participates in the asymmetry and demonstrates a partial cleft in the sphenoid body. In the figure on the right, a magnified view of the right inner ear demonstrates dysplasia with a large cavity containing the vestibule and semicircular canals. The ossicles are unremarkable. (Courtesy of Dr. Anton N. Hasso, Loma Linda, Calif.)

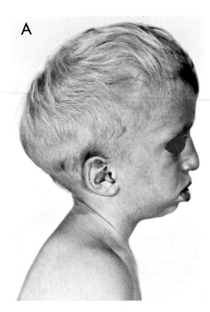
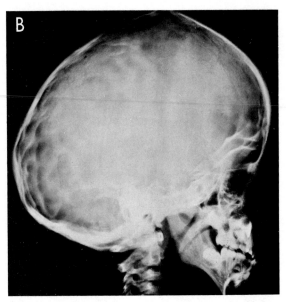

FIG 1–54.
Crouzon disease (craniofacial dysostosis). **A,** lateral photograph of the large calvaria and cranial cavity elongated ventrodorsally. The face is small, and the beaked nose is not seen completely in this view. There is also marked bilateral exophthalmos. **B,** in the lateral radiograph, the frontal squamosa is large, and the edges of the frontal and parietal bones bulge externally at the anterior fontanelle. Convolutional markings are heavy in the occipital squamosa. The facial segment is relatively and absolutely small, with a small maxilla and relatively larger mandible; the latter has a markedly increased obtuse angle. The anterior cranial fossa is small and shallow in comparison with the middle and posterior fossae.

tion. Procedures developed to separate the cantilevered facial mass from the base of the skull and move it forward have improved respiratory function as well as cosmetic appearance.

A form of generalized cranial synostosis associated with hydrocephaly is known by its German name *Kleeblattschädel,* or its anglicized form, "cloverleaf skull." Usually, the hydrocephaly develops in utero, deforming the very plastic skull into a superior portion related to the position of the dilated frontal lobes, and bilateral inferolateral portions corresponding to the dilated temporal lobes. Most patients do not survive infancy. Skeletal abnormalities indistinguishable from those of thanatophoric dysplasia may be present.

There is not complete agreement on the management of patients with craniosynostosis. Enthusiasm for surgical creation of sutures to allow expansion has waxed and waned. At present, the evidence is believed to support craniotomy in most instances. Prevention or improvement of mental retardation, as well as cosmetic improvement to avoid psychic trauma, have been cited as reasons for surgery. In competent hands, the surgical procedures are simpler in the early months of life. If the relief of constraints on a growing brain is a consideration, surgical therapy should be undertaken during the first 6 months when brain growth is most rapid. Mohr et

al. point out that the brain weight increases 130% during the first 12 months of life. Progressive deformity of the neurocranium indicates that the endocranial contents are increasing in size; US and CT can be of value in recognition of associated hydrocephalus, vascular compromise, and other contributing factors to assist in decisions.

CRANIOFACIAL SYNDROMES

The number of syndromes that include radiographic craniofacial features is large. Unlike Crouzon disease, many are not associated with craniosynostosis. Specialized reference texts such as those by Gorlin et al.; Smith; Taybi; and Warkany are important sources of information concerning them. Only a few of the more common that are likely to be referred to the pediatric radiologist are noted briefly in this section.

Stewart has divided craniofacial malformations into craniosynostosis syndromes, otocraniofacial syndromes, midface abnormalities, and craniofacial clefts. The first group is discussed above. The second is subdivided into conditions with bilateral, symmetric facial involvement and those with asymmetric involvement. The most common of the bilateral, symmetric forms is the Treacher Collins syndrome.

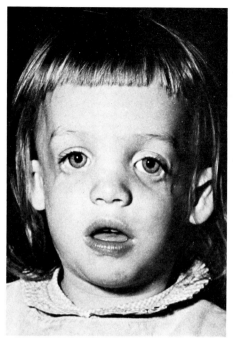
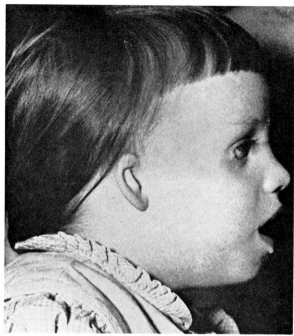

FIG 1–55.
Characteristic facies of Treacher Collins syndrome. The lateral angles of the palpebral fissures are lower than their medial angles, producing an antimongoloid tilt to them. The interorbital distance is increased, and the upper parts of the cheeks are depressed due to deficiencies of both malar bones. Both external ears are folded and misshapen. (From Stovin JJ, Lyon JA Jr, Clemens RL: *Radiology* 1968; 74:223–231. Used by permission.)

Treacher Collins mandibulofacial dysostosis is characterized clinically by flattened cheeks, an antimongoloid slant of the palpebral fissures with notching of the temporal segment of the lower eyelids, and reduced or absent eyelashes in the medial two thirds of the lower lids; deformities of the external ears; and micrognathia (Fig 1–55). The underlying skeletal abnormalities include hypoplasia to complete aplasia of the zygomatic processes of the temporal bones and of the frontal processes of the zygomatic bones, and hypoplasia of the mandible. The zygoma itself is only mildly affected. The pterygoid plates are usually also hypoplastic, the medial more frequently and severely than the lateral. Bony abnormalities of the ears occur in the external canals and in the ossicles, the latter sharing a developmental field with the zygomatic arch and the mandible, all arising from the first and second branchial arches (Fig 1–56). CT (Fig 1–57), often together with three-dimensional re-formation, has replaced conventional multidirectional tomography in the evaluation of the middle ear components, which is necessary if surgery is contemplated for management of defective hearing. The internal ear is usually normal. Treacher Collins syndrome is inherited as an autosomal dominant trait with complete penetrance but variable expressivity.

Two conditions confused with Treacher Collins syndrome are Nager acrofacial dysostosis, an autosomal recessive form of mandibulofacial dysostosis associated with preaxial upper limb deficiency (Fig 1–58), and the Wildervanck-Smith syndrome in which limb deficiencies are both preaxial and postax-

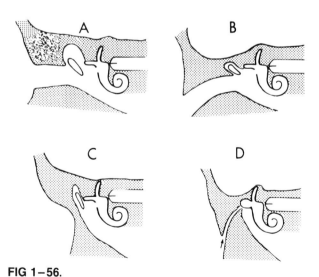

FIG 1–56.
Diagram of tomographic features of the external and internal ear abnormalities in Treacher Collins syndrome. **A,** normal coronal section; **B,** slit attic with ossicular mass; **C,** thin atretic plate and reduced middle ear cavity; **D,** thick atretic plate with anterior facial nerve, no attic, and descent of the tegmen. (From Lloyd GAS, Phelps PD: *Acta Radiol* 1979; 20:233–240. Used by permission.)

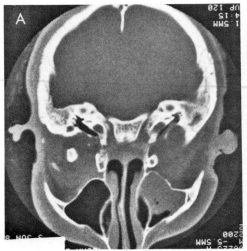

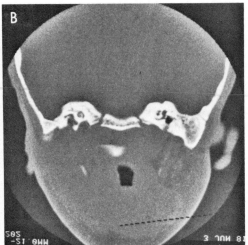

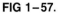

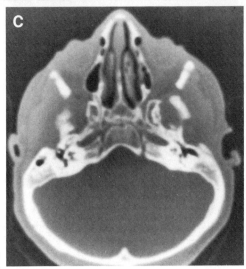

FIG 1–57.
CT in Treacher Collins syndrome. **A,** examination
in the axial plane demonstrates deformed auricles
with no external auditory canals; the middle ear
cavities are hypoplastic with malformed small ossicles. The left auditory tube is larger than the right.
Temporal bone structures are more medial than is
usual. The absence of zygomatic arches is clearly
demonstrated; asymmetry of the posterior walls of
the maxillary sinuses may be part of the malformation, although the opacification of the right is due
to incidental disease. **B,** a coronal plane examination is recorded. **C,** axial slice through the orbits
and petrous area in another patient reveals a
sharply sloping face with absent zygomatic
arches. Although the petrous anomalies are poorly
seen, the left ossicles and middle ear cavities are
hypoplastic. The mastoids are poorly developed
for a 7-year-old. (**A, B,** courtesy of Anton Hasso,
MD, Loma Linda, Calif; **C,** courtesy of Dr. Charles R.
Fitz, Washington, D.C.)

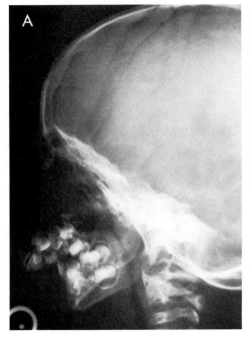

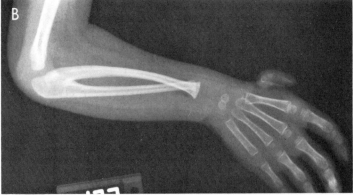

FIG 1–58.
Nager syndrome. The patient had clinical craniofacial features of mandibulofacial dysostosis and, in addition, upper limb anomalies. **A,** lateral skull
film shows marked micrognathia. **B,** radioulnar synostosis and hypoplasia
of the thumb clarify the diagnosis. (Courtesy of Dr. Fred Lee, Pasadena,
Calif.)

ial and occur in lower as well as upper limbs. The preaxial upper limb defect in the Nager syndrome usually involves the radius and thumb; the diagnosis has been made by prenatal US that demonstrated micrognathia in the facial profile together with absence of the thumb. The oculomandibulofacial syndrome (Hallermann-Streiff-François syndrome) was described in detail by François in 1958, although Hallermann and Streiff had independently identified it in earlier reports as a craniofacial malformation differing from mandibulofacial dysostosis. Affected patients have proportionate dwarfism that can be severe, but the diagnostic features are otherwise limited to the skull. The face is small in relation to the cranium, a relation that is exaggerated by the hypoplastic mandible and a narrow, beaked nose due to hypoplasia of the nasal cartilages. Dental anomalies include natal teeth, supernumerary teeth, hy-

podontia, and hypoplasia of the enamel. Alopecia is generally present and is predominantly frontotemporal in location and associated with hypotrichosis of eyelids and eyebrows and atrophy of the skin. Microphthalmia and bilateral congenital cataracts are the major ocular features. The mental status is usually normal. Most cases are sporadic, but some instances of familial involvement have been reported. The radiographic features are primarily those of micrognathia. The condition can be confused with oculodentoosseous dysplasia, but in the latter, the mandible is thickened rather than hypoplastic, soft tissue syndactyly of the fourth and fifth fingers is present, and hair abnormalities are much milder. Metaphyseal widening of the long bones in oculodentoosseous dysplasia has caused some confusion with Pyle disease, but sclerosis of bone is lacking.

In the asymmetric group of craniofacial malfor-

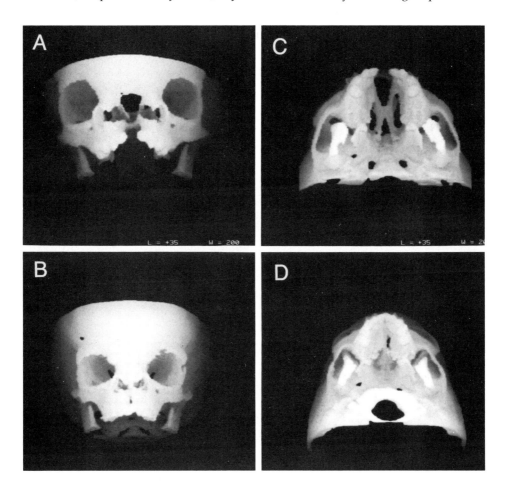

FIG 1–59.
Three-dimensional facial CT for evaluation of Tessier type 0–14 cleft malformation and its reconstruction. **A,** preoperative and **B,** postoperative views of the midline cleft that involves the frontal bone (median encephalocele), and the ethmoid bone with duplication of the crista galli. The nasal bone shows duplication of the septum and columnella. The maxilla has a central defect and hy-

pertelorism is present. The postoperative reconstruction shows correction of the defects and a marked reduction in the interorbital distance. **C,** preoperative and **D,** postoperative views of the palate from below. The patient also had absence of the corpus callosum. (Courtesy of Drs. D.H. and N.R. Altman, and Dr. S.A. Wolfe, Miami, Fla.)

mations, the most common conditions are the Gold-enhar syndrome and hemifacial microsomia. The former is also known as oculoauriculovertebral dysplasia and demonstrates microtia, mandibular hypoplasia, anomalies of the cervical spine, and epibulbar dermoids. External ear anomalies are usually associated with hypoplasia of the ossicles. The condyle and ramus of the mandible are deformed on the more severely affected side, and craniocervical fusions, as well as other vertebral malformations, occur in about 50% of patients. Hemifacial microsomia is similar to mandibular dysostosis but is asymmetric and zygomatic involvement is less marked. Hemifacial atrophy, a progressive acquired disorder, should be differentiated from hemifacial microsomia (Wartenberg).

A discussion of midface abnormalities and craniofacial clefts is outside the scope of this work, but an example depicting their complex anatomy by three-dimensional CT re-formation can indicate the quality of imaging currently available (Fig 1–59).

CONGENITAL DERMAL SINUS

One form of neural tube closure defect is a sinus tract extending from the surface of the body to the central nervous system. The continuity with skin elements explains the name *dermal sinus*. These may develop at any level along the neural axis in the midsagittal plane of the skull and spine, but are most frequent in the lumbosacral region; the second most frequent site is in the occipital area. In the latter case, a bony defect is usually demonstrable in the

midsagittal plane near the inion (Fig 1–60). Both AP and lateral projections are necessary for the satisfactory demonstration of the defect which should be sought roentgenographically when the clinical findings—dimpling of the skin, chronic discharge with or without signs of meningeal irritation—suggest the possibility of congenital dermal sinus. Shackelford and associates found that the bony defect could appear only as a narrow, radiolucent strip passing obliquely through the bone in the caudal direction. When a cyst forms, the defect tends to be circular. The frequency of channels for emissary veins in this region must be kept in mind when congenital dermal sinus is considered on radiographic grounds alone. In the less common glabellar or nasal dermal sinuses, deformity of the base of the skull is said to be characteristic and recognizable radiographically (Sessions).

ORBITAL (OCULAR) HYPERTELORISM

In 1924, Greig described a deformity of the anterior portion of the base of the cranium that he called ocular hypertelorism; the most conspicuous feature was an increase in the interpupillary distance clinically and the interorbital distance radiographically (Fig 1–61). The orbits tend to be circular and deep and are shifted toward the sides of the skull. The nasal bone is short. Greig stated that overgrowth of the lesser wings of the sphenoid and underdevelopment of the greater wings were responsible for the deformity. The ethmoid bone is also widened and probably participates in the basic malformation. Clinically, lateral displacement of the canthi (dystopia cantho-

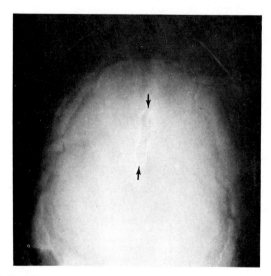

FIG 1–60.
Occipital defect associated with a congenital dermal sinus in an infant 5 months of age. This elongated radiolucent patch extends through the site of the torcular Herophili.

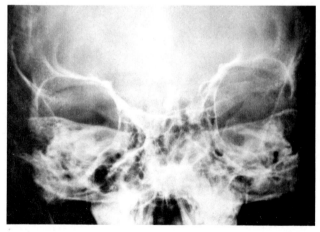

FIG 1–61.
Orbital hypertelorism in a patient 7 years of age. The interorbital distance is greatly increased, the nasal cavity is grossly malformed, and the orbits are shifted laterad in the skull. The volume of the ethmoid labyrinth is increased on each side.

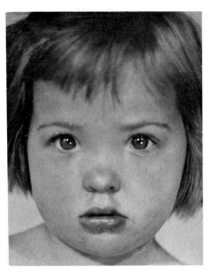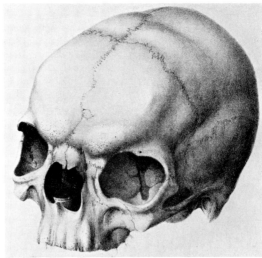

FIG 1–62.
Left, widening of the interpupillary space in ocular hypertelorism in the girl of 3 years. **Right,** orbital hypertelorism, its morbid anatomy shown in a dissection of Welcker. The nasofrontal process and nasal bones are widened, increasing the distance between the orbits. The last are displaced laterad and broadened horizontally. The metopic suture is open. (From Welcker H: *Untersuchungen über Wachstum und Bau des menschlichen Schädels.* Leipzig, W Engelmann, 1862.)

rum) may mimic mild forms of orbital hypertelorism. The gross anatomical changes are shown in Figure 1–62. Mental deficiency of varying degrees occurs in the severe types. Syndactyly and polysyndactyly have been recognized as part of the Greig syndrome. Recent reports of patients with severe digital defects (postaxial hand polydactyly and preaxial foot polydactyly) have been considered possible variant forms. Some show, in addition, absence of the corpus callosum, giving rise to labels of "acrocallosal syndrome" and "cephalopolysyndactyly." It is not yet clear if these forms represent a specific mutant gene syndrome or are phenotypic variants of the autosomal dominant gene causing the Greig syndrome. Orbital hypertelorism is a component of many dysmorphic syndromes including some associated with cranisynostosis.

REFERENCES

Cranioschisis or Cranium Bifidum and Lacunar Skull of the Newborn

Diebler D, Dulac O: Cephaloceles: Clinical and neuroradiological appearance. Associated cerebral malformation. *Neuroradiology* 1983; 25:188–216.

Eteson DJ, Steward RE: Craniofacial defects in the human skeletal dysplasias. *Birth Defects* 1984; 20:19–45.

Fishman MA, Palkes HS, Shackelford GD, et al: Lacunar skull deformity and intelligence. *Pediatrics* 1977; 25:296–299.

McRae DL: Observations on craniolacunia. *Acta Radiol* 1966; 5:55–64.

Marin-Padilla M: Study of the skull in human cranioschisis. *Acta Radiol* 1965; 62:1–20.

Pollack JA, Newton TH, Hoyt WF: Trans-sphenoidal and transethmoidal encephaloceles: A review of clinical and roentgen features in 8 cases. *Radiology* 1968; 90:442–453.

Terrafranca RJ, Zellis A: Congenital hereditary cranium bifidum occultum frontalis. With a review of anatomical variations in lower midsagittal region of frontal bones. *Radiology* 1953; 61:60–66.

Symmetric Parietal Foramina and Sinus Pericranii

Aoyagi M, Matsushima Y, Takei H, et al: Parietal foramina complicated by meningocele. *Childs Nerv Syst* 1985; 1:234–237.

Currarino G: Normal variants and congenital anomalies in the region of the obelion. *Am J Roentgenol* 1976; 127:487–494.

Golabi M, Carey J, Hall BD: Parietal foramina clavicular hypoplasia. An autosomal dominant syndrome. *Am J Dis Child* 1984; 138:596–599.

Goldsmith WM: Catlin mark: Inheritance of unusual opening in parietal bones. *J Hered* 1941; 32:301–309.

Nashold BS Jr, Netsky MG: Foramina, fenestrae and thinness of parietal bones. *J Neuropathol Exp Neurol* 1959; 18:432–441.

O'Rahilly R, Twohig MJ: Foramina parietalia permagna. *Am J Roentgenol* 1952; 67:551–561.

Pendergrass EP, Pepper OHP: Observations on the process of ossification in the formation of persistent enlarged parietal foramina. *Am J Roentgenol* 1939; 41:343–346.

Witrak BJ, Davis PC, Hoffman JC Jr: Sinus pericranii. A case report. *Pediatr Radiol* 1986; 16:55–56.

Premature Craniosynostosis

Andersson H, Paranhos G: Craniosynostosis: Review of the literature and indications for surgery. *Acta Paediatr Scand* 1968; 57:47–54.

Antley RM, Hwang DS, Theopold W, et al: Further delineation of the C (trigonocephaly) syndrome. *Am J Med Genet* 1981; 9:147–163.

Bertelsen TI: The premature synostosis of the cranial sutures. *Acta Ophthalmol Suppl (Copenh)* 1958; 51:1–174.

Carlsen NL, Krasilnikoff PA, Eiken M: Premature cranial synostosis in X-linked hypophosphatemic rickets: Possible precipitation by 1-alpha-OH-cholecalciferol intoxication. *Acta Paediatr Scand* 1984; 73:149–154.

Clarren SK: Plagiocephaly and torticollis: Etiology, natural history and helmet treatment. *J Pediatr* 1981; 98:92–95.

Cohen MM Jr (ed): *Craniosynostosis: Diagnosis, Evaluation, and Management,* New York, Raven Press, 1986.

Collmann H, Sorensen N, Krause J, et al: Hydrocephalus in craniosynostosis. *Childs Nerv Syst* 1988; 4:279–285.

Currarino G, Silverman FN: Orbital hypotelorism, arrhinencephaly and trigonocephaly. *Radiology* 1960; 74:206–217.

Currarino G: Premature closure of the frontozygomatic suture: Unusual fronto-orbital dysplasia mimicking unilateral coronal synostosis. *AJNR* 1985; 7:643–646.

Don M, Siggers DC: Cor pulmonale in Crouzon's disease. *Arch Dis Child* 1971; 46:394–396.

Eaton AP, Sommer A, Sayers MP: The Kleeblattschädel anomaly. *Birth Defects* 1975; 11:238–246.

Escobar V, Bixer D: On the classification of the acrocephalosyndactyly syndromes. *Clin Genet* 1977; 12:169–178.

Faber HK, Towne EB: Early craniectomy as a preventive measure in oxycephaly and allied conditions: With special reference to the prevention of blindness. *Am J Med Sci* 1927; 173:701–711.

Fernbach SL, Naidich TP: Radiologic evaluation of cranisynostosis, in Cohen MM Jr (ed): *Craniosynostosis: Diagnosis, Evaluation, and Management.* New York, Raven Press, 1986.

Furuya Y, Edwards MS, Alpers CE, et al: Computerized tomography of cranial sutures, Part 2: Abnormalities of sutures and skull deformity in craniosynostosis. *J Neurosurg* 1984; 61:59–70.

Gellad FE, Haney PJ, Son JC, et al: Imaging modalities of craniosynostosis with surgical and pathological correlation. *Pediatr Radiol* 1985; 15:285–290.

Graham JM, Badura JA, Smith DW: Coronal craniostenosis: Fetal head constraint as one possible cause. *Pediatrics* 1980; 65:995–999.

Marchandise X, Dhellemmes P, Pellerin P, et al: Bilan de la scintigraphie de la route crânienne. A propos de 85 cas de craniosténoses. *Ann Radiol* 1983; 26:505–509.

Marsh JL, Gado MH, Vannier MW, et al: Osseous anatomy of unilateral coronal synostosis. *Cleft Palate J* 1986; 23:87–100.

Marsh JL, Vannier MW: The anatomy of the cranio-orbital deformities of craniosynostosis: Insights from 3-D images of CT scans. *Clin Plast Surg* 1987; 14:49–60.

Mohr G, Hoffman HJ, Monro IR, et al: Surgical management of unilateral and bilateral coronal craniosynostosis: 21 years' experience. *Neurosurgery* 1978; 2:83–92.

Moss ML: The pathogenesis of premature cranial synostosis in man. *Acta Anat* 1959; 37:351–370.

Noetzel MJ, Marsh JL, Palkes H, et al: Hydrocephalus and mental retardation in craniosynostosis. *J Pediatr* 1985; 107:885–892.

Park EA, Powers GF: Acrocephaly and scaphocephaly with symmetrically distributed malformations of the extremities: A study of the so-called "acrocephalosyndactylism." *Am J Dis Child* 1920; 29:235–315.

Penfold JM, Simpson DA: Premature craniosynostosis: A complication of thyroid replacement. *J Pediatr* 1975; 86:360–363.

Reilly BJ, Leeming JM, Fraser D: Craniosynostosis in the rachitic spectrum. *J Pediatr* 1964; 64:396–405.

Saldino RM, Steinbach HL, Epstein CJ: Familial acrocephalosyndactyly (Pfeiffer's syndrome). *Am J Roentgenol* 1972; 116:609–622.

Sargent C, Burn J, Baraitser M, et al: Trigonocephaly and the Opitz C syndrome. *J Med Genet* 1985; 22:39–45.

Seeger JF, Gabrielsen TO: Premature closure of the fronto-sphenoidal suture in synostosis of the coronal suture. *Radiology* 1971; 101:631–635.

Smith DW, Töndury G: Origin of the calvaria and its sutures. *Am J Dis Child* 1978; 132:662–666.

Tait MV, Gilday DL, Ash JM, et al: Craniosynostosis: Correlation of bone scans, radiographs and surgical findings. *Radiology* 1971; 101:631–635.

Tessier P: The definitive plastic surgical treatment of the severe facial deformities of craniofacial dysostosis: Crouzon's and Apert's diseases. *Plast Reconstr Surg* 1971; 48:419–442.

Craniofacial Syndromes

Altman NR, Altman DH, Wolfe SA, et al: Three dimensional CT reformation in children. *Am J Roentgenol* 1986; 146:1261–1267.

Benson CB, Pober BR, Hirsh MP, et al: Sonography of Nager acrofacial dysostosis syndrome in utero. *J Ultrasound Med* 1988; 7:163–167.

François J: A new syndrome: Dyscephalia with bird face and dental anomalies, nanism, hypotrichosis, cutaneous atrophy, microphthalmia and congenital cataracts. *Arch Ophthalmol* 1958; 60:842–862.

Gorlin RJ, Pindborg JJ, Cohen MM Jr: *Syndromes of the Head and Neck,* ed 2. New York, McGraw-Hill, 1976.

Hallermann W: Vogelgesicht und Cataracta congenita. *Klin Monatsbl Augenheilkd* 1948; 113:315–318.

Herring SW, Rowlat UF, Pruzansky S: Anatomical abnormalities in mandibulofacial dysostosis. *Am J Med Genet* 1979; 3:225–259.

Kay ED, Kay CN: Dysmorphogenesis of the mandible, zygoma, and middle ear ossicles in hemifacial microsomia and mandibulofacial dysostosis. *Am J Med Genet* 1989; 32:27–31.

Lloyd GAS. Phelps PD: Radiology of the ear in mandibulofacial dysostosis Treacher Collins syndrome. *Acta Radiol* 1979; 20:233–240.

Mafee MF, Achild JA, Kumar A, et al: Radiographic features of the ear-related developmental anomalies in patients with mandibulofacial dysostosis. *Int J Pediatr Otorhinolaryngol* 1984; 7:229–238.

Marsh J, Celin DE, Vannier MW, et al: The skeletal anatomy of mandibulofacial dysostosis (Treacher Collins syndrome). *Plast Reconstr Surg* 1986; 78:460–470.

Meyerson MD, Nisbet JB: Nager syndrome: An update of speech and hearing characteristics. *Cleft Palate J* 1987; 24:142–151.

Smith DW: *Recognizable Patterns of Human Malformations,* ed 2. Philadelphia, WB Saunders, 1976.

Steele RW, Bass JW: Hallermann-Streiff syndrome. Clinical and prognostic considerations. *Am J Dis Child* 1970; 120:462–465.

Stewart RE: Craniofacial malformations: Clinical and genetic considerations. *Pediatr Clin North Am* 1978; 25:485–515.

Slovin JJ, Lyon JA Jr, Clemens RL: Mandibulofacial dysostosis. *Radiology* 1968; 74:223–231.

Streiff EB: Dysmorphie mandibulo-faciale (tête de oiseau) et altérations oculaires. *Ophthalmologica* 1950; 120:79–83.

Taybi H: *Radiology of Syndromes, Metabolic Disorders, and Skeletal Dysplasias,* ed 3. St Louis, Mosby–Year Book, 1989.

Warkany J: *Congenital Malformations.* St Louis, Mosby–Year Book, 1971.

Wartenberg R: Progressive facial hemiatrophy. *Arch Neurol Psychiatr* 1945; 54:75–96.

Congenital Dermal Sinus

Schijman E, Monges J, Cragnaz R: Congenital dermal sinuses, dermoid and epidermoid cysts of the posterior fossa. *Childs Nerv Syst* 1985; 2:83–89.

Sessions RB: Nasal dermal sinuses—new concepts and explanations. *Clin Neuropathol* 1982; 92(suppl 29):1–20.

Shackelford GD, Shackelford PG, Schwetschenau PR, et al.: Congenital occipital dermal sinus. *Radiology* 1974; 111:161–166.

Ocular Hypertelorism

Baraitser M, Winter RM, Brett EM: Greig cephalopolysyndactyly: Report of 13 affected individuals in three families. *Clin Genet* 1983; 24:257–265.

Greig DM: Hypertelorism. *Edinburgh Med J* 1924; 31:560–593.

Schinzel A, Schmid W: Hallux duplication, postaxial polydactyly, absence of the corpus callosum, severe mental retardation, and additional anomalies in two unrelated patients: A new syndrome. *Am J Med Genet* 1980; 6:241–249.

Schinzel A, Kaufmann U: The acrocallosal syndrome in sisters. *Clin Genet* 1986; 30:399–405.

SECTION 3

Traumatic Lesions

CONGENITAL DEPRESSIONS

Congenital depressions of the calvaria are due to mechanical factors that operate either before or during birth. They are usually satisfactorily visualized by direct inspection, but roentgenograms are often made in the search for associated fractures. During labor, depressions of the calvaria are caused by excessive localized pressure on the head by the bony prominences in the maternal pelvis such as the sacral promontory, pubic symphysis, and sciatic spines (Fig 1–63). Application of forceps to the fetal head and traction with excessive force is another, but less common, cause of congenital depressions that occur in labor.

Severe cranial deformities may also develop earlier during fetal life, long before labor sets in, owing to sustained abnormal fetal positions (Fig 1–64). Ac-

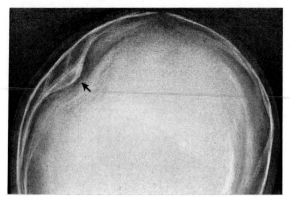

FIG 1–63.
Drawing of a film showing a congenital parietal depression in an infant 37 days of age.

cording to Brown, grooves in the calvaria and face may be caused by excessive pressure of an ectopic shoulder or limb. Lower as well as upper limb positions may be responsible and represent restrictions of the usual active movements of the fetus due to uncertain causes. Deformities may also arise secondary to pressure of amniotic bands. These asymmetries and depressions of the cranium in infants, children, and adults should be interpreted roentgenographically only after a birth history has been carefully obtained. Cranial depressions present at birth and not associated with edema or hemorrhage of the underlying soft tissues are usually due to long-

standing faulty fetal position rather than to recent birth injury. Axton and Levy reported spontaneous elevation of prenatal depressions during the first year after birth without adverse residual effects. Acute depressions secondary to the application of forceps, often called "Ping-Pong ball depressions" have been elevated by simple tangential digital pressure on opposite sides of the depression (Raynor and Parsa) and also by suction with a hand breast pump (Schrager).

CAPUT SUCCEDANEUM

Caput succedaneum is a local swelling of the scalp, usually a result of pressure on the presenting head, recognized at birth and disappearing after a few days. Contents of the caput—edema fluid and blood—cast a shadow of water density that disappears without residual bone production or destruction. In rare cases, the hemorrhagic edema can be so massive that it can be associated with shock. In such cases, intracranial hemorrhage is often present.

HEMORRHAGE

Hemorrhage in the neonatal scalp may occur at three different levels: the subcutaneous (as in caput succedaneum), the subaponeurotic (subgaleal), and the subperiosteal. The more superficial bleedings

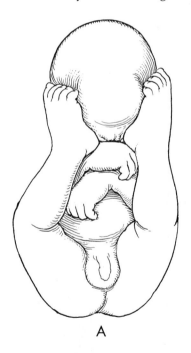

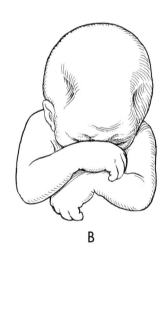

B

A

FIG 1–64.
Schematic drawing of the pathogenesis of congenital depressions in the cranium due to a faulty fetal posture. **A,** abnormal fetal position in which the feet indent the calvaria. **B,** lateral frontoparietal depressions in the calvaria after removal of the feet from the depressions.

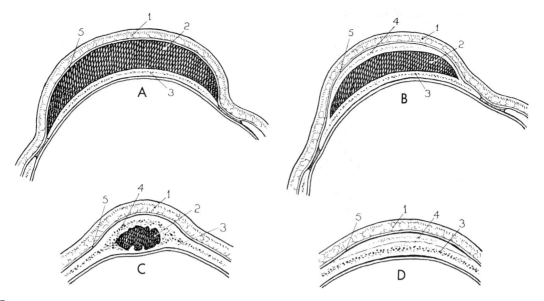

FIG 1–65.
Diagrammatic sketches of anatomical changes in cephalhematoma. **A,** fresh subperiosteal hematoma. **B,** healing phase that shows a new shell of subperiosteal bone over the hematoma. **C,** persistence of an organized hematoma in the diploic space. **D,** persistent residual external thickening of the outer table after complete resorption of subperiosteal blood. **C** and **D** represent late residuals that may persist into adult life. *1,* scalp; *2,* hematoma; *3,* normal calvaria; *4,* new subperiosteal bone; *5,* periosteum.

cross suture lines and may extend widely into the face ventrad, onto the neck dorsad, and onto the zygomatic arches and mastoid processes laterad. Subgaleal hemorrhages are known as cephalhematoceles and may contribute to the swelling and clinical findings in massive caput succedaneum. Subperiosteal hemorrhages are known as cephalhematomas. In contrast with the previous two conditions, cephalhematomas are confined sharply by the edges of the bones they overlie and shells of bone form over them during resolution, arising from the elevated periosteum that covers them externally (Fig 1–65). The usual cause is trauma to the fetal head during labor; cephalhematomas may, however, also develop following cephalic injuries during infancy and childhood. At birth, hemorrhagic disease of the newborn used to be an added predisposing factor. Fine linear fractures of the underlying bone are often found in the sites of cephalhematomas and are thought by some to be the principal cause of the bleeding of the pericranium. Kendall and Woloshin found 69 cephalhematomas in 2,774 newborn infants (2.49%). Of 64 examined roentgenographically, 16 (25%) had associated fractures. Zelson et al. found 111 cephalhematomas in 7,250 newborn infants (1.5%). Only 6 of the 111 had linear fractures under the cephalhematoma (5.4%). The incidence of forceps delivery in the two studies was 75% and 33% respectively, a probable explanation for the difference in incidence of fracture-associated lesions.

Clinically, subperiosteal cephalhematomas appear as localized swellings, usually over the parietal and occipital bone (Fig 1–66). The fresh tumors characteristically extend over the entire surface of the affected bone and are sharply limited at the edges of the bone where the periosteum is bound tightly to the membranous tissue of the sutures. The parietal bones are most often affected, but occipital lesions are by no means rare and are often confused with occipital meningoceles during the first days of life before the shell of subperiosteal bone begins to form. Frontal cephalhematomas are very rare.

The roentgen findings vary with the age of the

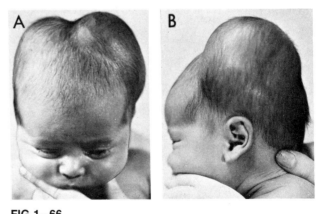

FIG 1–66.
Bilateral parietal cephalhematomas in an infant 13 days of age. Limitation of the edges of the tumors to the sutures is well shown at the sagittal, coronal, and lambdoidal sutures. The deep furrow between the two parietal tumors is due to fixation of the periosteum at the sagittal suture. **A,** frontal, and **B,** lateral views.

cephalhematomas. During the first 2 weeks, the lesion is made up of fluid blood and during this time it casts a shadow of water density (Fig 1–67,A). Near the end of the second week, bone begins to form under the elevated periosteum, first at the margins of the cephalhematoma, but soon the entire blood tumor is overlaid with a complete shell of bone (Figs 1–67,B and 1–68). Depending on their size, cephalhematomas are gradually absorbed during periods varying from 2 weeks to 3 months. Usually, the process of resorption requires 6 weeks as measured in the clinical examination. The roentgen findings, in contrast, persist long after the clinical signs have disappeared (Fig 1–69). The outer table usually remains thickened as a flat, irregular hyperostosis for several months and is gradually resorbed. Fresh cephalhematomas are prone to infection during bacteremias. US may be used for early diagnosis and avoids radiation (Fig 1–70). Associated fractures are generally of no clinical significance.

In some cases, the space between a new shell of bone and inner table remains widened for many years, and the space originally occupied by the hematoma becomes filled with normal diploic bone (Fig 1–71). In other cases, large and small cystlike defects persist in the sites of cepahalhematomas for

months (Fig 1–72) and years as described by Chorobski and Davis. Occasionally, infantile cephalhematoma persists into adult life, when large segments of bone production and destruction may still be visible in the calvaria (Fig 1–73), the cephalhematoma deformans of Schüller and Morgan. The cephalhematomas, according to the authors, remain unchanged and symptomless throughout life.

In the differential diagnosis of productive and destructive lesions of the cranium in children and even adults, the long-standing sequelae of neonatal cephalhematoma have not been adequately appreciated and given the importance that their frequency deserves. Actually, the possibility of residual bone destruction or production from neonatal cephalhematoma should be considered in practically all of the lesions of parietal and occipital bones in older infants, children, and adults. An adequate history of the neonatal state of the head should be taken before the final roentgen evaluation of lesions of the calvaria is made.

SUBGALEAL HYDROMA

Subgaleal hydroma, clinically, may simulate cephalhematoma and also caput succedaneum. Radio-

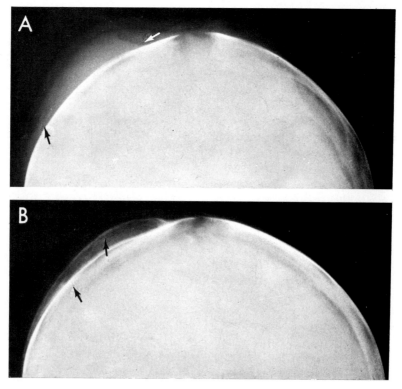

FIG 1–67.
Cephalhematoma. **A,** a rounded soft tissue swelling of water density over the left parietal bone at the age of 7 days. **B,** the same skull at 32 days of age shows a thin shell of newly formed subperiosteal bone overlying the margin of partially resorbed hematoma.

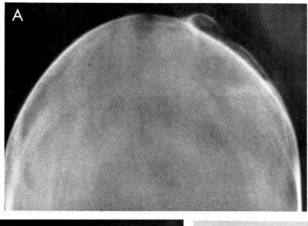

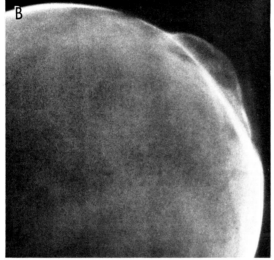

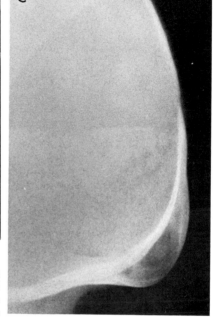

FIG 1–68.
Changes in an ossifying subperiosteal hematoma on the left parietal bone of an infant 6 weeks of age who had been delivered by forceps. **A,** frontal, and **B,** lateral projections. A thin but incomplete shell of bone covers the hematoma. **C,** occipital subperiosteal cephalhematoma with complete and thicker shell of bone over the radiolucent mass of organized hematoma, both sharply limited below at the level of the mendosal suture.

graphically, the swellings in the parietal regions usually are associated with underlying fracture of the bone (Fig 1–74). The scalp swells owing to the accumulation of cerebrospinal fluid and usually some blood beneath the epicranial aponeurosis. The abnormal fluid extends across the sutures, contrary to the pattern in cephalhematomas. Trauma from obstetric forceps is a common cause. In older children, it may result from hair-pulling stress in cases of child abuse or accidental entrapment of long hair in mechanical equipment. Subgaleal hematoma may occur without antecedent trauma in patients with hematologic abnormalities such as platelet defects.

NEONATAL CRANIAL FRACTURES

Occasionally, the vault of the skull is fractured during delivery. Fractures of the base are rare. Simple linear or fissure fractures are the rule, and in roentgenograms these appear as lines and strips of diminished density. In some cases, the fragments separate widely (Fig 1–75), and the soft tissue shadow between the fragments may simulate the wide sutures that normally separate the bones of the neonatal skull.

Among 270 infants who had head injury at birth, Harwood-Nash and associates found that 32, or 12%, had fractures of the skull, all depressed. Forceps were used for 28 of the 32. Virtually all the fractures were in the parietal and occipital bones.

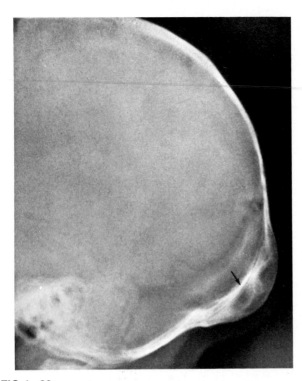

FIG 1–69.
Ossifying subperiosteal cephalhematoma on the occipital squamosa of an infant 4 months of age. The cephalhematoma extends from the lambdoidal suture above to the level of the mendosal suture below, which is already fused. The large radiolucent patches beneath the subperiosteal shell of newly formed bone are cast by masses of blood in varying degrees of organization and resorption.

One was associated with subdural hematoma and another with extradural hematoma. As in older patients, fractures in neonates are of less importance than associated intracranial reactions to trauma, invisible to conventional radiography. When clinical signs warrant, CT and MRI examinations are particularly informative. US via the wide sutures and large fontanelles, and even across the thin calvaria, may be diagnostic; alternatively, it can indicate the need for the special examinations or support their nonemployment.

CRANIAL FRACTURES IN INFANTS AND CHILDREN

Over the past two decades, separate studies on the role of radiographic diagnosis following head trauma in infants and children have indicated that plain radiographic examination of the skull has little to offer in the management of such injuries. In one study (Boulis et al.), 1,000 of 1,032 consecutive children under 12 years of age referred to an outpatient department because of head injury had radiographs; only 21 had fractures. The presence or absence of a fracture neither correlated with the clinical situation nor affected management. Attempts have been made to establish "high-yield" clinical criteria that, if present after head trauma, would warrant radiographic examination. It is suggested that such a program identifies patients needing special management and eliminates unnecessary examinations

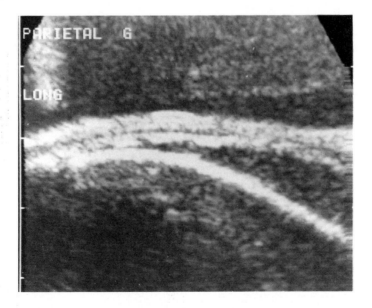

FIG 1–70.
US scan of edge of parietal cephalhematoma. Compare with Figure 1–65,B. The periosteum is raised by the sonolucent blood; its width and echogenicity result from subperiosteal bone formation that is too little to show on radiographs. (Courtesy of Dr. Daniel Nussle, Geneva, Switzerland.)

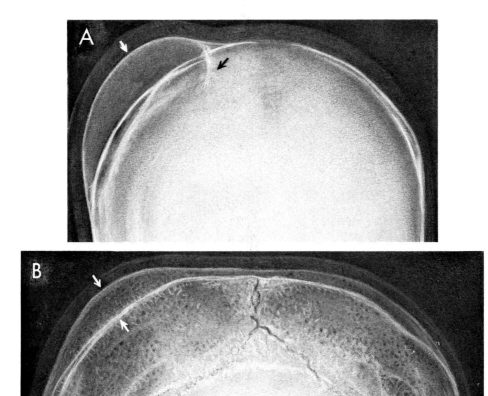

FIG 1–71.
Drawings of films that demonstrate late residual thickening of the calvaria due to neonatal cephalhematoma. **A,** at 7 weeks of age there is a large hematoma *(arrows)* covered by a thin osseous shell on the right parietal bone. **B,** at 3 years and 11 months there is now a widening of the diploic space *(arrows)* in the right parietal bone where the neonatal hematoma was located.

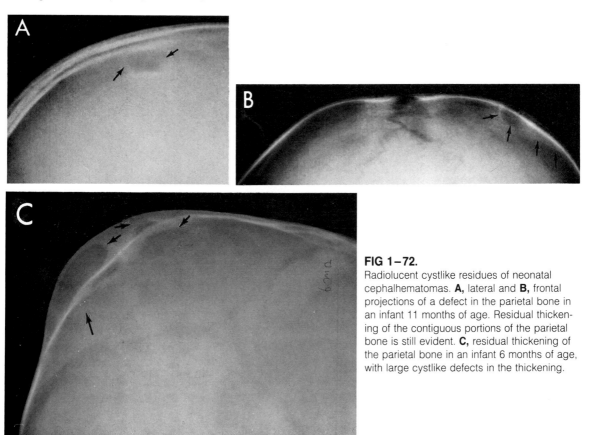

FIG 1–72.
Radiolucent cystlike residues of neonatal cephalhematomas. **A,** lateral and **B,** frontal projections of a defect in the parietal bone in an infant 11 months of age. Residual thickening of the contiguous portions of the parietal bone is still evident. **C,** residual thickening of the parietal bone in an infant 6 months of age, with large cystlike defects in the thickening.

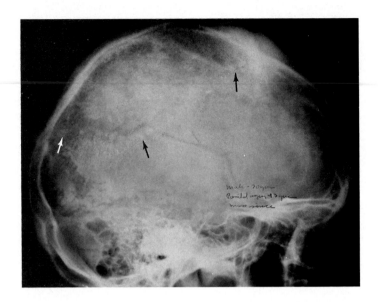

FIG 1–73.
Cephalhematoma deformans parietalis in a youth of 20 whose cranium was injured when he was 2 years old. A large segment of one parietal bone is irregularly dense and rarefied, with a heavy peripheral rim of sclerosis and thickening. (**Courtesy of Dr. Juan M. Taveras.**)

(Phillips). In fact, the studies suggest that if certain clinical criteria are present singly or in combination, CT or MRI examination is in order. These conclusions have been supported by a prospective study of over 7,000 patients with head trauma and can be considered established (Masters et al.). The selection criteria are (1) unconsciousness or documented decreasing level of consciousness; (2) history of previous craniotomy with shunt in place; (3) skull depression probable or identified by probe through laceration or a puncture wound; (4) blood in, or fluid discharge from, the ear; (5) cerebrospinal fluid discharge from the nose; (6) ecchymosis behind the ear (Battle sign); (7) bilateral orbital ecchymoses; and (8) unexplained focal neurologic signs. Leonidas and associates believe that these criteria are less useful in children than in adults. If cephalhematoma, drowsiness, and age less than 1 year were added, there would have been no missed fractures in their series.

The advantages of CT and MRI scanning of the head in trauma in terms of their contributions to patient management have delegated conventional skull radiography to a secondary procedure after the patient's condition is sufficiently stabilized. This is frequently accomplished days after injury and generally to corroborate or supplement equivocal special

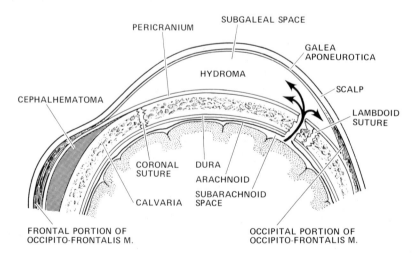

FIG 1–74.
Course of flow of the cerebrospinal fluid after fracture of the calvaria. Tears of the arachnoid and dura internally and the periosteum externally into the subgaleal (epicranial) space form a large subgaleal hydroma under the galea aponeurotica. (**Modified from Epstein JA, Epstein BS, Small M:** J Pediatr 1961; 59:562–566.)

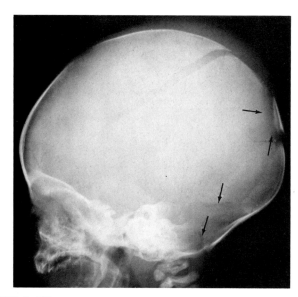

FIG 1–75.
Long diastatic fracture of the parietal bone in an infant 14 days of age caused by a fall from a nurse's arms. The *arrows* point to a large wormian bone in the posterior fontanelle and to the normal intraoccipital synchondrosis and the mendosal suture in the squamosa of the occipital bone.

special procedures are not available. Otherwise, CT is best for evaluation of skeletal structures and MRI for the intracranial contents and other soft tissue structures. Their use is discussed further in Chapter 3.

If neonatal fractures associated with forceps are excluded, depressed fractures of the skull occur most frequently when large vectors of force are involved, as in vehicular accidents or direct local trauma. Many are compounded by associated lacerations or communication with the nasal or aural cavities. They are often comminuted. In the study of Harwood-Nash and associates, dural tears were found in one third of the depressed fractures, whereas extradural and subdural hematomas were relatively uncommon.

In the examination for fractures in young persons, in whom the cranial sutures are conspicuously visible, it is necessary to keep in mind the great normal variability of these structures. In addition, sutures may widen radiographically as a possible disturbance of desmogenous ossification secondary to long-term prostaglandin E1 administration. The observation of sutural widening during recovery from deprivational dwarfism may involve similar mechanisms. The unclosed segment of the metopic suture superimposed on a sagittal suture in a frontal projection may give a false impression of a fracture (Fig 1–76). The linear shadows of diminished density

studies. Two reservations to this program must be made: one, for the unconscious patient in whom the cross-table lateral view to include the cervical spine can be of considerable importance to identify associated injuries; and two, for circumstances in which

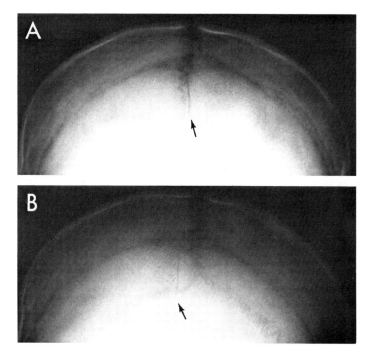

FIG 1–76.
Open cephalic segment of the metopic suture, superimposed on the sagittal, which falsely suggests an intrasutural fracture of the sagittal. In **A,** the short metopic segment is superimposed on the sagittal; but in **B,** in which the head is slightly rotated, the metopic segment is clearly not in the sagittal suture but in the frontal squamosa, extending off the anterior angle of the anterior fontanelle.

arising from fractures must be differentiated from linear vascular markings, particularly those of the grooves for the middle meningeal artery and its branches. Whether or not depressed, fractures may result in tears of dural sinuses, especially when located in areas through which they course. The position of the bone edges at the time of posttrauma examination may give no indication of how much displacement took place at the moment the fracture occurred. Oblique single-bevel fractures that interrupt the continuity of the inner and outer tables in different planes may be invisible or simulate two fractures in certain projections. In some cases, especially with depressed fractures, the edges of the fragments may overlap and thus cast linear shadows of increased density. CT is the optimal procedure for evaluating the depressed fragments and their relation to the underlying brain (Fig 1–77). Some of the roentgenographic characteristics of cranial fractures are shown in Figures 1–78 to 1–82.

Linear fractures in infants and children generally heal with few or no sequelae. The relatively sharp margins become hazy, and obliteration of the fracture line itself may occur between 3 and 6 months after the original injury. In some instances, where there has been considerable comminution, bone may be resorbed locally leaving a defect. If the dura has been disrupted at the time of fracture, there is a tendency for the bony edges of the fracture to separate. Leakage of the cerebrospinal fluid from damaged underlying pia-arachnoid into the area of fracture can result in the development of what has been called, apparently incorrectly, a leptomeningeal cyst. The leptomeninges disappear from the inner surface of the torn dura as well as over the underlying brain. Cysts are thought to be most common in fractures that involve the sutures as the dura is tightly bound there and likely to rupture when the bone edges separate. They have been reported following vacuum extraction when too anterior a placement of the cup was followed by widening of one coronal suture. CT demonstrated widening of the affected coronal suture on the second day of life with a hypodense area beneath it. Fifteen months later, a porencephalic cavity was found in the region.

Transmitting the pulsations of the brain, the cyst causes pressure atrophy of bone that is unprotected by dura, and a huge defect may develop after many months or years (Figs 1–83 and 1–84). The progressive changes are shown schematically in Figure 1–85. Prior to the development of a cyst, it is probably the pulsating brain that begins the erosion of the

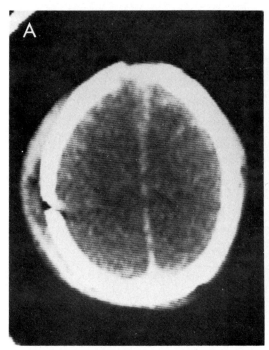
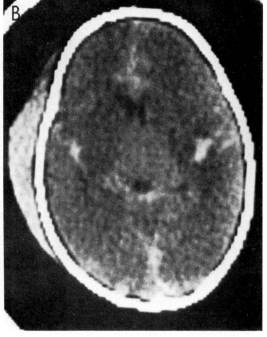

FIG 1–77.
Representative non–contrast-enhanced CT scans of the cranium of a 9-month-old infant with multiple skull fractures and a loss of consciousness following a motor vehicle accident. **A,** one of several fractures together with overlying subgaleal hemorrhage and cerebrospinal fluid as well as blood in the interhemispheric fissure.

B, at another level, blood is also present in both sylvian cisterns and in the quadrigeminal plate cistern. Other levels showed cerebral contusions as well as subarachnoid and intraventricular hemorrhage. (Courtesy of Dr. W. Marshall, Stanford, Calif.)

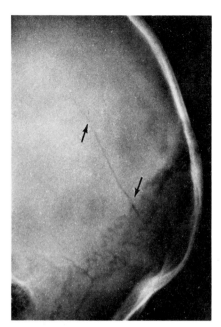

FIG 1–78.
Fine linear fracture of the parietal bone in an infant 15 months of age who fell from a highchair.

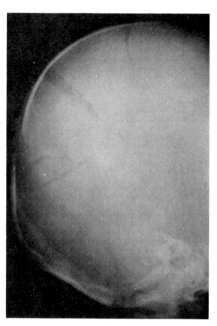

FIG 1–79.
Multiple fractures of the right parietal bone in an infant 9 months of age.

internal table, as suggested by Penfield and Erickson in 1941. Progressive enlargement of the calvarial defect has given rise to the term "growing fracture." The brain has been damaged by the trauma, and, also having lost its leptomeningeal cover, is in pro-

cess of becoming necrotic or gliotic, leading to the development of a porencephalic cavity that ultimately underlies the calvarial defect. The scalloped margin of the defect results from differential erosion of inner and outer tables. Occasionally, an intradip-

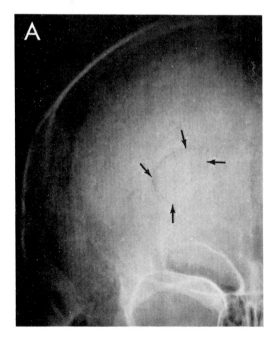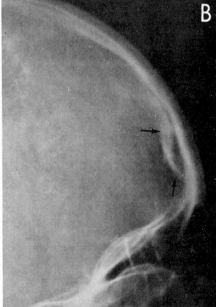

FIG 1–80.
Depressed fracture of the frontal bone in a child 9 years of age. **A,** PA projection. The fracture is indicated by the *arrows*. In the medial inferior segment, the arcuate shadow of diminished density is replaced by a curved linear shadow of increased density, caused by overlapping of the fragments in this segment. **B,** lateral projection. The depression of the tables is clearly seen in this position.

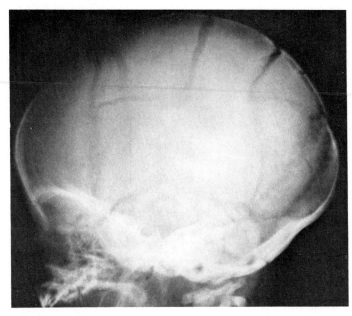

FIG 1–81.
Comminuted diastatic fractures of both parietal bones in an infant 2 months of age. Both ocular fundi contained hemorrhages, and there were bilateral subdural hematomas. Police investigation disclosed that the patient had been severely beaten by the mother.

loic cyst is present. These lesions generally occur following fractures in infancy and are seldom observed in those occurring after the fifth year.

Subdural hematomas are discussed in detail in Chapter 3. Their association with metaphyseal lesions was a feature noted by Caffey in his initial description of what was subsequently called "the battered child syndrome."

Gas may accumulate in the soft tissues of the skull contiguous to fractures, usually through breaks in paranasal air spaces or pneumatic cells of the temporal bone. If the air escapes from the sinuses externally into the subaponeurotic space of the scalp, the result is called extracranial traumatic pneumocephalus. Air may also leak into the cranial cavity, causing internal pneumocephalus. Intranasal manipula-

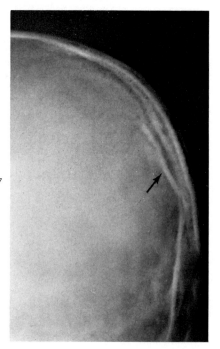

FIG 1–82.
Spurious depressed fracture of one parietal bone, due to hypoplasia and flattening of the left side of the calvaria, which produces a segment of the inner table of the smaller parietal bone that is centrad to the larger right parietal bone. The patient was an asymptomatic girl 7 years of age, with the left side of the calvaria smaller than the right, who had never suffered head injury.

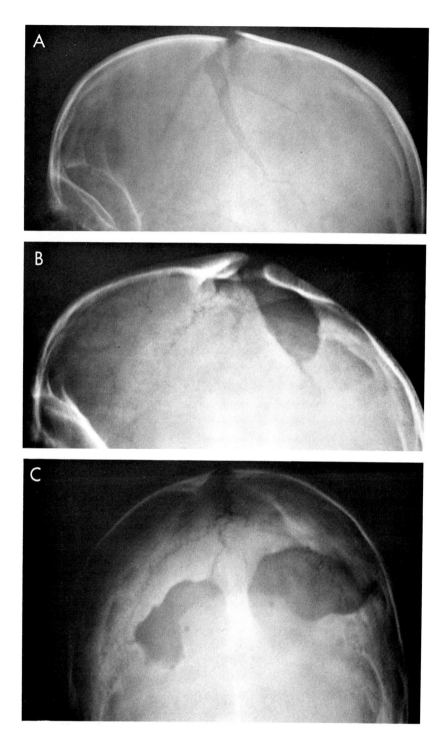

FIG 1–83.
Pulsating "leptomeningeal cyst" with residual bilateral large defects in the calvaria. **A,** diastatic bilateral comminuted parietal fractures after head injury during infancy. **B,** lateral and **C,** frontal projections 5 years later show large bilateral defects in the sites of the earlier parietal fractures. At surgery, the dura beneath the fractures was found to be torn. The bone on the margins of the defect is sclerotic and thickened. (Courtesy of Dr. Walter E. Berdon, New York, N.Y.)

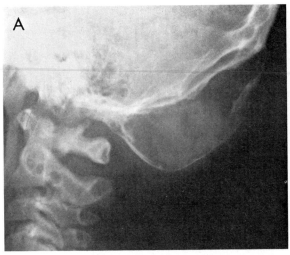
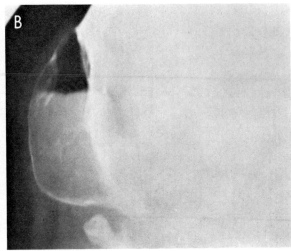

FIG 1–84.
Regional thinning and bulging of a large segment of the occipital squamosa over a pulsating leptomeningeal cyst several years after head injury with occipital fracture. **A,** left lateral projection. **B,** right lateral projection during pneumoencephalography, demonstrating cerebrospinal fluid–gas level in the cyst. A tear in the dura was found on surgical exploration. **(Courtesy of Dr. Walter E. Berdon, New York, N.Y.)**

tions, craniotomy, and erosions due to inflammatory destruction and to pressure atrophy arising from expanding neoplasms may result in pneumocephalus. Intraventricular pneumocephalus has been observed due to a congenital defect in the roof of the nasal cavity.

In a study of 100 "head bangers" in a hospital for the mentally retarded, Williams and associates found hematomas of the skull, thickenings of the calvaria, widening of cranial sutures, calcifications in the eyes, and a hematoma of the corpus callosum, in addition to external soft tissue signs of trauma. Subdural hematomas were not detected, but the observations were made before the availability of CT and MRI. Others have noted erosion of calvarial outer tables in similar cases. Helfer et al. reviewed records of 256 children under 5 years of age who fell out of bed at home or in the hospital. In only 3 were there skull fractures, and these were clinically insignificant. Serious injuries attributed to falls from a bed must be evaluated very carefully for possible child abuse factors.

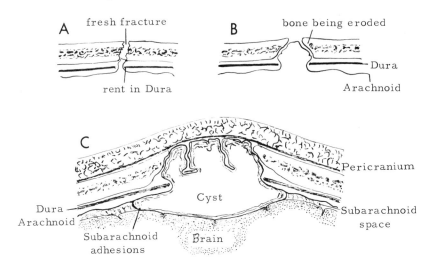

FIG 1–85.
Schematic drawing of the mechanism and progressive changes in the formation of a "leptomeningeal cyst." **A,** immediately after injury, fresh fractures of the parietal bone, a fresh rent in the underlying dura, and early protrusion of the arachnoid membrane into and through the fracture. **B,** later marginal erosion of bone and widening of the dural defect. **C,** later incomplete cyst formation in the arachnoid due to adhesions, depression and pressure atrophy of the underlying brain and leptomeninges, and increases in bony and dural defects. **(Courtesy of Dr. Juan M. Taveras.)**

REFERENCES

Axton JHM, Levy LF: Congenital moulding depressions of the skull. *Br J Med* 1965; 1:1644–1647.

Azar-Kia B, Sarwar M, Batnitzky S, et al: Radiology of intracranial gas. *AJR Am J Roentgenol* 1975; 124:315–323.

Beitzke A, Stein J: Pseudo-widening of cranial sutures as a feature of long-term prostaglandin E1 therapy. *Pediatr Radiol* 1986; 16:57–58.

Bonadio WA, Smith DS, Hillman S: Clinical indicators of intracranial lesion on computed tomographic scan in children with parietal skull fractures. *Am J Dis Child* 1989; 143:194–196.

Boulis ZF, Dick R, Barnes NR: Head injuries in children—aetiology, symptoms, physical findings and x-ray wastage. *Br J Radiol* 1978; 51:851–854.

Brown D: Congenital deformities of mechanical origin. *Proc R Soc Med* 1936; 29:1409–1421.

Caffey J: Multiple fractures in the long bones of infants suffering from chronic subdural hematoma. *Am J Roentgenol* 1946; 56:163–173.

Capitanio MA, Kirkpatrick JA: Widening of the cranial sutures: A roentgen observation during periods of accelerated growth in patients treated for deprivation dwarfism. *Radiology* 1969; 92:53–59.

Chorobski J, Davis L: Cyst formation of the skull. *Surg Gynecol Obstet* 1934; 58:12–31.

Hansen KN, Pedersen H, Pedersen MB: Growing skull fracture—rupture of coronal suture caused by vacuum extraction. *Neuroradiology* 1987; 29:502.

Harwood-Nash DC, Hendrick EB, Hudson AR: The significance of skull fractures in children: A study of 1,187 patients. *Radiology* 1971; 101:151–155.

Helfer RE, Slovis EL, Black M: Injuries resulting when small children fall out of bed. *Pediatrics* 1977; 60:533–535.

Kendall N, Woloshin H: Cephalhematoma associated with fracture of the skull. *J Pediatr* 1952; 41:125–132.

Leonidas JC, Ting W, Binkiewicz A, et al: Mild head trauma in children: When is a roentgenogram necessary? *Pediatrics* 1982; 69:139–143.

Masters SJ, McClean PM, Arcarese JS, et al: Skull x-ray examinations after head trauma. Recommendations by a multidisciplinary panel and validation study. *N Engl J Med* 1987; 316:84–91.

Penfield W, Erickson TC: *Epilepsy and Cerebral Localization.* Springfield, Ill, Charles C Thomas, 1941. pp 363–364.

Phillips LA: *A Study of the Effect of High Yield Criteria for Emergency Room Skull Radiography.* Washington, DC, US Government Printing Office, 1978, HEW Publication No. (FDA) 78–8069.

Raynor R, Parsa M: Nonsurgical elevation of depressed skull fracture in an infant. *J Pediatr* 1968; 72:262–264.

Roy S, Sarkar C, Tandon PN, et al: Cranio-cerebral erosion (growing fracture of the skull in children). Part I. Pathology. *Acta Neurochir* 1987; 87:112–118.

Schrager GO: Elevation of depressed skull fracture with a breast pump. *J Pediatr* 1970; 77:300–301.

Schüller A, Morgan F: Cephalhematoma deformans: Late developments of infantile cephalhematoma. *Surgery* 1946; 19:651–660.

Stuck K, Hernandez R: Large skull defect in a head banger. *Pediatr Radiol* 1979; 8:257–258.

Tandon PN, Banerji AK, Bhatia R, et al: Cranio-cerebral erosion (growing fracture of the skull in children). Part II. Clinical and pathological observations. *Acta Neurochir* 1987; 88:1–9.

Theander G, Thunander J: Congenital deformities of skull caused by fetal limbs. *Acta Radiol* 1980; 21:309–313.

Williams JP, Fowler GW, Pribram HF, et al: Roentgenographic changes in head bangers. *Acta Radiol* 1972; 13:37–42.

Zelson C, Lee SJ, Pearl M: The incidence of skull fractures underlying cephalhematomas in newborn infants. *J Pediatr* 1974; 85:371–373.

SECTION 4

Infections

OSTEOMYELITIS

Osteomyelitis of the skull is rare in children. Trauma is a common precursor. Pin site infection has been reported in patients treated with halo fixation devices, especially in those whose pins had become loose. Cranial injuries resulting from darts are often penetrating and result in intracranial infection following closure of the cutaneous puncture wounds; CT imaging must be considered for identification of intracranial penetration. Occasionally, the frontal bone is involved by direct extension of infection from the frontal sinus, or the sphenoid bone by extension from the sphenoid sinus. Hematogenous osteomyelitic foci may develop in the course of bacteremia, or the underlying bone may be infected by direct extension from cellulitis of the scalp or from compound fractures.

During the early stages of bone infection, the roentgen findings are negative. Later, when areas of inflammatory necrosis of sufficient size develop, they can be identified roentgenographically as areas of diminished density of variable size, shape, and position involving the inner and outer tables and diploë singly and in combination. These lesions may be single or multiple (Fig 1–86) and are more common in the frontal and parietal bones than elsewhere. In chronic osteomyelitis, productive changes in sclerosis of the affected bone are usually present; in disease secondary to paranasal sinusitis, the bony walls of the affected sinus are often sclerotic. Localized osteomyelitis may spread by contiguity or through the diploic veins; metastatic lesions first appear as fine foci of rarefaction, then enlarge and coalesce, sometimes giving rise to a moth-eaten rarefaction that involves the entire bone or even the entire calvaria. In infants, the avascular sutures interposed between the bones act as barriers to the exten-

sion of spreading infection. After the infection subsides, repair may begin on the margins or in the center of the necrotic areas; reossification is an exceedingly slow process and usually requires years for completion, even in young children. Nuclear scans may identify osteomyelitis before radiographic changes occur. The addition of white blood cell scans has proved valuable in some instances.

TUBERCULOSIS

Tuberculous infection of the skull is rarely encountered today in infants or children. Roentgenographically, tuberculous osteomyelitis resembles nonspecific osteomyelitis; it produces areas of diminished density with or without regional sclerosis (Fig 1–87). When destructive tuberculous foci in the calvaria are associated with destructive foci in other bones, especially in the ilium, the radiologic appearance may resemble that of skeletal neuroblastoma or of Langerhans cell histiocytosis.

SARCOIDOSIS

Microscopically proven sarcoidosis of the diploic space was found by Toomey and Bautista in a girl of 14 years with large radiolucent patches in the frontal, parietal, and occipital bones (Fig 1–88). The cal-

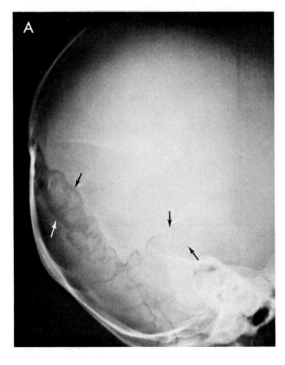 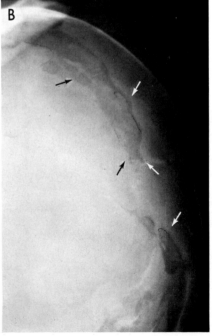

FIG 1–86.
Hematogenous osteomyelitis of the calvaria in an infant 8 months of age. **A,** lateral, and **B,** AP projections. The patient had bacteremia due to *Staphylococcus aureus*, with multiple osteomyelitic foci in the long tubular bones. The *arrows* point to multiple areas of de- struction in the margins of the parietal, occipital, and temporal bones. The patient recovered. The destructive areas were still evident in roentgenograms made 3½ years later.

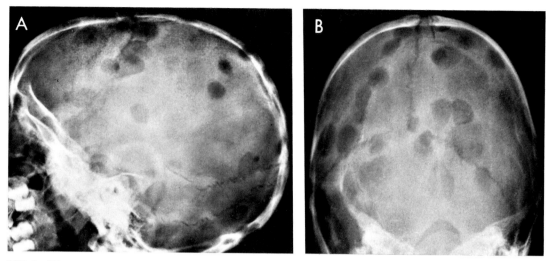

FIG 1–87.
Multiple destructive tuberculous foci in the calvaria of a girl 3 years of age. **A,** lateral, and **B,** frontal projections.

varial lesions diminished substantially during steroid treatment. Posner also found numerous radiolucent foci in the calvaria of an infant 28 months of age; these proved to be sarcoid granulomas in the diploic space with pressure necrosis of the overlying tables of the calvaria. Calvarial lesions may be demonstrated and response to treatment can be followed by bone scanning with^{99m}Tc MDP (Cinti et al.).

SYPHILIS

The cranium is commonly involved in infantile syphilis in association with severe syphilitic osteitis of the long bones. Both tables may show destructive and productive changes, usually in the parietal and frontal bones (Fig 1–89). In older children also,

syphilis of the skull causes a variety of destructive and productive changes. On roentgenographic grounds alone, one cannot make a conclusive differentiation between syphilitic and other types of osteomyelitis. Productive changes in the calvaria resemble rachitic bossing.

MYCOTIC OSTEOMYELITIS

The cranium is sometimes involved in the rare chronic infections: actinomycosis, blastomycosis, and coccidioidomycosis. The roentgenographic appearance of the lesions is similar to that of tuberculous, syphilitic, and chronic purulent osteomyelitis, and diagnosis requires identification of the responsible organism from lesions or from elsewhere in the

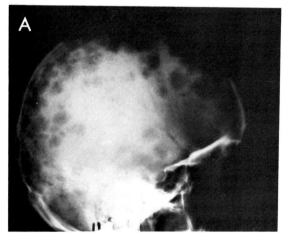

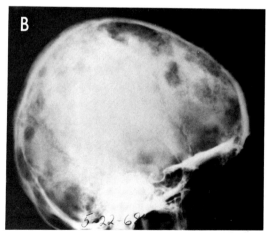

FIG 1–88.
Sarcoidosis of the diploic space in a girl 14 years of age, lateral projections. **A,** before treatment, multiple large and small radiolucent defects are scattered widely in the frontal, parietal, and occipital bones. Microscopically, the radiolucent patches represent focal destruction of internal and external tables that overlie expand-

ing sarcoid granulations in the diploic space. **B,** after 7 months of steroid therapy, some of the radiolucent patches have disappeared, and others have shrunk, presumably due to the treatment. (From Toomey F, Bautista A: *Radiology* 1970; 94:569–573. Used by permission.)

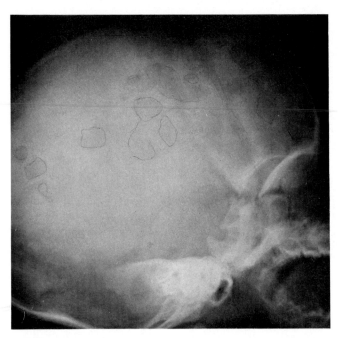

FIG 1–89.
Extensive syphilis of the frontal and parietal bones in an infant 2½ months of age. There are several large and small areas of diminished density in the frontal and parietal regions. A major portion of the outer table of the squamosa of the frontal bone is destroyed. The patient also had extensive destructive syphilitic osteitis of the long tubular bones. (Margins of several lesions retouched.)

body in the case of disseminated infection. In instances of unusual infection (e.g., *Candida* and other organisms of low virulence), the possibility of immunodeficiency must be considered.

RHEUMATOID STATE

Cystic bone lesions occur occasionally in the calvaria of children with rheumatoid arthritis and may be associated with overlying subcutaneous nodules; they may also develop in areas free of nodules. The lesions respond to steroid therapy but may recur when therapy is discontinued.

REFERENCES

Bouvier M, Lejeune E, Queneau P, et al: Sarcoidosis avec lacunes crâniennes. A propos d'une observation personelle et de sept observations relevées dans la littérature. *Rev Rhum Mal Osteoartic* 1972; 39:205–214.

Cinti DC, Hawkins HB, Slavin JD Jr: Radioisotope bone scanning in a case of sarcoidosis. *Clin Nucl Med* 1985; 10:82–84.

Garfin ST, Botte MJ, Waters RL, et al: Complication in the use of the halo fixation device. *J Bone Joint Surg [Am]* 1986; 68:320–325.

Ginsburg MH, Genant HK, Yu TF, et al: Rheumatoid nodulosis: An unusual variant of rheumatoid disease. *Arthritis Rheum* 1975; 18:49–50.

Hanigan WC, Olivero WC, Duffy JJ, et al: Lawn dart injury in children: Report of two cases. *Pediatr Emerg Care* 1986; 2:247–249.

Maurer AH, Chen DCP, Camlargo EE, et al: Utility of three-phase skeletal scintigraphy in suspected osteomyelitis: Concise communication. *J Nucl Med* 1981; 22:941–949.

Posner S: Sarcoidosis: Case report. *J Pediatr* 1942; 20:486–495.

Schlesinger BE, Forsythe CC, White RHR, et al: Observations on the clinical course and treatment of 100 cases of Still's disease. *Arch Dis Child* 1961; 36:65–76.

Toomey F, Bautista A: Rare manifestations of sarcoidosis in children. *Radiology* 1970; 94:569–573.

Turner OA, Weiss DR: Sarcoidosis of the skull; Report of a case. *Am J Roentgenol* 1969; 105:322–325.

Weber ML, Abela A, de Repentigny L, et al: Myeloperoxidase deficiency with extensive candidal osteomyelitis of the base of the skull. *Pediatrics* 1987; 80:876–879.

SECTION 5

Neoplasms

Primary neoplasms of the skull are rare. Ruge et al., in a review of 70 children with a solitary nontraumatic lump on the head, found 61% were dermoid tumors of the scalp, 9% were cephalhematoma deformans, 7% were eosinophilic granuloma, and 4% were occult meningoceles and encephaloceles.

Osteochondromas may arise from the cartilaginous bones of the skull base; osteoblastomas have been reported in the calvaria of infants, and aneurysmal bone cysts have been noted in the base and the calvaria (Fig 1–90). Osteomas are rare, small, and usually limited to the outer table, although osteoid osteomas may occur in the diploë. The latter may present the appearance of a button sequestrum. Angiomas and neurofibromas of the scalp may affect the underlying skull and cause deformities, bony defects, and regional hyperostoses. Cavernous hemangiomas of the skull are characterized by rounded areas of diminished density in which there may be a honeycomb or radial pattern of heavier density caused by spiculation of the part. Calvarial hemangiomas (Fig 1–91) usually thicken the outer table externally and are radially striated. They do not displace the inner table.

Lymphangiomas of the skull are rare and may produce radiologic changes resembling cephalhematoma deformans. Epidermoidomas (cholesteatomas) are ectodermal rests or inclusions that may be located in the scalp, in the diploic spaces, or between the internal surface of the inner table and the dura. They are usually benign and grow slowly. If they protrude into the cranial cavity, they may be the source of cerebral symptoms. When epidermoidomas grow within the bone or impinge on it, they produce local destruction of bone that appears roentgenographically as a sharply demarcated shadow of diminished density surrounded by a smooth sclerotic margin (Fig 1–92). The margin is due to flaring of the edge of the bone into a marginal ridge. Sometimes the periphery of the defect is scalloped. In the majority of cases, the lesions disappear within a few years of discovery (Holthusen et al.). Thirteen cases were found in 9,177 skull examinations of children up to 3 years of age contrasting with only one in 8,353 children between 3 and 10 years; one case was found in 5,323 children older than 10 years. In patients followed serially, a transient period of moderate enlargement occurred prior to spontaneous resolution.

Meningiomas are rare in children. The essential radiographic changes include hyperostosis, an increase in the caliber and number of grooves for regional blood vessels, and calcifications in the meningioma itself. The hyperostosis is made up of normal reactive bone with few or no neoplastic meningeal cells in it and is a complication rather than an integral part of the neoplasm. Occasionally, the overlying bone is destroyed, giving rise to radiolucent patches. Multiple meningiomas do occur, most commonly in association with neurofibromatosis. In the latter condition, congenital absence of portions of the walls of the orbit and defects in the region of the lambdoidal sutures are common lesions. Calvarial lesions, not unlike the defects in neurofibromatosis, can occur in congenital generalized fibromatosis. Chordomas are infrequent in children; they occur predominantly in the base with clinical signs of diplopia, palatal or tongue weakness, headaches, etc. Torticollis occasionally is present. MRI demonstrates its location and extent. The tumor is inhomogeneous in T1- and T2-weighted images and demonstrates septations (Fig 1–93).

A rare tumor of the skull is the melanotic progonoma, also called a retinal anlage tumor but currently bearing the label of melanotic neuroectodermal tumor of infancy. Over 90% of cases involve the head and neck region; 70% occur in the maxilla and about 13% in the calvaria where it has a predi-

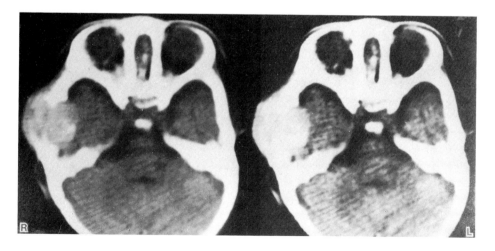

FIG 1–90.
Axial CT scans of osteoblastoma in temporal bone without and with contrast enhancement. The tumor demonstrates prominent enhancement. The patient was a 7-month-old girl with right temporal swelling, slowly increasing in size. (From Miyazaki S, Tsubokawa T, Katayama Y, et al: *Surg Neurol* 1987; 27:277–285. Used by permission.)

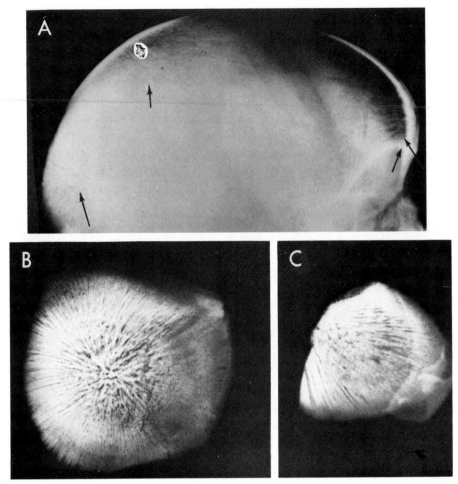

FIG 1–91.
Radially striated hemangiomas *(arrows)* in the frontal and occipital squamosae as well as in both parietal bones of a child who also had hemangiomas of the neck, shoulder, and upper portion of the thorax. **A,** lateral radiograph of the head; **B** and **C,** necropsy specimens from the occipital squamosa. **(Courtesy of Dr. Marie Capitanio, Philadelphia.)**

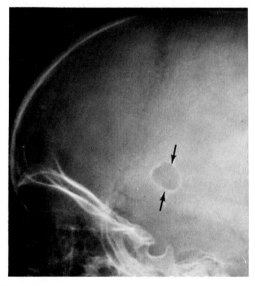

FIG 1–92.
Epidermoidoma in an infant 1 year of age. The *arrows* point to a small oval defect in the parietal bone with a sharply defined sclerotic border.

lection for the region of the anterior fontanelle (Fig 1–94), and about 6% in the mandible, with occasional cases occurring elsewhere in the body, especially the genital organs. Other calvarial sites are in the regions of the anterolateral and posterolateral fontanelles. In the calvaria, the tumor usually begins during the first year of life as a movable scalp nodule that subsequently invades the bone; becomes fixed to it, often adhering to the dura; and grows very rapidly. The bone is destroyed but reactive spicules develop internally and externally producing a sunburst appearance in films tangential to the mass (Fig 1–95). Occasionally, the mass is only of soft tissue density. CT and MRI can be helpful in evaluation of the extent and nature of the tumor. Local recurrences have been noted following surgical removal. Although malignancy has been noted in extracalvarial tumors, it has not been reported for those in the calvaria. The tumor is believed to be of neuroectodermal origin.

In all of these cranial tumors, and in others,

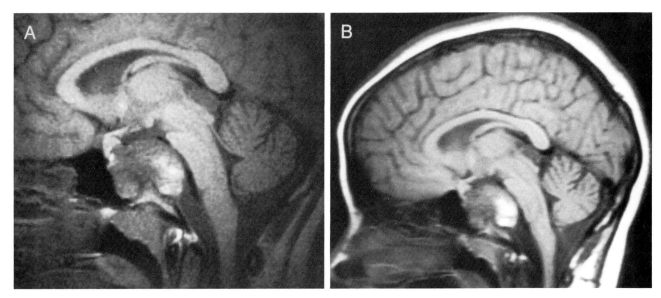

FIG 1–93.
A, midline sagittal T1-weighted (TR/TE = 500/20) image shows mass replacing the clivus, flattening the pons, and extending into the sphenoid sinus, sella, and suprasellar cistern. **B,** sagittal image (TR/TE = 520/20) displays a posterior region of high signal which corresponded to an area of old hemorrhage at surgery. (From Matsumoto J, Towbin RB, Ball WS Jr: *Pediatr Radiol* 1989; 20:28–32. Used by permission.)

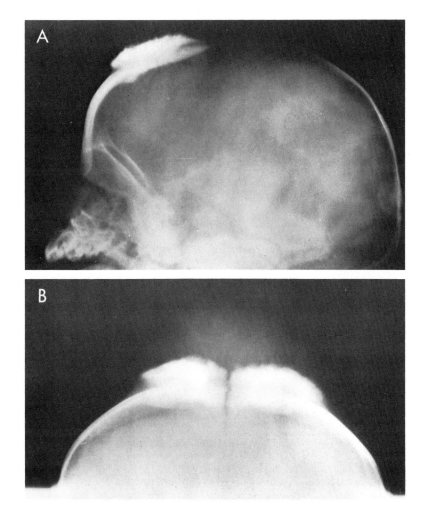

FIG 1–94.
Tangential projection of melanotic progonoma in the region of the anterior fontanelle in a 5-month-old infant. The superficial soft tumor mass is visible in the AP projection. (From Best PV: *J Pathol* 1972; 107:69–72. Used by permission.)

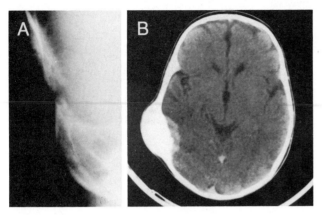

FIG 1–95.
Tangential projection of melanotic progonoma in the region of the posterolateral fontanelle. The spiculated nature of the tumor and the bone reaction is typical **(A).** The nonenhanced CT **(B)** demonstrates the internal expansion of the tumor as well as the massive bone reaction. (From Jones HH, Parker BR, Ballerio CG, et al.: *Skeletal Radiol* 1990; 19:317–318. Used by permission.)

plain film diagnosis is being superseded by CT for investigation and presurgical mapping of tumors of the head and neck, but it still plays a role in initial evaluation.

Keats and Holt reported 21 examples of rounded or oval radiolucent calvarial defects with a surrounding sclerotic halo or central bone density, or both. Royen and Ozonoff found similar, but multiple, radiographic "doughnut lesions" in a 13-year-old boy with increased serum alkaline phosphatase activity, dilatation of medullary cavities, and "squaring of the shafts" of all the metacarpal bones. Microscopic features in the calvarial lesions included fibrous tissue with clusters of foam cells or histiocytes and surrounding sclerotic bone. Bone marrow from the iliac crest and biopsy of a metacarpal bone showed no abnormalities. Familial doughnut lesions (Fig 1–96) of the skull have been reported and similar radiographic changes have been found in sickle cell anemia. However, a malignant calvarial doughnut lesion due to a metastatic carcinoma has been reported with features of a button sequestrum. Most of the conditions associated with button sequestrum are rare in children.

REFERENCES

Atkinson GO, Davis PC, Patrick LE, et al: Melanotic neuroectodermal tumour of infancy. MR findings and a review of the literature. *Pediatr Radiol* 1989; 20:20–22.

Bartlett JE, Kishore PRS: Familial "doughnut" lesions of the skull. *Radiology* 1976; 119:385–387.

Best PV: Pigmented tumor arising in the skull of an infant. *J Pathol* 1972; 107:69–72.

Braendli AF, Bulfamamte GP: Unusual osteoblastoma of the skull. *Helv Paediatr Acta* 1987; 41:505–508.

Briselli MF, Soule EH, Gilchrist DS: Congenital fibromatosis. Report of 18 cases of solitary and 4 cases of multiple tumors. *Mayo Clin Proc* 1980; 55:554–562.

Calliauw L, Roels H, Caemaert J: Aneurysmal bone cysts in the cranial vault and base of the skull. *Surg Neurol* 1985; 23:93–98.

Cutler LS, Chaudhry AP, Topazian R: Melanotic neuroectodermal tumor of infancy. An ultrastructural study, literature review, and revaluation. *Cancer* 1981; 48:257–270.

Holt JF: Neurofibromatosis in children. *Am J Roentgenol* 1978; 130:615–639.

Holthusen W, Lassrich MA, Steiner C: Epidermoids and dermoids of the calvarian bones in early childhood: Their behavior in the growing skull. *Pediatr Radiol* 1983; 13:189–194.

Joffe N: Calvarial bone defects involving the lambdoid suture in neurofibromatosis. *Br J Radiol* 1965; 381:23–27.

Johnson RE, Scheithauer BW, Dahlin DC: Melanotic neuroectodermal tumor of infancy. A review of 7 cases. *Cancer* 1983; 52:661–666.

Jones HH, Parker BR, Ballerio CG, et al: Case report 617; Melanotic neuroectodermal tumor of infancy in the calvaria. *Skeletal Radiol* 1990; 19:317–318.

Keats TE, Holt JF: The calvarial "doughnut lesion": A previously undescribed entity. *Am J Roentgenol* 1969; 105:314–318.

Matsumoto J, Towbin RB, Ball WS Jr: Cranial chordomas in infancy and childhood. A report of two cases and review of the literature. *Pediatr Radiol* 1989; 20:28–32.

Miyazaki S, Tsubokawa T, Katayama Y, et al: Benign os-

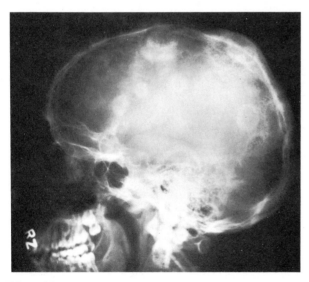

FIG 1–96.
"Doughnut" lesions observed as an incidental finding in the skull of a young man. (Courtesy of Dr. William S. Ball, Jr., Albuquerque, N.M.)

teoblastoma of the temporal bone in an infant. *Surg Neurol* 1987; 27:277–285.

Nolte K: Malignant intracranial chordoma and sarcoma of the clivus in infancy. *Pediatr Radiol* 1979; 8:1–6.

Prabhakar B, Reddy TR, Dayananda B, et al: Osteoid osteoma of the skull. *J Bone Joint Surg [Am]* 1972; 54:146–148.

Rawlings CE III, Wilkins RH: Solitary eosinophilic granuloma of the skull. *Neurosurgery* 1984; 15:155–161.

Rosen IW, Nadel HI: Button sequestrum of the skull. *Radiology* 1969; 92:969–971.

Royen PM, Ozonoff MB: Multiple calvarial "doughnut lesions: A case report. *Am J Roentgenol* 1974; 121:112–123.

Ruge JR, Tomila T, Naidich TP et al: Scalp and calvarial

masses of infants and children. *Neurosurgery* 1988; 22:1037–1042.

Russell EJ: The radiologic approach to malignant tumors of the head and neck, with emphasis on computed tomography. *Clin Plast Surg* 1985; 12:343–374.

Sebes JI, Diggs LW: Radiographic changes in the skull in sickle cell anemia. *Am J Roentgenol* 1979; 132:373–377.

Sholkoff SD, Mainzer F: Button sequestrum revisited. *Radiology* 1971; 100:649–652.

Smith RJ, Evans JM: Head and neck manifestations of histiocytosis-X. *Laryngoscope* 1984; 94:395–399.

Som PM, Anderson PJ, Wolf BS: A malignant calvarial doughnut lesion ("button sequestrum"?). *Mt Sinai J Med* 1978; 45:390–393.

SECTION 6

Miscellaneous Disorders

HYPOVITAMINOSES

Rickets

In some rachitic patients, concurrent with the failure of mineralization, excessive amounts of poorly mineralized bone (osteoid) are heaped up on the outer tables of the parietal and frontal eminences, separately or in combination, and cause regional thickening of the calvaria. During the active phase of the disease, when the mineral content of the bone is reduced, the thickenings are not well visualized roentgenographically. Clinically, they may produce local bosses that have given rise to the term "hot cross bun skull" (Fig 1–97). With healing of the rickets, the calcium content increases and the hyperostoses become more evident (Fig 1–98). Rachitic bossing of the skull persists throughout childhood and may endure into adult life. Kattan observed thickening of the calvaria in epileptic children after protracted treatment with an anticonvulsant for 3 or more years (Fig 1–99). This is a manifestation comparable to rachitic metaphyseal changes also observed in some cases and is believed to reflect intrahepatic competition with vitamin D for liver hydroxylation function required for metabolism of both pharmacologic agents.

Scurvy

Subperiosteal hemorrhages in scurvy may occur over the flat bones of the cranium, as well as on the surfaces of tubular bones, but scorbutic cranial subperiosteal hemorrhages are rare. They have roentgen characteristics similar to those of subperiosteal

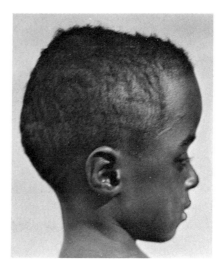

FIG 1–97.
External thickening of the parietal and frontal eminences in a boy 5 years of age with healed rickets.

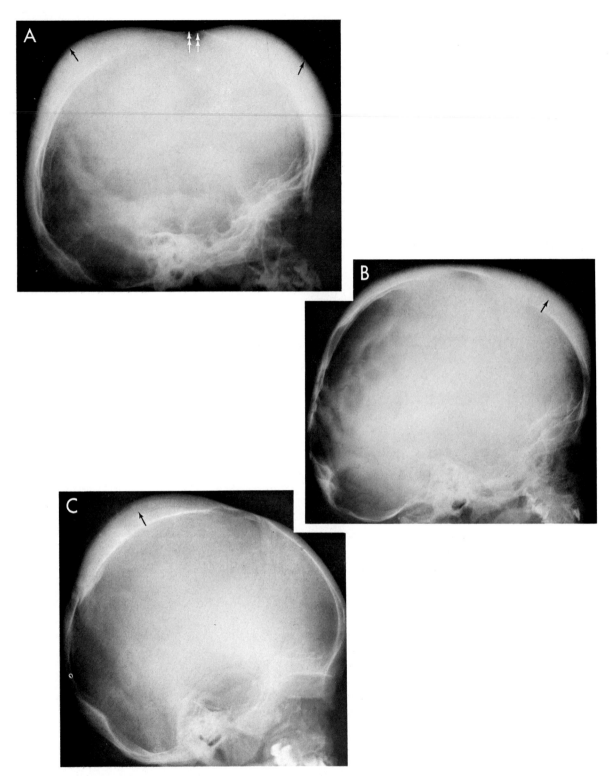

FIG 1–98.

A, healed rachitic hyperostosis (bossing) of the skull with external thickening of the frontal and parietal bones in the regions of the frontal and parietal eminences *(single arrows).* The edges of the bones are not thickened, which accounts for the wide deep groove at the coronal suture *(double arrows).* A similar groove was present at the sagittal suture but is not visible in this projection. The patient, 5 years of age, had the "hot cross bun" grooving of the external surface of the calvaria. It is noteworthy that the hyperostosis is limited to the outer table and that the diploic space and markings are obliterated. The inner table is normal. **B,** thickening limited to the eminences *(arrow)* of the frontal bone in a patient 3 years of age. **C,** hyperostosis of the parietal eminences *(arrow)* in a boy 4 years of age. The frontal bone is not affected.

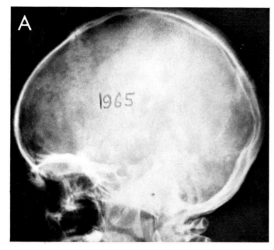

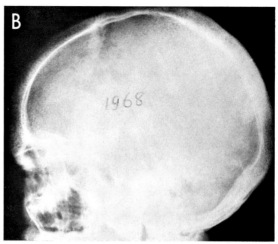

FIG 1–99.
Thickening of the calvaria during the administration of phenytoin (Dilantin) to an epileptic boy. **A,** at the age of 11 years, prior to treatment. **B,** thickened calvaria at 14 years of age. The diploic space is deepened, and both tables are thickened. (Courtesy of Dr. Kenneth Katten, Cincinnati, Ohio.)

hemorrhages elsewhere in the skeleton. Bleeding into the orbit in infantile scurvy may cause exophthalmos.

Vitamin K

Hemorrhagic disease of the newborn is rarely observed today; years ago it was a common contributing factor to the incidence of cephalhematoma, and may occasionally merit consideration when cephalhematomas are exceptionally large.

DISEASES OF ENDOCRINE GLANDS

Thyroid

Retardation of maturation of the skull occurs in untreated hypothyroidism analogous to that observed in the skeletal system elsewhere (Fig 1–100). Dental developmental delay is much less marked than that of the skeletal structures, but does occur. Macroglossia may be observed in lateral skull films.

In hypothyroidism of long standing, the pitu-

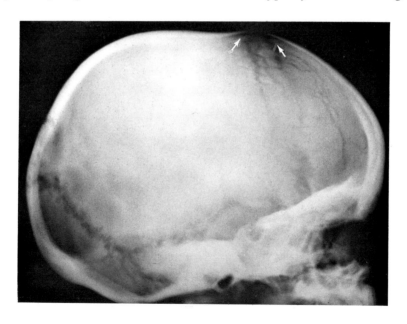

FIG 1–100.
The skull of a cretin 3½ years of age with marked retardation of development. The outer and inner tables and the diploic space are not differentiated. The anterior fontanelle is open *(arrows),* and the coronal lambdoidal and squamosal sutures are wide. The diploic and vascular markings are scanty. Pneumatization has not yet begun in the temporal bone.

itary fossa is commonly enlarged and rounded but not eroded (Fig 1–101). This feature appears to be more common in acquired hypothyroidism than in congenital, probably because the former may persist unrecognized for a longer period of time. Van Wyck and Grumbach described children with spurious precocious sexual development, manifested by lactorrhea, who had unrecognized hypothyroidism and whose enlarged pituitary fossa returned to normal size within weeks to months after the institution of appropriate therapy. In juvenile hyperthyroidism, conventional radiography may demonstrate early closure of cranial sutures as a manifestation of accelerated maturation. CT of the orbit is able to demonstrate the orbital changes responsible for some cases of exophthalmos and other eye signs resulting from infiltration of the ocular muscles, lacrimal glands, and retro-orbital fat; similar changes can be seen in some instances of leukemia (see Fig 1–164).

Pituitary

In primary hypopituitarism, the skull is usually normal; rarely, a small pituitary fossa is noted. The empty sella syndrome has been observed with conventional films and with CT in some children with growth hormone deficiency and other pituitary dysfunction syndromes. MRI studies suggest that a hypoplastic and, often, ectopic pituitary gland is usually present in such cases together with an abnormal or disrupted pituitary stalk. Secondary hypopituitarism and an empty sella can develop following hyperplasia consequent to hypothyroidism, and treatment of the latter with thyroid hormone. In psychosocial, or deprivational dwarfism, in which there is transient hypopituitarism, widening of sutures may be present or develop during recovery. Pseudowidening of cranial sutures may occur following prostaglandin E1 administration. Congenital absence of the pituitary gland is often, but not always, associated with a small sella. Association with endocrine disturbances and secondary clinical features (micropenis, neonatal hypoglycemia, diabetes insipidus, etc.) has been reported. One case has been observed in an infant with sacral agenesis.

Gonads and Adrenals

In hypergonadism and the adrenogenital syndrome, maturation of the skeleton is accelerated. The skull is involved in this acceleration, but the cranial changes are not as conspicuous as those in the appendicular skeleton. Pneumatization of the paranasal sinuses and the mastoid processes may be observed (Fig 1–102).

Parathyroids

Children with hyperparathyroidism demonstrate the granular mottling of osteoporosis in the skull only

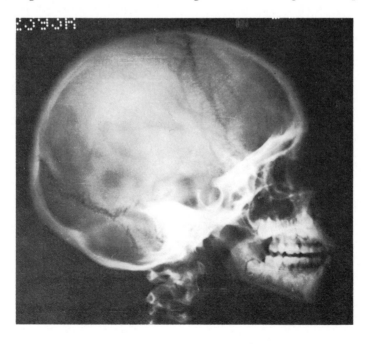

FIG 1–101.
Adolescent girl with acquired hypothyroidism of 5 years' duration. The pituitary fossa is large and rounded; the vertical density superimposed on it is in the squamosa of the temporal bone separating two convolutional markings. (From Silverman FN, Currarino G: *Metabolism* 1960; 9:248–283. Used by permission.)

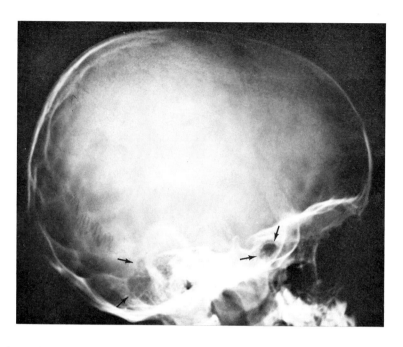

FIG 1–102.
The skull of a girl 4 years of age who exhibited accelerated heterosexual development and suffered from the adrenogenital syndrome. The *arrows* are directed to the extensive pneumatization of the sphenoid and temporal bones. Compare the advanced maturation in this skull with the retarded maturation of the hypothyroid skull in Figure 1–100.

rarely in comparison with adults. When it does occur, it is more frequent in the secondary form associated with renal rickets than in the primary form. Loss of the lamina dura of the teeth is occasionally noted and may assist in diagnosis. The skull may participate in the osteosclerosis occurring in hypoparathyroidism, but by itself would not call attention to the disorder.

DISEASES OF BLOOD

Hemolytic Anemias

In the major groups of chronic hemolytic anemias of infancy and childhood—thalassemia, sickle cell anemia, and spherocytosis—the bone marrow become hyperplastic. This overgrowth of hematopoietic tissue in the skull causes a widening of the diploic space owing to external displacement of the outer table (Figs 1–103 and 1–104), which also becomes atrophic (Figs 1–105, 1–106, and 1–107). In a small percentage of cases, the spicules of diploic bone are arranged in a radial pattern with their long axes extending across the widened diploic space and at right angles to the inner table. Owing to marrow hyperplasia and internal swelling of the temporal and paranasal bones, the air spaces in the temporal bones and in the paranasal sinuses are encroached upon and sometimes obliterated (see Fig 1–105). Swellings of the zygomas make the cheek bones

stand out and are responsible for the "mongoloid" or "rodent" facies, as it is variously characterized in some of the more severe cases. Expansion of maxilla and mandible may cause malposition of the teeth and malocclusion of the jaws, with protrusion of the maxilla that has stimulated the use of these uncomplimentary descriptions. The magnitude of the roentgen findings in the skull does not always parallel the changes in the rest of the skeleton or the changes in the blood. Some patients show no significant abnormality in the skull. The cranial changes are most marked and most frequent in thalassemia; they are least common in spherocytosis.

The similarity of the changes of cranial "symmetric osteoporosis" in prehistoric humans (Hrdlicka) and the cranial manifestations of hemoglobinopathies of current peoples is discussed by Moseley. He deemphasized the role of hereditary hemolytic disease and pointed to the possibility of iron deficiency anemia as a possible cause.

El-Najjar and associates found that, in Indian remains from the southwestern United States, more craniums from canyon botton sites were porotic and hyperostotic than were those from the plains. In the canyon bottoms, a major component of the diet was maize, which is low in iron and contains an inhibitor of iron absorption; the food of the Plains Indians included ample animal protein and was rich in absorbable iron. Children from the canyon bottoms had a higher incidence of porotic hyperostosis of the skull

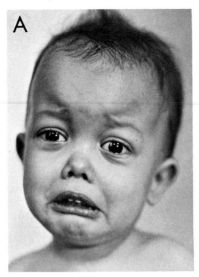
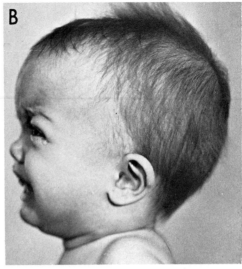

FIG 1–103.

β-Thalassemia (Mediterranean anemia, Cooley anemia). Mongoloid facies and diffuse thickening of the cranium of a Greek boy, aged 1 year and 10 months. The upper maxilla and zygomatic bones are disproportionately enlarged, and the upper teeth are turned upward and outward. The entire calvaria is thickened, but there are no furrows in the sites of the great sutures as in rickets. **A,** frontal, and **B,** lateral views.

than adults, an indication of their greater susceptibility to iron deficiency.

The hair-on-end pattern of calvarial bone has been reported, in addition to its occurrence in the common hemolytic anemias, in eliptocytosis (Moseley 1963), red cell enzyme deficiencies (Becker and associates), polycythemia vera (Dykstra and Halbertsma), and in cyanotic heart disease (Powell and associates). Similar changes have been observed in a child with dyserythropoietic anemia (Glader).

HISTIOCYTOSIS

Conditions falling into this category of disease are covered in more detail in Part VI; only their manifestations in the skull are presented here. Lesions in

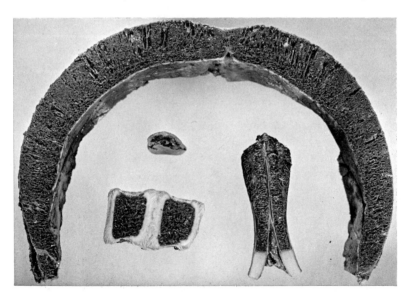

FIG 1–104.

β-Thalassemia: morbid anatomy of the bones studied at necropsy on an Italian girl 5 years of age. In all bones, overgrowth of the red elements in the marrow enlarges the marrow spaces and thins out the overlying cortical layers of bone. In the coronal section of the calvaria, the diploic space is increased to several times its normal depth, and the spongiosa is arranged in a radial pattern; the outer table is largely destroyed from pressure atrophy, while the inner table is relatively little affected. The ribs and vertebrae show similar changes. (From Whipple GH, Bradford WL: *Am J Dis Child* 1932; 44:336–365. Used by permission.)

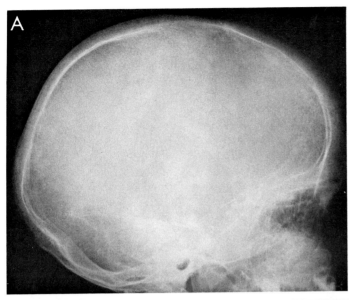

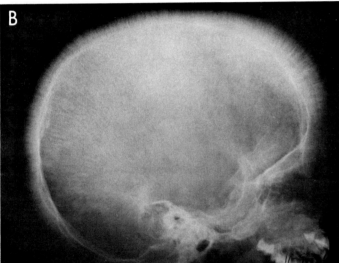

FIG 1–105.
β-Thalassemia. Variations in the cranial findings in two patients, approximately 3 years of age, with similar clinical
and hematologic findings. **A,** widening of the diploic space
and atrophy of the outer table, with granular osteoporosis
but no radial striation. The most marked changes are in the
frontal bone. The maxillary sinus is obliterated, as are the
air spaces in the temporal bone. **B,** widening of the diploic
space, absence of the outer table, and generalized radial
striation. The last two features have been present in fewer
than 20% of our cases.

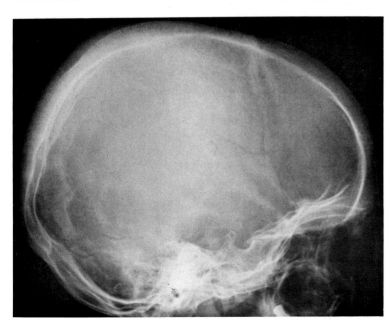

FIG 1–106.
Familial hemolytic icterus (spherocytic anemia) in a girl
13 years of age, showing widening of the diploic space
in the frontal and parietal bones and slight radial striation of the thickened parietal bones.

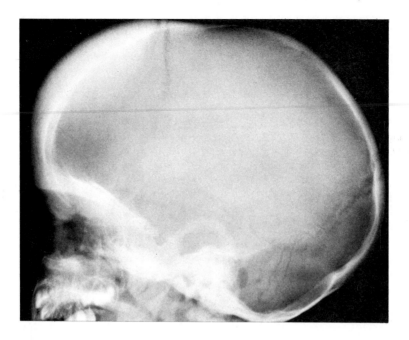

FIG 1–107.
Cranial changes in severe spherocytic anemia in a patient 23 months of age. The tables and the diploic space in the frontal squamosa and in the horizontal plates of the frontal bone are deepened and thickened. The maxillary sinuses are obliterated. The parietal, occipital, and temporal bones are not affected.

the skull are very common. Kirks and Taybi found 28% of 934 lesions in 542 patients in the literature to be located in the skull. The calvaria is more frequently affected than the base. The radiographic hallmark of the disease, here as well as elsewhere, is a bone-replacing radiolucent defect with little or no adjacent reaction. In the calvaria, it is generally described as being "punched out." Involvement of the external table to a greater degree than of the internal table by an enlarging lesion may produce a beveled edge. The lesion, however, may extend intracranially and across sutures. In the base, lesions occur in the mastoid portion of the temporal bone and adjacent petrous pyramids, in the sphenoid bone, and in

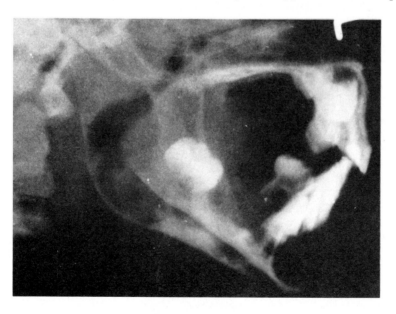

FIG 1–108.
"Floating teeth" in a 54-month-old child with histiocytosis X (Hand-Schüller-Christian disease). The mandibular granuloma has already resulted in destruction of alveolar bone and the loss of one deciduous molar; the remaining deciduous molar appears to "float" in the radiolucent granulomatous tissue. The unerupted first permanent molar is unaffected.

the bones of the orbit. Sphenoid bone involvement may be associated with diabetes insipidus, but this condition can supervene without skeletal changes. Exophthalmos may occur when the bones of the orbit are affected.

Histiocytosis X (Langerhans cell histiocytosis) is said to be the most common cause of the so-called button sequestrum (Rosen and Nadel). This lesion also occurs in infection, neoplastic disease, radiation necrosis, postsurgical defects, and in a variety of other conditions. Mandibular involvement is more common than maxillary and begins characteristically in the molar areas of the alveolar processes, where focal destruction of bone results in "floating teeth" (Fig 1–108); frequently, teeth are loose and spontaneous shedding of teeth is not uncommon. Multiple lesions (Fig 1–109) are more frequently associated with Hand-Schüller-Christian disease than with Letterer-Siwe disease and generally occur in children under 5 years of age. In the latter condition, focal skeletal lesions may be totally lacking, and only osteopenia and thin cortical bone may be observed. A

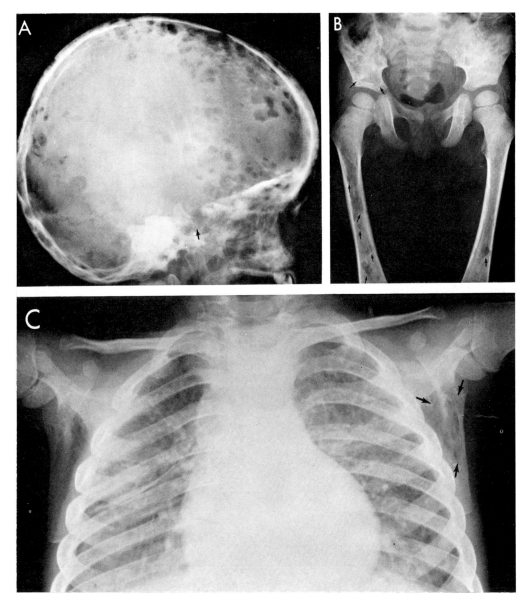

FIG 1–109.
Hand-Schüller-Christian disease (histiocytosis X) in a boy 3½ years old. **A,** the skull shows numerous small and large rounded defects in the calvaria and base *(arrow).* Necropsy disclosed a large part of the body of the sphenoid replaced by cholesterol-containing hyperplastic reticulum cells. **B,** large and small defects in the ilia and femora; the latter show erosions of the cortex, which indicates that destruction originates in the medullary cavity and not under the periosteum. **C,** defects in the scapulae and reticulosis of the lungs and pleura.

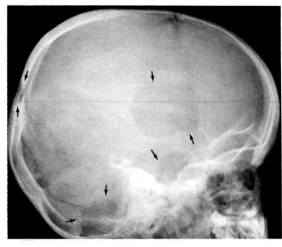

FIG 1–110.
This 3-year-old boy with calvarial lesions *(arrows)* had similar lesions in the ilium and femur, characteristic of Hand-Schüller-Christian disease, all of which regressed after roentgenotherapy. Microscopic diagnosis was eosinophilic granuloma. The validity of the term *histiocytosis X*, or better, *Langerhans cell histiocytosis*, is supported by this example of confusion of the disorders subsumed under the earlier terms.

solitary calvarial lesion in a child over 5 years of age (Fig 1–110) is likely to be associated with eosinophilic granulona of bone.

In the course of healing, the margins of the lesions lose their sharpness, and the disparity in opacity between the lesion and the adjacent bone diminishes to the point of disappearance.

REFERENCES

Hypovitaminoses

Hess AF: *Scurvy, Past and Present*. Philadelphia, Lippincott, 1920.

Hess AF: *Rickets, Osteomalacia and Tetany*. Philadelphia, Lea & Febiger, 1929.

Hunt PA, Wu-Chen ML, Handal NJ, et al.: Bone disease induced by anticonvulsant therapy and treatment with calcitriol (1,25-dihydroxyvitamin D_3). *Am J Dis Child* 1986; 140:715–718.

Kattan KR: Calvarial thickening after Dilantin medication. *Am J Roentgenol* 1970; 110:102–105.

Diseases of Endocrine Glands

Anderton JM, Owen R: Absence of the pituitary gland in a case of congenital sacral agenesis. *J Bone Joint Surg [Br]* 1983; 65B:182–183.

Beitzke A, Stein J: Pseudo-widening of cranial sutures as a feature of long-term prostaglandin E1 therapy. *Pediatr Radiol* 1986; 16:57–58.

Bellini MA, Neves J: The skull in childhood myxedema: Its roentgen appearance. *Am J Roentgenol* 1956; 76:495–498.

Bjernulf A, Hall K, Sjögren I, et al.: Primary hyperparathyroidism in children: Brief review of the literature and a case report. *Acta Paediatr Scand* 1970; 59:249–258.

Bourgeois MJ, Jones B, Weagner DC, et al: Micropenis and congenital adrenal hypoplasia. *Am J Perinatol* 1989; 6:69–71.

di Natale B, Scotti G, Pellini C, et al: Empty sella in children with pituitary dwarfism: Does it exist? *Pediatrician* 1987; 14:246–252.

Enzmann DR, Donaldson SS, Kriss JP: Appearance of Graves' disease on orbital computed tomography. *J Comput Assist Tomogr* 1979; 3:815–819.

Johnsonbaugh RE, Bryan RN, Hierlwimmer UR, et al: Premature cranial synostosis: A complication of thyroid replacement. *J Pediatr* 1978; 93:188–191.

LaFranchi SH, Hanna CE, Krainz PL: Primary hypothyroidism, empty sella, and hypopituitarism. *J Pediatr* 1986; 108:571–573.

Riggs W, Wilroy RS, Etteldorf JN: Neonatal hyperthyroidism with accelerated skeletal maturation, craniosynostosis and brachydactyly. *Radiology* 1972; 105:621–625.

Root AW, Martinez CR, Muroff LR: Subhypothalamic high-intensity signals identified by magnetic resonance imaging in children with idiopathic anterior hypopituitarism. Evidence suggestive of an "ectopic" posterior pituitary gland. *Am J Dis Child* 1989; 143:366–367.

Smith SP, Wolpert SM, Sadeghi-Najad A, et al: Value of computed tomographic scanning in patients with growth hormone deficiency. *Pediatrics* 1986; 78:601–605.

Van Wyk JJ, Grumbach MM: Syndrome of precocious menstruation and galactorrhea in juvenile hypothyroidism: An example of hormonal overlap in pituitary feedback. *J Pediatr* 1960; 57:416–422.

Diseases of Blood

Becker MH, Genieser N, Piomelli S, et al: Roentgenographic manifestations of pyruvate kinase deficiency hemolytic anemia. *Am J Roentgenol* 1971; 113:491–498.

Caffey J: Cooley's anemia: A review of the roentgenographic findings in the skeleton. *Am J Roentgenol* 1957; 78:381–391.

Dykstra OH, Halbertsma T: Polycythemia vera in childhood: Report of a case with changes in the skull. *Am J Dis Child* 1940; 60:907–916.

El-Najjar MY, Lozoff B, Ryan DJ: The paleoepidemiology of porotic hyperostosis in the American Southwest: Radiological and ecological considerations. *Am J Roentgenol* 1975; 125:918–924.

Glader BE: Personal communication.

Hrdlicka A: Cited by Moseley JE, 1965.

Moseley JE: *Bone Changes in Hemolytic Disorders*. Philadelphia, Grune & Stratton, 1963.

Moseley JE: The paleopathologic riddle of "symmetrical osteoporosis." *Am J Roentgenol* 1965; 95:135–142.

Powell JW, Weens S, Wenger NK: The skull roentgenogram in iron deficiency anemia and in secondary polycythemia. *Am J Roentgenol* 1965; 95:143–147.

Whipple GH, Bradford WL: Racial or familial anemia of children associated with fundamental disturbances of bone and pigment metabolism (Cooley-van Jaksch). *Am J Dis Child* 1932; 44:336–365.

Histiocytosis

Jones RO, Pillsbury HC: Histocytosis X of the head and neck. *Laryngoscope* 1984; 94:1031–1035.

Kirks DR, Taybi H: Histiocytosis X, in Parker BR, Castellino RA (eds): *Pediatric Oncologic Radiology.* St Louis, Mosby–Year Book, 1977.

Nesbit ME, Wolfson JJ, Lieffer SA, et al: Orbital sclerosis in histiocytosis X. *Am J Roentgenol* 1970; 110:123–128.

Rosen IW, Nadel HI: Button sequestrum of the skull. *Radiology* 1969; 92:969–971.

SECTION 7

Face and Individual Cranial Structures

In addition to conventional examinations, CT is used to clarify the unavoidable superimpositions of the many structures that constitute the complex anatomy of the face. The latter technique has rendered multiplanar tomography obsolete. Roentgen cephalometry, a technique used extensively by orthodontists and maxillofacial surgeons, provides excellent depiction of anatomical relations. It is particularly useful for evaluation of growth changes or results of surgical intervention because of its ability to provide exact registration, in serial films, of landmarks in relation to any constant reference point. As in the neurocranium and base, MRI, and CT with three-dimensional reformatted images, have become of major import in diagnosis and in the planning and control of surgical procedures.

THE NOSE

Some of the anatomical features of the normal nose are illustrated in Figures 1–111 and 1–112.

The external nose is best visualized roentgenographically in the lateral projection (Fig 1–113); for evaluation of the arch formed by the nasal bones (in suspected fracture), an exaggerated Waters projection is very helpful (see Fig 1–134). The posteroanterior (PA) projection is used for demonstration of the internal nose (Figs 1–114 and 1–115). The nasal septum is straight and thick at birth; the thinning and lateral deviation of later life (Fig 1–116) have been explained by buckling of the septum because it grows more rapidly than the lateral walls of the na-

sal fossa, and because the median incisor teeth erupt asymmetrically. The septal deviations are usually toward the right and are most common at the site of junction of the ethmoid bone and the vomer. Three-dimensional CT re-formation is taking the place of the above techniques for evaluation of congenital malformations as well as for the surgical approach to, and postoperative assessment of, craniofacial ab-

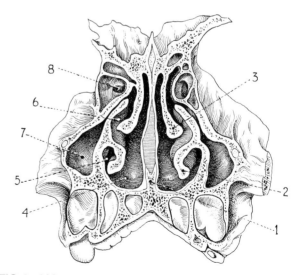

FIG 1–111.
A frontal section through the nasal fossa and paranasal sinuses at the level of the ostium of the maxillary sinus in a child 7 years of age. *1*, nasal septum; *2*, inferior turbinate; *3*, middle turbinate; *4*, nasal fossa; *5*, inferior meatus; *6*, middle meatus; *7*, maxillary sinus; *8*, ethmoid cells. **(Redrawn from Schaeffer JP:** *The Nose, Paranasal Sinuses, Naso-Lacrimal Passageways and the Olfactory Organ in Man.* **Philadelphia, P Blakiston's Sons & Co, 1920.)**

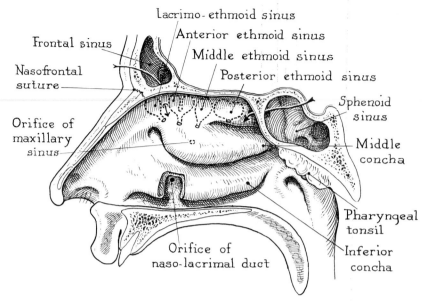

FIG 1–112.
Lateral wall of the right nasal fossa and nasopharynx.

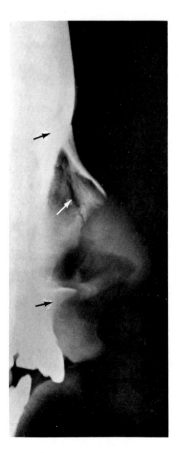

normalities of various types, but the more simple examinations remain valuable initial diagnostic tools and, not infrequently, the only ones needed for most investigations in this region.

Diseases of External Nose

Both the soft tissues and the bones of the external nose vary greatly in size and contour in different people. The paired nasal bones exhibit many normal variations; they may be divided into several separate ossicles by accessory sutures, and tiny intrasutural ossicles may develop in the normal sutures. These variant ossicles should be given appropriate consideration in the diagnosis of fractures. The normal sutures may be absent. The nasal bones are hypoplas-

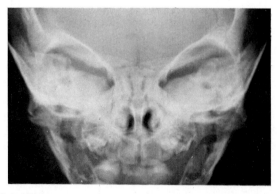

FIG 1–113.
The normal external nose, lateral projection. The two *upper arrows* point to the nasofrontal and nasomaxillary sutures where the nasal bone articulates with the frontal bone and the nasofrontal process of the maxillary bone. The *lowest arrow* is directed at the anterior nasal spine of the maxilla.

FIG 1–114.
The internal nose of an infant 2 days of age with a low, broad nasal fossa and a thick, straight septum. The turbinates are well developed and fill much of the space in the nasal cavities.

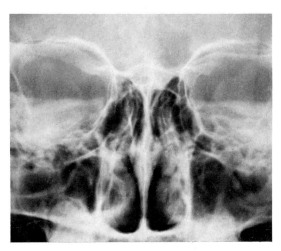

FIG 1–115.
The internal nose of a child 6 years of age. In comparison with that in Figure 1–114, the nasal cavities are heightened, and the nasal septum is thin. The frontal, maxillary, and ethmoid sinuses are pneumatized. The ethmoids are located in the medial walls of the orbits below the cribriform plate.

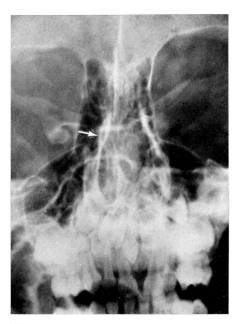

FIG 1–116.
Obliteration of the left nasal cavity in a patient with rhinitis. The turbinates are swollen; the lower segment of the nasal septum is deflected to the right *(arrow)*.

tic in Down syndrome and in chondrodysplasia punctata, and may even be absent in the latter. Elongation of the nasal bones has been observed in the trichorhinophalangeal syndrome. Complex malformations can occur in association with facial clefting syndromes.

Diseases of Internal Nose

Large inferior turbinates may protrude dorsad into the air column of the nasopharynx and be seen in lateral projection as rounded masses of water density (Fig 1–117). Atresia or stenosis of the posterior nares (choanae) is generally suspected in a newborn with respiratory distress and excessive nasal mucus in whom a nasal catheter could not be passed to the nasopharynx and esophagus.

Choanal atresia is due to failure of the normal rupture, on the 35th to 38th fetal days, of the partition (bucconasal membrane) that separates the bucconasal and the buccal cavities. The obstruction is bony or cartilaginous in 90% of cases and membranous in 10%. One third of the cases are bilateral. The lesion is more common in girls and more common on the right side, both in ratios of 2:1. The obstructive tissue varies from a thin diaphragm of soft tissue to a thick wall composed of bone, cartilage or soft tissues, singly or in combination. Radiographic confirmation can be made by instillation of an opaque medium into the nasal cavity with the patient supine, and a cross-table lateral projection. If this procedure is used, the nasal cavity should first be aspirated, and a nasal decongestant should be in-

stilled into each nostril to prevent misdiagnosis due to inflammatory swelling of the mucosa or as a consequence of maternal drug exposure, particularly to reserpine. Unilateral choanal atresia is usually benign; diagnosis and treatment are not emergent. Bilateral atresia may be fatal because newborn infants are usually obligate nasal breathers.

CT examination is the procedure of choice for evaluation of the anatomy and assists in determining the surgical approach (Fig 1–118). Narrowing of the posterior nasal airway occurs at the site of stenosis and is associated with enlargement of the vomer to which the medially bowed walls are fused. The skeletal changes are less marked or absent in nonosseous atresia, but the space between the vomer and the lateral walls is diminished in comparison with the normal. A clustering of abnormalities in association with choanal atresia has been reported under the acronym of CHARGE. It includes *c*oloboma, *h*eart disease, *a*tresia of choanae, *r*etarded growth and development, *g*enital hypoplasia, and *e*ar anomalies or deafness.

Bony stenosis of the nasal pyriform aperture (anterior nares) may clinically simulate posterior choanal obstruction. CT examination clearly differentiates the two conditions for which the surgical management is quite different.

Dermoid cysts of the nose are largely external but may have components that can involve not only the internal nose but even the intracranial struc-

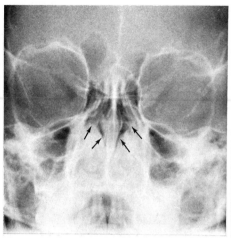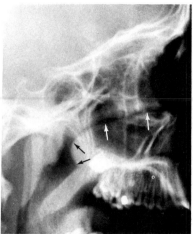

FIG 1–117.
Inflammatory swelling of the inferior turbinates. **A,** frontal projection. In **B,** a lateral projection, the dorsal end of the swollen inferior turbinate projects dorsad into the air column of the nasopharynx. A strip of gas *(arrows)* outlines the superior edge of the enlarged turbinates.

tures. When the cyst is large and in the frontal squamosa, the associated bony defect may simulate that of epidermoidoma or frontal encephalocele (Fig 1–119]). In about 20% of patients, an intracranial extension is present; in some cases, there is only a fibrous cord extending to the base of the foramen cecum. Preoperative imaging may indicate the need for neurosurgical standby or actual participation in treatment. CT is valuable in identifying associated skeletal features of intracranial extension; a bifid crista galli has been reported in some cases (Fig 1–120). MRI may assist in evaluation of soft tissue features, especially in differentiating nasal "gliomas," which may attach or arise from the brain, and encephaloceles (Fig 1–121).

Thickening of the soft tissue linings of the nasal fossae and of the turbinates, and inflammatory exudate in the air spaces, occlude the nasal passages in acute and chronic infections (see Fig 1–117). Similar features can be seen in allergic rhinitis and in the presence of radiolucent foreign bodies; in the latter case, a bloody discharge is often present. Opaque foreign bodies are usually seen but bony ones may be difficult to recognize (Fig 1–122).

Fractures of Facial Bones

Direct trauma is the common cause of fracture of the nasal bones; injuries to other parts of the head may be associated. Nasal fractures may be simple or comminuted (Fig 1–123). The fragments are usually displaced laterally; when the vertical plate of the ethmoid is also broken, the fragments are driven posteriorly. The Waters projection (see Fig 1–134) is use-

ful as it projects the nasal bones in an arch and displays depression of the bones if present. Extension of a fracture into the frontal or ethmoid sinuses can result in regional interstitial emphysema. Infection may be superimposed on the changes.

The complex bony structures of the face commonly fall into a special group of fractures that are subdivided into five major types: (1) fracture of the alveolar processes; (2) horizontal maxillary fracture (Le Fort type I); (3) pyramidal maxillary fracture (Le Fort type II); (4) craniomaxillary dysjunction (Le Fort type III); and (5) blow-out fracture of the orbit. The frequency of facial fractures tends to increase with age during childhood. Mandibular fractures are the most frequent and are described in Section 8. The zygomatic and nasal complexes are next in frequency, while fractures of the maxilla and middle third of the face are relatively rare in comparison with adults.

Alveolar process fractures occur more frequently in the maxilla than in the mandible because of the position of the anterior teeth and are more common in older children, partially because the bone-to-tooth ratio is higher in younger children. They are best demonstrated on intraoral films in which the horizontal radiolucent fracture lines are clearly recognized. They are also visible on conventional PA projections of the skull which may demonstrate associated dental injuries such as root fracture, displacements, and avulsions, and in pantomographic films as well. CT is the most informative technique to show the extent and nature of facial fractures.

Recognition of the Le Fort fractures often depends on careful evaluation of the bony borders to

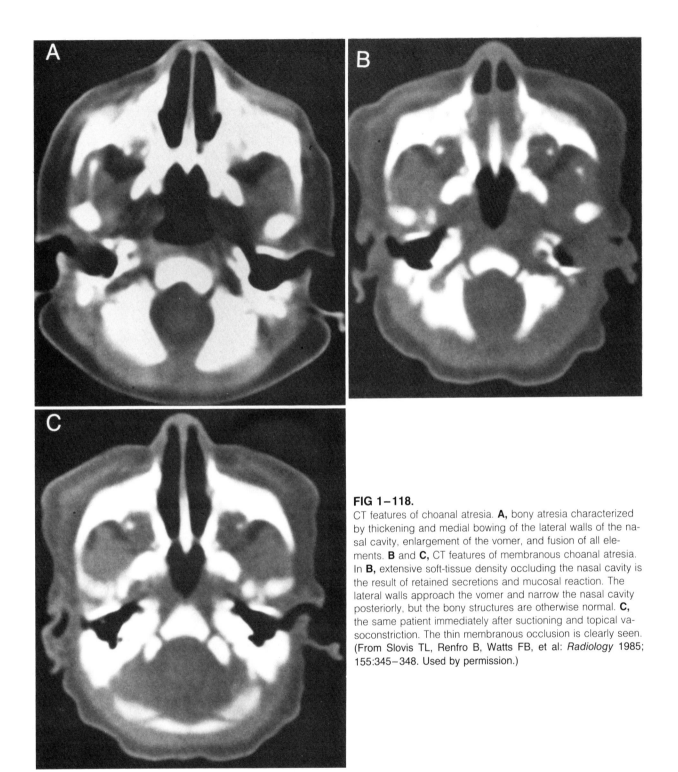

FIG 1–118.
CT features of choanal atresia. **A,** bony atresia characterized by thickening and medial bowing of the lateral walls of the nasal cavity, enlargement of the vomer, and fusion of all elements. **B** and **C,** CT features of membranous choanal atresia. In **B,** extensive soft-tissue density occluding the nasal cavity is the result of retained secretions and mucosal reaction. The lateral walls approach the vomer and narrow the nasal cavity posteriorly, but the bony structures are otherwise normal. **C,** the same patient immediately after suctioning and topical vasoconstriction. The thin membranous occlusion is clearly seen. (From Slovis TL, Renfro B, Watts FB, et al: *Radiology* 1985; 155:345–348. Used by permission.)

identify discontinuities and displacements. The Le Fort I fracture crosses the maxilla horizontally with discontinuities recognizable in the lateral and nasal walls of the antra and lower portions of the pterygoid plates. The affected segment is commonly displaced posteriorly and inferiorly. Because of proximity to the maxillary antra, hemorrhage into the cavities may obliterate the air space. Bony components of the nasal septum and the zygoma are frequently injured as well.

The Le Fort II fracture generally disrupts the suture lines between the maxilla and the zygomatic and frontal bones particularly. Here too, fracture of the zygoma with displacement is common. In the Le

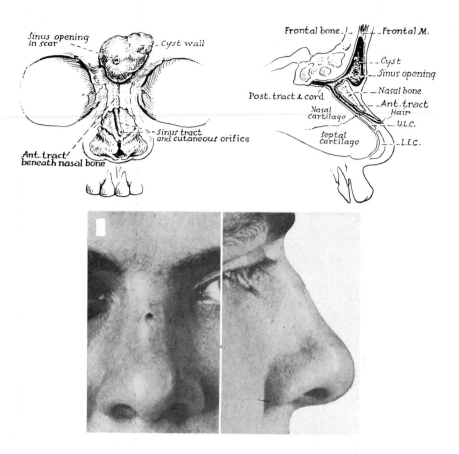

FIG 1–119.

Dermoid cyst of the nose. The schematic drawings above the photographs show a frontal defect containing a cyst with an epithelium-lined tube that extends caudad from the cyst to penetrate the nasal bones near the midsagittal plane and then to course caudad again and open on the skin surface. The photographs show the opening with localized swelling. (From Crawford JK, Webster JP: *Plast Reconstr Surg* 1952; 9:235–260. Used by permission.)

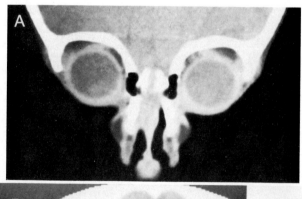
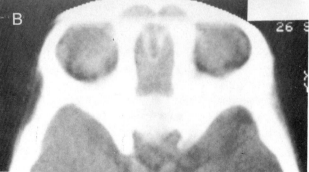

FIG 1–120.

High resolution CT of a 20-month-old boy with a nasal dermoid showing features of intracranial extension. **A,** there is deep involvement of the base of the skull indicated by the midline lucency; a bifid crista galli is shown in **B.** (From Clark WD, Bailey BJ, Stiernberg CM: *Otolaryngol Head Neck Surg* 1985; 93:102–104. Used by permission.)

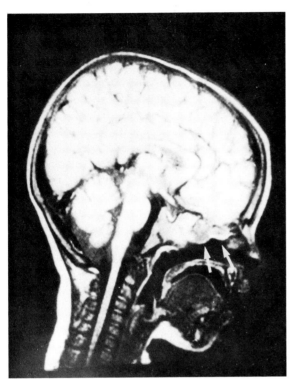

FIG 1–121.
Sagittal MRI of a 19-month-old boy with a congenital midline encephalocele *(arrows)* protruding into the roof of the nasal cavity. (From Lusk RP, Lee PC: *Otolaryngol Head Neck Surg* 1986; 95:303–306. Used by permission.)

Fort III fracture, the facial mass tends to be separated from the cranium, The orbits are usually traversed by the fracture line, In lateral projection, the entire midface often appears displaced posteriorly.

Pressure applied to the globe, directed from the base of the orbital cone toward the narrowing apex, causes a breakthrough in one of the walls of the orbit, most frequently the inferior, which is also the superior wall of the maxillary sinus, and results in the blow-out fracture of the orbit. Some of the inferior orbital contents, such as fat and a portion of the inferior rectus muscle, may herniate through the defect (Fig 1–124). The displacement of orbital contents results in characteristic enophthalmos (often not recognized until after the swelling has receded), impaired upward rotation of the eyeball, and diplopia that constitute the clinical signs of blow-out fracture. Recognition of the depressed bony fragments of the orbital floor and of herniation of contents is important, as atrophy of the intraorbital soft tissues may interfere with correction of the enophthalmos, and visual problems may arise if treatment is delayed. CT identifies not only the muscle and fat displacements of blow-out fractures of the orbits but also injury to the optic canal that may require optic nerve decompression to prevent blindness. Fractures of the lesser wing of the sphenoid, which are well demonstrated, are an important finding for decisions on management.

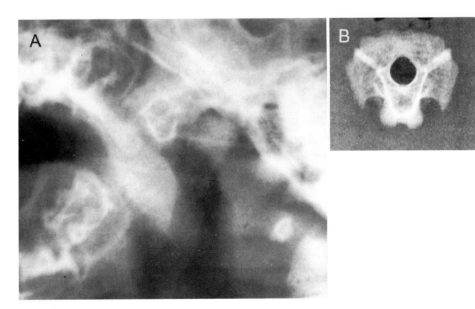

FIG 1–122.
A 10-month-old infant who developed respiratory distress while in the playpen. A sibling was reported to have given the infant a piece of a cooked chicken neck that was seen in the hypopharynx by a physician who was unable to retrieve it. A consultant was unable to confirm its presence, and a film of the neck and chest failed to reveal any foreign body. The next day, an attempt to pass a small nasogastric tube for administration of a barium examination of the esophagus and stomach was unsuccessful; a larger tube was passed, the child coughed, and spewed out a foreign body. A radiograph of the foreign body, **B,** permitted its recognition in review of the nasopharyngeal region, **A,** of the film of the previous day.

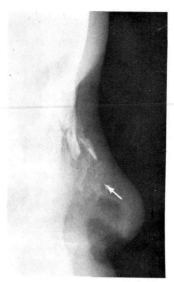

FIG 1–123.
Comminuted fracture of the nasal bones without a striking depression deformity of the nose in a boy 10 years of age.

Neoplasms

New growths, rare in infants and children, obliterate the air spaces of the nasal fossa. Unless the tumor is large or destroys contiguous bones, the roentgen findings simulate those of nasal inflammation. Respiratory distress may be the initial clinical sign. Antronasal polyps may be associated with cystic fibrosis of the pancreas (Fig 1–125); other tumors reported include fibrous histiocytoma and dermoid polyp. The juvenile nasopharyngeal angiofibroma is a be-

nign, highly vascular tumor that can be locally invasive, even extending intracranially. The tumor is included among the juvenile fibromatoses, a group of nonmetastasizing fibroblastic tumors. It may arise in the sphenoid sinus, maxillary antrum, or posterior end of the inferior turbinate. In its growth, it usually causes anterior bowing of the posterior wall of the maxillary antrum (Fig 1–126). It occurs in adolescents, almost always male, and presents with severe, often unilateral, nosebleeds, airway obstruction, and recurrent middle ear disease. CT is ideal for defining extent and, with selective angiography and preoperative embolization, greatly assists the surgical treatment. Preoperative steroids had been used to diminish the size of the tumor. Both CT (Figs 1–127 and 1–128) and MRI are extremely helpful in demonstrating the effects of neoplasms in and adjacent to the complex structures of the nasal and paranasal regions. Other tumors in this region are discussed in a series of papers by Fu and Perzin.

SINUSES

Paranasal Sinuses

The paranasal sinuses are paired pneumatic cavities that communicate with the nasal fossae and are situated in the paranasal bones: maxilla, ethmoid, frontal, and sphenoid (Fig 1–129). Because of the continuity of its air cell mucosa with that of the nasal cavity via the eustachian tubes, the mastoid cells can be

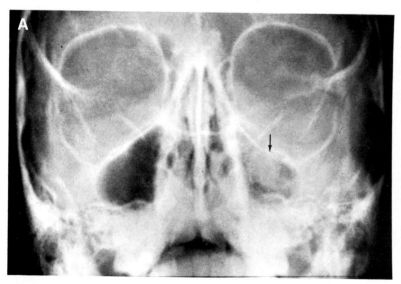

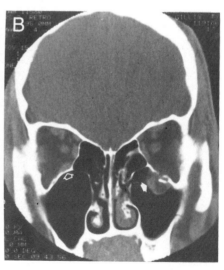

FIG 1–124.
A, blow-out fracture of the floor of the left orbit of a girl 9 years of age. The left maxillary sinus is partially obscured (arrow) by soft tissue displaced caudad from the left orbit. **B,** coronal CT in a blow-out fracture of the orbital floor. There is a fracture of the or-

bital floor with downward displacement of a fracture fragment and a mass protruding into the sinus. The mass contains orbital fat and the inferior rectus muscle (white arrow). Compare with the inferior rectus muscle (open arrow) on the normal right side.

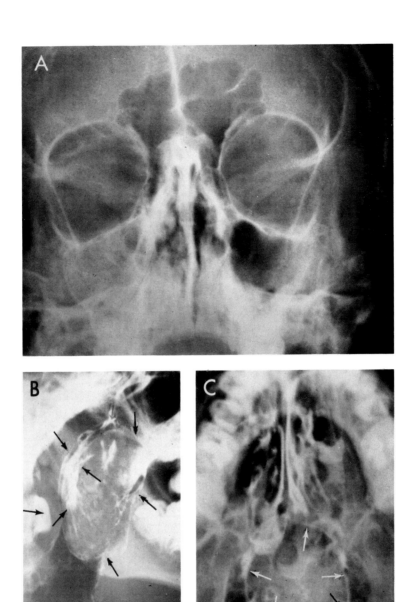

FIG 1–125.
Antronasal polyp in the nasopharynx with an opaque-looking maxillary sinus in the Waters projection **(A).** In the lateral projection **(B),** the large tumor in the nasopharynx *(arrows)* is outlined with a thin film of opaque contrast agent. In the basilar projection **(C),** the mass is also seen in the nasopharynx and is outlined *(arrows)* with a film of opaque contrast agent. There was no information about cystic fibrosis of the pancreas in this patient. **(Courtesy of Dr. Andrew Poznanski, Chicago.)**

considered an additional component. The size and shape of the cavities varies in different age periods, among individuals, and on the two sides of the same individual.

The sites of the openings of the sinuses into the nasal cavity are shown in Figure 1–112. The postnatal growth and extension of the sinuses are shown in Figure 1–130. The fully developed maxillary, frontal, and ethmoid sinuses are illustrated diagrammatically in Figures 1–131 and 1–132. The diagrams are based on conventional radiographic examinations; CT has demonstrated extension from adjacent sinuses into the orbital roofs and apices of the petrous temporal bone that is not easily recognized on conventional films.

Disease of the paranasal sinuses is characterized

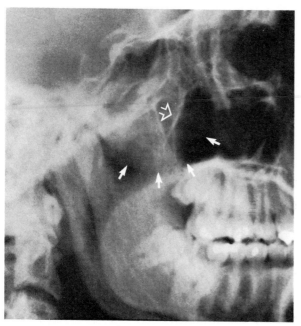

FIG 1–126.
Nasopharyngeal angiofibroma in a 20-year-old man. The *solid arrows* outline the mass where it projects into the nasopharynx and nasal cavity; the open *arrow* indicates the anterior bowing of the posterior wall of the maxillary sinus. (**Courtesy of Dr. Corning Benton, Cincinnati, Ohio.**)

roentgenographically by reduction of the air content of the sinus cavities and by changes in definition of the surrounding bony margins. Asymmetries of development (Fig 1–133) as well as thickening of the soft tissues of the face may simulate pathologic change, as may errors of positioning.

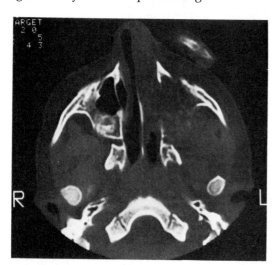

FIG 1–127.
CT scan at a level just below the roof of the maxillary sinuses in a child with neuroblastoma metastasized to the orbit. A tumor has invaded the left maxillary sinus, broken through its walls, and extended into the left nasal cavity. (**Courtesy of Dr. Robert Brasch, University of California, San Francisco.**)

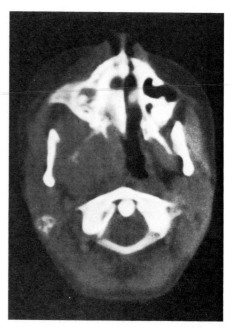

FIG 1–128.
CT scan of a child with a soft-tissue mass in the right tonsillar fossa; the clinical differential diagnosis was between an abscess and tumor. The destruction and displacement of the pterygoid plates clearly indicated the malignant nature of the mass, which was a rhabdomyosarcoma. (**Courtesy of Dr. Robert Brasch, University of California, San Francisco.**)

Maxillary Sinuses

Changes in size and configuration of the maxillary sinuses with age are shown in Figure 1–134. Variations in development include isolated unilateral hypoplasia and prominent septa that appear to com-

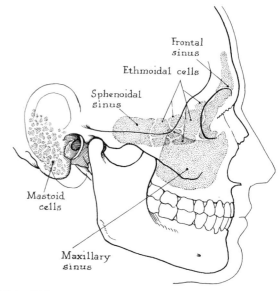

FIG 1–129.
Surface projection of the paranasal sinuses and mastoid cells.

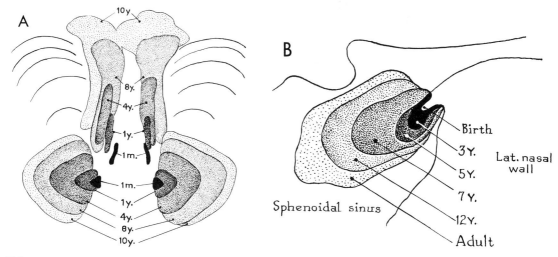

FIG 1–130.
A, composite drawing showing the changes in size and shape of the maxillary and frontal sinuses in one individual during infancy and childhood. *m* = month; *y* = year. (Modified from Maresh MM: *Am J Dis Child* 1940; 60:55–78.) **B,** diagram illustrating the post-natal growth of the sphenoid sinus from birth to maturity. (Redrawn from Scammon RE: A summary of the anatomy of the infant and child, in Abt IA (ed): *Pediatrics,* vol 1. Philadelphia, WB Saunders, 1923, pp 257–444.)

partmentalize the sinus cavity (see Fig 1–133). Occasionally, the roots of the maxillary molars impinge on the walls of the sinuses (Fig 1–135) and sometimes produce folds in the mucous membranes. In oblique ventrodorsal projections of the skull, the roots of the teeth may be superimposed on the sinuses and appear to project into them when no direct anatomical relations exist between the sinus cavity and the dental roots (see Fig 1–138). A molar that fails to migrate is found in its fetal position near the

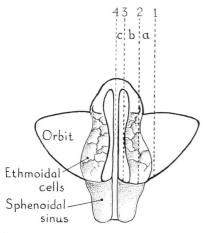

FIG 1–131.
Relations of the ethmoid labyrinths, sphenoid sinuses, and orbits as viewed in horizontal section. In segment *a* the posterior ethmoid cells are located on the margins of the orbit lying lateral to the anterior and middle groups and so are not superimposed on them or the sphenoid sinus in the dorsoventral roentgenographic projection. In segment *b*, the three groups of ethmoid cells lie in the same dorsoventral axis and are therefore superimposed on one another and on the sphenoid sinus in the dorsoventral roentgen projection. In segment *c*, a portion of the anterior wall of the sphenoid sinus lies medial to the ethmoid labyrinth and is not superimposed on it in the dorsoventral roentgenographic projection. (Redrawn from Koehler A: *Roentgenography: The Borderlands of the Normal and Early Pathological in the Skiagram.* New York, William Wood & Co, 1928.)

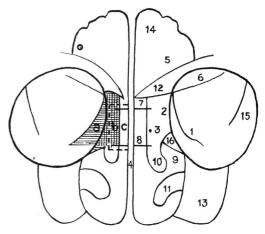

FIG 1–132.
The paranasal sinuses in a dorsoventral projection. *a,* posterior ethmoid cells; *b,* superimposed anterior, middle, and posterior ethmoid cells; *c,* sphenoid sinus without superimposed ethmoid cells. *1,* inner edge of the inferior orbital fissure; *2,* inner margin of the orbit; *3,* medial border of the lateral mass of the ethmoid bone; *4,* nasal septum; *5,* superciliary ridge; *6,* upper border of the superior orbital fissure; *7,* nasofrontal and nasomaxillary sutures; *8,* roof of the superior nasal meatus; *9,* uncinate process; *10,* middle turbinate; *11,* inferior turbinate; *12,* internal projection of the superior orbital margin; *13,* maxillary sinus; *14,* frontal sinus; *15,* sphenozygomatic suture; *16,* ethmoid bulla. (Redrawn from Koehler A: *Roentgenography: The Borderlands of the Normal and Early Pathological in the Skiagram.* New York, William Wood & Co, 1928.)

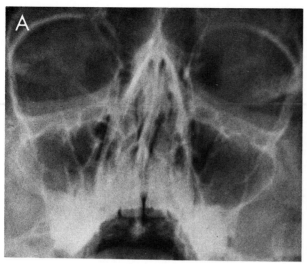
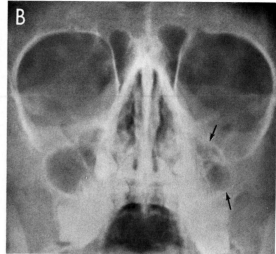

FIG 1–133.
Variants of the maxillary sinus. **A,** several septa and ridges dividing the maxillary sinus into several small cavities in a girl 11 years of age. **B,** hypoplasia of the left maxillary sinus in a boy 7 years of age.

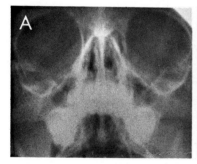
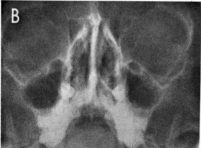
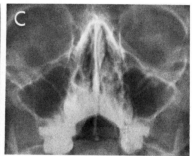

FIG 1–134.
Waters projection of normal maxillary sinuses in a child at age 4 **(A),** 7 **(B),** and 11 **(C)** years.

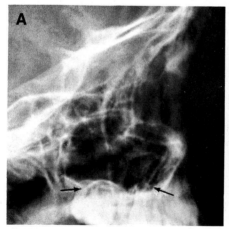
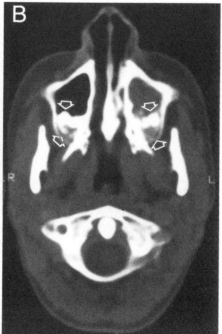

FIG 1–135.
A, a lateral view of the maxillary sinus shows the roots of the molars and bicuspids in contact with the floor of the maxillary sinus in a child 11 years of age. **B,** molar-indenting maxillary sinus in a 12-year-old with CT done for sinus disease. Unerupted molars indent the posterior aspects of both maxillary sinuses *(arrows).* The left sinus is opaque due to sinus disease.

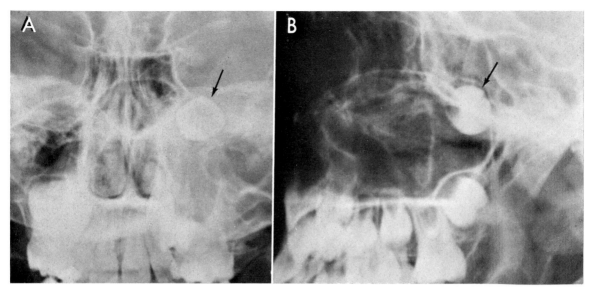

FIG 1–136.
Ectopic third molar *(arrows)* in the fetal position owing to a failure of normal migration. **A,** frontal, and **B,** lateral projections.

posterosuperomedial angle of the maxillary sinus (Figs 1–136 and 1–137).

Inflammation (Maxillary Sinusitis)

Inflammatory changes are similar in all of the paranasal sinuses, and this discussion of the morbid changes in maxillary sinusitis holds good for frontal, ethmoid, and sphenoid sinusitis as well. During the acute stage, the membranous linings become swollen owing to edema, congestion, and polymorphonuclear cellular infiltration. The air space of the sinus is reduced peripherally by the internal swelling of the walls and is partially or completely filled centrally with catarrhal or purulent exudate. These changes are reflected roentgenographically by reduction or disappearance of air content and clouding or opacification of the sinus (Fig 1–138). Air-fluid levels are not observed in infants as frequently as in older children and adults in whom exposures can be made with a horizontal beam while the patient is erect. The roentgenographic findings usually persist after the acute infection and the clinical manifestations

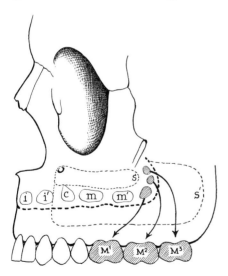

FIG 1–137.
The postnatal growth of the maxillary sinus, upper maxilla, and superior dental arch. The broken line outlines the maxilla at birth; the adult bone is drawn in solid line. *c,* deciduous canine; *i* and *i′,* deciduous incisors; *m* and *m′,* deciduous molars; *M¹, M², and M³,* permanent molars *(shaded); s,* maxillary sinus at birth; *s′,* maxillary sinus at maturity. (Redrawn from Keith A: *Human Embryology and Morphology,* ed 4. London, Edward Arnold & Co, 1921.)

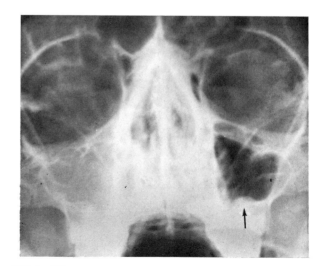

FIG 1–138.
Acute inflammation of the right maxillary sinus with obliteration of the air space by inflammatory exudate. The *arrow* points to the molar tooth roots that bulge into the floor of the sinus on the left side.

have disappeared. These features are usually diagnostic in children 5 years of age or older.

Nevertheless, there is no universal agreement on the significance of opaque sinuses in children under that age. Most pediatric radiologists, aware of the many times that opaque sinuses are observed in skull films obtained for clinical signs and symptoms unrelated to those ascribed to sinusitis are wary of making the diagnosis in children under 5 years old. Pediatricians and allergists, on the other hand, place considerable significance on the radiographic findings when signs of upper respiratory infection or reactive airway disease are present. Reports of radiographic and bacteriologic correlations in children suspect for sinusitis generally fail to indicate how frequently similar radiographic findings occur in apparently healthy children. Odita and associates found that maxillary sinus opacity in children was an unreliable index for the diagnosis of sinusitis. Several prospective and retrospective studies of sinus abnormalities found in children undergoing CT and MRI skull examinations for intracranial pathologic conditions with no clinical suspicion of sinus disease showed large numbers with features comparable to those generally associated with sinusitis. Examination of the paranasal sinuses in cranial CT scans undertaken for complaints that would not warrant sinus films disclosed high rates of maxillary opacification (Diament et al.). In another study, almost 50% of children whose skulls were examined by MRI for other indicated reasons had mucosal thickening in the sinuses as an incidental finding (Kuhn). An air-fluid level in an upright film of the sinuses is probably the most reliable feature to warrant the diagnosis. Otherwise, the radiographic diagnosis of sinusitis in children under 5 years of age should be advanced, only with compelling clinical and laboratory support.

In chronic sinusitis, fibrous thickening of the mucous membrane takes place; fluid exudate may or may not be present (Fig 1–139). Retention cysts in the mucous membrane may develop in long-standing infections. Occasionally, progressive enlargement of a retention cyst (mucocele) may enlarge a sinus, apparently erode its wall, and simulate a malignant tumor. Conventional films are usually adequate for the diagnosis and definition of the extent of mucoceles but, in uncertain cases, CT is desirable. Mucoceles and mucosal polyps are occasional manifestations of cystic fibrosis of the pancreas. We have seen proptosis as the presenting sign of an ethmoid mucocele in a 3½-year-old child with the disease (Fig 1–140). Erosion of the lateral wall of the opacified sinus suggested a malignancy but biopsy showed only a mucocele and further studies disclosed unsus-

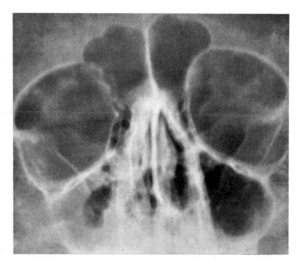

FIG 1–139.
Chronic inflammation of the right maxillary sinus with thickening of the mucous membrane without fluid inflammatory exudate.

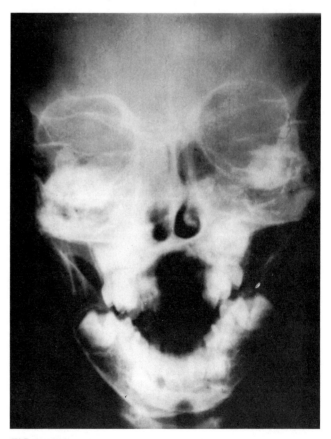

FIG 1–140.
This 3½-year-old child presented with proptosis of the right eye. Obliteration of the cavity of the right ethmoid labyrinth and bulging of its lateral wall into the orbit seen in tomograms suggested tumor, probably rhabdomyosarcoma. Biopsy showed mucocele, and further study indicated that the infant had cystic fibrosis of the pancreas. Chest films were normal. (From Strauss R, et al: *Pediatrics* 1969; 43:297–300. Used by permission.)

pected cystic fibrosis of the pancreas. Abnormal paranasal sinuses are so common in this condition that the observation of clear sinuses has been said to almost exclude the diagnosis (Ledesma-Medina et al.). This view has been supported by CT evaluation (Cuyler and Monaghan).

Obliteration of the sinus air space can result from trauma, especially fractures extending into a sinus. The maxillary sinuses are frequently obliterated by internal expansion of the swollen maxillary bone in thalassemia (Fig 1–141). Neoplasms are rare in infants and children; sinus opacification may reflect associated infection.

Frontal Sinuses

Marked variation in size and shape is the rule for the frontal sinuses as is asymmetry in development. They are not sufficiently developed for radiographic identification until they extend into the base of the vertical plate of the frontal bone between 2 and 6 years of age. By 6 to 8 years, they extend to the level of the orbital roofs. Some are actually extensions of anterior ethmoid cells. In some cases (especially in instances of hypoplasia of the frontal lobes of the brain), exaggerated extension into the horizontal plates of the frontal bones may occur. This extension is more easily recognized in lateral than in frontal projections.

Ethmoid Sinuses

The ethmoid sinuses are composed of a series of cells of variable number, forming paired bony labyrinths, suspended from the horizontal plate of the ethmoid bone, on each side of the vertical plate,

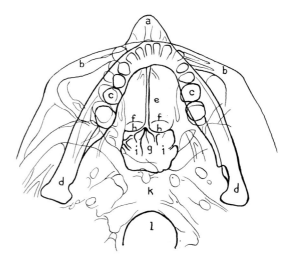

FIG 1–142.
The sphenoid sinus in a submentovertical projection. *a*, external nose; *b*, frontal bone; *c*, superimposed upper and lower teeth; *d*, mandible; *e*, hard palate; *f*, posterior margin of the hard palate; *g*, septum between the sphenoid sinuses; *h*, anterior wall of the sphenoid sinus; *i*, cavities of the sphenoid sinuses; *k*, basiocciput; *l*, foramen magnum. (Redrawn from Koehler A: *Roentgenography: The Borderlands of the Normal and Early Pathological in the Skiagram.* New York, William Wood & Co, 1928.)

with the lateral walls forming the medial walls of the orbits. They are separated by thin osseous septa covered with mucous membrane. They all communicate with the nasal cavities either directly by independent channels or indirectly through cells of the same group. They usually form three groups: the anterior, middle, and posterior (see Figs 1–112 and 1–132). The ethmoid cells often extend into the turbinates, crista galli, and the neighboring frontal, maxillary, sphenoid, and palate bones. Extension of infection from the sinus to the orbit can occur easily through the lamina papyracea.

Sphenoid Sinus

The paired cavities in the body of the sphenoid bone are separated by an osseous partition that may be displaced to one side so that the two cavities vary greatly in size and shape. They can be visualized superimposed in lateral projections or side by side in submentovertical projections (Fig 1–142). Ridges and septa sometimes divide each single cavity into separate compartments.

REFERENCES

The Nose

Altman NR, Altman DH, Wolfe SA, et al: Three dimensional CT reformation in children. *Am J Roentgenol* 1986; 146:1261–1267.

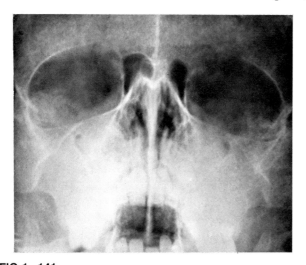

FIG 1–141.
Obliteration of the air spaces of the maxillary sinuses in β-thalassemia due to swelling of the maxillary bone.

Clark WD, Bailey BJ, Stiernberg CM: Nasal dermoid with intracranial involvement. *Otolaryngol Head Neck Surg* 1985; 93:102–104.

Crawford JK, Webster JP: Congenital dermoid cysts of the nose. *Plast Reconstr Surg* 1952; 9:235–260.

Cyran SE, Martinez R, Daniels S, et al: Spectrum of congenital heart disease in CHARGE association. *J Pediatr* 1987; 110:576–578.

Duvall AJ III, Moreano AE: Juvenile nasopharyngeal angiofibroma: Diagnosis and treatment. *Otolaryngol Head Neck Surg* 1987; 97:534–540.

Ey EH, Han BK, Towbin RB, et al: Bony inlet stenosis as a cause of nasal airway obstruction. *Radiology* 1988; 168:477–479.

Fu YS, Perzin KH: Non-epithelial tumors of the nasal cavity, paranasal sinuses, and nasopharynx: A clinicopathologic study. *Cancer* 1974–1980; 33–45.

Jacobsson M, Petruson B, Svendsen P, et al: Juvenile nasopharyngeal angiofibroma. A report of eighteen cases. *Acta Otolaryngol* 1988; 105:132–139.

Koltai PJ, Wood GW: Three dimensional CT reconstruction for the evaluation and surgical planning of facial fractures. *Otolaryngol Head Neck Surg* 1986; 95:10–15.

Levine RS, Grossman RI: Head and facial trauma. *Emerg Med Clin North Am* 1985; 3:447–473.

Lusk RP, Lee PC: Magnetic resonance imaging of congenital midline nasal masses. *Otolaryngol Head Neck Surg* 1986; 95:303–306.

Pagon RA, Graham JM Jr, Zonana J, et al: Coloboma, congenital heart disease, and choanal atresia with multiple anomalies: CHARGE association. *J Pediatr* 1981; 99:223–227.

Pensler JM, Bauer BS, Naidich TP: Craniofacial dermoids. *Plast Reconstr Surg* 1988; 82:953–958.

Slovis TL, Renfro B, Watts FB, et al: Choanal atresia: Precise CT evaluation. *Radiology* 1985; 155:345–348.

Sinuses

Cuyler JP, Monaghan AJ: Cystic fibrosis and sinusitis. *J Otolaryngol* 1989; 18:173–175.

Diament MJ, Senac MO, Gilsanz V, et al: Prevalence of incidental paranasal sinus opacification in pediatric patients: A CT study. *J Comput Assist Tomogr* 1987; 11:426–431.

Fujioka M, Young LW: The sphenoidal sinuses: Radiographic patterns of normal development and abnormal findings in infants and children. *Radiology* 1978; 129:133–136.

Glasier CM, Mallory GB Jr, Steele RW: Significance of opacifications of the maxillary and ethmoid sinuses in infants. *J Pediatr* 1989; 114:45–50.

Kuhn JP: Imaging of the paranasal sinuses: Current status. *J Allergy Clin Immunol* 1986; 77:6–8.

Ledesma-Medina J, Ozman MZ, Girdany BR: Abnormal paranasal sinuses in patients with cystic fibrosis of the pancreas: Radiologic findings. *Pediatr Radiol* 1980; 9:61–64.

Maresh MM: Paranasal sinuses from birth to late adolescence. I. Size of the paranasal sinuses as observed in routine posteroanterior roentgenograms. *Am J Dis Child* 1940; 60:55–78.

Odita JC, Akamaguna AI, Ogisi FO, et al: Pneumatisation of the maxillary sinus in normal and symptomatic children. *Pediatr Radiol* 1986; 16:365–367.

Rachelefsky GS, Katz RM, Siegel SC: Chronic sinus disease with associated reactive airway disease in children. *Pediatrics* 1984; 73:526–529.

Wald ER, Milmoe GJ, Bowen A, et al: Acute maxillary sinusitis in children *N Engl J Med* 1981; 304:749–754.

SECTION 8

Individual Bones, Orbit, Mandible, and Temporomandibular Joint

TEMPORAL BONE

Normal Anatomy

The temporal bone demonstrates a wide range of normal variation in size and external contour as well as the relations of its internal components. This is particularly true of the pattern, texture, and extent of its pneumatization. Some bones are extensively pneumatized with large, small, or medium-sized cells; in others, pneumatization is limited to the tympanic cavity and antrum with a few cells on the borders of the auditory tube. Between these extremes, various degrees of pneumatization occur. A minor variant that may simulate a fracture fragment in conventional radiographs is the os suprapetrosum (Fig 1–143).

Important anatomical features of the normal temporal bone are shown in Figures 1–144, 1–145, and 1–146. The normal temporal bone at birth is depicted in Figure 1–147. High resolution CT (HRCT) has become the examination of choice for evaluation of temporal bone diseases, particularly those of the middle ear and mastoid process. In addition, abnormalities in the inner ear affecting the cochlea, semicircular canals, and vestibular and cochlear aqueducts are demonstrated with excellent detail. MRI provides information relating to the soft tissues, particularly nervous tissue in the region of the temporal bone, but is not felt to be of any greater value for evaluation of inner ear disease.

Pneumatization

Pneumatization of the mastoid process, which can be considered a temporal sinus, takes place by extensions of epithelial evagination of the mastoid antrum; the cells thus formed are usually designated according to their position in relation to other structures (see Fig 1–144). The infantile form (up to 2 years) is characterized by limited air cell development; a transitional type extends to about 5 years with increasing pneumatization but may develop a diploic pattern with poor air cell formation. After that time, the gradual increase in number and size of air cells continues to maturity when pneumatization ceases. The diploic pattern is unrelated to infection in contrast to the sclerotic pattern, and may be a genetic variant. Pneumatization of the petrous pyramid occurs by extension from three primary cavities; cells therein may be of tubal, tympanic, or antral origin. The variability of pneumatization gives rise to many normal variants at different ages (Fig 1–148), in individuals of the same age, and in the two temporal bones of the same individual. Nevertheless, serious consideration should be given to asymmetric opacification that is not of a diploic character as infections during the period of cellular pneumatization are an important cause of slow and reduced pneumatization.

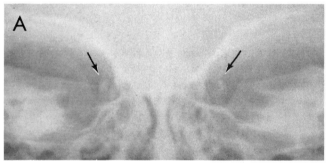

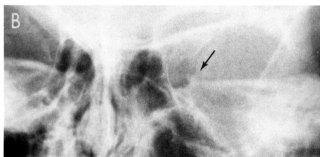

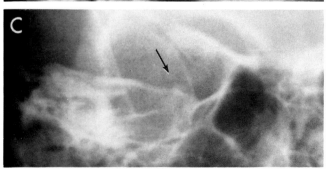

FIG 1–143.
A, bilateral os suprapetrosum *(arrows)* in a girl 2 years of age who had had convulsions. **B** and **C,** similar findings 3 years later. (From Currarino G, Weinberg A: *AJR Am J Roentgenol* 1974; 121: 139–142. Used by permission.)

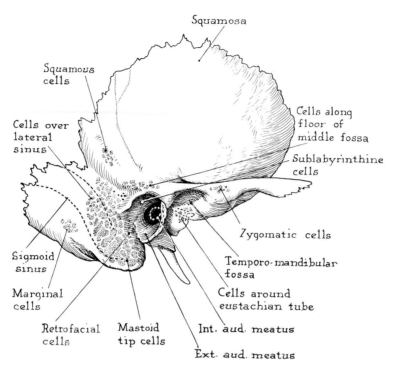

FIG 1–144.
Surface projection of the pneumatic cells and some of the internal structures of the normal temporal bone. The cells are grouped and labeled according to Tremble. (Tremble GE: *Arch Otolaryngol* 1934; 19:172.)

The spaces in the spongiosa of the temporal bone may be filled with red marrow and fatty marrow as well as with air. When there is only partial pneumatization of the mastoid process or the petrous pyramid, the pneumatic cells are relatively small, their cellular walls are relatively thicker, and the thin lining mucosa of the cells lies directly in the marrow-containing spaces without the layer of bone that usually separates the pneumatic cells from the marrow. The roentgen findings in the pneumatic and diploic types of pneumatization are shown in Figure 1–149.

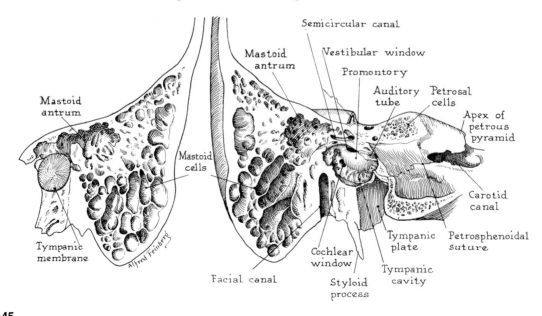

FIG 1–145.
Curved section of the temporal bone through the right mastoid process and petrous pyramid, illustrating the normal internal structures and their topographic relations. The anterior segment is turned outward and backward.

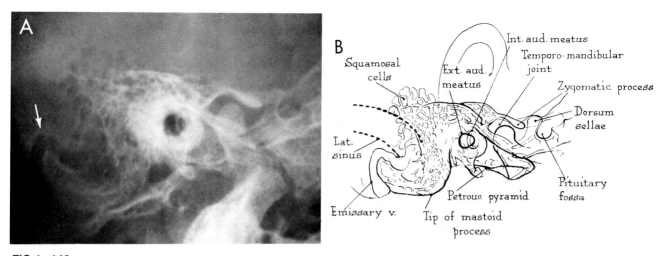

FIG 1–146.
Roentgenographic features of a normal temporal bone, lateral oblique projection of Law. **A,** roentgenogram of a boy 6 years of age. The *arrow* points to a large emissary vein. **B,** tracing of **A.**

Diseases of Temporal Bone

Malformations of the temporal bone of concern to pediatric radiologists are largely related to those affecting the complex structures of the external, middle, and inner ear, and particularly those related to hearing loss (Figs 1–150, 1–151, and 1–152). Generally, an obvious malformation in the external canal (e.g., atresia) is not accompanied by others in the middle or inner ear as development of the inner ear structures occurs independently of external ear structures. Several textbooks describing the indispensable CT aspects are currently available for those requiring detailed information concerning both diagnosis and surgical management (see References).

The earliest anatomical changes caused by acute infection in the temporal bone are hyperemia and edema of the mucosal lining of the pneumatic cells, followed by the accumulation of serous, then purulent exudate in the pneumatic cavities. A reduction of the air content results (Figs 1–153 and 1–154). This is followed by demineralization of the cellular walls and loss of definition (Fig 1–155). Chronic infection is uncommon today because of the efficacy of anti-infective therapy, but when it occurs it can result in persisting sclerosis (Figs 1–156 and 1–157) or cholesteatoma formation (Fig 1–158). The latter begins as an infolding or perforation of the Shrapnell membrane which becomes filled with desquamated epithelium and develops into a mass as the epithelium continues to proliferate and desquamate (Fig 1–159), extending into the tympanic cavity or mastoid process, or both, with infection and pressure necrosis of neighboring bone. Breakthrough into the cranial cavity is a rare, but not to be overlooked,

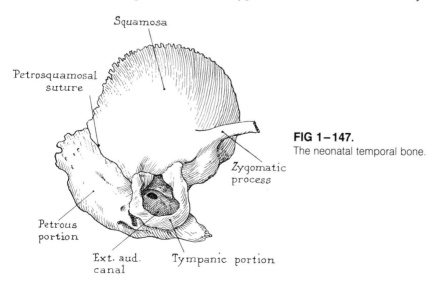

FIG 1–147.
The neonatal temporal bone.

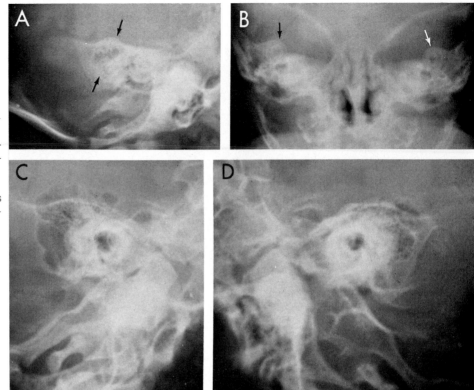

FIG 1–148.
Roentgenograms illustrating the normal variations in the extension of pneumatization in the temporal bone with advancing age in different patients. **A** and **B,** at 10 days of age there is no evidence of cellular structure, but the mastoid antrum is visible. The semicircular canals are visible because their bony walls are more dense than is the remainder of the petrous pyramid. **C,** at 14 months the mastoid process is completely pneumatized, and large pneumatic cells are already visible in the squamosa and the base of the zygomatic process. **D,** at 2 years, pneumatization is limited to the periantral region; the cells are small in this case.

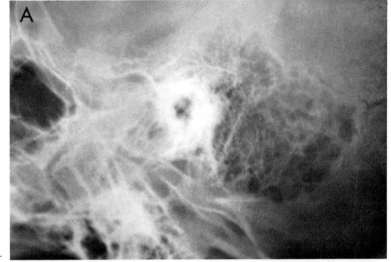

FIG 1–149.
Normal variants in pneumatization of the temporal bone. **A,** extensive pneumatization in a girl 6 years of age. The air cells are large and the cellular walls delicate. **B,** limited pneumatization in a boy 6 years of age. The cells are small and poorly defined and have relatively thick walls.

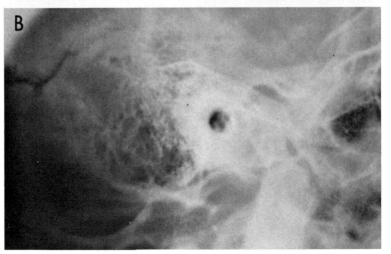

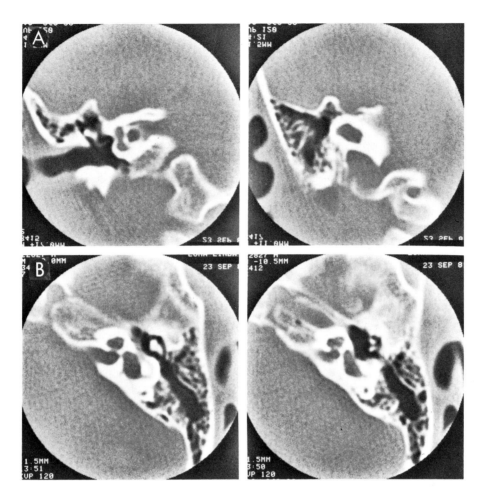

FIG 1–150.
CT scans of the temporal bones. This 5-year-old boy had severe bilateral neurosensory hearing loss. **A,** direct coronal, and **B,** direct axial sections of the right side. **A** is inverted and reversed in printing for anatomical orientation. Congenital anomalies were sim-ilar on both sides. The vestibules and portions of the lateral and posterior semicircular canals expand into a large vesicle. The cochlea is incompletely coiled (Mondini malformation). **(Courtesy of Dr. Anton N. Hasso, Loma Linda, Calif.)**

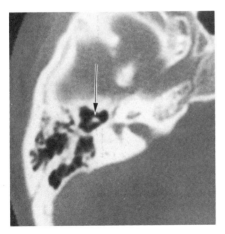

FIG 1–151.
Congenital malformations of the external and internal ears. Bony external auditory canal atresia in a 17-year-old girl. There is a thick, irregular atresia plate with a markedly deformed ossicular mass *(arrow).* The middle ear cavity is small. (From Swartz JD, Faerber EN: *Am J Roentgenol* 1985; 144:501–506. Used by permission.)

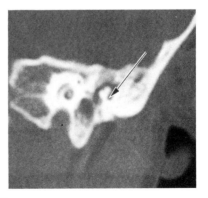

FIG 1–152.
Bony external ear atresia in a 3-year-old girl. The neck of the malleolus is fused to the atresia plate *(arrow).* (From Swartz JD, Faerber EN: *Am J Roentgenol* 1985; 144:501–506. Used by permission.)

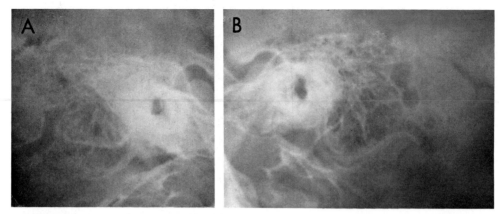

FIG 1-153.
Acute mastoiditis, without destruction of bone, in a patient 5 years of age. **A,** right temporal bone shows clouding of the pneumatic cavities and intact cellular structure. **B,** normal left temporal bone.

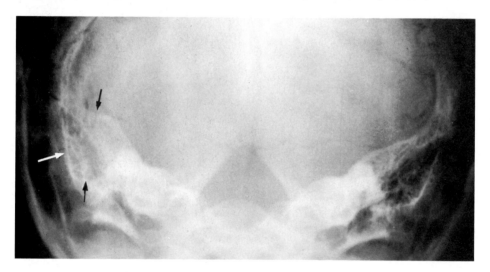

FIG 1-154.
Unilateral right acute mastoiditis in a 3-year-old boy viewed in Towne projection. Reduction of the air content of the right mastoid air cells is caused by replacement of air by edema of the mucosal lining and by acute purulent exudate. The Towne projection is very useful by virtue of the contrast it provides between the two sides in a single film. Because of the continuity of mucosa and the proximity of the middle ear and the mastoid air cells, there is very likely some "mastoiditis" in every child with otitis media.

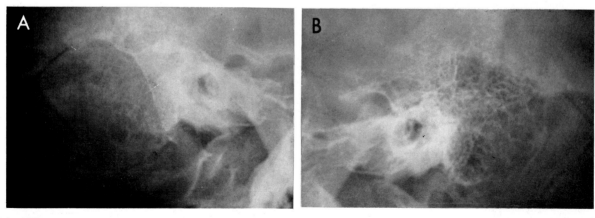

FIG 1-155.
Acute mastoiditis with generalized demineralization of the cellular walls and clouding of the air spaces in a patient 5 years of age. **A,** abnormal right temporal bone. **B,** normal left temporal bone. Note the sharpness of the groove for the sigmoid sinus in **A** due to the loss of the overlying pattern of bony cell walls and the air content.

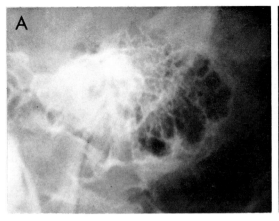

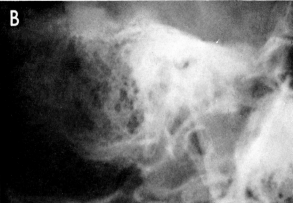

FIG 1–156.
Chronic mastoiditis with thickening of the cellular walls in a patient 11 years of age. **A,** normal right temporal bone. **B,** abnormal irregularly sclerotic left temporal bone. The cellular walls are thickened, and the pneumatic cavities are correspondingly diminished in volume.

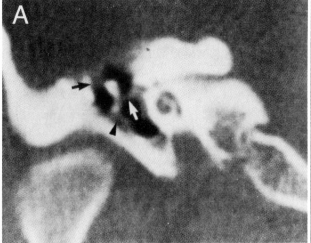

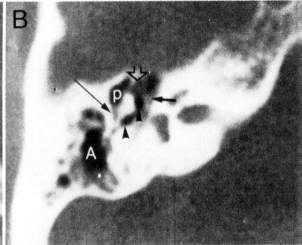

FIG 1–157.
Example of the detail available in CT of a middle ear with chronic otomastoiditis. **A,** a coronal scan shows thickening of the tensor tympani tendon *(white arrow)*, a thick superior malleolar mucosal fold *(black arrow)*, and a thick tympanic membrane *(arrowhead)*. The density with the meniscus in the hypotympanum is produced by a small amount of fluid. **B,** an axial scan in the same patient shows the tensor tympani tendon *(black arrow)*, the tensor fold *(open arrow)*, and the lateral incudal fold *(long arrow)*. A change in position has caused fluid to shift from the tympanic cavity into the antrum *(A)* where trabecular thickening of air cells indicates chronicity of the disease. *p* = Prussak space. **(From Mafee MF, Aimi K, Kahen HL, et al: *Radiology* 1986; 160:193–200. Used by permission.)**

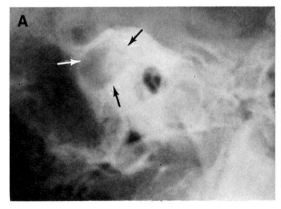

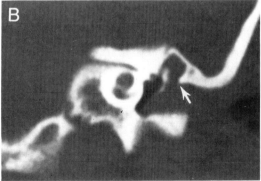

FIG 1–158.
A, chronic sclerotic mastoiditis and a large cholesteatoma *(arrows)* behind the tympanum and below the tegmen in an oblique lateral projection of Law. The patient, 11 years of age, had had an aural discharge for 9 years. **B,** inflammatory cholesteatoma: coronal CT of the left petrous bone. There is a soft-tissue mass extending down from the attic that is eroding the ossicles and the tip of the scutum *(arrow)* and filling the external canal.

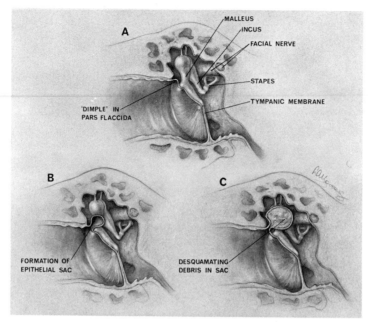

FIG 1–159.
Sequential changes in the formation of a cholesteatoma. (From Thomas GL: *Calif Med* 1968; 108:205–208. Used by permission.)

complication. CT is extremely helpful in the evaluation of infections of the middle ear providing micro-anatomical delineation of its soft tissue and ossicular components (see Fig 1–157). Fluid and granulation tissue can be identified and the latter can be differentiated from cholesteatoma. Intra- and extracranial complications of cholesteatoma can be identified and evaluated.

Fractures of the temporal bone are usually longitudinal, transverse, or complex in nature and are best evaluated with HRCT in axial and, occasionally, coronal scans (Fig 1–160). Longitudinal fractures are the most common and result from temporal or parietal blows. Transverse fractures, more or less perpendicular to the fracture shown in Figure 1–160, result from frontal or parietal blows and are often associated with facial fractures. Complications include facial paralysis from fractures in the region of the geniculate ganglion and otorhinoliquorrhea resulting from disruption of the dura in the region of the tegmen tympani. The latter may lead to meningitis. The site of dural rupture may be identified by the use of metrizamide with HRCT. In the case of basilar fractures involving the temporal bone, CT is mandatory for optimal demonstration of the extent of injury. Fractures in the region of the pterion may be associated with epidural hematoma. CT and MRI are both useful in evaluation of tumors; MRI is especially helpful when the cerebellopontine angle is involved.

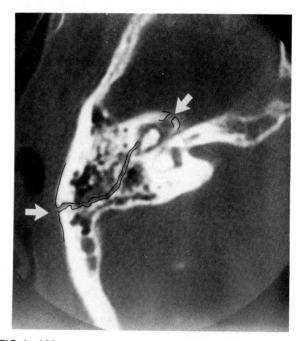

FIG 1–160.
High resolution axial CT examination of temporal bone fracture. The uncomplicated longitudinal fracture *(arrows)* passes from dorsolateral to anteromedial and ends in the anterior wall of the epitympanic space. The head of the malleus and the body of the incus show the typical configuration resembling an ice-cream cone with the ball on top produced by the malleus. A hemotympanum is present and only a few air cells still contain air. The course of the fracture has been retouched. (From Schubiger O, Vanavanis A, Stuckman G, et al: *Neuroradiology* 1986; 28:93–99. Used by permission.)

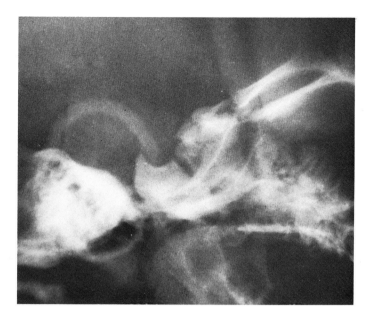

FIG 1–161.
Intrasphenoid synchondrosis between the presphenoid and basisphenoid portions of the sphenoid bone. Note its termination in the anterior portion of the pituitary fossa just beneath the tuberculum sellae.

SPHENOID BONE

The sphenoid bone develops from an anterior, or presphenoid, part and a posterior, or postsphenoid, part, each with its own appendages. Its image is usually based on its appearance as seen in lateral films with the pituitary fossa its most obvious landmark. A synchondrosis between the two parts (Fig 1–161) is observed in radiographs at birth and is often confused with the so-called persistent basipharyngeal canal (Fig 1–162). The former terminates superiorly anterior to the pituitary fossa in the tuberculum sellae; the latter ends superiorly in the floor of the pituitary fossa. According to Kier and Rothman, the intrasphenoid synchondrosis is actually the centrally located remnant of the cartilaginous presphenoid. Persistence of vascular channels in the postsphenoid ossification center is believed to be responsible for what has been called the basisphenoidal canal (Arey), notwithstanding the fact that the buccal ("pharyngeal") portion of the pituitary gland does traverse the basicranium in this region and may leave rests from which ectopic pituitary tumors can arise. Lowman and associates recommend the term *intrasphenoidal channel* to eliminate implications that the canal has a neurogenic embryonic origin.

During the neonatal period, the pituitary fossa tends to be rounded with smooth margins. In the dorsum sellae, the clinoid processes are poorly differentiated in comparison with later life (Fig 1–163). There is considerable variation in all the bony structures bordering on the pituitary fossa that contributes to the great variation in its size in healthy persons. Enlargement in long-standing hypothyroidism has been noted; it has been attributed to feedback to the pituitary from thyroid not responding to thyro-

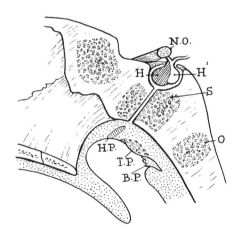

FIG 1–162.
Sagittal section through the pharynx and sphenoid bone, showing the pharyngeal remnant of the hypophysial duct in a newborn infant. *B.P.*, pharyngeal bursa; *T.P.*, pharyngeal tonsil; *H.P.*, pharyngeal hypophysis; *S*, ossification center for the body of the sphenoid; *H*, anterior lobe of the hypophysis; *H'*, posterior lobe of the hypophysis; *N.O.*, optic nerve; *O*, ossification center in the basioccipital portion. The basipharyngeal canal, which traverses the body of the sphenoid, is said to be present in about 5% of newborn infants. (Redrawn from Scammon RE: A summary of the anatomy of the infant and child, in Abt IA (ed): *Pediatrics*, vol 1. Philadelphia, WB Saunders, 1923.)

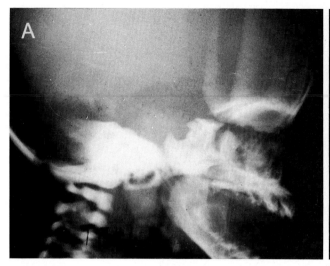

FIG 1–163.

The normal pituitary fossa; lateral projection. **A,** in the newborn, the fossa is round with smooth margins, and the dorsum sellae and clinoid processes are poorly developed. **B,** at 6 years, the fossa has lost its round, smooth contours and the bony processes are prominent. These features become exaggerated with the passage of time.

tropic hormone production (see Fig 1–101). Linear, area, and volume measurements of the pituitary fossa are available; volume measurements are considered more reliable for estimation of pituitary size than are sellar areas because of variations in sellar width. HRCT scanning permits evaluation of the actual size of the pituitary gland and correlation with clinical aspects of growth. Small volumes have been observed in children with growth hormone deficiencies.

Empty sella syndrome is a term describing the radiologic appearance of the sella turcica into which a cerebrospinal fluid–filled arachnoid hernia, arising in the chiasmatic area, partially or completely extends into the sella displacing or compressing the pituitary gland and its stalk. It is more common in middle-aged women but has been observed in children in association with visual disturbances and endocrinopathies, especially with growth hormone deficiencies. The radiologic features are said to be sellar enlargement, often with doubling of the floor and erosion of the clinoid processes. On CT the sella turcica may be flattened and small, the intrasellar contents are not always of fluid density, and though there may be penetration of spinal fluid and subarachnoid space within the sella, on MRI a hypoplastic pituitary gland may be present. The pituitary stalk may be widened or even interrupted. MRI has demonstrated ectopia of the pituitary gland, particularly the posterior portion that is identified by its high intensity signal. Familial instances have been reported. Enlargement of the pituitary fossa in hypothyroidism has been ascribed to secondary pituitary hyperplasia involving feedback mechanisms, but it may be associated with this syndrome in some cases.

ORBIT

The walls of the orbit are composed of the frontal, maxillary, sphenoid, ethmoid, lacrimal, and zygomatic bones. In addition to the eyeball and optic nerve, the orbit contains the extraocular muscles, other nerves, vessels, glands, and adipose tissue. It has the form of a cone with its base facing outward and its apex facing inward and somewhat medially. Hemorrhage, inflammation, and other agents that can alter the volume of its contents are potentially damaging to vision. Penetrating orbital injuries require a meticulous ophthalmologic examination and orbital and brain CT or MRI examination as the situation warrants. The common walls that the orbit shares with the paranasal sinuses, if breached, permit communication of these bony cavities to the outside; disease can extend intracranially, through the orbital roof, from infection in the orbit. Because of the variable densities of the orbital contents, CT and MRI are the procedures of choice for their evaluation, with CT oriented toward skeletal structures and foreign bodies (Fig 1–164), and MRI toward soft tissues (Fig 1–165). However, nonmetallic foreign bodies, such as some types of wood and plastic, may be difficult or impossible to identify if their density is similar to that of the surrounding tissues.

Congenital malformations such as defects of the

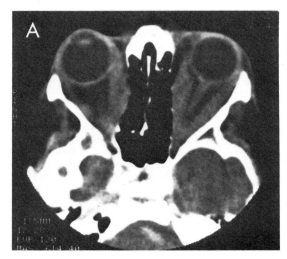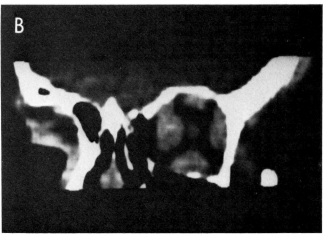

FIG 1–164.
Proptosis in a leukemic child due to infiltration of extraocular muscles. **A,** axial CT examination through both orbits. **B,** oblique trans- verse orbital reconstruction. **(Courtesy of Dr. Robert Brasch, Uni-** versity of California, San Francisco.)

greater wing of the sphenoid bone in neurofibromatosis, along with an intraorbital encephalocele, are clearly demonstrated. The extent of tumors is well shown and differentiation is facilitated. Burton et al. reported a 6-year-old patient with intraorbital sinus histiocytosis and proptosis. A homogeneously enhancing intraorbital lesion was demonstrated on CT; on MRI, the tumor was isodense to gray matter on T1-weighted, proton density, and T2-weighted images. Infections can be evaluated effectively. Preseptal inflammatory infection can be differentiated from

intraorbital infection, conditions for which treatment and prognosis are significantly different while the clinical presentations may be very similar.

MANDIBLE

Normal Anatomy

Some of the anatomical features of the mandible are shown in Figure 1–166. At birth the mandible consists of two lateral halves united in the midline at

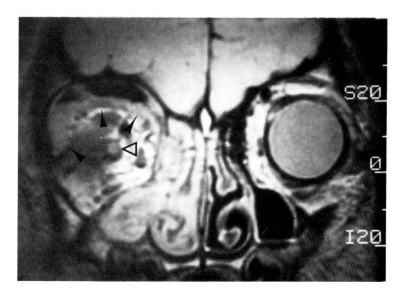

FIG 1–165.
MRI of orbital disease in a 4-year-old child with sinusitis: coronal proton density image. The right sinuses and nasal canal are opaque with fluid and swollen mucosa. There is an extraconal mass superiorly in the orbit *(arrowheads)* that has a lower signal than orbital fat does. Within this are two areas of low signal thought to be fresh hemorrhage within the abscess. The proptosis caused by the mass has displaced the right globe anteriorly. The optic nerve *(open arrowhead)* and adjacent extraocular muscles are well outlined by the fat. The low signal just lateral to the optic nerve is caused by the most posterior aspect of the right globe.

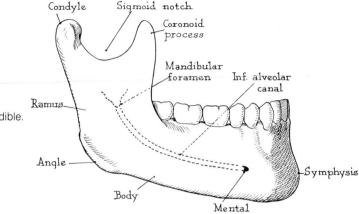

FIG 1–166.
Some important anatomical features of the normal mandible.

the symphysis by a bar of cartilage (see Fig 1–4). Bony fusion of the symphysis usually occurs before the second year, but segments of the fissures may persist beyond puberty. The body of the mandible is large at birth in comparison with the relatively short rami and poorly differentiated coronoid and condylar processes. The rami form an angle of about 160 degrees with the body at birth. As the rami grow, the angle with the body is reduced to about 130 degrees at adolescence and 120 degrees in adulthood (Fig 1–167). In old age, atrophy of the alveolar processes contributes to reversion to the infantile configuration.

The mandible is the only freely movable bone of the face; it articulates with the temporal bone in the temporomandibular fossa anterior to the external auditory canal (Fig 1–168). The range of motion is free in all directions, and the condyle moves forward in the articular fossa on opening of the jaw. The extent of the movement may simulate anterior dislocation of the condyle (Fig 1–169).

Standards for calcification and eruption of the deciduous and permanent teeth have been established by Moorrees, Fanning, and Hunt and an example of their rating scales is shown in Figure 1–170. In contrast to bone age, dental age is relatively little affected by endocrine aberrations. Prader and Perabo compared height age, bone age, and dental age in 58 children suffering from a variety of endocrinopathies. Variations in maturational status of the teeth were in the same direction as those of the skeleton, but the dental variations rarely fell out of the normal range for age. Kuhns and associates attempted to assess gestational age of premature infants by study of mineralization of the cusps of the first and second deciduous molar teeth as observed when the mandible was visible in a film of the chest. Beginning mineralization in the first molar tooth occurred between the 33rd and 34th weeks, and in the second, between the 36th and 37th weeks.

Natal teeth occur occasionally in normal chil-

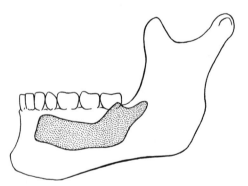

FIG 1–167.
Relative size and shape of the neonatal and adult mandibles. (Redrawn from Arey LB: *Developmental Anatomy.* Philadelphia, WB Saunders, 1942.)

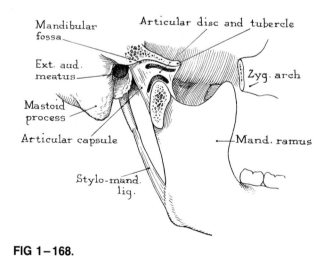

FIG 1–168.
Anatomy of the normal temporomandibular joint. The zygomatic arch and a portion of the ramus of the mandible are cut away to expose the articular disk.

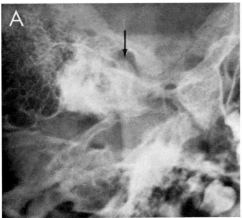 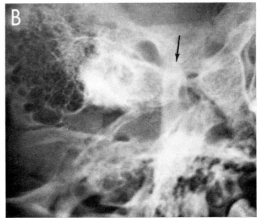

FIG 1–169.
The normal range of condylar motion in opening and closing the jaws. **A,** roentgenogram of the temporomandibular joint with the mouth closed and the condyle in the articular fossa. **B,** the same patient with the mouth open showing an anterior excursion of the condyle out of the fossa to a position below the articular tubercle.

dren. They are also seen in association with the following syndromes: Pena-Shokeir, chondroectodermal dysplasia, Hallermann-Streiff, and hypoglossia-hypodactylia; in the last, the tongue is small or even absent. All or only some of the teeth may be missing developmentally in anhidrotic ectodermal dysplasia which is characterized, in addition, by partial or total absence of hair, faulty fingernails, and scantiness or absence of sweat glands. The last may be a cause for fever when the ambient temperature is elevated. Because infants and children appear to have a plethora of teeth in radiographs including the jaws (deciduous *and* permanent dentitions), the condition may be recognized even in the newborn by the lack of dental buds (Fig 1–171). Evaluation of uneruptured and displaced teeth in older children is more effective by CT than by orthopantomographic films, and both were found superior to clinical examination.

Diseases of Mandible

Significant congenital malformations of the mandible are rare in contrast with the frequency of cleft palate in the maxilla. The anomaly of greatest pediatric interest is hypoplasia (micrognathia), which may be a cause of congenital stridor. The short, small mandible apparently causes a retrodisplacement of the tongue and obstruction to the flow of air to and from the larynx. The malposition of the tongue and the hypoplastic mandible can be demonstrated roentgenographically (Fig 1–172).

The combination of cleft palate and hypoplasia of the mandible defines the Pierre Robin syndrome (or anomalad) radiographically. The tongue, which may be overly large, may become impacted in the cleft of the palate. Failing disengagement, it may bulge backward into the nasopharynx. Here, it can act as a plug and produce signs of suffocation until, owing to hypoxia, it becomes limp and falls forward into the mouth. The tongue may also stimulate vomiting by its pressure on the posterior wall of the pharynx. In such cases, the infants lose weight and become cachectic. Dennison suggested that sudden death may result from vasovagal reflex when aspirated vomitus irritates the carina. The syndrome exists in both severe and mild types; the latter are often overlooked. Micrognathia occurs in a variety of dysmorphic syndromes. Cohen pointed out that the Pierre Robin anomalad is not a specific syndrome but occurs with several genetic syndromes, some drug-induced syndromes, and some loosely associated anomalies as well as an isolated symptom complex. In the cerebrocostomandibular syndrome, it is associated with defects in the ribs posteriorly, cleft palate, and, occasionally, mental retardation.

Elongation of the body of the mandible and widening of its arc occur in conditions associated with an enlarged tongue. These include lymphangioma of the tongue and the Beckwith-Wiedemann syndrome. Relative enlargement of the mandible is observed in several of the craniofacial syndromes. The angle of the mandible is markedly increased in pyknodysostosis. Rare cases of hyperplasia of the coronoid process are observed; the enlargement impinges on the zygomatic arch and interferes with normal opening of the jaw. CT demonstrates the abnormality to best advantage. The temporomandibular joints are frequently involved in juvenile rheuma-

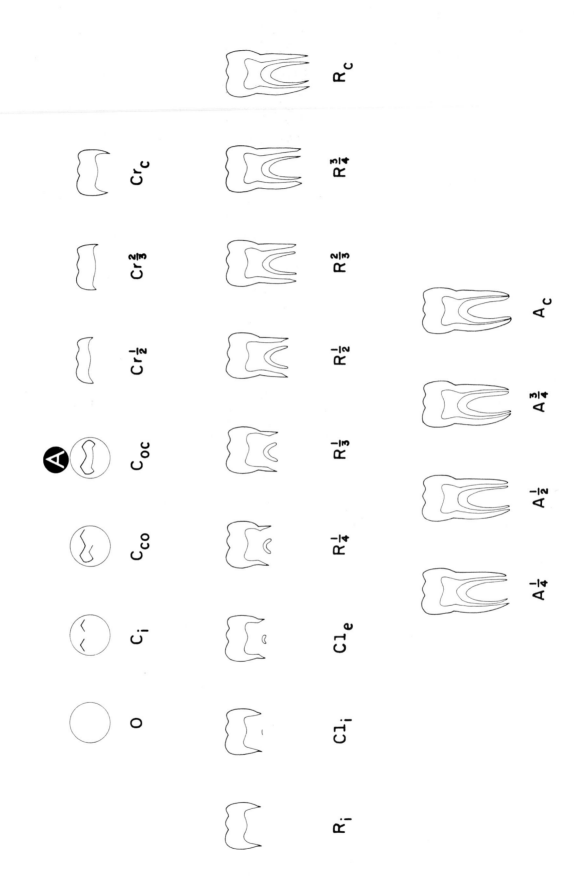

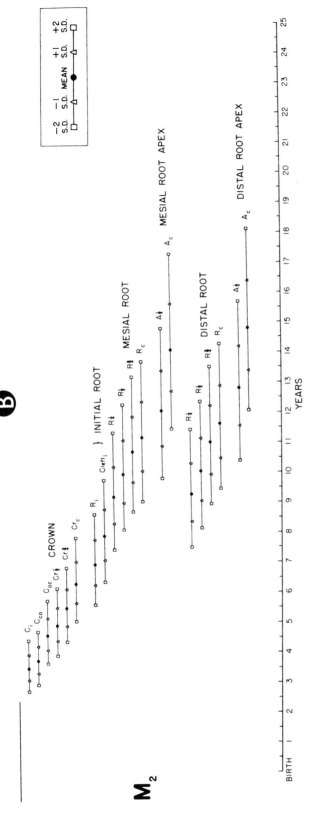

FIG 1–170.

A, stages for formation of molar teeth. C = cusps (subscripts indicate initial formation, coalescence, and outline completion); Cr = crown (subscripts indicate ½, ⅔, and completed formation); Cl = cleft formation (subscripts indicate initial and enlarging phases); R = root (subscripts indicate initial to complete formation); A = apex (subscripts indicate degrees of closure). **B,** norms for assessing development of the second permanent molar in boys. Data are available for males and females separately, and for permanent and deciduous dentition. (Modified from Moorhees CFA, Fanning EA, Hunt EE Jr: *J Dent Res* 1963; 42:1490–1502; and *Am J Phys Anthropol* 1963; 21:205–214.)

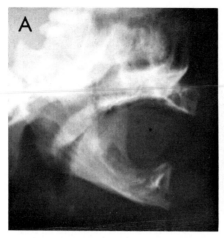
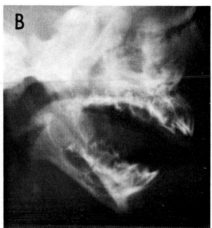

FIG 1–171.
A, the mandible in hereditary ectodermal dysplasia in an infant 8 weeks of age shows the failure of calcification of dental crowns and defective dental sacs. **B,** a roentgenogram of a normal infant 8 days of age shows normal dental development in the neonatal period.

toid arthritis. Becker and associates described variations in the upward curve of the lower border of the mandible anterior to its angle (gonion), known as antegonial notching. It occurs as a long, smooth arc extending from the gonion to the menton in congenital disorders, but as a fairly sharp notch in acquired disorders such as rheumatoid arthritis and trauma. Rarely, the mandible may be partially duplicated.

Fractures

Fractures high in the ramus are the ones most frequently overlooked in standard films but are clearly

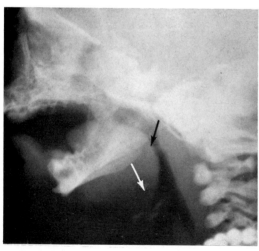

FIG 1–172.
Hypoplasia of the mandible in an infant 1 day old, lateral projection. The short dorsoventral diameter of the mandible is evident; the tongue is displaced posteriorly and fills the greater part of the pharynx (black arrow). The displaced tongue impinged on the epiglottis and interfered with the flow of air to and from the larynx (white arrow).

defined by multiplanar tomography (Fig 1–173) and especially by CT; occasionally, it can be useful to inspect the region fluoroscopically with the head slightly flexed and rotated. Panographic tomography can also be used (Fig 1–174). Direct trauma is the usual cause; pathologic fractures occur in association with cysts, destructive inflammations, and neoplasms. More than half of the traumatic fractures are found in the body of the mandible near the canine fossa. The radiographic criteria for healing of fractures in other bones are not applicable to mandibular fractures because strips of rarefaction may persist at the margins of the fracture long after satisfactory union has taken place.

Vehicular trauma is said to be responsible for 35% of mandibular fractures in children, and falls cause 28%. During childhood, the mandible contains teeth in different stages of eruption, and the pattern of the alveolar bone predisposes it to fractures along the lines of the developing dental crypts. The lack of cortical bone and the relative excess of cancellous bone are responsible for the frequency of incomplete, greenstick fractures with minimal destruction of the bone or cartilage. The condylar neck usually breaks before the condyle itself, owing to the vascularity and thickness of the latter. However, a blow to the tip of the chin will "mushroom" a condyle in its glenoid temporomandibular fossa. Injuries to the mandible during the period of rapid growth between the ages of 4 and 7 years have maximal residual deformities. During childhood, rapid union of mandibular fractures should be expected because of the rich blood supply, the high osteogenic potential of the periosteum, and the high local metabolic rate.

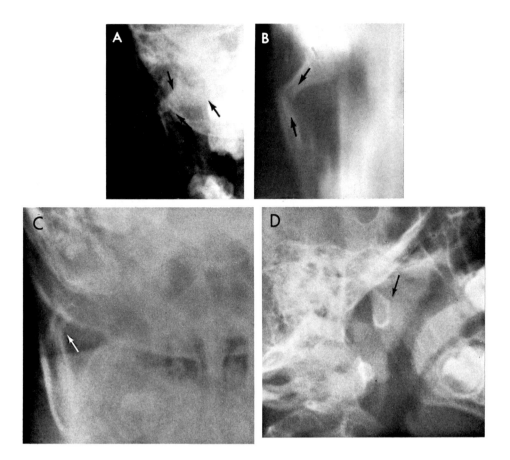

FIG 1–173.

Fracture of the right ramus of the mandible of a boy 5 years of age; it is barely visible in the standard frontal projection of the skull **(A),** but clearly visible in a coronal planigram **(B). C,** transverse fracture of the left ramus of the mandible *(arrow),* in which the proximal fragment is flexed mediad; in **D,** right lateral projection, it is seen on end *(arrow),* superimposed on the soft tissues of the posterior nasopharyngeal wall. This boy was 7 years of age.

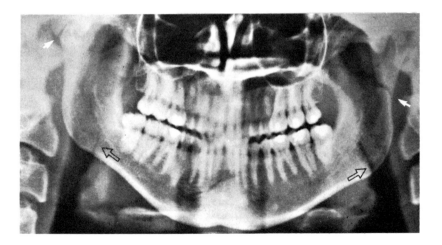

FIG 1–174.

Panoramic film demonstrating fractures of both condylar processes *(solid arrows).* The *open arrows* indicate artifacts produced by superimposition of the anterior border of the trachea on the portions of the mandible exposed during the lateral transit of the x-ray beam. Note the adjacent cervical vertebrae for orientation.

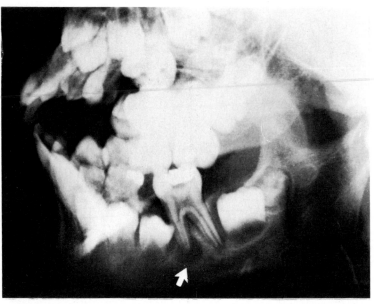

FIG 1–175.
Periapical abscess. Granulation tissue *(arrow)* has destroyed the bone surrounding the affected root.

Osteomyelitis

Because the mandible has no metaphyseal-epiphyseal junction structures, osteomyelitis occurs only rarely and is generally secondary to dental infection or local trauma. The inflammatory changes caused by different organisms are similar roentgenographically. Mandibular structure in childhood is so immature that inflammation extends easily and rapidly. Bone necrosis and sequestra formation are common; destructive changes may not be visible by conventional radiography until weeks after the onset of infection. Hyperplastic changes usually predominate and have been confused with the manifestations of infantile cortical hyperostoses, especially if only the mandible is examined or in the rare cases of the latter when only mandibular involvement is present. The osteomyelitis occurring in cases of osteopetrosis is probably secondary to fracture of the bone or extension from dental infection. Tuberculous osteomyelitis of the mandible usually occurs by hematogenous spread but may occur by direct inoculation or extension from other infected sites. Signs of chronic infection may be present with mixed destructive and reactive sclerotic changes.

Cysts and Neoplasms

Most primary mandibular cysts and neoplasms are of dental origin. Dental root cysts result from proliferation of paradental epithelial cells in the periapical granulation tissue of local infection (Fig 1–175). Dentigerous cysts are formed by the excessive accumulation of fluid between the enamel and the dental capsule, and demonstrate a well-formed dental crown without roots with its base close to the wall of a large cystic structure that surrounds its upper portion (Fig 1–176). Cystic adamantinomas or ameloblastomas result from the proliferation of ectopic ameloblasts derived from the enamel organ. Composite odontomas are tumors of increased density (Fig 1–177). Osteomas and giant cell tumors also occur and resemble similar lesions elsewhere, but tissue diagnosis is necessary in all cases unless diagnostic tissue is available from similar lesions elsewhere in a proper clinical setting. This applies to lesions of neuroblastoma, leukemia, and other metastatic neoplasms. Batsakis and Rice pointed out that giant cells are found in a variety of bone lesions in the jaws. Usually they are osteoclasts and are secondary to the primary disease involved. Radiographic findings alone do not provide adequate differential characteristics because a single radiographic pattern may be found in association with several different microscopic patterns. This diagnostic reservation also applies to CT and MRI examinations. Belkin and associates found that MRI was better than, or equal to, CT for ability to detect the lesion, define its margins, demonstrate soft tissue extension, and determine degree of bone involvement in the evaluation of malignant tumors of the jaws; in benign lesions, the same result obtained with respect to defi-

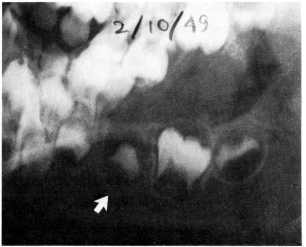 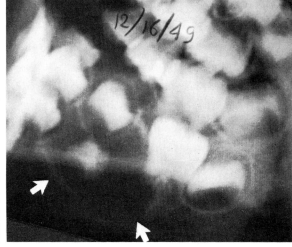

FIG 1–176.
Development of a dentigerous cyst over a period of 10 months in a 6-year-old girl. The excess fluid surrounding the developing crown was not recognized in the earlier film, but the typical enlarged follicle *(arrows)* is obvious 10 months later.

nition of margins and soft tissue extension, but MRI was equal or slightly inferior to CT in lesion detection and determining bone involvement. On CT, sharp, well-demarcated margins were generally related to benign lesions, while irregular, indistinct margins were found in malignant ones. There were no specific tumor characteristics on MRI that helped to distinguish benign from malignant lesions.

The "floating teeth" of histiocytosis X (Langerhans cell histiocytosis) is well known but not pathognomonic as it has been observed in metastatic neuroblastoma, lymphosarcoma, reticulum cell sarcoma, and Ewing sarcoma. The common pathologic factor is a destructive process that affects the supporting alveolar structures of the teeth. Benign os-

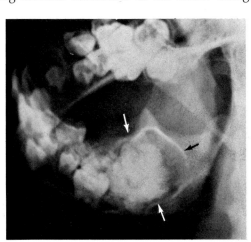

FIG 1–177.
Composite odontoma (dental embryoma) *(arrows)* with an intracystic mass in a patient 9 years of age.

teoblastoma has been reported in the mandible; desmoblastic fibroma and chondrosarcoma have also been described. Although the melanotic neuroectodermal tumor of infancy occurs most frequently in the maxilla, instances of mandibular localization are occasionally found. Osteomas of the mandible and other cranial bones may be a manifestation of Gardner syndrome in which they are associated with connective tissue tumors elsewhere and particularly with polyposis of the large bowel. Woods and associates, however, state that radiology of the jaw and skull have not been a useful screening tool in members of affected families. In the native children of equatorial Africa, Burkitt lymphoma of the jaw accounts for 30% to 50% of all lymphomas; this is rare in the non-African form of the disease.

Familial Fibrosis of Jaws (Cherubism)

Facial swellings that begin about the third year of life, are asymptomatic, and are unattended by any constitutional symptoms characterize this condition that is transmitted by autosomal dominant inheritance. The mandibles and maxillae are generally involved with multilocular cystic changes but other facial bones are spared and cystic lesions elsewhere have been reported rarely and only in the anterior ends of the ribs. Stretching of the skin, owing to maxillary involvement, tends to pull the lower eyelids down revealing a band of white sclerae between the eyelid and the iris (Fig 1–178,*A* and *B*). This cherubic "eyes-raised-to-heaven" expression induced Jones to coin the term *cherubism* in the first report of

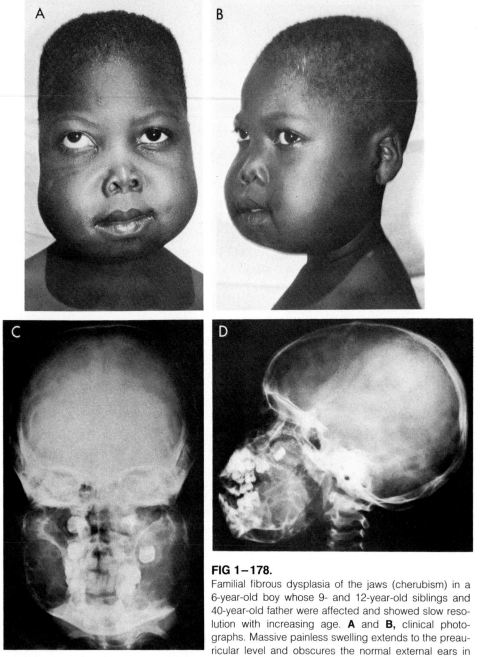

FIG 1–178.
Familial fibrous dysplasia of the jaws (cherubism) in a 6-year-old boy whose 9- and 12-year-old siblings and 40-year-old father were affected and showed slow resolution with increasing age. **A** and **B,** clinical photographs. Massive painless swelling extends to the preauricular level and obscures the normal external ears in the frontal view. The downward displacement of the lower lids explains the term "cherubism" ("eyes raised to heaven"). **C,** frontal, and **D,** lateral skull projections show cystic swelling of the mandible and, to a lesser degree, the maxilla. The teeth are displaced medially except for the unerupted left maxillary molar. The unerupted right molar and the swollen maxilla impinge on the right maxillary sinus, partially obliterating its cavity. The clouding of the left maxillary sinus extends to the left ethmoid as if the walls of both are involved in the fibrous dysplasia, although occlusion of the ostia could account for the opacification. (From Shuler RK, Silverman FN: *Ann Radiol* 1965; 8:45–52. Used by permission.)

the condition. Dentition is seriously disturbed; deciduous and permanent teeth are shed prematurely and irregularly, and some of the molar and premolar teeth are congenitally absent. Submandibular lymph nodes are usually enlarged. Radiographs disclose diffuse swelling and multiloculated rarefaction of the mandible (Fig 1–178,C and D); the maxilla is also swollen with, at least partial, obliteration of the sinuses. CT (Fig 1–179) has detected lesions of the upper jaws not observable in conventional radio-

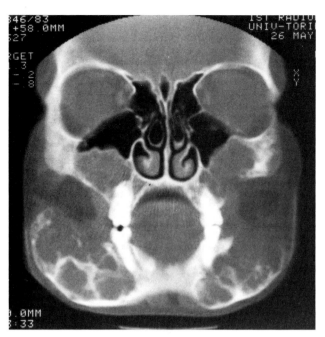

FIG 1–179.
CT features of cherubism in a 13-year-old boy. The obliteration of the maxillary air space and distortion of its walls are caused by involvement of the upper jaw. The mandibular condyle was also affected. (From Bianchi SD, Boccardi A, Mela F, et al: *Skeletal Radiol* 1987; 16:6–10. Used by permission.)

graphs, including involvement of the head of the condyle. Microscopic examination shows diffuse fibrosis of the affected bones, with replacement of bone by fibrous tissue that contains varying numbers of giant cells and blood vessels. Nonspecific hyperplasia has been found in submandibular lymph node biopsy. During the first 2 to 3 years after onset, the swellings increase in size rapidly, then remain stationary until puberty when spontaneous regression begins and continues through the second and third decades. Mandibular enlargement and some sclerosis may persist in later life.

Not all patients have the typical features and course; but with massive jaw swelling and similar dental abnormalities, most seem to be variants of the condition as no other satisfactory diagnosis can be made. Cornelius and McClendon reported two cases and found reports of 89 others that more or less followed the usual pattern. No definite relation with polyostotic fibrous dysplasia has been demonstrated.

Cystic changes of the jaw may be a manifestation of the basal cell nevus syndrome in which basal cell carcinomas, skeletal anomalies, ovarian and falx calcification, and pits in the palms and soles are also present. The jaw cysts may present in childhood and only later do the basal cell carcinomas develop.

Mandibular Involvement in Generalized Diseases of Skeleton

The sclerotic mandibular bone was frequently subject to osteomyelitis, sequestration, and even extrusion of large portions of the bone in the era before the availability of effective antibiotic therapy. In cleidocranial dysplasia, marked delay in shedding of the deciduous teeth is noted; early extraction has no effect on the subsequent eruption of the permanent dentition and may inflict a lengthy period of edentulous existence upon the affected child. Rheumatoid arthritis affects the mandible secondarily in about 15% of cases owing to the retardation of growth ventrad and caudad following temporomandibular arthritis. Deformity of the condyles is also present. Because of the smallness of the mandible, these patients have birdlike facies, and movements of the mandible are limited. A prominent antegonial notch can be noted immediately in front of the angle of the mandible.

In thalassemia, the changes in the mandible are similar to those in the calvaria and long bones and include swollen external contours, dilatation of the medullary spaces, cortical atrophy, and generalized osteoporosis. Fibrocystic changes in the mandible may be a feature of polyostotic fibrous dysplasia.

The disappearance of the lamina dura in hyperparathyroidism was considered a pathognomonic radiographic sign of the disease. More experience has shown that the lamina dura may also be resorbed (in part or in toto) in rickets, following dental extractions, in leukemia, myelomatosis, Cushing disease, Paget disease, idiopathic osteomalacia, idiopathic chronic familial hyperphosphatemia, and primary and metastatic malignancies. Berry emphasized that the bone of the alveolar processes is always affected when the lamina dura has disappeared and that the lamina dura does not disappear in the presence of normal alveolar bone. Mandibular involvement in infantile cortical hyperostosis is an important and almost diagnostic feature of this condition.

TEMPOROMANDIBULAR JOINT

The temporomandibular joint (see Figs 1–168 and 1–169) is a complex joint in which a biconcave fibrous disk divides the articular space between the temporal bone and the mandible into upper and lower compartments. Gliding movements occur in the upper compartment while the lower compartment functions as a true hinge joint. It has been classified as a hinge joint with a movable socket. The articulating surfaces of the bones are not covered by hyaline cartilage as in other joints, but by an avascular, fibrous tissue that is separated from the underlying bone of the condyle by growth cartilage. Signs and symptoms of internal derangement are almost seven times more common in girls than in boys. Radiographic examination requires special projections because of superimposition of other osseous structures and descriptions of these are given by Pruzansky and by Brunelle and Fauré. CT offers the most satisfactory technique to evaluate the structures that compose the joint but may not be necessary in all cases. It has proved of value in patients with juvenile rheumatoid arthritis, internal derangements of the joint, and, even in children, degenerative arthritis. Direct sagittal examination with jaws closed and open are most informative. MRI may provide additional information.

REFERENCES

Temporal Bone

Bergeron RT, Osborn AG, Som PM: *Head and Neck Imaging Excluding the Brain.* St Louis, Mosby–Year Book, 1984.

Currarino G, Weinberg A: Os supra petrosum of Meckel. *Am J Roentgenol* 1974; 131:139–142.

Fritz P, Rieden K, Lenarz T, et al: Radiological evaluation of temporal bone disease: High-resolution computed tomography versus conventional x-ray diagnosis. *Br J Radiol* 1989; 63:107–113.

Jackler RK, Dillon WP: Computed tomography and magnetic resonance imaging of the inner ear. *Otolaryngol Head Neck Surg* 1988; 99:494–504.

Mafee MF, Aimi K, Kahen HL, et al: Chronic otomastoiditis: A conceptual understanding of CT findings. *Radiology* 1986; 160:193–200.

Maslan MJ, Latack JT, Kemink JL, et al: Magnetic resonance imaging of temporal bone and cerebellopontine angle lesions. *Arch Otolaryngol Head Neck Surg* 1986; 112:410–415.

Schubiger O, Vanavanis A, Stuckmann G, et al: Temporal bone fractures and their complications. Examination with high resolution CT. *Neuroradiology* 1986; 28:93–99.

Vignaud J, Jardin C, Rosen L: *The Ear: Diagnostic Imaging. CT Scanner. Tomography, and MR.* New York, Masson Publ USA, 1986.

Virapongse C, Sarwar M, Bhimani S, et al: Computed tomography of temporal bone pneumatization: I. Normal pattern and morphology. *Am J Roentgenol* 1985; 145:473–481.

Sphenoid Bone

Arey LB: The cranial pharyngeal canal—reviewed and reinterpreted. *Anat Rec* 1950; 106:1–16.

Chow MH: Natal and neonatal teeth. *J Am Dent Assoc* 1980; 100:215–216.

Chilton LA, Dorst JP, Garn SM: The volume of the sella turcica in children: New standards. *AJR Am J Roentgenol* 1983; 140:797–801.

di Natale B, Scotti G, Pellini C, et al: Empty sella syndrome in children with pituitary dwarfism: Does it exist? *Pediatrician* 1987; 14:246–253.

Goldstein SJ, Lee C, Carr WA, et al: Magnetic resonance imaging of the sella turcica and parasellar region. A clinical-radiographic evaluation with computed tomography. *Surg Neurol* 1986; 26:330–337.

Kier EL, Rothman SLG: Radiologically significant anatomic variations of the developing sphenoid in humans, in Bosma JF (ed): *Symposium on Development of Basicranium.* Bethesda, Md, US Department of Health, Education, and Welfare, 1976, DHEW Publication No (NIH) 76–989, pp 107–140.

Lowman RM, Robinson F, McAllister WB: The craniopharyngeal canal. *Acta Radiol* 1966; 5:41–54.

Root AW, Martinez CR, Muroff LR: Subhypothalamic high-intensity signals identified by magnetic resonance imaging in children with idiopathic anterior hypopituitarism. Evidence suggestive of an "ectopic" posterior pituitary gland. *Am J Dis Child* 1989; 143:366–367.

Stanhope R, Hindmarsh P, Kendall B, et al: High resolution CT scanning of the pituitary gland in growth disorders. *Acta Paediatr Scand* 1986; 74:779–896.

Orbit

Burton EM, Hickman M, Boulden TF, et al: Orbital sinus histiocytosis: MR appearance. *J Comput Assist Tomogr* 1989; 13:696–699.

Fernbach SK, Naidich TP: CT diagnosis of orbital inflammation in children. *Neuroradiology* 1981; 22:7–13.

Goldberg F, Berne AS, Oski FA: Differentiation of orbital cellulitis from preseptal cellulitis by computed tomography. *Pediatrics* 1978; 62:1000–1005.

Hirsch M, Lifshitz T: Computerized tomography in the diagnosis and treatment of orbital cellulitis. *Pediatr Radiol* 1988; 18:302–305.

Messinger A, Radkowski MA, Greenwald MJ, et al: Orbital roof fractures in the pediatric population. *Plast Reconstr Surg* 1989; 85:213–215.

Myllyla V, Pyhtinen J, Paivansalo M, et al: CT detection and location of intraorbital foreign bodies. Experiments with wood and glass. *ROFO* 1987; 146:39–43.

Mandible: Normal Anatomy

Capitanio MA, Chen JTT, Arey JB, et al: Congenital anhydrotic ectodermal dysplasia. *Am J Roentgenol* 1968; 103:168–172.

Kuhns LR, Sherman MP, Poznanski AK: Determination of neonatal maturation on a chest radiograph. *Radiology* 1972; 102:597–603.

Leuno AK: Natal teeth. *Am J Dis Child* 1986; 140:249–251.

Moorrees CFA, Fanning EA, Hunt EE Jr: Formation and resorption of 3 deciduous teeth in children. *Am J Phys Anthropol* 1963; 21:105–214.

Moorrees CFA, Fanning EA, Hunt EE Jr: Age variation of formation stages for 10 permanent teeth. *J Dent Res* 1963; 42:1490–1502.

Prader VA, Perabo F: Körperwachstung, Knochen und Zahnentwicklung bei den Endokrinen-Erkrankung im Kindesalter. *Helv Paediatr Acta* 1952; 7:517–529.

Traxler M, Fezoulidis J, Schadelbauer D, et al: Unerupted and displaced teeth in CT-scan. *Int J Oral Maxillofac Surg* 1989; 18:184–186.

Diseases of the Mandible

Becker MH, Coccaro PJ, Converse JM: Antegonial notching of the mandible: An often overlooked mandibular deformity in congenital and acquired disorders. *Radiology* 1976; 121:149–151.

Cohen MM Jr: Pierre Robin anomalad—Its non-specificity and associated syndromes. *J Oral Surg* 1976; 34:587–593.

Dennison WM: The Pierre Robin syndrome. *Pediatrics* 1965; 36:336–341.

Maisels FO: Reduplication of the mouth and mandible. *Br J Plast Surg* 1981; 34:23–25.

Munk PL, Helms CA: Coronoid process hyperplasia: CT studies. *Radiology* 1989; 171:783–784.

Randall P: Micrognathia and glossoptosis with airway obstruction: The Pierre Robin syndrome, in Converse JM (ed): *Reconstructive Plastic Surgery,* vol 3. Philadelphia, WB Saunders, 1964.

Silverman FN, Streffling AM, Stevenson DK, et al: Cerebro-costomandibular syndrome. *J Pediatr* 1980; 97:406–416.

Fractures, Osteomyelitis, Cysts and Neoplasms, Familial Fibrosis of the Jaws (Cherubism), and Mandibular Involvement in Generalized Diseases of the Skeleton

Batsakis JG, Rice DH: Diseases affecting the jaws: III. Giant cell lesions and fibrous dysplasia of the jaws. *Univ Mich Med Cent J 1969;* 35:162–169.

Belkin BA, Papageorge MB, Fakitsas J, et al: A comparative study of magnetic resonance imaging versus computed tomography for the evaluation of maxillary and mandibular tumors. *J Oral Maxillofac Surg* 1988; 46:1039–1047.

Berry HM Jr: The lore and the lure of the lamina dura. *Radiology* 1973; 109:525–528.

Bianchi SD, Boccardi A, Mela F, et al: The computed tomographic appearances of cherubism. *Skeletal Radiol* 1987; 16:6–10.

Burkes EJ Jr, Kelley DR: Primary mandibular neuroblastoma. *J Oral Surg* 1980; 38:128–131.

Christianson R, Lufkin RB, Abemayor E, et al: MRI of the mandible. *Surg Radiol Anat* 1989; 11:163–169.

Cornelius EA, McClendon JL: Cherubism—a familial fibrous dysplasia of the jaws. *Am J Roentgenol* 1969; 106:136–143.

Eisenbud L, Kahn LB, Friedman E: Benign osteoblastoma of the mandible: Fifteen year follow-up showing spontaneous regression after biopsy. *J Oral Maxillofac Surg* 1987; 45:53–57.

Ferris RA, Hakkal HG, Cigtay OS: Radiologic manifestations of North American Burkitt's lymphoma. *J Laryngol Otol* 1975; 123:614–619.

Gunge M, Yamamoto H, Katoh T, et al: Suppurative osteomyelitis of the mandible in a child. *Int J Oral Maxillofac Surg* 1987; 16:99–103.

Gupta DS, Gupta MK, Borle RM: Osteomyelitis of the mandible in marble bone disease. *Int J Oral Maxillofac Surg* 1986; 15:201–205.

Jackson R, Gardere S: Nevoid basal cell carcinoma syndrome. *Can Med Assoc J* 1971; 125:850–862.

Jones WA: Familial multilocular cystic disease of the jaws. *Am J Cancer* 1933; 17:946–950.

Kozlowski K, Masel J, Sprague P, et al: Mandibular and paramandibular tumors in children: Report of 16 cases. *Pediatr Radiol* 1981; 11:183–192.

Mekek M, Lello GE: Desmoplastic fibroma of the mandible: Literature review and report of three cases. *J Oral Maxillofac Surg* 1986; 44:385–391.

Totten JR: The multiple nevoid basal cell carcinoma syndrome: Report of its occurrence in four generations of a family. *Cancer* 1980; 46:1456–1462.

Waite DE: Pediatric fractures of jaw and facial bones: Review of literature. *Pediatrics* 1973; 51:551–559.

Wood RE, Housego T, Nortjé CJ, et al: Tuberculous osteomyelitis in the mandible of a child. *Pediatr Dent* 1987; 9:317–320.

Woods RJ, Serra RG, Cteroteko GC, et al: Occult radiologic changes in the skull and jaw in familial adenomatous polyposis coli. *Dis Colon Rectum* 1989; 32:304–306.

Temporomandibular Joint

Avrahami E, Segel R, Solomon A, et al: Direct coronal high resolution computed tomography of the temporomandibular joints in patients with rheumatoid arthritis. *J Rheumatol* 1989; 18:298–301.

Brunelle F, Fauré C: L'articulation temporo-maxillaire chez l'enfant. *J Radiol Electrol Med Nucl* 1978; 59:697–701.

Pruzansky S: The temporomandibular joint. *Otolaryngol Clin North Am* 1973; 6:523–548.

Sanchez-Woodworth RE, Katzberg RW, Tallents RH, et al: Radiographic assessment of temporomandibular joint pain and dysfunction in the pediatric age group. *ASDC J Dent Child* 1988; 55:278–281.

2

Spine and Pelvis

SECTION 1

Introduction to the Spine

NORMAL ANATOMY

In this section we consider primarily the vertebral column and the pelvic segments of the axial skeleton. The vertebral column is derived from condensations of mesoderm that surround the neural tube and notochord. In the course of development, segmentation of the mesenchyme takes place and results in division into the approximately 32 to 34 units that compose the definitive vertebral column. Each unit is initially represented by a cartilaginous model within which ossification centers develop, enlarge, and unite. Remnants of the notochord contribute to the formation of the intervertebral disks that separate and unite the individual vertebral bodies, acting as shock absorbers and helping maintain the strength and mobility of the spine.

With few exceptions, a vertebral segment is composed of an anterior mass or body and a posterior ring or arch. Several appendages project from the arch: the paired transverse processes, the paired superior and inferior articulating processes, and the single spinous process (Fig 2–1; see also Figs 2–7, 2–8, and 2–9). The cartilaginous model forms from a right and left chondrification center for the body and one each for the right and left sides of the arch. Their coalescence forms the cartilaginous vertebra. Failure of development or hypoplasia of one of the two chondrification centers of the vertebral body is thought to be the principal cause of hemivertebra. The two sides of the arch unite posteriorly, around the spinal cord just after the end of the second fetal month. Ossification centers first make their appearance in the cartilaginous vertebrae at about the tenth fetal week. One or two centers appear in the body; when two centers occur, their relationships often differ from those of the side-by-side chondrification centers as one may be anterior and the other posterior. Single centers appear in the pedicles of each arch. These primary ossification centers continue to expand into the cartilaginous vertebrae during embryonic life but are still separated from one another by cartilaginous bridges at birth. Ossification centers make their appearance first in the bodies of the lower dorsal and upper lumbar area at about 3 months' gestation, and extend cephalad more rap-

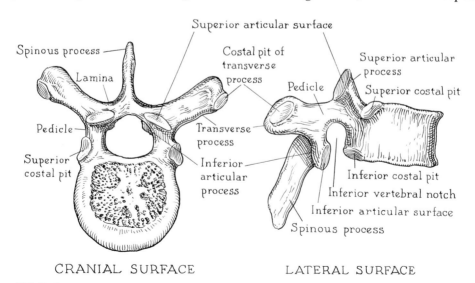

CRANIAL SURFACE   LATERAL SURFACE

FIG 2–1.
Normal thoracic vertebra: cranial and lateral aspects.

idly than caudad, paralleling roughly the pattern of closure of the neural tube. By the fifth month of fetal life, ossification centers are present in all of the bodies, and ossification of the neural arches has occurred independently beginning in the cervical region and progressing in a different pattern from that of the bodies. A large portion of the posterolateral aspects of the vertebral bodies is ossified by extension from the neural arches. Ossification centers that are present histologically, in cleared and stained preparations, or even radiographically in excised segments, may be invisible in radiographs of the intact subject.

The ossification center in the body fuses with the center in each side of the arch at the neurocentral sutures between the third and the sixth year. The two bony centers in the arch extend posteriorly toward the midline and complete the bony neural arch by ten years, after which little or no further growth of the encircled spinal canal occurs. Ossification centers appear in the cartilaginous rims (annular cartilages) of the bodies about the age of puberty; their development is advanced in the upper rims in comparison with the lower rims. Secondary ossification centers occur at the tips of the several bony appendages arising from the neural arch, the transverse processes, the articulating processes, and the spinous processes. These all appear approximately at puberty and fuse with their respective processes at approximately 25 years (Fig 2–2).

At birth, the vertebral column forms a single long shallow curve extending from the first cervical to the fifth lumbar segments with its concavity directed anteriorly. The cervical curve appears shortly after the head is held up during the first year. The lumbar curve develops when erect posture is assumed at about the beginning of the second year and gradually becomes more prominent during the years of childhood. The normal curves of the spine do not become fixed until after puberty.

The postnatal longitudinal growth of the spine is due exclusively to the proliferation of cartilage on the upper and lower zones of the primary ossification center in the vertebral body; according to Beadle, there is no growth and no trace of endochondral bone formation in the annular cartilages. This ring of cartilage, often miscalled an epiphysis, ossifies independently of the primary center, which constitutes the body of the vertebra, bears no direct relation to its longitudinal growth, and contributes nothing to its endochondral bone formation. It merely fuses with the body when growth of the body is complete.

The spongiosa of the vertebral bodies, a delicate wide-meshed reticulum, is surrounded by a thin cylindric wall of compact bone. Amstutz and Sissons demonstrated that the vertebral spongiosa consists of a complex network of bony plates perforated by round openings of varying size. These plates are oriented preferentially in the vertical and horizontal planes, and the amount of spongiosa is greatest near the upper and lower edges of the vertebral bodies and least in their central segments. The upper and lower surfaces of the body are not limited by a true closing plate of compact bone, as is the case in the ends of the tubular bones in the limbs. At these vertebral surfaces, the trabeculae of the spongiosa are concentrated transversely into a profusely perforated plate. The perforations afford direct contact of the marrow spaces with the articular plates and permit the direct transfer of fluids from the vertebral body into the contiguous intervertebral disks, thus serving as channels through which the disk is nourished and, at times, infected, from the body. The neural arch and its appendages are covered with a

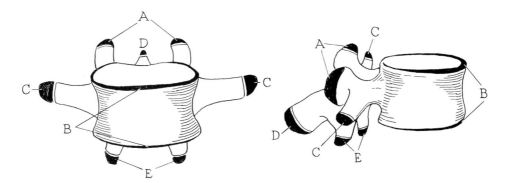

FIG 2–2.
The secondary vertebral ossification centers: *A*, superior articular processes; *C*, transverse processes; *D*, spinous processes; *E*, inferior articular processes. These all appear at approximately 16 years and fuse with their respective processes at approximately 25 years. *B*, the annular ossification centers; these appear as early as the seventh year in females and fuse with the main mass of the body at approximately 25 years.

layer of compact bone that is much thicker and stronger than the thin cortex in the cylindric wall of the vertebral body.

At birth, the average length of the spine without the sacrum is 20 cm; during the first 2 years, growth is rapid and the length increases to about 45 cm. The velocity of growth is greatly diminished thereafter; at puberty, the longitudinal axis measures about 50 cm. The final adult length of 60 to 75 cm is attained between the 22nd and the 24th year. There is a significant change in the relative length of the cervical and lumbar portions during growth. At birth, the cervical spine makes up one fourth of the total length of the spinal column, the thoracic spine one half, and the lumbar spine one fourth. In the adult, the cervical spine is reduced to one fifth or one sixth of the total length, while the lumbar segment is increased until it constitutes nearly one third of the whole (Scammon). The apparent shortness of the neck in infants is due to the fullness of the cervical soft tissues.

The longitudinal growth of each vertebral body and the total composite longitudinal growth of the whole spine are modified by the stress of weight-bearing. Gooding and Neuhauser demonstrated longitudinal overgrowth and transverse undergrowth of vertebral bodies in growing children whose spines had never been subjected to the stresses of gravity and weightbearing because of neuromuscular weaknesses and paralysis. In the lumbar levels, where the normal stress of weightbearing is greatest, excessive longitudinal growth and transverse hypoplasia of the vertebral bodies were maximal. The vertical elongation and the anteroposterior (AP) shortening cause the affected vertebral bodies to resemble those of the dog, and have been described as "caninization."

Each intervertebral disk contains three components: the paired cartilaginous articular plates, the fibrous ring or anulus fibrosus, and the nucleus pulposus (Fig 2–3). The anulus fibrosus is a homologue of the fibrous capsule of the freely movable joints of the limbs; it is made up of a series of connective tissue lamellae that run in wide curves from one vertebral surface to the adjacent vertebral surface. Compressed in the central portion of the disk, and surrounded by the anulus, is a highly elastic fluid-fibrous mass, the nucleus pulposus, which plays an outstanding role in many vertebral diseases. It is a segmental intervertebral remnant of the fetal notochord.

The principal change in the intervertebral disk during growth is the reduction of its fluid content, particularly in the nucleus pulposus which is, at birth, a mass of mucoid, gelatinous fluid dispersed

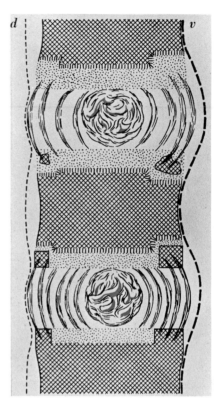

FIG 2–3.
Schematic drawing of sagittal section of the spine. Phases in progressive ossification and fusion of the vertebral rings. In the underedge of the uppermost vertebral body, the vertebral ring in the peripheral notch is made up entirely of cartilage *(stippled)*. In the upper edge of the middle vertebral body, an ossification center *(crosshatched)* is present in the vertebral ring, front and back. In the underedge of the same body, this ossification center is larger and occupies more of the cartilaginous ring. In the upper edge of the lowermost vertebral body, the ossification center occupies all of the notch and has fused with the main mass of the vertebral body. In all phases of its development, the vertebral ring is deeply penetrated by Sharpey fibers. The growth and ossification of the vertebral ring appears to contribute little or nothing to the growth of the vertebral body. The anterior longitudinal ligament *(heavy broken line)* is attached to the vertebral bodies but skips attachment to the intervertebral disks; the converse is true for the posterior longitudinal ligament. *d,* dorsal edge; *v,* ventral edge. (From Schmorl G, Junghanns H: *The Humal Spine in Health and Disease. Anatomicopathologic Studies.* Philadelphia, Grune & Stratton, 1957. Used by permission.)

through a widely meshed reticulum of mesenchymal cells derived from the notochord. With increasing age, the anulus fibrosus expands centrally into the margins of the cartilaginous plates, which, at the same time, are contracting peripherally. Physiologic calcification occurs occasionally, even in children.

ROENTGENOGRAPHIC APPEARANCE

There are generally seven cervical segments, 12 thoracic, five lumbar, five sacral, and four to five coccygeal, with variations at the upper three junction levels that are associated with excess or deficiency of articulations with lateral structures such as ribs or ilia (cervical ribs, absent 12th ribs, lumbarization of the first sacral segment, sacralization of the fifth lumbar segment). The first and second cervical vertebrae, the atlas and axis, differ from each other and from the remaining cervical vertebrae; in fact, phylogenetically, they represent the fifth and sixth axial segments, as the first four have been incorporated in the occipital bone of the skull. The sacral segments, although separated from one another prior to maturity, are fused to form a single bone in the adult. The coccygeal segments are rudimentary vertebrae consisting usually of just a body; the first through third are generally united with one another by fibrocartilage while the more caudal segments are united by bony substance. The distance between the medial borders of the vertebral pedicles in a true AP projection of the spine may provide information about localized constrictions or widenings when compared with curves based on measurements at different ages (Fig 2–4). The cervical and lumbar spaces are widest at all ages; their discrepancy with respect to thoracic measurements increases with age. Because the range at any age is great, the actual measurements are less important than local deviations from the basic curves of normal measurements.

During infancy and childhood, in comparison with adolescence, the intervertebral spaces appear proportionately thicker and the vertebral bodies smaller, owing to the radiolucent cartilage zones in the upper and lower surfaces of the vertebral bodies. These merge with the radiolucent shadows of the intervertebral disks and augment their apparent size. All portions of even a single vertebra cannot be satisfactorily visualized in a single projection because of superimposed shadows of the different vertebral components. Frontal, lateral, and often oblique projections are essential for complete visualization with conventional radiography. Computed tomography (CT) is ideal for study of the spine, and with three-dimensional displays can provide reasonably accurate models of the osseous structures and the spinal canal. Magnetic resonance imaging (MRI) is more effective for evaluation of the soft tissues within and adjacent to the spine. CT and MRI have become the gold standard for demonstrating these areas when the clinical situation warrants.

The vertebrae present widely different normal roentgen images at different ages. In the first weeks of life, the three primary ossification centers are still separated by radiolucent cartilaginous bridges (Fig 2–5). The radiolucent neurocentral synchondroses persist as longitudinal bands and, in older children, as lines of diminished density at the junctions of the body and the two sides of the neural arch until the third to sixth years. In lateral projections, the vertebral bodies exhibit paired notched defects in the middle third of the anterior and posterior walls. The anterior notch is produced by a large sinusoidal blood space within the ossification center; the posterior one represents an actual perforated indentation of the posterior wall of the body containing nutrient arteries and vertebral veins. Central radiodense patterns occur in the vertebral bodies of some normal infants under 2 months of age; they resemble the "bone-within-bone" pattern observed in patients with osteopetrosis but diminish and disappear within a few weeks. Brill and associates observed them in 19 of 30 infants under 6 weeks of age and in only 2 of 10 infants over 6 weeks of age.

With advancing age, the vertebral body loses its oval shape and becomes more rectangular. The anterior notch narrows, reflecting the presence of anterolateral vessels; it disappears late in childhood but may persist longer in some cases. Notched anterior defects become visible in the upper and lower ante-

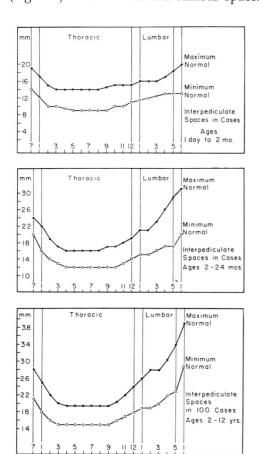

FIG 2–4.
Upper and lower limits of interpediculate distances from birth to 12 years. The curve for upper limits in adults is only slightly greater than that for 12-year-old children. (From Simril WA, Thurston D: *Radiology* 1955; 64:340–347. Used by permission.)

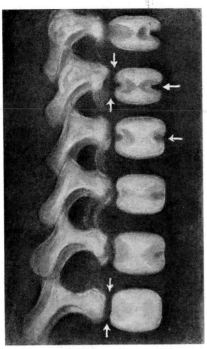

FIG 2–5.
The normal roentgen appearance at birth; drawing of a roentgenogram. The anterior and posterior "notch" shadows *(arrows)* in the vertebral body are noteworthy. The cartilaginous neurocentral synchondroses *(arrows)* between the body and the arch cast shadows of water density.

rior angles of the bodies (Fig 2–6); they indicate the position of the thick, furrowed cartilaginous rims of the annular cartilages in which secondary centers of ossification develop during late childhood.

CERVICAL SPINE

Ossification of the cervical vertebrae, except for that of the atlas and axis, proceeds as in other segments with centers in the body and the neural arches. The individual components of the first (atlas) and the second (axis) cervical vertebrae are shown in Figures 2–7 and 2–8. The components of a typical cervical vertebrae (C3 through C7) are shown in Figure 2–9. The dens of the axis is phylogenetically the body of the first cervical vertebra, but the small arch of bone in front of the dens, articulating with a convex articular facet on the anterior surface of the latter, is called the body of C1 by convention. It generally ossifies from its own center (or centers) but can ossify by extension from the centers in the lateral masses. The multiple components of the second cervical vertebra may result in horizontal, vertical, and oblique radiolucencies corresponding to the synchondroses shown in Figure 2–10. The "summit" ossification center, also known as the ossiculum terminale Bergman, may simulate a fracture fragment. Closure of

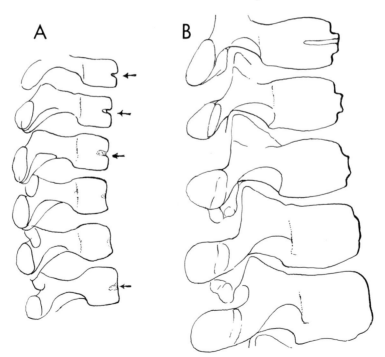

FIG 2–6.
A, tracing of a normal roentgenogram at 1 year of age. The bodies are more rectangular, and the intervertebral spaces are proportionately narrower than in the neonatal spine. Horizontal clefts in the midportion of the body are still visible. **B,** tracing of a normal roentgenogram of a child 6 years old. There are now notched de-

fects in the superior and inferior angles of the vertebral bodies, and a steplike shelf projects from the intervening portion of the anterior surface. A narrow anterior intrasegmental cleft is still evident in some of the bodies.

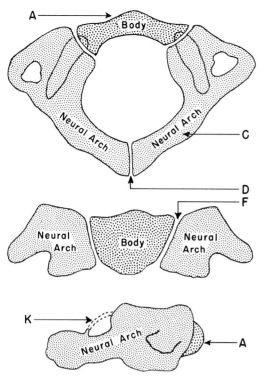

FIG 2–7.
Developmental components of the first cervical vertebra (atlas). *A*, ossification center for the anterior arch. This may normally appear during the last fetal months or the early postnatal months. *C*, components of the dorsal segment of the neural arch that may appear as ossification centers as early as the third fetal month. *D*, the synchondrosis that binds the neural arch together at its dorsal extremity in the midsagittal plane of the spinous process. Rarely, an independent ossification center may appear in this synchondrosis. *F*, the neurocentral synchondroses that bind the vertebral body (the anterior arch in C1) to the neural arches on both sides. These gradually diminish and disappear during the last half of childhood. *K*, the ligament that crosses behind the superior vertebral notch. In adults, this may ossify to form a superior vertebral foramen. (Redrawn from Bailey DK: *Radiology* 1952; 59:712–719.)

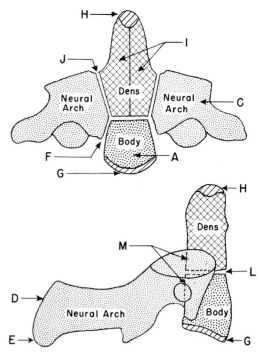

FIG 2–8.
Developmental elements in the second cervical vertebra (axis). *A*, body; a single ossification center usually appears during the fourth fetal month. *C*, neural arches appear in paired ossification centers by the sixth fetal month. *D*, neural arches that fuse posteriorly during the third and fourth years. *E*, bifid spinous process. *F*, neurocentral synchondroses that disappear when the body and pedicles fuse during the fourth to seventh years. *G*, inferior vertebral ring that ossifies during the late years of childhood and fuses with the body during early life. This ring is not part of an epiphysis and contributes nothing to growth of the vertebral body. *H*, "summit" ossification center of the odontoid that appears between the second and sixth years and then fuses with the main mass of the odontoid at 11 to 12 years. *I*, odontoid process or dens. Two independent ossification centers appear during the fifth fetal month and then usually fuse with each other during the seventh fetal month. *J*, synchondroses that bind the base of the dens on each side to the neural arches. They disappear between 3 and 7 years of age. *L*, synchondrosis between the dens and body that disappears between 3 and 7 years. *M*, posterior surfaces of the dens and body. (Redrawn from Bailey DK: *Radiology* 1952; 59:712–719.)

the neural arches of the atlas and axis are the last to take place so that apparent spina bifida may be suggested in oblique lateral projections, or when these neural arches are visualized in Towne projections of the skull, during the first decade. Ossification of the lateral edge of the posterior atlanto-occipital membrane behind the superior vertebral notch in the C1 segment (see *K*, Fig 2–7) sometimes forms a bony curved bridge that closes the notch and forms a foramen (Fig 2–11) that transmits the vertebral artery and first spinal nerve. This bridge, the ponticulus posticus, may be unilateral or bilateral.

The apophyseal joint spaces of the cervical vertebrae usually lie at an angle of 45 degrees from the coronal plane in lateral projection. Variations occur in the planes of the joints between C2 and C3 and may result in a barlike structure seeming to unite these two segments (Fig 2–12). The affected C2–3 joint spaces can be demonstrated in oblique projections.

Alignment of the vertebrae as seen in lateral projection varies with the position of the head and neck. In flexion, a distinct step-off can be observed, especially between C2 and C3, and C3 and C4 (Fig 2–13). The body of C1 may appear disproportionately remote from the anterior margin of the dens, in part because of the large amount of intervening unmineralized cartilage of both structures. In extension, with marked hyperextension of the head, the body of C1 may seem to ride over the tip of the ossified portion of the odontoid. The excess of move-

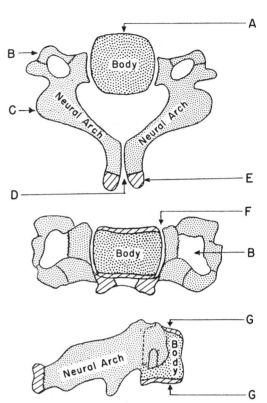

FIG 2–9.
Developmental parts of typical cervical vertebrae (C3 through C7). *A,* body. *B,* anterior segment of the costal portion of the transverse process; this may develop from a separate center that appears in the cartilage about the sixth fetal month and is fused with the main ossification center of the transverse process by the sixth year. *C,* neural arches whose ossification centers usually appear by the third fetal month. *D,* synchondrosis that binds the two sides of the spinous process; this usually disappears by the fourth year but may persist 2 or 3 years longer. *E,* secondary, separate ossification centers in the tips of the two sides of the spinous process. *F,* neurocentral synchondroses that bind the neural arches to each body on both sides; they usually disappear between 3 and 7 years of age. *G,* superior and inferior vertebral rings that may begin to ossify as early as age 7 years in girls and then fuse with their vertebral body at about 25 years. These rings are not parts of an epiphysis and contribute nothing to growth of the vertebral body. They also have no causal relationship to juvenile kyphosis. (Redrawn from Bailey DK: *Radiology* 1952; 59:712–719.)

ment of the body of C1 in relation to the odontoid in infants and children is probably related to increased ligamentous laxity that can, however, become pathologic in patients with conditions associated with excessive laxity, as in Down syndrome. The great range of movement of components of the cervical spine in normal children is an important consideration in the evaluation of trauma to the cervical

spine. The tip of the clivus is normally aligned with the odontoid tip; malalignment is an indication of, at least, potential cord impingement usually resulting from damage to the occipitoaxial ligament.

Defects in the pedicles of the second cervical vertebra occur occasionally in children with no history of trauma and without clinical signs or symptoms. The patient in Figure 2–14 was examined at 4

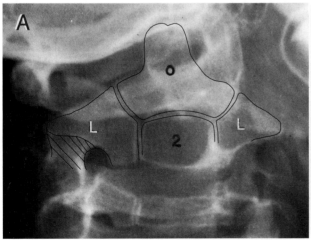

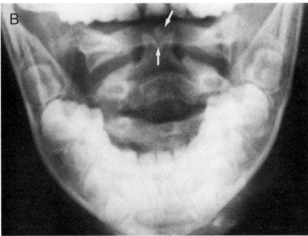

FIG 2–10.
Roentgen anatomy of the axis vertebra. **A,** oblique AP projection in a 7-year-old boy showing the synostoses between the body *(2)* and the lateral masses *(L)* of C2, and the body of C2 and the odontoid process *(O).* Note the slight V-shaped cleft at the tip of

the odontoid. **B,** AP projection of C2 in a 4-year-old girl; the synchondroses are not seen because of their oblique course, but a residual cleft is present in the tip of the odontoid in which an early summit ossification center can be seen. Compare with Figure 2–7

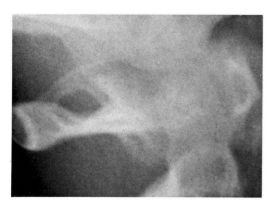

FIG 2–11.
Ponticulus posticus. Complete ossification of the atlanto-occipital membrane that completely bridges the arcuate notch of the C1 spinal segment to form a small posterior bridge (ponticulus posticus). This girl, 8 years of age, was asymptomatic.

months because of large fontanelles and found to have skeletal features characteristic of pyknodysostosis. No clinical signs related to the defects were detected over a period of 4 years' observation during which time little or no change occurred in the defect. One of two additional children with similar defects had Crouzon disease (Currarino). Among several other asymptomatic patients previously reported, one also had pyknodysostosis.

In the seventh cervical vertebra, variation in the size of the costal processes may simulate cervical ribs. A change in size relative to the transverse process that ultimately unites with it to form the costo-transverse foramen, together with the clearly downward curving and constant relative size and nature of the cervical ribs, serves to make the differentiation (Keating and Amberg).

Delayed mineralization of the cervical vertebral bodies, when thoracic and lumbar vertebral bodies appear better developed, occurs in achondrogenesis, thanatophoric dysplasia, spondyloepiphyseal dysplasia congenita, chondrodysplasia punctata, and the cerebrocostomandibular syndrome. In these conditions, delayed mineralization is usually found also in the lower lumbar and sacral vertebral bodies. At both levels, it is manifested by absent or small ossification centers, which may assume normal size in their cartilaginous precursors if the patient survives.

THORACOLUMBAR SPINE

The thoracic vertebrae are larger than the cervical, and the lumbar are larger than the thoracic, as if each segment were designed to support the progressively increasing weight of the body above it. In the

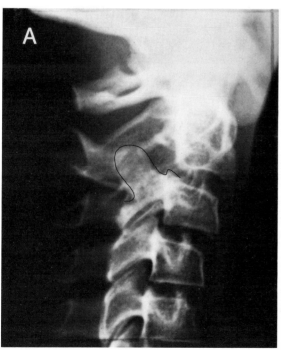

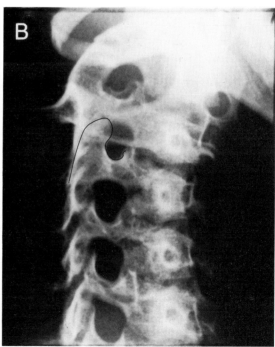

FIG 2–12.
Variant in orientation of the apophyseal joint at the C2–3 level simulating synostosis. **A,** in the lateral projection, the C2–3 apophyseal joint cannot be identified as can the joints below this level. A bony bar appears to arise from the neural arch of C3 and extend to, and possibly unite with, the neural arch of C2. In **B,** the "bar" is seen to be the superior articular process of C3, but the joint, though visible in this posterior oblique projection, is still ill-defined in comparison with those below C3. There were no clinical signs associated with this variant.

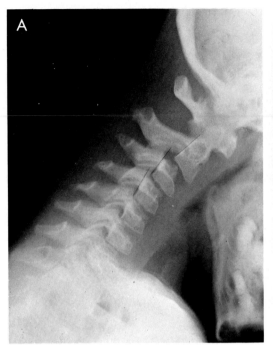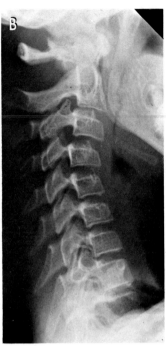

FIG 2–13.
Normal mobility of the cervical spine in children. **A,** normal forward shift of C2 on C3 in an asymptomatic girl 3 years old. **B,** normal forward shift of C3 on C4 (pseudoluxation) in an asymptomatic girl 5 years of age. (From Sullivan CR, Bruwer AJ, Harris LE: *Am J Surg* 1958; 95:636–640. Used by permission.)

thoracic levels, the pedicles and lamina are directed posteriorly and downward, with each one overlapping the neural arch below. In the lumbar segment, the pedicles and lamina are directed straight backward. The heads of the 1st, 11th, 12th, and sometimes the 10th ribs articulate with their corresponding vertebral bodies. All the other ribs articulate

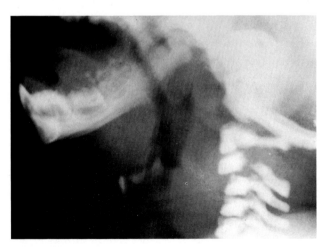

FIG 2–14.
Asymptomatic defect in the neural arch of C2 in a 4-month-old infant with large fontanelles and other features of pyknodystostosis. Note osteosclerosis and failure of development of the angle of the mandible. (From Currarino G: *Pediatr Radiol* 1989; 19:535–538. Used by permission.)

with two adjacent vertebral bodies, with the larger articulating surface at the upper lateral margin of the corresponding vertebral body and the smaller articulating surface at the lower margin of the vertebral body immediately above. The 1st through 10th ribs also articulate, by a costal tubercle, with a facet near the tip of the transverse process of the vertebrae. The articulating facets of the thoracic vertebrae proper lie in the coronal plane except for the inferior facets of the lower two thoracic vertebrae which approach the sagittal plane to correspond to the plane of the lumbar facets. In the fifth lumbar vertebral body, the plane of the inferior facets may be coronal, oblique, or even horizontal, and are frequently asymmetric.

Transitional areas exist in the vertebral column at the cervicothoracic, thoracolumbar, and lumbosacral levels. Variations that are not malformations occur in these levels, including cervical ribs, hypoplastic or absent 12th ribs and lumbarization of the first sacral segment, or 1st lumbar ribs and sacralization of the fifth lumbar segment, depending on a cranial or caudal "shift" of vertebral processes at each level. When shifts occur at any level, they tend to follow the same direction at the others. In a *cranial shift*, there is commonly present a cervical rib or a long transverse process at the cervicothoracic level, an absent or short 12th rib at the thoracolumbar level, and a short transverse process of the fourth lumbar vertebra with sacralization of the fifth. In a *caudal shift,* the seventh cervical vertebra has a short transverse process, the 12th rib is long and a 1st lumbar rib may be present, the transverse process of the fourth lumbar vertebra is long, and the first sacral segment is lumbarized. These shifts account for the approximately 30% of people who vary in number of segments, or composition, of individual regions. The greatest variations are in the thoracolumbar and lumbosacral levels.

Bands of increased density form on the upper and lower edges of the growing vertebral body under the same conditions in which Park's transverse lines appear in the ends of growing long bones (see Fig 4–136). In the vertebral body, however, the line formation is not as rapid or as marked owing to the limited slow growth in each segment of the spine. In experimental bismuth poisoning, heavy marginal lines have been produced in the vertebral bodies of young dogs.

REFERENCES

Anatomy and Roentgenographic Appearance
Amstutz HC, Sissons HA: The structure of the vertebral spongiosa. *J Bone Joint Surg [Br]* 1969; 51:540–550.

Bagnall KM, Harris PE, Jones PRM: A radiographic study of the human fetal spine. *J Anat* 1977; 124:791–802.

Beadle OA: *The Intervertbral Discs.* Special Report Series No 161, Medical Research Council. London, His Majesty's Stationery Office, 1931.

Brill PW, Baker DH, Ewing ML: "Bone-within-bone" in the neonatal spine: Stress change or normal development? *Radiology* 1973; 108:363–366.

Gooding CA, Neuhauser EBD: Growth and development of the normal vertebral body in the presence and the absence of stress. *Am J Roentgenol* 1965; 93:388–394.

Pate D, Resnick D, Sartoris DJ, et al: 3D CT of the spine: Practical applications. *Appl Radiol* 1987; May:86–94.

Pauchster DM, Modic MT, Masaryk TJ: Magnetic resonance imaging of the spine: Applications and limitations. *Radiol Clin North Am* 1985; 23:551–562.

Scammon RE: A summary of the anatomy of the infant and child, in Abt IA (ed): *Pediatrics.* Philadelphia, WB Saunders, 1923, pp 257–444.

Schmorl G, Junghanns H: *The Human Spine in Health and Disease. Anatomicopathologic Studies.* Philadelphia, Grune & Stratton, 1957.

Schwarz GS: Width of spinal canal in growing vertebra with special reference to sacrum; maximum interpediculate distances in adults and children. *Am J Roentgenol* 1956; 76:476–481.

Simril WA, Thurston D: Normal interpediculate space in the spines of infants and children. *Radiology* 1955; 64:340–347.

Cervical Spine
Bailey DK: The normal cervical spine in infants and children. *Radiology* 1952; 59:712–719.

Cattell HS, Filtzer DL: Pseudosubluxation and other normal variations in the cervical spine in children. A study of one hundred sixty children. *J Bone Joint Surg [Am]* 1965; 47:1295–1309.

Currarino G: Primary spondylolysis of the axis vertebra (C2) in three children, including one with pyknodysostosis. *Pediatr Radiol* 1989; 19:535–538.

Harwood-Nash DC, Fitz CR: *Neuroradiology in Infants and Children,* vol 1. St Louis, Mosby–Year Book, 1976, p 241.

Kattan KR: *"Trauma" and "No-Trauma" of the Cervical Spine.* Springfield, Ill, Charles C Thomas, 1975.

Kattan KR: Backward "displacement" of the spinolaminal line at C-2: A normal variation. *Am J Roentgenol* 1977; 129:289–290.

Keating DR, Amberg JR: A source of potential error in the roentgen diagnosis of cervical ribs. *Radiology* 1954; 62:688–894.

Overton LM, Grossman JW: Anatomical variations in the articulation between the second and third cervical vertebrae. *J Bone Joint Surg [Am]* 1952; 34:155–161.

Sullivan CR, Bruwer AJ, Harris LE: Hypermobility of the cervical spine in children: A pitfall in the diagnosis of cervical dislocation. *Am J Surg* 1958; 95:636–640.

von Torklus D, Gehle W: *The Upper Cervical Spine. Regional Anatomy, Pathology and Traumatology. A Systematic Radiological Atlas and Textbook.* Philadelphia, Grune & Stratton, 1972.

SECTION 2

Congenital Malformations of the Spine

CERVICAL SPINE ABNORMALITIES

Congenital malformations of the cervical spine vary from clinically insignificant ones recognized radiographically to those with potential or present signs and symptoms. Congenital absence of a portion of a cervical vertebra most frequently involves components of the neural arch (Fig 2–15). In a girl 13 years of age reported by Oestreich and Young, pain in the neck, shoulder, and arm was present on the same side on which a cervical pedicle was absent. The defect was best demonstrated in oblique films where a large common intervertebral foramen was observed on the affected side. A portion of the transverse process was also missing in this patient. Notwithstanding absence of all or part of the posterior arch, no instability at the level of the defect was observed in a patient reported by Garber. Over 50% of cases are asymptomatic and the defect is a chance finding. It is almost always unilateral and more frequently reported on the right side. In several reported instances, incorrect interpretation of the commonly observed enlarged intervertebral foramen has resulted in inappropriate management. Spina bifida, as in other levels, can be occult or manifest. In rare cases, cervical spina bifida, with protrusion of soft tissues of the spinal canal, is seen in association with occipital encephalocele.

Absence or hypoplasia of the odontoid process occurs in several skeletal dysplasias, particularly in spondyloepiphyseal dysplasia congenita and Morquio disease. The possibility of atlantoaxial instability in such patients should be kept in mind when procedures involving neck flexion or extension are required. It is worth noting that atlantoaxial instability can occur with a normal odontoid when ligamentous structures are lax, as in Down syndrome.

One structural abnormality of the dens is its appearance as an accessory ossicle moving with the body of C2, the os odontoideum (Fig 2–16). Early reports classified it as a malformation in which bony union between this center arising from the proatlas and the body of the atlas failed to occur. More recently, it has been considered an acquired lesion secondary to fracture of the odontoid, and numerous instances of this sequence of events have been reported. von Torklus and Gehle, however, favor the congenital origin of the os odontoideum on the basis of its deviation in shape from that of the usual odontoid process, although they do not deny that acquired separations can occur. Changes in shape of an obviously fractured segment have been observed and attributed to interference with blood supply to the dens following the injury. Support for this concept comes from the observation by Treadwell and O'Brien who noted avascular necrosis of the proximal portion of the dens as a complication of halopelvic distraction. They postulated that ligament disruption interfered with the blood supply to the dens. It is clear that both congenital and acquired mechanisms exist. Only in instances where a definitely normal dens has been observed prior to a known injury can the presence of a separate dens be identified as an acquired phenomenon. The occurrence of symptoms associated with an os odontoideum, congenital or acquired, is extremely variable notwithstanding significant displacement of the structure in flexion and extension of the head and

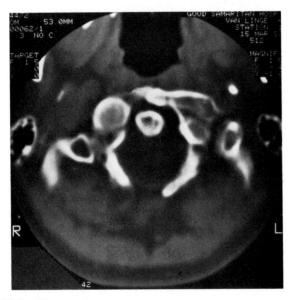

FIG 2–15.
CT examination demonstrating a congenital absence of portions of the anterior and posterior arches of the first cervical vertebra and deformity of the left lateral mass. Anatomical detail is exceptionally well demonstrated. (Courtesy of Dr. P. Moskowitz, Los Gatos, Calif.)

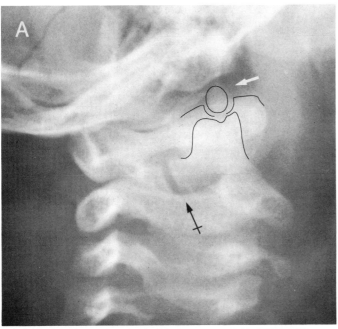

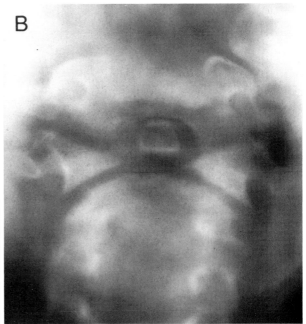

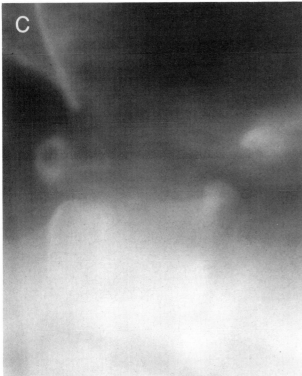

FIG 2–16.
A, oblique views of the upper cervical spine with either a large summit ossification center or an os odontoideum *(arrow)* in C2. The defect in the neural arch indicates the synchondrosis at its site of junction with the body of C2. **B** and **C,** AP and lateral tomograms of an os odontoideum. The dens itself is hypoplastic. (**B** and **C,** from Oestreich AE, Crawford AH: *Atlas of Pediatric Orthopedic Radiology,* New York, Georg Thieme, 1985, p 295. Used by permission.)

neck. Usually, the dens maintains its relation to the body of the atlas, probably indicating integrity of the posterior transverse ligament. Nevertheless, when symptoms such as neck pain and headaches, upper limb paresthesias, or transient quadriplegias occur, cervical spine fusion must be considered. CT and MRI may be helpful in evaluation.

Segmentation abnormalities of the cervical spine occur with both horizontal and vertical "fusions" and separations of varying degree. "Fusions" are actually failures of normal segmentation of preosseous embryonic components with subsequent bony continuity (Fig 2–17). They may be associated with separations, together causing comparable anomalies of the occipital bone, and include basilar fissures, accessory ossicles, occipital-vertebral and vertebro-ver-

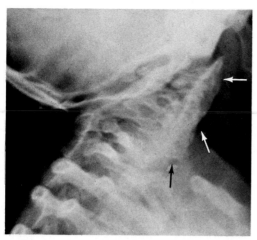

FIG 2–17.
Klippel-Feil anomaly in a girl 14 months of age. The *arrows* point to the short, unsegmented cervical spine. The occiput extends caudally to the level of the shoulders.

tebral synostoses, as well as hemivertebra malformations, singly or in combination. In 1912, Klippel and Feil reported an extreme example of fusion of vertebral segments at the cephalic end of the spine. The vertebral column between the occipital bone and the sacrum was composed of only 12 clearly differentiated vertebrae plus a bony mass at the cephalic end, bearing four pairs of ribs and articulating with the occipital base. The lower eight ribs were attached to typical dorsal vertebrae which continued, via four lumbar vertebrae and a transitional fifth lumbar vertebra, to join the sacrum. The portion of the fused mass above the four rib-bearing vertebrae was identified as cervical vertebrae by the presence of canals for the vertebral artery bilaterally. Since that time, almost any form of cervical vertebral fusion has been labeled the Klippel-Feil syndrome as if this morphologic abnormality constituted a single entity. The condition is usually associated, understandably, with shortness of the neck and a low hairline. It is not surprising that the Sprengel anomaly (failure of descent and lateral migration of the scapula) is frequently present. An interesting clinical observation in some cases has been the presence of mirror movements. A patient with the condition has been described who was so affected that he was unable to climb a ladder because he could not release one hand without releasing the other as well. Associated anomalies include scoliosis, unilateral absence of the kidney or hydronephrosis, or both, ureteropelvic obstruction, and ear malformations with deafness.

Cervical vertebral fusion is also a part of other syndromes including the cervico-oculo-acoustic or Wildervank syndrome, in which it is associated with congenital deafness, paralysis of the lateral rectus muscles, and retraction of the globe of the eye on attempted upward gaze. Another combination was described by Forney et al., in which a mother and two daughters with heart disease had conductive deafness, short stature, and cervical vertebral and carpal fusions. Heart disease or deafness was not reported in the patient, described by Jaffres et al., who also demonstrated cervical as well as dorsal vertebral fusions and carpal and tarsal synostoses. Mandibular hypoplasia was present and may indicate a link with the middle ear malformation found in the patient of Forney et al. It is obvious that fusion of cervical vertebrae can occur as an isolated malformation or in association with other conditions and that the eponymic term does not describe a disease but rather a component of several different malformation complexes. CT and MRI provide excellent depiction of complicated malformations of the cervical spine.

THORACOLUMBAR SPINE ABNORMALITIES

Variations in the number of the lumbar and thoracic vertebrae other than those described previously result from oversegmentation and undersegmentation (or fusion) during fetal life. Either teratologic or genetic factors are probably involved. Defects in the body may be due to undergrowth of one or both of the fetal chondrification centers (Figs 2–18 and 2–19). Occasionally the entire body may be absent when the arch is well developed. Asymmetric undergrowth of one of the paired fetal chondrification centers in the body gives rise to hemivertebrae, a common and sometimes disabling malformation. One or many spinal segments may be affected. In the case of thoracic hemivertebrae, errors in segmentation of the ribs are almost invariably associated (see Fig 2–29). Sprengel deformity may also be present (Fig 2–20). Congenital hypoplasia of one lung is often accompanied by hemivertebrae, and renal anomalies are also frequent. The spinal malformations are not necessarily at the same segmental level as the associated visceral malformations but there does appear to be some proximity, particularly when considering embryonic cranio-caudal growth patterns. Vertebral malformations are a prominent component of the so-called VATER (*v*ertebral defects, imperforate *a*nus, *t*racheo*e*sophageal fistula, *r*adial and *r*enal dysplasia) association, which includes other skeletal malformations as well as visceral ones. Cardiac malformations are common. Multiple hemivertebrae that affect the spine at many

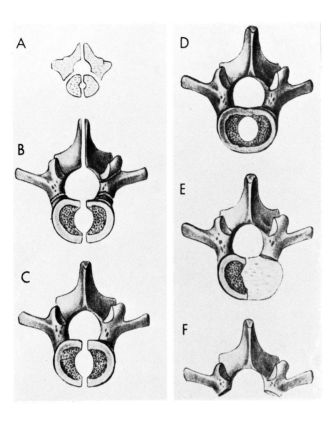

FIG 2–18.
Developmental errors in the vertebral segments in the chondrification stage. **A,** normal pattern during early chondrification stage. **B,** persistence of early midsagittal cleft. **C,** persistence of midsagittal cleft in the body only. **D,** persistence of chordal canal in the vertebral body. **E,** lateral hemivertebra only due to agenesis and hypoplasia of the right half of the chondrification center in the body. **F,** aplasia of the entire body due to failure of growth of both early paired cartilaginous masses. (From Köhler A, Zimmer EA: *Borderlands of the Normal and Early Pathologic in Skeletal Roentgenology,* ed 11. Philadelphia, Grune & Stratton, 1968. Used by permission.)

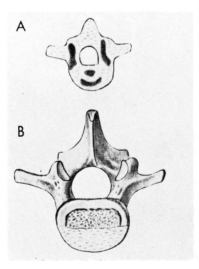

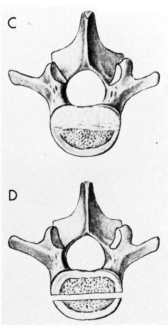

FIG 2–19.
Malformations secondary to developmental errors during the ossification stage. **A,** early normal ossification centers. In contrast to the two early chondrification centers in the body, which are lateral to each other, these ossification centers in the body are ventrodorsal to each other. **B,** dorsal transverse hemivertebra. **C,** ventral transverse hemivertebra. **D,** transverse fissure between the two tandem ossification centers of the vertebral body—coronal cleft in the vertebral body. (From Köhler A, Zimmer EA: *Borderlands of the Normal and Early Pathologic in Skeletal Roentgenology,* ed 11. Philadelphia, Grune & Stratton, 1968. Used by permission.)

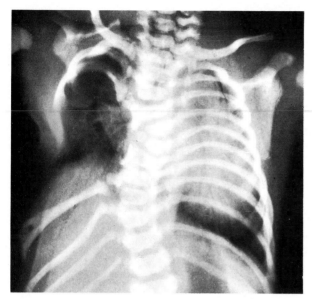

FIG 2–20.
Multiple thoracic hemivertebrae in a stillborn infant with congenital failure of descent of the right scapula; regional agenesis, hypoplasia, and failure in segmentation of ribs on the right; displacement of the heart leftward; and thoracic scoliosis.

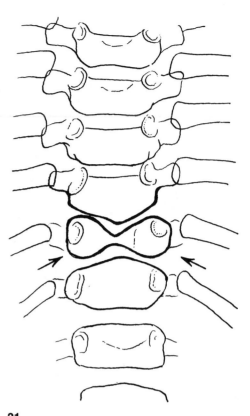

FIG 2–21.
"Butterfly" deformity of the vertebral body due to persistence of a remnant of the fetal notochord in the vertebral body in an infant 13 months of age. There are no associated errors in segmentation of the ribs, which are almost invariably present in hemivertebra. The diagnosis was not proved anatomically.

levels may cause marked dwarfism owing to shortening of the trunk when the limbs are of normal length, as in spondylocostal dysplasia. Vertebral anomalies occur in association with neurenteric communications. These lesions are discussed in greater detail in the sections on the spinal cord and on the gastrointestinal tract (split notochord syndrome).

Persistence of remnants of the fetal notochord in the center of a vertebral body results in a characteristic "butterfly" appearance in films exposed in the coronal plane (Fig 2–21). The soft tissue in the defect that is continuous with the disk tissue above and below the affected body has been demonstrated by both CT and MRI (Fig 2–22), and histologic proof of its notochordal origin has been provided in some cases. "Butterfly vertebra" has been a common finding in the Alagille syndrome (arteriohepatic dysplasia) which is associated with hyperbilirubinemia and other skeletal abnormalities. The vertebral anomaly has been noted in several infants with deletions involving chromosome 20.

A possibly related normal variation in the contour of the thoracolumbar vertebral bodies, particularly in lateral radiographs, is a widening of the intervertebral space posteriorly (Fig 2–23). The enlarged nuclei pulposi associated with this configuration have been given the name "megalonuclei pulposi" and "balloon disk." Similar findings can be observed in what has been called the "Cupid's bow contour" in AP projections as a result of symmetric parasagittal defects posteriorly in the inferior end

plates of the lower lumbar vertebrae. A relation of these variants to persistent notochordal structures has been postulated for these lesions too. Focal remnants of notochordal tissue are termed *ecchordosis physaliphora*; they have been considered potential precursors of chordomas.

Coronal cleft vertebrae, recognized in lateral projections in the newborn, are most likely examples of delay in fusion of ventral and dorsal ossification centers for vertebral bodies (Fig 2–24). The study by Schinz and Töndury showed that the coronal cleft is merely the normal mass of cartilage between these two centers. In rare instances, as in one of the cases of Wollin and Elliot, the coronal cleft represented persistence of an axial rod of notochord. Coronal clefts are often noted in association with other abnormalities, especially with chondrodysplasia punctata. One or several vertebral bodies may be affected, most commonly in the lumbar spine. Ordinarily the clefts disappear during the first weeks of life; they predominate in males in a ratio of about 10:1.

Congenital anomalies of the vertebral arches may be found in several sites (see Figs 2–18 and

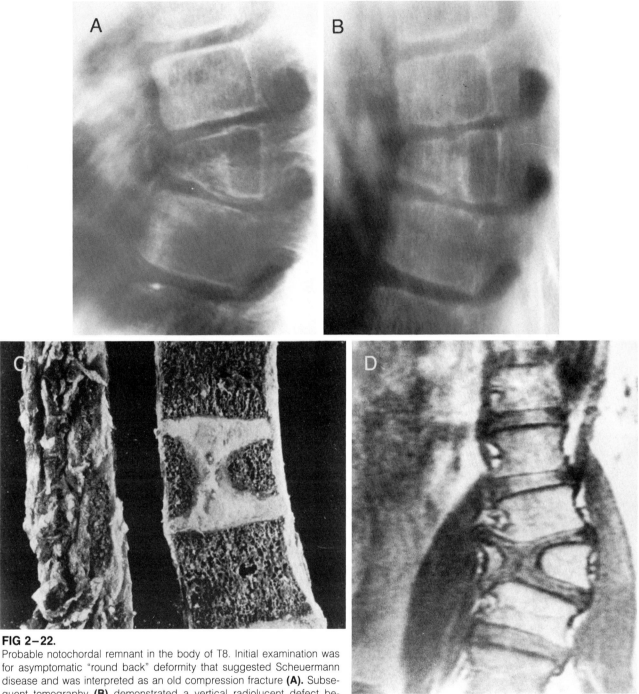

FIG 2–22.
Probable notochordal remnant in the body of T8. Initial examination was for asymptomatic "round back" deformity that suggested Scheuermann disease and was interpreted as an old compression fracture **(A).** Subsequent tomography **(B)** demonstrated a vertical radiolucent defect between the relatively dense anterior two thirds of the vertebral body and the relatively radiolucent posterior one third. Note narrow intervertebral disks above and below T8 and a defect in the end plate of T7 above the site of the vertical defect in T8 that is faintly visible in **A. C,** gross lateral section of a proven case of persistent notochordal remnant. **D,** coronal MRI of a similar lesion. (**C,** from Beadle OA: *The Intervertebral Disks.* Special Report Series No. 161, Medical Research Council. London, His Majesty's Stationery Office, 1931; **D,** from Duffern H, Auer R, Moolsintong P, et al: *Magn Reson Imaging* 1987; 5:499–503. Used by permission).

2–19); one or more of these defects may be present in a single arch. The roentgen defect results from absence of bone segments in different regions. A defect of continuity in the arch on one side is frequently associated with hypertrophy of the weight-bearing portions, and particularly the pedicle, on the opposite side. In addition to the enlargement and sclerosis of the compensating pedicle that is seen in AP projections, the spinous process of the affected arch may be observed to tilt toward the defective

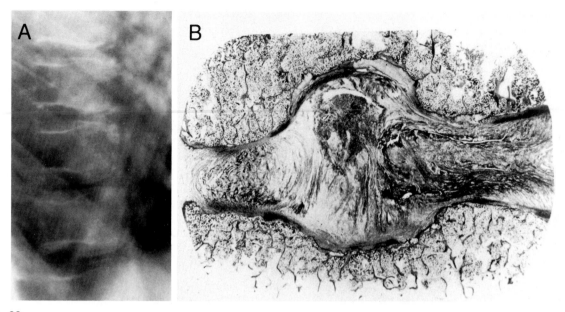

FIG 2–23.

A, posterior enlargement of intervertebral space (meganuclei pulposi or balloon disk) as an incidental finding in a young adolescent. **B,** section from posterior one third of the intervertebral disk and adjacent vertebral bodies showing persistent notochordal remnant. (**A,** courtesy of Dr. Virgil Condon, Salt Lake City; **B,** from Beadle OA: *The Intervertebral Discs,* Special Report Series No. 161, Medical Research Council. London, His Majesty's Stationery Office, 1931.)

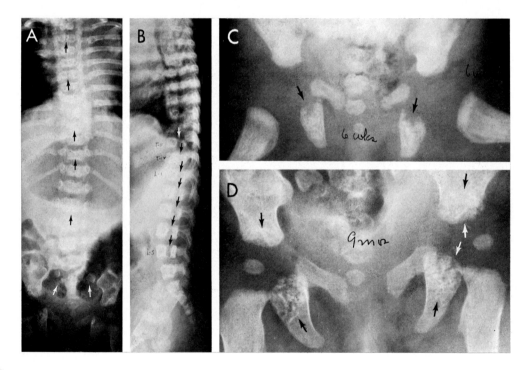

FIG 2–24.

Multiple coronal cleft vertebrae in a 7-month-old girl with multiple malformations. Other features included defective ossification in wrist and ankle metaphyses, the absence of several small tubular bones in her hand and one foot, a hypoplastic right tibia, an absent left tibia, and large accessory ossicles in the innominate synchondrosis of the occipital bone. Sagittal and coronal clefts in vertebral bodies are from the midthoracic to the lumbar levels in frontal **(A)** and lateral **(B)** projections, respectively. There are bilateral defects in the lateral masses of the sacrum and clusters of small ossification centers in the ischia. **C** and **D,** ossification irregularities in the ischia and ilia at 6 and 9 months of age. Aplasias and hypoplasias are atypical for chondrodysplasia punctata.

side of the arch. The tilt of the spinous process is believed to indicate rotational instability at the defective level (Fig 2–25). The role of defects in the neural arches in the causation of spondylolisthesis is discussed in Section 3.

Spina bifida (rachischisis, spinal dysraphism) is a congenital cleft in the neural arches (see Fig 2–18, *A* and *B*) that may permit external protrusion of the soft tissues and fluid of the spinal canal. Normal nonunion of arch ossification centers may simulate spina bifida up to the second decade. Failure of bony union or close proximity and overriding of one part of the spinous process over the other is a common observation of no clinical significance in the lumbosacral region. These are the mildest examples of spina bifida occulta where there is no protrusion of spinal canal contents beyond the confines of the neural arch. The incidence of spina bifida occulta diminishes in males from 22% in the seventh year to 4% in adults, and in females from 9% in the seventh year to 1% in adults (Sutow and Pryde). In spina bifida vera, the defect is usually appreciably wider and the distance between the pedicles at the level of the defect is abnormally great. Under these circumstances, there may be pigmentation or a patch of hair over the corresponding area of the skin, or a mass that represents a meningocele or a meningomyelocele. Protrusion of spinal canal contents through defects between the neural arch and the vertebral body, or through the vertebral body itself, may give rise to lateral and anterior meningoceles, respectively. Discontinuities in vertebral bodies and the sacrum anteriorly may be difficult to identify in simple films because of overlying viscera, especially

intestine, containing gas and gas mixed with other content. Since many patients with spina bifida vera present with signs of mass and, particularly, with neurologic symptoms, CT and metrizamide myelography has much to offer in place of multiple plain films or conventional tomography. MRI is becoming the procedure of choice by virtue of its ability to depict soft-tissue detail. According to Barson, lumbar kyphosis involving all the lumbar vertebrae is rare apart from its association with the more severe forms of spina bifida. In his study, lumbar kyphosis was always associated with paraplegia and the sac contained nerve tissue.

Diastematomyelia, in which a bony, cartilaginous, or fibrous septum transfixes the cord, may be suspected on plain films when there is a relatively local increase of interpediculate distances in several thoracic or lumbar levels with hemivertebrae deformity. The diagnosis is practically assured when an approximately midline, vertically oriented ossicle is seen at or near the midsagittal plane of the spinal canal. This bony septum, transfixing the cord, is attached anteriorly to the posterior surface of the vertebral body, posteriorly to the dura, and, occasionally, to the deformed vertebral arches as well (Fig 2–26). The spinal cord, consequently, cannot make its normal shift cephalad as the vertebral column lengthens with growth. The spicule may be located sufficiently low to transfix the filum terminale; in this case, failure of ascent of the cord also occurs. The septum may extend the length of several vertebral bodies. Rarely, two separate septa occur, usually in the same cleft. The two halves of the spinal cord are usually asymmetric, the cord uniting below

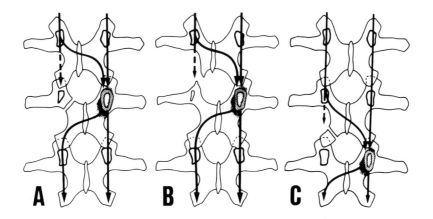

FIG 2–25.
Unilateral hypertrophy and sclerosis of a pedicle from several types of neural arch defects. **A,** the most common defect in the pars interarticularis as occurs in spondylolysis. **B,** facet joint hypoplasia above a pedicular hypoplasia. **C,** rare infralaminar defect. In **A** and **B,** the defects are supralaminar, and the stress is diverted to the contralateral pedicle at the same level; in **C,** the de-

fect is infralaminar, and the pedicle one level below is affected. The spinous process at the defective level in **A** and **B** tilts toward the defect and away from the sclerotic pedicle below. The *heavy lines* indicate the direction of the stresses. (From Maldague BE, Malghem JJ: *Radiology* 1976; 16:412–416. Used by permission.)

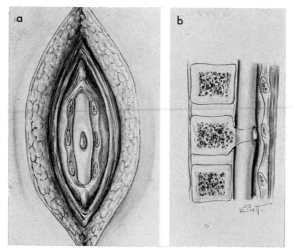

FIG 2–26.
Morbid anatomy of diastematomyelia exposed on surgical exploration. The spinal cord is widened and split by a transfixing ossicle that is continuous with the vertebral body ventrad and the dura dorsad. (Courtesy of Dr. E.D.B. Neuhauser, Boston.)

bodies, nonsegmented vertebral bodies, and single and double hemivertebrae deformities are often associated. CT demonstrates the bone components of the transfixing structure, often in a "belt buckle" configuration (Fig 2–28).

THE SPINE IN SKELETAL DYSPLASIAS

The vertebral bodies may act like short tubular bones exhibiting, in skeletal dysplasias, changes similar to those occurring in long tubular bones. The vertebral changes, however, are less marked because the amount of growth from endochondral bone formation is appreciably less on the growing surface of each vertebra than in the growing ends of a long bone. In achondroplasia, the bodies are relatively short vertically as well as sagittally, and in the AP projection the lack of widening of interpediculate distance, or actual narrowing in the lumbar area, is

the cleft. In some instances, union does not occur and the cleft extends through the filum terminale.

Conventional roentgenograms demonstrate dilatation of the spinal canal for several segments in the region of the split spinal cord (Fig 2–27). The bony spicule may be identified at the widest level in frontal plane projections. The pedicles are not flattened as in the case of an intraspinal mass. Small vertebral

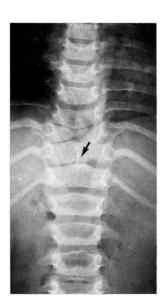

FIG 2–27.
Radiologic findings in diastematomyelia on a plain film in a frontal projection. The spinal canal is widened, and the interpediculate distances are increased from T9 through L2. The *arrow* points to the transfixing ossicle superimposed on T11. The body of T10 is deformed in a fashion consistent with bilateral hemivertebra or a notochordal remnant.

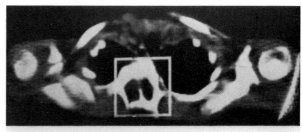

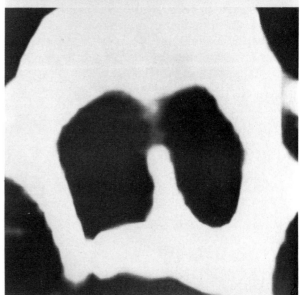

FIG 2–28.
CT scan in 6-year-old girl with diastematomyelia. **A,** the typical "belt-buckle" configuration produced by the bony spicule is shown. **B,** enlargement shows the osteocartilaginous anterior part of the septum. The lesion was at the T4 level. (From Lohkamp F, Claussen C, Schumacher G: *Prog Pediatr Radiol* 1978; 6:200–207. Used by permission.)

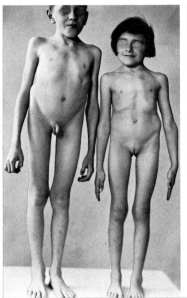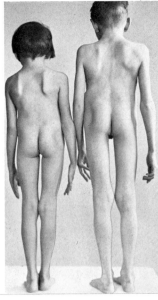

FIG 2–29.

Familial dwarfism in siblings due to multiple hemivertebrae. A brother and a sister, 10 and 8 years of age, show a short neck, thorax, abdomen, and pelvis in contrast to a normal length of the limbs. Roentgenographic examination revealed multiple hemiverte-brae at practically all levels of the spine in both children. Otherwise, the skeletons were normal. Clinically, these patients resemble patients with better-categorized forms of short-trunk dwarfism.

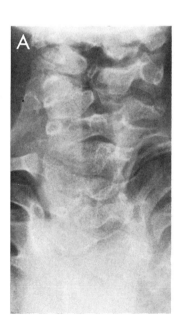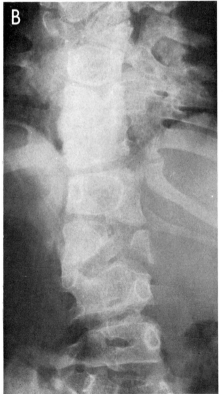

FIG 2–30.

Multiple hemivertebrae in the boy shown in Figure 2–29. **A,** in the cervical and superior thoracic segments. **B,** in the inferior thoracic and lumbosacral levels. The deformed vertebral bodies occupy practically the entire spine. The errors in segmentation of the ribs are noteworthy. The other bones were all normal roentgenographically.

helpful in diagnosis. The narrowing of interpediculate distances in the caudal portions of the vertebral column in achondroplasia is mimicked by what has been called the narrow lumbar spinal canal syndrome (Roberson et al.). It has also been described in patients with hypophosphatemic rickets. All such patients have been adults; relief of clinical symptoms, particularly back pain, has responded to lumbar laminectomy. Kyphosis is an occasional complication (see Fig 43–25).

Waferlike vertebral bodies separated by large interspaces are characteristic for thanatophoric dysplasia. Kyphosis of the cervical spine is a common finding in diastrophic dysplasia. Generalized platyspondyly is a characteristic feature of Morquio disease and occurs with exaggerated sagittal length in the Kniest syndrome and spondylometaphyseal dysplasia. Undulations of the borders of the vertebral plates in lateral projection of the spine are helpful in the diagnosis of the Dyggve-Clausen-Melchior syndrome. Various forms of irregularities of vertebral bodies occur in the group of spondyloepiphyseal dysplasias. The spine may be involved with multiple hereditary exostoses. The exostoses are of importance when they intrude on the spinal canal, as noted in Figure 42–25. A variant of enchondromatosis with platyspondyly has been reported under the term *spondyloenchondromatosis* (see Chapter 43); dysplasia epiphysealis hemimelica may have spinal manifestations. In the mucopolysaccharidoses, lumbar kyphosis is extremely common and is generally associated with a hypoplastic, hook-shaped vertebral body that results from extension of disk material into an anterior defect. The osteopenia of osteogenesis imperfecta is usually associated with multiple compression fractures or, at least, concave upper and lower vertebral plates. The vertebral bodies participate in the general sclerosis of osteopetrosis. In addition, their development is distinctly retarded and infantile characteristics may persist for many years. In many instances, an inset of a dense miniature vertebral body is surrounded by a zone of radiolucency within the larger dense vertebral body. Details of the radiographic features in skeletal dysplasias can be found in Chapter 43.

In most of these generalized diseases, the diagnosis is supported by the overall pattern of disorganized skeletal growth and development in addition to the vertebral changes. However, there is a group of conditions in which the disturbance is almost restricted to the spine and ribs to the degree that it conforms more to a dysostosis than a dysplasia (Figs 2–29 to 2–31), and that results in distinct short-trunk dwarfism. These conditions have been vari-

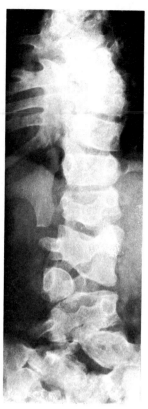

FIG 2–31.
Multiple hemivertebrae, scoliosis, and costal deformities in the dwarfed girl shown in Figure 2–29. The hemivertebra deformities are similar to, but not identical with, those of her brother (Fig 2–30). Her other bones were normal roentgenographically.

ously reported under the category of dysplasia or dysostosis, preceded by costovertebral, spondylocostal, or spondylothoracic. In addition, they are also found under the eponym Jarcho-Levin syndrome and the acronymic designation, COVESDEM syndrome (see below). The term *spondylocostal dysostosis* was preferred in the 1977 Paris nomenclature. Multiple horizontal and vertical segmentation deformities are present in the thoracolumbar spine with hemivertebra formation and fusions; the cervical spine is often spared. The ribs are usually affected with posterior fusions of varying degree so that their appearance may be fan-shaped. The appendicular skeleton is involved only in the COVESDEM syndrome in which mesomelic shortening occurs accounting for the acronym (*co*stovertebral *s*egmental *de*fect with *m*esomelia). Instances have been reported of associated visceral abnormalities, particularly in the urogenital system. A neonatal form of severe vertebral malformation has been reported under the term *dyssegmental dwarfism*.

Autosomal dominant and autosomal recessive inheritance have been postulated for this group of disorders, with both severe and mild cases. The majority of the severe cases with death in early infancy from respiratory failure are believed to belong to the dominant form, and those with the most variability, to the autosomal recessive form. In the mild cases of either form, normal life expectancy is the rule. Differential diagnosis includes dyssegmental dysplasia, the fetal face or Robinow syndrome (with respect to the cases with mesomelia), and, less often, the VATER anomalad. Prenatal diagnosis has been accomplished with ultrasound on the basis of thoracic and vertebral abnormalities in association with normal limbs.

REFERENCES

Cervical Spine Abnormalities

Cox HE, Bennett WF: Computed tomography of absent cervical pedicle. *J Comput Assist Tomogr* 1984; 8:537–539.

Dalinka MK, Rosenbaum AE, van Houton F: Congenital absence of the posterior arch of the atlas. *Radiology* 1972; 103:581–583.

Dawson EG, Smith L: Atlanto-axial subluxation in children due to vertebral anomalies. *J Bone Joint Surg [Am]* 1979; 61A:582–587.

Fielding JW, Griffin PP: Os odontoideum: An acquired lesion. *J Bone Joint Surg [Am]* 1974; 56:187–190.

Forney WR, Robinson SJ, Pascoe DJ: Congenital heart disease, deafness and skeletal malformations: A new syndrome? *J Pediatr* 1966; 68:14–26.

Garber JN: Abnormalities of the atlas and axis vertebrae—Congenital and acquired. *J Bone Joint Surg [Am]* 1964; 46A:1782–1791.

Hensinger RN, MacEwan GD, Pizzutillo PD: The Klippel-Feil syndrome. *J Bone Joint Surg [Am]* 1974; 56:1764.

Hungerford GD, Akkaraju V, Rawe SE, et al: Atlanto-occipital and atlanto-axial dislocations with spinal cord compression in Down's syndrome: A case report and review of the literature. *Br J Radiol* 1981; 54:758–761.

Jaffres R, Tatibouet L, Toudic L: Dysplasie poly-épiphysaire avec blocs vertébraux congéniteux, synostoses carpiènnes et tarsiènnes, hypoplasie mandibulaire. *Rev Rhum Mal Osteoartic* 1978; 45:655–659.

Kalamchi A, Yau ACMC, O'Brien JP, et al: Halo-pelvic distraction apparatus: An analysis of 150 consecutive patients. *J Bone Joint Surg [Am]* 1976; 58:1119–1124.

Klippel M, Feil A: Un cas d'absence des vertébres cervicales avec cage thoracique remontant jusqu'à la base du crâne (cage thoracique cervicale). *Nouv Icon Salpetriere* 1912; 25:223–250.

Kopits SE, Perovic MN, McKusick V, et al: Congenital atlanto-axial dislocation in various forms of dwarfism. *J Bone Joint Surg [Am]* 1972; 54:1349–1350.

Modic MT, Weinstein MA, Pavlicek W, et al: Magnetic resonance imaging of the cervical spine: Technical and clinical observations. *Am J Roentgenol* 1983; 141:1129–1136.

Nagib MG, Maxwell RE, Chou SN: Klippel-Feil syndrome in children: Clinical features and management. *Childs Nerv Syst* 1985; 1:255–263.

Oestreich AE, Young LW: The absent cervical pedicle syndrome: A case in childhood. *Am J Roentgenol* 1969; 107:505–510.

Ricciardi JE, Kaufer H, Louis DS: Acquired os odontoideum following acute ligament injury. Report of a case. *J Bone Joint Surg [Am]* 1976; 58:410–412.

Treadwell SJ, O'Brien JP: Avascular necrosis of the proximal pole of the dens: A complication of halo-pelvic distraction. *J Bone Joint Surg [Am]* 1975; 57:332–336.

van Dijk Azn R, Thijssen HOM, Merx JL, et al: The absent cervical pedicle syndrome. *Neuroradiology* 1987; 29:69–72.

Wildervank, KS, Hoeksema PE, Penning L: Radiological examination of the inner ear of deaf-mute presenting the cervico-oculo-acusticus syndrome. *Acta Otolaryngol (Stockh)* 1966; 61:445–453.

Thoracolumbar Spine Abnormalities

Ayme S, Preus M: Spondylocostal/spondylothoracic dysostosis: The clinical basis for prognosticating and genetic counseling. *Am J Med Genet* 1986; 24:599–606.

Barson AJ: Radiological studies of spina bifida cystica. The phenomenon of congenital lumbar kyphosis. *Br J Radiol* 1965; 38:294–300.

Bartsocas CS, Kiossoglou KA, Papas CV, et al: Costovertebral dysplasia. *Birth Defects* 1974; 10:221–226.

Beadle OA: *The Intervertebral Discs.* Special Report Series No. 161, Medical Research Council. London, His Majesty's Stationery Office, 1931.

Bethem D, Winter RB, Lutter L, et al: Spinal disorders of dwarfism: Review of the literature and report of eighty cases. *J Bone Joint Surg [Am]* 1981; 63:1412–1425.

Brunelle F, Estrada A, Dommergues P, et al: Skeletal anomalies in Alagille's syndrome. Radiographic study in 80 cases. *Ann Radiol* 1986; 29:687–690.

Cartwright DW, Latham SC, Masel JP, et al: Spinal canal stenosis in adults with hypophosphataemic vitamin D–resistant rickets. *Aust N Z J Med* 1979; 9:705–708.

Currarino G: Primary spondylolysis of the axis vertebra (C2) in three children, including one with pyknodysostosis. *Pediatr Radiol* 1989; 19:535–538.

Dietz GW, Christensen EE: Normal "Cupid's bow" contour of the lower lumbar vertebrae. *Radiology* 1976; 121:577–579.

Duffern H, Auer R, Moolsintong P, et al: MRI, CT, and plain film appearance of anterior spina bifida. *Magn Reson Imaging* 1987; 5:499–503.

Frager DH, Subbarao K: The 'bone within a bone." *JAMA* 1983; 249:77–79.

Franceschini P, Grassi E, Fabris C, et al: The autosomal recessive form of spondylocostal dysostosis. *Radiology* 1974; 112:673–675.

Gruhn JG, Gorlin RJ, Langer LO: Dyssegmental dwarfism. A lethal anisospondylic camptomicromelic dwarfism. *Am J Dis Child* 1978; 132:382–386.

Handmaker SD, Campbell JA, Robinson LD, et al: Dyssegmental dwarfism: a new syndrome of lethal dwarfism. *Birth Defects* 1977; 13:79–90.

Hilal SK, Marton D, Pollack E: Diastematomyelia in children. Radiographic study of 34 cases. *Radiology* 1974; 112:609–621.

Kozlowski K: Spondylo-costal dysplasia—severe and moderate types (report of 8 cases). *Aust Radiol* 1981; 25:81–90.

Maldague BE, Malghem JJ: Unilateral arch hypertrophy with spinous process tilt: A sign of arch deficiency. *Radiology* 1976; 121:567–574.

Neuhauser EBD, Harris GBC, Berrett A: Roentgenographic features of neurenteric cysts. *Am J Roentgenol* 1958; 79:235–240.

Ramirez H Jr, Navarro JE, Bennett WF: Cupid's bow contour of the lumbar vertebral end plates detected by computed tomography. *J Comput Assist Tomogr* 1984; 8:121–124.

Rimoin DL, Fletcher BD, McKusick V: Spondylocostal dysplasia. A dominantly inherited form of short-trunked dwarfism. *Am J Med* 1968; 45:948–953.

Roberson GH, Llewllyn HJ, Taveras JM: The narrow lumbar spinal canal syndrome. *Radiology* 1973; 107:89–97.

Roberts AP, Conner AN, Tolmie JL, et al: Spondylothoracic and spondylocostal dysostosis. Hereditary forms of spinal deformity. *J Bone Joint Surg [Br]* 1988; 70:123–126.

Romero R, Ghidini A, Eswara MS, et al: Prenatal findings in a case of spondylocostal dysplasia type I (Jarcho-Levin syndrome). *Obstet Gynecol* 1988; 71:988–991.

Roos RAC, Vielvoye GJ, Voormolen JHC, et al: Magnetic resonance imaging in occult spinal dysraphism. *Pediatr Radiol* 1986; 16:412–416.

Schinz HR, Töndury G: Zur Entwicklung der menschlichen Wirbelsäule: Die Frühossifikation der Wirbelkörper. *Fortschr Geb Roentgenstr* 1942; 66:253–289.

Silengo MC, Lopez-Bell G, Biagioli M, et al: Partial deletion of the short arm of chromosome 20: 46,XX,del(20)(p11)/46,XX mosaicism. *Clin Genet* 1988; 33:108–110.

Sutow WW, Pryde AW: Incidence of spina bifida occulta in relation to age. *Am J Dis Child* 1956; 91:211–217.

Temtamy SA, Miller JD: Extending the scope of the VATER association: Definition of the VATER syndrome. *J Pediatr* 1974; 85:345–349.

Tsuji H, Tsutomu Y, Sainah H: Developmental balloon disc of the lumbar spine in healthy subjects. *Spine* 1985; 10:907–911.

Wadia RS, Shirole DB, Dikshit MS: Recessively inherited costovertebral segmentation defect with mesomelia and peculiar facies (Covesdem syndrome): A new genetic entity: *J Med Genet* 1978; 15:123–127.

Wollin DG, Elliot GB: Coronal cleft vertebrae and persistant notochordal derivatives of infancy. *J Can Assoc Radiol* 1961; 12:78–81.

SECTION 3

Traumatic Spinal Lesions

CERVICAL SPINE INJURIES

Initial conventional AP and cross-table lateral films are the usual approach to examination of cervical spine injuries, but CT and MRI are practically indispensable for proper evaluation, especially of those patients in whom there is neurologic involvement. Apple and associates suggested that teen-agers be evaluated by an adult radiographic series including trauma oblique views. In infants and young children, evaluation for upper cervical injuries are in order after supine, horizontal-beam lateral, and verti- cal-beam AP films are obtained, if there is retropharyngeal swelling or clinical abnormality. Jaffe and associates found that 58 of 59 children with cervical spine injury would have been identified if the criteria for radiographic examination were positive findings in any one of eight variables. The variables were (1) neck pain, (2) neck tenderness, (3) limitation of neck mobility, (4) history of trauma to the neck, and abnormalities of (5) reflexes, (6) strength, (7) sensation, or (8) mental status.

In interpretation of conventional radiographs of the cervical spine, one must be aware of factors that may lead to overreading of normal variations. The mobility of the upper segments of the cervical spine in normal children may simulate displacements due to injury (see Section 2). In addition, the anterior height of cervical bodies may be greater than the posterior height and can simulate compression fractures. Apparent odontoid fracture must be evaluated with consideration for possible anatomical variation (see Section 2). Similar consideration should be given to the ossification centers in the superior and inferior rings of the vertebral bodies that can simulate avulsion fractures. Fractures may be superimposed on congenital malformations; differentiation may be difficult. In young children, careful attention to the presence or absence of prevertebral soft tissue swelling assists in the evaluation for trauma.

FRACTURES

Dislocations are most common in the flexible cervical spine and at the lumbosacral articulation and are discussed in the sections that relate to these regions. Dislocations usually accompany fractures, particularly those associated with vectors of force of significant magnitude.

Fractures may occur at one or more sites in a single vertebra, and more than one spinal segment may be affected. The vertebral body is fractured more frequently than the arch. As in other bones, a simple fracture casts an irregular linear shadow of diminished density between the separated fragments. The fracture line is usually obliterated and the overlap of the edges of the fragments may produce a border of increased density (Fig 2–32). Fracture lines in the vertebral body are usually best visualized in lateral projections. Fracture lines of the vertebral bodies, which are invisible with standard techniques in multiple positions, are usually clearly defined by CT (Fig 2–33). In crushing fractures, the body is deformed by compression; usually the body assumes the shape of a wedge sloping to one side or anteriorly. The intervertebral disks usually escape injury, but they may be lacerated and become narrow owing to collapse of the nucleus pulposus or loss of some of its substance by penetration through the vertebral plate into the body of the vertebra. In infants and children, the normal vascular channels and persistent intrasegmental cleft of the provertebrae can be mistaken for fracture lines. Similarly, in adolescents, the secondary ossification centers in the superior

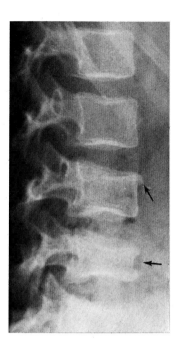

FIG 2–32.
Compression fractures of L3 and L4 bodies in a boy 7 years of age. There are no visible fracture lines. The edges of the broken bodies are compressed and mushroomed beyond normal limits, and the altitudes of the two affected bodies are diminished. There is a corresponding expansion of the contiguous intervertebral spaces owing to expansion of the nucleus pulposus against the weakened bodies. The greater compression of the bodies in their ventral axes produces the wedge-shaped deformities. The superior edge of the wedge-shaped body is usually displaced more than its inferior edge.

and inferior annular apophyses may simulate marginal chip fractures. External callus is rarely visible during the healing of fractures in the vertebral body. CT may be required for demonstration of fractures of the arch and its processes. Clinical judgment and the availability of techniques will determine the procedure or procedures to be used in individual cases.

Fractures of the cervical spine are frequently accompanied by dislocations. Cervical spinous processes are more delicate than those at lower spinal levels and fracture is more common. Avulsion of the tip of the large spinous process of C7 as a consequence of direct muscular pull was described by Weston in two adolescents and likened to "clayshoveler's disease" in adults. After hyperflexion injuries to the cervical spine in four adolescents, Keller found that the ossified vertebral rings for the vertebral bodies of C2 and C3 (Fig 2–34) were avulsed and displaced forward. In the same cases, later myelograms disclosed prolapses of the contiguous intervertebral disks. As in adults, bursting fractures (Jefferson fracture) occur in children secondary to

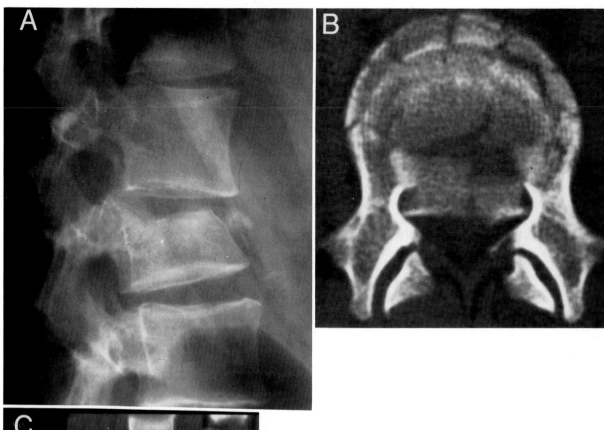

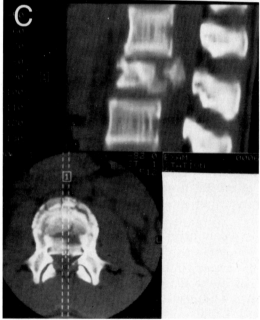

FIG 2–33.
Compression fracture of the lumbar vertebral body. **A,** lateral film; note the superior end-plate fracture with an anteriorly displaced fragment. **B,** axial CT shows that the fracture is comminuted and that a large fragment is displaced posteriorly into the spinal canal. **C,** sagittal re-formation depicts the position of the displaced fragment to better advantage. (From Moskowitz PS: *Diagn Radiol* 1986, pp 147–160. Used by permission.)

compression injuries of the cervical spine (Fig 2–35). Similarly, vertical fracture of the vertebral bodies may occur below C2.

Fractures of the spinous processes in the cervical and upper thoracic segments (Fig 2–36) can be seen clearly on both frontal and lateral projections when the terminal fracture fragment is displaced caudad.

CT provides better display of the neural canal, demonstrates injuries to other organ systems, and can be completed, without having to change the patient's position, in less time and with less radiation than is required with conventional tomography. A combination of standard radiographs and axial CT scans is accurate in evaluating most posterior element frac-

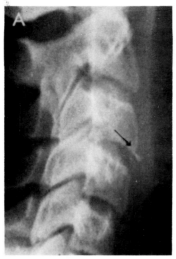 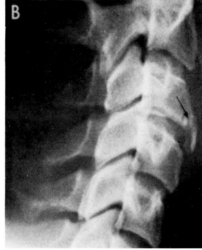

FIG 2–34.
A, avulsion of the partially ossified caudal rim of the vertebral body of C3, which is also displaced ventrad *(arrow)*. **B,** 22 months later, an osteophyte now elongates the avulsed fragment *(arrow)*. This boy was 17 years of age at the time of injury. Avulsion of the verte- bral rims in the cervical levels is due, in this case, to hyperflexion injury during tumbling gymnastics; it may also occur in motor car accidents. (From Keller RH: *Radiology* 1974; 110:21. Used by permission.)

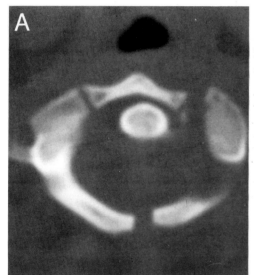

FIG 2–35.
A, axial CT scan of C1 in a 4-year-old boy with Jefferson "bursting" fracture after a fall on the vertex of his head but without symptoms. Lateral cervical spine film findings were normal. An open-mouth odontoid view showed displacement of the lateral masses of C1 relative to C2. Disruption of the posterior synchondrosis of C1 is clearly shown on CT together with an asymmetric prevertebral soft-tissue swelling not appreciated on the lateral film. (From Wirth RL, Zatz LM, Parker BR, et al: *Am J Roentgenol* 1987; 149:1001–1002. Used by permission.) **B** and **C,** axial CT of C1 in an asymptomatic 2½-year-old boy who fell out of a crib and landed "on the top of his head." Pseudospread of the atlas was shown on an AP tomogram. These are contiguous slices showing in **B,** an intact C1 ring with a narrow posterior synchondrosis; in **C,** there are asymmetric, tripartite ossification centers. (From Suss RA, Zimmerman RD, Leeds NE: *Am J Roentgenol* 1983; 140:1079–1082. Used by permission.)

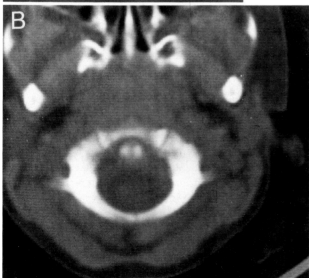 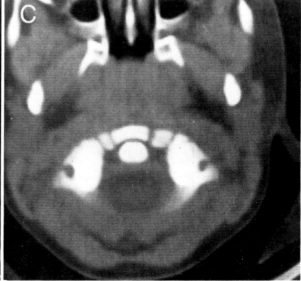

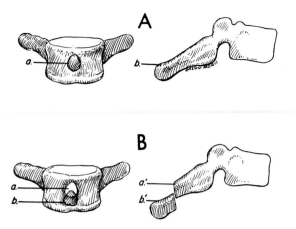

FIG 2–36.
Schematic representation of fractures of the spinous processes in the cervical and upper thoracic vertebrae. **A,** normal vertebra; **B,** vertebra with fractured spinous process. In **B,** the caudally displaced fragment of the spinous process *(b)* casts a separate image *(a)* in frontal projection. (From Zanca P, Lodmell EA: *Radiology* 1951; 56:427–428. Used by permission.)

tures. During the second decade of life, trophic changes of traumatic origin in the tips of the spinous processes may simulate those of osteochondrosis in other bones. It is likely that these changes represent necrosis following mechanical injury. Small fractures without displacement of the fragments can be satisfactorily identified only several weeks after the injury when callus formation becomes evident. Secondary ossification centers in the various processes of the arch during late adolescence may simulate fracture fragments.

ATLANTO-OCCIPITAL AND ATLANTOAXIAL INJURIES

The laxity of ligaments in infants and children results in displacements more frequently than in fractures. Atlanto-occipital dislocation carries a high immediate mortality but, if recognized in early survivors, this dislocation can be successfully treated. The lateral film permits recognition of malalignment of the odontoid and the anterior rim of the foramen magnum and of the posterior arch of the atlas and the posterior rim of the foramen. If displacement of the tip of the odontoid from its normal close alignment with the anterior rim of the foramen magnum is noted, fixed stabilization is indicated followed by atlanto-occipital fusion.

Atlantoaxial instability is so common in Down syndrome that recommendations have been made to evaluate its extent in those who wish to participate in sports that involve possible trauma to the head and neck. Restriction of such sports is said to be in-

dicated when the arch–dens distance exceeds 4.5 mm or when the odontoid is abnormal; in the absence of atlantoaxial instability, restriction of activity is not necessary. Davidson recommended a physical examination with careful attention to neurologic signs prior to participation in sports as more predictive of potential or impending dislocation than radiologic examination. In adult patients with Down syndrome, there is a high incidence of degenerative changes in the upper cervical levels in contrast with the lower levels seen in the general population.

Atlantoaxial rotary displacement (subluxation) is characterized by torticollis and apparent malposition of the first two cervical vertebrae with persistent pain and muscular spasm that, together with swollen joint capsules and synovial tissue, maintain the abnormal position. It is often a consequence of laxity of the transverse ligament, congenitally as in Down syndrome, or acquired as following nasopharyngeal or cervical infections, and occasionally following surgical procedures in the nasopharyngeal region. Inflammatory processes apparently can extend from these regions via pharyngovertebral veins to the ligamentous structures causing hyperemia and relaxation with even the possibility of bone resorption at their insertions. The gliding, opposing facets of the lateral atlantoaxial joints slip out of position, lock, and are held locked by muscular spasm. In these circumstances, the condition is known as Grisel syndrome and generally responds to conservative treatment with anti-infective agents and muscle relaxants, with or without traction. If resolution does not occur, the condition is designated atlantoaxial fixation rather than displacement. In instances of fixation following mechanical trauma for which surgical intervention is considered, concomitant rotation of the vertebral vessels and other vascular structures must be anticipated. The problem in diagnosis is that the malposition may be a consequence of the pain and spasm rather than a cause. Furthermore, the marked mobility of the cervical spine in childhood may permit identical malpositions to arise in the course of asymptomatic head and neck movement so that films exposed at appropriate times may mimic the features considered pathologic.

The usual radiographs obtained for evaluation of subluxation include, in addition to AP and lateral projections, an open-mouth AP view in the optimal degree of rotation to project the first and second cervical vertebrae so that the axis is in the coronal plane. If rotation has occurred on one lateral mass, the other forward-displaced mass appears wider and closer to the midline than the first. If the displacement is backward, the findings are reversed. In either event, the joint between C1 and C2 on the displaced side is obscured by overlapping bone. CT demonstrates the relations between the vertebrae to best advantage.

SPONDYLOLYSIS

Once considered a congenital discontinuity in the pars interarticularis of the neural arch, most frequently affecting the fifth lumbar vertebra, this condition is now believed by most investigators to be an acquired lesion. Some evidence has been presented supporting an autosomal dominant transmission of the risk for developing the condition, probably on the basis of a dysplasia involving the pedicles and the pars interarticularis. Spondylolysis becomes manifest by a thinning and elongation in some cases prior to the appearance of the lytic defect. The defect itself is otherwise considered to be a stress fracture related also to the stresses of the erect posture. Spondylolysis has not been demonstrated in embryos or the fetus, or at birth. It appears during infancy, childhood, or adolescence and has a frequency of 5% to 6% after the age of 10 years in the white population. Wiltse et al. reported an unquestioned lesion of the pars in an 8-month-old child whose father also had the same lesion. In one of Caffey's patients, the spine was normal at 9 months but there was a large defect in the pars interarticularis of the fourth lumbar vertebra at age 10 years (Fig 2–37). It occurs much more frequently in Eskimos, another argument for a hereditary predisposition. According to Taillard, fatigue fractures develop in the pars interarticularis of a lumbar vertebra above a fused segment of the lumbar spine between 18 months and 3 to 10 years after the fusion; this illustrates the role played by lumbar lordosis when mechanical stresses, normally present in the lumbosacral joint, become localized in a higher segment. Like fatigue fractures elsewhere, the lytic defect can heal spontaneously or after immobilization. Wilkinson and Hall observed hypertrophy of a pedicle in 12 children with pars interarticularis defects on the side opposite the hypertrophy, similar to the changes observed on the side opposite a congenital arch defect (see Section 2).

SPONDYLOLISTHESIS

This is the term applied to dislocation of a vertebra, usually at the lumbosacral junction, where the body of the fifth lumbar slips anteriorly and caudad over the body of the first sacral. It is most frequently a consequence of spondylolysis and is associated with separation of the arch from the body at the pars interarticularis defect, occasionally with elongation of the pedicles. Malformations of the lumbosacral articulations may result in spondylolisthesis without spondylolysis. In this case, the entire vertebra moves forward. This is the dysplastic form of spondylolisthesis (spondylolisthesis with intact neural arch) contrasted with the isthmic which is the more usual. In some cases of the more common type, the separated posterior segment of the fifth lumbar neural arch may be crowded backward and downward. Cozen observed two patients in whom neither slipping of the vertebral body nor defects in the pars interarticularis had been present at birth; in one of

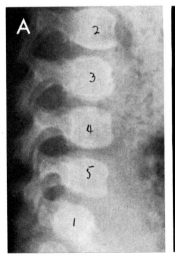 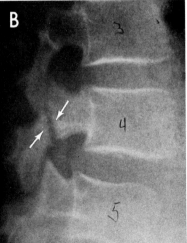

FIG 2–37.
A, normal spine at 9 months of age. **B,** spondylolysis in the L4 vertebra at 10 years of age.

these patients, both of these features developed between the 5th and 7th years, and in the other between the 10th and 13th years.

The roentgen signs of spondylolisthesis are best demonstrated in lateral projection; frontal projections are not to be depended on for a conclusive diagnosis. The most important single finding is the anterior displacement of the fifth lumbar body and the attached anterior segment of its divided neural arch in relation to the first sacral; this causes a break in the normal curved configuration that extends along the anterior and posterior surfaces of the vertebral bodies (Fig 2–38). The defect in the fifth lumbar arch appears as a wide gap between the anteriorly placed body and its neural arch. Oblique films may be the only ones that will demonstrate the defect when displacement is not present or not marked. The magnitude of the displacement varies considerably in different patients; Meyerding's technique for measuring the degree of displacement is a satisfactory method to follow the progress and estimate therapeutic results (Fig 2–39). The position of the posterior edge of the fifth lumbar body in relation to four equal divisions of the sagittal dimension of the upper border of the first sacral body indicates the degree of displacement. In long-standing cases, bony overgrowth may thicken the sacrum anteriorly. In frontal projections, the overlapping of the fifth lumbar and first sacral segments may be recognized by the curved edge, convex caudally, of the fifth lum-

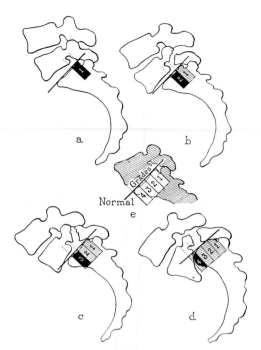

FIG 2–39.
Meyerding method of classifying degree of spondylolisthesis.

bar body; sometimes the transverse processes of the caudally luxated fifth lumbar can be seen superimposed on the wings of the sacrum.

COMPRESSION AND FULCRUM FRACTURES

Tetanic convulsions may be responsible for compression fractures of the vertebral bodies and secondary spinal deformity (Fig 2–40); these fractures were observed years ago in as many as 70% of a group of children who had recovered from tetanus. This incidence has probably declined appreciably with current management procedures.

A special type of distraction injury to the thoracolumbar spine (fulcrum fracture) is noted following injuries to persons wearing the lap type of seat belt in acute deceleration accidents. In adults and older children, the vertebral injuries are characterized by marked longitudinal distraction of adjacent posterior elements with relatively little anterior compression and wedging of associated vertebral bodies (Figs 2–41 and 2–42). The causal mechanism is illustrated in Figure 2–43. The addition of a shoulder strap component to the seat belt mechanism may introduce some shoulder girdle injuries, but should diminish the incidence and severity of the more serious spinal injuries. Some persons may also suffer a Chance fracture—a horizontal splitting through a vertebral body and its appendages without compression of the body itself. In young children, who have

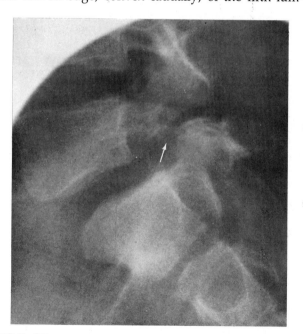

FIG 2–38.
Defect in the pars interarticularis *(arrow)* of the neural arch of L5 (spondylolysis) that has permitted the body of L5 to slip forward (spondylolisthesis) on the body of S1.

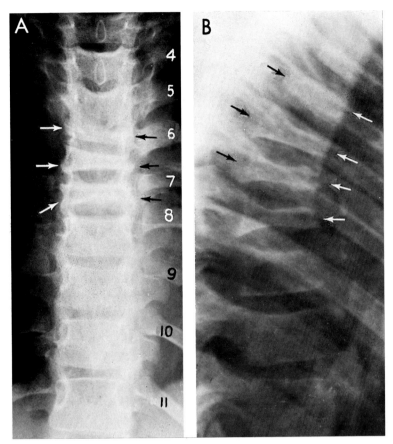

FIG 2–40.
Residual fractures and compression deformities of vertebral bodies due to tetanus in a boy 8 years of age. **A,** frontal, and **B,** lateral projections.

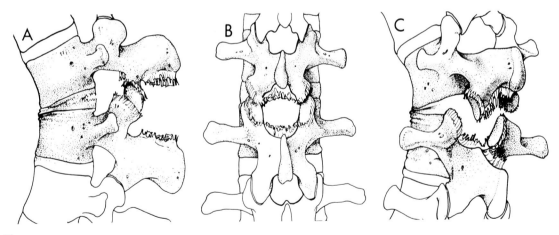

FIG 2–41.
Distraction injury to two lumbar vertebrae is the outstanding pattern of seat belt injuries. **A,** the posterior elements are widely separated with slight or no anterior compression. The lumbosacral fascia, interspinous ligaments, ligamentum flavum, posterior longitudinal ligament, and joint capsules are all lacerated. **B,** the neural arches of the two injured vertebrae are spread longitudinally, the intervening intervertebral foramen is enlarged longitudinally and ventrodorsally, the intervertebral disk is broken and wedged ventrad, but the lumbar bodies themselves are intact, although tipped counterclockwise (upper vertebral body) and clockwise (lower vertebral body). **C,** the intervertebral space is shallow ventrad and deepened dorsad. (From Smith WS, Kaufer H: *J Bone Joint Surg [Am]* 1969; 51:239–254. Used by permission.)

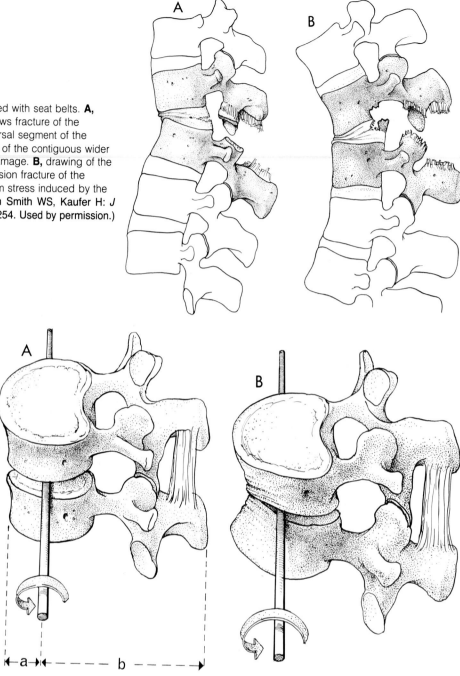

FIG 2–42.
Characteristic spinal injuries associated with seat belts. **A,** drawing of lateral radiograph that shows fracture of the articular process, laceration of the dorsal segment of the intervertebral disk, posterior widening of the contiguous wider vertebral spaces, and ligamentous damage. **B,** drawing of the lateral radiograph with additional avulsion fracture of the dorsal edge of the vertebral body from stress induced by the posterior longitudinal ligament. (From Smith WS, Kaufer H: *J Bone Joint Surg [Am]* 1969; 51:239–254. Used by permission.)

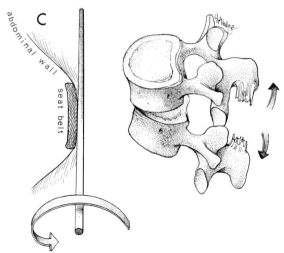

FIG 2–43.
Mechanism of distraction fracture from seat belt injury. **A,** in the usual flexion injury of an intact lumbar spine, the active force rotates the vertebral body counterclockwise around a transverse axis that passes through the nucleus pulposus. The distance from the transverse axis to the anterior edge of the vertebral body *(a)* is one fourth the distance from the transverse axis to the tip of the spinous process *(b).* According to the law of leverage, the anterior segment of the vertebral body will be subjected to a compression force four times greater than the stretch distraction force on the interspinous ligaments. **B,** hyperflexion around the normal transverse axis produces compression fracture of the anterior segment of the vertebral bodies without laceration of the intervertebral ligaments. **C,** with hyperflexion around the belt, the axis of flexion is far forward at the point of contact of the belt and abdominal wall anterior to the spine. Both bodies and neural arches are subjected to tension stress with laceration of the posterior ligaments and distraction of the neural arches and bodies, but no compression. (From Smith WS, Kaufer H: *J Bone Joint Surg [Am]* 1969; 51:239–254. Used by permission.)

a high center of gravity compared with adults, and a large, relatively heavy head, the spinal injuries tend to occur lower in the lumbar spine. Often, back pain is not an immediate complaint. Intra-abdominal injuries may be more obvious and lead to only causal inspection of the skeletal structures observed in conventional radiographs and even in abdominal CT examinations. In the latter, careful attention to the relations of articulating facets may indicate unsuspected dislocations (Fig 2–44), and subsequent review of conventional AP and lateral spine films may identify subtle compression fractures and posterior element distractions. Axial CT films may show lack of apposition of facets, the so-called naked facet sign.

In adult epileptics, the incidence of fractures and compression deformities in the vertebral bodies has been reported as high as 66% and as low as 7%. Detailed information on spinal fractures in juvenile epileptics is scarce. It is probable that their incidence is considerably lower than in adult epileptics owing to the protection afforded by the encasing layer of cartilage and the lesser degree of muscular development than in adults. In adult male epileptics, the incidence of spinal fracture is higher than in females owing to the stronger, heavier muscles.

Osteopenia of various types predisposes to compression fractures of vertebral bodies; these are seen in patients with osteogenesis imperfecta, hemolytic anemias, neoplasms involving the vertebral body,

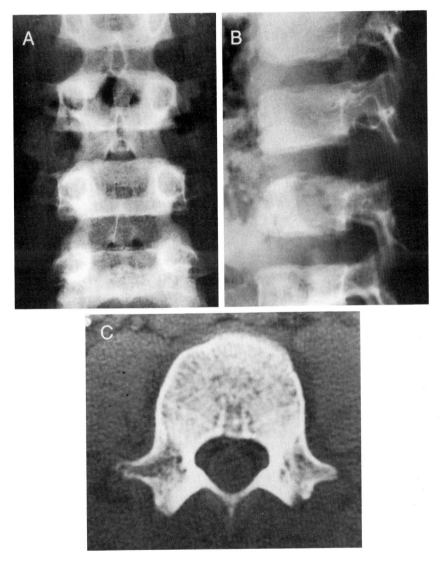

FIG 2–44.
Lap belt spine injury in a 9-year-old child. In **A,** an AP projection, the distance between the spinous processes of the two middle vertebrae is greater than that of the top two vertebrae. The posterior distraction is more obvious in **B.** In **C,** axial CT demonstrates the "naked facet" feature in which no facet apposition is visible. (From Taylor GA, Eggli KD: *Am J Roentgenol* 1988; 150:1355–1358. Used by permission.)

and following exposure to exogenous or endogenous corticosteroids.

REFERENCES

Cervical Spine Injuries

Apple JS, Kirks DR, Merten DF, et al: Cervical spine fractures and dislocations in children. *Pediatr Radiol* 1987; 17:45–49.

Jaffe DM, Binns H, Radkowski MA, et al: Developing a clinical algorithm for early management of cervical spine injury in child trauma victims. *Ann Emerg Med* 1987; 16:270–276.

Sherk HH, Schut L, Lane JM: Fractures and dislocations of the cervical spine in children. *Orthop Clin North Am* 1976; 7:593–604.

Silverman FN, Kattan K: "Trauma" and "no-trauma" of the cervical spine in pediatric patients, in Kattan KR (ed): *"Trauma" and "No-Trauma" of the Cervical Spine.* Springfield, Ill, Charles C Thomas, 1975, pp 206–241.

Fractures

Galinda MJ Jr, Francis WR: Atlantal fracture in a child through congenital anterior and posterior arch defects. A case report. *Clin Orthop* 1983; 178:220–222.

Gehweiler JA Jr, Daffner RH, Roberts L Jr: Malformations of the atlas vertebra simulating the Jefferson fracture. *Am J Roentgenol* 1983; 140:1083–1086.

Keller RH: Traumatic displacement of the cartilaginous vertebral rim: A sign of intervertebral disc prolapse. *Radiology* 1974; 110:21.

Richman S, Friedman RL: Vertical fracture of cervical vertebral bodies. *Radiology* 1954; 62:536–543.

Suss RA, Zimmerman RD, Leeds NE: Pseudospread of the atlas: False sign of Jefferson fracture in young children. *Am J Roentgenol* 1983; 140:1079–1082.

Weston WJ: Clay-shoveler's disease in adolescents (Schmitt's disease): A report of 2 cases. *Brit J Radiol* 1957; 30:378–380.

Zanca P, Lodmell EA: Fracture of the spinous processes: A "new" sign for the recognition of fractures of the cervical and upper dorsal spinous processes. *Radiology* 1951; 56:427–428.

Atlanto-occipital and Atlantoaxial Injuries

Boiton J, Hageman G, deGraaff R: The conservative treatment of patients presenting with Grisel's syndrome. *Clin Neurol Neurosurg* 1986; 88:95–99.

Davidson RG: Atlantoaxial instability in individuals with Down syndrome; a fresh look at the evidence. *Pediatrics* 1988; 81:857–865.

Miller JD, Capusten BM, Lampard R: Changes in the base of skull and cervical spine in Down syndrome. *J Can Assoc Radiol* 1986; 37:85–89.

Parke WW, Rothman RH, Brown MD: The pharyngovertebral veins: An anatomical rationale for Grisel's syndrome. *J Bone Joint Surg Am* 1984; 66:568–574.

Shaffer TE, Chairman: Committee on Sports Medicine, American Academy of Pediatrics: Atlantoaxial instability in Down syndrome. *Pediatrics* 1984; 74:152–154.

Swischuk LE: Anterior displacement of C-2 in children: Physiologic or pathologic? *Radiology* 1977; 122:759–763.

Wilson BC, Jarvis BK, Haydon RC III: Nontraumatic subluxation of the atlantoaxial joint: Grisel's syndrome. *Ann Otol Rhinol Laryngol* 1987; 96:705–708.

Spondylolysis and Spondylolisthesis

Cozen L: The developmental origin of spondylolisthesis: Two case reports. *J Bone Joint Surg [Am]* 1961; 43:180–184.

Haukipuro K, Keranen N, Koivisto E, et al: Familial occurrence of lumbar spondylolysis and spondylolisthesis. *Clin Genet* 1978; 13:471–476.

MacNab I: Spondylolisthesis with intact neural arch—the so-called pseudospondylolisthesis. *J Bone Joint Surg [Br]* 1950; 32:325–333.

Meyerding HW: Spondylolisthesis. *Surg Gynecol Obstet* 1932; 54:371–377.

Taillard WF: Etiology of spondylolisthesis. *Clin Orthop* 1976; 117:30–39.

Wilkinson RH, Hall JE: The sclerotic pedicle: Tumor or pseudotumor? *Radiology* 1974; 111:683–688.

Wiltse LL, Newman PH, MacNab I: Classification of spondylolysis and spondylolisthesis. *Clin Orthop* 1976; 117:23–29.

Wiltse LL, Widell EH, Jackson DW: Fatigue fracture: The basic lesion in isthmic spondylolisthesis. *J Bone Joint Surg [Am]* 1975; 57:17–22.

Compression and Fulcrum Fractures

Smith WS, Kaufer H: Patterns and mechanisms of lumbar injuries associated with lap seat belts. *J Bone Joint Surg [Am]* 1969; 51:239–254.

Sujoy E: Spinal lesions in tetanus in children. *Pediatrics* 1962; 29:629–635.

Taylor GA, Eggli KD: Lap-belt injuries of the lumbar spine in children: A pitfall in CT diagnosis. *Am J Roentgenol* 1988; 150:1355–1358.

SECTION 4

Infections of the Spine

CERVICAL SPINE INFECTIOUS PROCESSES

Inflammatory lesions of the cervical spine are rare in infants and children. Bacteria sometimes gain entrance to the spine through penetrating wounds of the neck or from direct extension from prevertebral abscesses, especially those associated with sharp foreign bodies in the pharynx. More frequently, as in other segments of the vertebral column, the route of entry is via the bloodstream. In addition, the destructive features of vertebral osteomyelitis are more obvious than is reactive sclerosis. Associated prevertebral abscesses may drain into the mediastinum and result in diagnostic confusion if the primary vertebral involvement is not recognized.

NONTUBERCULOUS INFECTIONS

Nontuberculous infections of the spinal column are rare during infancy and childhood, age periods when osteomyelitis occurs most frequently in the long bones. When appendicular bones are infected during staphylococcal or streptococcal bacteremias, the spine usually escapes concurrent infection. In rare instances, however, the vertebrae are affected and a wide variety of organisms may be causal agents: staphylococcus, streptococcus, *Salmonella typhosi* and *paratyphi*, pneumococcus, meningococcus, *Brucella melitensis,* and other organisms. These may be introduced into the spine via the vertebral arteries as suggested by Trueta or via the vertebral vein system, rediscovered and described so effectively by Batson. The high incidence of vertebral osteomyelitis in intravenous drug abusers may be explained by the availability of both routes. The Batson system of intercommunicating, intraspinal and extraspinal, valveless veins connects the upper and lower portions of the body, supplementing and, at times substituting for, the flow of blood in the venacaval system. When physiologic or pathologic pressure changes compromise the venacaval drainage, this system serves as a safety valve. It is probably responsible for the frequency of axial skeletal infections following surgery of the urinary tract, as well as during transient bacteremias from other sites.

Vertebral osteomyelitis may have an acute febrile presentation or an indolent one with a complaint only of back pain. Blood cultures are usually positive in the former and negative in the latter. CT-guided percutaneous biopsies have been suggested for early diagnosis in cases with typical radiographic features and negative blood cultures. Infection of the vertebrae produces the same changes that occur in other bones, namely, bone destruction and bone production, singly or in combination and in a variety of patterns (Fig 2–45). Destructive changes predominate during the early stage of acute infections; later, productive changes appear. In low-grade chronic infections, productive changes are the rule throughout the course of the disease. Either the margins of the bodies or their central portions may be infected first, and collapse of the body or the intervertebral disk may occur early or late. The roentgen findings in the different kinds of spondylitis are similar and etiologic differential diagnosis from the roentgen findings alone is uncertain. However, note must be taken of the unusual frequency of *Pseudomonas* infections in drug abusers. In the neonate, vertebral osteomyelitis tends to have severe sequelae, possibly because of delayed recognition and rapid progression of destructive changes.

CT demonstrates the skeletal features and, in addition, indicates the presence of soft tissue changes both outside and inside the vertebral canal. MRI has been found as accurate and as sensitive as radionuclide scanning, and both more so than conventional radiography (Fig 2–46). Spinal epidural abscesses have been clearly demonstrated (Fig 2–47). Kyphosis from anterior fusion of vertebral bodies, simulating congenital block vertebrae, or destruction of portions of the body simulating hemivertebrae, may cause confusion in diagnosis in later years if history of the acute infection is not provided.

Spondyloarthritis (diskitis) in children is very likely a vertebral osteomyelitis with disk involvement. A single level of involvement is the rule with the lumbar region most common. The route of infection may be through the valveless venous plexus; septic emboli entering via intraosseous arteries constitute an alternative route. The condition usually presents with back pain and stiffness, local tenderness, and

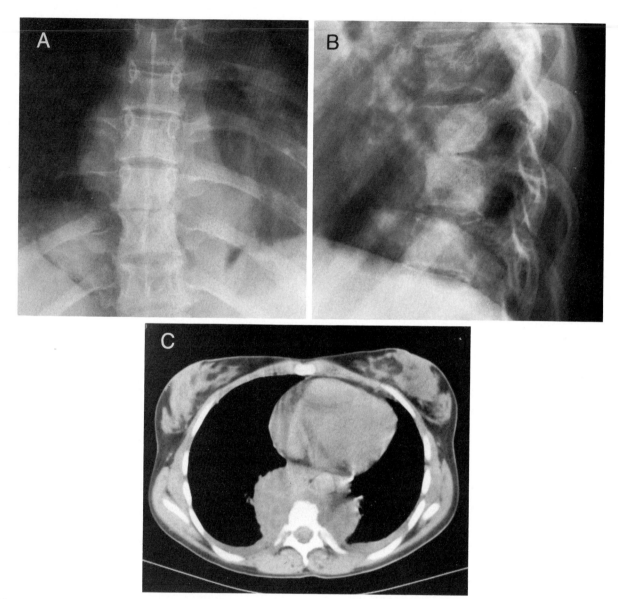

FIG 2–45.
Osteomyelitis and diskitis of the spine in a 16-year-old girl who, because of arthralgias, myalgias, fever, and back pain, together with an elevated erythrocyte sedimentation rate, was believed to have juvenile rheumatoid arthritis. After several weeks of progressive back pain, typical radiographic findings of vertebral infection were observed **(A** and **B).** The AP film **(A)** demonstrated a paraspinal abscess. This was confirmed and better evaluated by CT **(C)** which clearly demonstrated destructive foci in the margins of the body. Surgical proof was provided and *Staphylococcus aureus* was cultured from the septic area.

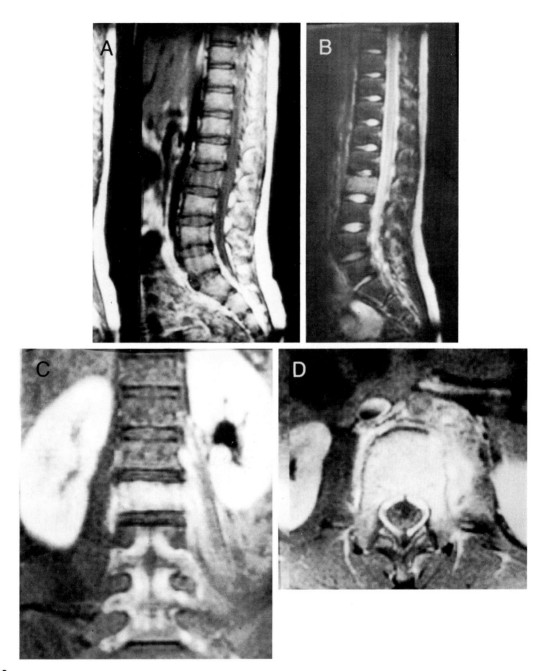

FIG 2–46.
MRI of vertebral osteomyelitis in a 10-year-old boy with back pain and fever. Sagittal T1-weighted image (TR/TE = 600/20) shows abnormal hypointense signal within the L3 vertebral body **(A)** that becomes hyperintense **(B)** on the T2-weighted image (TR/TE = 1,800/100). Adjacent intervertebral disks are relatively normal. Post-gadolinium coronal **(C)** and axial **(D)** images show diffuse signal enhancement within the L3 vertebral body that extends into the left and anterior soft tissues. The disks are not enhanced and there is no compression of the thecal sac. (From Prenger EC: *Semin Ultrasound CT MR* 1991; 12:410–428. Used by permission.)

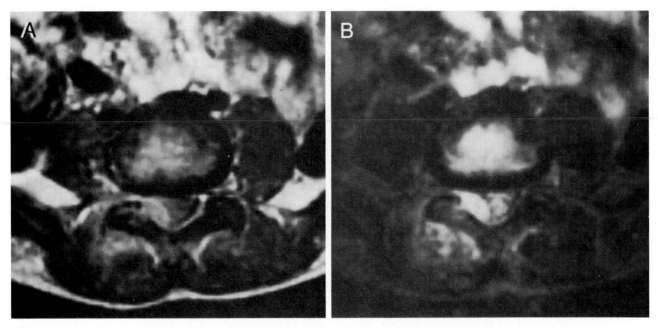

FIG 2–47.
MRI in spinal osteomyelitis. **A,** axial T2-weighted image (TR/TE = 2,000/80) through the L4–5 interspace shows a posterolateral epidural mass with increased signal intensity adjacent to the right lamina. The mass compresses the dural sac. Note indistinct increased signal in right paraspinal muscles. **B,** T1-weighted image corresponding to **A** shows clearly a lytic lesion of the right lamina and the adjacent epidural mass as well as the paraspinal muscle reaction. (From Angtuaco EJC, McConnell JR, Chadduck WM, et al: *Am J Roentgenol* 1987; 149:1249–1253. Used by permission.)

low-grade fever with elevated erythrocyte sedimentation rate. Occasionally, especially in young children, the patient refuses to walk; abdominal pain also is a frequent complaint. Trauma is often an apparent precursor. The radiographic changes are primarily those of narrowing of the intervertebral space, usually with some irregularity of the contiguous vertebral end plates (Fig 2–48). Some swelling of the adjacent soft tissues may be present. Sclerosis of the affected bodies may be noted shortly after the onset (1–2 weeks) and increases with time. CT and MRI demonstrate paravertebral soft tissue swelling and paravertebral abscesses; fragmentation or erosions of vertebral end plates are best shown by CT. Bone scans are generally positive but no modality is free from false-positive or false-negative results. An association with spondylolisthesis has been observed in some cases; a causal relation cannot be assured. Fusion of the sclerotic bodies may occur, but with rest and appropriate antibiotic treatment, and occasionally with rest alone, progressive healing is the rule. Aspiration biopsy under fluoroscopic control has resulted in recovery of pathogens; staphylococcus and *Escherichia coli* have been frequent in our experience. Rarely, other organisms have been obtained including *Mycobacterium tuberculosis*.

TUBERCULOUS SPONDYLITIS

Tuberculosis is the commonest vertebral infection in adults in many parts of the world, although its frequency has diminished in countries where public health standards are high. New immigrants from Third World countries, a high-risk group, have made necessary an awareness of tuberculous infection, skeletal as well as pulmonary, even in developed regions. Tuberculous spondylitis in infants and children may become manifest during the early stages of the primary pulmonary infection or years later after the primary infection has subsided in the lungs. Pain and stiffness are prominent, though nonspecific, symptoms. The diagnosis may first be suggested after radiographic examination. One or several vertebral segments may be involved at any level of the spine; the cervical and sacral portions are least commonly affected, although when cervical involvement occurs in children under 10 years of age, it tends to be more extensive than in older children. The disease is characteristically limited to the vertebral bodies but, on rare occasions, the neural arches may be affected.

The macroscopic, anatomical, and radiographic findings are characterized by destructive changes in

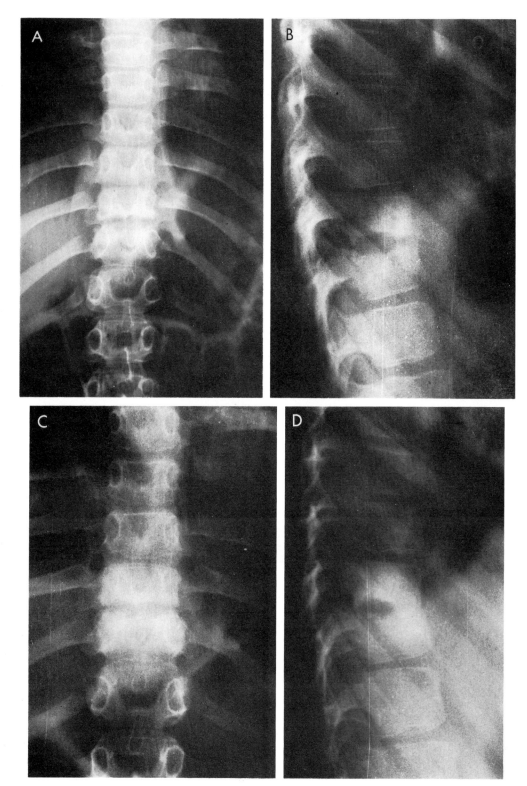

FIG 2–48.

Diskitis in a 9-year-old boy. The patient had had back pain for 2 weeks and a low-grade fever. **A** and **B,** AP and lateral projections. The tenth dorsal interspace is narrowed, the opposing vertebral end plates are irregular and sclerotic **(A)** and demonstrate focal bone destruction **(B),** and a paraspinal swelling is present in **A.** Fluoroscopically guided aspiration was performed 1½ weeks later, and *Staphylococcus aureus,* coagulase-positive, was recovered. **C** and **D,** 8 weeks after **A** and **B.** Sclerosis has increased, and autofusion of the anterior portions of the vertebral bodies has occurred.

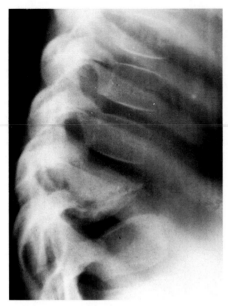

FIG 2–49.
Tuberculous spondylitis in a young boy. Notwithstanding the destruction of contiguous vertebral bodies and their common intervertebral disk, there is no extension to the adjacent vertebral bodies or the disks between each of them and its disk shared with the affected body.

the vertebral bodies, destruction of neighboring intervertebral disks, and formation of paraspinal abscesses. The lesions usually begin in the anteroinferior portion of a vertebral body and spread rapidly beneath the anterior longitudinal ligament to involve adjacent vertebral bodies (Fig 2–49). Narrowing of the intervertebral spaces may develop when destruction of vertebral end plates permits herniation of the disk into the affected vertebral bodies. Lesions are predominantly destructive; osteoblastic changes usually occur late in the disease. The bodies may be destroyed from secondary extension by contiguity from an overlying paraspinal abscess whose infection originated in bodies one or more segments distant. The paraspinal abscess casts a fusiform or rounded shadow of soft tissue density that is best visualized in the thoracic levels where air-filled lungs provide contrast density (Fig 2–50). The paraspinal abscess may become visible before destructive changes in the vertebral bodies are evident by conventional radiography. In long-standing cases, paraspinal and psoas abscesses may become calcified (Fig 2–51).

The roentgen findings of tuberculosis of the spinal column resemble those of nontuberculous infections and of several noninfectious diseases. Destruction and deformities of the bodies, narrowing and obliteration of the interspaces, and swelling of the

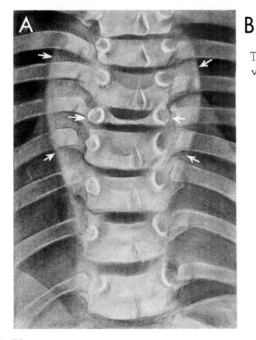

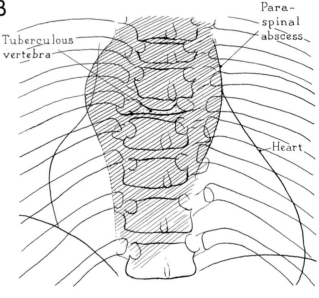

FIG 2–50.
Tuberculous paraspinal abscess in a boy 4 years of age. **A,** drawing of a roentgenogram; **B,** diagrammatic sketch of **A.** A fusiform soft-tissue mass surrounds the lower portion of the thoracic spine and has displaced the posterior portions of the lungs away from each side of the spine. The body of the T7 vertebra is collapsed, and the adjacent intervertebral spaces are narrowed.

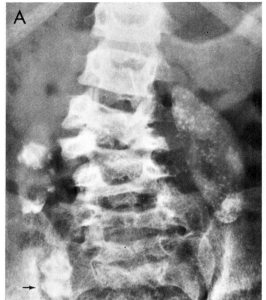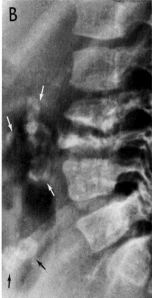

FIG 2–51.
Destructive tuberculosis and partial collapse of the vertebral bodies of L3 to L5 and the intervertebral disks, with calcifying bilateral paraspinal abscesses and calcification of some of the mesenteric lymph nodes in the right side. **A,** frontal, and **B,** lateral projections. This boy was 5 years of age.

paraspinal soft tissues occur in many spinal disorders, e.g., purulent spondylitis, trauma, neoplasms, histiocytosis. CT is more sensitive to the pathologic changes than is conventional radiography but is not diagnostically specific. Because of the lytic nature of the early lesions, bone scans may be negative even with the use of gallium. Consequently, a high index of suspicion for tuberculosis must be maintained when destructive lesions are observed together with interspace narrowing and soft tissue swelling, and appropriate additional procedures, including aspiration, merit consideration. The posterior elements of the spine are rarely affected in tuberculous disease.

Occasional cases of tuberculosis, including tuberculosis of the spine, have been reported with associated polyarthritis in which there is no evidence of microbacterial involvement of the joints themselves. A hypersensitivity reaction has been postulated and support for it claimed by the demonstration of increased purified protein derivative (PPD)–induced reactivity of synovial fluid lymphocytes compared with that of peripheral blood lymphocytes. The combination of the sterile joint reaction and active tuberculosis elsewhere has been called Poncet's disease.

RHEUMATOID ARTHRITIS

Although not primarily infectious in nature, rheumatoid arthritis commonly affects the cervical spine in girls; it is less common and produces much less severe disease in the remainder of the spine. The diarthroses of the cervical spine are the first joints involved. The clinical signs of juvenile rheumatoid arthritis in the cervical spine, especially stiffness, may precede the radiologic signs by many weeks and both are much more frequent in patients with polyarticular- or systemic-onset disease than those with pauciarticular-onset disease. Severe neck pain or torticollis is uncommon; its presence may suggest an intercurrent problem such as fracture or infection.

When there is dorsal or lumbosacral involvement, the changes are similar to those in the cervical spine but usually not so striking. The affected vertebral bodies ultimately demonstrate diminution in height and breadth in comparison with adjacent unaffected vertebrae, and the related intervertebral disk may be narrowed. Neurologic complications are less likely than in patients with adult rheumatoid arthritis.

As in other diarthrodial joints, rheumatoid disease in the joints of the articular processes of the vertebrae produces soft tissue swelling, destruction and obliteration of articular cartilages and their cartilage spaces, generalized rarefaction of bone, and local subchondral necrosis of bone. With subsequent bony fusion across the joints of the articular processes, the radiographic features in the cervical spine may resemble congenital failure of segmenta-

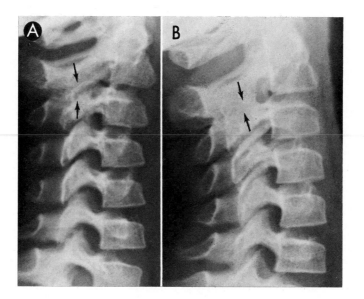

FIG 2–52.
Rheumatoid arthritis of the cervical spine. **A,** at 6 years of age, early destruction of the articular cartilages between the articular processes of C2 and C3 is already evident, but the cartilage spaces are still visible roentgenographically. **B,** at 8½ years of age, with complete destruction of the same cartilages and bony fusion of the articular processes between C2 and C3. The findings now simulate congenital failure of segmentation of the neural arches. The intervertebral disks between the affected vertebrae are, in contrast, normal roentgenographically.

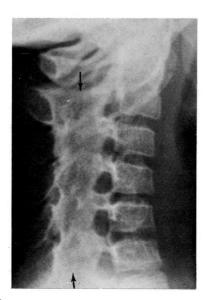

FIG 2–53.
Bony fusion of all the articular processes of the cervical spine in a girl 9 years of age who had had rheumatoid arthritis and a painful cervical spine for over 5 years. The joint spaces between the articular processes have been obliterated by bony ankylosis following complete destruction of the articular cartilages between the articular processes. Without the history, these acquired rheumatoid fusions of the neural arches might be mistaken for congenital failure of segmentation of the arches. It is noteworthy that the synchondroses between the vertebral bodies, the intervertebral disks, are not affected. This is a clear demonstration of the special vulnerability of the tissues of the true joints to rheumatoid disease in the presence of apparent immunity of the tissues of the synchondroses.

tion of the neural arches (Figs 2–52 and 2–53). CT and MRI have been used in adults to demonstrate bony abnormalities as well as effects of the disease on the spinal cord and brainstem and can have applications in children with the disease.

REFERENCES

Nontuberculous Infections

Angtuaco EJC, McConnell JR, Chadduck WM, et al: MR imaging of spinal epidural sepsis. *AJR Am J Roentgenol* 1987; 149:1249–1253.

Batson OV: The vertebral vein system. Caldwell Lecture, 1956. *Am J Roentgenol* 1957; 78:195–212.

Burke DR, Brandt-Zawadzki M: CT of pyogenic spine infection. *Neuroradiology* 1985; 27:131–137.

Digby JM, Kersley JB: Pyogenic non-tuberculous spinal infection. An analysis of thirty cases. *J Bone Joint Surg [Br]* 1979; 61:47–55.

Eismont FJ, Soni PL, Bohlman HH, et al: Vertebral osteomyelitis in infants. *J Bone Joint Surg [Br]* 1982; 64:32–35.

Ekengren K, Bergdahl S, Eriksson M: Neonatal osteomyelitis. Radiographic findings and prognosis in relation to site of involvement. *Acta Radiol* 1982; 23:305–311.

Forster A, Pothmann R, Winter K, et al: Magnetic resonance imaging in nonspecific discitis. *Pediatr Radiol* 1987; 17:162–163.

Hoffer FA, Strand RD, Gebhardt MC: Percutaneous biopsy

of pyogenic infection of the spine in children. *J Pediatr Orthop* 1988; 8:442–444.

Kopecky KK, Gilmor RL, Scott JA, et al: Pitfalls of computed tomography in diagnosis of discitis. *Neuroradiology* 1985; 27:57–66.

Loder RT, Birth JG, Johnston CE II: Concomitant discitis and spondylolisthesis at adjacent lumbar vertebrae. *Orthopedics* 1986; 9:283–285.

Modic MT, Feiglin DH, Piraino DW, et al: Vertebral osteomyelitis: Assessment using MR. *Radiology* 1985; 157:156–166.

Perloff KG, Clancy GL, Perloff JJ: False negative bone scans in pediatric sepsis of the axial skeleton. *Orthop Rev* 1988; 17:1218–1224.

Ratcliffe JF: Anatomic basis for the pathogenesis and radiologic features of vertebral osteomyelitis and its differentiation from childhood discitis. A microarteriographic investigation. *Acta Radiol* 1985; 26:137–143.

Wenger DR, Bobechko WP, Gilday DL: The spectrum of intervertebral disc-space infection in children. *J Bone Joint Surg [Am]* 1978; 60:100–108.

Wiley AM, Trueta J: The vascular anatomy of the spine and its relationship to pyogenic vertebral osteomyelitis. *J Bone Joint Surg [Br]* 1959; 41:796–809.

Tuberculous Spondylitis and Rheumatoid Arthritis

Bailey HL, Gabriel M, Hodgson AR, et al: Tuberculosis of the spine in children: Operative findings and results in one hundred consecutive patients treated by removal of the lesion and anterior grafting. *J Bone Joint Surg [Am]* 1972; 54:1633–1657.

Barkin RE, Stillman JS, Potter TA: The spondylitis of juvenile arthritis. *N Engl J Med* 1955; 253:1107–1110.

Fried JA, Athreya B, Gregg JR, et al: The cervical spine in juvenile rheumatoid arthritis. *Clin Orthop* 1983; 179:102–106.

Hensinger RN, DeVito PD, Ragsdale CG: Changes in the cervical spine in juvenile rheumatoid arthritis. *J Bone Joint Surg* 1986; 68:189–198.

Kumer K: A clinical study and classification of posterior spinal tuberculosis. *Int Orthop* 1985; 9:147–152.

Reynolds H, Carter SW, Murtagh FR, et al: Cervical rheumatoid arthritis: value of flexion and extension views in imaging. *Radiology* 1987; 164:215–218.

Southwood TR, Hancock EJ, Petty RE, et al: Tuberculous rheumatism (Poncet's disease) in a child, *Arthritis Rheum* 1988; 31:1311–1313.

SECTION 5

Spinal Neoplasms

TUMORS OF THE SPINE

Giant cell tumors have been described in cervical vertebrae in children, but in view of the usual age incidence of this tumor, some may well have been aneurysmal bone cysts comparable to that illustrated in Figure 2–54. When vertebral bodies are affected by such tumors, extensive destructive changes with collapse can occur. Osteoid osteoma and osteoblastoma are frequent in the spine; they may be associated with scoliosis and are best localized by nuclear scan and CT. Figure 2–55 is of an osteolytic-osteoblastic tumor in a 16-year-old girl that demonstrated histologic features of osteoblastoma and aneurysmal bone cyst. Hemangiomas are much more rare in the cervical spine than in thoracolumbar levels but, if present, have the same radiographic characteristics. The regional incidence probably reflects the number

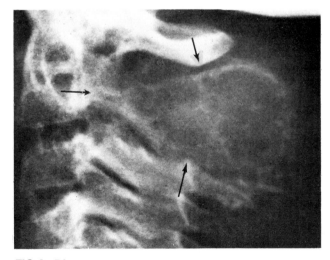

FIG 2–54.
Dilation and rarefaction of the spinous process of C2 of a boy of 8 years. Microscopic diagnosis was aneurysmal bone cyst.

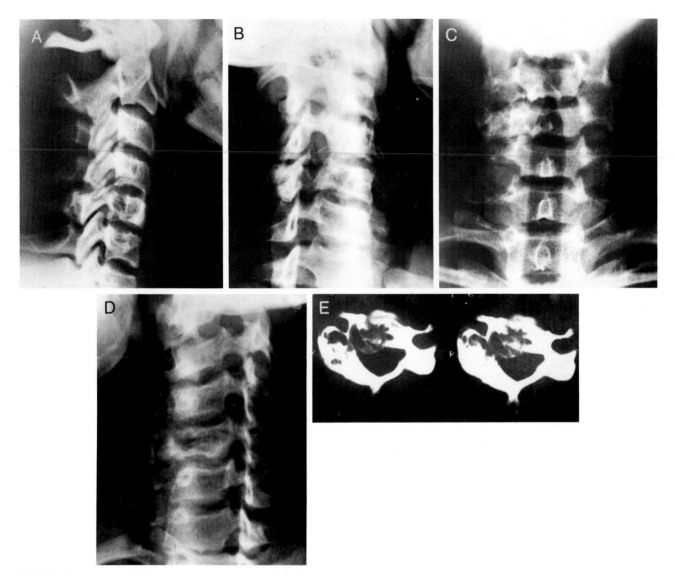

FIG 2–55.
Series of radiographs of a 16-year-old girl with neck pain following a minor accident; she had no neurologic complaints but had some swallowing problems. Films disclosed a mixed lytic and blastic lesion in the right lamina and the adjacent portion of the body of C5. **A,** left lateral projection; **B,** left posterior oblique projection of cervical spine; **C,** AP projection; **D,** right posterior oblique projection.

CT scan at the level of the fifth cervical vertebra, **E,** demonstrates the destructive and reactive productive reaction to best advantage. The preoperative diagnosis was aneurysmal bone cyst or osteoblastoma. Postoperative histologic study showed features of both conditions. **(Courtesy of Dr. Henry H. Jones, Stanford, Calif.)**

of elements available for tumor in the several spinal divisions. Intraspinal growth of an exostosis in multiple cartilaginous exostoses can produce cervical cord compression with motor and sensory signs and symptoms.

Tumors of the spinal nerves, neurofibromas and schwannomas, may grow through the intervertebral foramina and enlarge them into defects including the contiguous pedicles and lamina (Fig 2–56). Enlargement of the foramina can also occur with cervical neuroblastomas, although this feature is more common in instances with primary thoracic or lumbar sites. Sharply angulated kyphosis of the spine (Fig 2–57) is occasionally another manifestation of neurofibromatosis as is scalloping of the posterior walls of t7he vertebral bodies. Cervical instability, however, is not frequent.

Primary Lesions

Primary tumors of the vertebrae are rare in infants and children. The more common primary tumors in-

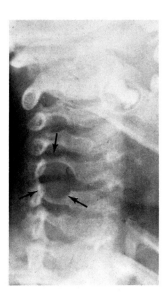

FIG 2–56.
Enlargement of the intervertebral foramen between C5 and C6 caused by a neurofibroma of the nerve root at this level that produced an hourglass-shaped tumor. Pressure atrophy of the laminae above and below resulted in this large circular defect *(arrows)*. This girl, 2 years of age, had neurologic deficits in the arm and leg on the same side as the enlarged foramen.

clude Ewing sarcoma, aneurysmal bone cyst, osteoblastoma, osteoid osteoma, and osteochondroma. Others reported are osteosarcoma, hemangioma, Langerhans cell histiocytosis, and giant cell tumor.

Ewing tumor is generally sclerotic or mixed lytic-sclerotic and often demonstrates adjacent soft tissue swelling (Fig 2–58,*A*). Neurologic deficit is fre-

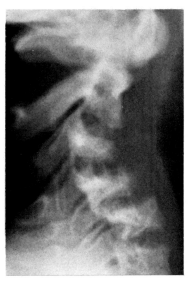

FIG 2–57.
Kyphosis of the cervical spine of a boy 10 years of age who had neurofibromatosis involving C3 through C6. This spine had also received x-radiation.

quently present; the pathologic anatomy of the bone and of the tumor in the spinal canal is well delineated by MRI (Fig 2–58,*B*). Metastatic disease is also frequent. Aneurysmal bone cyst presents radiographically as a radiolucent, expanding lesion, often blown-out or ballooned in appearance and usually located eccentrically in the affected vertebral structure. The borders of the tumor are usually well defined by a thin shell of cortical bone with occasional lamellar subperiosteal bone where the cortex is eroded. Ridges on the interior aspect of the shell result in a compartmentalized or honeycomb appearance. Osteoblastoma has a predilection for the vertebral column and particularly the posterior elements. It resembles a giant osteoid osteoma, presenting as a slightly expanding, radiolucent defect on one side of a vertebra with less reactive bone formation than the usual osteoid osteoma. It also differs from osteoid osteoma in lacking the typical pain pattern. Rarely, it may develop osteosarcomatous changes. In the cervical spine, either may produce radicular symptoms in the shoulders and arms. Osteoid osteoma should be suspected when back pain is worse at night than during the day and is associated with regional muscular spasm, paravertebral tenderness, and localized scoliosis. Aspirin often gives substantial relief from the pain. The radiographic findings are similar to those of the condition in other parts of the skeleton and consist of a sclerotic focus with a prominent central radiolucent nidus, located most often in the laminae (Fig 2–59). Bone scan is extremely accurate in localization and useful intraoperatively to assure total removal of the lesion. Surgical excision of the nidus usually results in immediate and permanent relief of the pain.

Rarely, vertebral and costal cartilaginous exostoses (osteochondromas) grow into the spinal canal, compress the spinal cord, and stretch the nerve roots (Fig 2–60). Twersky and associates described three such examples in children 11, 12, and 13 years of age. Osteogenic sarcomas cause extensive destruction of the bodies and neural arches; fragmentation and collapse of the body and spinal curvature may follow. A paraspinal neoplastic mass may produce a paraspinal shadow of water density that resembles the shadow cast by a paraspinal tuberculous abscess. Hemangiomas often produce no symptoms and are incidental findings. They are characterized radiographically by a spongy or honeycomb osteoporosis. Adjacent intervertebral spaces are normal in width. Langerhans cell histiocytosis is discussed under vertebra plana. Giant cell tumors may produce massive destruction of the vertebral body and col-

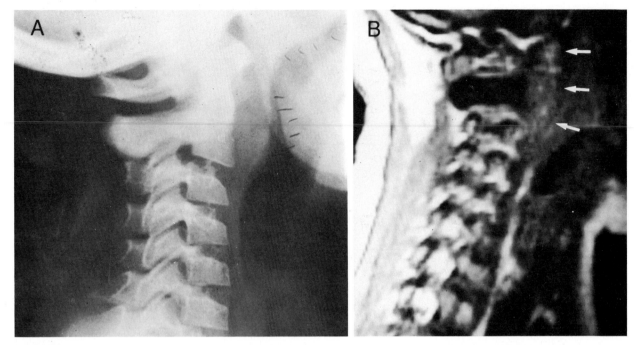

FIG 2–58.
Ewing tumor of C2 in a 4-year-old girl with 2 months of back and shoulder pain, mild fever, and cough. The immediate cause for evaluation was a stiff neck of 1 week's duration. Lateral film of the cervical spine **(A)** shows sclerotic and lytic reaction in the body and neural arch of C2 with a retropharyngeal soft tissue mass. Chest film showed multiple nodules in both lungs. Neurologic signs developed and progressed rapidly. Emergency MRI **(B)** shows complete destruction of bone and marrow in all of C2, and a soft tissue mass anterior to it as well as in the spinal canal causing a block at the C2 level. There was a good initial response to steroid and radiation therapy, followed by chemotherapy.

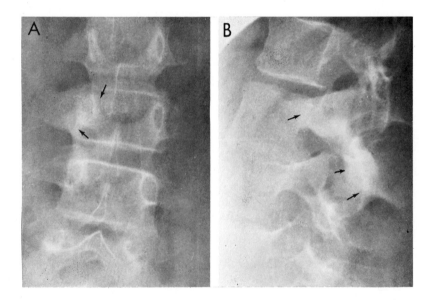

FIG 2–59.
Osteoid osteoma (microscopic diagnosis) of the right pedicle, lamina, superior and inferior articular processes, and the transverse process of the L3 vertebra of a girl 10 years of age who had had severe low back pain at night for 2 months. **A,** frontal, and **B,** lateral projections. The sclerotic changes *(arrows)* are confined to the right side of the neural arch and are better demonstrated in a lateral projection **(B).** The spinous process is not affected. The nidus was not demonstrable radiographically.

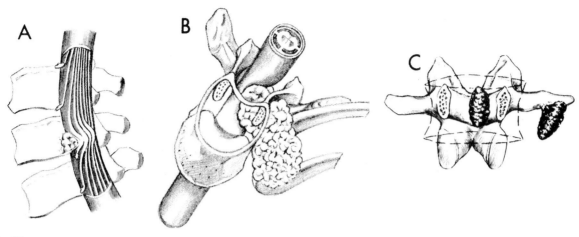

FIG 2–60.
Cartilaginous exostoses are rare in the vertebrae but occasionally cause significant compression of the spinal cord and its nerve roots. **A,** compression of the spinal cord and displacement of the nerve roots by extension of a cartilaginous exostosis from the dorsal inferior edge of the L4 body into the intervertebral foramen. **B,** extension of a cartilaginous exostosis from the dorsal end of a rib into the spinal canal, with severe compression and displacement of the spinal cord. **C,** intraspinal cartilaginous exostosis that grew ventrad from the dorsal edge of the neural arch to compress the underlying spinal cord. A second cartilaginous exostosis projects caudad off the underedge of a transverse process. (From Twersky J, Kassner EG, Tenner MS: *Am J Roentgenol* 1975; 124:124–128. Used by permission.)

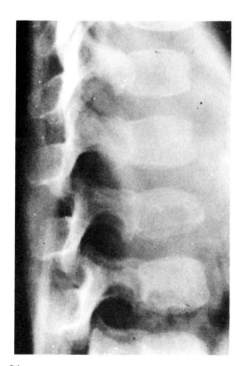

FIG 2–61.
Eosinophilic granuloma (not proved histologically) of the body of L2 in a 5-year-old boy. The body is elongated anteroposteriorly and diminished in height in comparison with adjacent bodies. Radiolucency in the lower half of the affected body has scalloped, nonreactive borders. The lack of obvious involvement of the extreme posterior portion of the body results from failure of the granuloma to pass across the cartilage between the body proper and the contribution made to it by the pedicles.

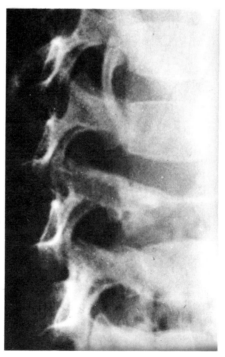

FIG 2–62.
Same patient as in Figure 2–61, 1 month later. Typical compression fracture resulting from the body destruction produced by the granuloma. Note the preservation of the height of the posterior portion of the body. The appearance was previously considered characteristic of Calvé disease.

lapse of the adjoining intervertebral spaces. Although it is probable that many of the earlier diagnoses of giant cell tumors of the spine were actually misdiagnoses of aneurysmal bone cysts, and the tumor is rare before the age of epiphyseal union, definite diagnosis has been made in some instances (Walker et al.). Chordomas, which arise from the primitive notochord or its remnants, destroy the intervertebral disks and later may extend into, and destroy, adjacent vertebral bodies. They are very rare. The rare sacrococcygeal chordoma, or chordoblastoma, is characterized by rapid growth and rapid destruction of the coccyx and lower sacral segments. The tumor is usually palpable per rectum and later may become visible as a swelling in the buttock and back. Although enlargement by direct extension is rapid, metastasis by blood or lymph is rare. Several chordoblastomas have occurred at the base of the skull in older children.

Vertebra Plana

Vertebra plana (Calvé disease) was originally considered to be an osteochondrosis of the primary ossification center of a vertebral body, comparable to that observed in the femoral head (Perthes disease) and other bone structures transforming from cartilage. For some time, it has been accepted, instead, as a manifestation of Langerhans cell histiocytosis (histiocytosis X), particularly the forms recognized as eosinophilic granuloma and Hand-Schüller-Christian disease. It results from proliferation of the granulomatous material in a vertebral body and its subsequent collapse. Usually a single vertebral body is affected. When there is more than one vertebral site, the affected bodies are usually separated by normal bodies. Symptoms may or may not be present locally.

Initially, the affected vertebral body may show only a faint, cystic appearance (Fig 2–61). When collapse occurs, the condensation of the bony tissue results in irregular sclerosis (Fig 2–62). The interspaces are not affected; pedicles may be involved in the destructive process, but generally the posterior elements are spared. Restoration of the body may begin after several months (Fig 2–63); deformity may persist for years. Because of the potential for disseminated disease in Langerhans cell histiocytosis, young children with vertebral collapse observed incidental to examination for apparently unrelated

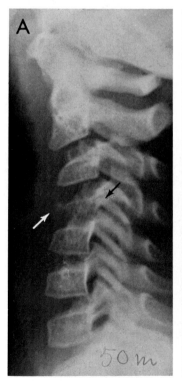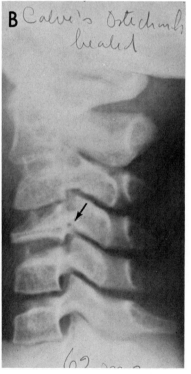

FIG 2–63.
A, vertebra plana of the body of the C4 segment of a girl 50 months of age. The body is rarefied and collapsed, with widening of the contiguous intervertebral spaces. **B,** at 60 months, the affected body is still flattened but has become sclerotic and is beginning to reexpand toward its normal thickness.

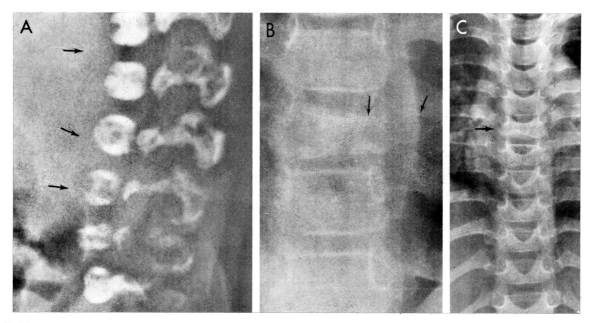

FIG 2–64.
Destruction of vertebrae by intraspinal neuroblastoma. **A,** extensive destruction of neural arches of the vertebral bodies of L3 to L5, with collapse of the body of L5, in an infant 5 months of age. **B,** partial destruction and collapse *(arrows)* with sclerosis of the left side of the vertebral body of a child 6 years of age. The *lateral arrow points* to a paraspinal swelling of soft tissue at the same level. **C,** bilateral collapse and sclerosis of the T6 vertebral body of a boy 5 years of age without paraspinal soft tissue swelling.

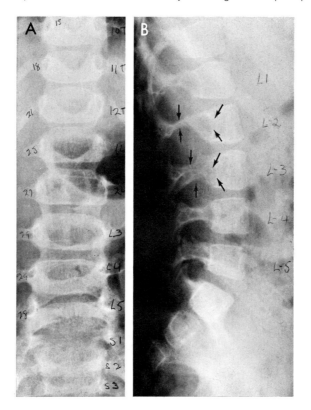

FIG 2–65.
Intraspinal extension of a neuroblastoma (microscopic diagnosis) in which the interpediculate spaces are increased and the pedicles eroded and elongated. Large portions of the pedicles of L2 and L3 are destroyed. In **A,** a frontal projection, the numbers on the right pedicles represent measurements in millimeters of the maximal interpediculate diameters; they are all enlarged in comparison with normal. **B,** lateral projection. Note the enlargement of the intervertebral foramina of L1–2 to L3–4 where "fingers" of the extraspinal neuroblastoma have extended into the intraspinal epidural space where they have coalesced.

complaints should have a skeletal survey to exclude other silent lesions whose presence might alter the management and prognosis.

Secondary Neoplasms

Metastatic or invasive lesions in the spine occur in neuroblastoma, rhabdomyosarcoma, lymphoma, and leukemia, as well as in other extravertebral tumors such as Ewing tumor, Wilms tumor, and osteosarcoma. Neuroblastoma of the vertebrae, metastatic or by direct extension, is generally destructive (Fig 2–64). Extension of tongues of neoplastic tissue into the extradural space through intervertebral foramina may be recognized by enlargement of the foramina and erosion of its osseous margins (Fig 2–65). Leukemia, lymphoma, and rhabdomyosarcoma (Fig 2–66) are also primarily destructive and may result in vertebral collapse, usually without changes in the intervertebral spaces. All of these, however, may be associ-

ated with reactive sclerosis and can result in a variably or uniformly dense vertebral body. Identification of the primary tumor or biopsy of the spinal lesion, or both, are necessary for diagnosis.

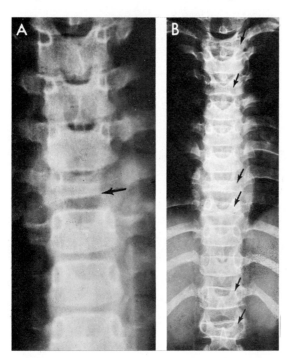

FIG 2–66.
Metastatic embryonal rhabdomyosarcoma of the spine. **A,** destruction and collapse of the vertebral body and left pedicle of the T6 vertebra of a boy 6½ years of age whose primary neoplasm was in the muscles above one ankle, with metastases to flat and long bones as well as this single vertebral body *(arrow)*. **B,** metastases in several vertebrae *(arrows)* with compression deformities in T2, T4, T8, T12, and L1 of a boy 52 months of age whose primary neoplasm was in the orbit. There were multiple skeletal metastases in several round and flat bones.

REFERENCES

Cervical Spine Tumors
Cohn RS, Fielding JW: Osteochondroma of the cervical spine. *J Pediatr Surg* 1986; 21:997–999.

Disch SP, Grubb RL Jr, Gado MH, et al: Aneurysmal bone cyst of the cervicothoracic spine: Computed tomographic evaluation of the value of preoperative embolization. Case report. *Neurosurgery* 1986; 19:290–293.

Ein SH, Shandling B, Humphreys R, et al: Osteomyelitis of the cervical spine presenting as a neurenteric cyst. *J Pediatr Surg* 1988; 23:779–781.

Madigan R, Worrall T, McClain EJ: Cervical cord compression in hereditary multiple exostosis: Review of the literature and report of a case. *J Bone Joint Surg [Am]* 1974; 56:401–404.

Polivy KD, Scott RM, Zimbler S: Osteoid osteoma of the cervical spine. *Orthopedics* 1986; 9:1101–1103.

Yong-Hing K, Kalmachi A, MacEwen GD: Cervical spine abnormalities in neurofibromatosis. *J Bone Joint Surg [Am]* 1979; 61:695–699.

Zwimpfer TJ, Tucker WS, Faulkner JF: Osteoid osteoma of the cervical spine: case reports and literature review. *Can J Surg* 1982; 25:637–641.

Thoracolumbar Spine Neoplasms
Hoeffel J-C, Brassi F, Schmitt M, et al: About one case of vertebral chondroblastoma. *Pediatr Radiol* 1987; 17:392–396.

Kozlowski K, Beluffi G, Masel J, et al: Primary vertebral tumours in children. Report of 20 cases with brief literature review. *Pediatr Radiol* 1984; 14:129–139.

Myles ST, MacRae ME: Benign osteoblastoma of the spine in childhood. *J Neurosurg* 1988; 68:884–888.

Pettine JA, Klassen RA: Osteoid osteoma and osteoblastoma of the spine. *J Bone Joint Surg [Am]* 1986; 68A:354–361.

Twersky J, Kassner RG, Tenner MS: Vertebral and costal osteochondromas causing cord compression. *Am J Roentgenol* 1975; 124:124–128.

Walker DR, Rankin RN, Anderson C, et al: Giant-cell tumour of the sacrum in a child. *Can J Surg* 1988; 31:47–49.

Weinstein JN, McLain RF: Primary tumors of the spine. *Spine* 1987; 12:843–851.

SECTION 6

Miscellaneous Spinal Disorders

ACQUIRED DISORDERS OF GROWTH

Adolescent Kyphosis (Scheuermann-Schmorl Disease)

Scheuermann (1921) called attention to kyphosis in adolescents associated with flattening and wedging of one or more vertebral bodies in the lower thoracic and lumbar levels, progressive deformity of the spine, and fragmentation of what he considered to be the epiphyseal ring together with narrowing of the intervertebral disk space. He called this syndrome "kyphosis deformans juvenilis" in the belief that it was similar pathogenetically to Perthes disease in the femur and Köhler disease in the tarsal navicular. Scheuermann hypothesized that the primary cause of the lesion was a disturbance in epiphyseal growth due to injury and ischemic necrosis of the marginal epiphyseal cartilaginous rings that rim the cartilaginous plates on the upper and lower edges of each vertebral body. The disorder has become known as Scheuermann disease.

In Schmorl's comprehensive studies of the spine, adolescent kyphosis was found to be due to an entirely different mechanism—protrusion of the nuclei pulposi into the marrow cavities of the neighboring vertebral bodies with narrowing of the intervertebral space or spaces between the affected bodies (Fig 2–67). According to Schmorl, the onset and progression of vertebral destruction and wedging are caused by excessively heavy stresses on the articular plates that permit the nuclei pulposi to break through these plates and extend into the vertebral body itself. During adolescence, these traumatic stresses are due to vigorous exercises, heavy manual labor, and habitual bending postures that weaken and break healthy cartilaginous plates. In many cases, however, these lesions develop in children who have undergone only normal activity, and in them it is believed that the cartilaginous plates are congenitally weak.

Schmorl expressed doubt that the so-called epiphyseal rings had anything to do with longitudinal growth of the vertebral body. The work of Ehrenhaft and of Bick and Copel confirmed Schmorl's view that longitudinal growth of the ver-

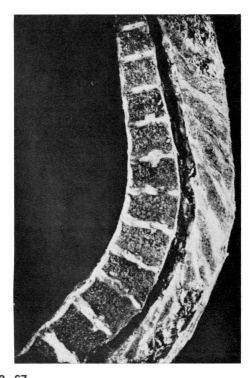

FIG 2–67.
Anatomic changes in adolescent kyphosis (Schmorl type). The disks are deformed and the vertebral bodies wedge shaped. Schmorl nodes, protrusions of the nuclei pulpusi into the spongiosa of the adjacent bodies, are seen at several levels. (From Beadle O: *The Intervertebral Discs*. Special Report Series no. 161, Medical Research Council. London, His Majesty's Stationery Office, 1931. Used by permission.)

tebra is exclusively the function of the cartilaginous plates, which are the counterparts of the proliferating cartilage and the provisional zones of calcification in the tubular bones. Actually the "epiphyseal" rings lie outside the zones of growth in the vertebral bodies, external to the growing cartilaginous plates. Ehrenhaft concluded that in adolescent kyphosis, nuclear prolapses into the body may occur at several sites in different bodies or in a single body, and this produces the uneven growth and marginal defects. It also causes a shift in the load on the vertebral body toward the ventral segment of the cartilaginous plate where growth is disproportionately retarded; and wedging, followed by kyphosis, develops. Fragmentation of the "epiphyseal" ring is a secondary compression phenomenon according to this hypothesis.

In careful roentgen studies, Begg found Schmorl nodes common in adolescent spines in the lower dorsal and lumbar segments and concurred with Schmorl's hypothesis concerning their pathogenesis. He suggested that anterior wedging also reflected protection of the dorsal portions of the body from compression stresses by the articular joints which maintain the intervertebral spaces posteriorly. Brauer found changes similar to those in Scheuermann disease in the spines of contortionists, supporting the traumatic hypothesis of the origin of the changes. The observations of typical anterior wedging without any radiologic evidence of injury to the cartilaginous ring or intervertebral disk have suggested that there may be other pathogenetic mechanisms for the deformity. Quantitative CT analysis of vertebral bone density showed that affected patients did not have osteopenic bone disease, but the advent of MRI has indicated associated changes in the intervertebral disks that bear on this problem. Patients (13–26 years of age) with typical clinical and radiographic changes have been found to show an increased frequency of reduced signal intensity in disks in affected levels (Fig 2–68). This feature reflects the water content of the disks, and the inference is that dessication is an index of disk degeneration, but it is not yet clear if the changes are a cause or an associated feature of the changes in the bodies and the clinical manifestations.

In one study, 55% of patients with Scheuermann disease were abnormal on MRI compared with 10% in asymptomatic controls. Narrowed disk spaces and alterations, generally attributed to lumbar Sheuermann disease, were always associated with disk degeneration on MRI.

The principal radiologic findings include progressive narrowing of the intervertebral space; deep irregularities on the edges of the vertebral body, sometimes even on the ventral edge; Schmorl nodes in the vertebral body; anterior wedging; and kyphosis (Figs 2–69 and 2–70). Actual fusion of the edges of the affected bodies in their ventral aspects, with complete obliteration of the intervertebral space, can be a late complication in some cases.

SCOLIOSIS

Scoliosis has been defined as the presence of one or more lateral-rotatory curvatures of the spine. It is generally described in relation to the convexity of the curve and is considered nonstructural or flexible if it corrects on bending toward the convexity, and structural if it is relatively rigid. Anatomical changes in affected vertebral bodies consist of wedging with rotation; the disks are only slightly affected, apart from adapting to the space available between adjacent bodies.

The deformity occurs in association with axial skeletal and, presumably soft tissue, malformations;

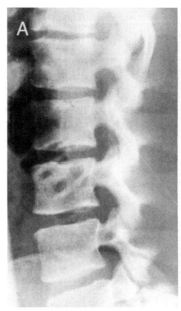
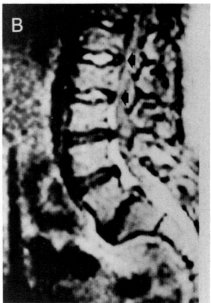

FIG 2–68.
Early Scheuermann disease in a young adult with clinical symptoms. **A,** lateral lumbar spine film demonstrates mild disk narrowing. **B,** T2-weighted MRI, however, demonstrates degeneration (water loss) at all levels except L1–3. Normal disks have high signal intensity. (From Paajanen H, Alanen A, Erkintalo M, et al: *Skeletal Radiol* 1989; 18:523–526. Used by permission.)

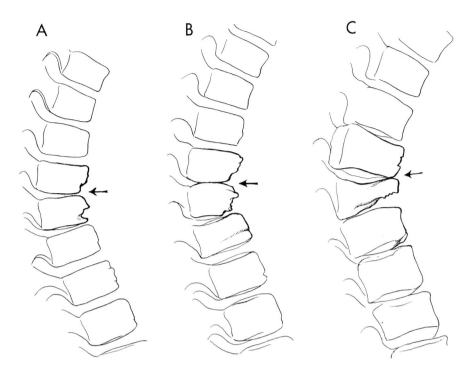

FIG 2–69.
Adolescent kyphosis (Scheuermann type), which developed in a nontuberculous child in the absence of recognized trauma. **A,** at 11 years the intervertebral spaces are narrowed, and the bodies of T6 and T7 show notched deformities on their anterior margins; ky- phosis is evident. **B** and **C,** progressive changes at 13 and 15 years, respectively. All of the changes can be explained on the basis of anterior herniation of the intervertebral disks followed by local compression atrophy of contiguous vertebral bodies.

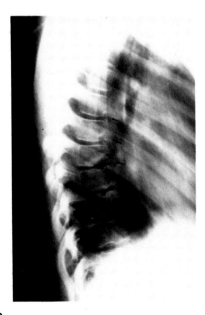

FIG 2–70.
Scheuermann-Schmorl disease. Disk herniations into the anterior portions of multiple dorsal vertebral bodies together with disk-space narrowing at affected levels are characteristic. In this case, the round-back deformity is very mild.

with skeletal dysplasias, particularly those whose name include the term *spondylo-;* and with various neuropathic, myopathic, metabolic, and other disorders. It can be congenital, presenting at birth or in later childhood, or acquired at any time during growth. Hemivertebrae or spinal segmental errors, and isolated or associated rib fusions are examples of congenital forms; neuropathic and myopathic forms may be congenital as in spinal dysraphic abnormalities or arthrogryposis syndromes. Scoliosis occurs in Marfan syndrome, neurofibromatosis, congenital torticollis, and is observed in some cases of congenital heart disease. It is acquired in cerebral palsy and in ocular torticollis secondary to extraocular muscle paralysis.

The most common form of scoliosis is the idiopathic form, which is subdivided into resolving or progressive infantile forms (usually thoracic with a left convexity, and more common in boys), a juvenile form, and the frequent adolescent form (thoracic right, lumbar left, and more frequent in girls). Neuromuscular curves are usually long and C-shaped; short, sharply angulated curves are common in neurofibromatosis. The etiology of most cases of scoliosis is uncertain and probably is multifactorial. Histochemical studies of erector spinae muscles have shown a decreased number of type 1 fibers on the concave side of curves in both girls and boys with adolescent idiopathic scoliosis, and an increased number on the convex side of patients with congenital scoliosis. In both groups, the number of type 1 fibers was normal on the opposite sides of the curves. Type 1 fibers are resistant to fatigue and are used during sustained tonic activities. The increased number in the congenital group has been considered secondary in the pathogenesis of the spinal curvature.

Adolescent idiopathic scoliosis is probably transmitted as an autosomal dominant trait. Because the curves tend to increase at a fairly steady rate up to the prepubertal growth spurt, when they can increase very rapidly, close periodic examination is recommended. Some structural scolioses can also worsen rapidly during this period.

Radiographic examination for scoliosis generally includes erect and recumbent AP films of the entire spine from the cervical level to the sacrum including both iliac crests, and a lateral film of the thoracolumbar spine. Occasionally, left and right bending films are requested to determine the degree of correction that can be obtained. Dickson and associates believe that flattening, or even reversal, of the normal thoracic kyphosis at the apex of the scoliosis is at fault, and can be demonstrated by lateral profile films at the apex of the thoracic scoliosis instead of the usual lateral films of the patient. Serial examinations quantitate the magnitude of the curves and their progression. The Cobb technique is most commonly used for measurement of the angles (Fig 2–71). Rotational deformity can be gauged by the position of the axially projected pedicles in relation to the bodies. Progression usually slows to disappearance at the time that the crestal centers of the ilium are completely fused to the body; however, Weinstein and associates reported that curves that had reached between 50 and 80 degrees at skeletal maturity tended to progress slightly in adult life.

The problem of constructing the lines to measure scoliosis is much greater than that of actual measurement of the angles they subtend. An angle of 20 to 50 degrees is considered to be an indication for the application of an orthosis, while angles of 50 degrees or over, prior to maturity, generally are considered an indication for fusion. In a carefully designed study, Oda and associates found that the angle must measure approximately 9 degrees greater than the critical angle to achieve 95% certainty that that particular critical angle has been reached.

The risks of exposure to x-rays for these examinations were investigated by Nash and associates who concluded that the diagnostic roentgenograms

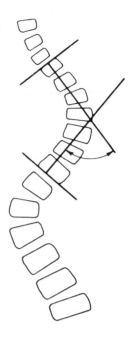

FIG 2–71.
Cobb technique for the measurement of scoliosis. The upper limit of a curve is defined by a line tangential to the upper border of the most cephalad body tilting toward the center of the radius of curvature; the lower limit is defined by a similar line related to the lower border of the most caudal body. The angle subtended between these lines (or perpendiculars constructed to them) measures the angle of scoliosis. (Modified from Cobb JR: *Am Acad Orthop Surg* 1948; 5:261–265.)

represented a minor risk to the patient with respect to any increased risk of carcinogenesis in any organ except for the breast. This particular risk can be greatly decreased by taking posteroanterior (PA) rather than AP films or by using lead breast shields. Information concerning dose to the thyroid was not provided. Nonvisualization of the cervical spine by shielding of the thyroid would protect this highly sensitive structure and not handicap the management in the great majority of patients.

Congenital Heart Defects and Scoliosis

Scoliosis is associated with congenital heart disease in a substantially higher incidence than in the general juvenile population, and has a higher incidence in cyanotic congenital heart disease than in acyanotic congenital heart disease. A high incidence of scoliosis has been found, however, in patients with coarctation of the aorta. The incidence in all cases of heart disease is greater in males than in females in contrast with the approximately 8:1 ratio of females to males in idiopathic scoliosis. The difference is not explained by the higher incidence of certain types of congenital heart disease in boys than in girls. In the group of Poitras et al., another differentiating feature was the fact that the scoliosis was convex to the left in three times as many patients as it was to the right. Although cyanotic patients tend to have more severe scoliosis than patients with acyanotic heart disease, there was no correlation between the severity of coarctation and the frequency or the degree of scoliosis in this group. The causal mechanism of the scoliosis is not known. Thoracotomy, of course, may be responsible for scoliosis in patients treated surgically.

The entire skeleton, especially the calvaria, may be thickened and dense as a result of long-standing hypoxia due to cardiac failure. In one patient, a peculiar patchy sclerosis of the vertebral bodies was observed (Fig 2–72).

ABNORMALITIES OF INTERVERTEBRAL DISKS

Traumatic Lesions

In severe compression fractures of the vertebral bodies, the intervertebral disks may also be injured and the nucleus pulposus dispersed or displaced. Direct

injury to the disk may be due to penetrating wounds of the verteral column. The commonest cause of direct injury to the disk in infants and children has been lumbar puncture when the needle is advanced the entire width of the spinal canal and beyond, anteriorly into the disk. During early life, when the nucleus pulposus is largely fluid, much of the nucleus may be aspirated back into the needle or may leak into the surrounding tissues. Thinning or obliteration of the affected intervertebral space may follow (Fig 2–73). The adjacent vertebral bodies may be injured or infected at the same time. Symptoms of lumbar pain, limitation of motion, and weakness of the back may appear immediately or as late as 2 weeks after the lumbar puncture. The normal lumbar lordosis is usually lost and, in severe cases, actual kyphosis may develop. Injuries to the intervertebral disks used to occur most frequently after repeated lumbar punctures made for the intrathecal injection of therapeutic agents in the preantibiotic era.

Prolapse of the nuclei pulposi through the articular plates into the spongiosa of contiguous vertebrae has been noted above in relation to adolescent kyphosis (Scheuermann disease). Protrusions of the intervertebral disks and their nuclei into the spinal canal and into the spinal nerve roots have apparently not been demonstrated as a cause of back pain in infants and younger children. In older children and adolescents, the typical disk syndrome has been found and demonstrated anatomically in several cases. The youngest patient reported was 3 years of age. Lumbar disks are affected most frequently; le-

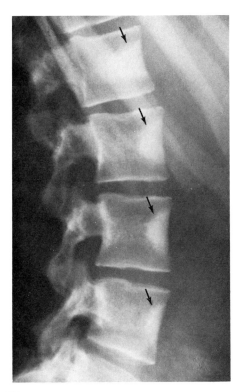

FIG 2–72.
Segmental sclerosis of the vertebral bodies in a boy 10 years of age associated with chronic hypoxia of a single-ventricle heart with transposition of the great arteries. The sclerotic segment in each body surrounds the canal of the nutrient artery. The calvaria and ribs were generally sclerotic and other bones were slightly sclerotic. (Courtesy of Dr. Marvin Daves, Denver, Colo.)

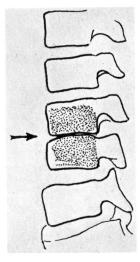

FIG 2–73.
Destruction of an intervertebral disk and sclerosis of the vertebral bodies after lumbar puncture. (Redrawn from Pease CN: *Am J Dis Child* 1935; 49:849–860.)

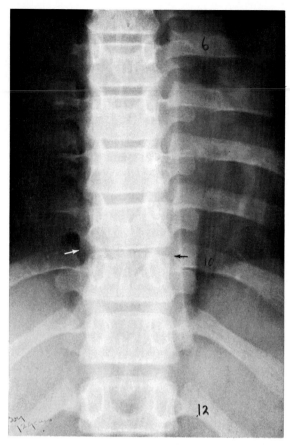

FIG 2–74.
Loss of intervertebral disk space *(arrows)* between T9 and T10 bodies after a boy 12 years of age had injured his back on a trampoline. His back became painful. Results of tuberculin skin tests were negative. (Courtesy of Dr. Arthur Robinson, Denver, Colo.)

sions are usually at the lumbosacral level and are associated with compression of the first sacral nerve. Plain films usually show normal findings but the protrusion and associated dessication of the disk can be seen on MRI. Diminution of the intervertebral space can result from trauma alone (Fig 2–74) but also occurs in infection (diskitis).

Calcification

Calcification of intervertebral disks is not uncommon in adults and is usually considered a sign of degeneration due to normal aging without specific clinical or anatomical significance. The incidence in infants and children is relatively small, although calciferous disk lesions are being described in them with increasing frequency. There are, of course, countless cases that have not been recorded. Usually, except when present in the cervical region, calcification is not associated with local clinical signs. Calcifications have been found in all of the components of the disk—in the cartilaginous plates, the nucleus pulposus, and the anulus fibrosus (Fig 2–75). The lesions may be single or multiple at different levels of the spine, with the highest incidence in the midthoracic levels. Histologic studies of the calcification in the nucleus pulposus of a 425-g fetus showed endochondral ossification with no signs of trauma, hemorrhage, or inflammation. Transitory disk calcifications have been reported in poisoning due to vitamin D, and an instance has been observed in an infant with I-cell disease.

Calcification of the nucleus pulposus in the cervical area is much more frequently associated with

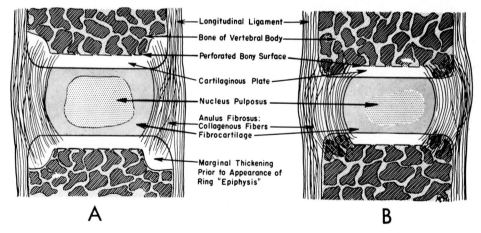

FIG 2–75.
Schematic drawings of the normal intervertebral disk. **A,** before the appearance of ossification centers in cartilaginous vertebral rings. **B,** after ossification of the vertebral rings and their fusion with the vertebral body. (From Silverman FN: *Radiology* 1954; 62:801–816. Used by permission.)

clinical signs and symptoms than when it occurs at other levels of the vertebral column. The calcified nucleus pulposus may herniate anteriorly into the prevertebral soft tissues or posteriorly into the spinal canal. As elsewhere, the calcifications usually disappear with no sequelae. Minor alterations of adjacent vertebral bodies as well as growth disturbances have been described.

Radiologic examination shows images of calcium density in the normally radiolucent intervertebral tissues (Fig 2–76). In AP and lateral projections, central and peripheral calcifications can be differentiated (Fig 2–77), but the exact components of the disk that carry the calcium cannot be identified with accuracy. As expected, the lesions demonstrate a high density on CT, and a low signal intensity on MRI. Urso and associates described alterations in the vertebral bodies adjacent to the calcified disk with changes more marked in the body above it than below. The change consisted of a decrease in vertical height in the anterior third or half of the body as seen in lateral projection. In two of our patients, 22 months and 5 years of age, the prevertebral tissues were calcified in a peculiar "bull's-eye" pattern (Fig 2–78). Clinical signs of fever and pain and stiffness in the neck disappeared after 2 to 3 weeks, and the calcification, after several months. Lesions may be

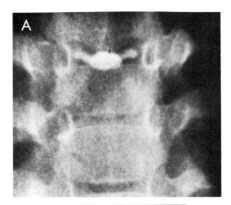

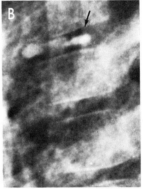

FIG 2–77.
Calcification of the intervertebral disk between T4 and T5 of an asymptomatic boy 5 years of age. In **A,** frontal projection, the central nucleus pulposus appears to be solidly calcified, with two lateral calcified wings that extend laterad into the fibrocartilage of the disk. In **B,** lateral projection, similar wings extend ventrad and dorsad into the fibrocartilage. The anterior borders of the vertebral bodies extend well beyond the superimposed border of the scapula.

transitory or permanent. The former are more frequent in the cervical spine and are usually associated with local pain, and often with torticollis. Anterior and posterior herniations of calcified nuclei pulposi into the spinal canal have been observed; these, too, are often located in the cervical levels. Posterior protrusions may have antecedent trauma, a feature seldom observed in anterior protrusions. Fever, leukocytosis, and elevated erythrocyte sedimentation rate occur in some cases, but the clinical course is generally benign, the calcifications tend to resorb spontaneously, and all clinical signs and symptoms subside.

ANEMIAS, ENDOCRINE DYSFUNCTION, AND OTHER DISORDERS

Hemolytic Anemias

Skeletal changes are largely limited to patients with hemolytic anemias and are more obvious in the

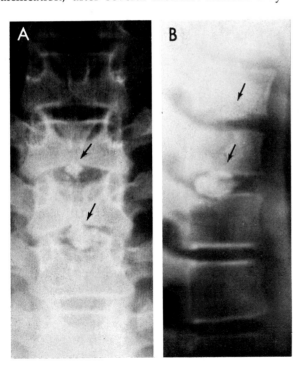

FIG 2–76.
Calcification of the nucleus pulposus in the third and fourth intervertebral disks of an asymptomatic girl 11 years of age. **A,** frontal, and **B,** lateral projections.

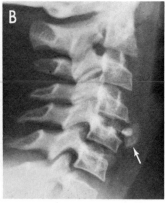

FIG 2–78.
Idiopathic transitory focal calcifications in the prevertebral ligaments and ventral segments of the intervertebral disks of the cervical spines of two young children who had fever and painful, tender necks. In both, the clinical signs disappeared after a few weeks and the calcifications after several months. **A,** in a boy 22 months of age most of the calcification is in front of the spine, and one must assume that the spinal ligaments, and possibly the disks, protrude forward to these levels. In the upper mass of calcification there is a distinct "bull's-eye" pattern. **B,** in a boy 5 years of age, there is a single focus of calcification with a "bull's-eye" pattern that seems to fit into the ventral segment of the intervertebral disk. In both cases the calciferous masses were in or near the midsagittal plane of the spine, and reactions to the tuberculin skin test were negative. There is a notable lack of thickening of the soft tissues at the levels of the calcifications.

bones of the limbs and the skull than in the vertebral column. The radiographic manifestations, in all regions, tend to be most severe in thalassemia major and progressively less marked in sickle cell anemia and familial hemolytic anemia (spherocytosis). In thalassemia, all parts of the vertebrae may become osteopenic and coarsely reticulated as a consequence of marrow hyperplasia. Associated growth disturbance may be reflected by hypoplasia of the bodies. Compression deformities are nevertheless rare. Hyperplastic marrow may extend through the thinned cortices of the vertebrae to present as paravertebral mass lesions (extramedullary hematopoiesis). Compression fractures are more common in sickle cell anemia, possibly partly the result of associated infarcts from intravertebral vascular occlusions. Focal central depressions in the end plates were thought to be indicative of this disease (see Fig 48–11) but have been observed in other types of anemia as well. Biconcave vertebral bodies, with smooth curves of the end plates resembling the changes in osteoporosis, are probably more common than the focal depressions in all types of marrow proliferative disorders.

Leukemia

In leukemia, destructive and productive changes may occur as in the long bones where they are more obvious. Wedging collapse of vertebral bodies may

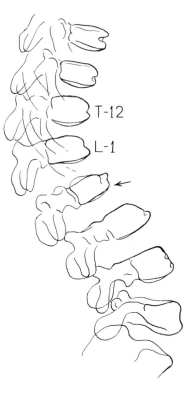

FIG 2–79.
The vertebral column of a hypothyroid boy 3 years of age. Maturation of the vertebrae is retarded, and the L1 body is hypoplastic. There is compensatory hyperplasia and deformity of the anterior portion of the L2 body. The kyphotic deformity persisted despite long-continued and otherwise effective thyroid therapy. In the 12th year, marked kyphosis, spondylolisthesis, and vertebral deformity were still evident.

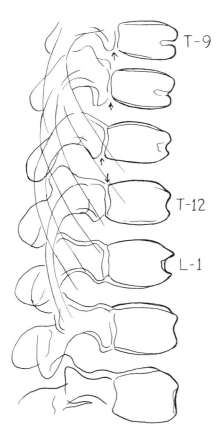

FIG 2–80.
Infantilism of the vertebral column in an untreated hypothyroid girl 8 years of age. The vertebrae have the oval anteriorly notched bodies characteristic of the first year of life. The *arrows* are directed at open neurocentral synchondroses.

occur when destructive changes are marked; more commonly, biconcave contours are noted. Rarely, these vertebral changes occur before the hematologic disorder has declared itself otherwise.

Endocrine Dysfunction

The maturation of the spine may be delayed or accelerated by endocrine dysfunction in the same way that the maturation of long bones is affected. In hypothyroidism, the development of the spine is retarded and individual vertebral bodies may be deformed (Figs 2–79 and 2–80).

REFERENCES

Acquired Disorders of Growth

Begg AC: Nuclear herniations of the intervertebral disc: Their radiological manifestations and significance. *J Bone Joint Surg [Br]* 1954; 36:180–193.

Bick EM, Copel JW: Longitudinal growth of human verte-bra; contribution to human ontogeny. *J Bone Joint Surg [Am]* 1950; 32:803–814.

Brauer W: Zur Atiologie der juvenilen Kyphose (M Scheuermann). *Fortschr Geb Roentgenstr* 1955; 83:839–843.

Ehrenhaft JL: Development of the vertebral column as related to certain congenital and pathological changes. *Surg Gynecol Obstet* 1943; 76:282–292.

Gilsanz V, Gibbons DT, Carlson M, et al: Vertebral bone density in Scheuermann disease. *J Bone Joint Surg [Am]* 1989; 71:894–897.

Paajenen H, Alanen A, Erkintalo M, et al: Disc degeneration in Scheuermann disease. *Skeletal Radiol* 1989; 18:523–526.

Resnick D, Niwayama G: Intervertebral disk herniations: Cartilaginous (Schmorl's) nodes. *Radiology* 1978; 126:57–65.

Scheuermann H: Kyphosis dorsalis juvenilis. *Z Orthop Chir* 1921; 41:305–317.

Schmorl G: Die Pathogenese der juvenilen Kyphose. *Fortschr Geb Roentgenstr* 1930; 41:359–383.

Scoliosis

Ardran GM, Coates R, Dickson RA, et al: Assessment of scoliosis in children: Low dose radiographic technique. *Br J Radiol* 1980; 53:146–147.

Bylund P, Jansson E, Dahlberg E, et al: Muscle fiber types in thoracic erector spinae muscles. Fiber types in idiopathic and other forms of scoliosis. *Clin Orthop* 1987; 214:222–228.

Cobb JR: Outline in the study of scoliosis. Instructional course lectures. *Am Acad Orthop Surg* 1948; 5:261–275.

Deacon P, Flood BM, Diskson RA: Idiopathic scoliosis in three dimensions. A radiographic and morphometric analysis. *J Bone Joint Surg [Br]* 1984; 66B:509–512.

Denton JR, Tietjen R, Gaerlan PF: Thoracic kyphosis in cystic fibrosis. *Clin Orthop* 1981; 55:71–74.

Dickson RA, Lawton JO, Archer IA, et al: The pathogenesis of idiopathic scoliosis. Biplanar spinal asymmetry. *J Bone Joint Surg [Br]* 1984; 66:8–15.

Dietrich DE, Slack WJ: Scoliosis secondary to unilateral extraocular muscle paresis (ocular torticollis). *Radiology* 1967; 88:538–542.

Holt JF: Neurofibromatosis in children. *Am J Roentgenol* 1978; 130:615–639.

Luke MJ, McDonnell EJ: Congenital heart disease in scoliosis. *J Pediatr* 1968; 73:725–733.

Micheli LJ, Hall JE, Wats HG: Spinal instability in Larsen's syndrome. Report of 3 cases. *J Bone Joint Surg [Am]* 1976; 58:562–565.

Nash CL Jr, Gregg EC, Brown RH, et al: Risks of exposure from x-rays in patients undergoing long-term treatment for scoliosis. *J Bone Joint Surg [Am]* 1979; 61:371–374.

Oda M, Rauh S, Gregory PB, et al: The significance of

roentgenographic measurement in scoliosis. *J Pediatr Orthop* 1982; 2:378–382.

Poitras B, Rosenthal A, Hall JE: Scoliosis and coarctation of the aorta (letter). *J Pediatr* 1975; 86:476–477.

Reckles LN, Peterson HA, Bianco AJ Jr, et al: The association of scoliosis and congenital heart defects. *J Bone Joint Surg [Am]* 1975; 57:449–455.

Rezaian SM: The incidence of scoliosis due to neurofibromatosis. *Acta Orthop Scand* 1976; 47:534–539.

Weinstein SL, Zavala DC, Ponseti IV: Idiopathic scoliosis. Long term follow-up and prognosis in untreated patients. *J Bone Joint Surg [Am]* 1981; 63:702–712.

Abnormalities of the Intervertebral Disks

Beadle OA: *The Intervertebral Disks.* Special Report Series No 161, Medical Research Council, London, His Majesty's Stationery Office, 1931.

Ho PS, Ho KC, Yu SW, et al: Calcification of the nucleus pulposus with pathologic confirmation in a premature infant. *AJNR* 1989; 10:201–202.

Jawish R, Rigault P, Padocani JP, et al: Calcifications discales inter-vertébrales chez l'enfant. *Rev Chir Orthop* 1989; 75:308–317.

Keene JS, Goletz TYH, Lilleas F, et al: Diagnosis of vertebral fractures. A comparison of conventional radiography, conventional tomography, and computed axial tomography. *J Bone Joint Surg [Am]* 1982; 64:586–595.

McGregor JC, Butler P: Disc calcification in childhood: Computed tomographic and magnetic resonance imaging appearances. *Br J Radiol* 1986; 58:180–182.

Mainzer F: Herniation of the nucleus pulposus: A rare complication of intervertebral-disk calcification in children. *Radiology* 1973; 107:167–170.

Melnick JC, Silverman FN: Intervertebral disk calcification in childhood. *Radiology* 1963; 80:399–408.

Mogle P, Amitai Y, Rotenberg M, et al: Calcification of intervertebral disks in I-cell disease. *Eur J Pediatr* 1986; 145:226–227.

Peacock A: Observations on the pre-natal development of the intervertebral disc in man. *J Anat* 1951; 85:260–274.

Urso S, Colajacoma M, Migliorini A, et al: Calcifying discopathy in infancy in the cervical spine: Evaluation of vertebral alterations over a period of time. *Pediatr Radiol* 1987; 17:387–391.

Wilkinson RH, Hall JE: The sclerotic pedicle: Tumor or pseudotumor? *Radiology* 1974; 111:683–688.

SECTION 7

Introduction to the Pelvis

NORMAL ANATOMY

The pelves of fetus, infant, and child are conspicuously small and funnel-shaped; during the neonatal period, the vertical diameter is elongated in proportion to the lateral and sagittal diameters. At birth, the acetabular cavities are relatively larger and shallower than in older children and the obturator foramina are proportionately smaller and situated nearer together. The sacrum makes up a larger segment of the pelvic girdle during the early years and is situated higher in relation to the ilia than later. The infantile sacral promontory is less marked than in the adult until the infant assumes an erect posture, when the sacrum descends between the ilia and tilts forward. Pelvic growth is rapid during the first 2 years, after which growth is slow until puberty.

Anatomists claim that sexual differences in pelves can be recognized as early as the fourth fetal month but, from the radiographic standpoint, the pelves of young boys and girls are practically indistinguishable. Later, the male pelves tend to be larger but the major sexual differences are not obvious until after puberty. In girls, the ossification centers for the iliac crests usually appear within 6 months of menarche. It is possible that similar changes in the ilia of boys represent an analogous level of maturation.

ROENTGENOGRAPHIC APPEARANCE

Normal Soft Tissues

In frontal projections, overlapping of the buttocks may be responsible for a vertical spindle-shaped shadow of increased density which is superimposed on the symphysis pubis at or near the midsagittal pelvic plane (Fig 2–81,*A*). Axial projection of the shaft and glans of the penis results in a surprisingly dense rounded shadow (Fig 2–81,*B*), which may

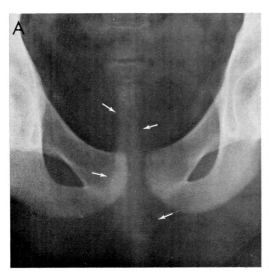
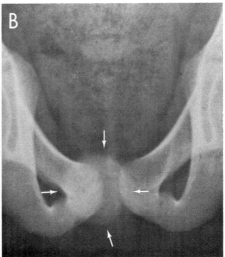

FIG 2–81.
A, spindle-shaped shadow of increased density in the midpelvic plane caused by overlapping buttocks.
B, heavy circular shadow cast by the penis projected in its axial plane.

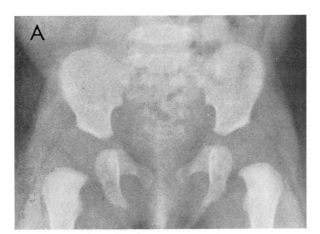

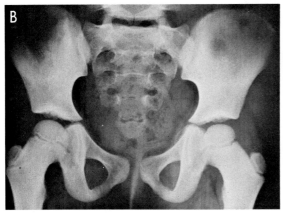
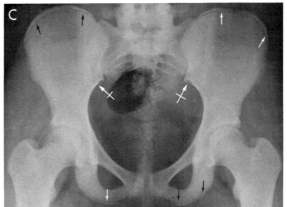

FIG 2–82.
Normal roentgen appearance of the pelvis at different ages. **A,** at 3 months of age in a girl, the ischiopubic synchondroses are widely opened. The symphysis pubis is normally wide. The ossification centers in the femoral epiphyses have not yet appeared. **B,** at 5 years, the ilia are still separated from the ischia and pubic bones, but the ischiopubic synchondroses are almost completely closed; the lateral masses of the sacrum have fused with their bodies; the acetabula are proportionately smaller and deeper than in **A. C,** at 14 years, the innominate bone is completely fused, and secondary centers are now visible in the crests of the ilia and in the inferior margins of the ischia *(arrows)*. A small paraglenoid fossa indents the top of each sciatic notch *(crossed arrows)*.

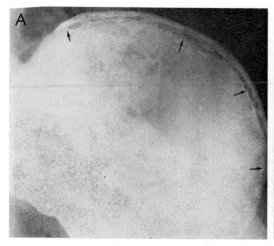
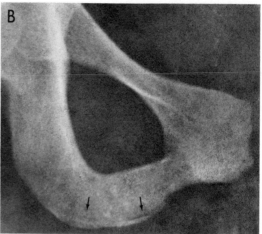

FIG 2–83.
A, normal secondary epiphyseal center in the crest of the ilium of a girl 12 years of age. The edges of the striplike crestal center and the contiguous edge of the ilium are both normally irregular—often more irregular than in this normal patient. **B,** apophyseal center on the inferior ramus of the ischium of an asymptomatic girl 15 years of age.

suggest to the inexperienced observer an opaque foreign body in the rectum or bladder, or even an intrapelvic calcification. Superimposition of the glans on the bones of the pubic arch may give rise to shadows suggestive of localized osteosclerosis.

Inconstant shadows of diminished density in the pelvis are cast by gas in the pelvic segments of the small intestine, colon, and rectum. Gas shadows superimposed on the pelvic bones produce local areas of diminished density which can simulate bone defects or bone destruction. Residual barium from earlier contrast examinations, foreign bodies, and fecaliths can result in confusing densities. After excretory urography, and after CT, MRI, or interventional procedures during which contrast material has been used, accumulations of radiodense material may produce confusing shadows in the lower abdomen and pelvis. Opaque myelographic medium may extend along lumbar nerve sheaths and persist in segments overlying the ilia.

Abnormal Soft Tissues

Dermoids are not infrequently located in the buttocks, and teratomas occur in that region as well as in the ovaries. Their skeletal components may be visualized but not clearly identified and lead to diagnostic concern during evaluation of pelvic roentgen-

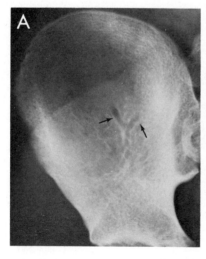
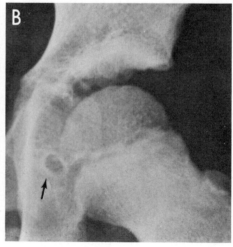

FIG 2–84.
Normal vascular markings in the pelvic bones. **A,** Y-shaped tubular shadow *(arrows)* in the ilium of a boy 4 years of age. **B,** circular vascular foramen *(arrow)* in the body of the ischium of an asymptomatic girl 4 years of age. Sometimes several small circular foramina are present in the same site instead of a single large foramen, as in this patient.

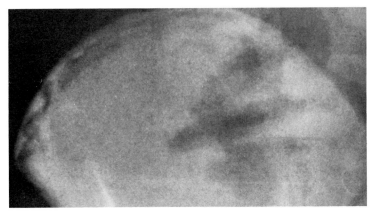

FIG 2–85.
Multiple independent ossification centers in the apophyseal cartilage of the crest of the ilium of a healthy girl 15 years of age, which simulate comminuted fracture fragments.

ograms. Opaque appendiceal fecaliths, urinary stones, and various medications should be considered when small, dense images are encountered. Granulomatous disorders affecting pelvic lymph nodes may result in calcification in the region. Pelvic phleboliths are rare in children but are occasionally seen in association with pelvic hemangiomas.

Normal and Variant Skeletal Structures

The normal pelvis at three different ages, and some of the normal secondary ossification centers, are shown in Figures 2–82 and 2–83. Grooves or channels for vascular structures can be seen in the ilium and ischium (Fig 2–84,*A* and *B*). The crestal center

of the ilium often develops from several foci that fuse with one another before fusing with the ala (Fig 2–85). Irregular extension of ossification into the cartilaginous roof of the acetabulum is a normal phenomenon during growth (Fig 2–86); the regularly smooth configuration of the roof develops from confluence of individual bony foci near the end of the first decade. Accessory centers of ossification may develop in cartilage in the spine of the ischium, and also in the rim of the acetabulum (the roentgenographic "os acetabuli"); they usually become visible between the 14th and 18th year (Figs 2–87 and 2–88), after which they fuse with the main body of the ischium and ilium, respectively. Rarely, the roentgenographic os acetabuli persists as a separate ossicle. The anatomical os acetabuli is an ossification center, or group of centers, that appears during pu-

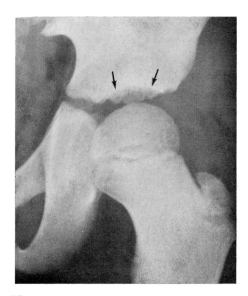

FIG 2–86.
Normal irregular margins of the acetabulum *(arrows)* in a boy 6 years of age.

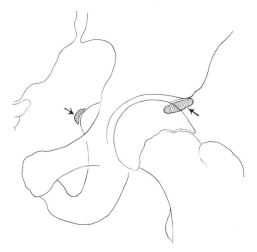

FIG 2–87.
Accessory secondary pelvic ossification centers; tracing of a roentgenogram. Ossicle in the rim of the acetabulum and in the tip of the ischial spine in a patient 14 years of age.

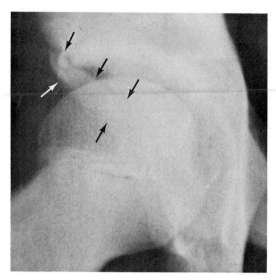

FIG 2–88.
Os acetabuli marginalis superior in the cartilaginous rim of the acetabulum of a girl 11 years of age. These normal separate marginal ossicles should not be mistaken for fracture fragments or calciferous foci in the soft tissues.

berty in the anterior segment of the Y cartilage in the wall of the acetabulum.

Ossification of the cartilage in the ischiopubic synchondrosis is extremely variable in both velocity and pattern. Caffey and Ross (1956) found that bilateral fusion of the ischiopubic synchondrosis is complete in about 6% of children at 4 years of age, and in 83% at 12 years. Unilateral swelling at the synchondrosis (Fig 2–89) was present in 18% of children at 7 years, and bilateral swelling in 47%. In some girls, the ischiopubic synchondrosis may close as early as the third year. They concluded that swelling preceded closure of the synchondrosis in most, and perhaps all, cases. The swellings lasted from 1 to 3 years. Irregular mineralization was present in

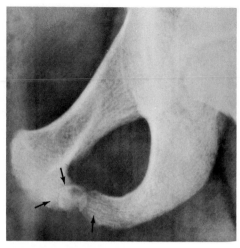

FIG 2–90.
Independent supernumerary circular ossification center in the ischiopubic synchondrosis of an asymptomatic boy 8 years of age.

about 42% of all subjects between ages 4 and 11; it was never present without swelling and tended to develop in the more pronounced examples of swelling. Occasionally, an independent supernumerary ossification center may develop in the ischiopubic synchondrosis (Fig 2–90). Kaufmann observed a similar center in an infant aged 6 months. Cawley and associates found accumulation of radionuclide to vary in intensity and, frequently, to be asymmetric in the ischiopubic synchondrosis area in healthy children during the period of beginning, but incomplete, fusion.

Cases have been reported in which regional pain and tenderness and impaired locomotion were associated with irregular mineralization and swelling of the ischiopubic synchondrosis; this clinical picture

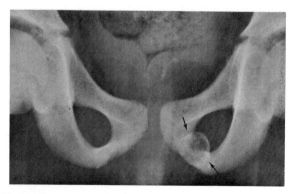

FIG 2–89.
Irregular mineralization and swelling of the left ischiopubic synchondrosis (arrows) in an asymptomatic boy 7 years of age. The osteoporotic swollen synchondrosis projects into the obturator foramen.

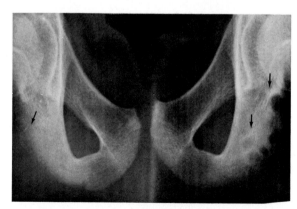

FIG 2–91.
Patchy, "soap-bubble" rarefaction of the ischial ramus and tuberosity on the left, with similar but much less marked changes at the same site on the right ischium of an asymptomatic boy 12 years of age. The possibility of prior, self-induced injury during play cannot be excluded. (Courtesy of Dr. R. Parker Allen, Denver, Colo.)

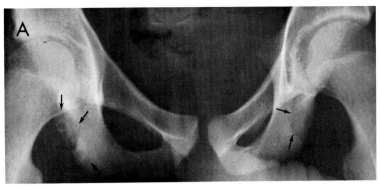
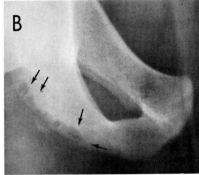

FIG 2–92.
Irregularities in both ischia of asymptomatic boys 12 and 11 years of age. In **A,** the right ischium is irregularly rarefied at the tuberosity and slightly caudad into the ramus. The tuberosity of the left is-chium is evenly rarefied. In **B,** there is "bubbly" rarefaction in the right tuberosity and caudad into the ramus.

and the associated roentgen findings have been called ischiopubic osteochondrosis (van Neck disease) in the belief that it is analogous anatomically and pathogenetically to ischemic necrosis of the skeleton, such as Perthes disease in the head of the femur and Köhler disease in the navicular bone. Junge and Heuck noted the considerable frequency with which the radiographic changes occur in asymptomatic school children, beginning about the age of 5 years. These authors, as well as Byers, report no evidence of inflammation or other pathologic change in material removed from a "swollen" ischiopubic synchondrosis. Apparently, the prognosis has always been favorable. Osteochondrosis is believed to arise, near the time of fusion, from microtrauma resulting from excessive or repeated activity of the adductor muscles that insert into the region of the synchondrosis. This region is also a classic site of stress fracture in the adult, and the lesion has been considered a pediatric equivalent of this in an appropriate clinical setting of local pain and progressive radiographic signs.

The diagnosis of osteomyelitis has also been made in some children with swelling of the ischiopubic junction. It is supported by positive blood cultures, elevated erythrocyte sedimentation rates, change from normal radiographs to focal irregularity before healing, and scintigraphic findings that differed from those in normal ischiopubic synchondroses. Histologic proof has not been demonstrated. In these cases, too, the prognosis has always been favorable following antibiotic treatment of 4½ to 12 weeks' duration.

Notwithstanding the above, it would seem that for the incidental observation of radiographic features, the normal irregular mineralization and vari-

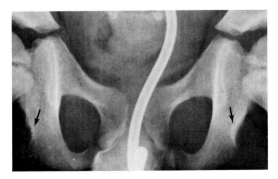

FIG 2–93.
Conspicuously deep and large lesser sciatic notches with sclerotic edges *(arrows)* in an asymptomatic boy 4 years of age.

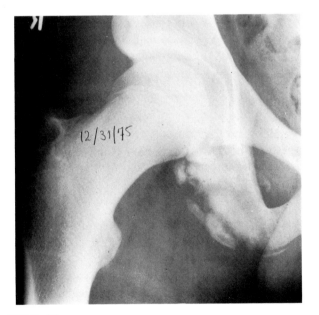

FIG 2–94.
New bone formation in avulsed cartilage from the ischium in a teen-age athlete who had been active in spite of moderate pain for over 6 months following an acute episode. **(From Silverman FN:** *Semin Roentgenol* 1978; 13:167–176. Used by permission.)

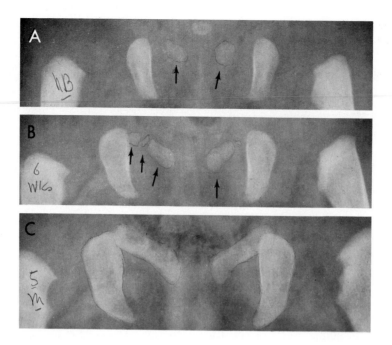

FIG 2–95.
Retarded and irregular mineralization of both superior pubic rami. **A,** neonatal. In the pubic rami, ossification is confined on each side to a round center; most of the superior pubic rami are entirely radiolucent because ossification has not yet occurred. **B,** at 6 weeks. Ossification is now increased in both superior rami, but it is still incomplete and irregular. On the right side there are at least three large independent ossification centers with radiolucent clefts between them. **C,** at 5 months. The superior rami are evenly and extensively ossified, but there is still cartilage between the dorsal ends of the rami and their ischial bodies. The changes in the pubic bones are chance findings in a patient who also had bilateral dysplasia and dislocation of the hips.

able scintigraphic features in this site should be kept in mind when the question of osteochondrosis or early osteomyelitic or neoplastic destruction at the ischiopubic synchondrosis is raised.

Irregularities in the posterolateral edge of the ischium may also be observed; occasionally during preadolescence, the lateral borders of the body of the ischium and its inferior ramus show marked irregularity both in the margin and in density (Fig 2–91); the two sides may be unequally affected (Fig 2–92). During growth and before fusion of the body of the ischium to its scalelike epiphysis along its under edge, this ischial edge is a provisional zone of calcification and is analogous to the provisional zones of calcification in the metaphyses of all the long bones; it is not cortical lamellar bone. The ischial spine, projecting posteriorly, usually is not visible in frontal radiographs of the pelvis. The lesser sciatic notch lies below it and sometimes appears as an indentation on the lateral margin of the ischium (Fig 2–93), at the region where the ischial irregularities are most common.

Some of the "variations" in mineralization are almost certainly sequelae to the normal vigorous activity of children and the response to minor tendon avulsions from sites where cartilage has yet to change to bone; they are comparable to minor

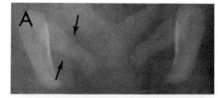

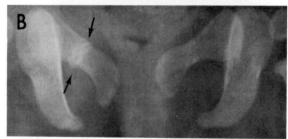

FIG 2–96.
Congenital "strip" defect in the superior ramus of the pubis; these lesions may be unilateral or bilaterally symmetric. **A,** at birth, there is a vertical band of diminished density in the middle third of the pubic ramus. **B,** at 6 months, at the same site there is a narrower radiolucent band, which is now bordered by strips of increased density. The patient was always asymptomatic, and palpation disclosed no signs of fracture at this site.

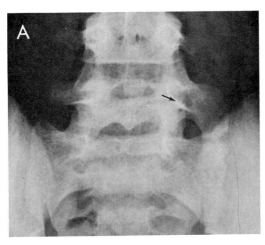
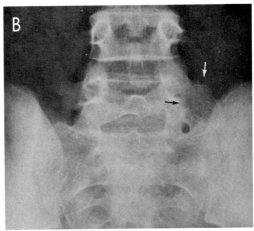

FIG 2–97.
Unilateral sacralization of the fifth lumbar vertebra. **A,** in a boy 6 years of age. **B,** in a boy 11 years of age.

epiphyseal separations. A few weeks of clinical observation during limited activity serves to resolve the significance of the observations when local symptoms were the reason for examination. The response to avulsions in more heavily muscled older children is illustrated in Figure 2–94 (see also Figs 2–113 to 2–116).

Delayed and irregular mineralization of the pubic rami may be present at birth with subsequent mineralization from several ossification centers (Fig 2–95). Vertical, radiolucent clefts occasionally noted as incidental findings in pelvis radiographs (Fig 2–96) probably represent bars of nonossified cartilage between expanding ossification centers. The medial edges of the bodies of the pubic bones are of-

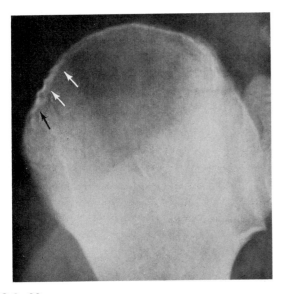

FIG 2–98.
Normal marginal scalloping in the ventral segment of the iliac crest of an asymptomatic girl 6 years of age.

ten irregularly mineralized during the growth period.

Failure of segmentation between the lateral masses of the first sacral and the fifth lumbar segments occurs in the variant known as sacralization of the fifth lumbar vertebra (Fig 2–97); it can be unilateral or bilateral and may be associated with narrowing of the lumbosacral interspace.

Defects in mineralization of the sacral neural arches are common in apparently normal infants and children (Fawcitt). The neural arches of the fourth and fifth lumbar segments are often similarly affected. These "defects" are not necessarily actual anatomical defects of the neural arches and, consequently, the term "spina bifida occulta" is often a misleading one. The arch is usually intact anatomically and the image defect represents a localized deficiency of ossification in cartilage rather than a gap in the arch itself. In many cases, the defects seen during the early years of life disappear in later childhood owing to ossification of the cartilaginous segment (Sutow and Pryde).

The iliac crest is smooth at birth but often becomes wavy and irregular after the second or third year (Fig 2–98). The ventral segment of the crest is always the most affected, and in many instances the scalloping of the crest is confined to the anterior portions. Such crestal irregularities may persist until puberty, after which they are obliterated by fusion of the crest of the ilium with the epiphyseal center.

REFERENCES

Bernard C, Sirinelli D, Timores, et al: Ostéochondrose ischio-pubiènne (cas radiologique du mois). *Arch Fr Pediatr* 1986; 43:505–506.

Byers PD: Ischio-pubic "osteochondritis": A report of a case and a review: *J Bone Joint Surg [Br]* 1963; 45:694–702.

Caffey J, Madell SH: Ossification of the pubic bones at birth. *Radiology* 1956; 67:346–350.

Caffey J, Ross SE: The ischiopubic synchondrosis in healthy children: Some normal roentgenographic findings. *Am J Roentgenol* 1956; 76:488–494.

Caffey J, Ross SE: Pelvic bones in infantile mongoloidism: Radiographic features. *Am J Roentgenol* 1958; 80:458–467.

Cawley KA, Dvorak AD, Wilmot MD: Normal anatomic variant: Scintigraphy of the ischiopubic synchondrosis. *J Nucl Med* 1983; 24:14–16.

Fawcitt J: Some radiological aspects of congenital anomalies of the spine in childhood and infancy. *Proc R Soc Med* 1959; 52:331–333.

Freedman E: Os acetabuli. *Am J Roentgenol* 1934; 32:492–495.

Jarvis J, McIntyre W, Udjus K, et al: Osteomyelitis of the ischiopubic synchondrosis. *J Pediatr Orthop* 1985; 5:163–166.

Junge H, Heuck F: Die Osteochondropathia ischiopubica (gleichzeitig ein Beitrag zur normalen Entwicklung der Scham-Sitzbeingrenze in Wachstumsalter). *Fortschr Geb Rontgenstr* 1953; 78:656–668.

Kaufmann HJ: *Röntgenbefunde am kindlichen Becken bei angeborenen Skelettaffektionen und chromosomalen Aberrationen.* Stuttgart, Georg Thieme Verlag, 1964.

Kloiber R, Udjus K, McIntyre W, et al: The scintigraphic and radiographic appearance of the ischiopubic synchondroses in normal children and in osteomyelitis. *Pediatr Radiol* 1988; 18:57–61.

Reynolds EL: The bony pelvic girdle in early infancy: A roentgenometric study. *Am J Phys Anthropol* 1945; 3:321–354.

Sutow WW, Pryde AW: Incidence of spina bifida occulta in relation to age. *Am J Dis Child* 1956; 91:211–217.

Van Neck M: Ostéochondrite du pubis. *Arch Franco-Belge Chir* 1924; 27:238–240.

Zander G: "Os acetabuli" and other bone nuclei: Periarticular calcifications at hip-joint. *Acta Radiol* 1943; 24:317–327.

SECTION 8

Congenital Malformations of the Pelvis

Aplasia and hypoplasia of the ischia or ilia are uncommon, but Kaufmann has described instances of total or partial reduction deformities involving ilium, ischium, and pubis in addition to the more common sacral and coccygeal abnormalities. The last-named are relatively frequent, varying from clinically insignificant absence of coccygeal segments to total sacral agenesis with associated visceral and neuromuscular manifestations. Other components of the pelvis may be dysplastic independently or as part of syndromic disorders. The pelvis also may participate in generalized dysplasias of the skeleton.

SACRAL AGENESIS

Because of associated spinal cord and spinal nerve abnormalities, most forms of sacral agenesis are accompanied by urinary tract abnormalities and disturbances of locomotion. Exceptions do occur. Vlachos reported a 5-year-old boy with partial sacral agenesis and crossed renal ectopia, but with no orthopedic signs or symptoms. One of the patients in the report

of Blumel and associates lacked the three lower sacral segments and the coccyx, but no orthopedic abnormalities were present, although urinary tract infection was a problem. Absence of part or all of the lumbar spine may accompany the more severe forms of sacral agenesis. Mongeau and LeClaire reported a patient in whom the ninth thoracic vertebra was the most caudal segment present.

Partial absence of the sacrum (Fig 2–99) may be recognized by sacral scoliosis. Also known as the "scimitar" deformity, it may be a marker for the "Currarino triad" where it is associated with anorectal malformations and a presacral mass, commonly an anterior meningocele, a presacral teratoma, an enteric cyst, or a combination thereof. The condition is often familial. Total agenesis is accompanied by a narrowed pelvis with the medial portions of the iliac alae in contact (Fig 2–100). Maternal diabetes occurs with considerable frequency in the sporadic cases (phocomelic diabetic embryopathy), but rare familial cases are recorded without such history. Sacral agenesis is included in the group of malformations

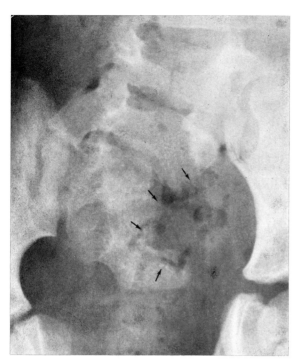

FIG 2–99.
Congenital regional hypoplasia of the left side of the sacrum *(arrows)* in a boy 6 years of age who had chronic pyuria.

known as the "caudal regression syndrome" that comprises malformations ranging from imperforate anus to sirenomelia and is believed to result from defects in embryonic development of the caudal mesoderm. Rarely, the lateral mass of the sacrum may be partially or completely absent; the adjacent ilium is usually displaced laterad and cephalad with resulting asymmetric pelvis. A widening of the symphysis may accompany this deformity.

SPINA BIFIDA

True spina bifida is most frequent in the lower levels of the vertebral column. Meningocele and meningomyelocele are usually associated together with the Arnold-Chiari group of malformations. Defects in the bodies or pedicles rather than the neural arches may give rise to anterior protrusion of intraspinal elements. The subject is discussed in more detail in Chapter 3.

OTHER PELVIC DYSPLASIAS

In exstrophy of the bladder, the pubic arch appears open and the centers of the pubic bones may be spread several inches apart. In some instances, the inferior pubic rami appear hypoplastic and their mineralization is delayed. Separation and incomplete ossification of the pubic bones have also been found in association with imperforate anus, diastasis of the recti muscles, deficiencies in the abdominal and pelvic musculature, and in epispadias. Persisting delayed ossification of the pubic bones is common in cleidocranial dysplasia.

Riblike structures occasionally arise from the sacrum or coccyx and are discovered incidental to examination of the pelvis for unassociated reasons (Fig 2–101). Sullivan and Cornwell identified a pelvic rib in films of a 15-year-old girl examined after a motor accident. The bone was curved and measured 6.0 × 2.5 × 1.8 cm. After excision, a normal medullary cavity, normal haversian cortical walls, and normal periosteum were demonstrated. There was no costal cartilage. The rib was attached to the right side of

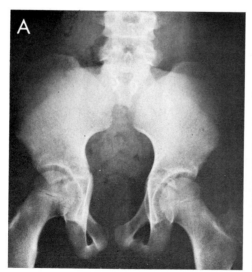
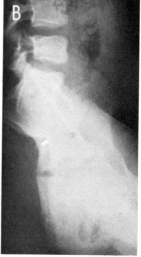

FIG 2–100.
Severe hypoplasia of the sacrum with bilaterally contracted pelvis in a girl 10 years of age. Only the first sacral segment is present. Both femoral necks demonstrate moderate coxa valga. **A,** frontal, and **B,** lateral projection.

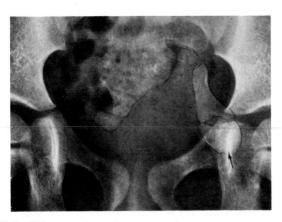

FIG 2–101.
Congenital left-sided pelvic rib with posterior attachment to the sacrum, which is deviated toward the right. This girl of 8 years was asymptomatic but had a palpable left-sided pelvic mass. The rib was excised without difficulty. (**Courtesy of Dr. Robert Wilkinson, Boston.**)

the junction of the sacrum and coccyx by ligaments and was freely movable. In two patients described by Pais et al., the bony masses arose from the coccyx or sacrococcygeal junction, were well differentiated in the form of ribs, and extended laterally and caudally into the gluteal region. Other cases have since been reported and likewise are asymptomatic.

Thirty-four cases of human "tails" have been reported according to Spiegelmann and associates. In all cases the "tail" lacked bone, cartilage, notochord, and spinal cord and in none were there any associated underlying spinal cord or vertebral abnormalities. If vertebral abnormalities are noted, lipomyeloschisis should be suspected.

The pelvic features of various skeletal dysplasias

are described in the section devoted to that group of disorders.

CONGENITAL DISLOCATION OF HIP

Congenital dislocation of the hip (CDH) varies greatly in incidence among different peoples and in different regions. It is more common in girls than in boys in the ratio of about 5:1; and it is ten times as common after breech deliveries as cephalic, but with the girl-to-boy ratio reduced to 2:1. It is more common in dizygotic twins, in the first-born girl, and in those born during winter months than in their opposites. Except for teratologic dislocations, as in some instances of proximal focal femoral deficiency, prenatal and perinatal relaxation of the capsule of the hip joint appears to be the primary cause of this often disabling condition that can be recognized in the newborn. Limitation of abduction by restrictive clothing or by actual binding of the legs in adduction, a practice still common in various cultures, may be responsible for postnatal onset of dislocation as late as the latter half of the first year. Dysplasia of the acetabulum (indicated by increased acetabular angle), elongation of the capsule, femoral anteversion, and contracture of the periarticular muscles are all secondary complications of primary hypotonia of the capsule and consequent malposition of the cartilaginous femoral head (Figs 2–102 and 2–103). Morphologic and histochemical studies of joint capsule and ligamentum teres biopsies during open reduction of CDH have demonstrated changes that were believed to be secondary to the mechanical stresses caused by the dislocation. The high incidence of

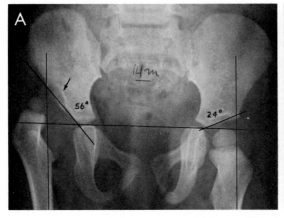

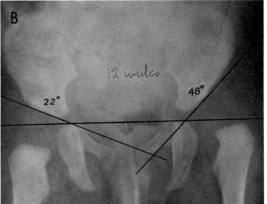

FIG 2–102.
A, unilateral CDH in a girl 14 months of age. On the right side all three elements in Putti's triad are visible: (1) hypoplasia of the acetabular roof with increase in its pitch; (2) hypoplasia of the femoral ossification center; (3) dislocation of the femur cephalad and laterad. The *arrow* points to a false acetabulum. **B,** dysplasia with dislocation of the left hip at 3 months of age. The left acetabular angle measures 48 degrees, and the left femur is dislocated cephalad and laterad.

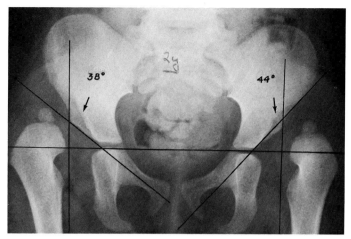

FIG 2–103.
Bilateral CDH in a girl 2 years of age. Putti's triad is present on both sides; the right acetabular angle is enlarged to 38 degrees, the left to 44 degrees. The *arrows* point to bilateral false acetabula.

CDH in girls suggested a hormonal factor (Andren) but no conclusive support for this has appeared. Thieme and colleagues measured the urinary estrogen content in 16 patients with CDH and 19 matched controls during the first 6 days of life and found no significant differences.

Initially, radiographic identification of congenital dislocation of the hip was made in late childhood. In 1925, Hilgenreiner described early radiographic diagnosis in infants by measurement of acetabular angles (Fig 2–104). The method was considered objective and was accepted with enthusiasm even after 1956 when Coleman and Caffey, independently, challenged the validity of the "standards" for acetabular angles. It was pointed out that the number of

patients previously evaluated was inadequate for a meaningful statistical value for the measurements. Furthermore, in practice, values reported as normal averages were used as limiting values between normal and abnormal. Caffey's study of over 600 infants indicated that radiographic examination, apart from demonstrating gross dislocation or malformation, had little to offer in the diagnosis of CDH in the newborn period. Nevertheless, radiographic methods (Andren and von Rosen) for identification of CDH has enjoyed considerable popularity among orthopedists even though strict adherence to the positioning standards is seldom accomplished. At present, US has become the procedure of choice for the diagnosis of congenital hip dislocation in the

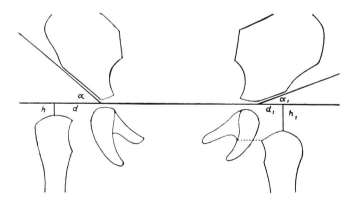

FIG 2–104.
Hilgenreiner's method for measuring the acetabular angles and degree of femoral dislocation before the femoral ossification centers appear. The horizontal line is drawn through the Y cartilages and is known as the Y–Y, or Hilgenreiner, line. The oblique line parallel to the acetabular roof is drawn to intersect the Y–Y line; the angle between these lines is the acetabular angle. Vertical lines *(h)* are dropped from the Y–Y line to the middle of the supe-

rior edge of each femoral shaft; their lengths measure the cephalad displacement if any is present. The distance *(d)* between the intersections of the roof lines and the *h* lines measures the lateral displacement of the femur. In this figure, the right acetabular angle is increased to 40 degrees, and the right femur is dislocated cephalad and laterad.

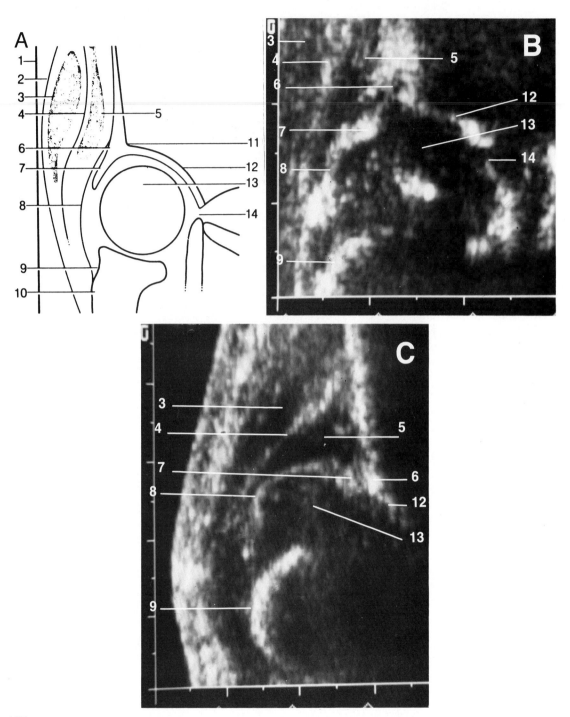

FIG 2–105.
Ultrasonographic features in the normal infant hip: *1,* skin; *2,* sub-cutaneous tissue; *3,* gluteus medius muscle; *4,* intermuscular sep-tum; *5,* gluteus minimus muscle; *6,* cartilaginous rim; *7,* acetabular limbus; *8,* articular capsule; *9,* osseocartilaginous border of femo-ral neck; *10,* greater trochanter; *11,* osseous rim of acetabulum; *12,* acetabular roof (ilium); *13,* cartilaginous head; *14,* triradiate cartilage. **A,** diagram of landmarks in longitudinal section. **B,** ultra-sonogram of the hip in a normal 7-week-old boy, with beginning calcification of the ossification center in the femoral head. **C,** ultra-sonogram in a 4-day-old girl with complete dislocation of the right hip. (**A** from Schulz RD, Zeiger M: *Radiol Today* 1987; 4:103–105. Used by permission. **B** and **C** courtesy of Dr. R.D. Schulz, Stuttgart, Germany.)

newborn and young infant (Zieger and Schulz). MRI and CT imaging have been used successfully, but are too elaborate for routine screening.

The monumental studies of CDH in the newborn by Andren and von Rosen, and by Palmen, indicated that a reliable, simple indication of CDH in the newborn period is clinical examination. The Ortolani maneuver, which detects the return of a dislocated femoral head to its acetabular cavity, coupled with the "subluxation provocation" maneuver (Palmen, Coleman), which recognizes dislocatability under appropriate physical stresses, have been utilized by trained examiners in studies of almost 500,000 children in Sweden and in over 62,000 children born during 1 year in Yugoslavia. In these and similar studies, all infants with positive tests were treated with devices maintaining constant, gentle abduction and external rotation of the hips for approximately 6 weeks, with the net result that gross dislocations and other sequelae of CDH in childhood have been virtually eliminated in infants so treated. Infants immobilized in plaster casts may develop necrosis of the femoral head ossification centers in the originally healthy femur as well as in the dislocated femur during treatment for unilateral CDH (Gore). Rarely, Perthes disease develops several years after apparently successful, uncomplicated closed reduction.

It is advisable to reexamine all infants during well-baby visits for clinical signs of hip abnormality up to the time of ambulation, as both Palmen, and Brecelj and associates, found that a small number of children, clinically and radiologically normal as newborns, may develop distinct dislocation by the second half of the first year. Closed reduction is still feasible with positional treatment in such cases, but for longer periods of time than in the newborn. In patients diagnosed late, especially those unresponsive to attempted closed reduction, arthrography may be helpful by demonstrating contraction of the capsule or interposition of the capsule and labrum between the head and the acetabular cavity preventing reduction. CT can demonstrate the exact location of the structures and can evaluate anterior or posterior malposition of the head, even through a plaster cast.

The application of US to the diagnosis of congenital dislocation of the hip has provided a noninvasive, nonionizing, repeatable, and sensitive method for evaluation of equivocal clinical signs of hip abnormality. The technique of Graf and his standards are used by many ultrasonographers with very satisfying results. Infants up to the age of 1 year can be examined satisfactorily with the usual 5-MHz transducers; in newborns, a 7.5-MHz transducer is recommended.

The cartilage components of the hip joint as well as the capsule and the margins of the bony structures can be visualized (Fig 2–105). US has been found to be 100% sensitive and highly specific for monitoring the position of the femoral head and the acetabular cavity in patients under treatment with the popular Pavlik harness.

Occasionally, newborn infants will have limitation of abduction and external rotation of the hip without clear-cut dislocation. Radiographs are normal except for adduction of the affected femur; the pelvis tends to be rotated and a true AP projection is difficult to obtain. It has been suggested that the adductor muscles on the affected side are "tight" because of the fetal position. Spontaneous resolution is the rule. Bowyer and associates reported a similar clinical finding, not present at birth, in older infants during the first year of life. Radiologic findings in these infants include acetabular angles greater on the affected than on the normal side, retardation of epiphyseal development of the ipsilateral femoral head, pelvic obliquity, and rotational deformity of the pelvis in the transaxial plane. Plagiocephaly was present in almost all cases. The authors believed that these features are due to postnatal postural habits and are self-correcting. None of 98 patients they examined had "clicks" (i.e., positive Ortolani or Palmen maneuvers).

Radiographic features similar to those described

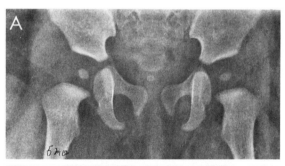
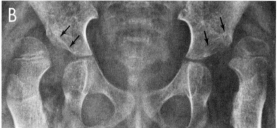

FIG 2–106.
Acquired bilateral dislocation of the hips in neuromuscular disease. **A,** normal at 5 months of age. **B,** bilateral dislocation of the hips at age 5 years. The patient had meningoencephalitis at 5 months of age, followed by persistent generalized spastic paraplegia.

for CDH (shallow acetabuli with highly angled roofs, lateral and cephalic displacement of the upper end of the femur, and small ossification center for the head) can be observed occasionally in congenital cretins. With improved tone and extension of ossification into the radiolucent cartilage of the acetabular roof following appropriate therapy, spontaneous resolution of the "dislocation" can occur. Recurrent dislocation has been observed in a 26-month-old girl with congenital indifference to pain.

Acquired traumatic dislocation of the hip is rare;

about four fifths of the cases occur in boys. Two thirds of them have complete recovery, and very few develop late coxa plana. Acquired nontraumatic dislocation may develop in neuromuscular disease (Fig 2–106) and is frequent in cerebral palsy. It can develop fairly rapidly in pyarthrosis of the hip; in such cases, clinical signs of infection and swelling of soft tissues may point to the proper diagnosis. Traumatic epiphyseal separation of the femoral head or fracture of the femoral neck in very young infants may simulate congenital dislocation as the head and

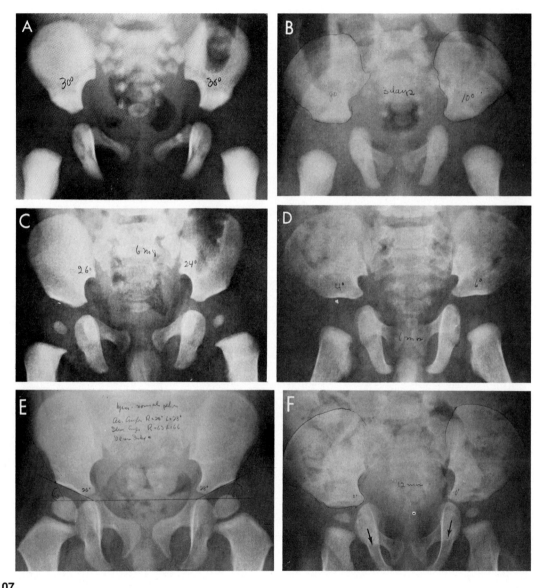

FIG 2–107.
Pelvic changes in infantile Down syndrome. **A** and **B,** normal and Down syndrome newborns; **C** and **D,** normal and Down syndrome children at 6 months, **E** and **F,** normal and Down syndrome children at 12 months. At all ages the ilia are large and flare laterad, and acetabular angles are small. In Down syndrome children older than 9 months, the ischial rami are usually hypoplastic, with small girth and a long taper to the ischiopubic synchondroses. Ossification centers in the proximal epiphyseal cartilages appear later and remain smaller in Down syndrome children than in normal children.

neck are still cartilaginous and not visible radiographicaly. With clinical or radiologic signs of abnormal orientation of the upper end of the femur and the adjacent acetabular cavity, this possibility must be entertained, especially when they are associated with a history of abnormal presentation and difficult delivery, or of other traumatic episodes.

DOWN SYNDROME

The pelvic features of Down syndrome during the first years of life can be diagnostic at a time when clinical findings may be equivocal (Fig 2–107). The acetabular slopes are flattened, and the ilia are large and flare laterad. After the sixth month, the ischial rami become hypoplastic; usually by the 12th month they are elongated and slender and have a long taper at their caudal ends. Kaufmann showed that the distinctive configuration of the ilia was produced by their having a greater parallelism with the coronal plane than the normal, and an outward and downward rotation on their sagittal axes. These changes can be quantitated by the method of Caffey and Ross (1958) (Fig 2–108). In affected infants, the size of the acetabular angles varied between 7 and 25 degrees (average, 16), and in normals between 12

and 37 (average, 28). The iliac angles varied between 30 and 56 degrees (average, 44) in comparison with normals in whom they measured between 44 and 66 degrees (average, 55). The less reliable iliac indices, which represent the sums of the two acetabular angles and the two iliac angles divided by 2, varied from 49 to 80 degrees (average, 60) in comparison with normals in whom the values ranged from 65 to 97 degrees (average, 81). These measurements proved diagnostic in about 80% of patients with Down syndrome, were suggestive in about 20%, and were normal in only 4%. The diagnostic significance and limitations of the method in the Caffey-Ross (1958) study have been corroborated by others.

Radiologic features outside the pelvis also occur in Down syndrome. The manubrial ossification center of the sternum is divided into two moieties, one above the other, best seen in lateral projection. In the study of Currarino and Swanson, this occurred in 90% of patients under 5 years of age and was found in only 20% of normal infants and children of the same age. The frequency of double manubrial centers in the newborn period was 80% in comparison with 9.6% in normal infants in a study by Edwards et al.; the frequency of 11 rib pairs was 33% and 5.2%, and of a bell-shaped thorax, 80% and 23.6%, respectively. When all three features were present in a newborn, the predictability was 58.4%. The pelvic configuration remains the best single radiographic feature of Down syndrome, but the definitive diagnosis is the karyotypic analysis. In the cranium, the interorbital distance is reduced in comparison with normals. The skeletal manifestations of Down syndrome, except for the interorbital distance, appear to be less marked in children with the mosaic form of the condition than in those with typical trisomy 21 or translocation.

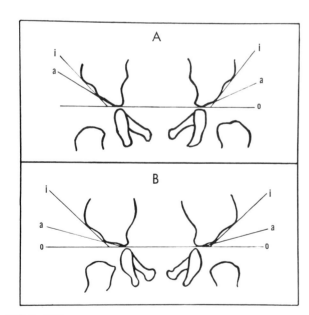

FIG 2–108.
Pelvic measurements in a normal newborn **(A)** and a newborn with Down syndrome. **(B).** The acetabular angle is enclosed in the lines *ao*, and the iliac angle in the lines *io*. In Down syndrome children, both of these angles are smaller than normal. Line *a* is drawn parallel to the face of the acetabular cavity. Line *i* is drawn through the two lateralmost points on the lateral edge of the ilial wing, below and above.

REFERENCES

Sacral Agenesis, Spina Bifida, and Other Pelvic Dysplasias
Blumel J, Evans EB, Eggers GWN: Partial and complete agenesis or malformation of the sacrum with associated anomalies. Etiologic and clinical study with special reference to heredity. A preliminary report. *J Bone Joint Surg [Am]* 1959; 41:497–518.

Currarino G, Coln D, Votteler T: A triad of anorectal, sacral and presacral anomalies. *Radiology* 1981; 137:395–398.

Kaufmann HJ: *Röntgenbefunde am kindlichen Becken bei*

angeborenen Skelettaffektionen und chromosomalen Aberrationen. Stuttgart, Georg Thieme Verlag, 1964.

Kirks DR, Merton DF, Filston HC, et al: The Currarino triad: Complex of anorectal malformation, sacral bony abnormality, and presacral mass. *Pediatr Radiol* 1984; 14:220–225.

Mongeau M, LeClaire R: Complete agenesis of the lumbosacral spine: A case report. *J Bone Joint Surg [Am]* 1972; 54:161–164.

Naidich TP, McLone DG, Mutluer S: A new understanding of dorsal dysraphism with lipoma (lipomyeloschisis): Radiologic evaluation and surgical correction. *Am J Roentgenol* 1983; 140:1065–1078.

Pais MJ, Levine A, Pais SO: Coccygeal ribs: Development and appearance in two cases. *Am J Roentgenol* 1978; 131:164–166.

Perrot LJ, Williamson S, Jimenez JF: The caudal regression syndrome in infants of diabetic mothers. *Ann Clin Lab Sci* 1987; 17:211–220.

Spiegelmann R, Schindler E, Mintz M, et al: The human tail: A benign stigma. Case report. *J Neurosurg* 1985; 63:461–462.

Sullivan D, Cornwell WS: Pelvic rib: Report of a case. *Radiology* 1974; 110:355–357.

Vlachos P: Asymptomatic sacral agenesis with crossed renal extopia. *Helv Paediatr Acta* 1976; 31:275–277.

Congenital Dislocation of the Hip

Andren L: Pelvic instability in newborns with special reference to congenital dislocation of the hip and hormonal factors: A roentgenologic study. *Acta Radiol Suppl (Stockh)* 1962; 212.

Andren L, von Rosen S: The diagnosis of dislocation of the hip in newborns and the preliminary results of immediate treatment. *Acta Radiol* 1958; 49:89–95.

Bowyer FM, Hoyle MD, McCall IW, et al: Radiological evaluation of asymmetrical limitation of hip abduction during the first year of life. *Br J Radiol* 1985; 58:935–939.

Brecelj B: *Congenital Dysplasia of the Hip. Final Report.* Department of Health, Education, and Welfare Project 02.477.2 (old grant SRS-YUGO-28-69). Ljubljana, Yugoslavia, May 1973.

Caffey J, Ames R, Silverman WA, et al: Contradiction of the congenital dysplasia-predislocation hypothesis of congenital dislocation of the hip through a study of the normal variation in acetabular angles at successive periods in infants. *Pediatrics* 1956; 17:632–641.

Coleman SS: Diagnosis of congenital dysplasia of the hip in a newborn infant. *JAMA* 1956; 162:548–554.

Donaldson WF Jr, Rodriguez EE, Skovron M, et al: Traumatic dislocation of the hip in children. Final report by the Scientific Research Committee of the Pennsylvania Orthopedic Society. *J Bone Joint Surg [Am]* 1968; 59:79–88.

Edelson JG, Hirsch M, Weinberg H, et al: Congenital dislo-

cation of the hip and computerised axial tomography. *J Bone Joint Surg [Br]* 1984; 66:472–478.

Gore DR: Iatrogenic avascular necrosis of the hip in young children: A review of 6 cases. *J Bone Joint Surg [Am]* 1974; 56:493–502.

Graf R: Fundamentals of sonographic diagnosis of infant hip dysplasia. *J Pediatr Orthop* 1984; 4:735–740.

Grissom LE, Harcke HT, Kumar SJ, et al: Ultrasound evaluation of hip position in the Pavlik harness. *J Ultrasound Med* 1988; 7:1–6.

Hilgenreiner H: Zur Frühdiagnose und Frühbehandlung der angegorenen Hüftgelenkverrenkung. *Med Klinik* 1925; 21:1385–1388, 1425–1429.

Ippolito E, Ishii Y, Ponseti IV: Histologic, histochemical, and ultrastructural studies of the hip joint capsule and ligamentum teres in congenital dislocation of the hip. *Clin Orthop* 1980; 146:246–258.

Palmen K: Preluxation of the hip joint: Diagnosis and treatment in a newborn and the diagnosis of congenital dislocation of the hip joint in Sweden during the years 1948–1960. *Acta Paediatr Suppl* 1961; 129:50.

Palmen K, von Rosen SS: Late diagnosis of dislocation of the hip joint in children. *Acta Orthop Scand* 1975; 46:90–101.

Roberts JM, Taylor J, Burke S: Recurrent dislocation of the hip in congenital indifference to pain. Case report with arthrographic and operative findings. *J Bone Joint Surg [Am]* 1980; 62:829–831.

Thieme WT, Winne-Davies R, Blair HAF, et al: Clinical examination and urinary oestrogen assays in newborn children with congenital dislocation of the hip. *J Bone Joint Surg [Br]* 1968; 59:546–550.

Yousefzadeh D, Ramilo JL: Normal hip in children: Correlation of ultrasound with anatomic and cryomicrotomic sections. *Radiology* 1987; 165:647–656.

Zieger M: Ultrasound of the infant hip. Part II. Validity of the method. *Pediatr Radiol* 1986; 16:488–492.

Zieger M, Hilpert S, Schulz RD: Ultrasound of the infant hip. Part I. Basic principles. *Pediatr Radiol* 1986; 16:483–487.

Zieger M, Schulz RD: Ultrasonography of the infant hip. Part III. Clinical application. *Pediatr Radiol* 1987; 17:226–232.

Down Syndrome

Astley R: Chromosomal abnormalities in childhood with particular reference to Turner's syndrome and Mongolism. *Br J Radiol* 1963; 36:2–10.

Caffey J, Ross SE: Mongolism (mongoloid deficiency) during early infancy—some newly recognized diagnostic changes in the pelvic bones. *Pediatrics* 1956; 17:642–560.

Caffey J, Ross SE: Pelvic bones in infantile mongoloidism: Radiographic features. *Am J Roentgenol* 1958; 80:458–467.

Currarino G, Swanson GE: A developmental variant of ossification of the manubrium sterni in mongolism. *Radiology* 1964; 82:916.

Edwards DK, Berry CC, Hilton SW: Trisomy 21 in newborn
infants: Chest radiographic diagnosis. *Radiology* 1988;
167:317–318.

SECTION 9

Traumatic Lesions, Infections, Neoplasms, and Other Pelvic Disorders

FRACTURES

Fractures of the pelvis may be single or multiple (Figs 2–109 and 2–110); multiple fractures are common in automobile accidents (Fig 2–111) and injuries to pelvic soft tissues, especially bladder and urethra, should not be overlooked. Athletic injuries in the pelvis are most commonly stress fractures and apophyseal avulsions. Secondary epiphyses in the region of the iliac crests, ischial tuberosities, ischial spine, and the rims of the acetabula can be mistaken for fracture fragments in adolescents (see Fig 2–88). Breaks in one portion of the bony ring surrounding the obturator foramen are usually accompanied by a fracture on another segment of the ring; a similar situation may be present in the pelvic ring as well. Traumatic separation of the symphysis or sacroiliac joints may accompany fractures. If there is little separation of the fragments and the plane of a fracture is oblique to the projection of the x-ray beam, it may be necessary to examine the pelvis in several projections before the fracture is visualized. Stereoscopic films are helpful in clarifying the problem, but CT is the method par excellence to demonstrate complex fractures and the position of the component parts (Figs 2–112 and 2–113). Various pathologic processes that are uncertain or even invisible on conventional examinations may be clearly defined with

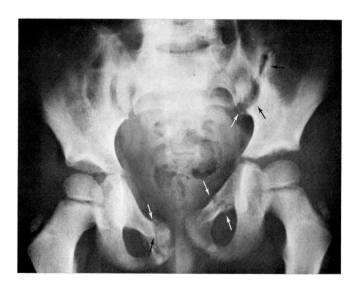

FIG 2–109.
Multiple fractures of the pelvis. *Arrows* indicate bilateral pubic fractures and sacroiliac separation as manifestations of the rule that the pelvic ring usually fractures in more than one site. Note the separation of the pubic bones at the synchondrosis.

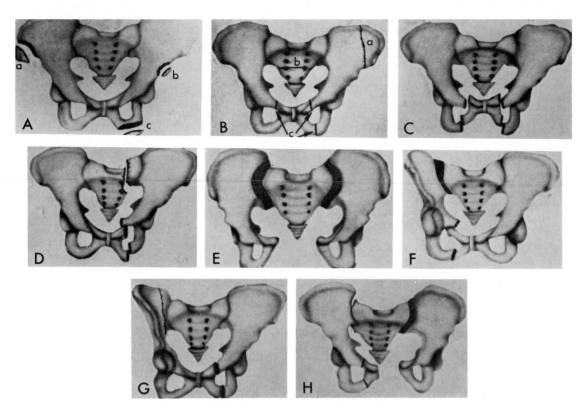

FIG 2–110.
Examples of pelvic fractures. **A,** avulsion fracture of the anterosuperior iliac spine *(a),* anteroinferior iliac spine *(b),* and ischial tuberosity *(c).* **B,** stable fractures of the wing of the ilium *(a),* body of the sacrum *(b),* and in the pubic rami *(c).* **C,** straddle fractures of the pubic rami with distraction of the fragments. **D,** longitudinal unilateral shear fractures of the lateral process of the sacrum and pubic rami on the left side. **E,** widening of both sacroiliac joints and separation of the symphysis pubis. **F,** lateral compression injury with fracture of the pubic rami on the side of the impact and widening of the sacroiliac joint on the same side. **G,** fracture (longitudinal) of the right iliac wing on the side of the impact and of the pubic rami on the opposite side. **H,** total pelvic disruption with stable fractures of the pubic rami on the side of the impact. (From Dunn AW, Morris HD: *J Bone Joint Surg [Am]* 1968; 50:1639–1648. Used with permission.)

FIG 2–111.
Fractures of the right pubic and ischial bones of a boy 7 years of age who was injured in an automobile accident. A substantial fragment is avulsed from the ischium *(lowest arrow).* (Courtesy of Dr. John Dorst, Baltimore, Md.)

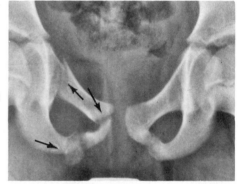

FIG 2–112.
This 7-year-old girl was injured in an automobile-pedestrian accident. Film of the pelvis shows disruption of the pubic symphysis, fracture of the body of the right pubis, possible separation of the left ischiopubic synchondrosis, and nondisplaced fractures of the inferior ramus of the left ischium and the superior ramus of the pubis. The left femoral head is displaced laterally in comparison with the right; traumatic dislocation had been reduced prior to this film. (Courtesy of Dr. Richard B. Jaffe, Salt Lake City, Utah.)

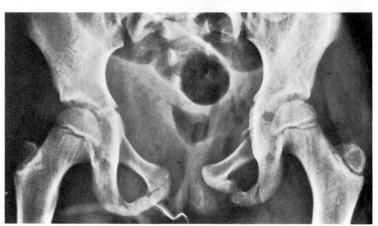

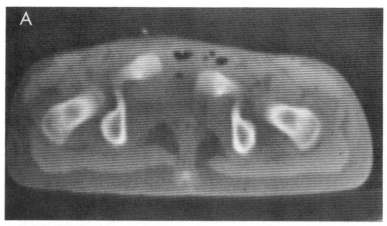

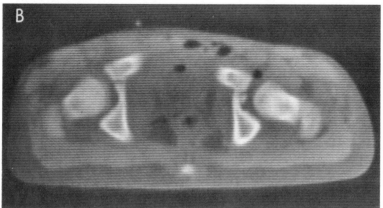

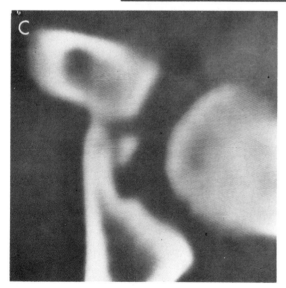

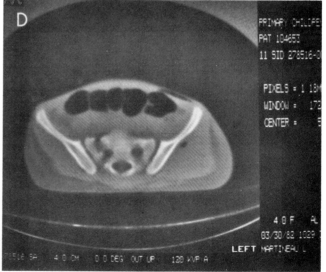

FIG 2–113.

Selected CT scans of the pelvis of the patient in the Figure 2–112. **A,** the diastasis pubis is clearly shown, and the left superior pubic ramus is depressed. **B,** the triradiate line is narrowed as a result of the left pubic ramus displacement. The left femoral head is displaced laterally in comparison with the right, and a small fragment of bone is noted in the cartilage space. **C,** reconstruction shows the fragment and a defect posteriorly from which it may have arisen. At surgery, no fragment was found in the joint, and the lesion was believed to be a subchondral fracture. **D,** an unsuspected fracture is shown in the right sacral ala. (Courtesy of Dr. Richard B. Jaffe, Salt Lake City, Utah.)

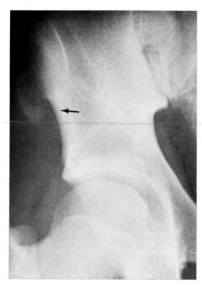

FIG 2–114.
Fracture and avulsion of a fragment of the iliac wing in a healthy boy 16 years of age who felt a sharp pain above his right hip as he left the starting block in a sprint.

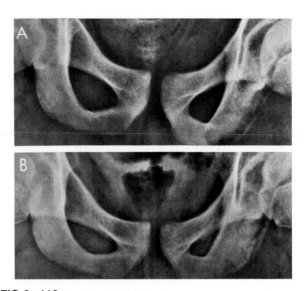

FIG 2–116.
Avulsion fracture of the apophysis of the ischium. **A,** this boy, 14 years of age, felt a sharp pain in the right buttock while jumping hurdles in a gymnasium. **B,** 10 days later, he tripped and fell and again had sharp pain in the right buttock.

CT. For example, it has demonstrated subchondral fractures previously unrecognized in sacroiliac joint trauma in children. Furthermore, CT demonstrates associated soft-tissue abnormalities, such as hematoma, not clinically obvious, within the bony pelvis or in the deep muscles of the upper thigh, and with three-dimensional reconstruction can demonstrate relations that are of importance for the orthopedic surgeon. Subtle diastasis and intra-articular fragments are best delineated by coronal reconstruc-

tions, sometimes coupled with sagittal reconstructions.

The ununited epiphyseal ossification centers of the pelvic bones may be torn away from the main mass during ordinary athletic activities, such as jumping and in sprinting races (Figs 2–114 and 2–115). Avulsion fractures of the ilia and ischia occur in a variety of patterns (Figs 2–116 and 2–117). The clinical features are not markedly different from those of slipped capital femoral epiphysis, toxic synovitis, or pathologic fractures, all of which must be

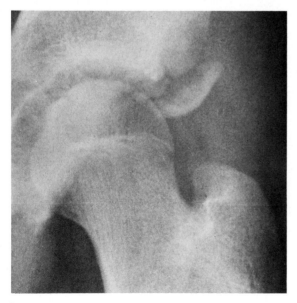

FIG 2–115.
Segmental avulsion fracture of the ilium at the site of the anteroinferior spine of a boy 13 years of age.

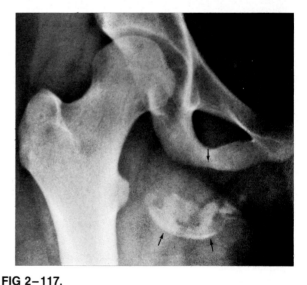

FIG 2–117.
Avulsion of the ischial apophysis *(upper arrow)* with a large comminuted fracture fragment widely displaced *(lower arrows).* The patient was a girl 15 years of age.

considered. In some instances, the avulsed osteocartilaginous mass undergoes a proliferative reaction but ultimate spontaneous resorption is the rule although it may be prolonged.

OSTEITIS AND OSTEOMYELITIS OF PELVIC BONES

Inflammatory disease of the pelvic bones is not uncommon; it may occur alone or as one of the sites of polyostotic infection. It is occasionally observed as a complication of a contiguous pelvic abscess, in which case intraosseous gas may be noted on CT examination. As in other bones, the anatomical changes consist of destructive and productive lesions with their usual bone density changes. The destructive features predominate in the early stages of infection. Gross destructive lesions in osteomyelitis of the ilium may simulate large, superimposed, gas-filled loops of bowel if there are no localizing symptoms. Symptoms are usually subacute in iliac infection apart from abdominal pain which may lead to overzealous search for gastrointestinal disease. In this and other pelvic bones, there is a history of fever and, often, an abnormal gait. Initial radiographs may be normal or demonstrate some soft-tissue swelling. The destructive radiographic changes are usually late in appearance being noted between 10 days to 10 weeks after clinical onset. Scintigraphy is much more sensitive for indicating bony involvement. MRI has a role in differentiating soft tissue infection with periostitis from osteomyelitis because of its ability to image the bone marrow. Tuberculous and nontuberculous inflammations are similar roentgenographically; Figure 2–118 illustrates an instance of cystic tuberculous destruction of the body of the ischium. Recurrent multifocal osteomyelitis (plasmacellular osteomyelitis) can also occur in the pelvic bones.

Pyogenic infections of the hip joints may accompany overt osteomyelitis but occur more frequently as an isolated pyarthrosis. Early diagnosis and management are imperative to prevent or minimize destruction of articular cartilage and compromise of joint function.

Osteitis pubis is found usually in adults following pelvic surgery. Rare cases are reported in children without prior surgery. The condition appears to be a self-limited disorder that goes through a cycle of local destruction and repair, usually with complete restitution of the pubic bones. However, ankylosis of the symphysis pubis has followed in some patients. The features are similar to those of spondyloarthritis (diskitis). Trauma has been postulated for

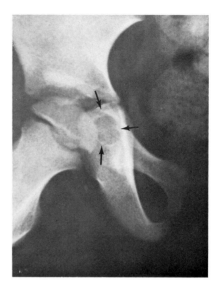

FIG 2–118.
Localized destructive tuberculous osteitis in the body of the ischium *(arrows)*.

some cases; others have occurred with purulent osteitis.

NEOPLASTIC DISEASE

The pelvic bones may be the site of primary benign and malignant osseous tumors as well as of metastatic malignancies from other sites with characteristics that are present when the tumors are located in other regions. One neoplasm with a higher frequency in the pelvis than elsewhere is the chordoma. It is infrequent in children but must enter into the differential diagnosis of mass lesions in the region of the sacrum and coccyx. Bony destruction and a soft tissue mass are its usual manifestations. In sacrococcygeal teratomas, which are much more common and occur predominantly in females in a ratio of 3:1, bone reaction is rare and the mass may contain foci of fat density, calcification, or actual bone. The diagnosis is usually clinical, with a mass in the sacrococcygeal region at birth or in early infancy. Prenatal diagnosis has been accomplished with US. Often, there is more tumor within the pelvis than is visible externally. CT is useful in neonates as their small size permits their placement in the scanner gantry so that direct sagittal scanning is possible; the internal extension of the tumor can be accurately assessed. When teratomas become malignant, the internal extension and the epithelial components are generally involved, giving rise to carcinomas and adenocarcinomas. Bale found 45 benign and 11 malignant sacrococcygeal teratomas in a group of 75 sacrococcygeal neoplasms. The clinical

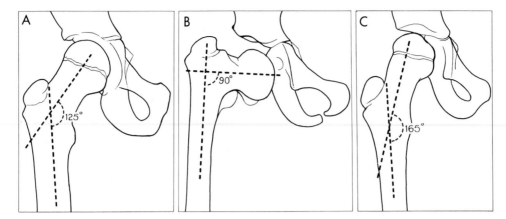

FIG 2–119.
Schematic drawing of coxa vara and coxa valga. **A,** normal angle of 125 degrees between the neck and the shaft. **B,** decreased an- gle of 90 degrees in coxa vara. **C,** increased angle of 165 degrees in coxa valga.

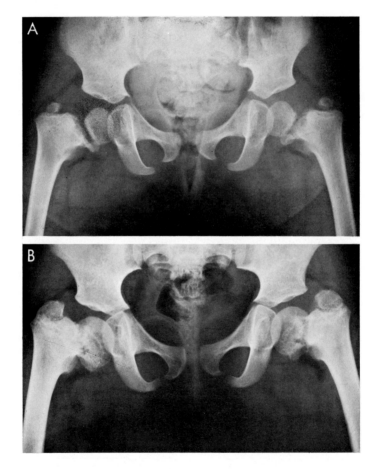

FIG 2–120.
Bilateral coxa vara. It is not known whether this patient had me- taphyseal chondrodysplasia in areas other than the hips. **A,** 3½- year-old girl. The nonmineralization of the femoral neck is respon- sible for the deformity from normal weight stresses. **B,** same pa- tient at age 6 years. The coxa vara has increased in comparison with **A,** notwithstanding diminution in the zone of nonmineralization. Similar findings might occur in rickets. The projected angle is also affected by anteversion of the femoral neck and less frequently by retroversion.

features most frequently associated with malignancy were age over 1 month at presentation, symptoms of pelvic obstruction, and elevated serum alpha-fetoprotein values. A rare cause of sacrococcygeal mass that may be confused initially with the more common teratoma is congenital ependymoblastoma. The diagnosis is made histologically.

OTHER PELVIC DISORDERS

Coxa vara is a deformity of the femur characterized by a decrease in the angle formed by the neck and the shaft to less than 120 degrees, owing to a caudal bowing in the region of the femoral neck (Fig 2–119), usually because of a primary femoral neck defect and resulting in shortening of the affected limb. Bilateral coxa vara is common in diseases associated with generalized weakening of the skeleton, such as rickets, osteomalacia, osteogenesis imperfecta, etc. It is also seen in several of the congenital generalized skeletal dysplasias: achondroplasia, metaphyseal chondrodysplasia, cleidocranial dysplasia, and others. Unilateral coxa vara may follow traumatic or pathologic fracture of the femoral neck, injury to the femoral head, or faulty intrauterine position with bowing deformity. In all types of coxa vara, a disturbed gait is a common symptom and anteversion of the femoral neck is a common associated deformity.

Limping gait is usually the principal clinical manifestation and may suggest congenital hip dislocation until appropriate imaging procedures are used. The degree of shortening of the limb varies with the degree of varus deformity. Limitation of movement at the hip is usually present. Radiographic examination demonstrates a shift caudad of the normal obliquely upright femoral neck toward the horizontal plane or beyond (Fig 2–120), together with a marked increase of the medial and downward inclination of the epiphyseal plate. There is a corresponding shift cephalad of the greater trochanter, which may ascend above the roof of the acetabulum in the more striking cases. In what is called idiopathic infantile coxa vara, the features in the femoral necks are practically identical to those observed in metaphyseal chondrodysplasias, especially the Schmid type (see Fig 42–76). The affected neck is wider than normal and, in unilateral cases, wider than its counterpart in the normal femur. Later, the femoral head and the acetabular cavity become enlarged and deformed. A triangular portion of metaphyseal bone usually appears at the medial end of

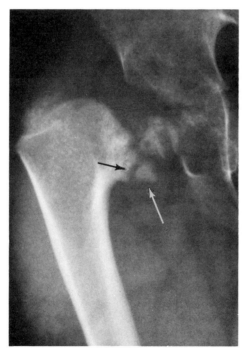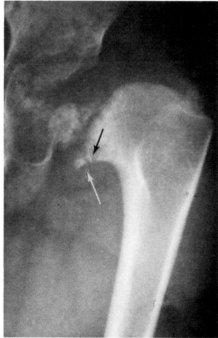

FIG 2–121.
Severe symmetric, bilateral, congenital coxa vara in a girl 5 years of age. Both femoral shaft-neck angles are less than 90 degrees. The short, bent femoral necks are thickened with small triangular ossicles at the medial aspects of their caudal ends *(arrows)*. The centers of the greater trochanters lie above the levels of the femoral necks.

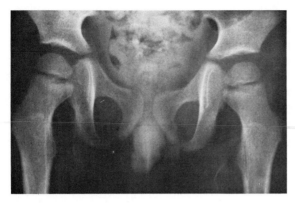

FIG 2–122.
Bilateral coxa valga simulated in a 3-year-old boy by external rotation of the lower limbs at the time of examination. Note the region of the greater trochanters superimposed on the base of the neck and the prominence of the lesser trochanters. The projected neckshaft angle in AP films is increased by external rotation and diminished by internal rotation from the value obtained when the knees and toes face forward during examination.

its junction with the epiphysis (Fig 2–121). The onset of the deformity in bilateral cases is often asynchronous. MRI studies have demonstrated expansion of the cartilaginous capital growth plate medially and distally at the site of attachment to the metaphysis with a low signal intensity on T1-weighted images and a high signal intensity on T2-weighted images. The triangular bone fragment could be identified. Histologic sections of the growth plate have shown a deficiency of cartilage cells with lack of normal columnar architecture and of longitudinal septa. These features have suggested a failure of proliferation, maturation, and hypertrophy of the chondrocytes of the growth plate and an apparent lack of osteoblast formation.

It is quite possible that some cases of the idio-

pathic variety of coxa vara actually were unrecognized instances of metaphyseal chondrodysplasia; with interest focused on the hips, roentgen examination of the full skeleton may not have been undertaken and the generalized nature of the deformity not been appreciated. Moreover, metaphyseal lesions and clinical signs, other than in the hips, may be extremely mild in the Schmid type.

Coxa valga is a deformity of the upper end of the femur in which the angle between the neck and the shaft is increased above 140 degrees. Partial lateral dislocation of the femoral head out of the acetabular cavity is an almost invariable associated finding in the more severe cases. Coxa valga is a persistence of the neonatal neck-shaft relations resulting from lack of normal muscular and gravity stresses that determine the form of the upper end of the femur. It is seen in paralytic and dystonic neuromuscular disorders such as poliomyelitis, cerebral palsy, spinal dysraphic deformity, and others. It also occurs in progeria, and some skeletal dysplasias in which bone growth factors may be disturbed. In a few cases, the coxa valga deformity diminishes after return of normal muscular function. Coxa valga may be simulated by external rotation of the lower limbs during radiography (Fig 2–122).

Protrusio acetabuli is a deformity in which the acetabular cavity is deepened to the point that it bulges into the pelvic cavity (Fig 2–123). It has been described radiographically by the lateral margin of the teardrop figure (the medial wall of the acetabulum) crossing the medial margin and has been noted in long-standing and demineralizing disorders such as rickets, rheumatoid arthritis, and hyperparathyroidism. It may be bilateral in association with osteomalacic diseases or unilateral in the case of local dis-

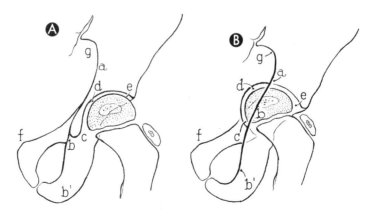

FIG 2–123.
A, normal acetabulum and **B,** protruded acetabulum. In **B,** the protruded acetabular floor juts into the pelvis well beyond the internal bony edge *(fg).* The "teardrop" figure *(ab-cd)* in **A** is obliterated in

B. (From McEwen C, Poppel MH, Poker N, et al: *Radiology* 1980; 135:631–640. Used by permission.)

ease in one hip. Marfan syndrome has been stated to demonstrate the deformity.

REFERENCES

Fractures

Donoghue V, Daneman A, Krajbich I, et al: CT appearance of sacroiliac joint trauma in children. *J Comput Assist Tomogr* 1985; 9:352–356.

Fishman EK, Magid D, Brooker AF, et al: Fractures of the sacrum and sacroiliac joint: Evaluation by computerized tomography with multiplanar reconstruction. *South Med J* 1988; 81:171–177.

Harley JD, Mack LA, Winquist RA: CT of acetabular fractures: Comparison with conventional radiography. *Am J Roentgenol* 1982; 138:407–412.

Torode I, Zieg D: Pelvic fractures in children. *J Pediatr Orthop* 1985; 5:76–84.

Waters, PM, Millis MB: Hip and pelvic injuries in the young athlete. *Clin Sports Med* 1988; 7:513–536.

Osteitis and Osteomyelitis of Pelvic Bones

Alperin LJ, Bender MJ: Osteitis pubis. *Am J Dis Child* 1954; 88:227–233.

Edwards MS, Baker CJ, Granberry WM, et al: Pelvic osteomyelitis in children. *Pediatrics* 1987; 61:62–67.

Modic MT, Pflanze W, Feiglin DH, et al: Magnetic resonance imaging of musculoskeletal infections. *Radiol Clin North Am* 1986; 24:247–259.

Zahran MH, Kaufmann HJ: Case report 336: Plasmacellular osteomyelitis of the iliac bone. *Skeletal Radiol* 1985; 14:296–300.

Neoplastic Disease

Bale PM: Sacrococcygeal developmental abnormalities and tumors in children *Perspect Pediatr Pathol* 1984; 8:9–56.

Ecklöf O: Roentgenologic findings in sacrococcygeal teratoma. *Acta Radiol* 1965; 3:41–48.

Murphy MN, Dhalla SS, Diocee M, et al: Congenital ependymoblastoma presenting as a sacrococcygeal mass in a newborn: An immunohistochemical, light and electronmicroscopic study. *Clin Neuropathol* 1987; 6:169–173.

Tam PK, Cha FL, Saing H: Direct sagittal CT scan: A new diagnostic approach for surgical neonates. *J Pediatr Surg* 1987; 22:397–400.

Utne JR, Pugh DG: The roentgenologic aspects of chordoma. *Am J Roentgenol* 1955; 74:593–608.

Other Pelvic Disorders

Blockley NJ: Observations of infantile coxa vara. *J Bone Joint Surg [Br]* 1969; 51:106–111.

Bos CFA, Sakkers RJB, Bloem L, et al: Histological, biochemical, and MRI studies of the growth plate in congenital coxa vara. *J Pediatr Orthop* 1989; 9:660–665.

Calhoun JD, Piesrret G: Infantile coxa vara. *Am J Roentgenol* 1972; 115:561–568.

McEwan C, Poppel MH, Poker N, et al: Protrusio acetabuli in rheumatoid arthritis. *Radiology* 1956; 66:33–40.

Pavlov H, Goldman AB, Freiberger RH: Infantile coxa vara. *Radiology* 1980; 135:631–640.

Weinstein JN, Kuo KN, Millar EA: Congenital coxa vara. A retrospective review. *J Pediatr Ortho* 1984; 4:70–77.

Wenger DR, Ditkoff TJ, Herring JA, et al: Protrusio acetabuli in Marfan's syndrome. *Clin Orthop* 1980; 147:134–138.

3

Brain and Spinal Cord

SECTION 1

Introduction to the Brain

DEFINITION AND NORMAL ANATOMY

The central nervous system (CNS) consists of the brain and spinal cord. The nervous system is composed of neurons (nerve cells) The neurons have a body and two types of processes that extend from the body; the processes that receive impulses are dendrites and the processes that conduct impulses away are the axons. The axons may vary in length and size. The thicker axons conduct impulses more rapidly than the thinner ones and are surrounded by a lipoprotein sheath (the myelin sheath). Large collections of myelinated axons compose the white matter of the CNS. The gray matter is composed predominantly of large collections of cell bodies.

The brain sits in the calvarial cavity and is covered by membranes. The dura mater lines the inner table of the calvaria. The pia mater surrounds the surface of the brain and the arachnoid mater is interposed between the pia and dura mater. The brain is surrounded by cerebrospinal fluid (CSF) and a prominent CSF space, the subarachnoid space, is situated between the pia and arachnoid mater.

The dura mater is a tough, fibrous membrane that divides the calvarial cavity into several connecting compartments. The tentorium cerebelli is a tent-like partition of dura; it is attached to the inner table of the occipital bones and extends across the cerebellum to attach to the petrous pyramids of the temporal bones. The opening within the midanterior portion of the tentorium is called its free edge (tentorial notch or incisure). The tentorium separates the calvarial cavity into supratentorial and infratentorial parts (Fig 3–1).

The infratentorial compartment is also called the posterior fossa and the hindbrain sits in this part. The hindbrain is composed of the cerebellum and brainstem. The cerebellum is composed of a midline structure, the vermis, and two lateral hemispheres; the cerebellar hemispheres contain the cerebellar tonsils (located inferomedially). The cerebellum has a peripheral surface of gray matter (the cortex) which is extensively folded into narrow elongated folia separated by furrows, or sulci (CSF spaces).

The brainstem is within the anterior compartment of the posterior fossa and is composed of three parts: inferiorly, the medulla oblongata; superiorly, the midbrain (mesencephalon); and between them, the pons. The medulla oblongata extends inferiorly to the foramen magnum and is connected to the cervical cord at this level (cervicomedullary junction). The midbrain is at the opening of the tentorium cerebelli and is connected to the thalamus at this level. Each part of the midbrain is connected to the cere-

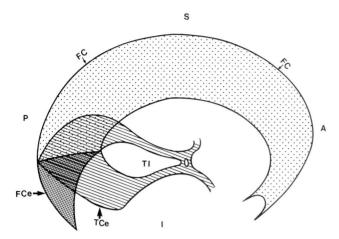

FIG 3–1.
The dura mater of the calvarial cavity: *FC*, falx cerebri; *FCe*, falx cerebelli; *TCe*, tentorium cerebelli; *TI*, tentorial incisure; *A*, anterior; *P*, posterior; *S*, superior; *I*, inferior.

bellum by compact bundles of fibers called peduncles. The superior cerebellar peduncle (brachium conjunctivum) connects the midbrain to the cerebellum. The middle cerebellar peduncle (brachium pontis) connects the pons to the cerebellum, and the inferior cerebellar peduncle connects the medulla oblongata to the cerebellum (Fig 3–2).

In the supratentorial region of the calvarial cavity lies the cerebrum, which is composed of two cerebral hemispheres (telencephalon) and a central area of deep gray matter structures: the basal gan-

glia, thalamus (diencephalon), and hypothalamus. The cerebrum has a peripheral surface of gray matter, the cortex, heavily folded into convolutions called gyri that are separated by grooves, the sulci. Underneath the cortex is a large intermediate area composed of white matter fibers. The central portion of the cerebrum is composed of the deep gray matter structures previously described (Fig 3–3).

The cerebral hemispheres are composed of four parts (the lobes): anteriorly, the frontal lobes; inferiorly, the temporal lobes; posteriorly, the occipital lobes; and superiorly, the parietal lobes. A large collection of white matter fiber tracts called the corpus callosum connects both cerebral hemispheres in the midline. Interposed between the upper halves of both cerebral hemispheres is a leaf of dura, the falx cerebri, which extends vertically down from its connection to the inner table of the parietal bone to connections anteriorly at the crista galli of the ethmoid bone and posteriorly to the tentorium cerebelli. The falx cerebri divides the supratentorial compartment into right and left sides.

The ventricular system consists of two lateral ventricles (right and left), the third ventricle, and the fourth ventricle. The lateral ventricles sit within the center of their respective cerebral hemispheres. The

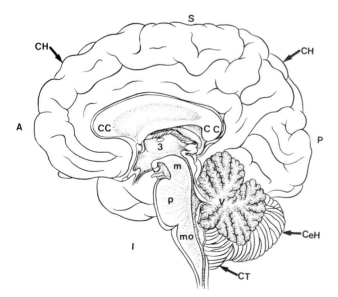

FIG 3–2.
The medial half of the brain. Brainstem (*m*, midbrain; *p*, pons, *mo*, medulla oblongata), *V*, vermis with folia and sulci; *CeH*, cerebellar hemisphere; *CT*, cerebellar tonsil; *CH*, cerebral hemisphere; *CC*, corpus callosum; *3*, third ventricle; *A*, anterior; *P*, posterior; *S*, superior; *I*, inferior.

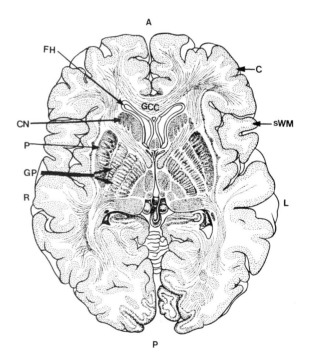

FIG 3–3.
Axial section through the brain at the level of the basal ganglia. *C*, cortex; *sWM*, interdigitation of subcortical white matter; *GCC*, genu of the corpus callosum; *FH*, frontal horn of lateral ventricle; *CN*, head of the caudate nucleus; *P*, putamen; *GP*, globus pallidus; *A*, anterior; *P*, posterior; *R*, right; *L*, left.

lateral ventricles are divided into parts: the frontal horn, body, atrium, occipital horn, and temporal horn. The third ventricle is within the middle of the thalamus. The fourth ventricle is within the posterior fossa surrounded by vermis posteriorly and the pons–medulla oblongata anteriorly. The ventricles contain CSF (Fig 3–4).

The formation of CSF is complex. A large portion of CSF is formed by the choroid plexus which sits in the lateral ventricles, the roof of the third ventricle, and the floor of the fourth ventricle. The CSF flows from the lateral ventricles through bilateral openings (foramen of Monro) into the third ventricle and through the aqueduct of Sylvius (in the midbrain) into the fourth ventricle. It then flows out of the fourth ventricle through three outlets, one midline (Magendie) and two lateral (Luschka), into the cisterna magna (an inferoposterior cistern) of the posterior fossa, down into the spinal canal and superiorly around the basal cisterns, and up over the convexities of the cerebral hemispheres to be reabsorbed by the arachnoid granulations projecting into the superior sagittal sinus.

EMBRYOLOGY

The normal development of the CNS is divided into four stages. The first stage is the primary inductive process (3rd to 6th week); the second stage is ventriculocisternal development (7th and 8th week); the third stage is cell proliferation (3rd to 6th week); and

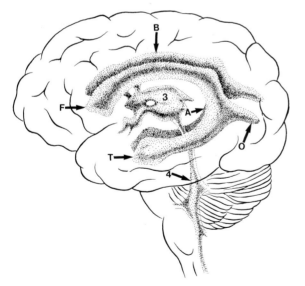

FIG 3–4.
The ventricular system. *F,* frontal horns; *B,* body; *A,* atrium; *O,* occipital horn; *T,* temporal horn of lateral ventricle; *3,* third ventricle; *4,* fourth ventricle.

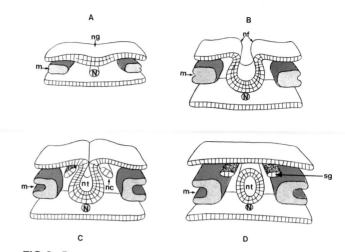

FIG 3–5.
Diagram of development of the neural tube. **A,** neural groove *(ng)*, notochord *(N)*, mesoderm *(m)*. **B,** neural fold *(nf)*. **C,** neural tube *(nt)*, neural crest *(nc)*. **D,** neural tube, spinal ganglion *(sg)*, notochord, mesoderm.

the fourth stage is neuronal migration (6th to 19th week).

First and Second Stages

The nervous system begins to develop at the third week of gestation with the formation of a thickened plate of ectoderm called the neural plate. The neural plate forms behind the primitive streak and Hensen's node and is above the notochord (Fig 3–5). Over the next several days the neural plate begins to form a groove (the neural groove) and two raised folds (neural folds). The neural folds continue to move toward the midline to fuse to form the neural tube. The neural folds fuse in the midline at the level of the fourth somite and then proceed to close craniad and caudad. The cranial end of the neural tube is called the anterior neuropore and the caudal end is the posterior neuropore. The anterior neuropore closes at about the 23rd day and the posterior neuropore 2 days later (Fig 3–6). At this stage, the nervous system is a closed neural tube with the brain developing from its cephalic end and the spinal cord from its caudal end. (The development of the spinal cord is discussed in Section 8).

During the 4th week of gestation, the cephalic end of the closed neural tube dilates into three primary brain vesicles: the anterior vesicle is the prosencephalon (forebrain); the middle vesicle is the mesencephalon (midbrain); and the posterior vesicle is the rhombencephalon (hindbrain) (Fig 3–7).

By the 5th week of gestation the prosencephalon has divided into the telencephalon (primitive cerebral hemispheres) and the diencephalon (primitive

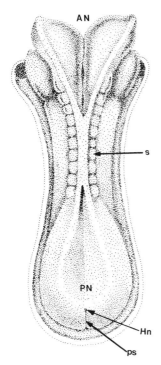

FIG 3–6.
Diagram of 22-day embryo. *AN*, anterior neuropore; *PN*, posterior neuropore; *Hn*, Hansen's node; *ps*, primitive streak; *s*, somites.

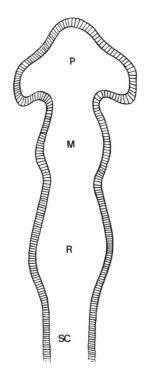

FIG 3–7.
The embryo during the fourth week with the three primary brain vesicles. *P*, prosencephalon; *M*, mesencephalon; *R*, rhombencephalon; *SC* spinal cord.

thalamus), and the rhombencephalon has divided into two parts: the anterior part, the metencephalon, later forms the cerebellum and pons; the posterior part, the myelencephalon, becomes the medulla oblongata.

The lumen of these three vesicles later develops into the ventricular system with the lateral ventricles in the telencephalon, the third ventricle in the thalamus, and the fourth ventricle in the metencephalon. The choroid plexus appears at the 7th week and begins to secrete CSF.

Third Stage

During the third week, the undifferentiated cells in the primitive ependymal zone that borders the embryonic ventricular system begin to proliferate and become the neuroblasts.

Fourth Stage

At about the 6th or 7th week of fetal gestation, the neuroblasts begin to migrate laterally in successive waves along a neuroglial glide to the periphery of the brain to form the cortex. By the 20th week of gestation the cortex and primary sulci are formed. The secondary and tertiary sulci are formed by the 36th week of gestation.

REFERENCES

Definition and Normal Anatomy
Clemente CD: *Gray's Anatomy.* Philadelphia, Lea & Febiger, 1985.
Grant JCB: *Grant's Anatomy* ed 5. Baltimore, Williams & Wilkins, 1962.
Heimer L: *The Human Brain and Spinal Cord.* New York, Springer-Verlag, 1983.
Last RJ: *Anatomy Regional and Applied*, ed 6. New York, Churchill Livingtone, 1978.
Pansky B, House EL. *Review of Gross Anatomy*, ed 2. London, MacMillan, 1970.

Embryology
Davies J: *Human Developmental Anatomy.* New York, Ronald Press, 1963.
Heimer L: *The Human Brain and Spinal Cord.* New York, Springer-Verlag, 1983.
Langman J: *Medical Embryology.* Baltimore, Williams & Wilkins, 1963.
Lemire RJ, Loeser JD, Leech RW, et al: *Normal and Abnormal Development of the Human Nervous System.* New York, Harper & Row, 1975.

SECTION 2

Imaging Modalities

The most common imaging modalities to evaluate the brain in infants and children are: (1) ultrasonography (US), (2) computed tomography (CT), (3) magnetic resonance (MR) imaging, and (4) cerebral angiography.

ULTRASONOGRAPHY

US is an excellent modality to evaluate the brain in the newborn and infant (Figs 3–8 to 3–14). It is most useful for demonstrating hemorrhage, ventricular size, pulsatility of the major cerebral vasculature, and for screening for congenital malformations (Figs 3–15 and 3–16). The advantage of US is its portability which allows the examination to be performed at the bedside in the critically ill and in premature newborns (Fig 3–17). The disadvantages are the relatively blind areas at the frontal and occipital poles and the lateral high convexity regions of the brain; its inability to differentiate a hemorrhagic from an ischemic infarction; its limited resolution of brain anatomy; and the need for an US window which limits performing US examinations after 1 year of age.

COMPUTED TOMOGRAPHY

CT is one of the best modalities for evaluating the pediatric brain. Since its medical debut in the early 1970s, it has become the most used and readily available imaging modality of the brain in children. It is the best modality to evaluate head trauma, cerebral infarction (in children under 2 years of age), and cerebral calcification.

During the first 2 years of life, there are some normal variations which can be seen on the CT im-

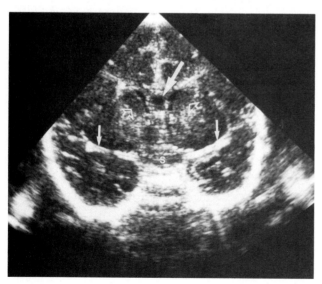

FIG 3–8.
Coronal US scan showing cavum septum pellucidum *(large arrow)* between frontal horns, suprasellar cistern *(s)*, vessels within sylvian fissure *(small arrows)*, and head of caudate nucleus *(open arrows)*.

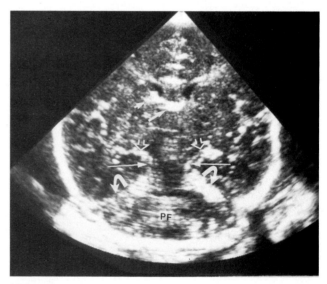

FIG 3–9.
Coronal US scan (posterior to Fig 3–8) demonstrating hyperechogenicity of the choroid plexus in the body of the right lateral ventricle *(small arrow)* and third ventricle *(thick arrow)*, the posterior fossa *(PF)* beneath the tentorium cerebelli *(curved arrows)*, and ambient cistern *(long arrows)*, leading to the choroidal fissure *(open arrows)*.

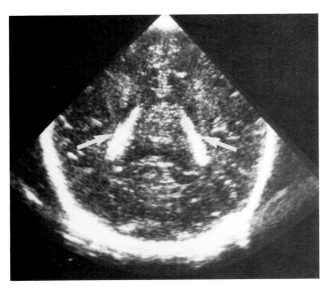

FIG 3–10.
Coronal US scan (posterior to Fig 3–9), showing increased echogenicity of the choroid plexuses of the bodies of the lateral ventricles (arrows).

ages. CT in newborns less than 34 weeks of gestation demonstrates large subarachnoid spaces, especially at the base of the brain at the sylvian fissures and middle cranial fossa. The cerebral cortex is thin and the secondary sulci development is limited. In both the premature and term infant, the normally high hematocrit in the venous sinuses may simulate a subarachnoid hemorrhage. Under 2 years of age, the CSF spaces (ventricular system and subarachnoid space) may be quite prominent simulating an

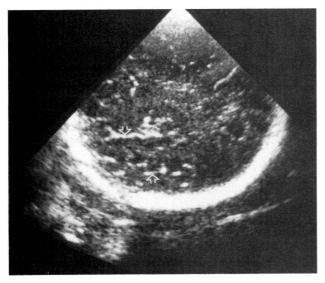

FIG 3–11.
Sagittal US scan (sector transducer) in a normal full-term neonate demonstrating normal increased echogenicity of secondary sulci at a far lateral level (arrows).

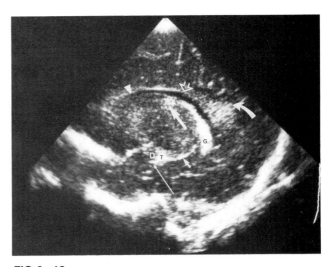

FIG 3–12.
Sagittal US scan demonstrating increased echogenicity of choroid plexus extending into the caudothalamic groove (thick arrow), at glomus (G) and in temporal horn (T); dentate gyrus (D); hippocampal fissure (long arrow); choroidal fissure (small arrow); sonolucent frontal horn (arrowhead) and body (open arrow) of lateral ventricle; and increased echogenicity of periventricular white matter (curved arrow).

early communicating hydrocephalus (Figs 3–18 and 3–19).

MAGNETIC RESONANCE IMAGING

At present, the best radiologic modality to evaluate the brain in infants and children is magnetic reso-

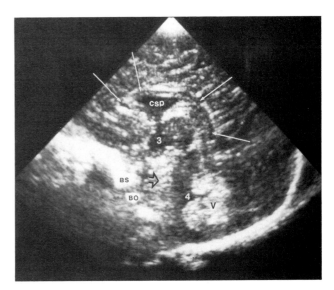

FIG 3–13.
Sagittal US scan (midline image). 3, sonolucent third ventricle; 4, fourth ventricle; csp, cavum septum pellucidum; V, increased echogenic vermis of cerebellum; hyperechogenicity of BS, basisphenoid, and BO, basiocciput bones; brainstem (open arrow) and decreased echogenic corpus callosum (long arrows).

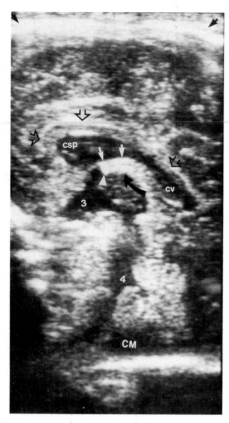

FIG 3–14.
Sagittal (midline) US scan (linear array transducer): top of calvaria *(black arrows)*; combination of choroid plexus *(small white arrows)* of the lateral ventricle extending to the ipsilateral foramen of Monro *(arrowhead)* and the choroid plexus of the roof of the third ventricle *(curved arrow)*; *3,* sonolucent third ventricle, *4,* fourth ventricle; *CM,* cisterna magna; *csp,* cavum septum pellucidum with posterior extension; *cv,* cavum vergae. Increased echogenicity of pericallosal cistern *(open arrows)* is demonstrated above the decreased echogenic corpus callosum.

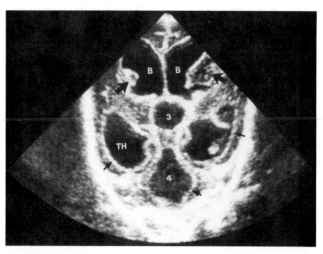

FIG 3–16.
Coronal sonogram (sector transducer) demonstrating hydrocephalus of all of the ventricles. *TH,* temporal horn; *B,* bodies of the lateral ventricles; *3,* third, and *4,* fourth ventricle, with increased echogenicity of the walls of the ventricles *(small arrows)* and hemorrhage into bodies of lateral ventricles *(large arrows).*

nance imaging (MRI). There are no known biological hazards, no ionizing radiation, and it produces exquisite anatomical detail of the CNS. MRI is a computer-generated image based on the principle of the alignment of the hydrogen nuclei of the body when the body is placed in a strong magnetic field and bombarded with high radiofrequency (RF) waves. The change in the alignment of the hydrogen nuclei when the RF waves are turned on and off generates a signal which by use of the Fourier transfer and a computer is reconstructed into an image of the body tissues.

A routine protocol for evaluation of the pediatric

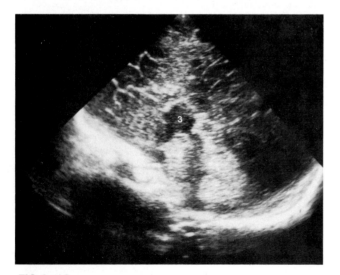

FIG 3–15.
Sagittal (midline) US scan (sector transducer) demonstrating absence of the corpus callosum which should normally be above the third *(3)* ventricle.

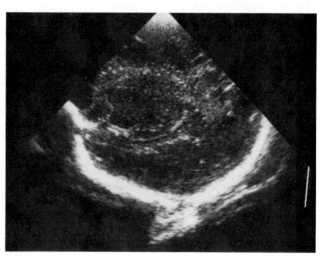

FIG 3–17.
Sagittal US scan (sector transducers) in premature (30 weeks' gestation) newborn with lack of development of the secondary sulci.

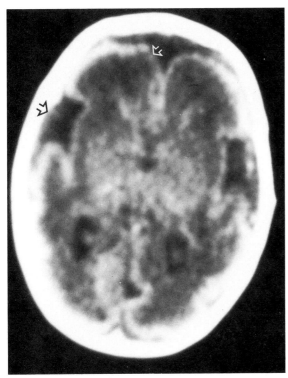

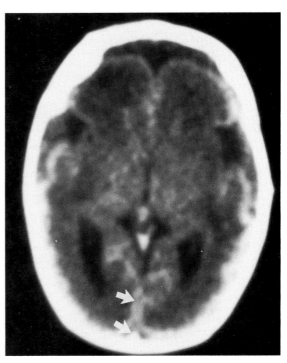

FIG 3–18.
Axial unenhanced CT scan obtained from a premature newborn (30 weeks' gestation) demonstrating thin cortex *(small arrow)* and large sylvian fissures *(large arrow)*.

FIG 3–19.
Axial unenhanced CT scan obtained from a premature newborn (30 weeks' gestation). High hematocrit of the blood in the normal venous sinuses *(arrows)* simulates subarachnoid hemorrhage.

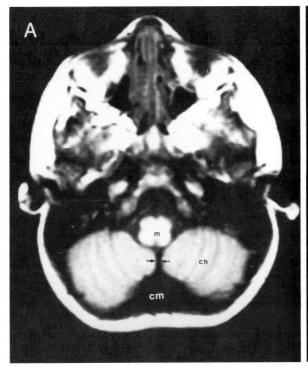

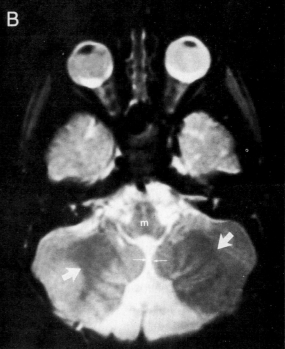

FIG 3–20.
A, axial T1-weighted MR image of a normal 3-year-old child, at the level of the medulla oblongata *(m)*, vallecula *(arrows)*, cerebellar hemispheres *(ch)*, and cisterna magna *(cm)*. **B,** axial T2-weighted image at a similar level as **A** showing medulla oblongata *(m)*, vallecula *(small arrows)*, and myelinated white matter *(large arrows)* of cerebellar hemispheres.

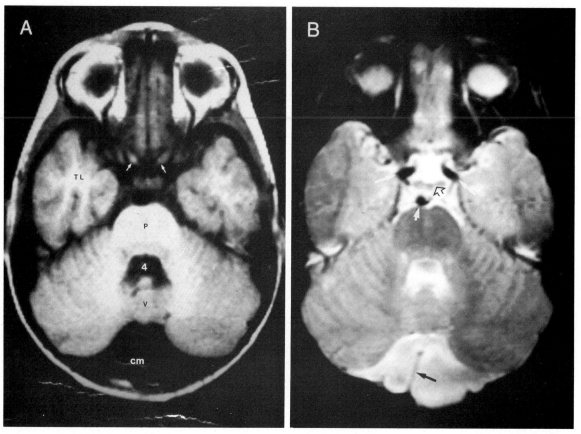

FIG 3–21.
MRI. **A,** axial T1-weighted image of a normal 3-year-old child, at level of pons *(p)*, fourth ventricle *(4)*, vermis *(V)*, cisterna magna *(cm)*, temporal lobes *(TL)* in middle cranial fossa, and optic nerves *(arrows)*. **B,** axial T2-weighted image at similar level as **A.** There is no signal of the internal carotid arteries *(large white arrows)* and basilar artery *(small white arrow)*, dorsum sellae *(open arrow)*, and falx cerebelli *(black arrow)* within the cisterna magna.

brain should consist of (1) T1-weighted images to evaluate anatomy, (2) T2-weighted images to evaluate for pathologic changes, and (3) T1-weighted gadolinium-enhanced images when searching for, or evaluating, a lesion (such as a neoplasm, vascular abnormalities, infarction, infection) (Figs 3–20 to 3–26). Gadolinium is a paramagnetic intravenous contrast agent approved by the Federal Drug Administration (FDA) for use with MRI. Gadolinium functions in the CNS in a manner similar to iodi-

TABLE 3–1.
MRI Protocol for Routine Evaluation of Pediatric Brain

	Age < 2 yr	Age >2 yr
Head coil	Yes	Yes
Spin-echo pulse sequences		
Sagittal T1-weighted	TR/TE=500–750/20–30	TR/TE=500–750/20–30
Axial T1/T2-weighted	TR/TE=3,000/30,100	TR/TE=2,000/30,80
Axial T1-weighted, post-Gd	0.2 mL/kg IV	0.2 mL/kg IV
Field of view	<24 cm²	24 cm²
Slice thickness	3 or 5 mm	5 mm
Interslice gap	0.5 or 1.0 mm	1 mm
No. of excitations	2 or 4	2 or 1
Matrix	192 × 256 or 256 × 256	192 × 256 or 256 × 256
Motion compensation		
parameters (cardiac gating for arterial and venous/CSF flow compensation	Yes	Yes

nated contrast agents used with CT. Enhancement with gadolinium is due to disruption of the blood-brain barrier by an abnormality (Table 3–1). The MR appearance of the pediatric brain must take into consideration the continued growth and development that occurs during the first 2 years of life. Since the MR signal is based on the water (hydrogen nucleus) of the body tissue, any dramatic changes in the water content of the brain will affect the MR image. During the first 2 years of life, the MRI appearance of the brain is due to two factors: (1) the changing water content of the gray and white matter, and (2) the myelination of the white matter. The myelination process begins at the eighth month of fetal gestation and is almost complete by 2 years of age. Ninety percent of the white matter is myelinated by 2 years of age with myelination of the remaining areas being completed by early adulthood. At birth, myelination is present in portions of the brainstem, middle cerebellar peduncle, posterior limb of the internal capsule, dorsal nuclei of the thalamus, and subcortical white matter of the postcentral gyrus (Fig 3–27).

By 1 year of age, myelination is present in the cerebellar hemispheres, all parts of the internal capsule, the corpus callosum, and portions of the subcortical white matter of the parietal, posterior frontal, posterior temporal, and calcarine cortex. By 2 years of age, myelination is present throughout the centrum semiovale, the subcortical white matter poles of the frontal, temporal, and occipital lobes of the brain (Fig 3–28, A).

Coinciding with the myelination process is the changing water content of the gray and white matter. At birth, the nonmyelinated white matter contains more water than gray matter, and therefore appears hypointense to gray matter on T1-weighted and hyperintense on T2-weighted images. During the first year of life, both the gray and white matter are rapidly losing water, with white matter losing water faster than gray matter. At about 1 year of life, the water content of the gray and white matter is about equal and an isointense MR appearance of gray and nonmyelinated white matter is seen. After 1 year of age, the myelination process predominates and by 2 years of age most of the white matter is myelinated, producing an MR appearance in which the white matter is hyperintense to gray matter on T1-weighted images and hypointense on T2-weighted images. Myelin, which is a lipid (fat), pro-

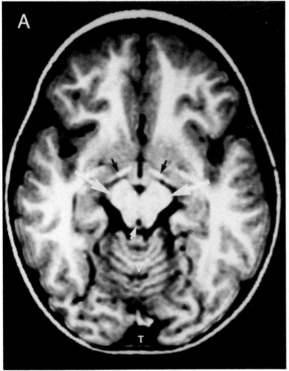
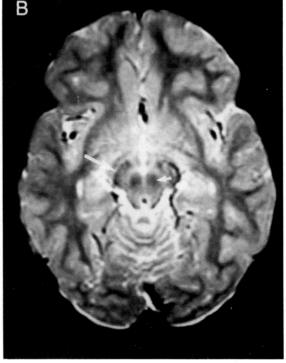

FIG 3–22.

A, axial T1-weighted image of a normal 3-year-old child, at midbrain, showing cerebral peduncles *(large white arrows)*, aqueduct *(small white arrow)*, superior vermis *(V)*, optic tracts *(small black arrows)*, and torcular Herophili *(T)*. **B,** axial T2-weighted image at similar level as **A.** There is no signal (iron) in red nucleus *(small white arrow)*, and substantia nigra *(large white arrow)*.

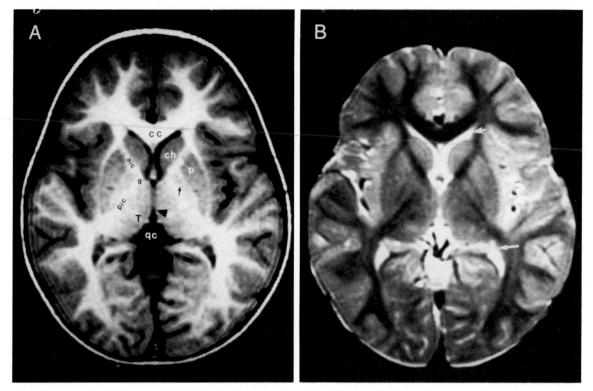

FIG 3–23.

MRI. **A,** axial T1-weighted image in a normal 3-year-old child, at level of basal ganglia. *ch,* head of caudate; *p,* putamen; globus pallidus *(small arrow); T,* thalamus; third ventricle *(arrowhead); C C,* genu of corpus callosum; *aic,* white matter of internal capsule, anterior limb; *g,* genu; *pic,* posterior limb; *qc,* quadrigeminal cis-

tern. **B,** axial T2-weighted image at similar level as **A** showing hypointense myelinated white matter fibers. Hyperintense CSF is seen within frontal horn *(small arrow)* and atrium *(large arrow)* of lateral ventricle.

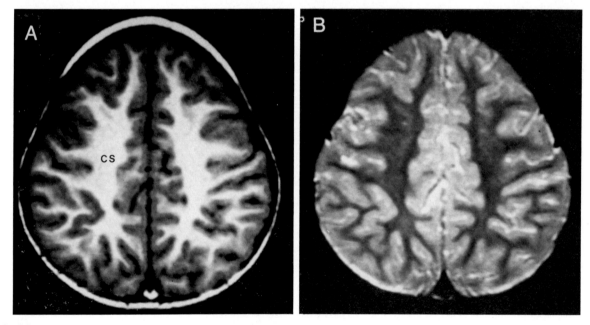

FIG 3–24.

A, axial T1-weighted image in normal 3-year-old child, at level of hyperintense white matter fibers of centrum semiovale *(CS).* **B,** axial T2-weighted image at similar level as **A** with marked hypointen-

sity of myelinated white matter fibers of centrum semiovale and isointense gray matter of cortex.

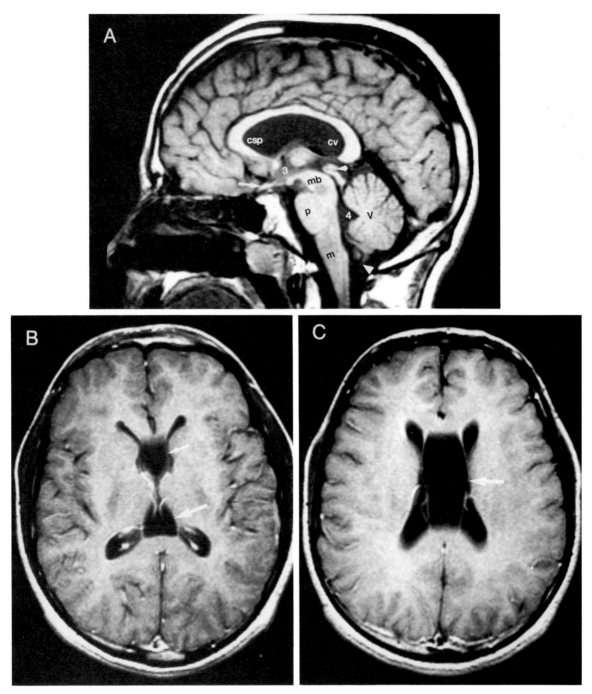

FIG 3–25.
A, sagittal (midline) T1-weighted image of a normal 8-year-old child. *csp,* cavum septum pellucidum; *cv,* cavum vergae; *cc,* hyperintense myelinated corpus callosum; pineal gland *(small white arrow);* optic chiasm *(large white arrow);* brainstem with components (*mb,* midbrain; *p,* pons; *m,* medulla oblongata), *3,* third, and *4,* fourth ventricles; *V,* vermis cerebellar tonsil *(arrowhead).* **B,** post-Gd axial T1-weighted image showing cavum septum pellucidum *(small arrow)* and cavum velum interpositum *(large arrow).* **C,** post-Gd axial T1-weighted scan showing cavum vergae *(arrow).*

duces an increased signal on T1-weighted images and a decreased signal on T2-weighted images (Fig 3–28, *B*) (Table 3–2).

For practical purposes, the brain of a 2-year-old can be used as the norm for the pediatric brain on MRI. T1-weighted images can be used to demonstrate normal anatomy. T2-weighted images, especially with long repetition times (TRs), are better at demonstrating mature myelin (TR = 3,000 ms <2 years of age and 2,000 ms >2 years).

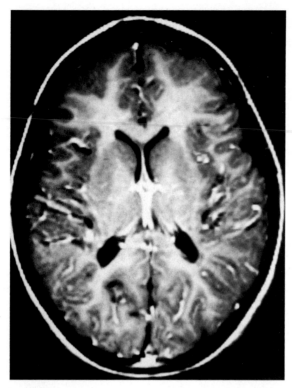

FIG 3–26.
Post-Gd axial T1-weighted image of a normal 4-year-old child demonstrating enhancement of veins and dural venous sinuses.

TABLE 3–2.

Timetable for Myelination of Specific Brain Structures

Posterior fossa	
Brainstem	Present at birth
Cerebrum	Present at birth
Cerebellar peduncles	Present at birth
Cerebellar hemispheres	Small amount present at birth
Thalamus	
Dorsal aspect	Small amount present at birth
Telencephalon	
Optic radiation	Present at birth
Internal capsule	
Posterior limb	Present at birth
Anterior limb	Present at 4 mo
Complete	8–12 mo
Corpus callosum	
Splenium	4–6 mo
Body	6–8 mo
Complete	12 mo
Postcentral gyrus	Present at birth
Precentral gyrus	2–3 wk
Lobes	
Occipital	6.5–15 mo
Temporal (posterior)	6.5–15 mo
Frontal (posterior)	6.5–15 mo
Parietal	6.5–15 mo
Temporal (mid and anterior)	21–27 mo
Frontal (anterior)	21–27 mo

Several fairly common normal variations and iron deposition areas can be seen in the pediatric brain on MRI. Iron begins to appear in the globus pallidus by 6 months, in the midbrain by 9 months, and in the dentate nucleus by 3 to 7 years of age. The cisterna magna can vary in size in children. A normal cisterna magna does not produce mass effect on the cerebellum or fourth ventricle. If there is a mass effect due to a large cisterna magna, then an arachnoid cyst of the cisterna magna is present. The cavum septum pellucidum, cavum vergae, and cavum velum interpositum are embryonic cavities which may not involute, but persist, after birth. The cavum septum pellucidum is a CSF space between the leaves of the septum pellucidum. The cavum vergae is the posterior extension of the cavum septum pellucidum. The cavum velum interpositum is a superior extension of the quadrigeminal cistern. Gadolinium-enhanced T1-weighted images demonstrate the normal enhancement of the circle of Willis, deep venous system, cortical veins, dural venous system, choroid plexuses, and dura (see Fig 3–25, B and C).

CEREBRAL ANGIOGRAPHY

The need for angiography has declined another notch owing to the ability of US and MRI to image vessels and blood flow better than did CT. Nonetheless, vascular disease often requires vascular studies, and familiarity with vascular anatomy remains useful. Infants and children have a faster circulation time, and cross-filling through patent anterior and posterior communicating arteries is common. The relative brachycephaly, large cisterns, and high tentorium in infants cause some differences in the position and course of the major arteries and veins of the cerebrum and cerebellum.

In infants, the sweep of the pericallosal vessels may be broader, more rounded, and closer to the vault than in older children. The middle cerebral vessels lie relatively high and are normally found above the clinoparietal line—a line drawn from the anterior clinoid process to a point 2 cm above the lambda in the lateral view. Both the anterior choroidal and posterior communicating arteries have a more upward sweep as they extend posteriorly (Fig 3–29). The basilar artery tip is located relatively higher; thus the posterior cerebral and superior cerebellar arteries are relatively higher as well.

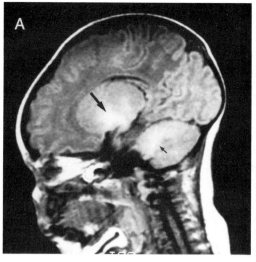

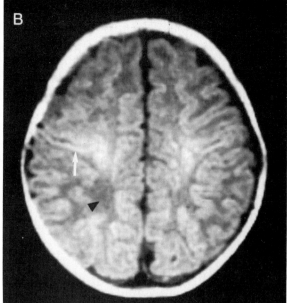

FIG 3–27.
A, sagittal T1-weighted image of a normal full-term newborn with hyperintense myelin present in middle cerebellar peduncle *(small arrow),* and white matter fiber tracts in dorsal thalamus and posterior limb of internal capsule *(large arrow).* **B,** axial T1-weighted scan in a normal newborn with hyperintense myelin *(arrow)* present in postcentral gyrus white matter. The majority of the white matter fibers are nonmyelinated and hypointense *(arrowhead).*

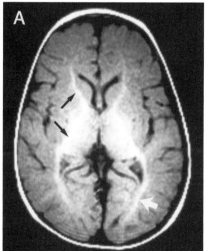

FIG 3–28.
A, axial T1-weighted image of a normal 8-month-old child showing myelinated white matter fibers in internal capsule *(black arrows)* and optic radiations *(white arrow).* **B,** axial T2-weighted image shows normal appearance of white matter fibers in a newborn with nonmyelinated hyperintense white matter fibers *(arrowhead); middle,* 1-year-old infant with isointense white and gray matter fibers *(arrowhead),* and hypointense myelinated fibers in the corpus callosum *(small arrow),* and internal capsule *(large arrow); right,* 2-year-old child with hypointense myelinated white matter fibers *(arrowhead).*

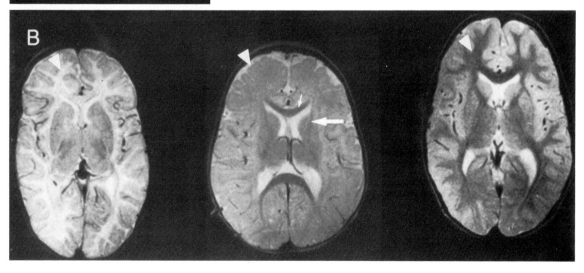

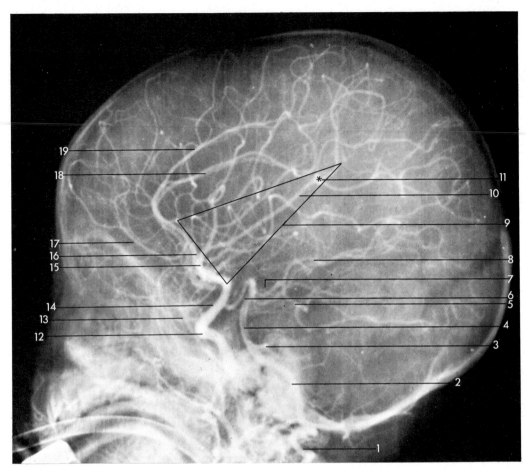

FIG 3–29.
Lateral view, arterial phase during brachial angiography, showing the internal carotid and basilar arteries and their major branches. *1,* extracranial portion of the vertebral artery; *2,* intracranial portion of the vertebral artery; *3,* posterior inferior cerebellar artery; *4,* basilar artery; *5,* posterior temporal artery; *6,* posterior communicating artery; *7,* posterior cerebral artery; *8,* medial occipital artery; *9,* insular arteries; *10,* angular artery; *11,* sylvian point; *12,* intracavernous portion of the internal carotid artery; *13,* ophthalmic artery; *14,* intradural portion of the internal carotid artery; *15,* middle cerebral artery; *16,* anterior cerebral artery; *17,* frontal polar artery; *18,* pericallosal artery; *19,* callosomarginal artery.

As the child matures, the upper carotid siphon becomes less vertical and is displaced downward toward the base of the skull. The pericallosal artery is less rounded in sweep and similarly lies closer to the base of the skull. The main axis of the middle cerebral vessels parallels the clinoparietal line.

On frontal projections, both the anterior and the middle cerebral arteries form less acute angles as they gradually ascend vertically from the carotid bifurcation; these should not be misinterpreted as upward displacement by a mass lesion. The middle cerebral vessels lie relatively more medial in relation to the midline in infancy, and some asymmetry of the sylvian vessels between the cerebral hemispheres is not uncommon. The posterior cerebral arteries lie closer to the midline in infancy and gradually splay out as the brainstem components grow.

Angiographers have assumed an important role in the treatment of vascular malformations and "inoperable" masses by selectively occluding pathologic vessels with injections of particulate emboli such as Gelfoam (absorbable gelatin sponge) or "glue" (isobutyl-2-cyanoacrylate) or by occluding the lumina of larger vessels with detachable balloons. Careful demonstration of the vessels to the lesion before manipulation is mandatory to avoid ischemic damage to normal brain tissue.

REFERENCES

Barkovich AJ, Kjos BO, Jackson DE, et al: Normal maturation of the neonatal and infant brain: MR imaging at 1.5T. *Radiology* 1988; 166:173–180.

Cohen MD, Edwardo MK: *Magnetic Resonance Imaging of Children.* Philadelphia BC Decker, 1990.

Dietrich RB, Bradley WG, Zaragoza EJ, et al: MR evaluation of early myelination patterns in normal and developmentally delayed infants. *AJNR* 1988; 9:69–76; *Am J Roentgenol* 1988; 150:889–896.

Harwood-Nash DC, Fitz CR: *Neuroradiology in Infants and Children.* St Louis, Mosby–Year Book, 1976.

Kirsch JE: Basic principles of magnetic resonance contrast agents. *Top Magn Reson Imaging* 1991; 3:1–18.

Lauffer RB: Magnetic resonance contrast media: Principles and progress. *Magn Reson Q* 1990; 6:65–84.

Runge VM: Clinical applications of magnetic resonance contrast media in the head. *Top Magn Imaging* 1991; 3:19–40.

SECTION 3

Congenital Brain Malformations

Congenital brain malformations result from abnormal formation and structure of the brain during intrauterine development. They can be classified into two main-types (Table 3–3). The first category consists of disorders of organogenesis in which some form of embryonic brain structure persists after birth. These disorders result in structural anomalies where parts of the brain are absent, partially developed, or malformed. Within this category are subtypes of disorders affecting closure, diverticulation, sulcation and migration, size, and destructive lesions of the brain.

The second category consists of disorders of histogenesis. They result from abnormal cell differentiation in which the brain appears relatively normal, but there are collections of deviant cell differentiation. The neurocutaneous abnormalities (phakomatosis) are disorders of histogenesis. MRI is the best imaging modality to evaluate the different types of congenital malformations of the brain.

DISORDERS OF ORGANOGENESIS

Migrational Disorders

The migrational disorders are anomalies of the cerebral wall and cortex which result from deranged migration of neuroblasts and deranged formation of gyri and sulci. These disorders arise during the 6th to 15th week of gestation when successive waves of neuroblasts migrate from the subependymal germinal matrix to the surface of the brain to form the standard six-layered cortex. The classic forms of migrational disorders are: lissencephaly (agyria with or without pachygyria), pachygyria (isolated), schizencephaly, heterotopia, polymicrogyria, and hemimegalencephaly.

Lissencephaly means "smooth brain," in which

TABLE 3–3.
Common Congenital Brain Malformations

I. Disorders of organogenesis
  A. Supratentorial
    1. Migrational disorders
      a. Classic forms
        (1) Lissencephaly (agyria with or without pachygyria)
        (2) Pachygyria (isolated)
        (3) Schizencephaly
        (4) Heterotopia
        (5) Polymicrogyria
        (6) Hemimegalencephaly
      b. Nonclassic forms
    2. Holoprosencephaly
    3. Syndrome of septo-optic dysplasia
    4. Dysgenesis of the corpus callosum
    5. Hydranencephaly
  B. Infratentorial
    1. Dandy-Walker malformations
    2. Cerebellar aplasia or hypoplasia
    3. Chiari malformation
  C. Mixed
    1. Cephaloceles
    2. Arachnoid cysts
II. Disorders of histogenesis
  A. Neurofibromatosis
  B. Tuberous sclerosis
  C. Encephalotrigeminal angiomatosis (Sturge-Weber syndrome)
  D. von Hippel–Lindau disease
  E. Ataxia-telangiectasia

there is a complete lack of gyri (agyria); pachygyria signifies too few, too broad, flattened gyri. In actuality, the lissencephalic brain may be completely smooth or show areas of both agyria and pachygyria. Although three clinical types of lissencephaly are recognized, the majority of children with lissencephaly do not have a specific clinical type. Type I is characterized by microcephaly and dysmorphic facies usually associated with heritable eponymic syndromes such as Miller-Dieker, Norman-Roberts, and Neu-Laxova (Fig 3–30). Type II lacks characteristic facies but exhibits macrocephaly due to hydrocephalus, retinal dysplasia, congenital muscular dystrophy, or posterior fossa abnormalities such as Dandy-Walker cyst and posterior cephalocele, individually or severally. Walker-Warburg and cerebro-ocular-muscular syndromes are associated with type II lissencephaly. Type III encompasses isolated cerebro-cerebellar lissencephaly with severe atrophy involving the posterior fossa. Lissencephaly is due to a deletion of part of chromosome 17. Affected children die in infancy or early childhood.

The characteristic MRI features of lissencephaly are an abnormal cerebral surface, cerebral contour, and gray or white matter distribution. The cerebral surface may be completely smooth and totally agyric (rare), almost agyric with a few areas of pachygyria, or nearly equally agyric and pachygyric. The cerebral contour is oval or hourglass-shaped (figure of eight) due to lack or incomplete opercularization of the brain with absent sylvian fissure or shallow sylvian grooves bilaterally. The distribution of gray and white matter is abnormal with a thickened cortex (increased gray matter), markedly reduced white matter, and loss of the normal cortical–white matter interdigitations. A smooth interface between cortical gray and white matter is present (Fig 3–31).

Pachygyria may be isolated in which there are no associated areas of agyria. This is a distinct type of migrational disorder and is different clinically and

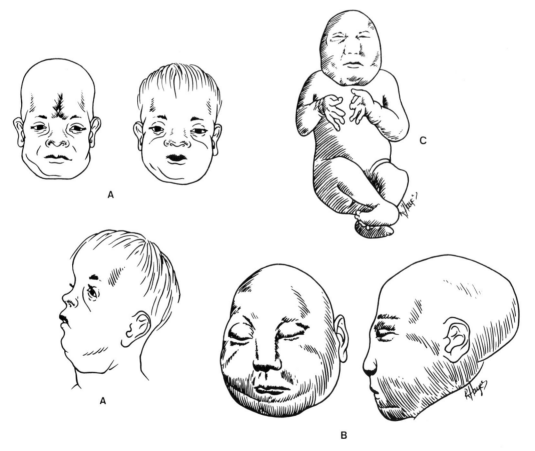

FIG 3–30.
Diagram of the dysmorphic features of type I lissencephaly. **A,** Miller-Dieker: microcephaly with bitemporal hollowing, prominent occiput, high forehead with vertical midline wrinkling, anteverted nares, low-set ears, and micrognathia. **B,** Norman-Roberts: microcephaly, bitemporal hollowing, and prominent occiput. Nares are not anteverted and the ears are normal, but the eyes are widely set with a prominent nasal bridge and micrognathia. (C) Neu-Laxova: microcephaly, low-set ears, receding forehead, grotesque facial appearance, and syndactyly of fingers and toes.

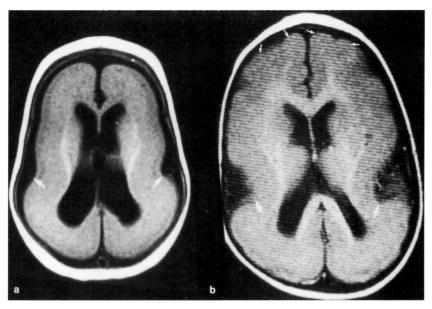

FIG 3–31.
Axial T1-weighted image showing lissencephaly *(a)*, total agyria *(b)*, almost total agyria with a few areas of pachygyria *(small ar-* *rows)* frontally, incomplete formation of sylvian fissures *(large arrows)*, and marked increased gray matter.

radiologically from lissencephaly. The symptoms are microcephaly, seizures, delayed development, mental retardation, and focal neurologic deficits. Affected children may or may not have associated dysmorphic facies. The dysmorphic facies in children with isolated pachygyria are not characteristic of any specific clinical syndrome. MRI shows a cerebral surface with either focal or diffuse areas of pachygyria without areas of agyria. The pachygyric areas consist of gyri that are broad-based, flat, thick, and coarse, with shallow intervening sulci. The cerebral contour is normal. The pachygyric areas consist of increased cortical gray matter with loss of the normal cortical–white matter interdigitations (smooth interface between cortex and subcortical white matter) (Fig 3–32).

Polymicrogyria is characterized by a cerebral cortex composed of numerous microscopic gyri. Since the gyri are microscopic, the diagnosis can only be made on the basis of histologic analysis of cerebral tissue. The symptoms may be mild, or there may be severe delay in development, seizures, and focal neurologic deficits. There is a high association with infections due to cytomegalovirus (CMV) or toxoplasmosis. Although polymicrogyria is a histologic diagnosis, it is possible to suspect the diagnosis on MRI because it resembles pachygyria. MRI demonstrates abnormal cortical areas which resemble long areas of pachygyria. The outer surface of these gyri, however, have an irregular, "nubby" appearance with increased gray matter, decreased white matter,

and loss of normal cortical–white matter interdigitation (smooth cortical–subcortical white matter interface). A few small intervening sulci may be seen (Fig 3–33).

Hemimegalencephaly is a migrational disorder resulting in hemihypertrophy of the brain. It may be idiopathic or result from a variety of causes including storage diseases, neurocutaneous syndromes (especially with neurofibromatosis type I), and con-

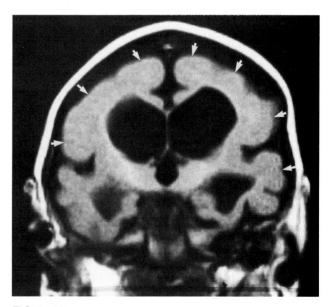

FIG 3–32.
Coronal T1-weighted image demonstrating multiple areas of pachygyria *(arrows).*

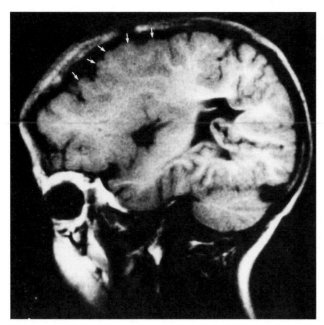

FIG 3–33.
Sagittal T1-weighted image. Polymicrogyria involves the frontal lobe with small irregular gyri *(arrows)* and increased gray matter.

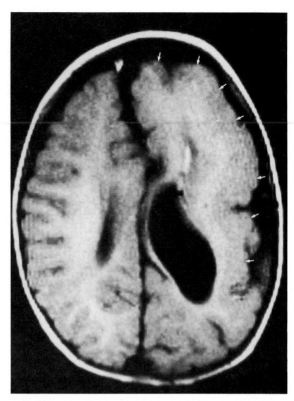

FIG 3–34.
Axial T1-weighted image demonstrating hemimegalencephaly of the left calvaria and cerebral hemisphere with abnormal pachygyric-appearing cortex *(arrows)*.

genital infection such as CMV and toxoplasmosis. MRI demonstrates a thickened, pachygyric, or agyric cortex, a smooth gray–white matter interface, and ipsilateral ventricular enlargement. Heterotopias may also be identified (Fig 3–34).

Heterotopia is a term used to describe collections of nerve cells (gray matter) in abnormal locations within the brain. The most common locations are the subependymal area of the ventricular system, especially the walls of the lateral ventricles and within the subcortical white matter. Children with heterotopia may be asymptomatic or present clinically with seizures. Heterotopia can be an isolated entity, part of more diffuse migrational disorders such as lissencephaly and schizencephaly, or occur in other malformations such as dysgenesis of the corpus callosum. MRI findings consist of single or multiple masses of gray matter of variable size and shape in the subependymal layer of the lateral ventricles or subcortical white matter. These masses maintain the same signal intensity as cortical gray matter on all pulse sequences. The heterotopias may be single or multiple and range in size from 0.5 to 3.0 cm (Fig 3–35).

Schizencephaly is a form of disordered migration characterized by abnormal transcerebral columns of gray matter. The basic abnormality in schizencephaly is a pial-ependymal seam (a gray matter–lined cleft) which extends across the full thickness of the cerebral hemispheres from the ventricular surface (ependyma) to the periphery (pial surface) of the brain.

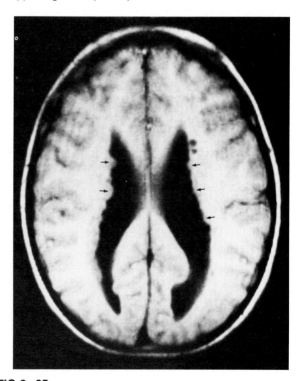

FIG 3–35.
Axial T1-weighted image demonstrating heterotopia with multiple nodules of gray matter *(arrows)* involving the subependymal region of the lateral ventricle.

Schizencephaly can be divided into two types depending on whether the cleft is totally fused or opened by a CSF cavity. Type I, or fused-lip schizencephaly, is characterized by a gray matter–lined pial-ependymal seam without an intervening CSF cavity. Patients with type I schizencephaly usually present with a history of seizures, delayed development, and a normal or microcephalic calvaria. The MRI findings consist of a gray matter–lined cleft which commonly involves the sylvian regions of the parietal and temporal lobes of the brain; the cleft is usually bilateral and fairly symmetric but it may be unilateral. The gray matter cleft may be thin or thick in width. It may be lined either totally or in part by gray matter, but there is always some gray matter within the cleft. The common site of involvement is the roof or lateral borders of the lateral ventricles. Small diverticula may extend from the lateral ventricles where they are joined by the cleft (Fig 3–36).

In type II, or open-lip schizencephaly, the pial-ependymal seam is opened by a CSF cavity. Patients present with a seizure disorder, failure to thrive, developmental delay, mental retardation, and a large percentage will also have hydrocephalus. MRI demonstrates a cleft which extends from the ventricular system to the pial surface of the brain opened by a CSF cavity. The CSF cavity may vary in size from small to large and is usually bilateral and symmetric; however, it may be asymmetric or even unilateral.

The ventricular system may be mild, moderately or markedly enlarged, and may or not communicate with the CSF cavity. Severe forms of open-lip schizencephaly present with massive CSF cavities which communicate with the ventricular system and have an appearance which is called "basket brain." In this form of open-lip schizencephaly, there is a relatively sparse amount of brain parenchyma involving the high convexity midline and base of the brain. Type II schizencephaly is at times difficult to differentiate from mild and massive hydrocephalus (Fig 3–37).

The septum pellucidum is commonly absent in both forms of schizencephaly and there is a high association with other congenital abnormalities such as heterotopia, polymicrogyria, arachnoid cyst, and septo-optic dysplasia.

Holoprosencephaly

Holoprosencephaly is a congenital malformation characterized by incomplete separation of the primitive forebrain into the cerebral hemispheres. The result is an abnormal continuation of gray and white matter across the midline of the brain. It is believed to be due to a primary disorder of the cephalic end of the notochord which leads to incomplete or defective telencephalic vesicles during the fourth to eighth week of gestation. Since the prosencephalon

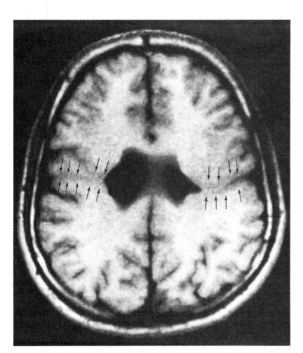

FIG 3–36.
Axial T1-weighted image showing type 1 schizencephaly with gray matter clefts *(arrows)* extending from the lateral ventricles to the cortex.

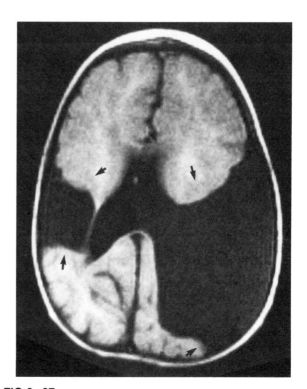

FIG 3–37.
Axial T1-weighted image showing type 2 schizencephaly with gray matter–lined clefts *(arrows)* separated by large CSF spaces.

remains undivided, the disorder is called holoprosencephaly.

Holoprosencephaly is always associated with orbital hypotelorism. The most extreme forms of holoprosencephaly are associated with dysmorphic facies which are characteristic and include cyclopia, cebocephaly, ethmocephaly, and midline midface cleft. The most commonly observed facies is absence of midline structures at the level of the upper lip which includes absence of the intermaxillary segment with absence of the middle of the upper lip, the central incisors, the primary palate, and a cleft within the secondary palate. Patients with trisomies of chromosomes 13 to 15 and 16 to 18 may exhibit holoprosencephaly. Patients with holoprosencephaly may have a trigonencephalic appearance to the calvaria (Fig 3–38).

Depending on the severity of the disorder, holoprosencephaly may be subdivided into three types. The most severe type is called alobar holoprosencephaly in which there is complete failure to form separate cerebral hemispheres; a less severe form is semilobar holoprosencephaly in which the posterior portions of the hemispheres develop partially; and the least severe form is lobar in which the hemispheres are nearly normal, but remain connected to

each other anteriorly and inferiorly at the level of the frontal lobes.

MRI in patients with alobar holoprosencephaly demonstrates a single, unlobed holoprosencephalon that contains a single monoventricle. There is no corpus callosum, interhemispheric fissure, falx, or crista galli. The diencephalon is also fused so that the thalami remain as a single central mass of gray matter with no midline slitlike third ventricle. This fused diencephalon indents the monoventricle giving it a horseshoe shape. The membranous roof of the third ventricle may balloon out into a "dorsal cyst" or "dorsal sac." The origin of the dorsal sac is not understood. One theory suggests that the dorsal sac may be a rudimentary third ventricle or a distorted velum interpositum. When the dorsal cyst is present, these patients commonly present with macrocephaly and hydrocephalus. The majority of patients with holoprosencephaly are normocephalic or microcephalic except for the 10% that present with hydrocephalus secondary to an enlarged dorsal cyst (Fig 3–39, *A* and *B*).

On MRI, a single midline arterial branch called the azygos artery may be seen coursing in the midline in the distribution where the normal pericallosal arteries should be. The internal cerebral veins, straight sinus, and superior sagittal sinus are absent.

MRI findings in patients with semilobar holoprosencephaly demonstrate an incomplete separation of the prosencephalon into lobes of the brain. Occipital or temporal lobes, or both, may be present with a rudimentary or absent corpus callosum. There is the beginning of differentiation of the monoventricle into occipital and temporal horns. A single ventricle is still present, but formation of the occipital or temporal horns, or both, is incomplete. There is partial cleavage of the diencephalon into thalami with partial formation of the third ventricle. Posteriorly, there is incomplete formation of the posterior aspect of the interhemispheric fissure, falx, and associated posterior dural venous sinuses (Fig 3–40).

In children with the lobar form of holoprosencephaly, the MRI findings are usually very subtle. MRI displays a more nearly normal cerebral hemisphere and thalami. However, there is still an area of gray and white matter that remains fused across the midline along the inferior anterior aspect of the frontal lobes. The ventricles, interhemispheric fissure, falx, arteries, and veins are nearly normal. The frontal horns of the lateral ventricles have a "squared-off" appearance instead of their normal semilunar appearance and the septum pellucidum is absent.

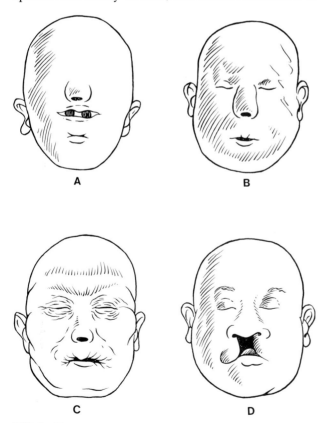

FIG 3–38.
The typical dysmorphic facies of holoprosencephaly. **A,** cyclopia; **B,** ethmocephaly; **C,** cebocephaly; **D,** premaxillary agenesis.

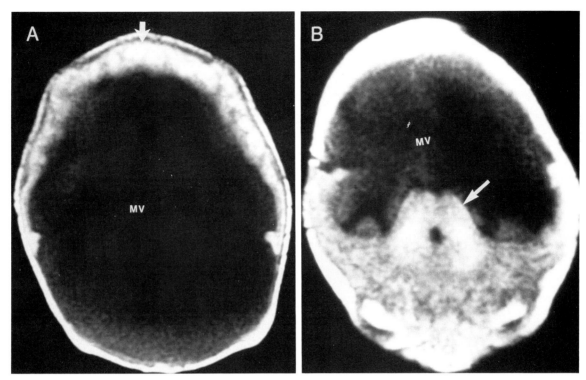

FIG 3–39.
Axial T1-weighted images. **A,** alobar holoprosencephaly with large monoventricle *(MV)* and small rim of cerebral tissue *(arrow)* anteriorly without cleavage by an interhemispheric fissure. **B,** alobar holoprosencephaly with monoventricle *(MV)* and fused thalamus *(arrow).*

Syndrome of Septo-optic Dysplasia

Septo-optic dysplasia (SOD) consists of optic nerve hypoplasia, absence of the septum pellucidum, and pituitary or hypothalamic insufficiency. The corpus callosum, fornix, and infundibulum may also be abnormal. SOD is felt to result from an insult which occurs during the 5th to the 7th week of fetal gestation. At this time, there is a failure of differentiation of the optic vesicle, retinal ganglionic cells, and ante-

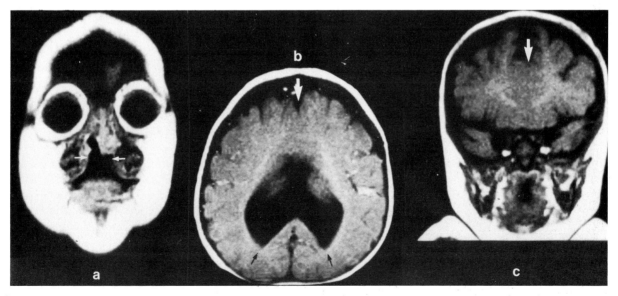

FIG 3–40.
T1-weighted MR images of semilobar holoprosencephaly. *a,* coronal image of the face showing midline facial cleft *(arrows). b,* axial image of the brain reveals incomplete formation of occipital horns *(small black arrows)* of the monoventricle and lack of cleavage of the anterior half of the brain *(white arrow) c,* coronal image of brain shows lack of cleavage of frontal lobes *(arrow).*

rior wall of the diencephalon. Patients usually present early clinically with visual abnormalities or blindness. Later they develop pituitary or hypothalamic abnormalities with deficiency of growth hormone resulting in a short stature, corticosteroid production, and inhibition of antidiuretic hormone resulting in polyuria or polydipsia.

MRI findings are absence of the septum pellucidum (seen in only 50% to 75% of patients with SOD), flattening of the roofs of the frontal horns, pointing of the floors of the lateral ventricles, dilatation of the suprasellar cistern and anterior third ventricle, small optic nerves, and a small optic chiasm. The corpus callosum is usually dysplastic or partially absent. In order to make the diagnosis of SOD the following have to be demonstrated: optic nerve hypoplasia, absence of the septum pellucidum, and pituitary hypothalamic insufficiency (Fig 3–41).

Dysgenesis of Corpus Callosum

Dysgenesis of the corpus callosum designates a spectrum of abnormalities affecting the corpus callosum. The corpus callosum may be congenitally absent (true agenesis); absent secondary to acquired intrauterine infarction of the anterior cerebral artery; or hypoplastic. The corpus callosum begins to de-

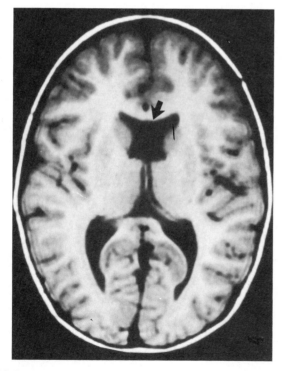

FIG 3–41.
Axial T1-weighted image revealing absence of septum pellucidum *(arrow).*

velop by the 10th to 12th week and is fully formed by the 20th week of gestation. It develops in a posteroanterior direction with the splenium forming first followed by the body, genu, and rostrum. Depending on the time of the insult there may be absence of all or only portions of the corpus callosum.

In true agenesis the abnormality is failure of formation of the commissural plate which allows axons to grow from side to side and across the midline to establish the corpus callosum. Since in true agenesis, the axons from the hemispheres cannot cross the midline due to absence of the commissural plate, they course longitudinally instead and establish paired longitudinal callosal bundles which run along the medial borders of the lateral ventricles. These bundles are called the bundles of Probst and are pathognomonic for true agenesis.

Eighty percent to 90% of children with dysgenesis (absence) of the corpus callosum are symptomatic, usually presenting at 3 years of age with seizures. Aicardi syndrome is associated with dysgenesis of the corpus callosum occurring in females and is characterized by chorioretinopathy (chorioretinal lacunae), infantile spasms, callosal agenesis, and mental retardation.

Dysgenesis of the corpus callosum may present as an isolated anomaly or in association with other malformations such as interhemispheric cyst and hydrocephalus, Dandy-Walker malformations, migrational disorders, absence of the inferior vermis, cephaloceles (anterior and basal), calvarial and facial dysmorphic anomalies (Apert disease, midline facial clefts, hypertelorism, and calvarial synostosis), holoprosencephaly, lipoma of the interhemispheric fissure (falx cerebri), and the Chiari II malformation.

The MRI findings in absence of the corpus callosum are best demonstrated on the sagittal projection. The normal C-shaped appearance of the corpus callosum is absent, totally or partially (Fig 3–42). The third ventricle is high-riding and interposed between the bodies of the lateral ventricles.

In true agenesis, on axial and coronal images, longitudinal callosal bundles of Probst are seen running along the medial walls of the lateral ventricles in a posteroanterior direction. The lateral ventricles may have a colpocephalic appearance in which there is a localized dilatation of the atria and occipital horns. The medial borders of the frontal horns appear concave because they are indented by Probst bundles (Fig 3–43).

A large percentage of patients with dysgenesis of the corpus callosum have a large interhemispheric cyst which may or may not communicate with the

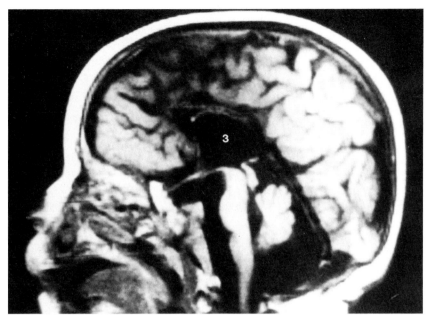

FIG 3–42.
Sagittal T1-weighted image. Note absence of corpus callosum with lack of the normal C-shaped corpus callosum over the third ventricle *(3)*, which is enlarged and superiorly elevated.

ventricular system. The cyst is frequently associated with hydrocephalus. The exact origin of the cyst is not known. Some authors suggest that it is a dilated third ventricle or a true arachnoid cyst. At autopsy, the lining of the cyst may contain ependymal or arachnoid cells. On MRI, the cyst usually maintains the same signal intensities with CSF. However, there may be bleeding into the cyst or high protein content, in which case the signal intensity on the T1-weighted image will be greater than CSF (Figs 3–44 and 3–45).

Dandy-Walker Malformations

Dandy-Walker malformations are of two types: the Dandy-Walker cyst and the Dandy-Walker variant. This disorder is believed to arise between the 7th to 10th week of fetal gestation due to defective development of the roof of the fourth ventricle and adjacent meninges. These infants present at birth or early infancy with an enlarged head with a localized bulging of the occiput. The majority present with raised intracranial pressure secondary to hydrocephalus.

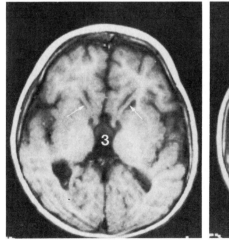
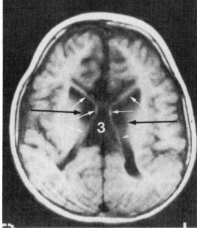
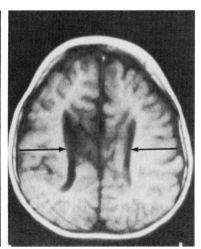

FIG 3–43.
Axial T1-weighted image demonstrating agenesis of the corpus callosum with Probst bundles *(white arrows)* along the medial borders of the lateral ventricle; the bundles are widely separated *(black arrows)* with the third ventricle *(3)* interposed.

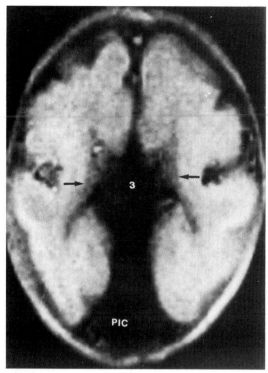

FIG 3–44.
Axial T1-weighted image showing dysgenesis (absence) of the corpus callosum with posterior interhemispheric cyst (PIC) communicating with the third ventricle (3), widely separated lateral ventricles (arrows), and diffuse pachygyria.

The Dandy-Walker cyst is characterized by absence of the foramen of Magendie with massive dilatation of the fourth ventricle and absence of the inferior vermis. The massive dilatation of the fourth ventricle presents as a posterior fossa cyst compressing and displacing the cerebellar hemispheres anterolaterally and the superior vermis upward. The posterior fossa is enlarged. The tentorium is elevated as the torcular lies superior to the lambdoid sutures producing the classic torcular-lambdoid inversion as described on plain skull radiographs of the condition.

The MRI appearance of the Dandy-Walker cyst consists of a large posterior fossa cyst without any appearance of a fourth ventricle. There is absence of the inferior vermis and the superior vermis may or may not be present. The torcular is elevated and the occiput is ballooned posteriorly. Hydrocephalus may be present with dilatation of the third and lateral ventricles. The Dandy-Walker cyst is associated with other congenital malformations such as dysgenesis of the corpus callosum, holoprosencephaly, migrational disorders, and posterior cephaloceles (Figs 3–46 and 3–47).

The Dandy-Walker variant is a less exaggerated form of the Dandy-Walker cyst. It is characterized by absence of the inferior vermis, and a less dilated and better-formed fourth ventricle which communicates with a retrocerebellar cyst. MRI in the Dandy-Walker variant demonstrates a moderately dilated

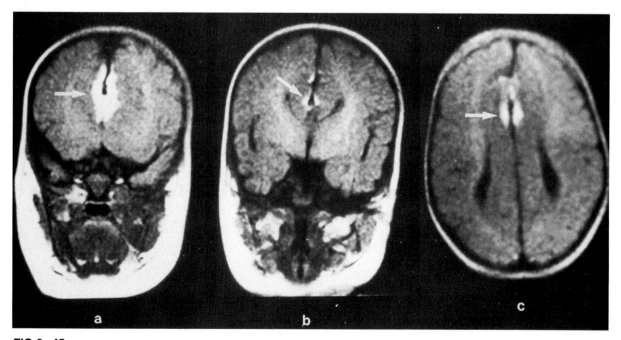

FIG 3–45.
Coronal (a, b) and axial (c) T1-weighted images revealing dysgenesis (absence) of the corpus callosum with interhemispheric lipoma (arrow).

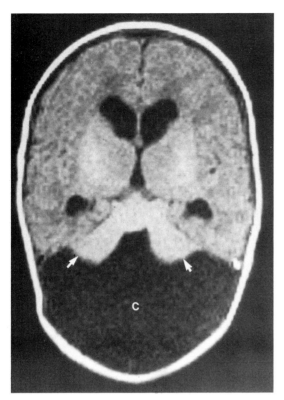

FIG 3–46.
Axial T1-weighted image showing Dandy-Walker cyst. A large posterior fossa cyst *(c)* compresses the cerebellar hemispheres *(arrows)*.

fourth ventricle which opens posteriorly into a retrocerebellar cyst with absence of the inferior vermis. The retrocerebellar cyst may compress and displace the cerebellar hemispheres anterolaterally. The cyst of the Dandy-Walker variant is not nearly as massive as the Dandy-Walker cyst. The Dandy-Walker variant is also associated with other congenital malformations such as dysgenesis of the corpus callosum, holoprosencephaly, migrational disorders, and posterior cephaloceles (Figs 3–48 and 3–49).

Cerebellar and Vermian Hypoplasia

The cerebellum develops from two lateral and one midline primordia. Complete failure to develop the primordia results in cerebellar aplasia. Lesser derangements produce variable degrees of hypoplasia of the vermis and cerebellar hemispheres. The most common finding is absence of part or all of the inferior vermis. This may occur as an isolated anomaly as part of Down syndrome (trisomy 21) or Jobert syndrome (familial vermian agenesis with episodic hyperpnea, ataxia, abnormal eye movements, and mental retardation). The Chiari IV malformation is extreme cerebellar hypoplasia. This is discussed under Chiari Malformations.

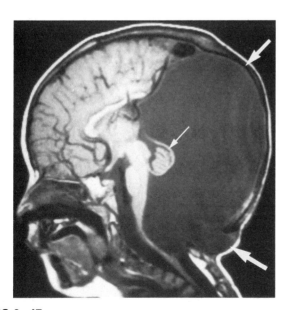

FIG 3–47.
Sagittal T1-weighted image showing Dandy-Walker cyst *(large arrows)* with absence of the inferior vermis and a small remnant of the superior vermis *(small arrow)* present.

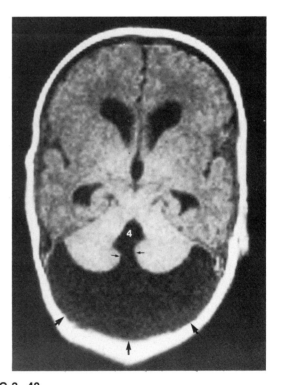

FIG 3–48.
Axial T1-weighted image showing Dandy-Walker variant with a fourth ventricle *(4)*, leading into a retrocerebellar cyst *(large arrows)*, and absence of the inferior vermis *(small arrows)*.

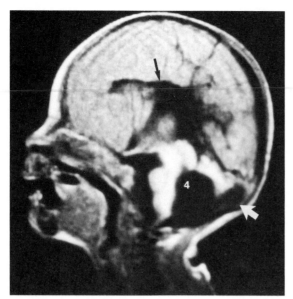

FIG 3–49.
Axial T1-weighted image showing Dandy-Walker variant with a fourth ventricle *(4)* communicating with a retrocerebellar cyst *(white arrow)*; absence of the inferior vermis; absence of the corpus callosum *(black arrow)*; and lissencephaly.

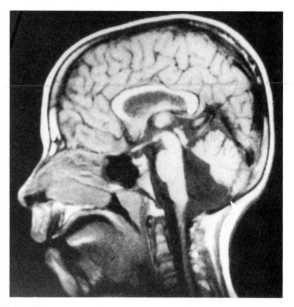

FIG 3–50.
Sagittal T1-weighted image demonstrating absence of the inferior vermis *(arrow)*.

MRI in patients with cerebellar hypoplasia reveals absence of parts of the vermis or of the cerebellar hemispheres, or of both. Cerebellar aplasia is an extremely rare congenital abnormality. Hypoplasia of the cerebellum may be mild, moderate, or extreme. The amount of cerebellar tissue present will determine the degree of hypoplasia. On MRI, there is no evidence of a mass effect associated with cerebellar hypoplasia. The CSF cisterns are enlarged secondary to absence of the adjacent cerebellar tissue. In children with severe cerebellar hypoplasia, the brainstem is thin and the pons is small owing to absence of, or a small, middle cerebellar peduncle (which normally forms the major part of the belly of the pons) (Fig 3–50).

Chiari Malformations

The Chiari malformations are four unrelated anomalies of the hindbrain which were classified by Chiari in 1891 and 1895. Cleland first described the complex anomaly of the lower brainstem and cerebellum in 1883. Chiari in 1891 described three types of cerebellar malformations based on pathologic studies of congenital hydrocephalus and in 1895 added cerebellar hypoplasia as type IV. The Chiari malformations consist of four subtypes: in Chiari I there is downward displacement of the tonsils through the foramen magnum into the upper cervical canal; in Chiari II, downward displacement of the tonsils, in-

ferior cerebellum, fourth ventricle, and medulla oblongata through the foramen magnum into the cervical canal in association with a myelomeningocele; in Chiari III, herniation of virtually all of the cerebellum into an infraoccipital–high cervical cephalocele; and in Chiari IV, there is severe cerebellar hypoplasia.

Chiari I
The Chiari I malformation consists of protrusion of the cerebellar tonsils and, at times, adjacent parts of the inferior cerebellum through the foramen magnum into the upper cervical canal with obliteration of the cisterna magnum. It is not considered an abnormality of closure of the neural tube but rather a dysplasia of the base of the calvaria and cervical vertebrae. The Chiari I malformation is associated with hydromyelia (60%–80%), hydrocephalus (20%–25%), and segmental abnormalities of the craniovertebral junction which include basilar impression (25%), assimilation of C1 to the occiput (10%), Klippel-Feil syndrome (10%), and incomplete ossification of the C1 ring (5%). It is not associated with a myelomeningocele. Clinically, children present with headaches, and occasionally raised intracranial pressure due to hydrocephalus. This condition is more commonly seen in children over 10 years of age and in young adults.

The MRI findings in Chiari I malformation are: (1) downward displacement of the cerebellar tonsils into the upper cervical canal; (2) obliteration of the cisterna magna; (3) occasionally mild to moderate hydrocephalus; and (4) occasionally hydromyelia of the spinal cord (localized dilatation of the central canal) (Fig 3–51).

Chiari II

The Chiari II malformation affects the calvaria, dura, and hindbrain. It is almost always associated with a myelomeningocele (99.99%) and is considered a disorder of closure. The embryogenesis of this malformation is complex and various theories include: (1) traction on the hindbrain by fixation of the spinal cord at the myelomeningocele; (2) tissue pressure gradients between the intracranial contents and the spinal theca; and (3) primary overgrowth of the entire CNS with persistent embryonic hydrocephalus and inferior displacement of the hindbrain.

Symptoms in these children are primarily related to the myelomeningocele. The incidence of myelomeningocele is 3 in 100 births in North America. Most cases are sporadic with a female predominance of 2:1 over males. These patients present clinically at birth with a myelomeningocele with sensory and motor deficits of the lower extremities and hydrocephalus. If the hydrocephalus is controlled by shunting, these patients go on to develop normal or near-normal intelligence.

The MRI findings are numerous and complex. The primary findings are necessary to make a diagnosis and classify this entity. They include the following: (1) The upper cervical cord is displaced caudad by the downward extension of the medulla (and at times the pons) into the cervical canal posterior to the upper cervical cord producing a cervicomedullary kink, usually located between C2 and C4, but occasionally as low as T1. A cervicomedullary kink is demonstrated in 70% of cases on MRI. In 30% of cases, the medulla descends into the cervical canal, but it remains in correct alignment and the pathognomonic kink is not seen. (2) The dysplastic cerebellum is elongated caudad so that it protrudes through the foramen magnum to rest on the upper border of C1. (3) There is further protrusion of a narrow tongue or peg of inferior cerebellar tissue (composed of parts of the dysplastic inferior vermis and cerebellar tonsils) into the upper cervical canal behind the herniated medulla (usually to the C2–4 level). (4) The fourth ventricle is elongated craniad and caudad and narrowed transversely to form a bent tube; it nearly always protrudes below the foramen magnum into the upper cervical canal. The distal aspect of the fourth ventricle may form a teardrop diverticulum that protrudes caudal to the medulla behind the upper cord (Fig 3–52). The secondary findings include tectal beaking, hydromyelia

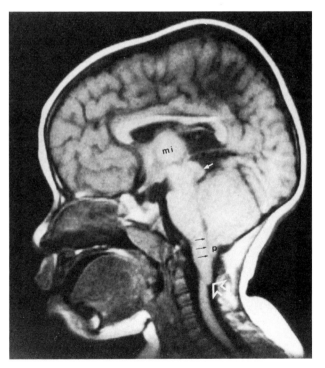

FIG 3–52.
Sagittal T1-weighted image demonstrating Chiari II malformation. Primary characteristics: downward herniation of the medulla behind the cervical cord (cervicomedullary kink, *open arrow*), fourth ventricle *(black arrows)*, and the inferior aspect of the cerebellum (cerebellar peg, *P*) into the upper cervical canal. Secondary characteristics: tectal beaking *(white arrow)*, large massa intermedia *(mi)*, and polygyria (posteriorly).

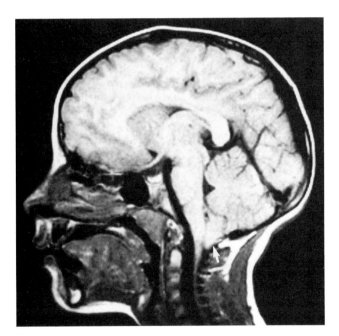

FIG 3–51.
Sagittal T1-weighted image demonstrating Chiari I malformation with downward herniation of the cerebellar tonsil *(arrow)* into the upper cervical canal.

(40%–60%), hydrocephalus (98%) colpocephaly (10%–25%), large massa intermedia, dysplasia involving the falx cerebri and tentorium cerebelli, low insertion of the tentorium, small posterior fossa, enlargement of the foramen magnum and ring of C1, and dysgenesis of the corpus callosum (Fig 3–53).

Chiari III

The Chiari III malformation is a low occipital–high cervical cephalocele, consisting of a bony defect involving the infraocciput, the posterior rim of the foramen magnum, the posterior arch of C1 and at times C2 with herniation of almost all of the cerebellum, as well as portions of the brainstem, fourth ventricle, and upper cervical cord through these defects. It may result from defective tissue induction producing simultaneous abnormalities of the brain, spinal cord, cranial vault, and upper cervical canal.

Children with this malformation are usually microcephalic and present at birth with a posterior calvarial-cervical mass of varying size and consistency. Symptoms depend on the amount and type of herniated posterior fossa–cervical tissue. The MRI findings are specific and consist of: (1) bony defects in the infraocciput, the posterior rim of the foramen magnum, and the posterior arch of C1 and at times

C2; (2) herniation of a sac with intracranial contents containing portions of meninges, CSF, cerebellum, brainstem, fourth ventricle, and upper cervical cord; and (3) protrusion of parts of the infratentorial dural venous sinuses, which may also herniate through the bony defects (Fig 3–54).

Chiari IV

The Chiari IV malformation is severe cerebellar hypoplasia. It is classified as part of the cerebellar hypoplastic anomalies occurring during the 8th to 13th week of fetal gestation. It is a rare condition which is seen in infancy and early childhood. Children present with the typical signs of cerebellar malfunction (ataxia, incoordination). MRI findings are: (1) almost complete absence of the cerebellum; (2) large posterior fossa CSF spaces without evidence of pressure or mass effect; and (3) a small brainstem. The small pons results from lack of formation of the cerebellar peduncles (Fig 3–55).

Cephaloceles

Congenital cephaloceles are considered disorders of closure. They are a broad category of malformations characterized by herniation of intracranial contents through a defect in the calvaria. Classification depends on the type of intracranial contents within the herniated sac. A cranial meningocele is a herniation of the leptomeninges. An encephalocele is herniation of the meninges and brain tissue, but not the

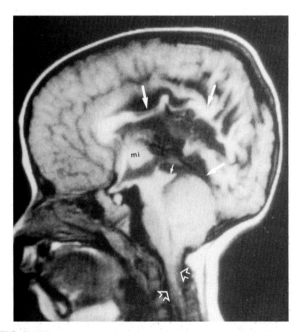

FIG 3–53.
Sagittal T1-weighted image showing Chiari II malformation with primary findings of downward displacement of medulla (without kink), inferior aspect of fourth ventricle, and inferior cerebellum (open arrows) into upper cervical cord. Secondary findings are tectal beaking (small white arrow), large massa intermedia (mi), and dysplastic corpus callosum, falx cerebri, and tentorium cerebelli (large white arrows), and polygyria.

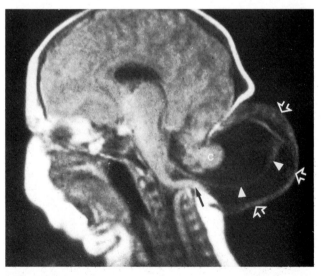

FIG 3–54.
Sagittal T1-weighted image demonstrating Chiari III malformation. Large herniated sac (open arrows) with enlarged portion of fourth ventricle (arrowheads), cerebellum (c), and cervical cord (black arrow) are seen.

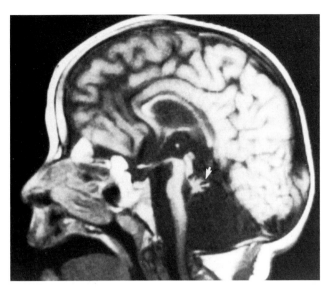

FIG 3–55.
Sagittal T1-weighted image demonstrating Chiari IV malformation with thin brainstem. The only part of the cerebrum is a small portion of the superior vermis *(arrow).*

ventricles. An encephalocystomeningocele is herniation of meninges, brain, and ventricles.

Cephaloceles can also be classified by location. In Europe and North America, cephaloceles are more commonly found posteriorly in the following order of decreasing frequency: occipital (71%), parietal (10%), frontal (9%), nasal (9%), and nasopharyngeal (1%). In Southeast Asia, nasal cephaloceles are the most common form.

Congenital cephaloceles may result from defective tissular induction, producing simultaneous abnormalities of the brain and cranial vault, or from defective formation of the chondrocranium at its junction with the membranous cranial capsule or at an isolated point.

Occipital cephaloceles may protrude through a defect in the occipital bone above the foramen magnum (high occipital cephalocele), through a defect in the occipital bone that extends into the foramen magnum (low occipital cephalocele), or through a cervico-occipital defect that includes the posterior arches of C1, C2, and so on (cervico-occipital cephalocele). The occipital lobes are encountered more frequently in the herniated sac in the high occipital cephalocele. The term *Chiari III malformation* is applied to a congenital malformation in which there is a cervico-occipital cephalocele that contains nearly all of the cerebellum. This entity is discussed above (see Fig 3–54).

Parietal cephaloceles herniate in the midline just superior to the lambda, near the middle of the sagittal suture and just posterior to the anterior fontanelle. The posterior part of the interhemispheric fissure frequently enlarges and communicates with the sac. Callosal dysgenesis and Dandy-Walker cysts may be associated with parietal cephaloceles.

Nasal frontal cephaloceles herniate between two deformed orbits through a defect in the region of the bregma, producing hypertelorism and a glabellar mass. The herniated portions typically include the meninges, olfactory tracts, and anterior aspects of the frontal lobes.

Nasal orbital cephaloceles extend through a defect in the ethmoids to enter the medial parts of one or both orbits. Interfrontal cephaloceles usually herniate through a defect in the lower portions of the metopic suture; frontal cephaloceles may extend through the frontal bones more superiorly and may coexist with a frontal subcutaneous lipoma or a lipoma in the interhemispheric fissure.

Anterior cephaloceles, which include the frontal, nasofrontal-ethmoid, and nasal-orbital-frontal cephaloceles, have a higher incidence of being associated with absence or dysgenesis of the corpus callosum, interhemispheric lipoma, and hypertelorism.

MRI demonstrates the site of herniation, the specific contents of the sac, and the structures from which the sac contents arise. Typically the head is microcephalic. The residual intracranial structures appear distorted and drawn toward the site of herniation. Not only are brain parenchyma, meninges, and ventricular parts herniated in the sac, but parts of the cerebral vasculature may pass into the herniated sac with the brain. The sphenoid and sphenoid-ethmoid cephaloceles constitute a special group and are considered occult cephaloceles. They present with signs of hypertelorism, nasal stuffiness, endocrine dysfunction, and mental retardation. Nearly two thirds have true midline clefts of the nose, upper lip, or both. Approximately 40% have some form of optic nerve dysplasia. MRI demonstrates brain herniated through the floor of the sella turcica just anterior to the dorsum sellae and medial to the two cavernous sinuses. The anterior edge of the herniated defect is variable accounting for both pure sphenoid and sphenoid-ethmoid types. The cephalocele thus protrudes inferiorly to occupy the nasal fossa or herniate further downward through a cleft palate into the oral cavity. The sac nearly always contains a third ventricle and hypothalamus. The pituitary gland is variable in location within this cephalocele. The optic chiasm and nerves usually extend inferiorly. Callosal dysgenesis is present in about 40% of cases (Figs. 3–56 and 3–57).

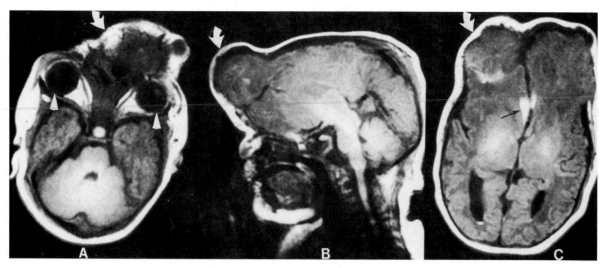

FIG 3–56.
T1-weighted MR images of anterior cephalocele. **A,** axial image, showing hypertelorism *(arrowheads)* with defect in ethmoid bone with herniation of frontal lobe *(curved arrow).* **B,** sagittal image, showing defect in frontal bone with herniation of frontal lobe *(curved arrow)* and absence of the corpus callosum. *C,* axial image, showing defect in frontal bone with herniation of frontal lobes *(curved arrow)* into an anterior sac, and lipoma of the interhemispheric fissure *(black arrow).*

Arachnoid Cysts

True arachnoid cysts are congenital cavities containing CSF lined by arachnoid cells which develop within the arachnoid membrane. Arachnoid cysts are believed to arise from aberrations in the formation of the subarachnoid space. They may or may not communicate with the normal CSF spaces of the brain. Symptoms vary depending on the size and location of the cysts. Small cysts are usually asymptomatic when they are situated within the middle cranial fossa. If the cysts are large, or in an area where

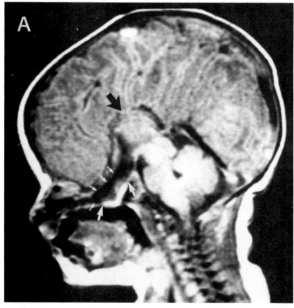

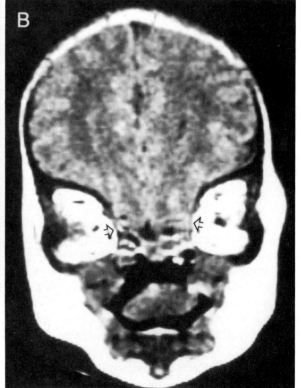

FIG 3–57.
A, sagittal T1-weighted image demonstrating basal (sphenoidal) cephalocele. Note defect in the sphenoid bone including the sella turcica *(large white arrows)* with downward herniation of the third ventricle *(small white arrows)* into the nasal cavity, and absence of the corpus callosum *(black arrow).* **B,** coronal T1-weighted image in the same patient as **B** showing herniation of frontal lobes *(arrows)* through a defect in the ethmoid bones. Also note hypertelorism.

they are adjacent to vital brain structures, the patient may present with headaches, seizures, psychomotor retardation, and raised intracranial pressure secondary to either the cysts themselves or to hydrocephalus. There may also be calvarial asymmetry with ballooning of part of the calvaria adjacent to the large arachnoid cysts.

Arachnoid cysts are more common in males with two thirds supratentorial and one third infratentorial. In the supratentorial area of the brain, the common locations can be divided into the following: sylvian fissure areas of the middle cranial fossa (50%), suprasellar (10%), interhemispheric fissure (4%), and cerebral convexity (3%). In the infratentorial area, the common locations are cerebellopontine angle (12%), superior vermian cistern (10%), cisterna magna (10%), and clival-interpeduncular space (2%). Arachnoid cysts of the middle cranial fossa have a higher tendency to bleed internally or to produce subdural hematomas. There is an association of arachnoid cysts with neoplasms (astrocytomas, meningiomas) of the brain.

On MR evaluation, T1- and T2-weighted images are necessary in order to follow the changing intensities of the cysts with the CSF of the ventricular system. When the fluid in the arachnoid cysts is of a similar consistency to CSF, the signal intensities are the same on all of the different pulse sequences. However, there may be a high content of protein within arachnoid cysts or they may bleed within their cavities, in which case the signal intensity will be different from that of the normal CSF of the ventricular system.

MRI of middle cranial fossa and sylvian fissure arachnoid cysts demonstrates a cystic mass in the anteroinferior region of the middle cranial fossa with posterior and superior displacement of the inferior aspect of the temporal lobe. The cyst may be large and in this case, there is ballooning and thinning of the middle cranial fossa. Hemorrhage within the cyst or subdural hemorrhage may be seen in this area (Fig 3–58).

Suprasellar cysts extend superiorly to compress the floor of the third ventricle and the pituitary stalk. They also commonly extend into the sella turcica as well as behind the dorsum sellae and into the anterior cranial fossa. Arachnoid cysts in an area of high convexity, produce effacement, displacement, and compression of the gyri and sulci adjacent to the cysts.

Posterior fossa cysts erode portions of the petrous bone above the cerebellopontine angle with displacement of structures adjacent to the cerebellopontine angle. Clival arachnoid cysts displace the brainstem and basilar artery posteriorly. Superior vermian arachnoid cysts displace the superior aspect of the vermis downward and may extend into the quadrigeminal cistern with compression of the colliculi producing aqueductal stenosis. Arachnoid cysts of the cisterna magna are divided into two types. The true arachnoid cyst does not communicate with the fourth ventricle or other adjacent CSF spaces. There is evidence of mass effect with compression and displacement of the fourth ventricle anteriorly. A Blake's pouch cyst of the cisterna magna communicates with the fourth ventricle through the foramen of Magendie and adjacent CSF spaces. On MRI, it is impossible to differentiate a

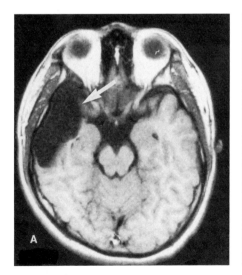 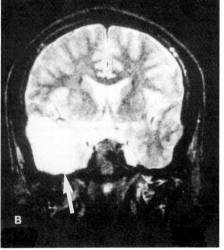

FIG 3–58.
MRI of arachnoid cyst. **A,** axial T1-weighted image shows hypointense cyst in the right middle cranial fossa *(arrow)* **B,** coronal T2-weighted image shows hyperintense cyst *(arrow)*.

true arachnoid cyst from a Blake's pouch cyst of the cisterna magna.

DISORDERS OF HISTIOGENESIS

Neurocutaneous Syndromes

The term *neurocutaneous syndromes* describes a group of congenital malformations that share neurologic and cutaneous manifestations. The classification consists of entities originally described by Van de Hoeve as phakomatoses to indicate their frequent association with cutaneous birthmarks and the potential of both types of lesions for later growth and even malignant degeneration: (1) neurofibromatosis (NF) or von Recklinghausen disease, (2) tuberous sclerosis (TS) or Bourneville disease, (3) Sturge-Weber (SW) syndrome, (4) von Hippel-Lindau (VHL) disease, and (5) the recent addition of ataxia-telangiectasia (AT) (see Table 3–3). The manifestations of the neurocutaneous syndromes are predominantly dysplastic or neoplastic, or both, and involve ectodermal structures (skin, eye, CNS, and peripheral nervous system); the mesoderm (bone and blood vessels) and endoderm (body organs) are involved to a lesser degree. The majority of diseases within the neurocutaneous syndromes are inherited as autosomal dominant or autosomal recessive disorders except for SW syndrome, which is sporadic, although familial cases have been reported. MRI is the best modality to evaluate the CNS abnormalities seen in the neurocutaneous syndromes. T1-weighted, T2-weighted, and Gd-enhanced T1-weighted sequences are needed.

Neurofibromatosis

Neurofibromatosis (NF) is the most common of the neurocutaneous syndromes. The classification has changed over the preceding years. Recently, the National Institutes of Health consensus development conference classified NF as two main types—type 1 (NF-1) and type 2 (NF-2).

Neurofibromatosis Type 1. NF-1 is inherited as an autosomal dominant disease with the genetic defect related to the long arm of the chromosome 17. It occurs in 1 in 3,000 in the general population and is commonly referred to as the childhood, peripheral, or von Recklinghausen form of NF.

The most reliable diagnostic criteria are the demonstration of six or more café-au-lait spots of 1.5 cm or more in size, Lesch spots (pigmented iris hamartomas), and a familial history. Patients with NF-1 may also have seizures, kyphoscoliosis, pseudarthrosis, and gastrointestinal, endocrine, genitourinary, and pulmonary abnormalities. The CNS and calvarial manifestations of NF-1 consist of the following: gliomas (optic nerves, optic chiasm, hypothalamus, thalamus, basal ganglia, brainstem, and cerebral hemispheres); neuromas, neurofibromas, or schwannomas of the cranial (II–XII), spinal, and peripheral nerves; dysplasia of the sphenoid bone and orbit; buphthalmos; plexiform neurofibroma of the scalp; macrocephaly secondary to megalencephaly or hemimegalencephaly; hydrocephalus secondary to aqueductal stenosis; kyphoscoliosis; and miscellaneous hyperintense brain lesions demonstrated on T2-weighted MR images.

Glioma of the optic nerve occurs in 30% to 90% of patients with NF-1. The average age of presentation is 3 to 7 years. Ten percent to 20% are bilateral. The enlargement and anatomical detail of the optic nerves is best demonstrated with fat suppression pulse sequences of the orbits. The optic nerve glioma (ONG) enlarges the optic nerve and is fusiform in appearance. It may show enhancement with Gd. The optic nerves in NF-1 may demonstrate an irregularity in outline without enlargement and this is believed to represent the dural ectasia which can be seen in NF-1. The optic nerves are normally not larger than 5 mm in diameter in children and 7 mm in adults. An ONG may commonly extend and infiltrate the optic chiasm, hypothalamus, thalamus, basal ganglia, brainstem, and occipital lobe. Ten percent to 15% of patients with NF-1 have a primary glioma of the chiasm, hypothalamus, thalamus, basal ganglia, occipital lobe, or brainstem without extension from an ONG. These gliomas have mass effect and demonstrate the classic MR appearance of isointensity or hypointensity on T1-weighted images and hyperintensity on T2-weighted images with homogeneous enhancement after Gd administration (Figs 3–59 and 3–60).

Meningiomas and acoustic neuromas can occur in NF-1, but they are rare and occur predominantly in NF-2. Although neuromas or schwannomas affecting the other cranial nerves (II–VII and IX–XII) commonly occur with NF-1, the nerve most commonly involved is cranial nerve V.

Dysplasia of the sphenoid bone (mainly the greater wing) with enlargement of the middle cranial fossa and possible herniation of the temporal lobe into the orbit is common in NF-1. The orbital involvement in NF-1 consists of buphthalmos (enlargement of the globe due to congenital glaucoma) with or without bony orbital enlargement. Osseous dysplasia frequently involves the bony orbit with enlargement.

Plexiform neurofibromas frequently involve the

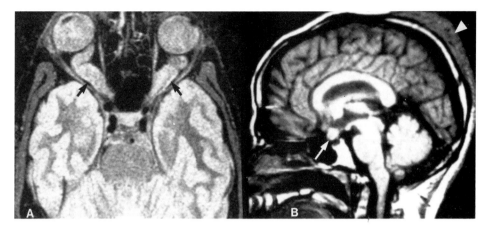

FIG 3–59.
Neurofibromatosis type 1. **A,** MRI of the orbits obtained with inversion recovery sequence showing bilateral optic nerve gliomas *(ar-* *rows).* **B,** chiasmatic glioma *(arrow)* and neurofibroma of scalp *(ar-* *rowhead).*

scalp. When the plexiform neurofibroma involves the temporal area of the scalp with extension into the frontal area and eyelid, it is often associated with ipsilateral dysplasia of the bony orbit and sphenoid bone with enlargement of the bony orbit and buphthalmos (Fig 3–61). Macrocephaly is seen in NF-1 patients and is due to megalencephaly or hemimegalencephaly. Hydrocephalus may be secondary to ob-

struction of CSF by associated neoplasm or aqueductal stenosis.

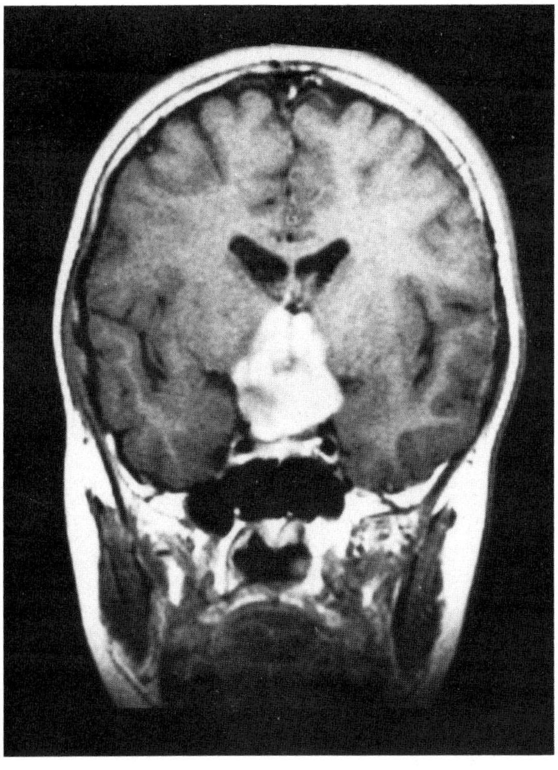

In 50% or more of patients with NF-1, there are abnormal areas of hyperintensity on T2-weighted images commonly seen in certain regions of the brain: basal ganglia, thalamus, cerebellum, and brainstem. These areas of hyperintensity are usually multiple and bilateral, although they can be single or unilateral. They are usually isointense with gray or white matter on T1-weighted images without mass effect and do not enhance with Gd. The exact cause of these abnormal hyperintense lesions is not known. They may represent atypical glial cells or hamartomas. If these lesions show enhancement with Gd and have mass effect, then they are be-

FIG 3–60.
Post-Gd coronal T1-weighted image demonstrating NF-1 with enhancement of chiasmatic-hypothalamic glioma.

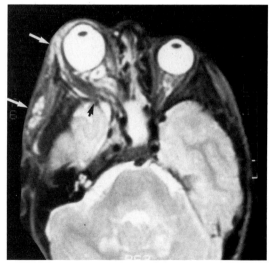

FIG 3–61.
Axial T2-weighted image: NF-1 with buphthalmos of the right orbit, dysplasia of the anterior wing of the sphenoid *(black arrow),* and neurofibromas of the temporal area of the scalp *(white arrows).*

lieved to represent low-grade gliomas (Figs 3–62 to 3–64).

The common spinal abnormalities that are seen in NF-1 consist of scoliosis (kyphoscoliosis), bony dysplasia, dural ectasia, neurofibromas and schwannomas of the spinal and paraspinal nerves, extensive plexiform neurofibromatosis of the spinal and paraspinal nerves, neurofibrosarcoma, and lateral thoracic meningocele. Ependymoma of the spinal cord is more common in NF-2. The bony abnormalities consist of dysplastic and abnormal development of the vertebral bodies, hypoplasia of the posterior elements (pedicles, transverse and spinous processes), and scalloping of the posterior aspect of the vertebral bodies. About one third of children with NF-1 have scoliosis or kyphoscoliosis of the thoracolumbosacral spine. Although CT and conventional pleuridirectional tomography (CPT) are better imaging modalities to evaluate bony detail, MRI can adequately evaluate the bony abnormalities. Neurofibromas of the spine are discussed in Section Thirteen.

Neurofibromatosis Type 2. NF-2 is commonly seen in young and middle-aged adults with a frequency of 1 in 50,000. It is a dominant disease with the abnormality located on chromosome 22 and is also called central neurofibromatosis. The diagnostic

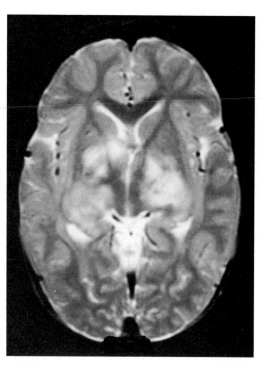

FIG 3–63.
Axial T2-weighted image: NF-1, with multiple hyperintense lesions involving the basal ganglia and thalamus with distortion of the third ventricle. Findings are compatible with degeneration into gliomas.

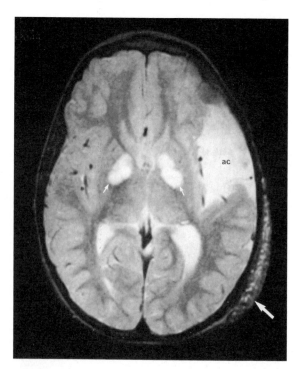

FIG 3–62.
Axial T2-weighted image: NF-1, with typical hyperintense lesions *(small white arrows)* of the globi pallidi bilaterally, neurofibroma of the scalp *(large white arrow)*, and an incidental left arachnoid cyst *(ac)*.

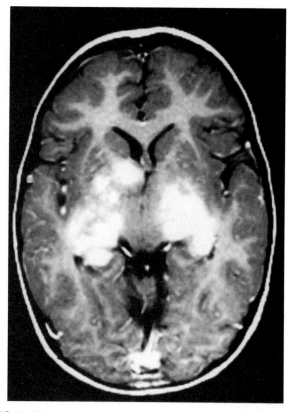

FIG 3–64.
Post-Gd axial T1-weighted image of a patient with NF-1 showing enhanced gliomas of the basal ganglia and thalamus.

criteria for NF-2 are the presence of a bilateral or a unilateral schwannoma of cranial nerve VIII plus two of the following: neurofibroma or schwannoma (in other locations), meningioma, glioma, and a relative with NF-2 (Fig 3–65).

NF-2 is a different disease from NF-1. The patients may have café-au-lait spots, but Lesch nodules, cutaneous neurofibromas, ONG, and skeletal dysplasias are rare. NF-2 is commonly associated with other cranial nerve schwannomas, cranial and spinal meningiomas, paraspinal neurofibromas, and spinal cord ependymomas.

Tuberous Sclerosis (TS)

TS is an autosomal dominant disease that occurs with a frequency of 1 in 20,000 of the general population. It is a disorder of cellular differentiation in which the clinical manifestations are secondary to hamartomatous malformations of the skin, brain, heart, and kidneys. TS is more commonly seen in children with the classic symptoms of mental retardation, epilepsy (seizures), sebaceous adenomas of the face (especially the nasolabial region), depigmented nevi, and various tumors. The most common and earliest cutaneous sign of TS is depigmented nevi (flat, well-delineated, round, or oval vitiliginous lesions of the skin).

The main CNS site of involvement is the brain.

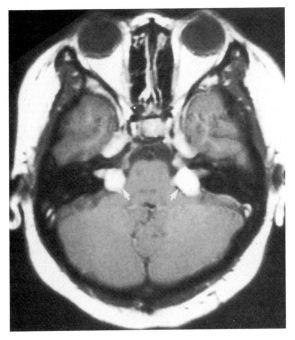

FIG 3–65.
Post-Gd axial T1-weighted image of a young adult with NF-2 showing enhancement of bilateral eighth cranial nerve schwannomas *(arrows).*

Findings are hamartomas (tubers), with or without calcium, involving the cortical and adjacent subcortical white matter, the white matter, and the subependymal region of the lateral ventricles; linear abnormalities within the white matter extending from the ventricular surface toward the cortex; and giant cell astrocytoma. The histologic features are an increase in the number of fibrillary astrocytes and large, oval, plump cells with two or three nuclei, some of which may resemble astrocytes or neurons. There is also dense fibrillary gliosis, abnormal myelination, and, at times foci of calcification. The MR evaluation should consist of T1-weighted, T2-weighted, and Gd-enhanced sequences to evaluate for hamartoma, neoplasm (giant cell astrocytoma), and calcification (although CT is still the best modality for demonstrating calcification). On MRI the cortical hamartomas flatten the gyri, giving them a more pachygyric appearance. Gross calcification within these hamartomas is extremely rare in infants but can be seen in children 2 years and older and in adults. These cortical hamartomas involve the cortex and at times the adjacent subcortical white matter. They can be solitary but are usually multiple and are isointense or hypointense on T1-weighted images and hyperintense on T2-weighted images.

Subependymal hamartomas commonly occur at the head of the caudate nucleus just posterior to the foramen of Monro, the lateral borders of the bodies of the lateral ventricles, and the anterior aspect of the atrium of the lateral ventricle. They are usually multiple and bilateral and they may vary in size from 1 to 10 mm. The hamartoma located near the foramen of Monro is usually the largest and commonly contains calcification. The subependymal hamartomas contain calcifications more frequently than either the cortical or white matter hamartomas. Subependymal hamartomas are usually isointense with, or slightly hyperintense to, gray matter on T1-weighted images, and hyperintense on T1-weighted images. If the calcification is large, it may be seen as hypointensity or hyperintensity on T1-weighted and hypointense on T2-weighted images (Fig 3–66).

Hamartomas can occur in the white matter of the cerebral hemispheres and, to a lesser extent, the cerebellar hemispheres. These lesions demonstrate hyperintensity on T2-weighted images (Fig 3–67).

The hamartoma can degenerate into a giant cell astrocytoma or astroblastoma. The most common location is the head of the caudate nucleus at the foramen of Monro. A giant cell astrocytoma commonly enlarges and grows faster than a benign hamartoma. A giant cell astrocytoma shows enhancement with

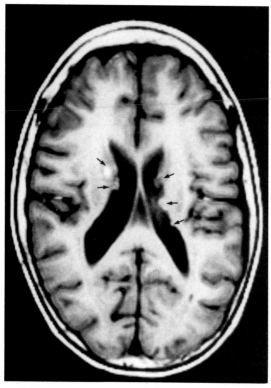

FIG 3–66.
Axial T1-weighted image of a patient with tuberous sclerosis. Subependymal calcified hamartomas demonstrate hyperintensity and hypointensity (arrows).

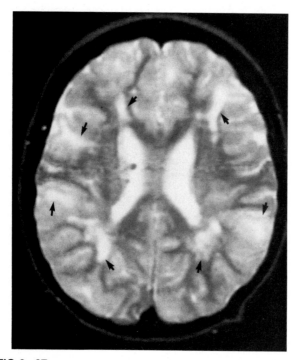

FIG 3–67.
Axial T2-weighted image of a patient with tuberous sclerosis showing hyperintense hamartomas (arrows) scattered throughout the brain.

Gd and frequently contains calcification (Figs 3–68 and 3–69).

On MR with T2-weighted images, linear areas of hyperintensity can be seen within the white matter extending from the region of the lateral borders toward the cortex. These areas are believed to represent regions of fibrillary gliosis or disturbances in myelination.

Sturge-Weber (SW) Syndrome

SW syndrome (encephalotrigeminal angiomatosis) is considered to be a sporadic, noninherited abnormality, although familial cases have been reported. It is congenital and characterized by angiomatous malformation affecting the skin, eye, and brain. Its two main manifestations consist of a port wine nevus involving the skin of the face (region of the eyelid, forehead, and cheek) and angiomatosis of the pia

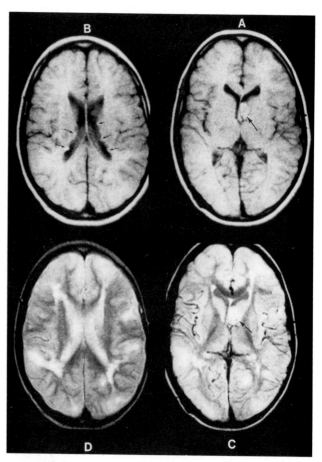

FIG 3–68.
MR axial images in a patient with tuberous sclerosis. **A,** T1-weighted image demonstrating subependymal giant cell astrocytoma (arrow). **B,** T1-weighted image, showing subependymal hamartomas (arrows). **C,** proton density image showing hyperintensity of subependymal giant cell astrocytoma (arrow). **D,** T2-weighted image showing multiple hyperintense hamartomas.

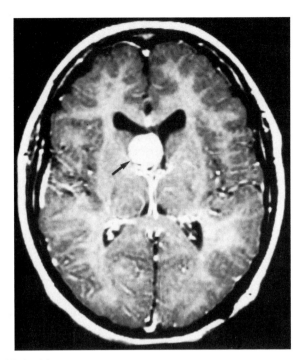

FIG 3–69.
Post-Gd axial T1-weighted image of a patient with tuberous sclerosis; showing enhancement of giant cell astrocytoma *(arrow)*.

mater in the occipital and occipitoparietal region. Over 90% of these patients have seizures with additional symptoms such as hemiparesis, hemianopsia, mental retardation, and glaucoma. The angiomatosis consists of small multiple tortuous venous vessels.

The CNS manifestations involve the (1) brain (pia mater angiomatosis, cortical calcification, hemiatrophy, parenchymal gliosis or demyelination, prominent deep venous system, enlarged choroid plexus); (2) the cranium (ipsilateral calvarial bone and paranasal sinus enlargement); and (3) the eyes (buphthalmos).

The main findings on MRI are abnormalities involving the brain. The classic changes of SW are demonstrated in older children and adults. There is fusiform serpentine calcification involving the cortex of the brain which is commonly unilateral in the occipital or occipitoparietal lobes, although a whole hemisphere or both hemispheres may be involved. There is cortical atrophy on the involved side, especially in the area of the calcification, with resultant hemihypertrophy of the ipsilateral calvaria, paranasal sinuses, mastoid air cells, and an elevated petrous ridge. The cortical calcifications are best demonstrated on T2-weighted images. However, CT remains the most sensitive modality for evaluating calcification in SW. The pia mater angiomatosis is not demonstrated with MRI. After administration of Gd, enhancement of the abnormal cortex may be seen.

The gyral enhancement is fusiform, serpentine, and is believed to be a result of anoxic ischemic changes that occur within the cortex underlying the angiomatous malformation of the pia mater. The pial angiomatous malformation steals blood from the underlying cortex with resultant ischemic infarction within the cortical layers (Fig 3–70).

In young children (usually 2 years and younger), an infantile form of SW can be seen on MRI. Calcification is not present. On the involved side, the sulci are smaller and the cortical gray matter is hypointense on T1-weighted images and slightly hyperintense on T2-weighted images. If Gd is given, there may be cortical enhancement on the involved side (Fig 3–71).

von Hippel-Lindau (VHL) Syndrome

VHL syndrome is an autosomal dominant disease that is characterized by CNS angiomatosis. In 1926, Lindau recognized the association of angiomatous retinal tumors (von Hippel disease) and angiomatous tumors of the CNS. VHL syndrome is commonly associated with cerebellar (40%–60%) and retinal (50%–70%) hemangioblastomas, cysts, and angiomas of the liver and kidney, renal cell carcinoma (20%–40%), and pheochromocytoma (10%). The diagnosis is based on the presence of one of the fol-

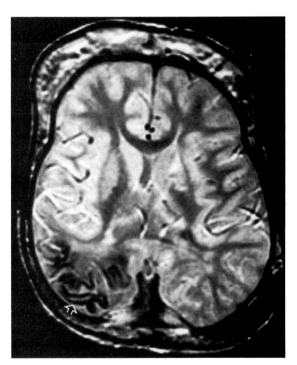

FIG 3–70.
Axial T2-weighted image of a patient with Sturge-Weber syndrome shows hypointense serpentine calcification of the cortex of the right occipital lobe *(arrow)*.

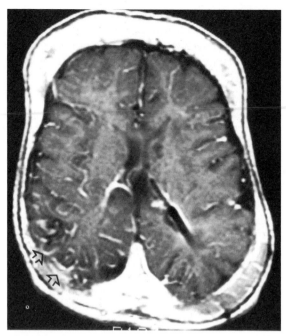

FIG 3–71.
Post-Gd axial T1-weighted image in a patient with Sturge-Weber syndrome demonstrating enhancement of the cortex of the right occipital lobe *(arrows)* and thickened calvaria.

lowing: (1) one or more hemangioblastomas of the CNS, (2) one hemangioblastoma of the CNS with a visceral manifestation, and (3) hemangioblastoma of CNS or a visceral manifestation with a known family history of the disease.

Patients with VHL present at about the third decade with raised intracranial pressure and cerebellar abnormalities. The primary CNS finding in VHL is a hemangioblastoma predominantly involving the cerebellum, the medulla, and spinal cord. The hemangioblastoma is usually unilateral but may be multiple. The neoplasm consists of a vascular solid nodule surrounded by a very large cystic component. The fluid of the tumor cyst may have increased protein or blood.

Ataxia-Telangiectasia (AT)

AT is an autosomal recessive disorder described by Louis-Bar in 1941. It is a progressive disorder with involvement of the CNS, skin, and respiratory and immune systems. It is characterized by telangiectasias involving the skin (face) and eyes, with cerebellar ataxia, immunodeficiencies, and infections of the paranasal sinuses and lungs. It occurs in children and produces progressive ataxia. The telangiectasia commonly involves the pia mater and white matter

of the brain, predominantly the cerebellum. The major MR finding is severe atrophy of the cerebellum.

INHERITED METABOLIC BRAIN DISORDERS

The term *metabolic brain disorders* refers to a group of inherited diseases in which a specific enzyme defect has been identified. Clinically, children with inborn errors of metabolism present with much variation in phenotype and symptoms which often makes diagnosis difficult. Although in recent years our knowledge of the specific enzymatic defect in many of these inherited metabolic brain disorders has increased, there remain many diseases in this group that share genetic transmission with progressive symptoms and metabolic abnormalities, but in which the precise enzymatic defect is unknown.

Children with inherited metabolic brain disorders frequently have neurologic manifestations. They also may have other visceral abnormalities. It is a combination of neurologic symptoms with and without visceral manifestation and age at onset of symptoms, that often leads to suspicion of an underlying inherited metabolic brain disorder. The diagnosis is made by laboratory analysis and tissue biopsy. Inherited metabolic brain disorders can be classified into four main groups and the characteristic findings may be demonstrated on MRI and CT depending on the specific disorder. The four groups consist of: (1) diseases involving only the white matter, the so-called leukodystrophies, which include sudanophilic leukodystrophy (Cockayne and Pelizaeus-Merzbacher diseases), metachromatic leukodystrophy, adrenoleukodystrophy, Canavan disease, Alexander disease, and globoid cell leukodystrophy (Krabbe disease); (2) diseases affecting predominantly the gray matter—the poliodystrophies ceroid lipofuscinosis and trichopoliodystrophy (Menke disease); (3) basal ganglia disorders: Huntington, Wilson, and Leigh diseases; and (4) the mucopolysaccharidoses, predominantly Hurler, Hunter, and Morquio diseases. Only the leukodystrophies are discussed in this chapter (Table 3–4).

TABLE 3–4.
Leukodystrophies

Metachromic leukodystrophy
Adrenoleukodystrophy
Globoid cell leukodystrophy (Krabbe disease)
Alexander disease
Canavan (van Bogaert) disease
Cockayne disease
Pelizaeus-Merzbacher disease

Leukodystrophies

The known leukodystrophies are genetic diseases involving defects in oligodendroglia function and myelinogenesis. The term *leukodystrophy* describes a chronic progressive destructive process of the myelin of the CNS characterized by a metabolic disorder of myelin sheath maintenance and formation. It belongs to a larger group of so-called degenerative processes of the nervous system. These disorders are characterized by a slow, but progressive loss of nervous structures and are caused by endogenous metabolic disorders of the nervous system. The course of clinical signs is progressive and includes mental retardation with signs of long tract dysfunction such as pyramidal and cerebellar disturbances with abnormal conduction of visual, auditory, and somatic sensory input measured by evoked potentials.

MR evaluation of patients with leukodystrophies should consist of T1-weighted images and T2-weighted images but with the emphasis on the latter. In young children, more heavily T2-weighted sequences with TRs of 2,500 to 3,500 ms and echo time (TEs) of 100 to 120 ms should be obtained, especially in children under 5 years of age. It is difficult to evaluate the degree of dysmyelination in children under 2 years of age because the normal myelination process does not begin until the eighth month of fetal gestation and proceeds rapidly during the first 2 years of life. By 2 years of age, 90% of all the white matter fiber tracts have become myelinated. In children under 2 years of age, the destructive process cannot be adequately demonstrated on T2-weighted images. However, by 2 years of age and older, the process, in which there is hyperintensity of the white matter fibers on long T2-weighted images is demonstrated in the leukodystrophies instead of the normal hypointensity. Under 2 years of age, CT is a better modality to demonstrate the marked abnormality of the white matter fibers. Unenhanced CT demonstrates marked hypodensity to the white matter fibers. The majority of leukodystrophies do not demonstrate enhancement except for adrenoleukodystrophy. The end state appearance of all the leukodystrophies on CT or MRI is marked generalized atrophy.

Metachromatic Leukodystrophy

Metachromatic leukodystrophy (MLD) is inherited as a recessive disorder. The frequency of MLD is 1 in 40,000 to 50,000 in the general population. There are four subtypes: congenital, late infantile, juvenile, and adult. The late infantile subtype is the most common and presents from around 14 months to 4 years of age. The early presentations are: an unsteady gait that progresses to severe ataxia and flaccid paralysis, dysarthria, mental retardation, and decerebrate posturing.

The enzymatic defect is secondary to a deficiency of the lysosome arylsulfatase A (cerebroside-3-sulfatase). The diagnosis is made by a build-up of sulfatide in the urine as well as low levels of arylsulfatase A in the urine and in the leukocytes of nervous tissue. Histologic analysis of the abnormal nervous tissue demonstrates a complete loss of myelin (demyelination) followed by axonal degeneration.

The MR findings are well demonstrated on T2-weighted images. There is marked hyperintensity of the white matter fiber tracts involving the cerebral hemispheres which may extend to the cerebellum, brainstem, and spinal cord. On T1-weighted images, the white matter fibers may be isointense with, or hypointense to, gray matter. The end stage of the disease demonstrates generalized cerebral and spinal cord atrophy (Fig 3–72, *A* and *B*).

Adrenoleukodystrophy

Adrenoleukodystrophy (ALD) is an X-linked recessive disorder involving predominantly the white matter of the CNS and the adrenal cortex. There are several subtypes and the most common is a childhood form which is commonly seen between 5 and 10 years of age. The neurologic symptoms are homonymous hemianopsia evolving to blindness with behavioral changes progressing to mental retardation and dementia. There are also gait disturbances starting with clumsiness and incoordination progressing to severe ataxia and then to spastic quadriplegia.

The underlying disorder of ALD is the abnormal accumulation of long-chain fatty acids in the plasma as well as in the brain (white matter), peripheral nerves, spinal cord, and adrenal glands. The basic metabolic defect is the impaired capacity to degrade very long-chain fatty acids (predominantly involving carbon chains of 24 to 30 atoms, but especially 25 to 26) caused by a defect in peroxisomal beta-oxidation. It is located at the level of acyl coenzyme A (acyl-CoA) synthetase. There is histologic evidence of myelin degeneration of the periventricular white matter beginning at the occipital and (posterior) temporal lobes, extending in an anterior direction eventually to involve the parietal and frontal lobes. An inflammatory reaction is seen along this spreading area of myelin degeneration.

The MRI changes are related to the locations of

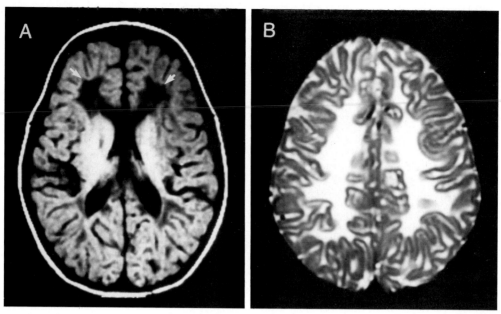

FIG 3–72.
Axial MR images of a patient with metachromatic leukodystrophy. **A,** T1-weighted image, shows periventricular *(arrows)* and subcortical areas of hypointensity and generalized cortical atrophy. **B,** T2- weighted image at the level of the centrum semiovale demonstrating diffuse hyperintensity of all the white matter fibers.

the beginning areas of degeneration. The first changes are increased hyperintensity on T2-weighted images involving predominantly the periventricular white matter along the occipital horns and atrial areas of the lateral ventricles, and subsequently involving the posterior temporal and parietal aspects of the lobes of the cerebral hemispheres. Eventually, this process extends to the remaining parts of the cerebral hemispheres, brainstem, and cerebellum. The long white matter tracts of the spinal cord eventually become involved and, with high resolution technique, either increased signal in this area or degenerative changes may be visualized. After administration of Gd there may be some enhancement along the peripheral aspect of the areas of myelin degeneration (Fig 3–73).

Globoid Cell Leukodystrophy (Krabbe Disease)
Globoid cell leukodystrophy (GLD) is an autosomal recessive disorder. The frequency of GLD is 2 in 100,000 in a series reported from Sweden. It is seen predominantly in young children and infants. The infantile form is the most common. Onset of symptoms usually begins a few months after birth with irritability. The disease continues to progress with development of encephalitis-like symptoms with motor deterioration and atypical seizures. At the end stage of the disease, the child is in a vegetative state with decerebrate posturing. Pathologically, the disease involves predominantly the white matter of the cere-

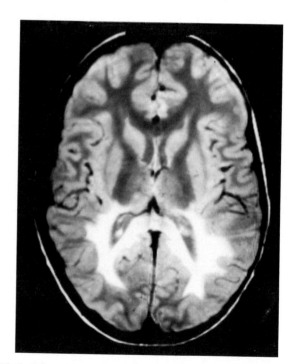

FIG 3–73.
Axial T2-weighted image in a patient with adrenoleukodystrophy showing hyperintensity of the white matter along the posterior horns of the lateral ventricles. (Courtesy of Joseph Levy, M.D., Lutheran General Hospital, Chicago.)

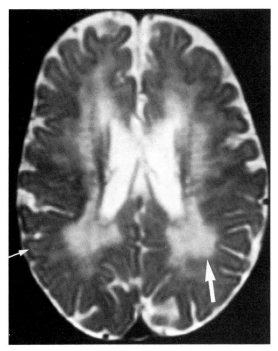

FIG 3–74.
Axial T1-weighted image of a patient with Krabbe disease showing greater hyperintensity of the central white matter *(large arrow)* in relation to the also involved peripheral (U) white matter fibers *(small arrow).*

bral hemispheres, cerebellum, and spinal cord. Histologically, the presence of globoid cells within the white matter is pathognomonic. These globoid cells are macrophages (histiocytes rather than glial cells). The primary defect in GLD is galactocerebroside

β-galactosidase deficiency. This enzyme degrades cerebroside to galactose and ceramide. It is a lysosomal enzyme, and the crystalline deposits in the globoid cells that are found within the white matter are composed of cerebroside. T2-weighted images show hyperintensity of the white matter of the cerebral hemispheres (centrum semiovale and periventricular), which is diffuse and symmetric. At times, changes within the cerebellar white matter can also be seen, with hyperintensity on T2-weighted images. The changes within the spinal cord are not as readily apparent and the usual MR findings are atrophic changes (Fig 3–74).

Alexander Disease

Alexander disease (AD) is a rare disorder. Although familial cases have been reported, its mode of transmission remains uncertain. Three clinical types exist: infantile, juvenile, and adult. The infantile type is the most common. The onset of symptoms is from birth, with delay in development, hypotonia, seizures, and progressive macrocephaly.

The diagnosis is made through biopsy of the brain. The histologic feature is a considerable amount of Rosenthal fibers within the white matter. Most commonly the disease begins in the periventricular white matter, usually involving the frontal lobes and then extending into the parietotemporal and then the occipital regions. Eventually, there is involvement of the cerebellar white matter and spinal cord.

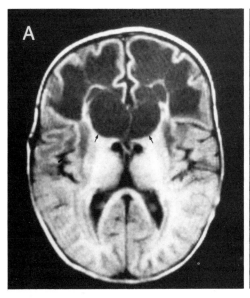 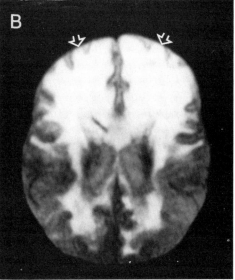

FIG 3–75.
Axial MR images in Alexander disease. **A,** T1-weighted image shows marked hypointensity of the white matter of both frontal lobes with dilatation of the frontal horns of the lateral ventricles *(ar-*rows). **B,** there is marked hyperintensity of the white matter fibers, especially within the frontal lobes *(arrows in T2-weighted images).*

The MR findings demonstrate macrocephaly with hyperintensity on T2-weighted images involving the white matter areas commonly seen in the frontal areas with progression posteriorly to involve other parts of the cerebral hemispheres (Fig 3–75, *A* and *B*).

Canavan Disease

Canavan disease (CD) is an autosomal recessive disorder that is also referred to as spongy degeneration of the CNS (van Bogaert-Bertrand). There are three clinical subtypes: infantile, juvenile, and adult. The most common is the infantile type which usually presents within the first 6 months of life. The infants present with hypotonia, irritability, and enlarging head size. The symptoms progress and lead to spasticity, blindness, choreoathetoid movement, and myoclonic seizures.

The diagnosis is made by demonstrating increased amounts of *N*-acetylaspartic acid in the urine and plasma. On histologic examination, the disease is seen to begin in a peripheral location involving the U-fibers of the subcortical white matter of the cerebral hemispheres. Later, the abnormality involves the deep white matter structures of both cerebral hemispheres and eventually it extends to the cerebellum and spinal cord. The involvement of the U-fibers of the white matter is diffuse and in the early histologic analysis, there is evidence of vacuoles within the subcortical white matter and extending into the adjacent cortex. The vacuolization gives the disease its characteristic name of spongy degenera-

tion of the CNS. Canavan disease, unlike the other white matter diseases, typically begins in the peripheral subcortical U-fibers of the white matter and only in the later stages of the disease extends to involve the deep white matter structures of the brain. There is a deficiency of the enzyme aspartoacylase with associated build-up of *N*-acetylaspartic acid. The MR findings are related to the myelin degeneration of the white matter fiber tracts; the first changes seen are subcortical U-fibers with hyperintensity on T2-weighted images. Eventually, there is diffuse involvement of all the white matter fiber tracts in both cerebral hemispheres. In the later stages of the disease, there is atrophy of the cerebral hemispheres (Fig 3–76).

Cockayne Disease

Cockayne disease (CoD) is a rare autosomal recessive disorder due to a defect in DNA repair. Its clinical manifestations begin at around 6 to 12 months of age and the disease is characterized by severe psychomotor retardation with dwarfism, kyphosis, loss of adipose tissue producing facies characteristic of an old person, hypoplasia of the mandible with maldeveloped ears, sensorineural hearing loss, ocular lesions leading to cataracts, optic atrophy and blindness, cerebellar ataxia with choreoathetoid movement, muscular atrophy, and cerebellar ataxia.

On histologic examination, there is a marked reduction in the white matter with a loss of myelin, lipids, and increase of cholesterol esters. The cerebral hemispheric white matter fiber tracts, including

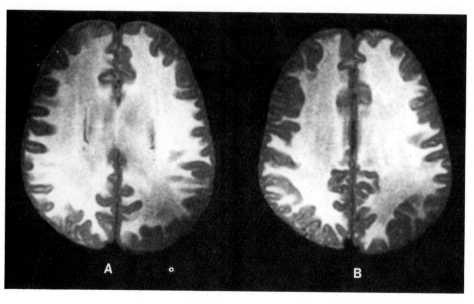

FIG 3–76.
Axial T2-weighted images. **A,** Canavan disease at the superior borders of the lateral ventricles and, **B,** at the centrum semiovale demonstrating macrocephaly with marked hyperintensity of all of the white matter fibers.

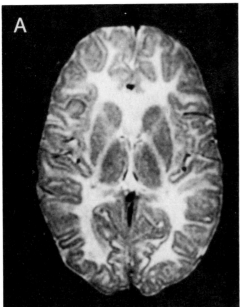
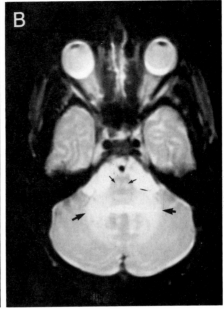

FIG 3–77.
Axial T2-weighted images. **A,** Pelizaeus-Merzbacher disease at the level of the internal capsule demonstrating diffuse hyperintensity of all the white matter fibers. **B,** same patient, at the level of the pons, demonstrating hyperintensity of white matter fibers within a small pons *(small black arrows)* and also within the white matter of the cerebellum *(large black arrows).*

the U-fibers, are involved as well as the cerebellar hemispheric white matter tracts. There is a marked decrease in the white matter with calcification involving the basal ganglia and at times the white matter and cortex. There is a diffuse dysmyelination process throughout the brain. The end stage consists of marked cerebral and cerebellar atrophy with calcification within the basal ganglia and, at times, the dentate nucleus. There is microcephaly.

The MR changes consist of hyperintensity involving the white matter fiber tracts of the cerebral and cerebellar hemispheres on T2-weighted images. Hypointensity is demonstrated involving the basal ganglia and dentate nucleus if calcification is present, and long TR and TE sequences. If the calcification is severe, it may also be seen within the white of the cerebral hemispheres. CT is the best modality to evaluate the calcification.

Pelizaeus-Merzbacher Disease

Pelizaeus-Merzbacher disease (PMD) is a rare white matter disorder in which the metabolic defect is unknown. It is familial. Three subtypes (depending on the presentation and clinical symptoms) exist: classic, connatal, and transitional.

The most common type is the classic, which occurs in late infancy. It is an X-linked recessive disorder. The early symptoms are wandering (pendular) eye movements with failure to develop normal head control. Eventually, the child develops spasticity

with choreoathetoid movement, cerebellar ataxia, and mental retardation with optic atrophy and blindness. Kyphoscoliosis is also common. The course is progressive with death in late adolescence or early adulthood.

The diagnosis is made on the basis of exclusion of other metabolic brain disorders as well as of the clinical signs and presentation. Laboratory investigations are of little help in the diagnosis except for the brainstem evoked response which is abnormal. On histologic examination, there is evidence of diffuse loss of myelin throughout the brain, involving both the cerebral and cerebellar hemispheres including the long white matter fiber tracts of the spinal cord and brainstem (Fig 3–77, *A* and *B*).

REFERENCES

Disorders of Organogenesis

Arslanian SA, Rothfus WE, Foley TP Jr, et al: Hormonal, metabolic and neuroradiologic abnormalities associated with septo-optic dysplasia. *Acta Endocrinol* 1984; 107:282–288.

Barth PG: Disorders of neuronal migration. *Can J Neurol Sci* 1987; 14:1–16.

Bignami A, Palladini G, Zappella M: Unilateral megalencephaly with nerve cell hypertrophy: An anatomical and quantitative histochemical study. *Brain Res* 1968; 9:103–114.

Bull J: The corpus callosum. *Clin Radiol* 1967; 18:2–18.

Byrd SE, Osborn RE, Bohan TP, et al: The CT and MR evaluation of migrational disorders of the brain. Part I. *Pediatr Radiol* 1989 19:219:222.

Cohen MM, Jirasek JE, Guzman RT, et al: Holoprosencephaly and facial dysmorphia nosology, etiology and pathogenesis. *Birth Defects* 1971; 7:125–135.

Curnes JT, Laster DW, Koubek TD, et al: MRI of corpus callosal syndromes. *AJNR* 1986; 7:617–622.

Davidoff LM, Dyke CC: Agenesis of the corpus callosum. *Am J Roentgenol* 1934; 32:1–25.

Deeb ZL, Rothfus WE, Maroon JC: MR imaging of heterotopic gray matter. *J Comput Assist Tomogr* 1985; 9:1140–1141.

DeMeyer W: Classification of cerebral malformations. *Birth Defects* 1971; 7:78–93.

DeMeyer W, Zeman G: Alobar holoprosencephaly (arhinencephaly) with median cleft lip and palate: Clinical, electroencephalographic and nosologic considerations. *Confin Neurol* 1963; 23:1–36.

DeMeyer W, Zeman W, Palmer CG: The face predicts the brain: Diagnostic significance of median anomalies for holoprosencephaly (arhinencephaly). *Pediatrics* 1964; 34:256–263.

Diebler C, Dulac O: Cephaloceles: Clinical and neuroradiological appearance. *Neuroradiology* 1983; 25:199–216.

Dobyns WB: Developmental aspects of lissencephaly and the lissencephaly syndromes. *Birth Defects* 1987; 23:225–241.

Dobyns WB, Gilbert EF, Opitz JM: Further comments on the lissencephaly syndrome. *Am J Med Genet* 1985; 22:197–211.

Dobyns WB, Stratton RF, Parke JT, et al: Miller-Dieker syndrome: Lissencephaly and monosomy y17p. *J Pediatr* 1983; 69:552–558.

Fitz CR: Holoprosencephaly and related entities. *Neuroradiology* 1983; 25:225–238.

Friede RL, Mikolasek J: Postencephalitic porencephaly, hydranencephaly and polymicrogyria: A review. *Acta Neuropathol* 1978; 43:161–168.

Hale BR, Rice P: Septo-optic dysplasia: Clinical and embryological aspects. *Dev Med Child Neurol* 1970; 16:812–820.

Hanaway J, Lee SI, Netsky MG: Pachygyria, relation of findings to modern embryologic concepts. *Neurology* 1968; 18:791–799.

Harwood-Nash DC, Fitz CR: *Neuroradiology in Infants and Children.* St Louis, Mosby–Year Book, 1976.

Jellinger K, Rett A: Agyria-pachygyria (lissencephaly syndrome). *Neuropediatrie* 1976; 7:66–91.

Kendall BE: Dysgenesis of the corpus callosum. *Neuroradiology* 1983; 25:239–256.

Lacey DJ: Agenesis of the corpus callosum clinical features in 40 children. *Am J Dis Child* 1985; 139:953–955.

Manz HJ, Phillips TM, Rowden G, et al: Unilateral megalencephaly, cerebral cortical dysplasia, neuronal hypertrophy, and heterotopia: Cytomorphometric, fluorometric, cytochemical, and biochemical analysis. *Acta Neuropathol* 1979; 45:97–103.

Naidich TP, McLone DG, Fulling KH: The Chiari II malformation: Part IV. The hindbrain deformity. *Neuroradiology* 1983; 25:179–197.

Naidich TP, Radkowski MA, Bernstein RA, et al: Congenital malformation of the posterior fossa, in Taveras JM, Ferucci JT (eds): *Radiology.* Philadelphia, JB Lippincott, 1986, pp 1–17.

Naidich TP, Zimmerman RA: Common congenital malformations of the brain, in Brandt-Zawadzki M, Normal D (eds): *Magnetic Resonance Imaging of the Central Nervous System.* New York, Raven Press 1987, pp 131–150.

Osborn RE, Byrd SE, Naidich TP, et al: MR Imaging of neuronal migrational disorders. *AJNR* 1988; 9:1101-1106.

Probst FP: Congenital defects of the corpus callosum: morphology and encephalographic appearance. *Acta Radiol* 1973; 1–52.

Radkowski MA, Naidich TP, McLone DG: Intracranial arachnoid cysts. *Pediatr Neurosci* 1986; 12:112–122.

Stewart RM, Richman DP, Caviness VS Jr: Lissencephaly and pachygyria. *Acta neuropathol (Berl)* 1975; 31:1–12.

Townsend JJ, Nielsen SL, Malamud N: Unilateral megalencephaly: Harmatoma or neoplasm? *Neurology* 1975; 25:448–453.

Yakovlev PI: Pathoarchitectonic studies of cerebral malformations. III Arrhinencephalies cholotelencephalies. *J Neuropathol Exp Neurol* 1959; 18:22.

Yakovlev PI, Wadsworth RC: Schizencephalies. A study of the congenital clefts in the cerebral mantle. I. Clefts with fused lips. *J Neuropathol Exp Neurol* 1946; 5:116–130.

Yakovlev PI, Wadsworth RC: Schizencephalies. A study of the congenital clefts in the cerebral mantle. II. Clefts with hydrocephalus and lips separated. *J Neuropathol Exp Neurol* 1946; 5:169–203.

Disorders of Histiogenesis

Altman NR, Purser RK, Post MSD: Tuberous sclerosis: Characteristics at CT and MR imaging. *Radiology* 1988; 167:527–532.

Atlas SW, Grossman RI, Hackney DB, et al: Calcified intracranial lesions, detection with gradient echo acquisition rapid MR imaging. *AJNR* 1987; 8:932–933.

Bognanno JR, Edwards MK, Lee TA, et al: Cranial MR imaging in neurofibromatosis. *AJNR* 1988; 9:461–468.

Braffman BH, Bilaniuk LT, Zimmerman RA: The central nervous system manifestations of the phakomatosis on MR. *Radiol Clin North Am* 1988; 26:773–800.

Burk DL Jr, Brunberg JA, Kanal E, et al: Spinal and paraspinal neurofibromatosis: Surface coil MR imaging at 1–5 T. *Radiology* 1987: 162:797–801.

Conference statement, neurofibromatosis. National Institutes of Health Consensus Development Conference. *Arch Neurol* 1988; 45:575–578.

Diebler C, Dulac O. *Pediatric Neurology and Neuroradiology.* New York, Springer-Verlag, 1987.

Harwood-Wash DC, Fitz CR. *Neuroradiology in Infants and Children.* St Louis, Mosby–Year Book, 1976.

Huson SM, Harper PS, Hourihan MD, et al: Cerebellar hemangioblastoma and von Hippel-Lindau disease. *Brain* 1986; 109:1297–1310.

Mirowitz SA, Sartor K, Gado M: High-intensity basal ganglia lesions on T1-weighted MR images in neurofibromatosis. *AJR* 1990; 154:369–373.

Monaghan HP, Krafchik BR, Mac Gregor DL, et al: Tuberous sclerosis complex in children. *Am J Dis Child* 1981; 135:912–917.

Paller A: Ataxia-telangiectasia. *Neurol Clin* 1987; 3:447–449.

Riccardi VM: Von Recklinghausen neurofibromatosis. *N Engl J Med* 1981; 305:1617–1628.

Roach ES, Williams DP, Laster D: Magnetic resonance imaging in tuberous sclerosis. *Arch Neurol* 1987; 44:301–303.

Sato Y, Waziri M, Smith W, et al: Hippel-Lindau disease: MR imaging. *Radiology* 1988; 166:241–246.

Terwey B, Doose H: Tuberous sclerosis: Magnetic imaging of the brain. *Neuropediatrics* 1987; 18:67–69.

Van der Hoeve J: Augenqeschwülste bei dem tuberösen Hirnsklerose (Bourneville) und verwandten Krankheiten. *Arch Ophthalmol* 1923; 111:1–16.

Van der Hoeve J: Les phakomatoses de Bourneville, de Recklinghausen et de von Hippel-Lindau. *J Belge Neurol Psychiatr* 1933; 33:752–762.

Wasenko JJ, Rosenbloom SA, Duchesneau PM, et al: The Sturge-Weber Syndrome: Comparison of MR and CT characteristics. *AJNR* 1990; 11:131–134.

Yakovlev PI, Guthrie RH. Congenital ectodermoses (neurocutaneous syndromes) in epileptic patients. *Arch Neurol Psychiatry* 1931; 26:1145–1197.

Inherited Metabolic Brain Disorders

Aubourg P. Scotti J, Rocchiccioli F, et al: Neonatal adreno-leukodystrophy. *J Neurol Neurosurg Psychiatry* 1986; 49:77–86.

Baram TZ, Goldman AM, Percy AK: Krabbe's disease: Specific MRI and CT findings. *Neurology* 1986; 36:111.

Lenard HG: Adrenoleukodystrophy. *Neuropediatrics* 1984; 15:16–19.

McKhann GM: Metachromatic leukodystrophy: Clinical and enzymatic parameters. *Neuropediatrics* 1984; 15:4–10.

Morrell P: A correlative synopsis of the leukodystrophies. *Neuropediatrics* 1984; 15:62–65.

Norton WT: Some thoughts on the neurobiology of leukodystrophies. *Neuropediatrics.* 1984; 15:28–31.

Seitelberg F: Structural manifestations of leukodystrophies. *Neuropediatrics* 1984; 15:53–61.

Soila KP: MRI of demyelinating and other white matter diseases, in Pomeranz SJ (ed): *Craniospinal Magnetic Resonance Imaging.* Philadelphia, WB Saunders, 1989, pp 459–488.

Valk J, van der Knaap MS: *Magnetic Resonance of Myelin, Myelination and Myelin Disorders.* New York, Springer-Verlag, 1990.

van der Knaap MS, Valk J: The reflection of histology in MR imaging of Pelizaeus-Merzbacher disease. *AJNR* 1989; 10:99–103.

Wende S, Ludwig B, Kishikawa T, et al: The value of CT in diagnosis and prognosis of different inborn neurogenerative disorders in children. *J Neurol* 1984; 231:57–70.

Zeman W, Demeyer W: Pelizaeus-Merzbacher disease. *Neuropathol Exp Neurol* 1964; 23:334–354.

SECTION 4

Trauma

HEAD TRAUMA

Head trauma is a significant cause of morbidity and mortality in infants and children. The common causes of trauma in the pediatric population are difficult birth, motor vehicle accident, fall, and child abuse. The trauma may involve the scalp, skull, intracerebral compartments, or brain. With acute head trauma, lacerations, contusions, hematomas, and edema are seen. The late sequelae of trauma consist of chronic hematomas and atrophy. CT is still the best radiologic modality to evaluate head trauma. CT allows excellent evaluation of scalp, and extracerebral and intracerebral hemorrhage. Acute, subacute, and chronic hemorrhage on CT is hyperdense, isodense, and hypodense to brain parenchyma. CT and plain skull radiographs are the best modalities to evaluate skull fractures, which are discussed in Chapter 1.

Although MRI is being used increasingly to evaluate the hemorrhage and edema associated with head trauma, it has certain limitations. There are a variety of factors that influence the appearance of hemorrhage on MRI. First are operator-dependent factors, which affect the signal intensity of hemorrhage. These factors consist of pulse sequence parameters and the field strength of the magnet. The signal intensity of hemorrhage will vary with low- and high-field-strength magnets. Second are the physiologic properties that influence the signal intensity of hemorrhage: the age of the hemorrhage, the size of the hematoma, the degree of oxygenation of the local surrounding tissue, and the amount of clot formation and retraction. The most important of the physiologic factors that affect the signal intensity of hemorrhage on MRI is the oxygen state of hemoglobin and its degree of metabolic change and breakdown. As a hematoma changes from the acute to the subacute to the chronic stage, the hemoglobin changes from oxyhemoglobin to deoxyhemoglobin to methemoglobin and, finally, with the loss of integrity of the red blood cell, the intracellular methemoglobin becomes extracellular with breakdown into ferritin and hemosiderin.

For an MRI 1.5 T scanner, the appearance of hemorrhage is as follows: (1) A hyperacute hemorrhage occurring within 4 to 6 hours is in the biochemical form of oxyhemoglobin and is isointense or hypointense on T1-weighted and hyperintense on T2-weighted images. (2) An acute hemorrhage 6 hours to 3 days old is in the deoxyhemoglobin form

and is isointense or hypointense on T1-weighted and hypointense on T2-weighted images. (3) The early subacute stage of the hemorrhage occurs within the first week. The hemoglobin is in an intracellular methemoglobin stage and demonstrates hyperintensity on T1-weighted and hypointensity on T2-weighted images. (4) This is followed by the late subacute stage which occurs within the second week to 3 months. At this stage, the hemoglobin is in the extracellular methemoglobin form and demonstrates hyperintensity on T1-weighted and hyperintensity on T2-weighted images. (5) This is followed by the chronic stage which occurs from 2 weeks to months or indefinitely. There has been rupture of the red cell with deposition of ferritin and hemosiderin that may be phagocytized by cells. This chronic stage demonstrates isointensity or hypointensity on T1-weighted images and hypointensity or hyperintensity with a hypointense rim on T2-weighted images (Table 3–5).

Other factors which influence the usefulness of MRI in the severely traumatized child are the difficulty in scanning severely injured children that require ancillary life support machines which are usually composed of ferromagnetic material, and the longer scan time required with MRI. However, with development of nonferromagnetic equipment, self-shielding magnets, very low-field-strength magnets, and the increasing expertise of radiologists in understanding the MR appearance of hemorrhage, there will be an increased role for MRI in the evaluation of head trauma.

The type of cerebral injury seen in head trauma depends upon the mechanism of the head injury. There are two fundamental types of injury. The first is direct injury to the skull with resultant skull distortion and localized fracture due to inbending of the skull and direct injury to adjacent brain paren-

TABLE 3–5.

MRI (1.5 T) Signal Intensity of Hemorrhage on Different Pulse Sequences

Type of Hemorrhage	Time Frame	Hemoglobin State	T1-Weighted Appearance	T2-Weighted Appearance
Hyperacute	4–6 hr	Oxyhemoglobin (intracellular)	Isointense or hypointense	Hyperintense
Acute	6 hr–3 days	Deoxyhemoglobin (intracellular)	Isointense or hypointense	Hypointense
Early subacute	First week (>3 days)	Methemoglobin (intracellular)	Hyperintense	Hypointense
Late subacute	Second week to 3 mo (>7 days)	Methemoglobin (extracellular)	Hyperintense	Hyperintense
Chronic	2 wk to months (>14 days)	Ferritin and hemosiderin (within phagocytes)	Isointense or hypointense	Hypointense or hyperintense with a hypointense rim

chyma. This type of injury can cause scalp lacerations and hematomas, cortical lacerations, and epidural or subdural hematoma secondary to a tear in the middle meningeal artery, venous sinus, or emissary veins, or, in the case of a subdural hematoma, a tear of the bridging veins.

The second type of head trauma is indirect and produces extensive neural damage. This may or may not be associated with skull distortion. This type of injury is most commonly due to a linear and rotational acceleration force and produces the classic shearing injury. Shearing injuries may be primarily intraaxial and arise as a result of the shearing force produced by the linear and rotational acceleration of the head with resultant damage to either the neurons or blood vessels. The most common types of intraaxial shearing injuries are: (1) diffuse axonal injuries, (2) cortical contusions, (3) deep gray matter injury, and (4) primary brainstem injury.

Diffuse axonal injuries consist of multiple small focal lesions scattered throughout the white matter. These lesions normally are nonhemorrhagic. The common locations are the subcortical white matter lobes of the brain (usually the parietal and frontal lobes); the corpus callosum (commonly the splenium and posterior aspect of the body), and the brainstem (Fig 3–78, *A* and *B*).

Cortical contusions are typically hemorrhagic. They are commonly associated with edema and produce mass effect. The most common locations are the frontal and temporal poles and, less frequently, the parietal and occipital lobes. Cerebellar contusions are less common and when found usually occur in the superior vermis or inferior cerebellar hemispheres (Figs 3–79 and 3–80).

Hemorrhage can be seen within the deep gray matter areas of the brain, mainly the basal ganglia, thalamus, and upper brainstem. These lesions are secondary to a dramatic shearing of the small perforating blood vessels that supply this area (lenticulostriate and thalamoperforate arteries).

Hemorrhage may also occur independently within the brainstem. Diffuse axonal injury is more common in children than was previously believed and is seen about as frequently as cortical contusions.

Injury to the cerebral vessels produce typical intracerebral, intraventricular, extracerebral, and subarachnoid hemorrhage. Intraventricular hemorrhages are secondary to tearing of subependymal veins and may be seen isolated within one of the ventricles or within all (Fig 3–81). Subarachnoid hemorrhages are difficult to demonstrate on MRI; depending on the series, they can be seen in 10% to 90% of children with head trauma on CT.

Epidural hematomas are commonly seen in adults secondary to a fracture across the middle meningeal artery. In children, epidural hematomas

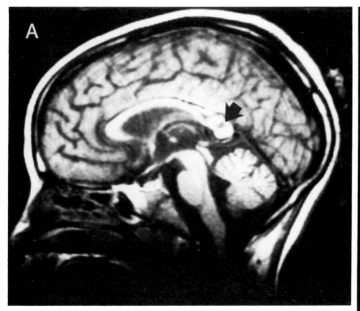
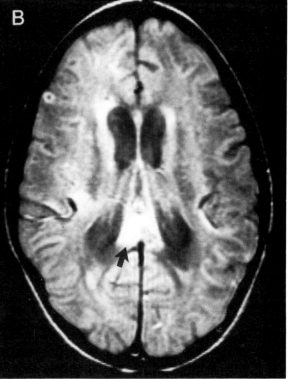

FIG 3–78.
A, sagittal T1-weighted image of axonal injury to the splenium of the corpus callosum with enlargement of the splenium and a central area of hypointensity *(arrow).* **B,** MR sagittal proton density image (same patient as **A**) shows hyperintensity of the splenium *(arrow).*

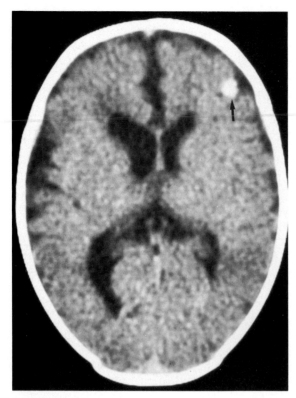

FIG 3–79.
Axial unenhanced CT scan showing small area of acute hemorrhage (contusion) *(arrow)* in the left frontal lobe.

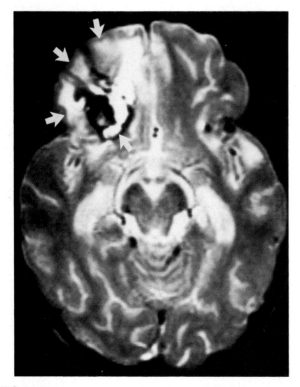

FIG 3–80.
Axial T2-weighted image demonstrating hyperacute and acute hemorrhagic contusion *(arrows)* of the right frontal lobe.

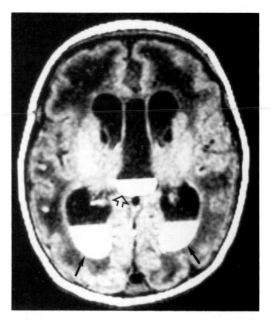

FIG 3–81.
Axial T1-weighted image demonstrating subacute hemorrhage within the lateral ventricles *(black arrows)* and cavum vergae *(open arrow)*.

are more often caused by tears in emissary veins, venous sinuses, or the middle meningeal artery. Epidural hematomas are typically lens-shaped; they are commonly temporal and parietal (Fig 3–82, A–C).

Subdural hematomas are caused by tearing of veins that traverse the subdural space. These are the bridging veins which leave the cortical surface of the brain to drain into the dural sinuses. Subdural hematomas are crescent-shaped and, depending on the size, produce distortion and compression of the ipsilateral ventricle. Common sites are the parietal, frontal, and parasagittal areas (Figs. 3–83, *A* and *B*, and 3–84, *A* and *B*). There is a form of subdural hematoma which occurs in the interhemispheric fissure and tentorial leaves. These are commonly seen in children that have been abused by violent shaking (the shaken baby syndrome). When interhemispheric and tentorial subdural hematomas are seen, as well as diffuse axonal shearing injuries within the subcortical white matter, the physician should be suspicious about the possibility of child abuse (Fig 3–85, *A* and *B*). Subdural hematomas may be produced by shunting of the ventricular system with too rapid a decompression of the ventricles that results in tearing of bridging veins (Figs 3–86 and 3–87). Subdural hygromas may also be produced by a traumatic tear within the subdural space with leakage of CSF into, and expansion of, this space.

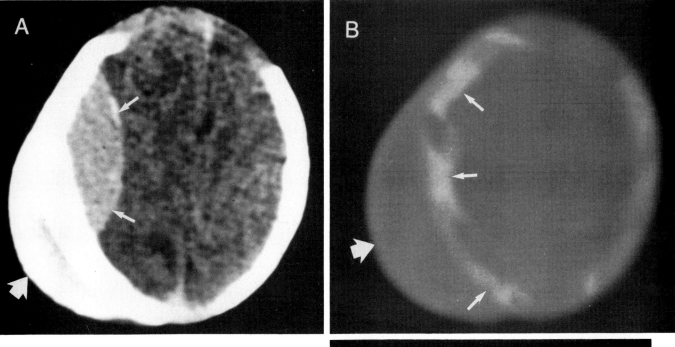

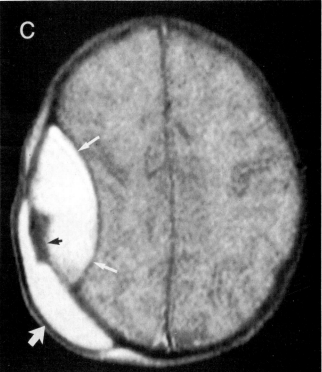

FIG 3–82.
A, axial unenhanced CT scan demonstrating acute epidural
hematoma *(small white arrows)* and right subgaleal hematoma
(large white arrow). **B,** axial unenhanced CT scan (bone
settings) in the same patient as **A** demonstrates multiple linear
and depressed fractures *(small arrows)* of the right parietal
bone and a subgaleal hematoma *(large arrow)*. **C,** axial MR
T2-weighted image of the same patient as in **A** and **B**)
demonstrates subacute epidural hematoma *(small white arrows)*
of the right-convexity parietal region of the brain, a subgaleal
hematoma *(large white arrow)* of the scalp, and depressed
bone fracture *(black arrow)*.

CEREBRAL EDEMA

Cerebral edema is a local or diffuse increase in brain
water. Since cerebral edema is commonly associated
with brain trauma, an understanding of its two
forms is necessary. The two forms are dry edema
and vasogenic edema. Dry edema is mainly intracellular water (when the surface of the brain is cut at
autopsy it appears dry). This form, also called cytotoxic edema by Klatzo, is predominantly limited to
the gray matter and is associated with metabolic insult such as hypoxia, hyperpyrexia, hypoglycemia,
seizures, and toxic states (Fig 3–88). Vasogenic
edema is mostly extracellular (the brain appears to
sweat when it is cut at autopsy). It involves predominantly the white matter and occurs as a response to

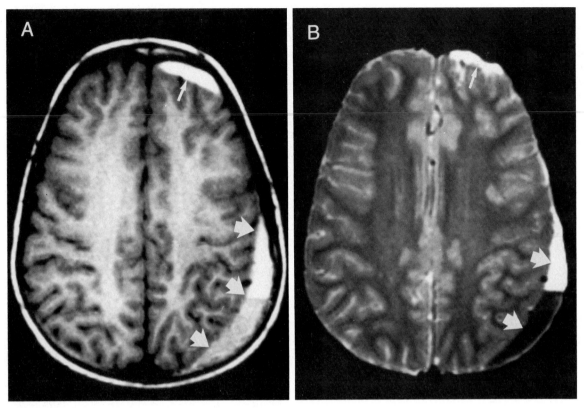

FIG 3–83.
A, axial T1-weighted image demonstrating subacute subdural hematoma *(small arrow)* in the left frontal area and mixed acute–subacute subdural hematomas *(large arrows)* in the left pa-

rieto-occipital area. **B,** axial T2-weighted image in the same patient as in **A** demonstrating subdural hematomas *(arrows)*.

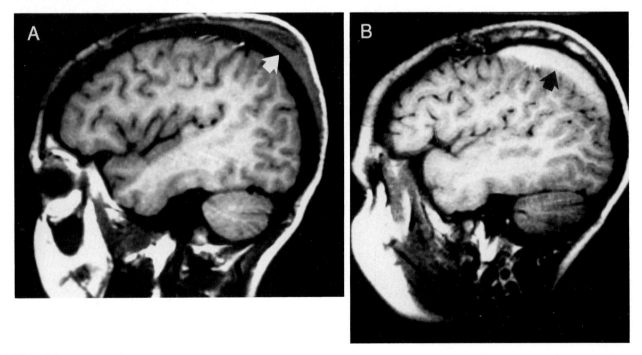

FIG 3–84.
A, sagittal T1-weighted image demonstrating hyperacute subgaleal hematoma *(arrow)* of the right parietal scalp. **B,** sagittal T1-

weighted image demonstrating subacute subdural hematoma *(arrow)* at the right high-convexity parietal area.

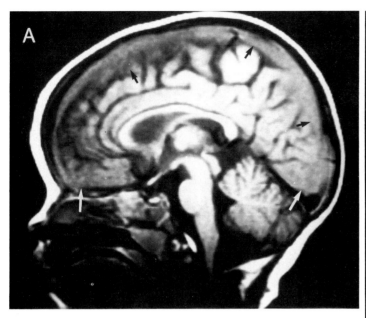

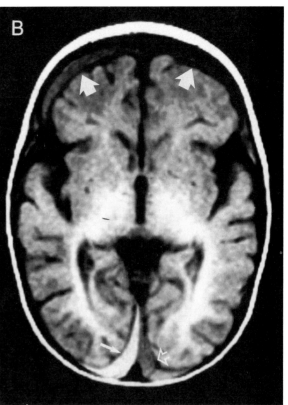

FIG 3–85.

A, sagittal T1-weighted image demonstrating isointense subdural hematomas in the interhemispheric fissure, high-convexity frontal, parietal, and occipital areas *(black arrows),* and the subfrontal and occipital regions *(white arrow).* **B,** axial T1-weighted image demonstrating isointense bilateral frontal acute subdural hematomas *(large arrows),* subacute hyperintense right occipital subdural hematomas *(small arrow),* and acute isointense left occipital subdural hematoma *(open arrow)* within the posterior interhemispheric fissure.

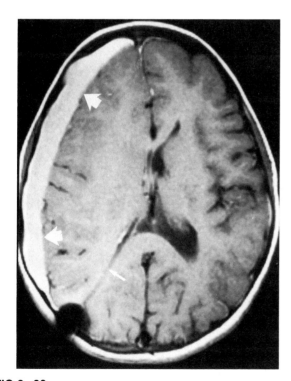

FIG 3–86.

Axial T1-weighted image demonstrating subacute hyperintense right subdural hematomas *(large arrows)* secondary to shunting *(small arrow)* of the ventricular system.

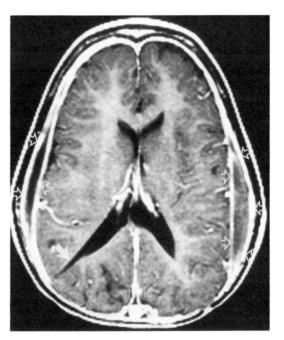

FIG 3–87.

Post-Gd axial T1-weighted image demonstrating enhancement of subdural membranes *(open arrows)* surrounding bilateral chronic subdural hematomas secondary to shunting *(closed arrow)* of the ventricular system.

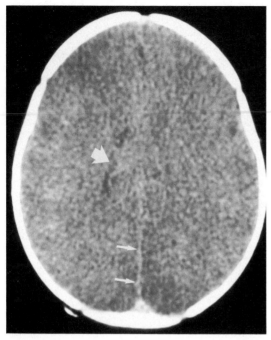

FIG 3–88.
Axial unenhanced CT scan of a patient with head trauma with cytotoxic edema, and diffuse swelling of the brain with compression of the ventricular system. Only small portions of the body of the right lateral ventricle *(large arrow)* are visualized. Acute subarachnoid hemorrhage is seen within the posterior aspect of the interhemispheric fissure *(small arrows).*

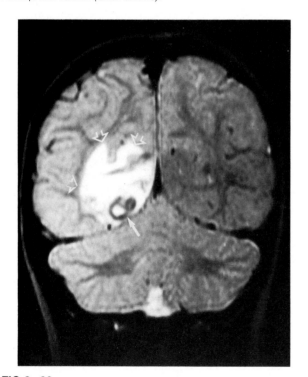

FIG 3–89.
Coronal T2-weighted image demonstrating vasogenic edema: hyperintensity indicated by *(open arrows)* surrounding a cysticercosis cyst *(closed arrow).*

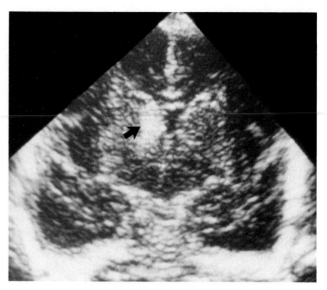

FIG 3–90.
Coronal sonogram (5-MHz sector transducer) demonstrating grade I isolated subependymal hemorrhage at the right frontal horn region (area of increased echogenicity indicated by *arrow*).

injury to the blood-brain barrier when the damage is secondary to tumors, traumatic injury, thermal injury, or other physically disruptive processes (Fig 3–89).

HEMORRHAGE IN PRETERM AND TERM INFANT

The most common types of hemorrhage in the preterm infant are subependymal, intraventricular, parenchymal, and subarachnoid. The most common

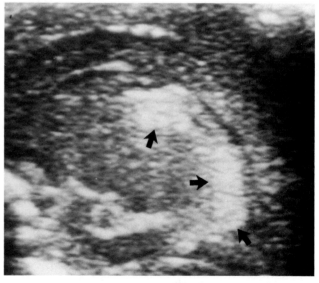

FIG 3–91.
Sagittal sonogram (5-MHz sector) demonstrating grade II choroid plexus hemorrhage with area of increased echogenicity *(arrows)* within the left lateral ventricle without ventricular dilatation.

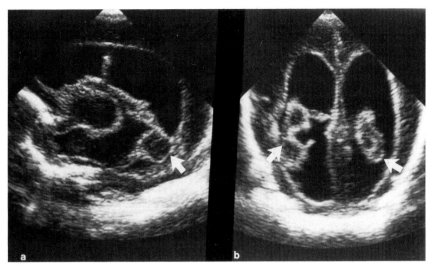

FIG 3–92.
Sagittal *(a)* and coronal *(b)* sonograms (5-MHz sector) demonstrating grade III intraventricular hemorrhage with areas of increased echogenicity *(arrows)* with lateral ventricular dilatation.

factors associated with hemorrhage in the preterm infant are presence of the germinal matrix, gestational age (<34 weeks), low birth weight (<1,500 g), and a severe hypoxic or anoxic episode. The hemorrhage commonly begins within the germinal matrix. The germinal matrix is an embryonic highly vascular, loosely supported membrane composed of spongioblasts and neuroblasts. The germinal matrix is located inferolateral to the ependyma lining the floor of the lateral ventricles. It is largest from 24 to 32 weeks of gestation, involutes during gestational life

(after 32 weeks), and is absent in the term infant.

The germinal matrix hemorrhage can be spontaneous, due to a severe hypoxic-anoxic episode(s) or to physiologic and hemodynamic changes in the brain of the fetus. The hemorrhage begins in the subependymal germinal matrix. There may be further extension of the hemorrhage into the choroid plexuses, ventricles, and brain parenchyma. The hemorrhage can be unilateral or bilateral with eventual involvement of all of the ventricular system and subarachnoid spaces. Subependymal, ventricular,

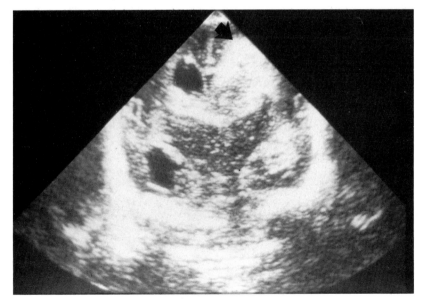

FIG 3–93.
Coronal sonogram (5-MHz sector) demonstrating grade IV hemorrhage in left lateral ventricle with extension to adjacent brain parenchyma *(arrow).*

and parenchymal hemorrhage is best appreciated on US with the hemorrhage being hyperechoic.

A simplified grading (I–IV) system for the location of the intracranial hemorrhage in the preterm infant has been developed. (Table 3–6) Grade I is isolated subependymal hemorrhage (Fig 3–90). Grade II is subependymal or choroid plexus hemorrhage with intraventricular hemorrhage without ventricular dilatation (Fig 3–91). In grade III there is intraventricular hemorrhage with ventricular dilatation (Fig 3–92), and in grade IV the hemorrhage extends into the adjacent brain parenchyma (Fig 3–93). Infants with grades I and II hemorrhage have the best prognosis and minimal or no neurologic sequelae. Fifty percent of infants with grades III and IV hemorrhage will have neurologic deficits. These infants may go on to have late changes of atrophy, porencephaly, and cystic or noncystic encephalomalacia of the brain. Subarachnoid hemorrhage is difficult to diagnose on US; the best modality for diagnosis is CT.

In the term infant, the most common types of hemorrhage are subarachnoid, epidural, subdural, and parenchymal. The hemorrhage is usually due to a traumatic or difficult birth (prolonged labor, forceps application, bleeding diathesis, or underlying vascular malformation. CT and MRI are the best radiologic modalities to evaluate these hemorrhages (Fig 3–94).

TABLE 3–6.

Ultrasound Grading of Intracranial Hemorrhage

Grade	Type
I	Isolated subependymal hemorrhage
II	Subependymal or choroid plexus hemorrhage with intraventricular hemorrhage without ventricular dilatation
III	Subependymal or choroid plexus hemorrhage with intraventricular hemorrhage and ventricular dilatation
IV	Subependymal or choroid plexus hemorrhage with intraventricular hemorrhage and intraparenchymal hemorrhage

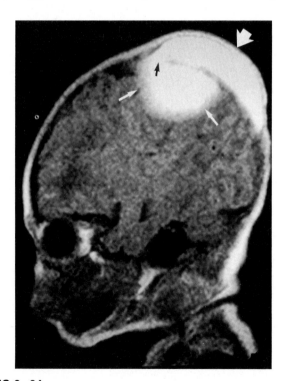

FIG 3–94.
Sagittal T1-weighted image obtained after traumatic forceps delivery in a term newborn illustrating subacute epidural hematoma *(small white arrows)*, parietal calvarial fracture *(black arrow)*, and cephalohematoma *(large white arrow).*

REFERENCES

Head Trauma and Cerebral Edema

Bradley WG: Hemorrhage, in Bradley WG, Bydder G (eds): *MRI Atlas of the Brain.* New York, Raven Press, 1990, p 205.

Clark RA, Watanabe AT, Bradley WG, et al: Acute hematomas: Effects of deoxygenation, hematocrit, and fibrous-clot formation and retraction on T2 shortening. *Radiology* 1990; 174:201–206.

Cohen RA, Kaufman RA, Myers PA, et al: Cranial computed tomography in the abused child with head injury. *AJNR* 1985; 6:883–888.

Cohen MD, McGuire W, Cory DA, et al: MR appearance of blood and blood products: An in vitro study. *Am J Roentgenol* 1986; 146:1293–1297.

Edelman RR, Johnson K, Buxton R, et al: MR of hemorrhage: A new approach. *AJNR* 1986; 7:751–756.

Gennarelli TA, Spielman GM, Langfitt TW, et al: Influence of the type of intracranial lesion on outcome from severe head injury. *J Neurosurg* 1982; 56:26–32.

Gentry LR, Godersky JC, Thompson B: MR imaging of head trauma: Review of the distribution and radiopathologic features of traumatic lesions. *AJNR* 1988; 9:101–110.

Gomori JM, Grossman RI: Mechanics responsible for the appearance and evaluation of intracranial hemorrhage. *Radiographics* 1988; 8:427–451.

Gomori JM, Grossman RI, Girton ME, et al: Sequential MR studies of intracerebral hematomas: Imaging by high-field MR. *Radiology* 1985; 157:87–93.

Gomori JM, Grossman RI, Goldberg HI, et al: Intracranial hematomas: Imaging by high field MR. *Radiology* 1985; 157:87–93.

Gomori JM, Grossman RI, Hackney DB, et al: Variable appearance of subacute intracranial hematomas on high-field spin-echo MR. *AJNR* 1987; 8:1019–1026.

Gomori JM, Grossman RI, Yu-Ip C, et al: NMR relaxation times of blood: Dependence on field strength, oxidation state and cell integrity. *J Comput Assist Tomogr* 1987; 11:684–690.

Hans JS, Kaufman B, Alfidi RJ: Head trauma evaluated by magnetic resonance and computed tomography: A comparison. *Radiology* 1984; 150:71–77.

Holbourn AHS: Mechanics of head injuries. *Lancet* 1943; 2:438–441.

Holbourn AHS: Mechanics of head injuries. *Br Med Bull* 1945; 3:147–149.

Klatzo I: Pathophysiological aspects of brain edema. *Acta Neuropathologica* 1987; 72:236–239.

Sato Y, Yuh WTC, Smith WL, et al: Head injury in child abuse; evaluation with MR imaging. *Radiology* 1989; 173:653–657.

Hemorrhage in Preterm and Term Infant

Babcock DS, Han BK: *Cranial Ultrasonography of Infants.* Baltimore, Williams & Wilkins, 1981.

Fisher AQ, Anderson JC, Shuman RM, et al: *Pediatric Neurosonography.* New York, John Wiley & Sons, 1985.

Grant EG: *Neurosonography of the Pre-Term Neonate.* New York, Springer-Verlag, 1986.

Naidich TP, Quencer RM: *Clinical Neurosonography.* New York, Springer-Verlag, 1987.

Rumack CM, Johnson M: *Perinatal and Infant Brain Imaging.* St Louis, Mosby–Year Book, 1984.

Rorke LB: *Pathology of Perinatal Brain Imaging.* New York, Raven Press, 1982.

SECTION 5

Infections

BACTERIAL INFECTIONS

Infants and children with brain infections present different clinical and imaging features depending on the type of infecting organism. Bacterial organisms produce cerebritis and meningitis. The cerebritis may progress to an organized abscess cavity (a localized collagen capsule with a liquefied purulent center). The common bacterial organisms are staphylococcus, streptococcus, *Escherichia coli, Listeria monocytogenes,* and *Haemophilus influenzae.* The organisms may spread to the brain by the hematogenous route, directly by paranasal sinus infection or mastoiditis, or by trauma.

The CT and MRI findings in early cerebritis consist of focal or diffuse swelling (hypodense on CT, and hypointense on T1-weighted and hyperintense T2-weighted MR images) with mass effect. Enhancement of the area of cerebritis usually does not occur until after 1 week. By 2 to 3 weeks, the cerebritis may have progressed to a localized abscess cavity with an outer collagen capsule which shows enhancement with contrast on both CT and MRI, and a central cavity of purulent material.

If meningitis is present, loss of cisterns and sulci is visualized on CT and MRI. The inflamed lepto-meninges show enhancement with contrast on both CT and MRI. There may be associated hydrocephalus secondary to obstruction of the flow of CSF at the basal cisterns and convexity areas, or with reabsorption at the superior sagittal sinus. There also may be secondary arterial or venous infarction.

Haemophilus influenzae infection is seen in children between 2 months and 10 years of age. It produces a leptomeningeal inflammation that may involve the superior sagittal sinus, subdural empyema (usually the frontal region), communicating hydrocephalus, and, occasionally, venous infarction (Fig 3–95).

If bacterial infections are successfully treated, then the imaging scans may be normal or may have sequelae such as atrophy, hydrocephalus, and infarction.

GRANULOMATOUS INFECTIONS

Granulomatous infections are similar in appearance to bacterial infections. They produce a cerebritis or meningitis, or both. However, cerebritis, if it progresses to an abscess cavity, is composed of caseous rather than purulent material. The most common organisms are *Mycobacterium tuberculosis* and

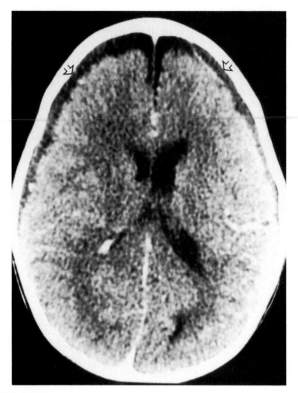

FIG 3–95.
Axial contrast-enhanced CT scan of a patient with *Haemophilus influenzae* infection, demonstrating bilateral frontal subdural effusions *(arrows)*.

fungi *(Coccidioides immitis, Cryptococcus neoformans,* and *Histoplasma capsulatum)*. They spread most commonly by the hematogenous route.

Tuberculous infection commonly produces a thick leptomeningeal inflammation predominantly at the base of the brain (basal cisterns). The leptomeninges become thickened and show enhancement with contrast on CT and MRI. Secondary communicating hydrocephalus may develop as well as arteritis with infarction of the brain. Tuberculous abscess may also form. The common sites are the cerebellar and cerebral hemispheres. The abscesses may be associated with a large amount of edema, and may be solitary or multiple. The fungal organisms may produce an image that is similar to that of tuberculosis. Although the basal leptomeningeal enhancement may not be as prominent, their abscesses are usually multiple and are not associated with as much edema as in tuberculous infection. During the early cerebritis stage, multiple lesions show enhancement (CT and MRI) by the second week. During the abscess stage, the capsule of the abscess is enhanced. The lesions appear hypodense on plain CT and, hypointense on T1-weighted and hyperintense on T2-weighted MR images. The end-stage brain may ap-

pear normal or demonstrate areas of atrophy, hydrocephalus, infarction, and encephalomalacia (Fig 3–96).

PARASITIC INFECTIONS

The most common parasitic infection to affect the brain in children that is now seen in the United States is cysticercosis. Neurocysticercosis develops when humans become the intermediate, rather than the definitive, host for the organism *Taenia solium.* The eggs of this organism are ingested and reach the stomach where the gastric juices liberate the oncospheres. The oncospheres travel by the blood and are disseminated to body organs. They have an affinity for the brain. The oncospheres develop into cysticercus larvae. The cysticercus larvae (cyst) can occur in the brain parenchyma, subarachnoid spaces (leptomeninges), or the ventricular system. The cysticercus larva has a head (scolex) and body (a bladder which becomes the cyst).

The parenchymal form consists of solitary or multiple small cystic lesions in the gray matter (cortex) or gray–white matter junction. The wall of the cyst is thin and shows enhancement with contrast on CT or MRI. Edema is present around the cyst and the center of the cyst may have a small eccentric dot

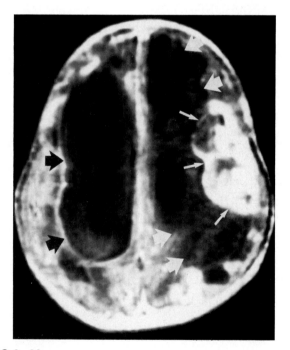

FIG 3–96.
Post-Gd axial T1-weighted image of a patient with tuberculous meningitis showing hydrocephalus *(large black arrows)* and vasogenic edema *(large white arrows)* with enhancement of an abscess *(small white arrows)* in the left cerebral hemisphere.

of calcification. The cyst is composed of serous fluid. CT is the best modality to demonstrate the small dot of calcification within the cyst. This may be missed on MRI. In the early stages of infection, both CT and MRI demonstrate the edema (hypodense on CT, and hypointense on T1-weighted and hyperintense on T2-weighted MR images). The capsule wall is isodense or hyperdense on CT, isointense on T1-weighted and hypointense on T2-weighted MR images. The cyst fluid is hypodense on CT, and, hypointense on T1-weighted and hyperintense on T2-weighted MR images. When the organisms die, some may calcify. This, the most common imaging appearance, consists of solitary or multiple small calcifications, 2 to 4 mm in size, within the brain. CT is the best imaging modality for demonstrating the calcifications (Figs 3–97 and 3–98).

The cysticercus cyst that occurs in the ventricular system (most commonly in the fourth ventricle) enlarges the involved ventricle and produces hydrocephalus. These cysts do not show enhancement with contrast.

A cysticercus cyst in the subarachnoid space may enlarge the involved portion of the space. It does not show enhancement. These are the most difficult lesions to identify, and both the CT and MRI scans may appear normal. The cysticerci in this location may die and produce an inflammatory leptomeningeal reaction with resultant hydrocephalus. The leptomeninges may be thickened and show marked enhancement with contrast.

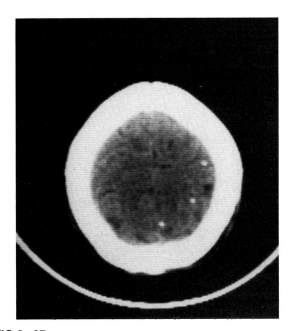

FIG 3–97.
CT scan without contrast showing three small calcified cysticercosis cysts of the cortex of the left cerebral hemispheres.

VIRAL INFECTIONS

Viral infections of the CNS produce an encephalitis as opposed to a cerebritis. An encephalitis is a diffuse infiltration of the brain parenchyma by inflammatory cells, whereas a cerebritis is inflammation of the perivascular areas of the brain. The early changes of infection produce a diffuse swelling of the brain. Damage to the blood-brain barrier with resultant enhancement with contrast may occur after the first week. The end stage may consist of generalized atrophy, encephalomalacia with or without cyst, gliosis, and demyelination. The gliosis and demyelination are better demonstrated on T2-weighted images as hyperintensity of the brain parenchyma (focal or diffuse).

Congenital Infections: TORCH

Congenital infections of the CNS are most commonly due to the TORCH organisms (*to*xoplasma, *r*ubella, *c*ytomegalovirus, and *h*erpes simplex). These infections are acquired by the maternal hematogenous-transplacental route or through the birth canal. If the infection occurs during the first or second trimester of pregnancy, then destructive or developmental brain anomalies may occur. If the infection occurs during the last trimester, then either a destructive process or no abnormality results. These organisms produce a necrotizing, calcifying meningoencephalitis with a particular predilection for periventricular tissue.

Toxoplasmosis and Cytomegalovirus

Toxoplasmosis is produced by a coccidian parasitic protozoan *(Toxoplasma gondii)* and cytomegalic disease is produced by CMV. The typical triad of findings in infants with congenital toxoplasmosis meningoencephalitis is hydrocephalus, chorioretinitis, and intracranial calcifications. Hydrocephalus is common and it is due to infection and gliosis in the region of the aqueduct of Sylvius. The calcifications have a predilection for the subependymal areas and basal ganglia but they may occur anywhere in the brain and tend to be more diffuse than CMV (Fig 3–99).

CMV infection also produces chorioretinitis, meningoencephalitis, and intracranial calcifications. The calcifications tend to be more periventricular and less diffuse. Both organisms may produce infarction of the brain which may become very extensive, producing hydranencephaly; atrophy may be seen as an end stage with calcification and microcephaly; and there is demyelination with gliosis. CT

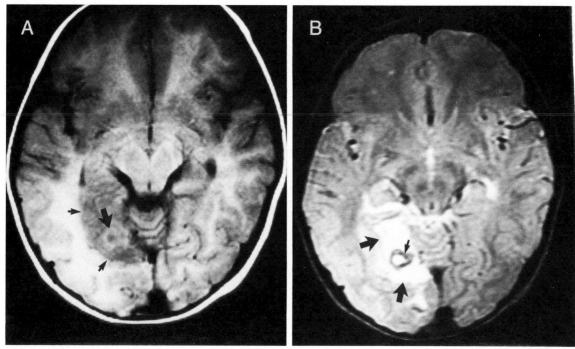

FIG 3–98.
A, axial T1-weighted image of a cysticercosis cyst *(large arrow)* in the right temporo-occipital lobe surrounded by hypointense edema *(small arrows)*. **B,** axial T2-weighted image obtained from the same child as in **A** demonstrating a cysticercosis cyst with hypointense capsule *(small arrow)* and a central area of hyperintensity with surrounding vasogenic edema *(large arrows)*.

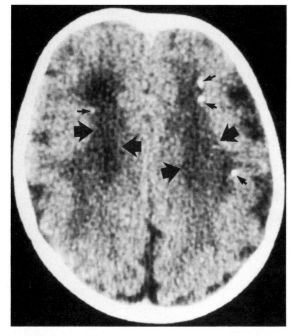

FIG 3–99.
Axial unenhanced CT scan at the centrum semiovale of a patient with toxoplasmosis revealing multiple small areas of calcification *(small arrows)*, hypodensity of the white matter *(large arrows)*, and pachygyric-appearing cortex.

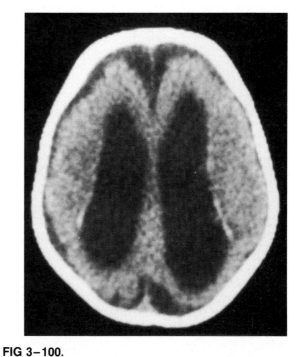

FIG 3–100.
Axial unenhanced CT scan of a patient with CMV infection shows central atrophy (enlarged lateral ventricles) and periventricular calcification.

is the best modality to evaluate the calcification (Fig 3–100), whereas MRI is best to demonstrate the areas of demyelination and gliosis in the brain which appear as hyperintense on T2-weighted images (Figs 3–101 and 3–102).

If infections with CMV or toxoplasmosis occur during the second trimester, neuronal migrational anomalies are produced. The most common forms are polymicrogyria and hemimegalencephaly. These MRI characteristics are described in Section 3.

Herpes Simplex Virus

There are two serotypes of herpes simplex virus (HSV), types 1 and 2. HSV-2 is more commonly seen in the fetus and neonate. It spreads to the fetus from the mother through the hematogenous-placental route. If the infection occurs during the first trimester, it may produce microcephaly, cerebral and cerebellar atrophy, hydranencephaly, and intracranial calcifications. HSV-2 is most commonly spread to the neonate from the mother when the baby traverses the birth canal. It produces a diffuse meningoencephalitis with diffuse swelling of the brain. There is a breakdown of the blood-brain barrier with enhancement of the brain (after the first week) demonstrated on CT or MRI. This type is not associated

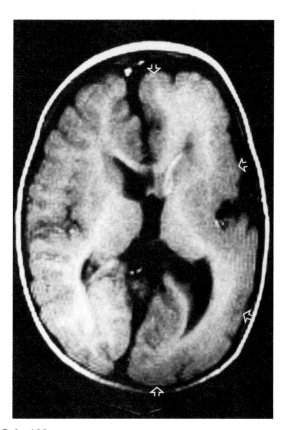

FIG 3–102.
Axial T1-weighted image of a patient with CMV infection with left cerebral hemimegalencephaly and pachygyric-appearing cortex *(arrows)* which represent polymicrogyria.

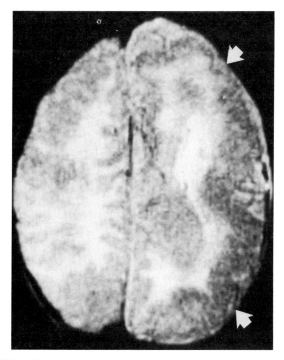

FIG 3–101.
Axial T2-weighted image at the level of the centrum semiovale of a patient with CMV infection demonstrating hemimegalencephaly of the left cerebral hemisphere *(arrows)* and abnormal patchy areas of hyperintensity of white matter fibers.

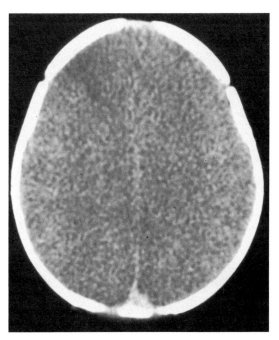

FIG 3–103.
Unenhanced CT scan at the level of the centrum semiovale demonstrating diffuse cerebral edema (loss of normal appearance of the sulci and gyri) in herpes simplex type 1 infection.

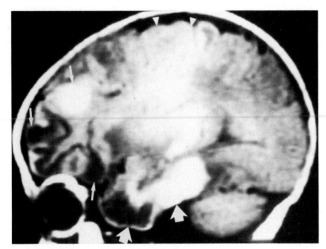

FIG 3–104.
Sagittal T1-weighted image in a patient with herpes simplex type 2 demonstrating hemorrhage (hyperintense and hypointense areas) involving the temporal *(large arrows)*, frontal *(small arrows)*, and parietal lobes *(arrowheads)*.

with focal areas of involvement or hemorrhage. The disease may progress to produce ischemic infarction of parts or all of the brain, necrosis, atrophy, encephalomalacia, demyelination, and gliosis (Fig 3–103).

HSV-1 is seen more often in adults and children. It produces a more focal, localized meningoencephalitic involvement with a predilection for the temporal lobes (unilateral or bilateral). There is swelling with mass effect. The patient may present with a recent change in personality. There is a greater tendency for hemorrhage or hemorrhagic infarction to develop with HSV-1 infection. On CT, the early stages of the infection demonstrate unilateral or bilateral enlargement of the temporal lobes with local or diffuse hemorrhage (hyperdensity) and mass effect. There is enhancement with contrast after several days of the infection. The MRI appearance depends on the stage of the hemorrhage (Fig 3–104). T1-weighted images demonstrate hypointensity or hyperintensity and T2-weighted images are hyperintense. There is enhancement after administration of Gd. The end stage of the disease demonstrates some areas of atrophy of the temporal lobes with or without encephalomalacia, demyelination, and gliosis.

Rubella

Rubella infections are rare in the United States as a result of the immunization program and current screening methods.

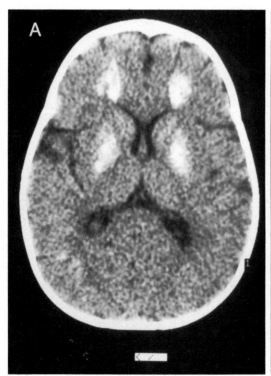

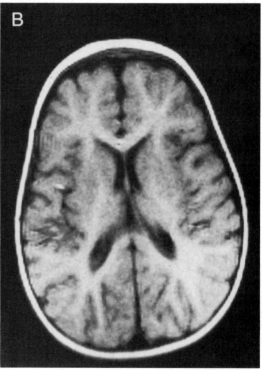

FIG 3–105.
Axial unenhanced CT scan of a child with HIV infection. Note calcification in the basal ganglia and white matter of the frontal lobes. **B,** axial T1-weighted image of the same child. Areas of calcification within the basal ganglia and white matter of the frontal lobes are not seen.

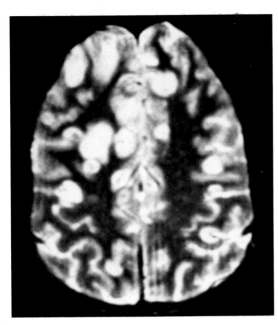

FIG 3–106.
Axial T2-weighted image at the level of the centrum semiovale in a child with HIV infection. Multiple round areas of hyperintensity represent toxoplasmosis infection.

Human Immunodeficiency Virus

Human immunodeficiency virus (HIV) infections in infants and children are due to hematogenous-placental transmission from an infected mother or, in older children, through blood or blood by-products in transfusions (especially in hemophilic children). The most common imaging appearance is diffuse atrophy, followed by basal ganglia calcifications and calcification in the white matter. Toxoplasmosis infection and progressive multifocal leukoencephalopathy (PML) are extremely rare in children. PML is secondary to a papovavirus which can produce demyelination and necrosis of the white matter. The calcification in HIV infections in children is best imaged on CT (Fig 3–105). Toxoplasmosis infection is well seen on MRI with multiple or solitary areas of hyperintensity on T2-weighted images which demonstrate some enhancement on post-Gd T1-weighted images (Fig 3–106). PML is best seen on T2-weighted images as solitary or multiple large areas of hyperintensity involving the white matter.

REFERENCES

Alford CA, Stagno S, Pass RF, et al: Congenital and perinatal cytomegalovirus infections. *Rev Infect Dis* 1990; 12:S745.

Anders BJ, Lauer BA, Foley LC: Computerized tomography to define CNS involvement in congenital cytomegalovirus infection. *Am J Dis Child* 1980; 134:795.

Bakski SS, Cooper LZ: Rubella. *Clin Dermatol* 1989; 7:8.

Bale JF: Human cytomegalovirus infection and disorders of the nervous system. *Arch Neurol* 1984; 41:310.

Bale JF, Andersen RD, Grose C: Magnetic resonance imaging of the brain in childhood herpesvirus. *Pediatr Infect Dis J* 1987; 6:644–647.

Bale JF, Bray PF, Bell WE: Neuroradiographic abnormalities in congenital cytomegalovirus infection. *Pediatr Neurol* 1985; 1:42.

Brewer NS, McCarty CS, Wellman WE: Brain abscess: Review of recent experience. *Ann Intern Med* 1975; 82:571–576.

Britt RH: Brain abscess, in Wilkins RH, Rengachary SS (eds): *Neurosurgery.* McGraw-Hill, New York, 1984.

Byrd SE, Locke GE, Bigges S, et al: The computed tomographic appearance of cerebral cysticercosis in adults and children. *Radiology* 1982; 144:819–823.

Davis LE, Johnson RT: An explanation for the localization of herpes simplex encephalitis? *Ann Neurol* 1979; 5:2–5.

Dennis JP, Alvord EC: Microcephaly with intracerebral calcification and subependymal ossification: Radiologic and clinico-pathologic correlation. *J Neuropathol Exp Neurol* 1961; 20:412.

Diebler C, Dusser A, Dulac O: Congenital toxoplasmosis: Clinical and neuroradiological evaluation of the cerebral lesions. *Neuroradiology* 1985; 27:125.

Enzmann DR (ed): *Imaging of Infections and Inflammation of the Central Nervous System: Computed Tomography, Ultrasound, and Nuclear Magnetic Resonance.* New York, Raven Press, 1984.

Fischer EG, McLennan JE, Suzuki Y: Cerebral abscess in children. *Am J Dis Child* 1981; 135:746–749.

Fitz CR: Inflammatory diseases, in Gonzalez CF, Grossman CB, Masdeu JC (eds): *Head and Spine imaging.* New York, John Wiley & Sons, 1985, p 537.

Freij BJ, Sever JL: Herpesvirus infections in pregnancy: Risks to embryo, fetus, and neonate. *Clin Perinatol* 1988; 15:203.

Friede RL, Mikolasek J: Post encephalitic porencephaly, hydranencephaly or polymicrogyria. A review. *Acta Neurol Pathol* 1978; 43:161.

Galloway PG, Roessman U: Diffuse dysplasia of cerebral hemispheres in the fetus: Possible viral cause? *Arch Pathol Lab Med* 1987; 111:143–145.

Hirsch MS: Herpes simplex virus, in Mandell GL, Boufor RG Jr, Bennett JE (eds): *Principles and practice of infectious diseases,* ed 2. New York, John Wiley & Sons, 1985, pp 945–952.

Johnson MA, Pennock JM, Bydden GM, et al: Clinical

NMR imaging of the brain in children. *AJNR* 1983; 4:1013–1026.

Levy R, Rosenbloom S, Perett LV: Neuroradiologic findings in AIDS: A review of 200 cases. *AJNR* 1986; 7:833–839.

Liske E, Weikers NJ: Changing aspects of brain abscess.

Review of cases in Wisconsin 1940 through 1962. *Neurology* 1964; 14:294–300.

Rodriquez-Carbajal J, Salgado P, Gutierrez-Alvarado R, et al: The acute encephalitic phase of neurocysticercosis computed tomographic manifestations. *AJNR* 1983; 4:51–55.

SECTION 6

Intracranial Neoplasms

Brain tumors are common lesions in children. The incidence is 2 to 3 per 100,000 in the United States. Brain tumor is the second most common neoplasm of childhood. Depending on the literature quoted, 50% to 60% of brain tumors occur in the supratentorial location and the remainder are infratentorial. A variety of classifications exist for brain tumors. Brain tumors may be classified on the basis of the degree of anaplasia within the tumor (Kernohan classification). Malignancy is graded from I to IV with grade I being benign and grade IV being a highly anaplastic, malignant tumor.

Other classifications are based on the aggressiveness of the clinical course and survival time of the tumor. The World Health Organization (WHO) classification of tumors is based on clinical course (Table 3–7). Additional classifications are based on the location of the tumor within the brain as brain tumors arise from a specific cell type within the brain or adjacent covering. The classification of Harwood-Nash and Fitz is used in this chapter (Table 3–8).

Children with brain tumors may present with signs of an expanding mass, raised intracranial pressure, and focal neurologic deficits.

POSTERIOR FOSSA NEOPLASMS

The most common intraaxial posterior fossa neoplasms consist of medulloblastomas, astrocytomas, and primitive neuroectodermal tumors (PNETs). The common extraaxial lesions consist of metastases from primary brain tumors, epidermoids, dermoids, and neuromas.

TABLE 3–7.

WHO Classification of Intracranial Tumors

A. Tumors of neuroepithelial tissue
   1. Astrocytic tumors
      a. Astrocytoma
      b. Pilocytic astrocytoma
      c. Subependymal giant cell astrocytomas (ventricular tumors of tuberous sclerosis)
      d. Astroblastomas
   2. Oligodendroglia tumors
      a. Glioblastoma
      b. Medulloblastoma
      c. Medulloepithelioma
      d. Primitive polar spongioblastoma
      e. Gliomatosis cerebri
   3. Ependymal and choroid plexus tumors
      a. Ependymoma
      b. Anaplastic ependymoma
      c. Choroid plexus papilloma
      d. Anaplastic choroid plexus papillomas (carcinomas)
   4. Pineal cell tumors
      a. Pineocytoma
      b. Pineoblastoma
      c. Pinealoma, germinoma
      d. Embryonal carcinomas
   5. Neuronal tumors
      a. Gangliocytoma
      b. Ganglioglioma
      c. Ganglioneuroblastoma
      d. Anaplastic (malignant) gangliocytomas and gangliogliomas
      e. Neuroblastoma
      f. Primitive neuroectodermal tumors (PNETs)
B. Tumors of the nerve sheath cells
   1. Neurilemoma
   2. Anaplastic (malignant) neurilemoma
   3. Neurofibromas
   4. Anaplastic (malignant) neurofibroma

C. Tumors of meningeal and related tissues
1. Meningioma
2. Meningeal sarcoma
3. Primary melanotic tumors (melanomas and meningeal melanomatosis)
D. Primary malignant lymphomas
1. Primary tumors of lymphoreticular system
E. Tumors of blood vessel origin
1. Hemangioblastoma
2. Monstrocellular sarcomas
F. Germ cell tumors
1. Germinoma
2. Embryonal carcinoma
3. Teratomas
G. Other malformative tumors and tumorlike lesions
1. Craniopharyngioma
2. Rathke's cleft cysts
3. Epidermoid and dermoid
4. Colloid cysts
5. Enterogenous cysts
6. Ependymal cysts
7. Lipomas
8. Hypothalamic neuronal hamartomas
9. Nasal glial heterotopias
H. Tumors of the pituitary
1. Tumors of the anterior pituitary
a. Pituitary adenoma
b. Pituitary adenocarcinom
2. Lesions of the posterior lobe
I. Local extension from regional tumors

Medulloblastoma

Medulloblastoma is the most common posterior fossa neoplasm. It is slightly more common in males and usually presents around 5 to 7 years of age. The presenting symptoms are signs of raised intracranial pressure (nausea, vomiting, headache) and cerebellar signs. Medulloblastomas are malignant lesions. Their 5-year survival with complete surgical resection followed by local and whole brain radiation ranges from 40% to 80%. Recurrence usually occurs within 3 to 5 years after diagnosis; however, there are reports of recurrence as late as 10 to 15 years. The recurrence may be local at the resected tumor bed or diffuse, secondary to spread via CSF to the spine and other portions of the brain. Medulloblastomas are the most frequent primary brain tumors to spread via CSF. Medulloblastomas may also spread outside of the CNS via the hematogenous route to bone, bone marrow, lymph nodes, and, occasionally, liver and lungs.

Medulloblastomas originate from germ cells of the medullary epithelium. The most common location is from a rest of primitive cells within the posterior medullary velum of the vermis of the cerebellum (90%–95%). A small percentage of medulloblastomas may occur within the cerebellar hemispheres.

TABLE 3–8.

Common Childhood Intracranial Tumors Based on Location*

I. Posterior fossa
  A. Intra-axial
    1. Vermis
      a. Medulloblastoma
      b. Astrocytoma
    2. Cerebellar hemisphere
      a. Astrocytoma
      b. PNET
    3. Brainstem
      a. Astrocytoma
      b. PNET
    4. Fourth ventricular
      a. Ependymoma
      b. Choroid plexus papilloma
  B. Extra-axial
    1. Cisterns
      a. Metastases from primary brain tumors
      b. Epidermoid (dermoid)
      c. Neuromas
II. Supratentorial
  A. Extra-axial
    1. Pineal region (quadrigeminal cistern)
      a. Pineal gland tumors
      b. Atypical teratomas
      c. Germinomas
      d. Teratomas and germ cell tumors
    2. Suprasellar (chiasmatic cistern)
      a. Craniopharyngioma
      b. Chiasmatic glioma
  B. Intra-axial
    1. Hemispheric
      a. Astrocytoma
      b. Oligodengioglioma
      c. Ependymoma
      d. PNET (neuroblastoma)
    2. Ventricular
      a. Choroid plexus papilloma (carcinoma)
      b. Meningioma
    3. Deep gray matter (basal ganglia, thalamus, hypothalamus)
      a. Astrocytoma
III. Meninges
  A. Leptomeningeal metastases
  B. Meningioma
  C. Melanoma

*Modified from Harwood-Nash DC, Fitz CR: *Neuroradiology in Infants and Children.* St Louis, Mosby–Year Book, 1976.

This is uncommon in children. Medulloblastomas may also be classified under the category of PNETs. Other tumors within this category are pineoblastomas and neuroblastomas. The best imaging modality to diagnose and evaluate medulloblastomas is MR. MR should be performed with T1-weighted, T2-weighted, and post-Gd T1-weighted images. Medulloblastomas present as a mass lesion within the vermis producing compression of the fourth ventricle with resultant hydrocephalus. On T1-weighted images, the medulloblastoma is usually hypointense to adjacent cerebellar parenchyma and on T2-weighted images, it demonstrates hyperintensity. After administration of Gd, there is usually homogeneous enhancement. Cysts and calcification are extremely rare, although they occur. Medulloblastomas commonly outgrow their blood supply and produce hemorrhagic infarction. Depending on the degree and age of the hemorrhage, the MR signal may be either isointense or slightly hyperintense on T1-weighted images. A small percentage of medulloblastomas may have seeded at the time of diagnosis. In these circumstances, there may also be enhancement of the leptomeninges with small nodules or masses within the cisterns of the posterior fossa and supratentorial area, and also within the thecal sac. Although medulloblastomas typically occur in the vermis, a very small percentage originate wholly within the fourth ventricle, contain calcifications with areas of necrosis, and simulate an ependymoma. This is rare and occurs in less than 3% of medulloblastomas (Figs 3–107 and 3–108).

Astrocytoma

Astrocytoma is the next most common posterior fossa neoplasm. Thirty percent occur within the cerebellar hemispheres, 30% within the vermis, and 30% within the brainstem. Astrocytomas are glial tumors that arise from astrocytes and have varying degrees of malignancy ranging from grades I to IV. Grade I is considered benign. The most common is the pilocytic astrocytoma. Grade IV is a highly malignant astrocytoma, also called glioblastoma multiforme. Cerebellar astrocytomas are seen within two age groups: the childhood form, which occurs around 5 to 6 years of age, and the juvenile form, which is seen in older children around 10 to 12 years of age. These children present with signs of raised intracranial pressure secondary to hydrocephalus resulting from compression of the fourth ventricle by the neoplasm. They also may have signs of cerebellar dysfunction such as ataxia. Eighty-five percent of cerebellar astrocytomas are pilocytic, which are considered benign tumors, and 15% are of the fibrillary type. Cerebellar astrocytomas may have a solid or cystic component, or both. Eighty percent have a cystic component. Calcification is rare, but hemorrhage may occur within the solid or cystic component of the tumor. Cerebellar astrocytomas have an excellent prognosis with 94% having a 10-year survival.

High-grade astrocytomas can recur. Recurrence is usually 3 to 5 years after initial diagnosis and treatment (surgery and radiation). The recurrence may be local but usually the recurrence is via lepto-

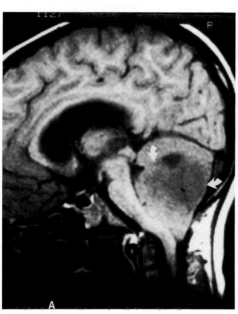
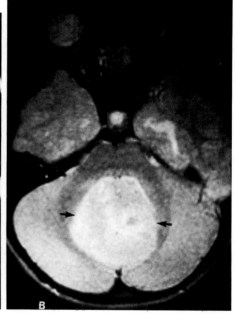

FIG 3–107.
MRI in medulloblastoma. **A,** sagittal T1-weighted image shows hypointense mass involving the vermis *(white arrows).* **B,** axial T2-weighted image shows hyperintense mass *(black arrows)* with areas of hypointensity representing acute hemorrhagic infarction within the medulloblastoma involving the vermis.

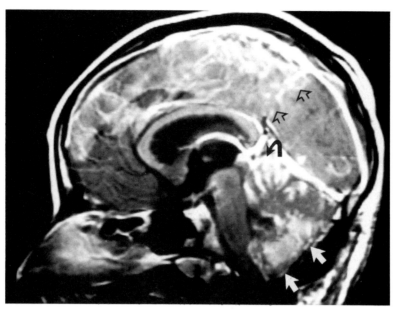

FIG 3–108.
Post-Gd sagittal T1-weighted image demonstrating enhancement of medulloblastoma involving the inferior vermis *(white arrows)* with leptomeningeal spread to the superior vermian cistern *(curved black arrow)* and interhemispheric fissure *(open arrows).*

meningeal CSF seeding. The recurrence is commonly within the spinal canal and also in sites within the brain independent of the primary tumor bed.

MRI is the best modality to evaluate these lesions. The lesion is usually either eccentric within the cerebellar hemisphere or involves the vermis or is a combination of both. The lesion usually contains solid and cystic components, although it is usual to see totally solid lesions commonly involving the vermis. The cystic component is usually large and only a small tumor nodule may be present when the tumor involves the cerebellar hemisphere. There is anterior displacement of the fourth ventricle when the tumor involves the vermis predominantly, and anterior and contralateral displacement of the fourth ventricle when a cerebellar hemisphere is predominantly involved. The MR signal characteristics are related to the solid and cystic components. The cystic component is usually hypointense on T1-weighted images; however, if there is increased proteinaceous material within the cyst or if there is hemorrhage, the signal intensity on T1-weighted images may be isointense or hyperintense. The solid component is usually isointense with, or hypointense to, adjacent cerebellar tissue. On the T2-weighted image, the cystic and solid components will show hyperintensity. After administration of Gd, the solid portion of the tumor demonstrates homogeneous enhancement. There also may be en-

hancement of the wall of the cyst. The solid component of benign or low-grade astrocytomas may not show enhancement after administration of Gd, but will also show a slight increase in signal on the T2-weighted image. Ninety percent of solid cerebellar astrocytomas show marked enhancement after administration of Gd. If the tumor recurs, the recurrence shows enhancement after administration of Gd. The recurrence consists of drop metastases spreading throughout the CSF spaces within the spine and brain. There also may be local recurrence of the tumor at the original site (Figs 3–109 and 3–110).

Brainstem Glioma

Ninety percent to 95% of neoplasms involving the brainstem are astrocytomas. The astrocytomas may be of the fibrillary or pilocytic type or the more malignant glioblastoma multiforme. Children with brainstem glioma usually present between 5 and 14 years, with a slight male predominance. The majority of these children present with lower cranial nerve palsies. Hydrocephalus is late in appearance. The brainstem glioma commonly occurs within the pons, followed by extension into the midbrain and then into the medulla. However, a small percentage of brainstem gliomas may originate wholly within the medulla or midbrain. When the tumor originates predominantly within the medulla, respiratory prob-

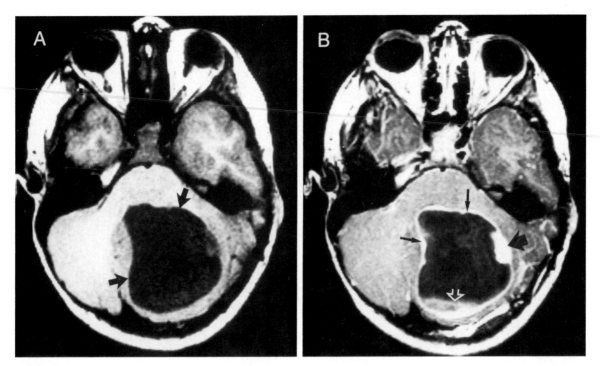

FIG 3–109.
A, axial T1-weighted image of a patient with cerebellar pilocytic astrocytoma, demonstrating predominantly cystic (hypointense) component *(arrows)* involving the left cerebellar hemisphere and vermis. **B,** post-Gd axial T1-weighted image in the same child demonstrates enhancement of the solid component *(large arrow)*, enhancement of the capsule *(small arrows)*, and layering of contrast material *(open arrow)* at the bottom of the cyst.

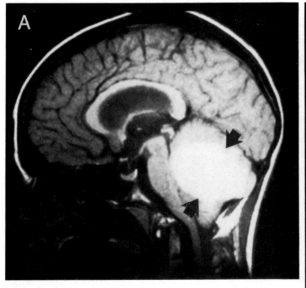
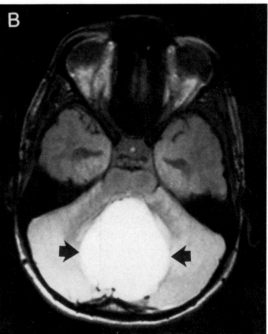

FIG 3–110.
A, sagittal T1-weighted image of cystic subacute hemorrhagic vermian astrocytoma demonstrating diffuse hyperintensity *(arrows)*. **B,** axial proton density MR image in the same child demonstrating subacute hemorrhagic cystic vermian astrocytoma *(arrows)*.

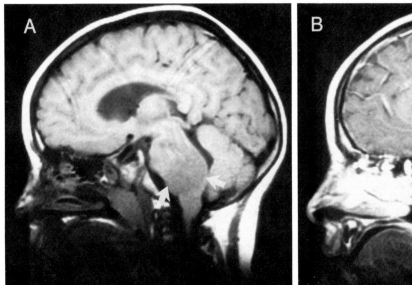

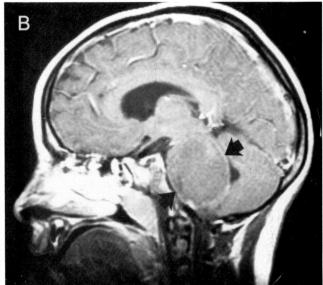

FIG 3–111.
A, sagittal T1-weighted image demonstrating brainstem astrocytoma with enlargement of the pons by a slightly hypointense mass *(arrows)*. **B,** post-Gd sagittal T1-weighted image demonstrating brainstem astrocytoma, without enhancement, and slightly hypointense mass *(arrows)* enlarging the pons.

lems, such as cyanosis or sleep apnea, may be the presenting symptoms. Brainstem gliomas infiltrate and grow up and down the brainstem, into the thalamus from the midbrain, and into the upper cervical cord from the medulla. From 5% to 10% of brainstem gliomas are classified as PNETs. Brainstem gliomas may be totally solid or solid with a cystic, necrotic, or hemorrhagic component. Survival is poor and death usually occurs within 6 months to 2 years after initial diagnosis. Treatment is usually local and whole brain radiation, and chemotherapy if there is recurrence or metastatic spread. The overall 5-year

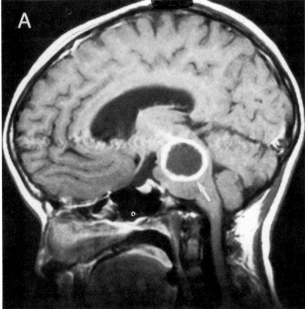

FIG 3–112.
A, post-Gd sagittal T1-weighted image demonstrating brainstem astrocytoma with enhancement of capsule *(arrow)* and a large cystic (hypointense) center enlarging the pons. **B,** sagittal T2-weighted image demonstrating brainstem astrocytoma with marked hyperintensity *(arrow)* enlarging the pons.

survival for brainstem glioma is 20% to 30%. Calcification may occur but is rare.

The best diagnostic radiologic modality is MRI with Gd. On the T1-weighted image, the MR appearance is either isointense or hypointense. If a cyst is present, the signal intensity will be hypointense if the cyst contains the same fluid as CSF; if there is proteinaceous material or hemorrhage, it may be isointense or hyperintense on T1-weighted images. On the T2-weighted image, there is a hyperintensity of both solid and cystic components. The solid component commonly will show enhancement either homogeneously or inhomogeneously after administration of Gd. Low-grade astrocytomas of the brainstem may not show enhancement after administration of Gd; however, there is slight hyperintensity on T2-weighted images (Figs 3–111, 3–112, and 3–113).

Brainstem gliomas may spread by infiltrating to other portions of the brain or spinal cord or outside of the brain parenchyma via the CSF-leptomeningeal route to other parts of the brain and spinal canal.

Ependymoma

About 10% of posterior fossa intra-axial tumors are ependymomas. They occur in a young age group (children <5 years of age, usually 2 to 3 at the time

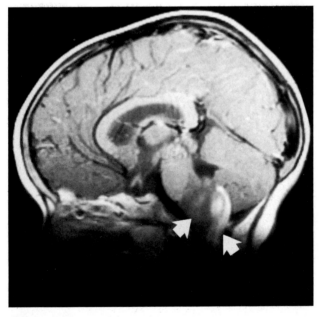

FIG 3–113.
Post-Gd sagittal T1-weighted image demonstrating brainstem astrocytoma involving predominantly the medulla oblongata with enlargement and partial enhancement *(arrows)*.

of diagnosis). They arise from the ependyma of the fourth ventricle and present as intraventricular masses with calcification. Children present with signs of raised intracranial pressure due to obstruction of the fourth ventricle from the intraventricular mass. Ependymomas within the supratentorial region arise from ependymal rests of cells within the cerebral hemispheres. Ninety-five percent of posterior fossa ependymomas occur within the fourth ventricle. A small percentage may originate within the cerebellopontine angle.

Overall survival is poor. The 5-year survival is 20% to 30%. There is increased frequency of local and CSF recurrence. Ependymomas are the second most common neoplasm to spread via the CSF. They commonly spread to the cisterns around the brain: the cerebellopontine angle, the cistern, suprasellar, and also into the spinal canal (lumbosacral area). These tumors frequently metastasize to other portions of the ventricular system, the most common site being the frontal horns of the lateral ventricles. The recurrence of ependymomas is usually earlier than that of other posterior fossa neoplasms, usually within 3 to 15 months after initial diagnosis and treatment. Ependymomas may rarely spread outside of the CNS to bone marrow, liver, and lung. They are the second most common brain tumor to spread outside of the CNS, medulloblastoma being the most common.

MR is the imaging modality of choice to evaluate primary and secondary spread of ependymomas. Posterior fossa ependymomas present as an intraventricular mass with areas of calcification. The calcification may be hypointense or hyperintense on T1-weighted and hypointense on T2-weighted images. The solid, noncalcified portion of the tumor is isointense with adjacent cerebellar parenchyma on T1-weighted and hyperintense on T2-weighted images. The solid portion will show enhancement either homogeneously or inhomogeneously after administration of Gd. Ependymomas may grow to be very large, expand the fourth ventricle, and spread outside of the outlets of the fourth ventricle. They commonly spread out of the lateral recesses of Luschka to the cerebellopontine angle, and from the midline foramen of Magendie down into the upper cervical canal. Ependymomas may have a "candle-dripping," lobulated appearance. Recurrence is either local within the resected tumor bed of the fourth ventricle or in the form of drop metastases throughout the spinal canal and within the cisterns or lateral ventricles of the brain (Figs. 3–114, 3–115, and 3–116).

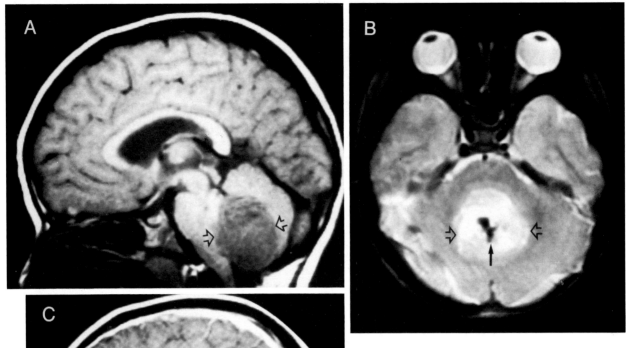

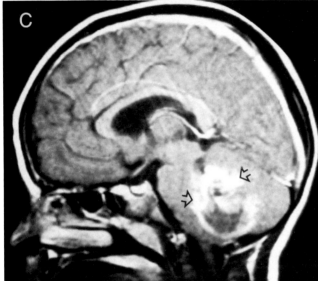

FIG 3–114.
A, sagittal T1-weighted image of a patient with ependymoma, demonstrating a hypointense mass *(arrows),* within the fourth ventricle. **B,** axial T2-weighted image of an ependymoma showing a hyperintense mass *(open arrows),* and a hypointense central area of calcification *(closed arrow)* within the fourth ventricle. **C,** post-Gd sagittal T1-weighted image demonstrating an ependymoma *(arrows).*

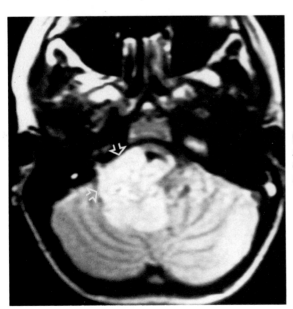

FIG 3–115.
Axial T1-weighted image: ependymoma within the fourth ventricle demonstrating hyperintensity and extension to the right cerebellopontine angle *(arrows).*

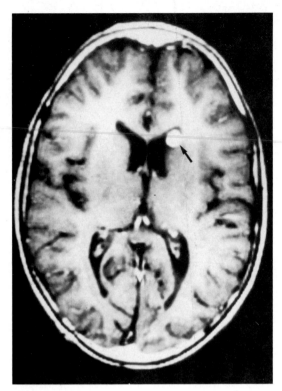

FIG 3–116.
Post-Gd axial T1-weighted image demonstrating metastatic spread of an ependymoma of the fourth ventricle to the left frontal horn. The mass shows enhancement *(arrow)*.

Extra-axial Posterior Fossa Neoplasms

The most common posterior fossa neoplasms within the cisterns are due to CSF metastatic spread from posterior fossa medulloblastomas, ependymomas, and high-grade astrocytomas. These lesions are usually multiple, round masses occurring within the CPA, pontine cistern, medullary cistern, or cisterna magna. The lesions vary in size from a few millimeters to 2 cm. They are usually isointense with adjacent brain parenchyma on T1-weighted images and demonstrate some slight increased signal on T2-weighted images. However, the lesions may be missed on T2-weighted images, because they are in cisterns with CSF which also demonstrate hyperintensity. The lesions enhance after administration of Gd (Figs 3–117 and 3–118).

Epidermoid tumors and cysts are benign lesions that consist of a collagen capsule lined with squamous epithelium with a center of keratin and cholesterol material. Epidermoids commonly occur within the CPA cisterns, sylvian fissure, cisterna magna, suprasellar cistern, and quadrigeminal cistern. They are usually hypointense to cerebellar parenchyma on T1-weighted images, usually do not demonstrate enhancement after administration of Gd, and may show some slight hyperintensity on T2-weighted images. They have a "popcorn" appearance.

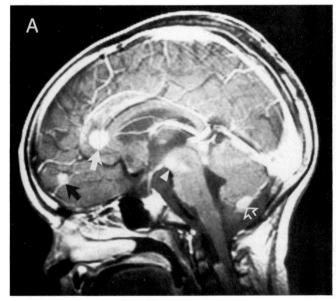

FIG 3–117.
A, post-Gd sagittal T1-weighted image demonstrating metastatic spread from the medulloblastoma of the posterior fossa to the cisterns and fissures of the brain. There is enhancement of multiple metastatic nodules in the inferior vermian cistern *(open arrow)*, interpeduncular cistern *(arrowhead)*, and interhemispheric fissure *(white* and *black arrows)*. **B,** Gd-enhanced axial image shows multiple metastatic nodules in the posterior fossa secondary to vermian medulloblastoma. The nodules demonstrate enhancement within cisterns *(black arrows)* and internal auditory canals *(white arrows)*.

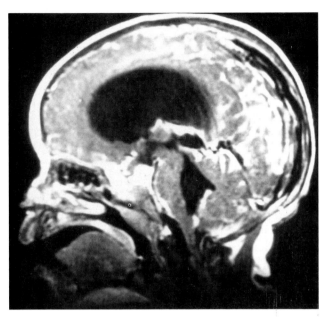

FIG 3–118.
Post-Gd sagittal T1-weighted image demonstrating diffuse lepto-meningeal enhancement secondary to metastatic spread from a vermian medulloblastoma.

Dermoids are similar to epidermoids. Dermoid tumors and cysts are benign tumors that contain hair, fat follicles, sebaceous gland, skin appendages, and keratin. They do not contain cholesterol. They may show a mixed signal intensity on T1-weighted images with increased signal from fat and with areas of isointensity and hypointensity. On T2-weighted images, there is a portion which demonstrates hyperintensity. They may or may not show enhancement after administration of Gd. Common sites are the cisterna magna, and suprasellar and quadrigeminal cisterns (Fig 3–119). They may be associated with a dermal sinus and with a tract extending from the scalp to the torcular. The lesions have a high incidence of infection and patients may present with meningitis.

Neuromas, neurolemomas, and schwannomas are benign tumors that arise from nerve root sheaths. They occur within the posterior fossa and may be seen in children with neurofibromatosis. A neuroma of cranial nerve VIII occurs in the cerebellopontine angle in association with NF-2. NF-2 is rare in children. When seen, it is usually in older children and teen-agers. Cranial nerves IX, X, XI, and XII are at the lower aspect of the posterior fossa and are commonly involved with neuromas in children with both forms of NF. Neurofibromas do not occur as tumors in the cranial nerves, even in NF. This is due to the leptomeninx of the nerve root cells of the cranial nerves which prevents the accumulation of mucoid material and thus the development of neurofibromas.

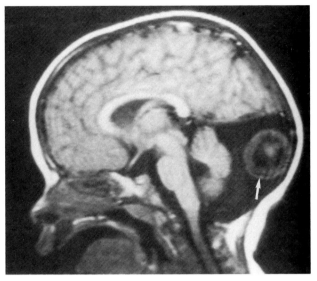

FIG 3–119.
Sagittal T1-weighted image revealing dermoid *(arrow)* within the cisterna magna.

SUPRATENTORIAL NEOPLASMS

Pineal Region Quadrigeminal Cistern Neoplasms

Tumors that occur within the pineal region quadrigeminal cistern can be classified into three main groups. Fifty percent of the tumors are germ cell tumors. These tumors originate from rests of primordial germ cells. Tumors within the germ cell category include germinomas, which are also called atypical teratomas and dysgerminomas. They are highly radiosensitive. Other tumors are teratomas, both the benign and malignant types; embryonal carcinoma; choriocarcinoma; endodermal sinus tumors (also called yolk sac tumors); and chorioepithelioma. A second category comprises about 20% of tumors in this location and are the true pineal gland tumors. In this category are the pineocytoma (also called the pinealoma) and the pineoblastoma. The third category includes tumors that extend into this area from adjacent infratentorial lesions such as an astrocytoma or medulloblastoma as well as miscellaneous tumors, such as hamartomas and lipomas.

It is important to differentiate neoplastic lesions that occur within the quadrigeminal cistern from a benign pineal cyst. The pineal gland normally should not be greater than 1 cm in size. Calcification within the pineal gland is rare before 10 years of age. Physiologic calcification begins between 10 and 12 years of age and is commonly seen in children after 12 years of age. Therefore, any calcified mass in a child under 10 years of age involving the pineal gland is highly suspicious for a germ cell or pineal tumor. A pineal cyst does not produce distortion or compression of the posterior recesses of the third ventricle. There may be calcification or enhancement of the wall of the cyst. On CT, the calcified rim of the pineal cyst can be seen easily, with the cyst fluid being similar to CSF although the cyst fluid may contain proteinaceous material and demonstrate a slightly increased density. On MRI, the pineal cyst may contain a rim of hypointensity that indicates calcification and is best seen on T2-weighted images. Increased signal involving the cystic material is seen on T2-weighted images. On T1-weighted images, the cyst fluid is isointense with, or slightly hyperintense to, CSF (Fig 3–120).

Pineal quadrigeminal cistern tumors present with hydrocephalus secondary to compression and distortion of the aqueduct and posterior aspect of the third ventricle, or with Parinaud's syndrome (paralysis of upward gaze).

Germ Cell Tumors

The most common germ cell tumor is the germinoma, accounting for 50% of germ cell tumors. The most common site is the quadrigeminal cistern, although suprasellar tumors are also common. Germ cell tumors of the pineal region have an increased incidence in males (about 90%) and are commonly seen within the first decade of life. Germ cell tumors may commonly produce abnormal levels of certain hormones. The most common are human chorionic gonadotropin, and luteinizing hormone. These two hormones are more commonly seen with germino-

mas or malignant teratomas. Alpha-fetoprotein is commonly seen in the CSF in malignant teratomas and yolk sac carcinomas. Germinomas and malignant teratomas may metastasize throughout the CSF to the spine as well as to the cisterns of the brain. They may also commonly invade the midbrain, thalamus, and hypothalamus.

Germinomas have a high incidence of calcification and are seen typically on CT as a solid mass with calcification. The solid portion of this mass usually shows homogeneous enhancement after administration of iodinated contrast. On MRI, both the solid and calcified portions are seen; the calcified portion is usually hypointense and the solid portion is usually isointense on T1-weighted images. On T2-weighted images, the calcified portion demonstrates hypointensity and the solid portion is hyperintense. The solid portion demonstrates relatively homogeneous enhancement after administration of Gd. When these lesions become large, the solid portion may also have a necrotic component and a hemorrhagic infarct. Hemorrhage is seen more frequently in the choriocarcinomas. Germinomas are very radiosensitive, whereas other germ cell tumors and pineal gland tumors are less responsive to radiation (Fig 3 121).

Teratomas in this area are usually malignant; they are more common in boys over 10 years old and in young adults. Benign teratomas may have subcomponents of epidermoid or dermoid cyst, and the MR and CT appearance is more like the epidermoid or dermoid component (Fig 3–122).

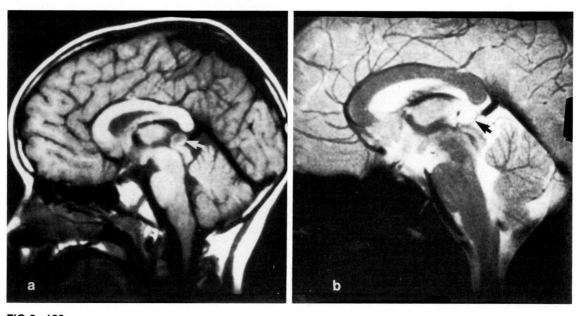

FIG 3–120.
Sagittal MR images. (a) T1-weighted image illustrating a hypointense pineal cyst (white arrow). (b) T2-weighted image illustrating a hyperintense pineal cyst with a hypointense rim (black arrow).

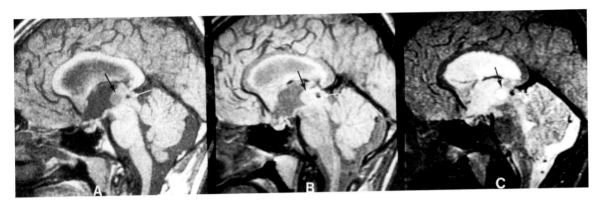

FIG 3–121.
Sagittal MR images of a quadrigeminal cistern mass germinoma. **A,** on the T1-weighted image, the mass is isointense and hypointense *(black arrow)*. **B,** on the proton density image, the mass is isointense and hypointense *(black arrow)*. **C,** on the T2-weighted image, the mass is hyperintense *(black arrow)* with calcification *(white arrow indicates no signal)*.

Pineal Gland Tumors

True tumors of the pineal gland are the pineocytoma (also called pinealoma), and the pineoblastoma. The pineocytoma is usually a more benign, less aggressive lesion, and the pineoblastoma is a more aggressive, highly malignant lesion that is also classified under the category of PNET. Pineoblastomas frequently metastasize throughout the CSF. There is an association of pineoblastomas with bilateral retinoblastomas. The combination is called the trilateral retinoblastoma and consists of bilateral retinoblastomas and pineoblastomas. The pineoblastoma usually occurs after treatment for bilateral retinoblastoma, although, rarely, all three tumors may be present at the time of diagnosis. The pineocytoma and pineoblastoma arise from pineal gland cells. Pineocytomas are more likely to contain calcifications, although calcification is seen less often than in germinomas. The pineoblastoma usually does not contain calcium. Pineoblastomas are more common in males and are extremely aggressive. Pineocytomas are usually solid tumors with or without calcium. They are

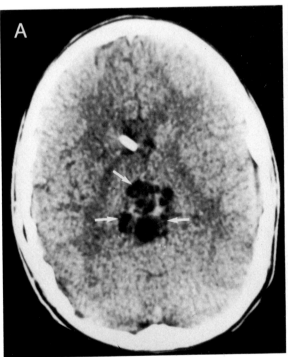 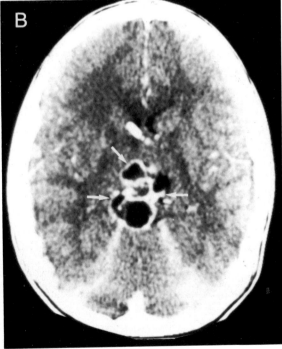

FIG 3–122.
A, axial unenhanced CT scan demonstrates quadrigeminal cistern teratoma with multiple hypodense components *(arrows)*. **B,** axial CT scan with contrast of the same child as in **A** shows enhancement of the solid components of the teratoma *(arrows)*.

hypointense or isointense on T1-weighted and hyperintense on T2-weighted images. They produce distortion of the third ventricle (posterior aspect) and show enhancement homogeneously after administration of Gd. They are usually fairly well-circumscribed, round lesions. Pineoblastomas may present a variable appearance on MR. They are usually isointense or hypointense on T1-weighted images and may be very large, round, or lobulated. When large, they have areas of necrosis or a more "popcorn" appearance. On T2-weighted images, they demonstrate hyperintensity and usually show enhancement marked after administration of Gd. The enhancement may be homogeneous or inhomogeneous (Fig 3–123).

Suprasellar Brain Tumors

The most common suprasellar brain tumors in children are craniopharyngioma, chiasmatic glioma, and suprasellar epidermoid, dermoid, teratoma, and germinoma.

Craniopharyngioma

Craniopharyngioma is the most common suprasellar tumor in childhood. Craniopharyngiomas arise from epithelial remnants of Rathke's pouch, which is an embryonic tract between the pharynx and pituitary gland. There are two age peaks for craniopharyngiomas: the childhood form that occurs between 5 to 12 years of age and the adult form that occurs in the fourth and fifth decade. Depending on the series, there is an equal incidence of boys and girls; however, some series report a slight predominance in boys. Children with craniopharyngioma present with the following signs, individually or in combination: raised intracranial pressure (headaches, nausea, vomiting), visual field defects, and hypothalamic pituitary dysfunction (e.g., diabetes insipidus, growth retardation, delayed puberty).

Craniopharyngiomas in children commonly present with three components: solid, cystic, and calcified. It is not unusual in children to see very large cystic components with relatively smaller solid components. Cystic components are rare in the adult form and these tumors usually present only with the calcium deposits and solid components.

In the childhood form of craniopharyngioma, the solid component is composed of cords of columnar or squamous epithelium often with small or large areas of calcification. The calcification may be within the walls of the cystic component which is composed of a combination of cholesterol material, keratin debris, and proteinaceous fluid. MRI is the best radiologic modality to evaluate children with craniopharyngiomas. The MRI should be performed with T1-weighted, T2-weighted, and post-Gd T1-weighted images. The MRI appearance of craniopharyngiomas varies depending on the type of cystic ma-

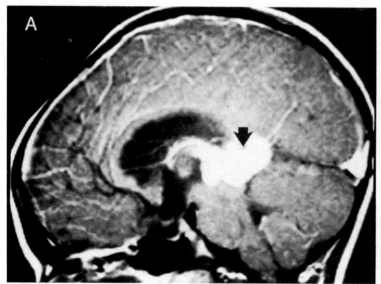
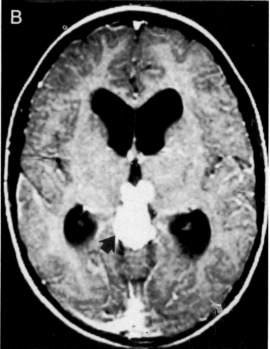

FIG 3–123.
A, post-Gd sagittal T1-weighted image demonstrating pineoblastoma with homogeneous enhancement of the solid quadrigeminal cistern mass *(arrow).*
B, post-Gd axial T1-weighted image of the same child as in **A** shows enhancement of the pineoblastoma *(arrow)* of the quadrigeminal cistern compressing the third ventricle and producing hydrocephalus.

terial present, whether it is cholesterol, keratin debris, or proteinaceous material, as well as on the amount of debris and calcification, and the size of the noncalcified solid component. Calcifications may be present either in the wall of the cyst or localized within the solid component. The cystic component on T1-weighted MRI demonstrates hypointensity, isointensity, or hyperintensity depending on the amount of keratin, proteinaceous material, and cholesterol present as well as on the state of hydration of the cholesterol. On T2-weighted images, the cyst is hypointense, isointense, or hyperintense. A common MRI appearance of the cystic component is hyperintensity on T1-weighted and T2-weighted images. After administration of Gd, the wall of the cyst may show enhancement. The solid component of the craniopharyngioma may be hypointense or isointense on T1-weighted images and usually hyperintense on T2-weighted images. However, calcification may be hypointense or hyperintense on T1-weighted and hypointense on T2-weighted images. If calcification is scattered throughout the solid component of the tumor, it will alter the signal characteristics of the solid portion. After administration of Gd, there is usually homogeneous or inhomogeneous enhancement of the solid component of the tumor.

Craniopharyngiomas will commonly extend superiorly to the area of the hypothalamus and third ventricle, and posteriorly into the posterior cranial fossa anterior to the midbrain and pons. Eighty-five percent to 95% of craniopharyngiomas are suprasellar and commonly extend into the sella turcica. They may also extend into the anterior cranial fossa. Craniopharyngiomas are benign tumors; however, because they are adherent to adjacent brain structures, surgery may often be incomplete, leaving with small residuals of the tumor. The recurrence of craniopharyngiomas is local and usually consists of the cystic component. The 5-year survival for craniopharyngiomas is 80%; however, local recurrence is common and radiotherapy is often necessary (Figs 3–124 and 3–125).

Chiasmatic Gliomas

Gliomas may originate within the optic chiasm. More commonly, they are extensions to the optic chiasm from an optic nerve glioma. If the optic chiasmatic glioma is large, it is often difficult to deter-

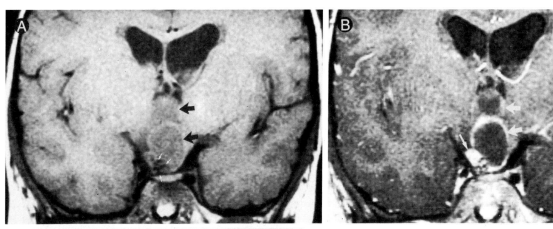

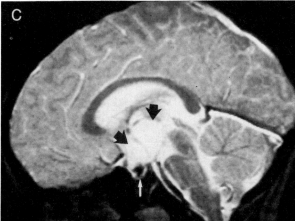

FIG 3–124.
A, coronal T1-weighted image demonstrating craniopharyngioma with an isointense cystic suprasellar-sellar component *(black arrows)* with a small hypointense calcified component *(white arrows)* within the sella. **B,** post-Gd coronal T1-weighted image (same child as in **A** shows enhancement of the solid component *(small arrow)* and capsule of the cystic components *(large arrows)*. **C,** sagittal T2-weighted image (same child as in **A** and **B**) demonstrates hyperintensity of the cystic components *(black arrows)* and hypointensity of the calcified component *(white arrow)*.

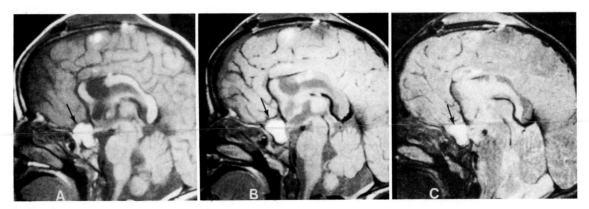

FIG 3–125.
Sagittal MR images of craniopharyngioma with suprasellar-intrasellar mass *(arrow)* demonstrating hyperintensity on **A,** T1-weighted, **B,** proton density, and **C,** T2-weighted sequences.

mine if it originated within the optic chiasm or within the hypothalamus with extension into the optic chiasm. Seventy-five percent of chiasmatic gliomas present within the first decade of life, usually between 2 and 6 years of age. These tumors are usually low grade or benign pilocystic astrocytomas although a small percentage may be highly anaplastic (grade IV). They are usually solid without cystic components, but the higher grades may demonstrate necrotic components. They often extend into the hypothalamus when large.

The clinical findings depend on the size of the tumor and consist of visual field defects with later extension into the hypothalamus, and endocrine abnormalities such as diabetes insipidus, growth failure, obesity, and precocious or delayed puberty. Occasionally, the diencephalic syndrome is seen. This syndrome can be seen with any hypothalamic lesion. It is characterized by a euphoria, emaciation, (typically in children <5 years of age), and a voracious appetite.

The MRI appearance consists of a solid suprasellar mass that is isointense or hypointense on T1-weighted and hyperintense on T2-weighted images. After administration of Gd, there may or may not be enhancement. The low-grade tumors may not show enhancement but the higher-grade tumors will demonstrate homogeneous or inhomogeneous enhancement depending on whether or not there is necrosis. Calcification is extremely rare.

Other Suprasellar Mass Lesions

Other lesions which may occur in the suprasellar region in children are epidermoids, dermoids, teratomas, and germinomas. Their MRI appearance has been described previously.

Intrasellar tumors are rare in children. The ma-

jority are secondary to an intrasellar spread from a suprasellar mass. Pituitary adenomas arise predominantly within the sella turcica. They are benign tumors arising from the anterior lobe of the pituitary gland. Pituitary adenomas are extremely rare in children. When they do occur, they do so in children 12 years and older. When pituitary adenomas occur in children, they are commonly functioning and these children present with endocrine abnormalities (increased prolactin, growth hormone, or adrenocortical hormone) (Fig 3–126). The lesions present as microadenomas or macroadenomas. The normal pituitary gland may be as large as 10 mm in teen-age girls (Fig 3–127). On T1-weighted images, the anterior lobe of the pituitary gland is isointense with brain parenchyma, whereas the posterior lobe is hy-

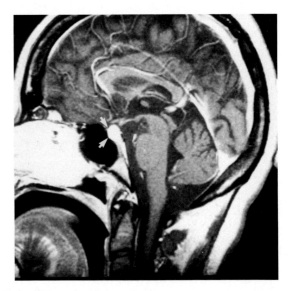

FIG 3–126.
Post-Gd sagittal T1-weighted image showing normal enhancement of a prominent pituitary gland *(arrows)* in a 17-year-old girl.

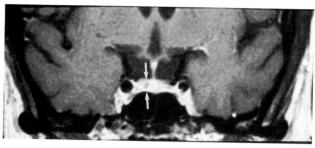

FIG 3–127.
Post-Gd coronal T1-weighted image: microadenoma *(arrows)* of the pituitary gland does not show enhancement.

perintense. This finding may be seen in the newborn.

Macroadenomas are pituitary adenomas greater than 10 mm in size. They usually have a suprasellar component and may compress adjacent brain structures, especially the optic chiasm. Microadenomas are usually hypointense or isointense on T1-weighted images and may demonstrate some increased signal on T2-weighted images. They do not show enhancement after administration of Gd; however, the remainder of the pituitary gland, the infundibulum, and the cavernous sinus do show enhancement and demonstrate the microadenoma as a hypointense lesion.

Macroadenomas commonly show enhancement after administration of Gd. They may contain necrotic or hemorrhagic foci. Although pituitary apoplexy (hemorrhagic infarction) is rare in children, there may be areas of hemorrhage and necrosis within these macroadenomas that are infrequently demonstrated in the older (teen-age) child. On T1-weighted images, macroadenomas are isointense or hypointense and on T2-weighted images they demonstrate varying degrees of hyperintensity.

Hemispheric Tumors

Astrocytoma

The most common supratentorial hemispheric tumor is the astrocytoma. This tumor represents 55% to 65% of all primary CNS tumors in children. Astrocytomas are seen in all childhood age groups. Clinically, children present with signs of raised intracranial pressure, such as headache, nausea, and vomiting, or with seizures or focal neurologic deficit.

Astrocytomas range from benign to malignant and are graded from I to IV with grade IV being highly malignant (glioblastoma multiforme). The cell types are usually fibrillary, protoplasmic, gemistocytic, or pilocytic. The pilocytic astrocytoma more commonly involves the cerebellar hemispheres. The

cerebral astrocytoma may also demonstrate a form that is called gliomatosis cerebri. This is a diffuse infiltrating lesion involving almost all or large portions of one or both cerebral hemispheres. These tumors are usually grade II or III.

The diagnosis can be made on CT and MRI. The lesions are usually large with solid and cystic components. Calcification is rare. The common locations are the parietal, frontal, and temporal lobes. The solid component of the lesion is isointense with gray matter with a cystic component that is hypointense or isointense depending on the contents of the cyst, i.e., the amount of proteinaceous material. After contrast administration, there is a marked, fairly homogeneous enhancement involving the solid component of the lesion with enhancement of the wall of the cyst. The 5-year survival for low-grade astrocytomas is 40% to 50% with less than 20% survival for grade III astrocytomas and less than 5% survival for grade IV astrocytomas and glioblastoma multiforme. High-grade astrocytomas commonly spread to other portions of the brain and spine via the CSF. The treatment is surgery with localized and whole brain radiation, depending on the age of the child. In children 2 years old and under, treatment is surgery with chemotherapy (Figs 3–128 and 3–129).

Oligodendroglioma

Oligodendrogliomas commonly occur within the cerebral hemispheres (the parietal lobe is a common site). They may be low grade or highly anaplastic. Seventy percent contain calcium which makes them the most common cerebral hemispheric tumor in children to calcify. They usually do not attain as large a size within the cerebral hemispheres as astrocytomas. The solid, noncalcified portion of this tumor is isodense with, or hypodense to, brain on unenhanced CT scans. The solid portion may or may not show enhancement after administration of iodinated contrast material. On MRI, oligodendrogliomas are usually solid, associated with edema around the periphery. The solid noncalcified part is isointense or slightly hypointense on T1-weighted images, and may be isointense or slightly hyperintense, on T2-weighted images. There may or may not be enhancement after administration of intravenous Gd (Fig 3–130).

Ganglioglioma

Gangliogliomas are tumors that contain components of neuronal cells (ganglion cells) and glioma cells (astrocytic neoplastic elements). They commonly in-

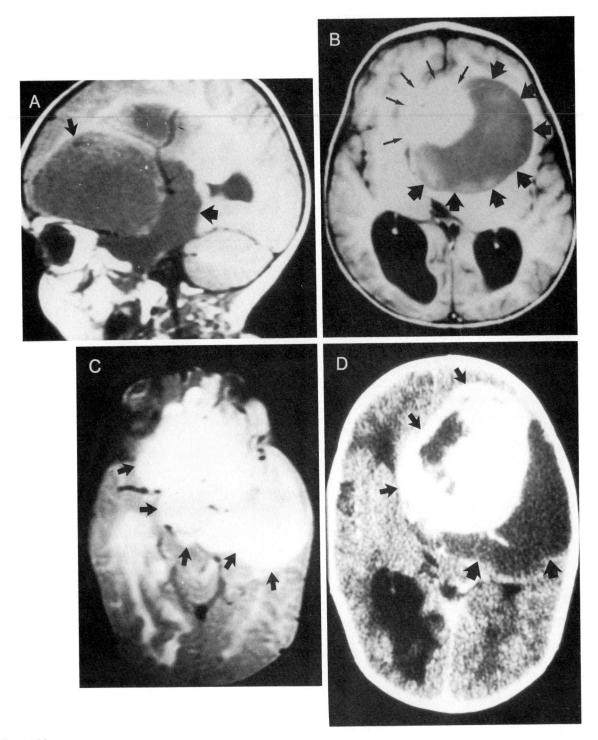

FIG 3–128.
A, sagittal T1-weighted image of astrocytoma (grade II) shows a large left frontal lobe neoplasm with hypointense solid *(small arrow)* and cystic *(large arrow)* components. **B,** post-Gd T1-weighted image (same child as in **A**) shows large tumor with cystic component *(large arrows)* and enhanced solid component *(small arrows)* of the left frontal lobe extending across the midline to the right. **C,** on axial T2-weighted image (same child as in **A** and **B**), hyperintensity is demonstrated in both the solid and cystic components of the large left frontal lobe astrocytoma (grade II) *(arrows)*. **D,** axial contrast-enhanced CT scan (same child) shows partial enhancement of the solid component *(small arrows)* of the solid-cystic *(large arrows)* astrocytoma.

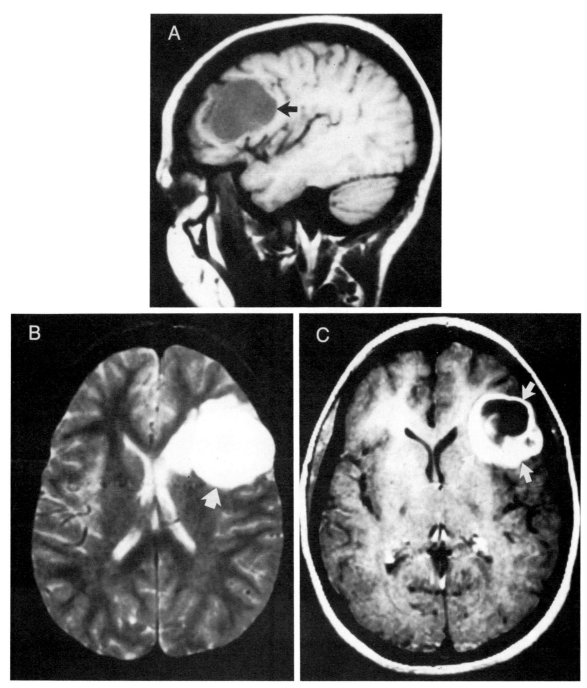

FIG 3–129.
A, sagittal T1-weighted image of astrocytoma (grade III) shows a hypointense cystic mass *(arrow)* within the left frontal lobe. **B,** axial T2-weighted image (same child as in **A**) demonstrating hyperintense solid-cystic astrocytoma (grade III) *(arrow)* of the left frontal lobe. **C,** post-Gd axial T1-weighted image (same child as in **A** and **B**) demonstrating solid-cystic astrocytoma with enhancement of the solid component and capsule *(arrows).*

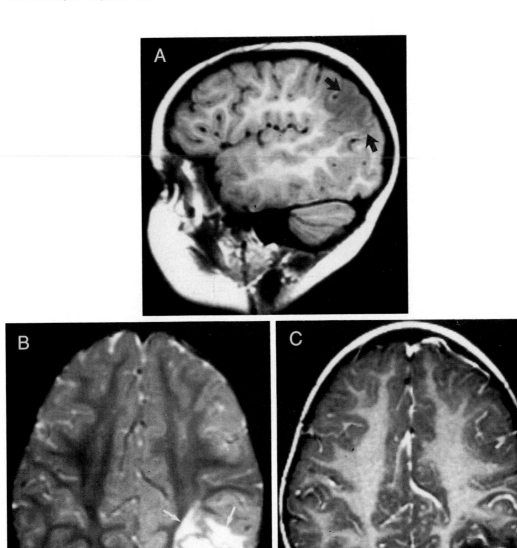

FIG 3–130.
A, sagittal T1-weighted image of oligodendroglioma showing a hypointense mass in the left parietal lobe *(arrows).* **B,** axial T2-weighted image (same child as in **A**) demonstrating a solid hyperintense mass *(large arrow)* with hyperintense peripheral edema *(small arrows).* **C,** post-Gd axial T1-weighted image (same child as in **A** and **B**) demonstrating a nonenhanced solid hypointense mass *(arrows)* surrounded by enhanced cortical vessels.

volve the temporal lobe (uncus region). They may present as solid or solid and cystic lesions. Calcification can be seen in these tumors, although it is rare. On MRI, the solid component is hypointense or isointense on T1-weighted images, hyperintense on T2-weighted images, and shows enhancement on post-Gd T1-weighted images. The cystic component follows the same intensity as CSF on the different pulse sequences (Fig 3–131).

Neuroblastoma

Neuroblastomas are classified under the category of PNET and represent the spectrum of anaplasia of the ganglionic cell. Neuroblastomas arise from rests of the ganglionic cell called the neuroblast. The neuroblast is an embryonic cell. It migrates from the subependymal layer of the ventricular system to the periphery of the brain to form the cerebral cortex. The neuroblast is a gray matter cell. Depending on

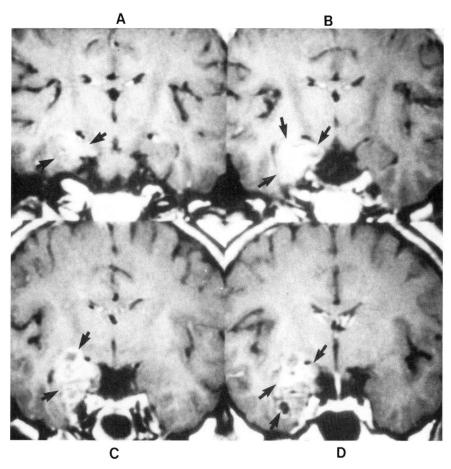

FIG 3–131.
Post-Gd coronal T1-weighted images at the level of the temporal lobe demonstrating inhomogeneous enhancement of the ganglio- glioma of the right temporal lobe extending into the uncus *(arrows).*

the degree of anaplasia (malignancy), tumors may develop into the highly malignant, aggressive neuroblastoma. The spectrum of malignancy of this ganglionic cell extends from the benign ganglioneuroma to the malignant ganglioneuroblastoma to the highly malignant neuroblastoma.

Neuroblastomas may originate as primary brain tumors or they may metastasize from neuroblastomas within the adrenal gland or the sympathetic paraspinal ganglionic chain.

Primary neuroblastomas commonly occur in the frontal and parietal lobes. They are malignant, aggressive lesions that may be associated with edematous, necrotic, and cystic components. They have a mixed signal intensity on T1-weighted images and demonstrate increased signal on T2-weighted images. The solid component may show enhancement after administration of Gd. Neuroblastomas may erode adjacent cortical bone or they may extend from metastatic foci within the cortical bone into the brain and present more as extra-axial brain tumors

that may eventually invade the brain. They have a propensity to bleed and commonly occur in children under 5 years of age. They are very aggressive tumors and may spread to other portions of the brain and spinal canal. Children present with signs of raised intracranial pressure; survival is poor, with death occurring within 6 months to 3 years (Fig 3–132).

Hemispheric Ependymoma:

When ependymomas occur in the supratentorial area, they commonly arise within the parenchyma of the cerebral hemispheres secondary to rests of ependymal cells. They are less likely to contain calcium, unlike their fourth ventricular counterparts which commonly do contain calcium. They are large tumors in the cerebral hemispheres with a large solid and cystic or necrotic component, usually adjacent to the lateral wall of the lateral ventricles and most commonly, in the temporal and parietal lobes. They may extend into the adjacent ventricular sys-

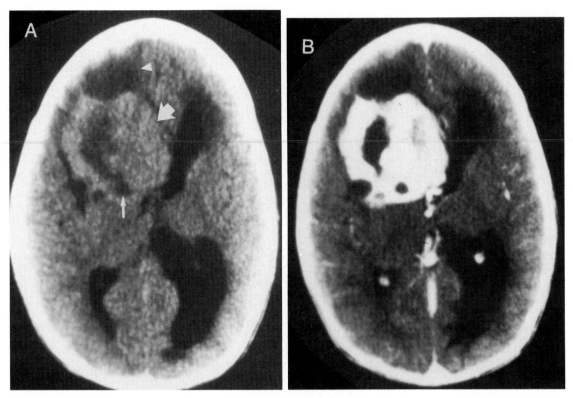

FIG 3–132.

A, axial unenhanced CT scan reveals a large isodense mass *(large arrow)* with a necrotic component *(small arrow)* and adjacent edema *(arrowhead)* in neuroblastoma of the right frontal lobe.

B, axial CT scan with contrast (same child) shows enhancement of the neuroblastoma.

tem and may be highly malignant with spread via dissemination through the CSF. They are rare in the supratentorial region. The majority occur within the posterior fossa in the fourth ventricle.

Ependymomas in the cerebral hemispheres can be imaged with both CT and MRI. On CT, the noncalcified solid portion is isodense with, or hypodense to, brain parenchyma. There is enhancement with iodinated contrast material. If calcium is present, it may be missed on MRI. The noncalcified solid part is isointense or hypointense on T1-weighted, hyperintense on T2-weighted, and shows enhancement with post-Gd T1-weighted images (Fig 3–133).

Intraventricular Neoplasms

Choroid Plexus Papillomas and Carcinomas

Choroid plexus papillomas are rare tumors of childhood. They usually occur within the first decade of life and 20% to 30% occur during the first year of life. They are most common in the neonate. Choroid plexus papillomas are benign lesions that arise from the epithelium of the choroid plexus. The most common site is the lateral ventricle. Ninety percent arise from the glomus of the lateral ventricle. The remaining papillomas arise from the fourth and third ventricles in order of decreasing frequency. Five percent to 10% of choroid plexus papillomas degenerate into carcinomas. Choroid plexus carcinomas may enlarge and extend into the ventricular system, but the majority are parenchymal, arising from rests of choroid plexus epithelium within the brain parenchyma. Choroid plexus papillomas are large lobulated lesions containing calcification and, occasionally, hemorrhage.

The symptoms are related to the large size of the lesion that produces a form of obstructive hydrocephalus. The literature states that choroid plexus papillomas produce an excess of CSF which contributes to the hydrocephalus. This is extremely rare. In the majority of cases, the hydrocephalus from choroid plexus papillomas is secondary to obstruction by the large mass effect of the lesion or results from hemorrhage and adhesions developing in the pathway of the flow of CSF. Choroid plexus papillomas on MRI appear as an intraventricular lobulated mass isointense or hypointense on T1-weighted images and hypointense, isointense, or hyperintense on T2-weighted images. If hemorrhage is present, the MRI

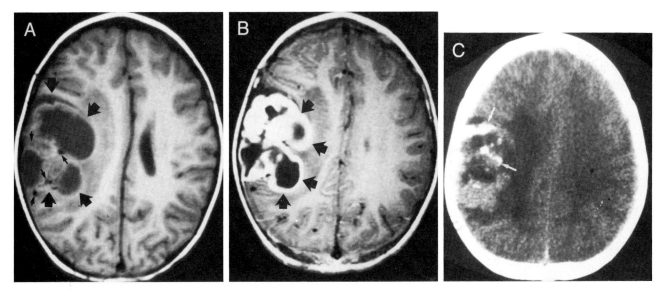

FIG 3-133.
A, axial T1-weighted image of an ependymoma of the right cerebral hemisphere demonstrating a large solid-cystic mass *(large arrows)* with calcification *(small arrows)* involving the temporoparietal region. **B,** post-Gd axial T1-weighted image of the same child demonstrating enhancement of the solid components and capsule *(arrows)* **C,** axial CT scan without contrast is better at demonstrating calcification *(arrows)* within the solid-cystic ependymoma.

signal intensity will depend upon the age and degree of hemorrhage. After administration of Gd, there is marked homogeneous enhancement. Choroid plexus papillomas have a lobulated appearance and can be partially differentiated from intraventricular meningiomas based on this appearance. Intraventricular meningiomas are round, well-circumscribed lesions, whereas choroid plexus papillomas demonstrate a more lobulated appearance (Figs 3-134 and 3-135).

Choroid plexus carcinomas are large lesions with cystic and necrotic components. They have a very

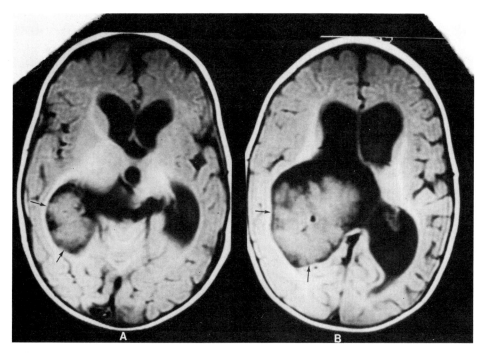

FIG 3-134.
Axial T1-weighted images of choroid plexus papilloma. Lobulated mass *(arrows)* is seen within the right lateral ventricle with hydrocephalus.

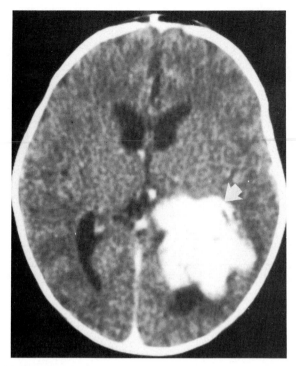

FIG 3–135.
Axial contrast-enhanced CT scan of choroid plexus papilloma *(arrow)* of the left lateral ventricle.

poor prognosis and frequently metastasize to other parts of the CNS via CSF by the time of diagnosis or within 3 to 6 months after diagnosis. The MRI appearance depends on the degree of necrotic involvement of the solid portion of the tumor and also on the degree of hemorrhagic infarction. On T1-weighted images, the tumor is hypointense and isointense; on T2-weighted images, both the solid and cystic components demonstrate increased signal; and after Gd administration, the solid portion will show an inhomogeneous enhancement. Choroid plexus carcinomas occur within the brain parenchyma adjacent to the walls of the lateral ventricles, but may extend into the lateral ventricle (Figs 3–136 and 3–137).

Deep Gray Matter Neoplasms (Basal Ganglia, Thalamus, Hypothalamus)

The most common neoplasm to affect the deep gray matter structures of the brain is the astrocytoma. It varies in grades of malignancy from benign (grade I) to the highly anaplastic (grade IV) astrocytoma and glioblastoma multiforme. When the lesion involves the hypothalamus, it is difficult to differentiate a hypothalamic glioma from a chiasmatic glioma. Hypo-

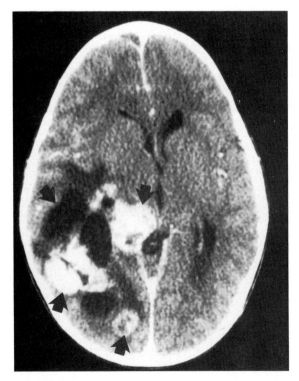

FIG 3–136.
Axial contrast-enhanced CT scan of choroid plexus carcinoma shows lobulated enhanced solid-cystic mass extraventricular *(arrows)* with compression of the atrium of the right lateral ventricle.

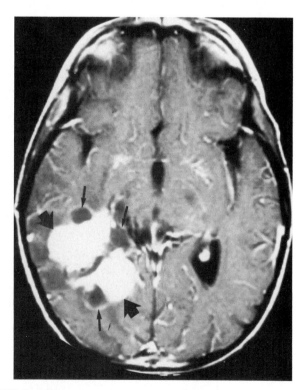

FIG 3–137.
Post-Gd axial T1-weighted MR image showing extraventricular choroid plexus carcinoma with enhancement of the solid components *(large arrows)* and of the capsule of the cystic components *(small arrows)*.

thalamic gliomas are midline lesions within the hypothalamus. They are solid tumors but after treatment with radiation or chemotherapy, they may have necrotic components. The neoplasm, depending on its degree of anaplasia, is isointense or hypointense on T1-weighted and hyperintense on T2-weighted images. The lesions may or may not show enhancement after administration of intravenous Gd. Grade I astrocytomas usually are not enhanced with Gd; however, the more anaplastic highly aggressive neoplasms will demonstrate marked enhancement after administration of Gd. The clinical signs are those of any lesion affecting the hypothalamus. Children may develop the diencephalic syndrome and have visual abnormalities and hydrocephalus.

Basal ganglia astrocytomas are usually unilateral. They distort and displace the third ventricle to the contralateral side. The lesions are round and may be solid, solid and cystic, or have a necrotic center. They are isointense or hyperintense on T1-weighted and hyperintense on T2-weighted images. There is usually diffuse enhancement after administration of Gd. The symptoms are related to the mass effect from the lesion and hydrocephalus. However, there may be specific signs related to the basal ganglia such as behavioral changes, emotional lability, memory loss, speech difficulties, and movement disorders such as choreiform movement or tremors.

Thalamic gliomas are similar in appearance to basal ganglia gliomas. However, they are within the thalamus, usually unilateral, with distortion and displacement of the third ventricle to the contralateral side. They may invade the adjacent basal ganglia or extend down into the hypothalamus or back into the midbrain. Gliomas that involve the hypothalamus, basal ganglia, and thalamus exhibit different cell types and degrees of anaplasia. The most common cell type is the fibrillary although the pilocytic type can also be seen (Figs 3–138, 3–139, and 3–140).

Miscellaneous Lesions

Dermoid and epidermoid tumors are benign lesions of ectodermal origin due to aberrant inclusions at the neural groove closure occurring in the third to fifth fetal week. Dermoids contain squamous epithelium and collagen as well as keratin material and skin appendages such as hair, fat, and sebaceous glands. They are usually midline in location and may be associated with a dermoid tract. They may occur in the posterior fossa, usually in the cisterna magna at the base of the brain, or at the anterior fontanelle. They are cystic lesions containing mucinous material and keratin debris. Epidermoids com-

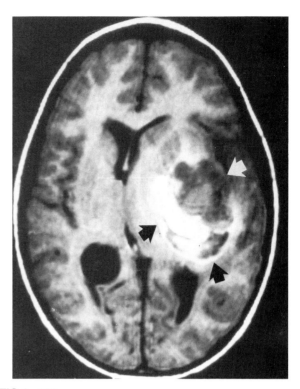

FIG 3–138.
Axial T1-weighted image of grade IV astrocytoma of the left basal ganglia with acute and subacute hemorrhagic components *(arrows).*

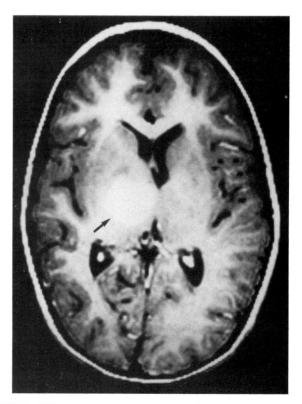

FIG 3–139.
Post-Gd axial T1-weighted image of grade III astrocytoma of the right thalamus demonstrating diffuse enhancement *(arrow).*

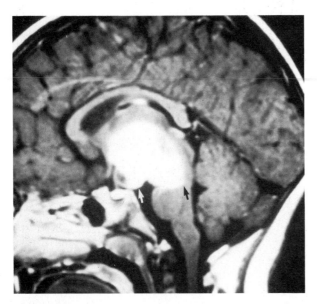

FIG 3–140.
Post-Gd sagittal T1-weighted image showing enhancement of grade III astrocytoma of the thalamus with extension into the midbrain *(black arrow)* and hypothalamus *(white arrow)*.

monly are cystic, containing keratin material, but also cholesterol. Collagen and epithelium line the walls of the cyst. The tumors are more lateral in location than dermoids and the most common sites are the cerebellopontine angle, the suprasellar cistern, sylvian fissure, and the calvaria.

MENINGEAL TUMORS

The common meningeal tumors in children are secondary to leptomeningeal spread from primary brain tumors. Other common lesions are meningiomas, lymphomas, meningeal sarcomas, and melanomas. The most common primary brain tumors are medulloblastomas, ependymomas, high-grade astrocytomas (glioblastoma multiforme), and PNETs, which also includes medulloblastomas, pineoblastomas, germinomas, and choroid plexus carcinomas. Other tumors that may spread to the leptomeninges from outside the CNS are the neuroblastomas. Leptomeningeal spread consists of thickening and enlargement of the leptomeninges. It is usually diffuse in appearance; however, the most common locations are at the level of the tentorium, base of the brain, and over the mid- and high-convexity areas of the cerebral hemispheres. These lesions are frequently nodular (round or oval) within the cisterns or scattered over the surface of the brain and spinal cord. On T1-weighted images, the dural involvement is difficult to delineate; however, after the administration of Gd, there is diffuse or localized enhancement

of the leptomeninges where they are thickened. Leptomeningeal involvement usually occurs 3 to 5 years after diagnosis of the primary brain tumor. Melanosis is discussed in the spinal cord section on meningeal lesions.

Meningioma

Meningiomas are rare in children. They represent less than 1% of intracranial childhood tumors. Meningiomas in children usually occur in the second decade; however, it is not unusual to see meningiomas in the first decade. There is an association between childhood meningiomas, which are usually multiple, and NF. However, the majority of children with meningiomas do not have NF. There is no sex predilection in children and the majority of meningiomas (99%) are benign. Malignant meningiomas are extremely rare in children. The childhood meningiomas are very similar to their adult counterparts. They have the same signal intensities and distribution. Meningiomas arise from the arachnoid cell of the arachnoid mater. Their most common locations are along the dural attachments at the convexity area of the brain, parasagittal in location, as well as in the middle cranial fossa, sylvian fissure region, sphenoid wings, and within the posterior fossa at the level of the tentorium, the cerebellopontine angle, and clivus. Intraventricular meningiomas may occur in children and, when they do occur, the most common site is the lateral ventricle. There are four common cell types of meningiomas: (1) meningothelial syncytial, (2) angioblastic, (3) fibroblastic, and (4) transitional. The MRI and CT appearances depend upon the cell type. There is a wealth of literature on the CT diagnosis of meningiomas. Meningiomas on CT are isodense with, or hyperdense to, brain, they are extra-axial in location, and the majority of meningiomas demonstrate diffuse homogeneous enhancement after administration of iodinated contrast material. They may contain calcification, microcysts, and fat (Fig 3–141). Rarely, they may bleed. The bony changes such as hyperostosis or bone erosion are better demonstrated on CT than on MRI. However, MRI, with high-field-strength magnets, is extremely accurate in diagnosing and delineating meningiomas. MRI with Gd provides excellent delineation of the location of the meningioma, its extent, its degree of vascularity, and whether or not there is arterial encasement and venous sinus invasion. Depending on the cell type, the following MR signal intensities are demonstrated: syncytial and angioblastic meningiomas demonstrate hypointensity on T2-weighted images in relation to cerebral cortex; transitional and fibroblastic

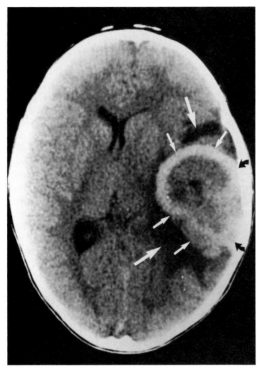

FIG 3–141.
Axial unenhanced CT scan shows meningothelial meningioma arising from the inner table of the left temporal bone *(black arrows)*. The meningioma is dense *(small white arrows)* secondary to calcification, with surrounding edema *(large white arrows)*.

meningiomas are isointense on T2-weighted images, although half of the fibroblastic meningiomas may demonstrate hypointensity; on T1-weighted images, the appearance of meningiomas varies depending on the amount of calcium, vascularity, and cystic formation.

Angioblastic meningiomas are highly vascular. They may bleed, in which case the signal intensity on MR will change depending on the age of the hematoma. Angioblastic meningiomas may also demonstrate fatty changes (the xanthomatous type) which consist of multiple fatty droplets scattered throughout the tumor. Microcysts may be seen in all types of meningiomas with coalescence into larger cysts so that a very small percentage of meningiomas appear more cystic than solid. About 20% of meningiomas have calcium. Calcium in meningiomas is diffuse, producing a fine, punctate appearance. The calcium may show increased or decreased intensity on T1-weighted images and demonstrates hypointensity if large enough on T2-weighted images. Gradient-echo accession (GEA) is more sensitive in demonstrating the magnetic susceptibility of calcium on MRI. Meningiomas present as extra-axial masses with variance in signal intensity depending on the cell type. The majority of meningiomas show enhancement after administration of Gd. The enhancement is either homogeneous or inhomoge-

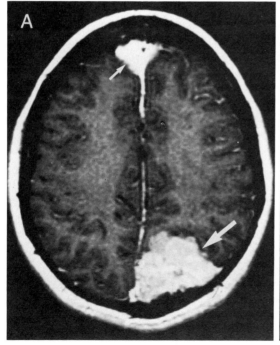

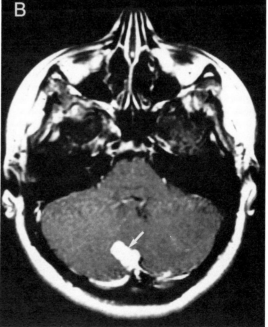

FIG 3–142.
A, on post-Gd axial T1-weighted image, parasagittal-convexity meningothelial meningiomas show enhancement in the frontal *(small arrow)* and parieto-occipital *(large arrow)* regions. **B,** en-

hanced meningioma *(arrow)* arising from the internal occipital protuberance.

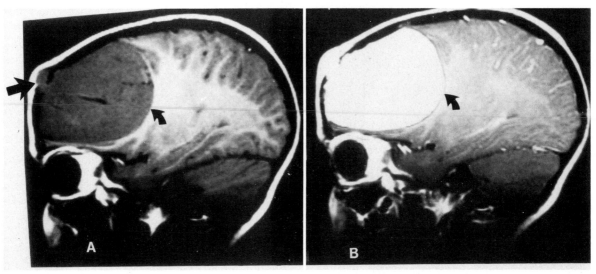

FIG 3–143.
Sagittal T1-weighted image of fibroblastic meningioma. **A,** on un-enhanced image, a large hypointense mass *(small arrow)* arises from the inner table of the right frontal bone with an area of bony erosion *(large arrow).* **B,** post-Gd image shows enhancement of tumor.

neous depending on other components of the tumor. Fifty percent of meningiomas produce brain edema. This is more commonly seen in the angioblastic and syncytial types. The majority of meningiomas are extra-axial dural base lesions. Intraventricular meningiomas (10%) arise from arachnoid cells of the tela choroidea or from cell rests within the stroma of the choroid plexus. The most common location is the lateral ventricles; 80% to 90% of intraventricular meningiomas occur within the lateral ventricles, 10% to 15% occur within the fourth ventricle, and less than 5% occur within the third ventricle in children. Intraventricular meningiomas are round lesions as opposed to the choroid plexus papillomas which have a more lobulated appearance. The signal intensity of intraventricular meningiomas depends on the degree of vascularity and calcium present. They are usually isointense or hypointense to cortex on T1-weighted images, and either hypointense or slightly hyperintense on T2-weighted images. They are markedly enhanced, either homogeneously or inhomogeneously, after administration of intravenous Gd (Figs 3–142 and 3–143).

REFERENCES

Al-Mefty O: *Meningiomas.* New York, Raven Press, 1991.

Baierl P, Muhlsteffen A, Haustein J, et al: Comparison of plain and Gd-DTPA-enhanced MR-imaging in children. *Pediatr Radiol* 1990; 20:515–519.

Berens ME, Rutka JT, Rosenblum ML: Brain tumor epidemiology, growth and invasion. *Neurosurg Clin North Am* 1990; 1:1–18.

Carpenter DB, Michelson WJ, Hays AP: Carcinoma of the choroid plexus. Case report. *J Neurosurg* 1982; 56:722–727.

Cohen MD, Edwards MK: *Magnetic Resonance Imaging of Children.* Philadelphia, BC Decker, 1990.

Cohen ME, Duffner PK: *Brain Tumors in Children. Neurologic Clinics.* Philadelphia, WB Saunders, 1991.

Diebler C, Dulac O: *Pediatric Neurology and Neuroradiology. Cerebral and Cranial Disease.* Berlin, Springer-Verlag, 1987.

Dohrmann GJ, Farwell JR, Flannery JT: Ependymomas and ependymoblastomas in children. *J Neurosurg* 1976; 45:273–283.

Duffner PK, Cohen ME, Freeman AI: Pediatrics brain tumors: an overview. *CA* 1985; 35:287–301.

Farwell JR, Dohrmann GH, Flannery JT: Central nervous system tumors in children. *Cancer* 1977; 40:3123–3132.

Farwell JR, Dohrmann GJ, Flannery JT: Medulloblastoma in childhood: An epidemiological study. *J Neurosurg* 1984; 61:657–664.

Gutin PH, Leibel SA, Sheline GE: *Radiation Injury to the Nervous System.* New York, Raven Press, 1991.

Halperin EC, Kun LE, Constine LS, et al: *Pediatric Radiation Oncology.* New York, Raven Press, 1989.

Harwood-Nash DC, Fitz CR: *Neuroradiology in Infants and Children.* St Louis, Mosby–Year Book, 1976.

Rorke LB, Gilles FN, Davis RL, et al: Revision of the World Health Organization classification of brain tumors for childhood brain tumors. *Cancer* 1985; 56:1869–1886.

Russell EJ, Geremia GK, Johnson CE, et al: Multiple cerebral metastases: Detectability with Gd-DTPA−enhanced MR imaging. *Radiology* 1987; 165:609−617.

Russell DS, Rubinstein LJ. *Pathology of Tumors of the Nervous System*, ed 5. Baltimore, Williams & Wilkins, 1989

Wara WM, Jenkin RDT, Evans A, et al: Tumors of the pineal and suprasellar regions: Children's cancer study group treatment results 1960−1975. *Cancer* 1979; 43:698−701.

SECTION 7

Miscellaneous Lesions

VASCULAR MALFORMATIONS AND ANEURYSMS

Vascular malformations are fairly common in children and account for about 20% of all vascular malformations seen, whereas aneurysms are extremely rare in children. Children with vascular malformations usually present with hemorrhage or seizure disorder, or both. Vascular malformations in children have a high tendency to bleed. They are classified into four major types: (1) arteriovenous malformations, (2) cavernous angioma, (3) capillary telangiectasia, and (4) venous angioma. The most common malformation encountered is the true arteriovenous malformation (AVM). These are congenital anomalies that result from direct communication between arteries and veins without intervening capillaries. They can be scattered throughout the brain but the supratentorial location is far more common (85%).

AVMs can be divided into a pial type that involves the intracranial circulation; a dural type that receives its circulation from the arteries that supply the meninges; and a pial-dural (mixed) type that receives circulation from the intracranial arteries (internal carotid or vertebral-basilar) and dural vessels as well. At autopsy, AVMs consist of a cluster of dilated tortuous vessels with hemosiderin and other blood products as well as either recent or old hemorrhage and adjacent areas of atrophy, infarction, and gliosis. The vein of Galen aneurysm is a form of AVM in which the venous component is a large vein of Galen and the arteries drain either directly into the vein of Galen or into veins which do so, such as the internal cerebral vein or basal vein of Rosenthal. Children with vein of Galen aneurysms are seen during the neonatal and infancy periods. They may present with congestive heart failure and hydrocephalus. Hydrocephalus is secondary to obstruction of the aqueduct by pressure from the large vein of Galen (Fig 3−144).

The definitive imaging modality to evaluate vascular malformation is cerebral angiography. Conventional cerebral angiography will accurately delineate the vascular components in 90% of cases (Fig 3−145). In a small percentage (10%), the vascular component is not demonstrated angiographically and these are the so-called occult vascular malformations.

MRI is an excellent modality for demonstrating vascular malformations with their associated complications such as hemorrhage, infarction, edema, and atrophy. Although MRI may not completely delineate the arteriovenous components and drainage of the vascular malformation, it will demonstrate all of the types of vascular malformations, including the occult vascular malformations. The MRI appearance of true AVMs consists of either linear or multiple serpentine areas of signal void seen on T1-weighted and T2-weighted images. After administration of Gd, there is enhancement within these abnormal vascular channels. If hemorrhage is present, depending on the amount and age of the hematoma, the signal characteristics will vary. There may be associated gliosis and infarction with these vascular malformations and these changes are demonstrated on MRI. It may be difficult to demonstrate calcium within the vessels or within old areas of hemorrhage; however, the typical characteristics of the vascular malformation will be demonstrated (Figs 3−146 and 3−147).

Other vascular malformations consist of venous angiomas which commonly involve the posterior fossa although they can also be seen within the su-

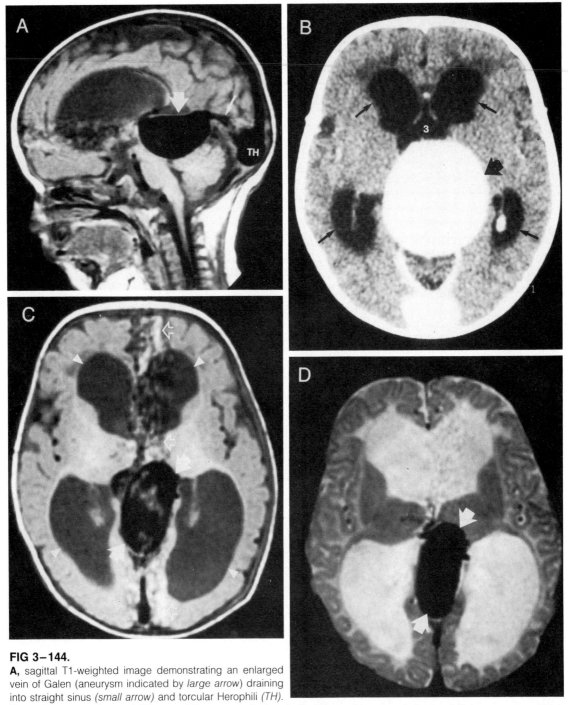

FIG 3–144.
A, sagittal T1-weighted image demonstrating an enlarged vein of Galen (aneurysm indicated by *large arrow*) draining into straight sinus *(small arrow)* and torcular Herophili *(TH).*
B, axial contrast-enhanced CT scan of the same patient as in **A** shows enhancement of vein of Galen aneurysm *(thick arrow)* producing hydrocephalus enlargement of the third *(3)* and lateral ventricles *(small arrows).* **C,** axial T1-weighted image (same patient as in **A** and **B**) of the aneurysm *(closed arrow)* producing flow artifact across the midline of the image *(open arrows)* and hydrocephalus of the lateral ventricles *(arrowheads).* **D,** axial T2-weighted image (same patient) shows that vein of Galen aneurysm *(arrows)* and hydrocephalus are present.

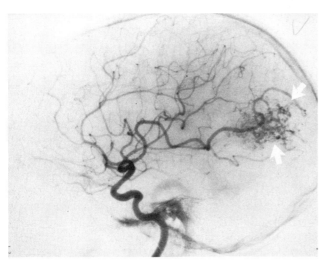

FIG 3–145.
Left carotid cerebral angiogram (arterial phase, lateral projection) reveals arteriovenous malformation. An abnormal collection of arteries and veins *(arrows)* involves the left posterior parietal area.

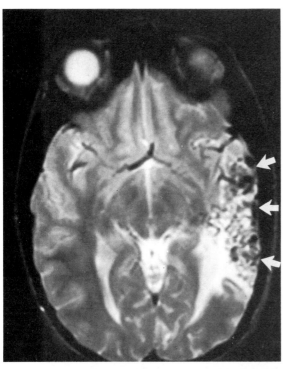

FIG 3–146.
Axial T2-weighted image showing arteriovenous malformation of the left temporal lobe with multiple vessels of mixed signal intensities *(arrows).*

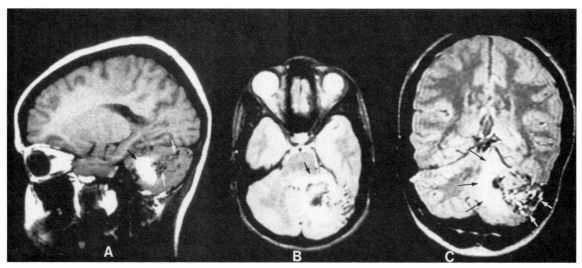

FIG 3–147.
MR of arteriovenous malformation. **A,** sagittal T1-weighted image shows subacute hyperintensive hemorrhage *(black arrow)* and multiple abnormal vessels in the left cerebellar hemisphere *(white arrows).* **B,** axial T2-weighted image shows vasogenic edema (hyperintensity indicated by *arrow*) surrounding hypointense hemor-

rhage and abnormal vessels. **C,** coronal T2-weighted image shows vasogenic edema (hyperintensity indicated by *black arrows*) surrounding hypointense hematoma with mixed signal intensities of vessels *(white arrows).*

pratentorial area. The typical appearance is of a large draining vein. The signal intensity of this vein usually will demonstrate a signal void on T1-weighted images. However, on T2-weighted images, there may be either a signal void or increased signal depending on how fast the blood is flowing within this large venous angioma. There is also noted on the T2-weighted image a chemical shift at the level of this anomalous vein. After administration of Gd, there is enhancement of the vessel. Venous angiomas usually are incidental findings and are well demonstrated on MRI and CT (Fig 3–148). A very small percentage may be associated with hemorrhage or infarction.

Cavernous hemangioma is a vascular tumor that is a honeycombed, epithelial-lined, sinusoidal vascular space containing stagnant blood. Thrombosis, calcification, and hemorrhage are frequent. They usually produce gliosis of the surrounding brain parenchyma and are more common in the cerebral hemispheres than elsewhere (Fig 3–149).

Capillary telangiectasias, also called capillary angiomas, are small solitary lesions which represent a collection of dilated capillaries with intervening brain parenchyma. Hemorrhage as well as associated areas of gliosis around adjacent brain tissue may be associated with this lesion. Cavernous hemangiomas and capillary telangiectasias are difficult to differentiate on MR. They are usually occult lesions which are picked up as incidental findings on MRI.

Although both forms of vascular malformation

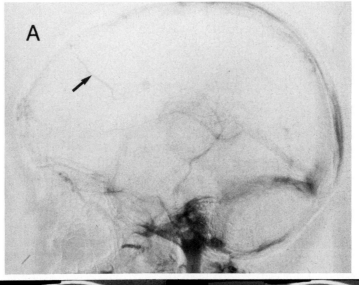

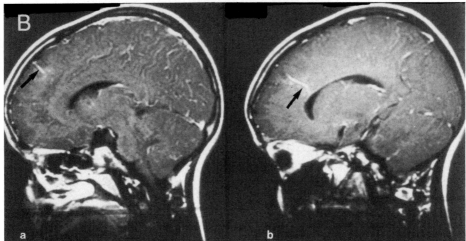

FIG 3–148.
A, right carotid cerebral angiogram (venous phase, lateral projection) reveals venous angioma, with abnormal left frontal vein *(arrow)*. **B,** post-Gd sagittal T1-weighted of image venous angiogram *(a)* shows linear enhancement extending from the right frontal lobe *(arrow)* superior sagittal sinus *(b)* to the lateral ventricle *(arrow)*.

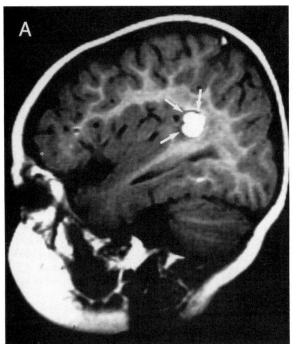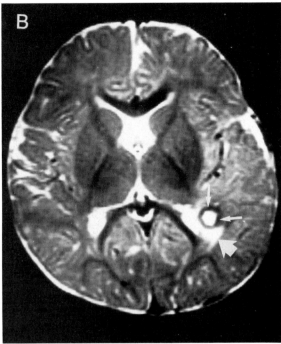

FIG 3-149.
A, sagittal T1-weighted image of cavernous hemangioma reveals small round lesion demonstrating hyperintensity with a partial hypointense rim *(arrows).* **B,** axial T2-weighted image (same patient as in **A**) showing cavernous hemangioma with small area of hyper- intense gliosis *(large arrow).* Central area of hyperintense subacute hemorrhage shows hypointense hemosiderin rim *(small arrows).*

may bleed within themselves, they do not bleed outside. They typically do not produce hemorrhagic rupture outside of the vascular malformation into adjacent brain parenchyma as do the true AVMs. The MRI findings on T1-weighted images consist of a round, oval, or lobulated mass with a peripheral ring of hypointensity that usually represents hemosiderin; the center of this lesion shows mixed signal intensities. On T2-weighted images, there are mixed signals of hyperintensity and hypointensity with a peripheral rim of hypointensity. The mixed signal intensities represent different stages of hemorrhage. Calcium may also be present within the vascular spaces of these lesions. A rim of adjacent gliotic brain may be present just beyond the hemosiderin ring. It may be very difficult to differentiate cavernous hemangioma and capillary telangiectasia vascular malformations from very small true AVMs that have bled and formed infarcts in portions of their vascular supply. These small occult vascular malformations can be demonstrated on MR, but cannot be differentiated from cavernous hemangioma and capillary telangiectasia. The cavernous hemangioma lesions are frequently multiple in children.

Intracranial aneurysms are extremely rare in children. When they do occur, they are usually associated with other predisposing factors such as coarc- tation of the aorta, polycystic kidney disease, and Ehlers-Danlos syndrome. These aneurysms may involve any portion of the internal carotid arterial or the vertebral basilar circulation. They usually occur along the distal branches of the intracranial arteries. Giant intracranial aneurysms are fairly common in children. They are greater than 2.5 cm in size. The common sites are the tip of the basilar artery, the horizontal portion of the middle cerebral artery, and the supraclinoid portion of the internal carotid artery (Fig 3-150). The aneurysms can attain a very large size. They have thrombi within the walls that narrow the lumen. They can expand by bleeding within their walls and thereby produce a pseudocapsule. They usually present as a mass with signs of either raised intracranial pressure or focal neurologic deficits. The diagnosis is made with a combination of imaging modalities. A cerebral arteriogram will demonstrate the patent lumen of the giant intracranial aneurysm. MRI is excellent at delineating the full extent of the aneurysm with its pseudocapsule, the thrombi present within its wall, and its lumen. There will be mixed signal intensities with a serpentine central area of signal void on both the T1-weighted and T2-weighted images that represents the fast-flowing blood within the patent portion of the lumen. Thrombi demonstrate mixed signal in-

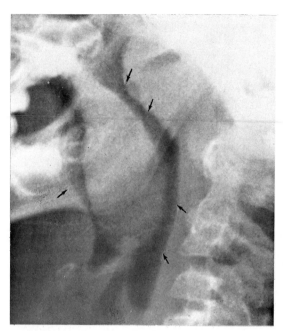

FIG 3–150.
Vertebral angiogram of the brain (lateral) reveals a giant intracranial aneurysm *(arrow)* of the tip of the basilar artery.

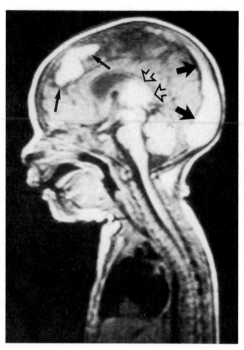

FIG 3–151.
Sagittal T1-weighted image reveals thrombosis of the superior sagittal sinus (hyperintensity indicated by *large black arrows*) and deep venous thrombosis secondary to severe dehydration with resultant subacute hemorrhagic infarction of the right frontal lobe (hyperintensity indicated by *small black arrows*) and thalamus *(open arrows).*

tensities that are concentric and give the giant intracranial aneurysm an onion appearance with layers of hyperintensity and hypointensity on both the T1-weighted and T2-weighted images.

CEREBRAL INFARCTION

Cerebral ischemia can be due to decreased blood flow to the brain or decreased oxygen content of the blood. Cerebral ischemia, if severe or persistent, may progress to cerebral infarction with irreversible damage to brain cells. Arterial infarction (focal or diffuse) may be due to trauma to the neck with occlusion of the carotid artery, arteritis, sickle cell anemia, meningitis (at the base of the brain), or congenital heart disease with a right-to-left shunt. Venous infarction may be due to thrombosis of the major venous sinuses (superior sagittal sinus) due to dehydration, trauma, or meningitis. There is a diffuse form of infarction that is seen in newborns and young children in which there is a global, severe, hypoxic or anoxic episode with infarction of the cortex and subcortical white matter of both cerebral hemispheres. Most infarcts are ischemic or bland. However, hemorrhagic infarction can be seen in children with bleeding diatheses, venous thrombosis, or disseminated intravascular coagulopathy (Fig 3–151).

The type and location of the infarction also de-

pends on the maturity of the vascular supply to the newborn brain. In the premature infant, the arterial blood supply is directed centrally with the watershed area being present within the periventricular white matter of the lateral ventricles. Cerebral infarction in the premature brain occurs within the periventricular white matter of the lateral ventricles producing periventricular leukomalacia. This is better seen on US as increased echogenicity in the periventricular white matter of the lateral ventricles. The later stage consists of periventricular cystic formation (Fig 3–152).

In the full-term infant the arterial blood supply has matured into its normal location with the watershed area being peripheral at the cortex of the brain. Infarction in the full-term infant has the normal arterial distribution, as in the adult.

CT and MRI are both useful modalities in the evaluation of brain infarction. The early stages of an ischemic infarct are better seen on CT in young children (<2 years of age) owing to the prominent water content of both gray and white matter. With MRI there may be difficulty in delineating the edema seen in early infarction from the water normally present in the gray and white matter. After 2 years

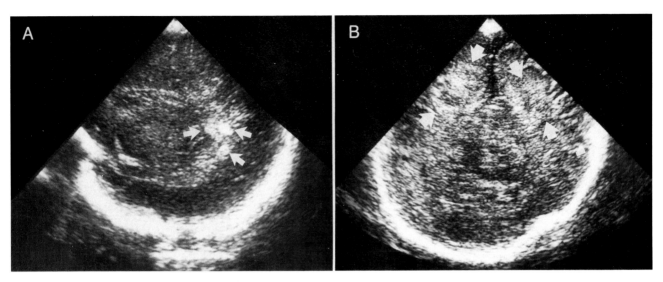

FIG 3–152.
A, sagittal US (sector transducer) scan of a preterm newborn with periventricular leukomalacia shows increased echogenicity *(arrows)* involving the adjacent white matter of the right lateral ventricle. **B,** Coronal US (sector transducer) scan of a preterm newborn with bilateral periventricular leukomalacia shows areas of increased echogenicity *(arrows)* involving the white matter adjacent to the posterior aspect of the bodies of the lateral ventricles.

of age, with the myelination process almost completed, the early edema is readily appreciated. In children aged 2 years and older, MRI is more sensitive in demonstrating early infarction with the infarction being seen within 6 hours after the initial insult, while early infarction may not be seen on CT until 3 days after the insult. If the infarction is large, then the mass effect from the edema may compress parts of the ventricles or sulci (Figs 3–153 and 3–154).

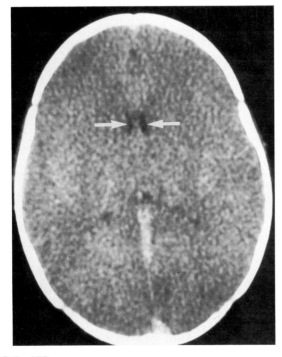

FIG 3–153.
Axial contrast-enhanced CT scan of an infant with a severe anoxic episode with diffuse cerebral edema (cytotoxic) compressing the frontal horns *(arrows)* of the lateral ventricles toward the midline.

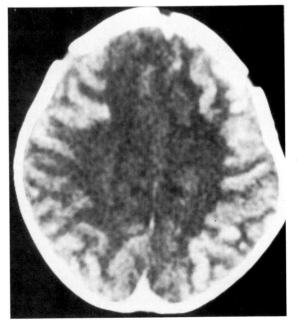

FIG 3–154.
Axial unenhanced CT scan obtained from an infant 3 days after a prolonged anoxic episode demonstrates damage to the blood-brain barrier with extravasation of blood into the perivascular, extracellular, and intracellular spaces of the cortex (increased density is seen involving the gyri).

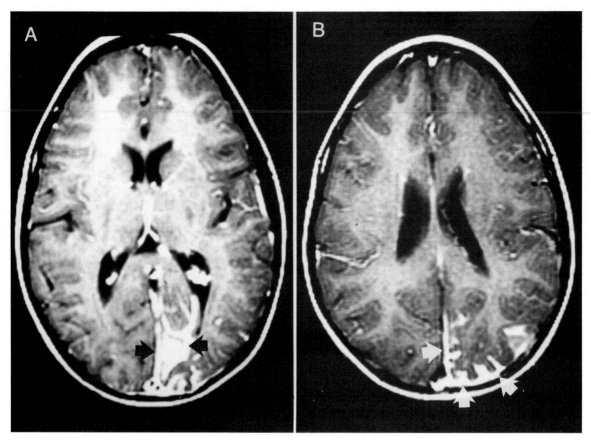

FIG 3–155.
A, post-Gd axial T1-weighted image shows acute ischemic infarction of the left occipital lobe with enhancement *(arrows).* **B,** post-

Gd axial T1-weighted image shows acute ischemic infarc tion of the left occipital lobe with enhancement of the cortex *(arrows).*

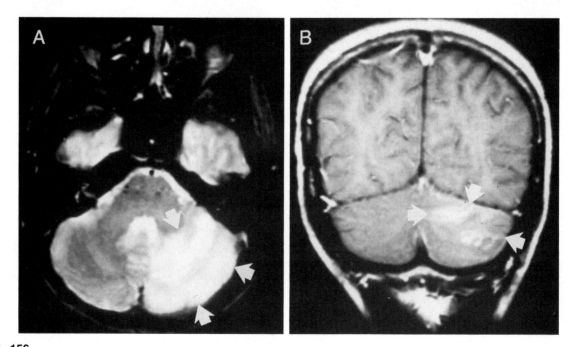

FIG 3–156.
A, axial T2-weighted image shows acute ischemic infarction of the left cerebellar hemisphere area of hyperintensity *(arrows).* **B,** post-Gd coronal T1-weighted image (same patient as in **A**) shows acute

ischemic infarction of the left cerebellar hemisphere with enhancement *(arrows).*

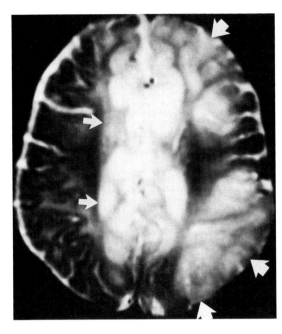

FIG 3–157.
Axial T2-weighted image obtained from an infant with granulomatous meningitis and occlusion of portions of the left side of the circle of Willis with acute ischemic infarction in the distribution of the left internal carotid artery and its branches. Hyperintensity involves the left cerebral hemisphere *(large white arrows)* and the medial aspect of the right cerebral hemisphere *(small white arrows).*

Enhancement with contrast may not be seen on CT or MRI within the first week of the infarction. Recent infarcts are hypodense on CT; and on MRI, they are hypointense on T1-weighted and hyperintense on T2-weighted images. Arterial infarction is wedge-shaped and in an arterial distribution within the brain.

Peripheral areas of infarction involve both gray and white matter (cortex and subcortical white matter) (Figs 3–155, 3–156, and 3–157). Venous infarction is usually not wedge-shaped. Infarction may be focal, unilateral, multiple, bilateral, or diffuse, involving any part of the brain.

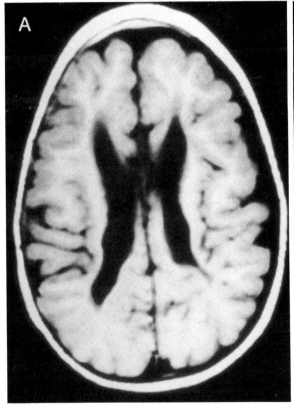

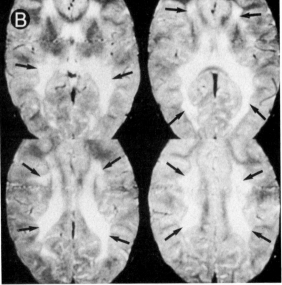

FIG 3–158.
A, axial T1-weighted image of a child with cerebral palsy. The child was premature with periventricular infarction. Note loss of periventricular white matter and irregularity of the lateral walls of the lateral ventricles. **B,** axial T2-weighted images (same child as in **A** show hyperintensity of the periventricular white matter (old infarction).

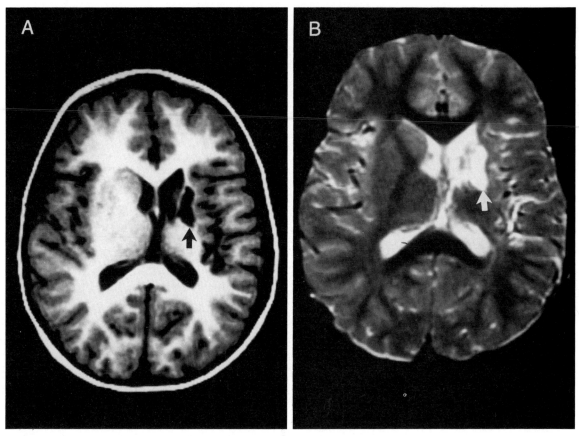

FIG 3–159.
A, axial T1-weighted image shows old lacunar infarct of the left basal ganglia (area of hypointensity indicated by *arrow*). **B,** axial T2-weighted image shows hyperintensity of the area of lacunar infarction *(arrow).*

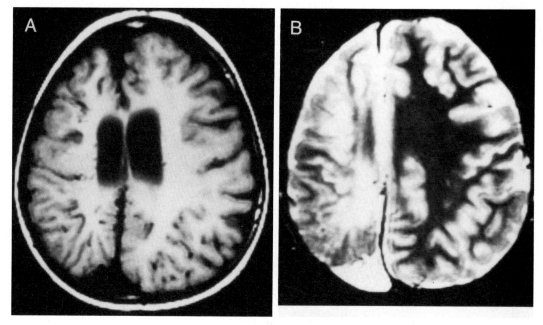

FIG 3–160.
A, axial T1-weighted image shows an old infarction of the right cerebral hemisphere which is small and atrophic. **B,** axial T2-weighted image (same child as in **A**) reveals infarction (hyperintensity) of the small atrophic right cerebral hemisphere.

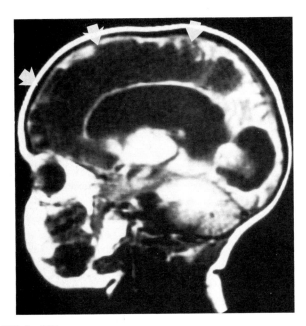

FIG 3–161.
Sagittal T1-weighted image shows old infarction involving the left cerebral hemisphere with multicystic encephalomalacia (hypointensity indicated by *arrows*).

The end stage of infarction may show a spectrum of findings. The brain may appear normal or atrophic with or without areas of gliosis, encephalomalacia, porencephaly, and cystic cavities. Severe asphyxia in the infant and young child may produce an end-stage brain that is almost totally destroyed (multicystic encephalomalacia). The CT and MRI findings in the chronic stage of infarction may show enlargement of parts or all of the ventricular system and sulci (atrophy). If encephalomalacia is present without cyst formation, then CT will demonstrate an area of hypodensity without mass effect and no enhancement. On MRI, encephalomalacia will be hypointense on T1-weighted and hyperintense (gliosis) on T2-weighted images. There is no enhancement of old lacunar infarcts with Gd. Cysts are lucent on CT and on MRI have the same signal as CSF (hypointense on T1-weighted and hyperintense on T2-weighted images) (Figs 3–158 to 3–161).

Hemorrhagic infarction is easily recognized on CT by areas of hemorrhage and edema. The MRI appearance of hemorrhagic infarction depends on the stage of the hemoglobin.

REFERENCES

Vascular Malformations and Aneurysms
Atlas SW: *Magnetic Resonance Imaging of the Brain and Spine.* New York, Raven Press 1990, pp 379–396.

Atlas SW, Grossman RI, Goldberg HI, et al: Partially thrombosed giant intracranial aneurysms: Correlation of MR and pathologic findings. *Radiology* 1987; 162:111–114.

Celli P, Ferrante L, Palmal, et al: Cerebral arteriovenous malformations in children. *Surg Neurol* 1984; 22:43–49.

Diebler C, Dulac O, Renier D, et al: Aneurysms of the vein of Galen in infants aged 2 to 15 months. Diagnosis and natural evaluation. *Neuroradiology* 1981; 21:185–197.

Gerosa MA, Cappellotto P, Licata C, et al: Cerebral arteriovenous malformations in children (56 cases). *Childs Brain* 1981; 8:356–371.

Locksley HB: Natural history of subarachnoid hemorrhage, intracranial aneurysms and arterio-venous malformations. *J Neurosurg* 1966; 25:219–239.

Olsen WL, Brant-Zawadzki M, Hodes J, et al: Giant intracranial aneurysms: MR imaging. *Radiology* 1987; 163:431–435.

Rigamonti D, Drayer BP, Johnson PC, et al: The MRI appearance of cavernous malformations (angiomas). *J Neurosurg* 1987; 67:518–524.

Rigamonti D, Spetzler RF, Drayer BP, et al: Appearance of venous malformations on magnetic resonance imaging. *J Neurosurg* 1988; 69:535–539.

Sakai NK, Sakate K, Yomada H, et al: Familial occurrence of intracranial aneurysms. *J Neurosurg* 1966; 25:593–600.

Cerebral Infarction
Baram TZ, Butler IJ, Nelson MD, et al: Transverse sinus thromboses in newborns: Clinical and magnetic resonance imaging findings. *Ann Neurol* 1988; 24:792–794.

Brown JJ, Hesselink JR, Rothrock JF: MR and CT of lacunar infarcts. *Am J Roentgenol* 1988; 151:367–372.

Bryan RN, Wilcott MR, Schneiders NJ, et al: Nuclear magnetic resonance evaluation of stroke. *Radiology* 1983; 149:189–192.

Cohen MD, Edwards MK: *Magnetic Resonance Imaging of Children.* Philadelphia, BC Decker, 1990, pp 277–290.

DeReuk J, Chatha AS, Richardson EP: Pathogenesis and evaluation of periventricular leukomalacia in infancy. *Arch Neurol* 1971; 27:220–236.

Diebler C, Dulac O: Prenatal and perinatal vascular lesions of circulatory origin, in *Pediatric Neurology and Neuroradiology.* New York, Springer-Verlag, 1987; pp 185–211.

El Gammal T, Adams RJ, Nichols FT, et al: MR and CT investigation of cerebrovascular disease in sickle cell patients. *AJNR* 1986; 7:1043–1049.

Humphreys RP, Hendrick EB, Hoffman HJ: Cerebrovascular disease in children. *Can Med Assoc J* 1974; 107:774–781.

Imakita S, Nishimura T, Naito H, et al: Magnetic resonance imaging of human cerebral infarction: Enhancement with Gd-DTPA. *Neuroradiology* 1987; 29:422–429.

Leblanc R, O'Gorman AM: Neonatal intracranial hemorrhage: A clinical and serial computerized tomographic study. *J Neurosurg* 1980; 53:642–651.

Moore JB, Parker CP, Smith RJ, et al: Concealment of neonatal cerebral infarction on MRI by normal brain water. *Pediatr Radiol* 1987; 17:314–315.

Sankaran K, Peters K, Finer N: Estimated cerebral blood flow in term infants with hypoxic encephalopathy. *Pediatr Res* 1981; 15:1415–1418.

Shuman RM, Seledrik TK: Periventricular leukomalacia. A one year autopsy study. *Arch Neurol* 1980; 37:231–235.

SECTION 8

Introduction to the Spinal Cord

DEFINITION AND NORMAL ANATOMY

The spinal cord is a cylindric column of nervous tissue composed of a central core of gray matter surrounded peripherally by white matter. It contains a small central CSF canal called the *central canal* which extends from the cervicomedullary junction to the lower end of the spinal cord, the *conus medullaris*. The spinal cord is divided into three parts: *cervical*, *thoracic*, and *lumbar*. The conus medullaris is cone-shaped and normally ends at the level of the L1–2 vertebrae. The *filum terminale* is a strand of nervous tissue (the terminal aspect of the spinal cord) that extends from the tip of the conus medullaris to pierce the dura of the thecal sac to end extradurally at the coccyx (Fig 3–162). Two continuous rows of nerve roots emerge on either side of the spinal cord (ventral and dorsal roots) to join distally to form 31 pairs of spinal nerves which exit through the intervertebral foramina. The spinal nerves distribute sensory and motor fibers to all parts of the body. The cord demonstrates normal enlargement in the midcervical and midlumbar spine due to the large number of nerve fibers at these levels, which are necessary to innervate the arms and legs (Fig 3–163). After the third month of gestation, the vertebral column grows faster than the spinal cord. This results in the distal aspect of the spinal cord being more superior than the distal aspect of the spinal canal and spine with the lower spinal nerve roots (lumbar and sacral) having to descend further to exit from the spinal cord through their respective intervertebral foramen. This produces a large collection of nerve roots extending below the conus medullaris called the *cauda equina* (owing to its resemblance to a horse's tail). The spinal cord is enveloped by a thin covering membrane (the *pia mater*) and it sits within

a CSF space called the *subarachnoid space*. This space in turn is surrounded by an *arachnoid membrane* which in turn is surrounded by a dural membrane covering called the *thecal sac*. The thecal sac is within the spinal canal, and the spinal cord is within the thecal sac, fixed to its walls by the dentate ligaments (Fig 3–164).

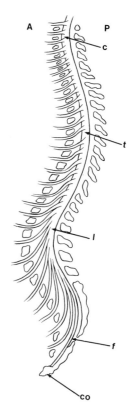

FIG 3–162.
Diagram of lateral view of the spinal cord with nerve roots: *A,* anterior; *P* posterior; *c,* cervical; *t,* thoracic; *l,* lumbar; *f,* filum terminale; *co,* coccyx.

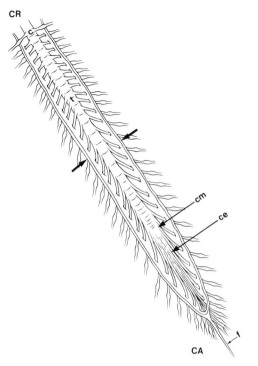

FIG 3–163.
Diagram of dorsal view of the spinal cord and nerve roots and nerves: *CR,* cranial; *CA,* caudal; *c,* cervical; *t,* thoracic; *cm,* conus medullaris; *ce,* cauda equina; *f,* filum terminale; thecal sac *(thick arrows).*

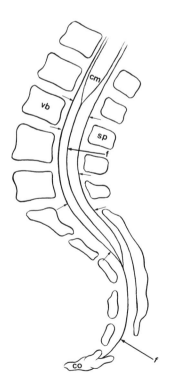

FIG 3–164.
Diagram of lateral view of the lumbosacrococcygeal spine: *cm,* conus medullaris; *f,* filum terminale; thecal sac *(small arrows); co,* coccyx; *vb,* vertebral body; *sp,* spinous process.

EMBRYOGENESIS

A basic overview of the development of the spine and spinal cord will aid in the understanding of the MRI appearance of the infant spine and the dysraphic conditions that commonly occur.

The formation of the fetal vertebral column begins at approximately 3 weeks' gestation, at which time two events occur. The first is the separation of the notochord (which develops from Hensen's node) from the overlying neural tube and underlying yolk sac. The notochord forms the framework for the developing spine and induces and controls the formation of the vertebral bodies and nucleus pulposus of the intervertebral disks (Fig 3–165). The second event is the division of the paraxial mesoderm (which arises from mesenchyme lateral to the closing neural tube) into somites. The somites separate into an anteromedial group, the sclerotomes, which, over the framework of the notochord, develop into the vertebral bodies and adjacent ribs. The posterolateral groups of somites, the dermomyotomes, develop into the paraspinal musculature (Fig 3–166). As each sclerotome proliferates, it divides into halves. The caudal half becomes denser than the rostral half. The intervertebral disk (the anulus fibrosus) is formed from the anterior surface of the caudal half. The next step is the joining of the caudal half of each sclerotome with the rostral half of the next most caudal one to form the vertebral body. The intersegmental vessels that were between the somites are now within the center of the developing vertebral body. This area of fusion with the vessels within the middle of the vertebral body is called the Hahn notch.

The development of the spinal cord occurs during three stages: neurulation, canalization, and retrogressive differentiation. The spinal cord develops from ectoderm. During the first week of gestation, there is a proliferation of ectodermal cells along the surface of the embryo to form the primitive streak. At the cephalic end of the primitive streak, a rapidly developing group of pluripotential cells forms the primitive node, or Hensen's node. The primitive streak which is the neural plate forms a groove in the midline and during the third week of gestation this groove forms folds laterally. The right and left neural folds begin to approach each other dorsally near the midline at the neural groove (Fig 3–167).

This is the beginning of the stage of neurulation, the closing of the neural plate into the neural tube. The neural plate closes at its midpoint dorsally and then proceeds to close from this midpoint craniad and caudad. Finally, at its cranial end, the anterior

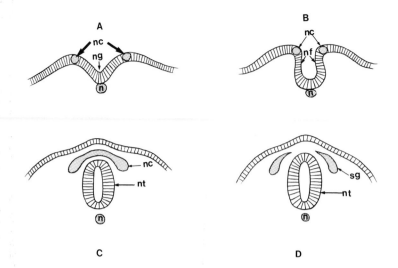

FIG 3–165.
Diagram of the development of the neural tube. **A,** neural groove (ng); notochord (n), neural crest (nc, arrows). **B,** neural folds (nf, small arrows); neural crest. **C,** neural tube (nt), neural crest (nc). **D,** neural tube (nt), spinal ganglion (sg).

neuropore closes at about the 25th day of gestation; its caudal end, the posterior neuropore, closes last at about the 28th day. This completes the stage of neurulation (Fig 3–168).

Simultaneous with the stage of neurulation, the overlying ectoderm of the skin separates from the neural tube and fuses in the midline and the perineural mesenchyme grows around the neural tube to form the meninges, bone, and muscle. It is believed that most of the spinal dysraphic states occur around this stage of development of the spine and spinal cord, most notably the myelomeningocele or myelocele and the lipomyelomeningocele. The dorsal dermal sinus is believed to be the result of focal incomplete separation of the ectodermal-neuroectodermal-mesenchymal adhesions.

The next stage, canalization, begins at about the 30th day of fetal life. During this stage, the caudal end of the neural tube elongates just distal to the posterior closure into a caudal cell mass, and ependyma lines a central tubular structure. It is be-

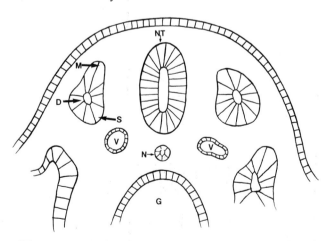

FIG 3–166.
Diagram of the relationship of the sclerotome to the neural tube: NT, neural tube; N, notochord; V, blood vessels; G, gut; M, myotome; D, dermatome; S, sclerotome.

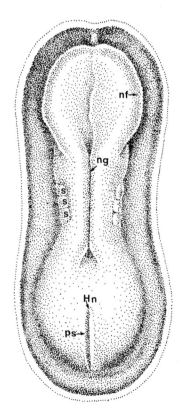

FIG 3–167.
Diagram of the dorsal aspect of a human embryo of 3 weeks: nf, neural fold; ng, neural groove; s, somites; Hn, Hensen's node; ps, primitive streak.

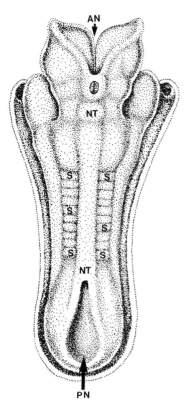

FIG 3–168.
Human embryo of 23 days: *AN,* anterior neuropore; *PN,* posterior neuropore; *S,* somites; *NT,* neural tube.

lieved that persistence of portions or abnormal development of the caudal cell mass may produce the sacral teratoma, intradural lipoma, and tethered low-lying spinal cord.

Finally, at 5½ weeks, during retrogressive differentiation, there is a decrease in the size of the central lumen and a decrease in the cell mass of the distal end of the neural tube, with formation of the spinal cord, filum terminale, conus medullaris, and central canal.

Although there are a variety of theories as to the causes of the different types of spinal dysraphism, the underlying cause is the result of an insult (whether genetic or acquired) which interferes with the normal process of neurulation, canalization, or retrogressive differentiation.

REFERENCES

Spinal Cord: Definition and Normal Anatomy
Clemente CD: *Gray's Anatomy.* Philadelphia, Lea & Febiger, 1985, pp 933–1148.
Grant JCB: *Grant's Anatomy,* ed 5. Baltimore, Williams & Wilkins, 1962.
Heimer L: *The Human Brain and Spinal Cord.* New York, Springer-Verlag, 1983.
Last RJ: *Anatomy Regional and Applied,* ed 6. New York, Churchill Livingstone, 1978.
Pansky B, House EL: *Review of Gross Anatomy,* ed 2. London, Macmillan, 1970.

Embryogenesis
Davies J: *Human Developmental Anatomy.* New York, Ronald Press, 1963, pp 199–224.
Heimer L: *The Human Brain and Spinal Cord.* New York, Springer-Verlag, 1983.
Langman J: *Medical Embryology.* Baltimore, William & Wilkins, 1963, pp 246–283.

SECTION 9

Imaging Modalities

The most important radiologic modalities in the evaluation of the pediatric spinal cord are MRI, CT, real-time US, and myelography with water-soluble contrast, singly and with follow-through CT (intrathecal contrast CT). The determination of which to use depends on the child's clinical presentation and the common pathologic conditions which affect the pediatric spinal cord. The common abnormalities are congenital malformations, neoplasms, infection, and trauma.

ULTRASOUND

US is increasingly being used to evaluate the spinal cord, canal, and thecal sac in newborns and infants. Real-time US is used predominantly in newborns

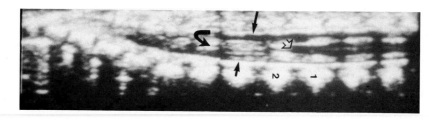

FIG 3–169.

Sagittal US scan through lower thoracic lumbosacral spine of a normal newborn showing the conus medullaris *(open arrow)* ending at the bodies of L1–2, the anterior *(short arrow)* and posterior *(long arrow)* walls of the thecal sac, and the cauda equina (nerve roots indicated by *curved arrow)* extending from the distal end of the spinal cord.

with a skin-covered back mass, or abnormal cutaneous manifestations of the back such as a hemangioma, hairy tuft, dimple, or sinus tract to look for spinal dysraphic states with intraspinal abnormality such as a dermal sinus, dermoid tumor, lipoma, tethered cord, or diastematomyelia. Excellent images of the spinal cord, canal, and thecal sac can be seen in children up to 3 to 6 months of age. A real-time US scanner with a 5-mHz linear-array transducer is used, and scans in the sagittal and axial planes are routinely obtained. The static US images of the normal spine show the increased echogenicity of the vertebrae with less echogenicity demonstrated by the spinal cord and nerve roots with the sonolucent CSF (Figs 3–169 through 3–171). Intraspinal lipomas show increased echogenicity, and intraspinal dermoid tumors and sinus tracts show isoechogenicity or hypoechogenicity with the spinal cord or nerve roots (Figs 3–172 and 3–173). Primary spinal cord neoplasms demonstrate widening of the involved portion of the spinal cord with increased or inhomogeneous echogenicity (Fig 3–174). The conus of the spinal cord may normally be at the body of the L3 vertebra in children up to 3 months of age. After

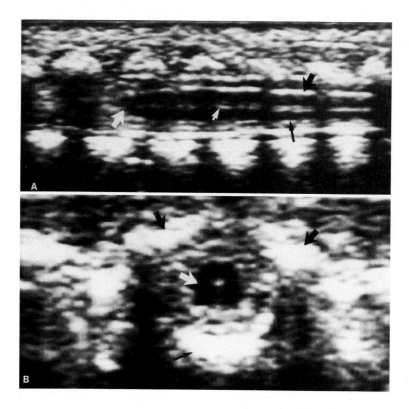

FIG 3–170.

Sonograms. **A,** sagittal scan of the lower thoracolumbar spine showing normal hypoechoic distal spinal cord with areas of hyperechogenicity along the anterior border *(thin black arrow)*, posterior border *(thick black arrow)*, and center *(small white arrow)*, the conus medullaris *(large white arrow)* at the bodies of the L1–2 vertebrae, and the nerve roots of the cauda equina extending from the conus as linear areas of hyperechogenicity. **B,** axial scan of the lower thoracic spine showing hypoechoic spinal cord *(white arrow)* with a central area of increased echogenicity, vertebral body *(thin black arrow)*, and laminae *(large black arrows)*.

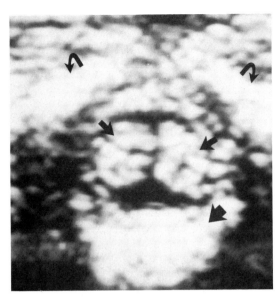

FIG 3–171.
Axial US scan at the level of the cauda equina with normal anatomy demonstrating two separate bundles of nerve roots *(small arrows)* within the spinal canal, vertebral body *(thick arrow)*, and laminae *(curved arrows)*.

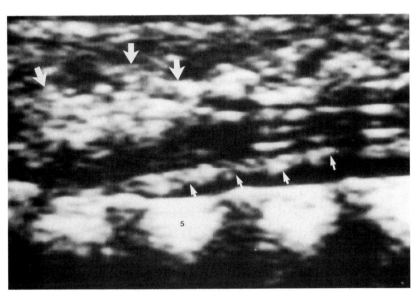

FIG 3–172.
Sagittal US scan of lumbosacral spine. Intradural lipoma demonstrating hyperechogenicity *(large arrows)* tethering a low-lying spinal cord *(small arrows)*; 5, L5 vertebral body.

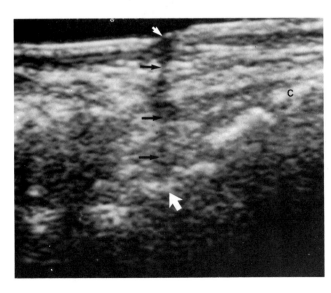

FIG 3–173.
Sagittal US scan of distal lumbosacral spine showing dermal sinus tract *(black arrows)* extending from the skin surface of the back *(small white arrow)* to the distal end of the spinal canal at S1 *(large white arrow). C, Coccyx.*

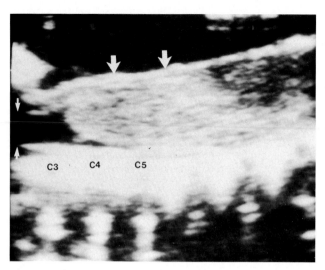

FIG 3–174.
Sagittal US scan of the cervical spine. Intraoperative sonogram (lamina removed posteriorly) demonstrates enlargement and hyperechogenicity of a cervical cord astrocytoma *(large arrows)*, normal hypoechogenic portion of the upper cervical cord at C3 *(small arrows)*, and hyperechogenicity of the anterior cervical vertebral bodies *C3, C4,* and *C5.*

However, in children who have bony dysraphic defects and postoperative laminectomy defects, it is possible to obtain a US window through the defect to evaluate intraspinal contents at the specific level. Real-time US has an important role in the evaluation of the postoperative spine in children for indications of spinal cord tethering (Fig 3–175). Normal cord pulsations are seen routinely with real-time US. If the pulsations are significantly diminished or absent in the neutral position or when the spine is flexed, then significant cord tethering is present.

Intraoperative US guidance is being used increasingly by neurosurgeons to help localize and determine the extent of spinal cord neoplasms. After a surgical laminectomy has been performed, the sterile US transducer is placed on the dura of the spinal canal to obtain the exact location of the neoplasm. Intraoperative US allows accurate delineation of the involvement of the spinal cord by neoplasm for biopsy, excision, or both (see Fig 3–174).

COMPUTED TOMOGRAPHY

CT with intravenous iodinated contrast material allows evaluation of some intraspinal abnormalities. The spinal cord, nerve roots, and thecal sac are demonstrated. The dura enhances with intravenous contrast, allowing better delineation of the spinal cord from dura (Fig 3–176). CT allows excellent evaluation of intraspinal lipomas, which are lucent on the scans. Intraspinal neoplasms may show enhancement with contrast. CT is excellent at evaluating paraspinal and bony abnormalities, which may extend into the spinal canal and compress the spinal cord or nerve roots. However, MRI is far superior

3 months the conus should be at the L1–2 level.

After 3 to 6 months of age, continued ossification of the posterior elements of the spine makes it exceedingly difficult to obtain adequate penetration of the bony spine with the 5-mHz transducer. At times, it may be possible to use the 3-mHz transducer and scan the spine at an oblique (off-lateral) angle and obtain images of the intraspinal contents in children up to about 3 to 4 years of age. Usually, after 1 year of age, adequate US images of the pediatric intraspinal contents are not possible because of the normal ossification process of the bony spine.

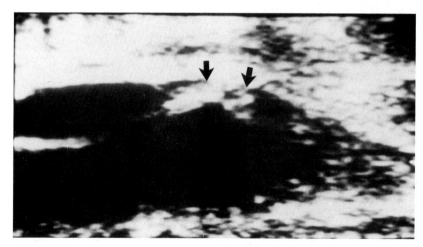

FIG 3–175.
Sagittal US scan of the distal lumbosacral spine reveals repaired myelomeningocele with retethering of a low-lying spinal cord *(arrows)* at the posterior wall of the distal lumbar thecal sac.

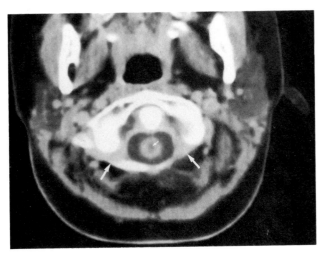

FIG 3–176.
Axial contrast-enhanced CT scan of the cervical spine shows enhancement of the dura *(large arrows)* with a small area of hydromyelia *(small arrow)* within the center of the spinal cord.

for evaluating intraspinal contents and pathologic conditions.

MYELOGRAPHY

Myelography with water-soluble contrast material is used predominantly to evaluate the spinal canal and intraspinal contents. This procedure is performed in the conventional manner under sterile technique, with the child sedated or under general anesthesia with a lumbar or C1–2 puncture. The water-soluble contrast material is instilled into the subarachnoid space, and views are obtained in the anteroposterior, lateral, and oblique projections. Follow-through CT should be employed routinely to evaluate subtle suspicious areas on conventional myelograms. My-

elography and CT are routinely used to evaluate spinal metastases from primary brain tumors, very subtle areas of tethering, severe scoliosis that cannot be adequately imaged with MRI, or subtle cases of diastematomyelia. In subtle cases of hydromyelia or syringomyelia, delayed CT performed 4 to 6 hours after myelography is necessary to see contrast material within the syringomyelic or hydromyelic area (Fig 3–177). Myelography has been almost totally replaced by MRI in the evaluation of pediatric spinal disorders.

ANGIOGRAPHY

Spinal angiography is used predominantly to evaluate vascular malformations of the spinal cord or to further outline the vessels in highly vascular spinal cord neoplasms in children. It is a time-consuming procedure owing to the need to selectively catheterize the multiple vessels that provide the arterial supply to the spinal cord. It is the modality of choice in evaluating the vascular supply to spinal cord vascular malformations.

MAGNETIC RESONANCE IMAGING

MRI is the modality of choice in evaluating intraspinal abnormalities. MRI can be used as an adjunct in further evaluation of bony abnormalities in children to determine if there is compression or extension into the spinal canal. However, its greatest role is in the evaluation of abnormalities affecting the soft tissues of the pediatric spine. Because real-time US is highly dependent on technical skill, the best overall noninvasive diagnostic imaging modality for evalu-

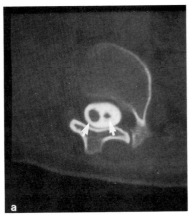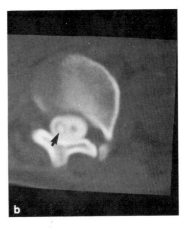

FIG 3–177.
Axial CT scan with intrathecal injection of contrast shows diastematomyelia of the upper lumbar spine. *(a)* Two asymmetric hemicords *(arrows)*. *(b)* Delayed scan with contrast within center *(arrow)* of the larger hemicord.

ating soft tissues of the pediatric spine in all age groups is MRI.

MRI is highly dependent on a variety of factors that affect resolution (signal-to-noise ratio). These factors include the technical parameters to use on the MR scanners, as well as the problems of physiologic and voluntary patient motion. Voluntary patient motion is an extremely important factor in degrading the MR image. Routinely, in children under 5 years of age and in some children between ages 5 and 12, sedation is necessary to prevent voluntary motion. Physiologic motion from CSF pulsations and vascular flow also creates a problem with image degradation. Various parameters are available to suppress arterial, venous, or CSF flow. Presaturation pulses can be used to suppress arterial flow, which may be significant on T1-weighted images. Certain flow compensation parameters are used on the T2-weighted images to suppress venous and CSF flow. Motion artifacts are more pronounced with high-field-strength MR scanners.

It is extremely important when imaging the pediatric spine to use surface coils and to tailor the type and size of the coil to the body part to be im-aged. Small slice thickness and interslice gaps should be used. Because decreasing the slice thickness and field of view decreases the signal-to-noise ratio, the number of excitations should be increased. This change increases the imaging time. A thorough knowledge of the factors that influence resolution in MRI will aid in appropriately evaluating the pediatric spine.

In the evaluation of the pediatric spine, it is important in most instances to obtain T1-weighted and T2-weighted images. The former allow for evaluation of anatomical detail (Figs 3–178 and 3–179). The latter allow further evaluation of intraspinal abnormalities. In certain instances, T2-weighted GEA may be substituted for true T2-weighted images. Gradient-echo sequences allow evaluation of the spine by reducing the time involved. However, the trade-off is a slight decrease in resolution, and this may interfere with evaluating subtle intraspinal abnormalities. For imaging obvious lesions and evaluating the CSF spaces, T2-weighted GEA is usually adequate. If detailed evaluation of an intraspinal abnormality is necessary, then true T2-weighted images should be obtained (Fig 3–180).

Intravenous Gd contrast agents play a role in

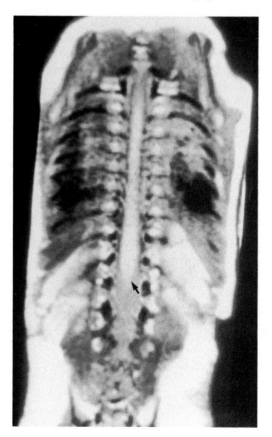

FIG 3–178.
Coronal T1-weighted image of the thoracolumbar spine of a normal newborn showing bulbous conus medullaris (arrow).

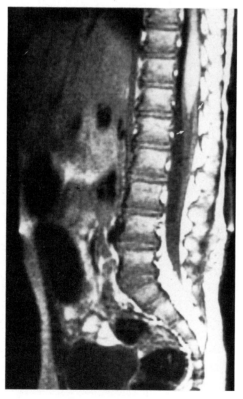

FIG 3–179.
Sagittal T1-weighted image of the lower thoracolumbosacral spine of a normal 1-year-old infant with conus medullaris and cauda equina (arrows) seen as two bundles of nerve roots.

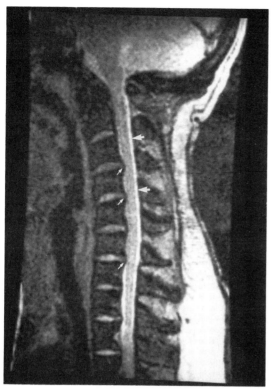

FIG 3–180.
Sagittal T2-weighted image of the cervical–upper thoracic spine illustrating achondroplasia with a narrow spinal canal; compression of the anterior aspect of the cervical spinal cord by bulging disks *(small arrows);* and almost complete loss of the normally hyperintense CSF *(large arrows)* subarachnoid space.

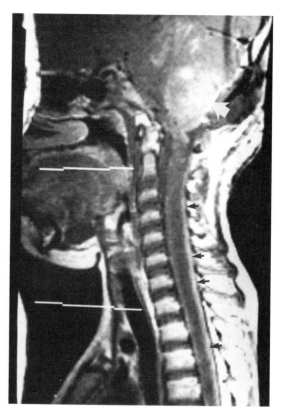

FIG 3–181.
Post-Gd sagittal T1-weighted image of the cervical spine shows recurrent enhancement of medulloblastoma *(large arrow)* and metastatic spread to the leptomeninges of the cervical cord with enhancement of the anterior and posterior borders *(small arrows).*

MRI: in evaluating primary or secondary spinal canal, cord, nerve root, or meningeal neoplasms, and in evaluating the spinal cord for infections, infarctions, vascular malformations, or trauma (Fig 3–181). It is important to obtain two projections of the spine in children when evaluating spinal abnormalities with MRI. The sagittal and axial projections are the most common. However, in some children with severe scoliosis or paravertebral masses with spinal canal extension, the coronal projection may also have to be obtained.

Because MRI is the noninvasive imaging modality of choice in the evaluation of the soft tissues of the pediatric spine, its role and usefulness in evaluating certain common pediatric spinal abnormalities is discussed in the remainder of this section.

Normal Spinal Cord

The spinal cord has the same signal intensity as the cerebrum. However, unlike brain, differentiation of gray and white matter in the spinal cord of young children is usually not possible with routine pulse sequences. At birth the conus medullaris may be slightly bulbous, with a low, central CSF cavity that represents the ventriculus terminalis (distal end of the central canal) which can be prominent in the neonate. The conus may normally extend to the body of the L3 vertebra in infants 3 months old and younger. After 3 months, the conus should normally lie at L1–2 level. The appearance of the cauda equina may vary from a "horse's tail" to two main bundles descending from the conus (see Fig 3–179). The filum terminale is best visualized on the axial view. It should not be greater than 2 mm in diameter, it runs along the posterior wall of the thecal sac, and it is the same signal intensity as the spinal cord or nerve roots. The curvature of the spinal cord follows that of the bony spine. At birth the spinal cord is relatively straight owing to the straight appearance of the bony spine (see Fig 3–178). The normal curvature of the bony spine begins with weightbearing and at 2 years of age the child's spine has its normal curvature; the cervical cord has a slight lordosis and the thoracic cord a slight kyphosis. The cervical cord has a slight enlargement in its midportion which is caused by the normal development of the nerves of the brachial plexus that innervate the arms. The central canal should not be greater than 2 mm in diameter.

REFERENCES

Imaging Modalities

Atlas C: *Magnetic Resonance Imaging of the Brain and Spine.* New York, Raven Press, 1991.

Epstein BS: *The Spine. A Radiological Text and Atlas,* ed 4. Philadelphia, Lea & Febiger, 1976.

Grossman CB: *Magnetic Resonance Imaging and Computed Tomography. Head and Spine.* Baltimore, Williams & Wilkins, 1991.

Harwood-Nash DC, Fitz CR: *Neuroradiology in Infants and Children.* St Louis, Mosby–Year Book, 1976.

Kirsch JE: Basic Principles of magnetic resonance contrast agents. *Top Magn Reson Imaging* 1991; 3:1–18.

Lauffer RB: Magnetic resonance contrast media: Principles and progress. *Magn Reson Q.* 1990; 6:65–84.

Maravilla KR, Cohen WA: *MRI Atlas of the Spine.* New York, Raven Press, 1991.

Naidich TP, Quenca RM: *Clinical Neurosonography.* New York, Springer-Verlag, 1987.

Swischuk LE: *Imaging of the Newborn, Infant and Young Child,* ed 3. Baltimore, Williams & Wilkins, 1988.

SECTION 10

Spinal Dysraphism

Spinal dysraphism is used as a broad term to encompass a variety of disorders which have as a common feature an abnormality in the formation of the pediatric spine. Spinal dysraphism is defined as incomplete or absent fusion of midline mesenchymal, bony, and neural structures. This term refers to large defects which involve the spine and not to the simple spina bifida occulta in which there is only a small cleft within the spinous process or only minor un-united laminae at L5 or S1.

The bone abnormalities associated with spinal dysraphism involve multiple vertebrae. Spina bifida, which means cleft into two parts, is characterized by incomplete fusion of the neural arch. There is absence of all or parts of the posterior elements (laminae and spinous processes). Associated segmental changes of the vertebral bodies such as hemivertebrae, butterfly vertebrae, and block vertebrae are usually present. Children with spinal dysraphism present with a back mass, abnormal cutaneous manifestations, gait disturbance, and bowel and bladder incontinence.

Spinal dysraphism can be classified into three categories based on the presence or absence of a back mass. The first category is spinal dysraphism associated with a back mass that is not covered by skin; the anomalies are the myelomeningocele and myelocele. The second category is spinal dysraphism associated with a skin-covered back mass; the anomalies are the lipomyelomeningocele, myelocystocele, and posterior meningocele. The third category is spinal dysraphism without an associated back mass (occult spinal dysraphism) which encompasses the largest group of anomalies: diastematomyelia, dorsal dermal sinus, spinal lipoma, tight filum terminale, anterior sacral meningocele, lateral thoracic meningocele, hydromyelia, split notochord syndrome, and syndrome of caudal regression (Table 3–9).

SPINAL DYSRAPHISM ASSOCIATED WITH BACK MASS NOT COVERED BY SKIN

Myelomeningocele and Myelocele

A myelomeningocele (meningomyelocele) is a back mass of exposed spinal cord, without a covering of skin, that resembles the primitive neural plate (Fig 3–182). The spinal cord is split dorsally, splayed open (myeloschisis), and herniated through a large posterior dysraphic defect in the bone and dura onto the back. Also herniated onto the back with the exposed spinal cord is CSF with pia and arachnoid. This exposed herniated sac protrudes beyond the

TABLE 3–9.

Classification of Common Types of Spinal Dysraphism

Spinal dysraphism associated with a back mass not covered by
    skin (spina bifida aperta)
    Myelomeningocele and myelocele
Spinal dysraphism associated with a skin-covered back mass
    (spina bifida cystica)
    Lipomyelomeningocele
    Myelocystocele
    Meningocele (posterior)
Occult spinal dysraphism (spina bifida occulta)
    Diastematomyelia
    Dorsal dermal sinus
    Spinal lipoma
    Tight filum terminale
    Anterior sacral meningocele
    Lateral thoracic meningocele
    Hydromyelia
    Split notochord syndrome
    Syndrome of caudal regression

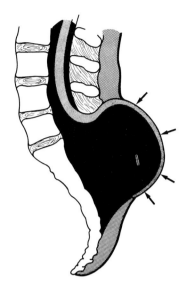

FIG 3–183.
Diagram (sagittal section) of the components of a myelomeningocele with exposed spinal cord *(black arrows)* and CSF herniated through a larger posterior dysraphic defect in the lumbosacral spine.

surface plane of the back and the cord is tethered at this level (Fig 3–183). The myelocele is similar to the myelomeningocele except that its herniated sac of exposed spinal cord is flush with the plane of the back. The most common site for the myelomeningocele or myelocele, in decreasing order of frequency, is the lumbosacral, lumbar, thoracolumbar, and thoracic spine.

The myelomeningocele is one of the most common congenital anomalies of the CNS, occurring in approximately 2 in 1,000 live births in North America. It is slightly more common in females than in males (1.3:1); it usually affects the first-born; and other children within the family have a higher incidence of other neural tube disorders such as encephalocele, anencephaly, meningocele, and myelomeningocele.

Children with a myelomeningocele present at birth with a back mass that is not covered by skin. Symptoms are severe paraparesis, or paralysis of the lower extremities, with sensory deficits and bowel and bladder dysfunction. Later symptoms may include scoliosis, kyphoscoliosis, and renal dysfunction. Ninety-eight percent of children with a myelomeningocele develop hydrocephalus and 95% require some form of shunting of the ventricular system. The spinal cord is low-lying and tethered distally as it extends into, and becomes part of, the herniated sac.

Children with a myelomeningocele have associated anomalies of the brain consisting of the Chiari II malformation (99%) (downward herniation of portions of the medulla oblongata, fourth ventricle, and inferior cerebellum into the upper cervical canal posterior to the cervical cord); dysgenesis of the corpus callosum; and dysplasia of the calvaria (Lückenschädel), meninges, cerebral hemispheres, and cerebellum (Fig 3–184). These children also have hydromyelia (40%–80%), arachnoid cyst of the spinal canal (20%), and diastematomyelia (30%–40%). They

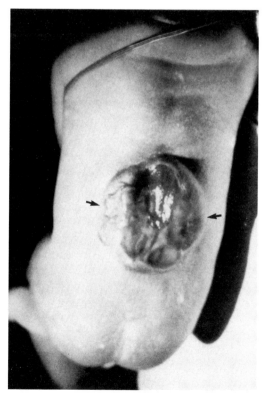

FIG 3–182.
The back of a newborn with a myelomeningocele *(black arrows).*

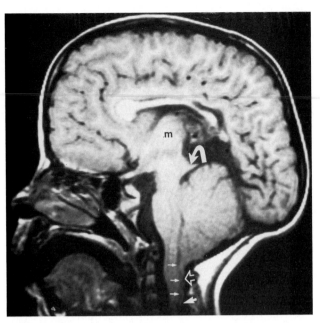

FIG 3–184.
Sagittal T1-weighted image of Chiari II malformation with cervicomedullary kink at C2–3 *(large white arrow)*, downward extension of the fourth ventricle *(small white arrows)*, and cerebellar peg *(open arrow)*. Secondary features include polygyria of the cortex of the cerebral hemispheres, large massa intermedia *(m)*, and tectal beaking *(curved white arrow)*.

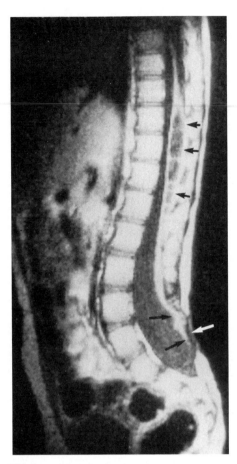

FIG 3–185.
Sagittal T1-weighted image showing repaired myelomeningocele in lumbosacral area *(white arrow)* with low-lying spinal cord *(long black arrows)* tethered by scar, and hydromyelia *(short black arrows)* of the lower thoracic spinal cord.

have or may develop scoliosis or kyphoscoliosis, which may be secondary to the large dysraphic defects of the neural arches, abnormal neuromuscular imbalance, hydromyelia, or retethering of the spinal cord if it has been repaired (Fig 3–185).

Children who have had surgical repair of their myelomeningocele may later develop retethering of the cord secondary to scar formation (adhesions), inclusion lipoma, or inclusion epidermoid (Figs 3–185 and 3–186).

Radiologically, the diagnosis is based on the demonstration of the characteristic features of this anomaly. MRI demonstrates the dysraphic defect with a large herniated sac with CSF and spinal cord forming the posterior wall of the herniated sac. The Chiari II malformation, hydrocephalus, hydromyelia, arachnoid cyst, and diastematomyelia are all well demonstrated on MRI (see Figs 3–184, 3–185, and 3–186). If the scoliosis or kyphoscoliosis is severe or if subtle findings or anomalies are questioned on MRI, then water-soluble myelography with CT should be obtained. A 4- to 6-hour delayed CT-myelogram will help to differentiate areas of localized hydromyelia from an arachnoid cyst or a localized area of cord atrophy with a large CSF space. The bony anomalies are better appreciated on CT.

SPINAL DYSRAPHISM ASSOCIATED WITH SKIN-COVERED BACK MASS

Lipomyelomeningocele

A lipomyelomeningocele is a skin-covered back mass that contains fat, spinal cord, CSF, and meninges herniated through a large defect within the posterior elements of the vertebrae (Fig 3–187). The back mass protrudes beyond the plane of the back. The distinguishing feature of this anomaly is a lipoma or lipomatous tissue which extends from the subcutaneous fat of the back as part of this back mass into the spinal cord. The spinal cord is cleft dorsally and tethered at this level by the fatty tissue growing into the spinal canal and spinal cord (Fig 3–188). The lumbosacral, lumbar, and lumbothoracic spine are the most common sites.

There are multiple large areas of spina bifida at the lipomyelomeningocele with segmentation anom-

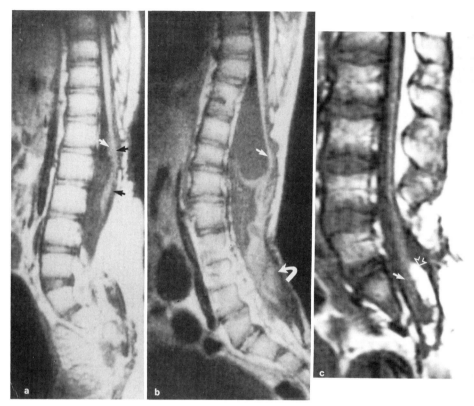

FIG 3–186.
Sagittal T1-weighted image of the distal spine showing repaired myelomeningocele with the spinal cord *(small white arrows)* teth-ered by *(a)* scar formation *(black arrows)*, *(b)* inclusion epidermoid tumor *(curved white arrow)*, and *(c)* inclusion lipoma *(open arrow)*.

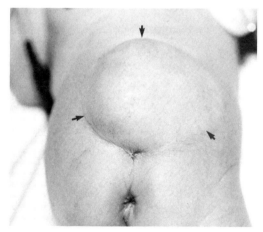

FIG 3–187.
The back of an infant with a lipomyelomeningocele with a skin-cov-ered back mass *(arrows)*.

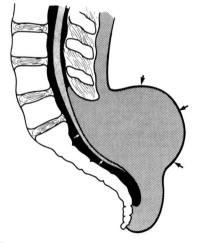

FIG 3–188.
Diagram (sagittal section) shows the components of a lipomyelo-meningocele. The skin-covered back mass *(black arrows)* of fat is contiguous with subcutaneous fat growing into the spinal canal and cord *(white arrows)* through a large posterior dysraphic defect in the bony spine. The spinal cord is low-lying and tethered by the fatty mass.

alies such as hemivertebra and butterfly vertebra (40%) and sacral asymmetry with partial sacral agenesis. Lipomyelomeningocele is associated with the Chiari I malformation (10%) and hydromyelia (10%).

Children with a lipomyelomeningocele usually present at birth with a slightly firm skin-covered back mass. Lipomyelomeningocele is more common in females than males and about half of these children exhibit some cutaneous manifestations such as skin tags or dimples, areas of telangiectasia, or hypertrichosis, and they usually manifest some sensory loss in the lower extremities, bladder dysfunction, motor loss with later development of orthopedic deformities, and leg or foot pain.

Radiologically, the anatomical derangement of the lipomyelomeningocele can be well demonstrated on MRI. The high signal of the fat of the back mass extending into the dorsal aspect of the low-lying tethered spinal cord is seen well on T1 images. There is no tissue plane within this back mass separating the subcutaneous fat from the lipomatous tissue growing into the dorsal area of myeloschisis.

The fat of the lipomyelomeningocele is the subcutaneous tissue. There is no conus present. The distal end of the spinal cord consists of an area of dorsal myeloschisis with fat growing into it (Fig 3–189). US demonstrates the increased echogenicity of the fat in relation to the lesser echogenicity of the low-lying spinal cord. CT demonstrates the dysraphic bony defect with the low-lying spinal cord tethered by lucent fatty tissue.

Myelocystocele

A myelocystocele is a localized cystic dilatation of the distal end of a low-lying spinal cord that has herniated through a posterior bony defect into a skin-covered mass which protrudes from the plane of the back. The lumbosacral area is the most common site. The cystic mass is actually the dilated terminal end of the central canal. The herniated sac consists of distal spinal cord, CSF, and meninges (Fig 3–190).

Children with a myelocystocele present at birth with a soft, cystic skin-covered back mass in the lumbosacral area, bowel and bladder dysfunction, and sensory and motor deficits in the lower extremities. There is a high association with cloacal exstrophy and partial sacral agenesis and hydromyelia within the noninvolved parts of the spinal cord.

Radiologically, US demonstrates a low-lying spinal cord extending into the cystic back mass; the bony abnormalities are well demonstrated with CT (Fig 3–191). T1-weighted MR images allow excellent delineation of all of the soft tissue components of

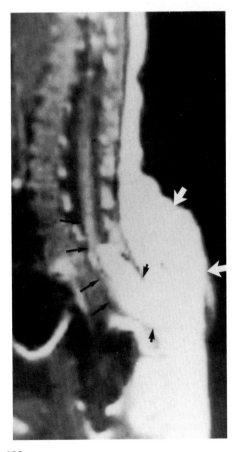

FIG 3–189.
Sagittal T1-weighted image of an MR lipomyelomeningocele. Fatty back mass *(white arrows)* extends into the spinal canal through a posterior dysraphic bony defect *(short black arrows)* tethering the spinal cord *(long black arrows).*

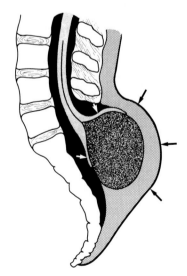

FIG 3–190.
Diagram (sagittal section) of the components of a myelocystocele showing skin-covered back mass *(black arrows)* with herniation of a cystic dilated spinal cord *(white arrows)* through a large posterior bony dysraphic defect.

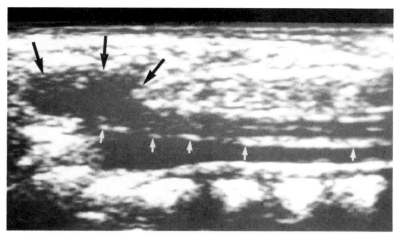

FIG 3–191.
Sagittal sonogram of the lumbosacral spine revealing myelocystocele with the spinal cord *(white arrows)* extending down and ending as a cyst *(black arrows)* in the distal sacral region.

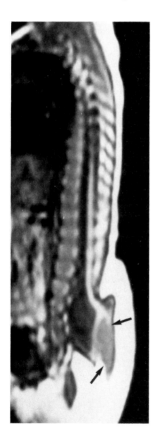

FIG 3–192.
Sagittal T1-weighted image of the lower thoracic lumbosacral spine showing a myelocystocele with cystic dilatation *(black arrows)* of the distal end of a low-lying spinal cord that has herniated through a large posterior dysraphic defect in the lumbosacral spine.

the myelocystocele, with the hypointensity of the cyst of the terminal spinal cord usually being slightly greater in signal from adjacent CSF of the thecal sac. The splaying of the distal end of the spinal cord, if present, as well as the associated hydromyelia, may be demonstrated on MRI (Fig 3–192).

Simple Posterior Meningocele

A meningocele is a herniated sac of meninges containing CSF that extends through a bony defect in the spine (Fig 3–193). The bony defect may involve the anterior aspect of the sacrum (anterior sacral me-

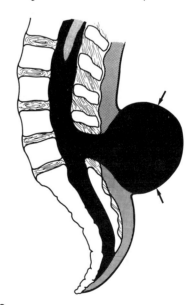

FIG 3–193.
Diagram (sagittal section) of the components of a simple posterior lumbosacral meningocele with herniation of a CSF sac *(arrows)* through a bony dysraphic defect.

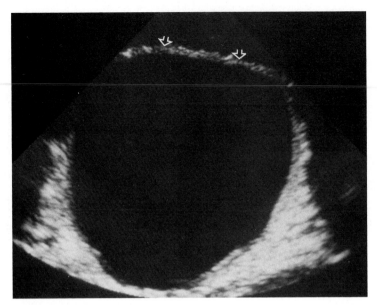

FIG 3–194.
Axial US scan of a total sonolucent simple meningocele of the lumbosacral spine (posterior wall indicated by *arrows*).

ningocele); the lateral aspect of the spine and intervertebral foramen (lateral thoracic meningocele), which is commonly seen in association with NF-I; the distal sacrum (intrasacral meningocele); and the posterior elements (the posterior meningocele). The meningocele by definition does not contain neural tissue. All of the meningoceles except the posterior meningocele are classified under occult spinal dysraphism. The posterior meningocele consists of a skin-covered mass in the lumbosacral, cervical, or thoracic areas of the back.

Radiologically, there is a posterior bony defect with herniation of a posterior CSF sac. The spinal cord with conus is in its normal position. US can easily demonstrate the cystic (sonolucent) posteriorly herniated CSF sac and the normal position of the conus (Fig 3–194). T1-weighted MR images provide good detail of the normal spinal cord and herniated CSF sac. The bony defect may be demonstrated on MR, but not as well as on CT.

OCCULT SPINAL DYSRAPHISM

Diastematomyelia

Diastematomyelia is characterized by partial or complete sagittal splitting (clefting) of the spinal cord (Fig 3–195). The clefting is usually located in the lumbar and thoracic regions. Segmental anomalies involving the vertebral bodies such as hemivertebra, butterfly vertebra, and block vertebra are usually present.

Fifty percent of patients with diastematomyelia are symptomatic. These are usually children, who have a form of diastematomyelia in which there is duplication of the dura and arachnoid at the level of the spinal cord clefting. There is always present a

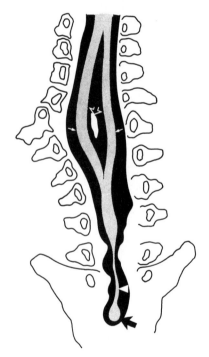

FIG 3–195.
Diagram (coronal section) of the lower thoracolumbosacral spine showing the components of diastematomyelia with splitting of the spinal cord *(small white arrows)* into halves, bony spur *(open arrow)*, thickened filum *(arrowhead)*, and distal lipoma *(black arrow)*.

cartilaginous, bony, or fibrous spur with this type of diastematomyelia and the cord is tethered. The symptoms consist of motor weakness and sensory deficits in the lower extremities, bowel and bladder dysfunction, gait disturbance, and scoliosis.

Fifty percent of patients with diastematomyelia are asymptomatic, have no spur present, and have no duplication of the arachnoid or dura. A single dura-arachnoid tube exists at the level of the clefting. The area of diastematomyelia occurs between T9 and S1 with the most common sites being the lumbar, thoracolumbar, and lower thoracic spine. The two hemicords typically reunite below the cleft, and the conus is usually low-lying.

Patients with diastematomyelia commonly manifest abnormal cutaneous stigmata on the skin of the back such as a large hairy tuft, hemangioma, nevus, and pilonidal cyst. Diastematomyelia occurs more frequently in females (85%) than in males. There is a high association with hydromyelia, lipoma of the filum terminale, intradural lipoma, and fibrous bands.

If a spur is present, the spinal cord is tethered at the level of the spur. However, if a lipoma of the filum terminale, intradural lipoma, or fibrous band is present, the spinal cord may be tethered at other levels by these lesions.

Radiologically, the diagnosis is made by demonstration of sagittal clefting of the cord. T1-weighted MR images demonstrate clefting of the cord and associated soft tissue abnormalities, but the spur (if it is

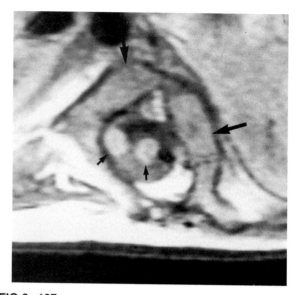

FIG 3–197.
Axial T1-weighted image of the thoracic spine showing diastematomyelia with two hemicords *(small arrows)* and abnormal segmentation of the vertebral body *(large arrows)*.

not composed of cartilage or bone marrow) and fibrous bands may be missed on MRI and is better demonstrated on CT (Figs 3–196, 3–197, and 3–198).

Dorsal Dermal Sinus

A dorsal dermal sinus consists of an epithelial tube which extends downward and inward from the skin surface of the back with extension at times into the spinal canal and distal spinal cord (Fig 3–199). The sites of the dermal sinus in decreasing order of frequency are the sacrococcygeal, lumbosacral, occipital, thoracic, and cervical levels. The sacrococcygeal dermal sinus rarely extends into the spinal canal. If the sinus is above the sacrococcygeal level, it frequently extends into and terminates in the spinal canal or onto the distal spinal cord. Fifty percent of dermal sinuses terminate as a tumor or dermoid cyst in the spinal canal or spinal cord (conus). The spinal cord is usually tethered by these cysts.

Patients with a dorsal dermoid sinus may present in childhood or early adulthood. A dimple may be present in the skin of the back or there may be associated cutaneous manifestations, such as a local area of hyperpigmentation, hairy nevus, or hemangioma. Sixty percent of these patients present with infection such as meningitis, or spinal or subcutaneous abscess. Vertebral anomalies are uncommon except for an occasional spina bifida involving one or two levels.

The simple pilonidal sinus is an epithelial-lined tube that extends from the skin surface inward. It only occurs in the sacrococcygeal region and does

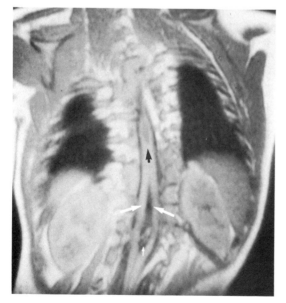

FIG 3–196.
Coronal T1-weighted image of the thoracolumbosacral spine showing diastematomyelia with two hemicords *(large white arrows)*, cartilaginous spur *(small white arrow)*, and localized hydromyelia *(black arrow)*.

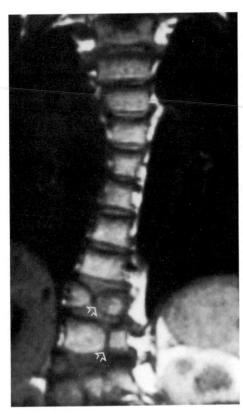

FIG 3–198.
Coronal T1-weighted image showing segmental abnormalities of the vertebrae *(arrows)* in a scoliotic, diastematomyelic thoracic spine.

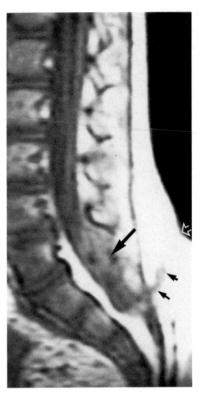

FIG 3–200.
Sagittal T1-weighted image of the lumbosacral spine showing part of the tract of a dermal sinus *(small arrows)* in the subcutaneous tissue extending from a dimple in the skin *(open arrow)* and ending in a dermoid tumor *(large arrow)* in the distal spinal canal.

not extend into the spinal canal. This is also called simple sacrococcygeal dimple.

Radiologically, MRI provides delineation of the sinus tract in the subcutaneous tissue and, if present, the dermoid cyst or tumor (Fig 3–200). The

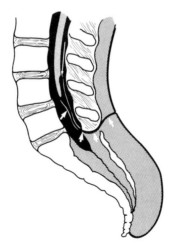

FIG 3–199.
Diagram (sagittal section) of the lumbosacral spine showing the components of a dorsal dermal sinus tract *(short arrows)* extending from the skin surface of the back to end as a small dermoid *(long arrow)* on the conus of the spinal cord.

dermoid is isointense or hypointense on the T1-weighted image and hyperintense on the T2-weighted image. US may also demonstrate the tract if it is large (Fig 3–173). The diagnosis is made by the demonstration of the dermal skin tract extending from the skin surface of the back downward through the subcutaneous fat of the back.

Tight Filum Terminale Syndrome

This syndrome is due to tethering of the spinal cord by a filum terminale which may be thickened by lipomatous or fibrous tissue (Fig 3–201). The normal location of the conus medullaris can be as low as the body of L3 in newborns and in infants up to 3 months of age. After 3 months of age, the conus should be at L1–2. The filum terminale should normally not be greater than 2 mm in diameter. The symptoms in this syndrome are due to stretching of the spinal cord with vascular insufficiency. The symptoms are orthopedic deformities such as clubfoot; atrophy of the lower extremities; difficulty in walking; shortening of one leg; and bladder dysfunction, such as enuresis.

If there is an associated vertebral anomaly, it is

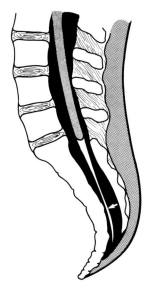

FIG 3–201.
Diagram (sagittal section) of the lumbosacral spine demonstrating the spinal cord conus tethered by a thickened fatty filum *(arrow)*.

usually only the simple spina bifida involving one or two vertebrae at the lumbosacral levels. The spinal cord may be in a normal position in half of patients, and below its normal level in the other half. The filum terminale is thickened, measuring over 2 mm in diameter, in all patients.

Radiologically, the conus is in normal position or abnormally low with an enlarged filum. T1-weighted MR images demonstrate the high signal of the enlarged filum if it is due to fatty infiltration; if the filum is thickened by fibrous tissue, it will be isointense with the spinal cord (Figs 3–202, 3–203, and 3–204).

Intradural Lipoma

Intradural lipoma consists of a localized collection of fat within the intradural space of the spinal canal connected to the spinal cord (Fig 3–205), which is tethered by the lipoma. The common locations are cervical, thoracic, and lumbosacral. The dura is commonly intact with a clear separation (tissue plane) between the intradural lipoma and the subcutaneous fat. The associated vertebral anomaly is spina bifida at one or several levels.

An intradural lipoma is more common in males than females and occurs in infancy and early childhood. The child may present with signs of paresis, paralysis, or bowel and bladder incontinence. T1-

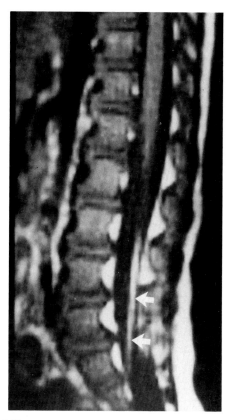

FIG 3–202.
Sagittal T1-weighted image of the lumbosacral spine demonstrating a thickened (hyperintense) fatty filum *(arrows)*.

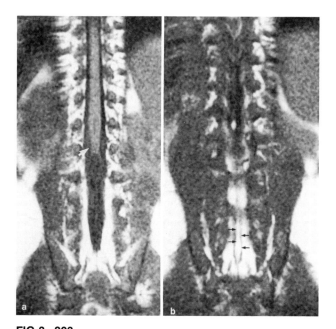

FIG 3–203.
Coronal T1-weighted image of the lower thoracic lumbosacral spine. *(a)* Image at the level of the normal conus *(white arrow)*. *(b)* Image 3 mm posterior to *(a)* demonstrating thickened (hyperintense) fatty filum *(black arrows)*.

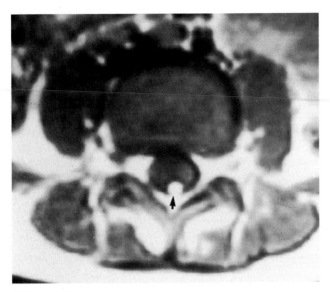

FIG 3–204.
Axial T1-weighted image of the lower lumbar spine. Note enlarged fatty filum *(arrow)*.

weighted MR images demonstrate the high signal of fat, the soft tissue plane between the subcutaneous fat and the lipoma, and the location and appearance of the tethered spinal cord (Fig 3–206). CT without intrathecal contrast demonstrates the bony defects, the lucent fatty mass (the lipoma), and the spinal cord. US demonstrates the marked increased echogenicity of the lipoma in the spinal canal.

Split Notochord Syndrome

The split notochord syndrome describes a group of anomalies which are believed to be due to abnormal splitting or deviation of the notochord with a persistent connection between the gut and dorsal skin. This persistent connection (the tract) can extend from any area of the gastrointestinal tract (most commonly the intestines) to the skin of the back (Fig 3–207). The tract can extend in any direction from the gut through the chest, posterior mediastinum, thoracic spine, or abdominal cavity, and lumbar area to the skin of the back.

If the tract becomes obliterated at any point or length along its course, a cyst, diverticulum, fistula, sinus, or fibrous band may develop. The classification of these entities depends on the location of the lesion. If they extend or are within the chest or posterior mediastinum, they are called mediastinal cysts, diverticula, fistulas, or sinuses. If they extend or are within the abdomen, they are called abdominal cysts, diverticula, fistulas, or sinuses. The nature of the gut connection determines the classification.

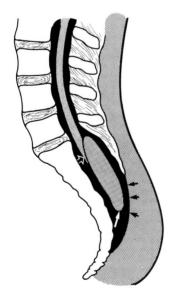

FIG 3–205.
Diagram (sagittal section) of the lumbosacral spine showing intradural lipoma *(white arrow)* tethering the spinal cord *(open arrow)* and separated from the subcutaneous fat by a tissue plane *(black arrows)*.

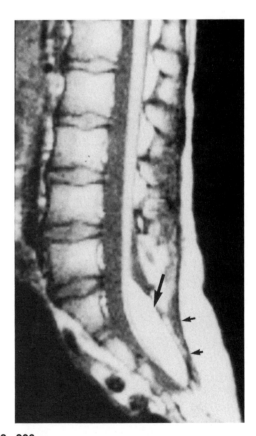

FIG 3–206.
Sagittal T1-weighted image of the lumbosacral spine. The spinal cord is low-lying and tethered by an intradural lipoma *(large arrow)* which is separated from the subcutaneous fat of the back by a tissue plane *(small arrows)*.

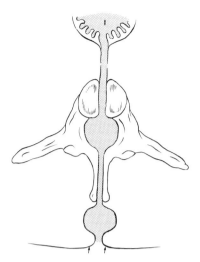

FIG 3–207.
Diagram illustrating the split notochord syndrome. The tract extends from the intestines *(I)* through a defect in the spine and spinal canal to the skin of the back *(arrows)*.

Since the most common gut connection is with the intestines, most of these lesions are called enteric cysts, diverticula, fistulas, or sinuses. The most common anomalies within the group are dorsal enteric cysts and diverticula. Other terms used for entities within the split notochord syndrome are neurenteric cyst, foregut cyst, gastroenteric cyst, and enteric duplication cyst.

The most common anomaly to occur with the split notochord syndrome is the mediastinal dorsal enteric cyst. The enteric cyst may be wholly within the chest or posterior mediastinum, or in a combined abdominal-mediastinal location through a defect in the diaphragm. It is seen in infancy and early childhood, and the presenting signs are dyspnea, cyanosis, and pulmonary infection. Males are more commonly affected (75%–80%) than females. The vertebrae are involved with anomalies such as hemivertebra and sagittal clefts within the vertebral body, laminae, and spinous process. The ribs at the level of the mediastinal dorsal enteric cyst may be fused or absent. A component of the cyst may extend into the spinal canal.

Segmentation anomalies and clefts involve the associated vertebrae. The spinal cord may be involved with a fistula or sinus. Radiologically, segmentation anomalies of the vertebrae with a cyst in the spinal canal are best demonstrated on T1-weighted MR images (Fig 3–208).

Caudal Regression Syndrome

Caudal regression syndrome refers to a spectrum of findings comprising absence of the lower portion of

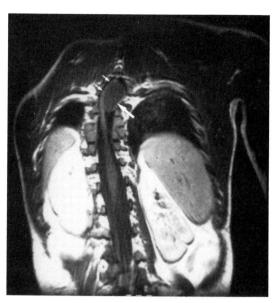

FIG 3–208.
Coronal T1-weighted image of the thoracic–upper lumbar spine showing a neurenteric cyst *(large arrow)* and compression of adjacent spinal cord *(small arrows)* within the thoracic spinal canal.

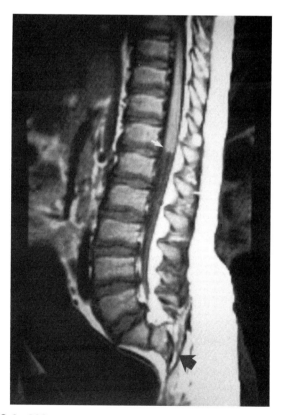

FIG 3–209.
Sagittal T1-weighted image of the lower thoracic–lumbosacral spine showing regression caudad with absence of the distal sacrum and coccyx of the bony spine *(black arrow)* and high-lying (T12) wedged-shaped conus *(white arrow)*.

the caudal spine; urologic abnormalities such as renal aplasia or dysplasia and neurogenic bladder; malformed external genitalia; anal atresia; and sirenomelia (fusion of the lower extremities).

The main findings involving the bony spine and spinal cord are absence of the lower end of the bony spine and of the spinal canal below T9. Failure of the coccyx to form, without other parts of the bony spine being involved, is an incidental finding and patients are asymptomatic. The distal end of the spinal cord may be abnormal with the conus having a bulbous or wedge-shaped appearance instead of the normal conical shape, and the conus may be abnormal in location (anywhere from the level of the beginning of the absence to as high as T8 or T9).

Children with caudal regression syndrome present with a combination of urologic, orthopedic, and neurologic symptoms. The syndrome is more common in males than in females (2.5:1).

The radiologic diagnosis and evaluation is best performed with plain radiographs of the spine and CT to evaluate the bony absence. T1-weighted MR images will provide detail of the abnormal conus and the absence of the distal spine (Fig 3–209).

Hydromyelia

Hydromyelia is abnormal dilatation of the central canal. It may be focal, localized, multiple, or diffuse. It may occur as an isolated anomaly, but is usually seen in association with other dysraphic states such as myelomeningocele, diastematomyelia, and the Chiari I and II malformations (see Fig 3–185).

REFERENCES

Spinal Dysraphism
Anderson FM: Occult spinal dysraphism: Diagnosis and management. *J Pediatr* 1968; 73:163–177.

Barkovich AJ, Raghavan N, Chuang S, et al: The wedge-shaped cord terminus: A radiographic sign of caudal regression. *AJNR* 1989; 10:1223–1231.

Bentley JFR, Smith JR: Developmental posterior enteric remnants and spinal malformations: The split notochord syndrome. *Arch Dis Child* 1960; 35:76–86.

Boldrey EB, Elvidge AR: Dermoid cysts of the vertebral canal. *Ann Surg* 1939; 220:273–284.

Duhamel B: From the mermaid to anal imperforation: The syndrome of caudal regression. *Arch Dis Child* 1961; 36:152–155.

Fitz CF: Diagnostic imaging in children with spinal disorder. *Pediatr Clin North Am* 1985; 32:1537–1558.

Flannigan-Sprague BD, Modic MT: The pediatric spine: Normal anatomy and spinal dysraphism, in Modic MT, Masaryk TJ, Ross JS (eds): *Magnetic Resonance Imaging of the Spine.* St Louis, Mosby–Year Book, 1989, pp 240–256.

Gammal TE, Mark EK, Brooks BS: MR imaging of Chiari II malformation. *AJNR* 1987; 8:1037–1044.

Garceau GJ: The filum terminale syndrome (the cord-traction syndrome). *J Bone Joint Surg [Am]* 1953; 35:711–716.

Hardwood-Nash DC, Fitz CR: *Neuroradiology in Infants and Children.* St Louis, Mosby–Year Book, 1976.

Kangarloo H, Gold RH, Diament MR, et al: High resolution spinal sonography in infants. *Am J Roentgenol* 1984; 142:1243–1247.

Karrer FM, Flannery AM, Nelson MD Jr, et al: Anorectal malformations: Evaluation of associated spinal dysraphic syndromes. *J Pediatr Surg* 1988; 23:45–48.

Lemire RJ, Loeser JD, Leech RW, et al: *Normal and Abnormal Development of the Human Nervous System.* Hagerstown, Md, Harper & Row, 1975, pp 54–83.

Miller JH, Reid BS, Kemberling CR: Ultrasound: Utilization of ultrasound in the evaluation of spinal dysraphism in children. *Radiology* 1982; 143:737–740.

Moore KL: *The Developing Human.* Philadelphia, WB Saunders, 1988.

Naidich TP, Harwood-Nash DC, McLone DG: Radiology of spinal dysraphism. *Clin Neurosurg* 1983; 30:341–365.

Naidich TP, McLone DG: Congenital pathology of the spine and spinal cord, in Taveras JM, Ferrucci JT (eds): *Radiology.* Philadelphia, JB Lippincott, 1986, pp 1–23.

Naidich TP, McLone DG, Harwood-Nash DC: Spinal dysraphism, in Newton TH, Potts DG (eds): *Computed Tomography of the Spine and Spinal Cord.* San Anselmo, Calif, Clavadel Press, 1983, pp 299–353.

SECTION *11*

Spinal Cord Injuries

Spinal cord injuries in children may occur independently or in combination with head trauma. Common causes of spinal cord injury in children are motor vehicular accidents, falls, firearms or knives, and sporting and recreational activities such as football and diving. Spinal cord injuries can result from penetrating direct wounds from guns or knives or may be secondary to indirect trauma from hyperextension and hyperflexion of the spine. Hyperextension and hyperflexion produce injuries of the bony spine and spinal cord. Among the bony injuries are fractures and ligamentous tears with secondary subluxations and dislocations of the spine and compression of the spinal cord.

Spinal cord injury, with or without bony and ligamentous derangement, produces intramedullary changes consisting of (1) spinal concussion, which is a reversible condition with normal radiologic studies; (2) spinal cord contusion, which may be secondary to shearing injuries of the cord with rupture of the small intramedullary vessels with resultant petechiae and edema, that may progress to larger areas of hemorrhage within the cord and vascular compromise; and (3) axonal injury without hemorrhage, with swelling and edema of the spinal cord. Both types of spinal cord injury—the contusion and axonal injuries—may produce necrosis with vacuolization and, depending on the degree and severity of the injury, later development of chronic changes of gliosis, demyelination, and atrophy with or without myelomalacia.

The best radiologic modalities to evaluate fracture, subluxations, and dislocations of the bony spine are plain films of the spine and CT. The best modalities to evaluate spinal cord injury are CT and MRI. There are technical and physical restrictions with MRI in evaluating the critically ill, traumatized patient. These factors were discussed in Section 4.

On CT, in the early stages of spinal cord injury, an enlarged hypodense (if edema is present) or hyperdense (if hemorrhage is present) cord is demonstrated. On MRI, an enlarged isointense, hypointense, or hyperintense (edema or hemorrhage, or both) area may be present (Figs 3–210 and 3–211). There may be some mild enhancement with Gd, de-

pending on the damage to the blood–spinal cord barrier. The chronic stage of injury on CT may demonstrate a small atrophic cord with or without a traumatic cyst (syringomyelia) or an area of hypodensity (myelomalacia). On MRI, the chronic changes may demonstrate a thin cord with or without an area of hypointensity on T1-weighted (myelomalacia-gliosis or syringomyelia) and hyperintensity of these areas on T2-weighted images (Fig 3–212). Gliosis and myelomalacia do not show enhancement with Gd.

Vascular injury to the spinal cord may compress the anterior spinal artery with resultant spinal cord infarction or vascular compromise secondary to tear-

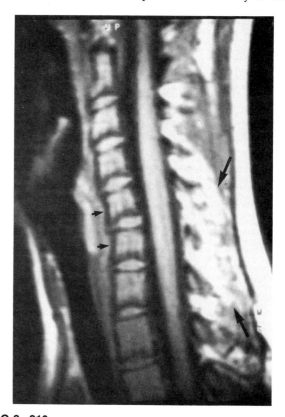

FIG 3–210.
Sagittal T1-weighted image of the spine showing cervical flexion-extension injury of the neck with subluxated locked facets at C5–6 on plain films. There is slight kyphosis at C5–6 *(small arrows)* and subacute hemorrhage (hyperintensity) of the paraspinal soft tissue *(large arrows).*

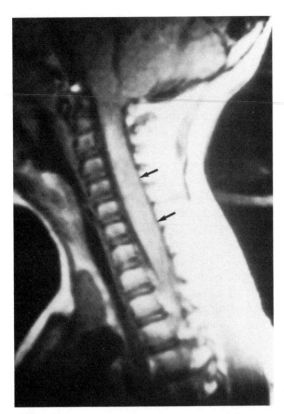

FIG 3–211.
Sagittal T1-weighted image of the cervical spine showing enlargement of the cervical cord secondary to subacute hemorrhage (hyperintensity is indicated by *arrows*).

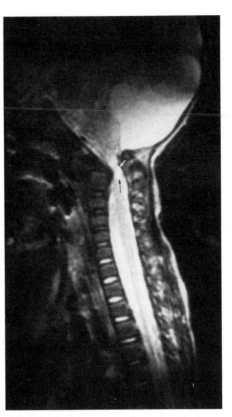

FIG 3–212.
Sagittal T2-weighted image of the cervical spine showing posterior subluxation of C2 with compression of the upper cervical cord and a myelomalacic area of hyperintensity *(arrows).*

ing of small intramedullary vessels. If the trauma is severe, there may be total disruption of the spinal cord (Fig 3–213). This can commonly be seen in the newborn at the time of birth if there was either a difficult birth with the use of forceps or a breech presentation. Depending on the type of injury and the location of the damage, the symptoms in these children may consist of motor or sensory deficits with variable degrees of quadriplegia, paraplegia, or paresis.

Spinal cord injury may be secondary to extramedullary compromise due to a traumatic disc herniation with compression or to extracerebral hematomas (epidural or subdural). Spinal epidural hematomas are more common than subdural hematomas and are believed to be secondary to the large number of vessels within the epidural compartment. The CT findings are an extradural mass compressing the spinal cord or nerve roots; the most common location is thoracic with increased density on the unenhanced CT scan. Depending on the age of the hemorrhage, the MRI appearance on T1-weighted images is hypointense, isointense, or hyperintense

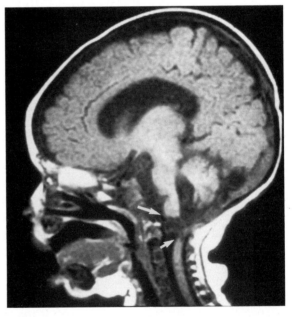

FIG 3–213.
Sagittal T1-weighted image showing traumatic complete transection of the brainstem *(long arrow)* from the cervical cord *(short arrow).*

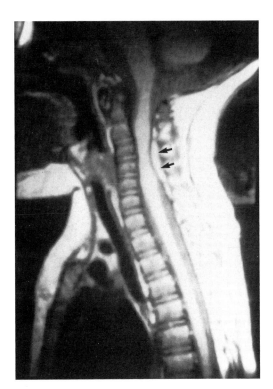

FIG 3–214.
Sagittal T1-weighted image of the MR cervical spine showing hyperintense epidural hematoma *(arrows)* compressing the spinal cord.

(Fig 3–214). Hemorrhage within the spine, either intramedullary or extramedullary, has the same signal characteristics as those described for hemorrhage within the brain. An additional injury that may occur with spine trauma is nerve root avulsion with development of a pseudo–nerve root sheath.

REFERENCES

Spinal Cord Injuries
Byers RK: Spinal cord injuries during birth. *Dev Med Child Neurol* 1975; 17:103–110.

Enzmann DR, DeLa Paz RL: Trauma, in Enzmann DR, DeLa Paz RL, Rubin JB (eds): *Magnetic Resonance of the Spine.* St Louis, Mosby–Year Book, 1990, pp 237–259.

Hackney DB, Asato D, Joseph PM, et al: Hemorrhage and edema in acute spinal cord compression: Demonstration by MR imaging. *Radiology* 1986, 161:387–390.

Hadley MN, Sabramski JM, Browner CM, et al: Pediatric spinal trauma: Review of 122 cases of spinal cord and vertebral column injuries. *J Neurosurg* 1988; 68:18–25.

Jellinger K: Neuropathology of spinal cord injuries, in Vinken PJ, Brayn GW (eds): *Handbook of Clinical Neurology.* New York, John Wiley & Sons, 1976, pp 43–121.

Kulkarni MV, McArdle CB, Kopanicky D, et al: Acute spinal cord injury MR imaging at 1-5T. *Radiology* 1987, 164:837–843.

Lanska MJ, Roessmann U, Wiznitzer M: Magnetic resonance imaging in cervical cord birth injury. *Pediatrics* 1990; 85:760–764.

Quences RM, Sheldon JJ, Post MJD, et al: MRI of the chronically injured cervical spinal cord. *Am J Roentgenol* 1986; 147:125–132.

Rothfus WE, Chedid MK, Deeb ZL, et al: MR imaging in the diagnosis of spontaneous spinal epidural hematomas. *J Comput Assist Tomogr* 1987; 11:851–854.

SECTION 12

Infections

Infection of the spinal cord is rare. It can occur as a result of hematogenous spread or direct penetrating injury. The common agents are viral, bacterial, and granulomatous. MRI is the best modality to evaluate the spinal cord for infection. The cord is isointense or hypointense on T1-weighted images and hyperintense on T2-weighted images. MRI with Gd may show enhancement (Fig 3–215). The cord may be enlarged during the early stages of the infection because of edema. Infection of the spinal cord may also produce a hemorrhagic component. The MRI appearance depends on the stage of the hemorrhage. During the chronic or end stage of the infection, the cord may be small with or without areas of myelomalacia.

Epidural abscesses, either from hematogenous

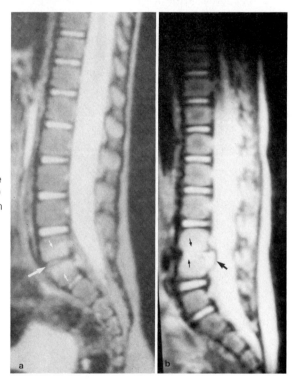

FIG 3–215.
Sagittal MR image of the spinal cord of a patient with a T1-weighted viral infection. *(a)* image shows hyperintense area *(arrow)* within the distal cervical cord. *(b)* Post-Gd T1-weighted image demonstrates diffuse enhancement of the distal cervical and upper thoracic spinal cord *(arrows).*

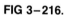

FIG 3–216.
Sagittal T2-weighted image of the MR lower thoracic–lumbosacral spine of a patient with diskitis. *(a)* Decreased signal and narrowing of the disk *(large arrow)* at the L5–S1 level with hyperintensity of bone marrow *(small arrows)* in adjacent vertebral bodies. *(b)* Posteriorly herniated disk *(large arrow)* with loss of disk space and hyperintensity *(small arrows)* of bone marrow in adjacent vertebral bodies.

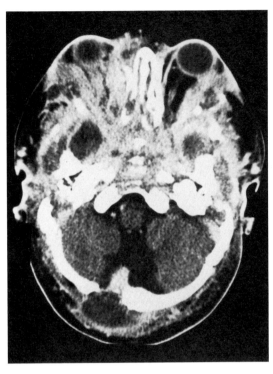

FIG 3–217.
Axial contrast-enhanced CT scan of the base of the skull and orbits of a patient with Langerhans' cell histiocytosis showing diffuse infiltration of Langerhans cells in the base of skull and orbits, with enhancement and bone destruction.

spread or from diskitis, are more commonly seen. On CT and MR an extradural mass is seen. Depending on its location and size, there may be compression of either the spinal cord or the nerve roots. If the infection is secondary to diskitis, the mass is at the level of the disk space. It is not unusual to see isolated diskitis in children. Involvement of the adjacent vertebral bodies can commonly be seen in children with diskitis. On T1-weighted images the epidural abscess demonstrates hypointensity, the disc space is usually narrow, and the disk, if there is diskitis, demonstrates greater hypointensity than the adjacent disk. On T2, increased signal is noted involving the disk and the epidural abscess (Fig 3–216).

HISTIOCYTOSIS

Histiocytosis is a nonmalignant proliferation of lipid-containing reticulum cells (Langerhans) of the reticuloendothelial system. It is classified into three clinical types. *Letterer-Siwe disease* is seen in infants and is characterized by skin petechiae, anemia, hepatosplenomegaly, lytic osseous lesions, and lymphadenopathy. *Hand-Schüller*-Christian disease is seen in young children and adults and is associated with a triad of findings: osteolytic bone defects, diabetes insipidus, and exophthalmos. This triad is only seen in 10% of patients; the most common finding is osteolytic skull lesions (50%). Cutaneous and visceral lesions are also seen, but less frequently. *Eosinophilic*

granuloma is the most benign form of this disease. It is seen in children (usually 3–10 years of age) and is characterized mainly by osteolytic bone involvement.

Radiologic involvement of the brain and spine consists of lytic lesions involving the calvarial vault, base of skull, orbits, and spine, best seen on CT and plain films. There may be a soft tissue component (histiocytoma) associated with lytic lesions at the

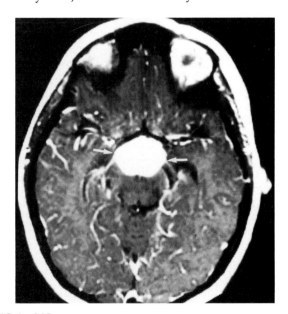

FIG 3–218.
Post-Gd axial T1-weighted image shows enhancement of suprasellar mass (*arrows* point to histiocytoma).

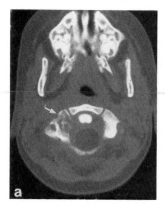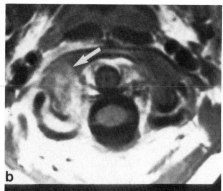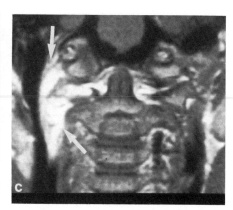

FIG 3–219.
Langerhans cell histiocytosis of the cervical spine. *(a)* Axial unenhanced CT scan shows lytic destruction of the right lateral mass *(arrow)* of C1. *(b)* Post-Gd axial T1-weighted image shows enhancement of the mass *(arrow)* and bony destruction of the right lateral mass of C1. *(c)* Post-Gd coronal T1-weighted image illustrates enhancing histiocytoma *(arrows)*.

base of the skull (temporal bone), orbits (infiltration of the ocular muscle cone), and spine (vertebral body or neural arch with an extradural component). A localized soft tissue mass (histiocytoma) can be seen without bony lesions in the suprasellar-hypothalamic region of the brain.

CT, with and without intravenous iodinated contrast, is the best modality for evaluating the calvarial, facial, and spinal lytic lesions and their associated soft tissue components (which show enhancement with contrast) (Fig 3–217). Although MRI is not as sensitive as CT in evaluating the bony lesions, if the bony destruction is large then it will be hypointense on T1-weighted and hyperintense on T2-weighted images. The soft tissue component will show enhancement with Gd (Fig 3–218 and 3–219).

REFERENCES

Infections

Enzmann DR: Infection and inflammation, in Enzmann DR, DeLa Paz RL, Rubin JB (eds): *Magnetic Resonance of the Spine.* St Louis, Mosby–Year Book, 1990, pp 260–300.

Rocco HD, Eyring EJ: Intervertebral disk infections in children. *Am J Dis Child* 1972; 123:448–451.

Smith RF, Taylor TKF: Inflammatory lesions of intervertebral discs in children. *J Bone Joint Surg [Am]* 1967; 49:1508–1520.

Wenger DR, Bobechko WP, Gilday DL: The spectrum of intervertebral disc-space infection in children. *J Bone Joint Surg [Am]* 1978; 60:100–108.

Histiocytosis

Cohen MD, Edwards MK: *Magnetic Resonance Imaging of Children.* Philadelphia, BC Decker, 1990.

Diebler C, Dulac O: *Pediatric Neurology and Neuroradiology.* New York, Springer-Verlag, 1987.

Edeiken J, Dalinka M, Karasick D: *Disease of Bone,* ed 4. Baltimore, Williams & Wilkins, 1990, Chap 18.

Epstein BS: *The Spine. A Radiological Text and Atlas,* ed 4. Philadelphia, Lea & Febiger, 1976.

Huk WJ, Gademann G, Friedmann G: *MRI of Central Nervous System Diseases.* New York, Springer-Verlag, 1990.

Stern MB, Cassidy R, Mirra J: Eosenophilic granuloma of the proximal tibial epiphysis. *Clin Orthop* 1976; 118:153–156.

SECTION 13

Spinal Tumors

Spinal cord tumors are 20 times less frequent than brain tumors in the pediatric population. They occur with about equal frequency in all three intraspinal compartments (30% intramedullary, 30% intradural-extramedullary, and 30% extradural). The onset of symptoms in children with an intraspinal tumor is usually acute in contrast to the insidious onset of symptoms in children with spinal dysraphism. Children with intraspinal tumors may present acutely with severe paresis or paralysis or, more commonly, with symptoms which persist over 3 to 6 months such as pain, gait disturbance, developing scoliosis (or kyphosis or torticollis), motor weakness, or bowel and bladder dysfunction. The radiologic modalities which are important in diagnosing and evaluating children with intraspinal tumors are CT, MRI, and water-soluble myelography with follow through CT. The modality of choice is MRI with T1-weighted, T2-weighted, and post-Gd, and T1-weighted images. CT with intravenous contrast will better define the bony changes associated with these tumors as well as the relationship to the spinal cord. Water-soluble myelography with CT is used as an adjunct to better define very small lesions within the spinal canal, such as drop metastases, from primary brain tumors.

The most common childhood intraspinal tumors are as follows: (1) in the intramedullary compartments, astrocytomas and ependymomas predominate; (2) of the intradural extramedullary tumors, the most common types are drop metastases (leptomeningeal spread) from primary brain tumors and neurofibromas; and (3) the most common extramedullary tumors are direct extension from neuroblastomas and Wilms tumors, histiocytosis, lymphoma, and sacrococcygeal teratomas.

INTRAMEDULLARY LESIONS

Astrocytoma

From 50% to 60% of intramedullary spinal cord lesions are astrocytomas. They usually present in children around 10 years of age with an equal predilection for males and females. They may be seen in neonates and infants. They arise from astrocytes and range from benign to malignant lesions, grades I through IV. The relatively benign lesions are the grade I astrocytomas, spongioblastomas, and pilocytic astrocytomas. The more malignant neoplastic lesions are the high-grade astrocytomas: grade IV astrocytomas and glioblastoma multiforme. The most common site is the cervical cord followed by the thoracic and lumbar regions. However, astrocytomas can involve the whole spinal cord and frequently astrocytomas in the cervical area extend to the cervicomedullary junction and into the medulla oblongata of the brainstem. Astrocytomas may be totally cystic; mixed with a combination of cystic and solid components; totally solid; or consist of solid, cystic, and necrotic components. The tumor may be small or large. When it is malignant, it may have neoplastic vascularity and simulate a large vascular malformation of the cord. Malignant neoplasms with neoplastic vascularity may bleed. Complete involvement of the spinal cord by a malignant astrocytoma is more commonly seen during the first year of life. Astrocytomas expand the involved portion of the spinal cord. There may be resultant expansion of the spinal canal and erosion of the bony spine.

The bony erosion and expansion of the spine are better seen on plain films and unenhanced CT scans. The solid portion of this tumor may show enhancement on CT after intravenous administration of iodinated contrast material. The modality of choice in evaluating spinal cord astrocytomas is MRI. The lesion will show enlargement of the involved portion of the cord with isointensity or hypointensity on T1-weighted images. If a cyst is present, it will be hypointense to, or isointense with, the spinal cord on T1-weighted images. On T2-weighted images, there is increased signal (hyperintensity) of the solid, cystic, or necrotic components of the tumor (Figs 3–220 and 3–221). After administration of intravenous Gd, the solid portions of the tumor may show enhancement. The enhancement may be homogeneous or inhomogeneous. Benign and relatively low-grade astrocytomas may not show enhancement after administration of Gd. However, these tumors will almost always demonstrate varying degrees of increased signal on

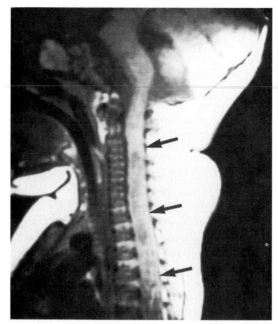

FIG 3–220.
Sagittal T1-weighted image of the cervical spine shows glioblastoma multiforme *(arrows)* involving the entire cord with areas of isointensity and hypointensity.

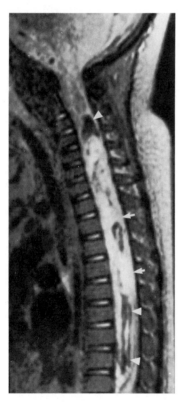

FIG 3–221.
Sagittal T2-weighted image of the cervical spine. Glioblastoma multiforme involves the entire cord with areas of mixed signal intensities representing solid tumor hyperintensity *(arrows)* and malignant vascularity *(arrowheads).*

T2-weighted images. Prominent neovascularity frequently will demonstrate serpentine enhancement after administration of Gd. If the tumor has bled, the signal intensity of the hematoma will depend upon its age.

Spinal Cord Ependymomas

Ependymomas account for 30% of intramedullary spinal cord tumors. They usually present in a slightly older age group than astrocytomas, usually at 13 or 14 years of age, with a slight predilection for girls. The most common location is the distal aspect of the spinal cord, conus, and filum terminale. Ependymomas arise from ependymal cell rests within the spinal cord parenchyma. They may expand the distal aspect of the spinal cord in a fusiform or eccentric shape with or without an exophytic component. They are usually solid and rarely have calcification, as opposed to the ependymomas of the posterior fossa, which commonly are calcified. The ependymomas that involve the filum terminale may bleed and produce subarachnoid hemorrhage.

MRI is the best imaging modality to evaluate this tumor. There is enlargement of the involved portion of the spinal cord, which is hypointense or isointense on T1-weighted and hyperintense on T2-weighted images. There is usually enhancement after administration of intravenous Gd (Figs 3–222 and 3–223). Spinal ependymomas commonly metastasize via CSF to other portions of the spine and brain. Although MR with Gd is excellent at demonstrating the small drop metastases from CSF spread of spinal cord ependymomas, if the lesions are very small, water-soluble myelography with follow-through CT may be necessary to demonstrate them. On myelography, solitary or multiple small filling defects are demonstrated, usually within the lower lumbosacral area of the spinal canal. The lesions may be seen in the thoracic and cervical regions as well as the cisterns of the brain. CT with intrathecal contrast material will demonstrate these small lesions coating the nerve roots, the surface of the spinal cord, and scattered throughout the CSF of the thecal sac.

INTRADURAL EXTRAMEDULLARY SPINAL TUMORS

Leptomeningeal Metastases

Metastatic spread to the spinal canal most commonly occurs secondary to drop metastases from

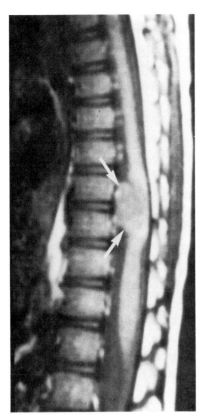

FIG 3–222.
Sagittal T1-weighted image of the lower thoracic–upper lumbar spine. Ependymoma of the distal spinal cord with an exophytic component (arrows) is illustrated.

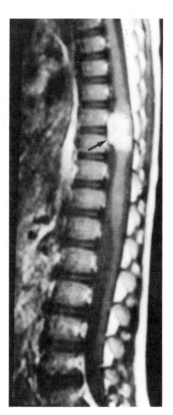

FIG 3–223.
Post-Gd sagittal T1-weighted image of the lower thoracic–upper lumbar spine shows enhancement of an ependymoma (arrow) of the distal cord.

primary brain tumors. The most common tumors of the posterior fossa that spread via the CSF are medulloblastomas, ependymomas, high-grade astrocytomas (glioblastoma multiforme), and PNETs. The common supratentorial brain tumors that spread via the CSF are pineoblastomas, high-grade astrocytomas, choroid plexus carcinomas, and PNETs. The type of primary brain tumor correlates with the age of the child at the time of presentation of intraspinal metastases. Leptomeningeal metastases usually develop 3 to 5 years after diagnosis of the primary brain tumor. However, metastases from posterior fossa ependymomas usually occur earlier, within 3 to 15 months after diagnosis of the primary tumor. Certain tumors, most notably choroid plexus carcinomas and posterior fossa ependymomas, may have already metastasized at the time of diagnosis. The most common tumor to metastasize via the CSF is the medulloblastoma.

CSF metastases may be solitary, multiple, or too numerous to count. They may range in size from a few millimeters to 1 to 2 cm. They may produce complete blockage of the flow of CSF. The most

common site is the distal aspect of the thecal sac in the lumbosacral area. They may involve coating of the conus of the spinal cord as well as the nerve roots of the cauda equina. The next most common site is the thoracic spine, followed by the cervical spine. When lesions occur in the thoracic area, they are usually dorsal. These metastatic lesions are round or oval.

The radiologic modality of choice to evaluate metastatic spread is MR. Metastatic lesions demonstrate isointensity or hypointensity on T1-weighted images and slight hyperintensity on T2-weighted images. The majority almost always show enhancement after administration of intravenous Gd. The most common MR appearance is hyperintense, enhanced, multiple small nodules scattered throughout the intradural aspect of the thecal sac, usually in the lumbosacral area (Fig 3–224). Diffuse leptomeningeal enhancement of the surface of the spinal cord occurs in 30% to 40% of patients with metastatic nodules (Fig 3–225). Although 95% of drop metastases can be diagnosed with Gd-enhanced MR, if CSF study is positive for metastatic disease and MR with

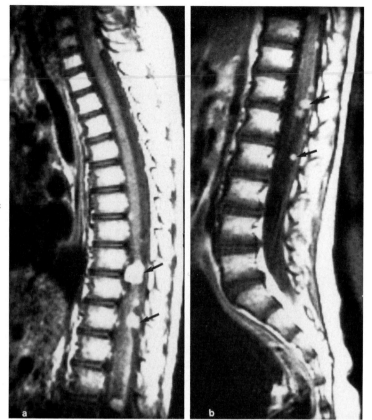

FIG 3–224.
Post-Gd sagittal T1-weighted images showing *(a)* thoracic and *(b)* lumbosacral CSF seeding of metastatic nodules *(arrows)* from a primary choroid plexus carcinoma.

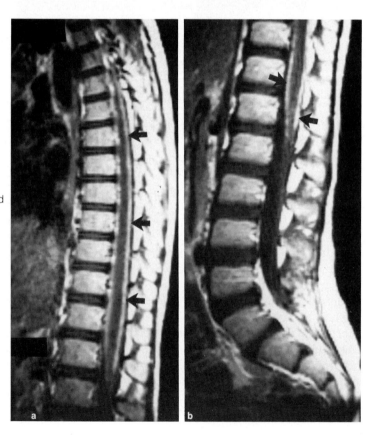

FIG 3–225.
Post-Gd sagittal T1-weighted image of *(a)* the thoracic and *(b)* the lumbosacral spine demonstrating leptomeningeal enhancement of the surface of the spinal cord *(arrows)* secondary to CSF seeding from medulloblastoma of the brain.

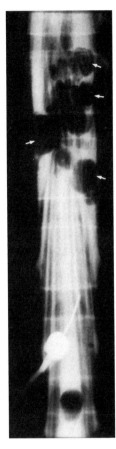

FIG 3–226.
AP myelogram with water-soluble contrast of the lumbar spine shows CSF metastatic seeding with multiple nodular filling defects (arrows).

Gd is negative, then water-soluble myelography with CT should be performed. On myelography, multiple small nodular filling defects are demonstrated. A complete block to the flow of contrast material is rare but may be seen (Fig 3–226). On follow-through CT, small round nodules may be demonstrated with filling of the subarachnoid space.

Neurofibroma

The majority of neurofibromas are intradural-extramedullary, although a small percentage may be totally extradural. Neurofibromas are benign tumors that arise from Schwann cells. The lesions may be single, multiple, or diffuse. Fifty percent of patients with NF have neurofibromas involving the spine. The most common site is the cervical area, although they may be scattered diffusely through the thoracic and lumbar area as well. There is also a higher incidence of an associated spinal cord ependymoma in patients with NF-2. Neurofibromas are different from the other Schwann cell and nerve sheath tumors, which are variously called neurinoma, neurilemoma, and schwannoma. Neurofibromas are composed of a proliferation of Schwann cells with a large amount of mucoid material containing mucopolysaccharides. Although 50% of patients that have neurofibromas of the spine also have NF, which is inherited as an autosomal dominant trait, 50% occur sporadically. Neurofibromas may occur in early childhood but they commonly present in later childhood and during the teen-age years. Malignant degeneration of these neurofibromas is very uncommon; only 1% to 2% degenerate into a neurofibrosarcoma. Additional spinal abnormalities that are seen in patients with neurofibromatosis consist of scoliosis or kyphoscoliosis, widening of the neuroforamina, dural ectasia, posterior scalloping of the bodies of the vertebrae, and lateral thoracic meningoceles.

The best imaging modality is MRI. Neurofibromas are situated at the level of the nerve root. There is widening of the intravertebral foramina, which is better appreciated on CT and plain radiographs than on MRI. Neurofibromas can be isointense with, or hypo- or hyperintense to the spinal cord on T1-weighted images. On T2-weighted images and GEA, they are hyperintense. These lesions show enhancement after administration of Gd (Fig 3–227). The enhancement may be homogeneous or inhomogeneous. The lesions may be single, multiple, or diffuse. Diffuse neurofibromas may spread symmetrically and bilaterally down the spine. They may involve the nerve roots with extension into the spinal canal and outside the intervertebral foramina to the level of the spinal nerves, producing the so-called dumbbell neurofibroma (Fig 3–228). Large plexiform neurofibromas may extend along the paraspinal regions, commonly in the cervical and thoracic area. Neurofibromas may extend to involve the spinal nerves of the pelvic, abdominal, thoracic, and cervical regions of the body. Neurofibrosarcomas are difficult to differentiate from benign neurofibromas. They are usually larger, demonstrate greater bone destruction, have areas of necrosis, and show inhomogeneous enhancement with Gd (Figs 3–229 and 3–230).

Meningioma

Intraspinal meningiomas are rare. When they do occur, the common locations are intradural, extramedullary, and extradural. They have the same MRI characteristics as neurofibromas and at times are difficult to differentiate from them (Fig 3–231). When seen in children they are usually multiple.

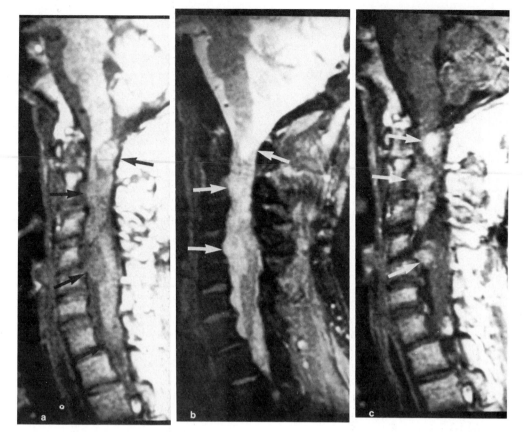

FIG 3–227.
Sagittal images of the cervical spine showing multiple neurofibromas. *(a)* On T1-weighted image, neurofibromas are isointense and hypointense *(arrows)*. *(b)* On T2-weighted gradient echo acces-sion (GEA) neurofibromas are hyperintense *(arrows)*. *(c)* On post-Gd T1-weighted image, neurofibromas are enhanced *(arrows)*.

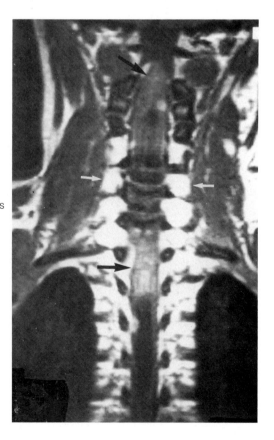

FIG 3–228.
Post-Gd coronal T1-weighted image of the cervical spine of a neurofibromatosis type 2 patient showing enhancement of multiple neurofibromas *(white arrows)* involving the cervical nerve roots. Note enhancement of ependymoma in the cervical cord *(black arrows)*.

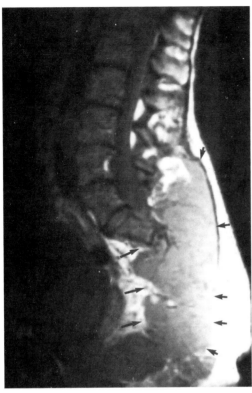

FIG 3–229.
Sagittal T1-weighted image of the lumbosacral spine showing neurofibrosarcoma *(arrows)* of the sacrococcygeal spine with bony destruction.

Intradural Tumors Associated With Spinal Dysraphism

Dermoids and lipomas are benign intradural tumors that are commonly associated with spinal dysraphism. These tumors were discussed in Section 10.

EXTRAMEDULLARY INTRASPINAL TUMORS

Neuroblastoma, Ganglioneuroblastoma, and Ganglioneuroma

Neuroblastomas are one of the common neoplasms of childhood. They present in early childhood, in children 5 years and younger, with 50% occurring in children 2 years and younger. Neuroblastomas originate from primitive neural crest cells called neuroblasts. Neuroblasts are found not only within the CNS but also within the adrenal medulla and the paraspinal sympathetic chain. Neuroblastomas commonly occur within the chest as a posterior mediastinal mass or within the retroperitoneum of the abdomen. They may metastasize to bone, liver, lymph node, and brain. Neuroblastomas are classified under the category of PNET when they involve the CNS. The most common spread of neuroblastoma to

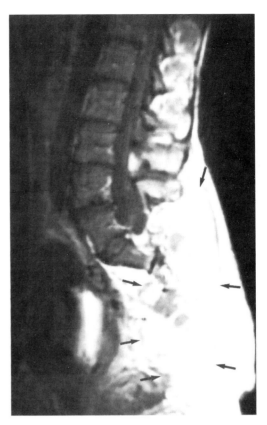

FIG 3–230.
Post-Gd sagittal T1-weighted image of the lumbosacral spine showing enhancement of the large neurofibrosarcoma *(arrows).*

the spine is either by bony metastasis with extradural extension or as an infiltrating mass along the paraspinal sympathetic chain through the neuroforamina. There may be associated bony destruction or enlargement of the neuroforamina. The lesions may infiltrate along the dura and produce spinal cord compression. When the tumor is large, it may have areas of hemorrhage and necrosis. The best diagnostic radiologic modality is MRI with Gd. Bony involvement is better evaluated with plain films and CT. On MRI, the neuroblastoma presents as a paraspinal mass in either the thoracic or lumbar area with extension into the spinal canal. The mass is isointense with, or hypointense to, the spinal cord. There may be areas of necrosis with inhomogeneity. On T2-weighted images, the lesion may demonstrate some hypointensity or hyperintensity (Fig 3–232). There may be areas of hypointensity secondary to calcification, although this is rare. After administration of Gd, the lesion shows homogeneous or inhomogeneous enhancement. This lesion also shows enhancement after administration of intravenous contrast material on CT.

A ganglioneuroblastoma is a less malignant form of neuroblastoma. It contains areas of neuroblas-

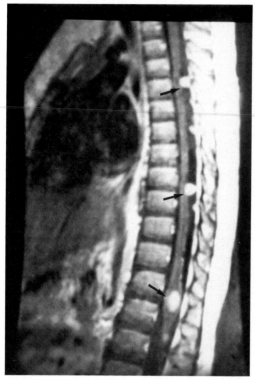

FIG 3–231.
Post-Gd sagittal T1-weighted image of the thoracic spine showing enhancement of meningiomas *(arrows).*

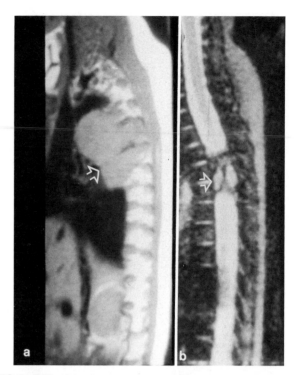

FIG 3–232.
Sagittal MR of the thoracic spine. *(a)* T1-weighted image and *(b)* T2-weighted GEA show isointense chest mass (neuroblastoma, indicated by *arrow*) extending into the thoracic spine *(arrow).*

toma as well as mature areas of ganglion cells (Fig 3–233). A ganglioneuroma is a benign lesion composed of a mixture of mature ganglion cells.

Sacrococcygeal Teratomas

Sacrococcygeal teratomas are neoplasms composed of all three germ layers that arise from multipotential cells of Hensen's node. Some of these multipotential cells of Hensen's node come to lie within the coccyx and give rise to the sacrococcygeal teratoma of childhood. This lesion may present with a predominantly external or internal component. The external sacrococcygeal teratoma presents as a mass at the level of the buttocks and extends below the gluteal fold. The location of the back mass will help to differentiate spinal dysraphic conditions with a back mass from a sacrococcygeal teratoma; spinal dysraphic lesions are typically above the gluteal fold whereas the mass of the sacrococcygeal teratoma is commonly below the gluteal fold. Sacrococcygeal teratomas can be classified into four types. Type 1 is external, type 2 is predominantly external with a small portion that extends into the pelvis, type 3 is predominantly intrapelvic, and type 4 is completely intrapelvic with no external component. Teratomas can be totally

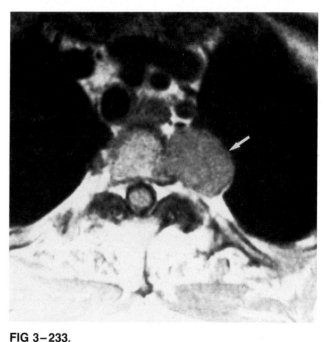

FIG 3–233.
Axial T1-weighted image of the thoracic spine (T3) showing left paraspinal hypointense ganglioneuroblastoma *(arrow)* with erosion of the left side of the vertebral body.

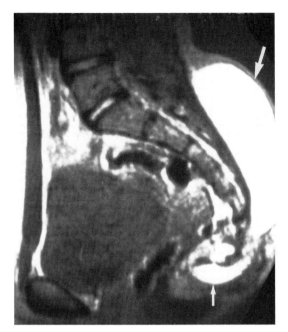

FIG 3–234.
Sagittal T1-weighted image of the sacrum showing a hyperintense (hemorrhagic and cystic) sacrococcygeal teratoma *(large arrow)* of the back with small intrapelvic extension *(small arrow).*

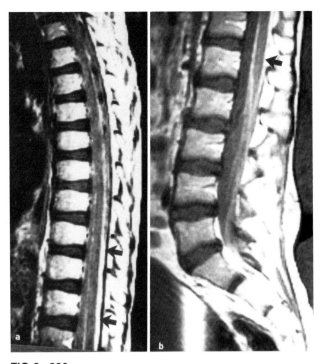

FIG 3–236.
Post-Gd sagittal T1-weighted images of a patient with leptomeningeal melanosis showing diffuse enhancement of the leptomeninges of the *(a)* thoracic and *(b)* lumbosacral spinal cord *(arrows).*

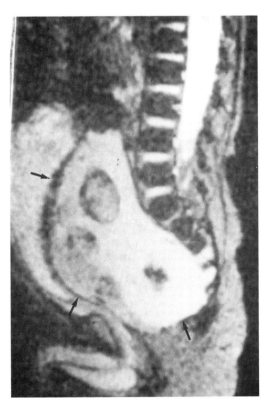

FIG 3–235.
Sagittal T2-weighted image of the lumbosacral coccygeal spine showing solid teratoma *(arrows)* with calcium and hemorrhage that is presacral and intrapelvic extending into the distal sacrum and coccyx.

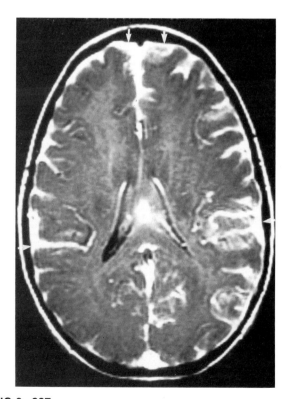

FIG 3–237.
Post-Gd axial T1-weighted image of a patient with leptomeningeal melanosis shows diffuse enhancement of the leptomeninges *(arrows).*

cystic, a combination of cystic and solid, or totally solid lesions. As already stated, they are composed of all three germ layers and contain neural elements, squamous and intestinal epithelium, skin appendages, teeth, and, at times, calcium. They may be associated with bony erosion of the coccyx and portions of the sacrum and extend into the spinal canal as an extradural mass. The lesions may be benign or malignant. The more solid the lesion and the greater the internal component, the more likely the lesion is malignant. Calcium is more commonly seen in benign lesions.

The best radiologic modalities to evaluate sacrococcygeal teratomas are CT and MRI. CT demonstrates bony destruction when there is involvement of the sacrum and coccyx. The cystic component is easily demonstrated on CT, and the solid component shows enhancement on contrast-enhanced scans. On MRI, bony destruction is not as well appreciated. However, the cystic component is well demonstrated and is hypointense on T1-weighted and hyperintense on T2-weighted images. The solid component may contain flakes of calcium in which there will be hypointensity that is inhomogeneous on T1-weighted images, and a combination of hypointensity of the calcium and hyperintensity of the solid component on T2-weighted images. The cystic component may bleed and contain hemorrhagic areas, in which case the signal intensity corresponds to the intensity of blood, depending on the age of the hemorrhage. The solid component of the teratoma may show enhancement after administration of Gd (Figs 3–234 and 3–235).

Lymphoma

Lymphomas rarely involve the spine. More commonly they involve bone, bone marrow, and lymph nodes. Lymphomas may involve the extradural component of the spine and present as an extradural mass. They may diffusely infiltrate the dura or present as localized masses of the dura or spinal cord. They are rare and usually occur in children 5 to 12 years of age.

Leptomeningeal Melanosis

Neurocutaneous melanosis is a rare and less known member of the phakomatoses (neurocutaneous syndromes). It is a nonfamilial disease characterized by large cutaneous pigmented nevi and melanosis of the leptomeninges. A forme fuste may occur in which only leptomeningeal involvement is present

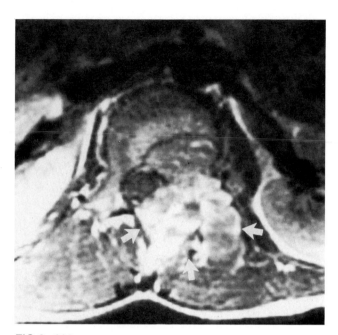

FIG 3–238.
Post-Gd axial T1-weighted image of the lumbar spine showing enhancement of an aneurysmal bone cyst (arrows) involving the left neural arch with extension into the spinal cord.

without cutaneous manifestations. It is seen in infants, young children, and teen-agers. It is due to melanocyte proliferation within the epidermis and leptomeninges. Patients present with signs of raised intracranial pressure and hydrocephalus secondary to the proliferation of melanocytes within the dura. This diffuse form of leptomeningeal melanosis can be demonstrated with MRI. Hyperintensity on T1-weighted images of the dura may be seen secondary to the melanin itself or to hemorrhage of the melanocyte. However, the most common MR appearance is diffuse thickening and enhancement of the leptomeninges demonstrated only on post-Gd T1-weighted images of the spine and brain (Figs 3–236 and 3–237).

EXTRADURAL BONY LESIONS

A host of vertebral bone abnormalities may extend outside of the bony framework of the spine and produce extradural lesions. Metastatic lesions to the vertebrae are rare in children, but they can be seen with neuroblastoma, Wilms tumor, and sarcomas as well as primary vertebral bone tumors such as aneurysmal bone cyst and osteoblastoma. Aneurysmal bone cysts and osteoblastomas usually involve the neural arches but may extend into the pedicles and adjacent body. They are lytic, expansive, highly vas-

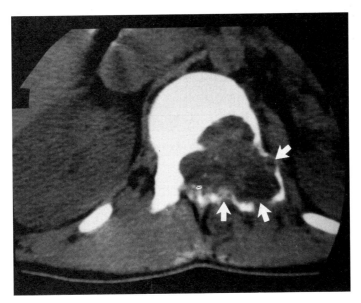

FIG 3–239.
Axial unenhanced CT scan of the lumbar spine reveals an aneurysmal bone cyst (arrows).

cular lesions. On MRI, they are hypointense on T1-weighted images, hyperintense on T2-weighted images, and they may or may not show enhancement after intravenous Gd. They expand all or part of the neural arch and may extend into the body or extradurally into the spinal canal (Figs 3–238 and 3–239). The bony abnormalities are discussed in Chapter 2.

REFERENCES

Spinal Tumors

Arcomano JP, Barnett JC, Wunderlich HO: Histiocytosis. *Am J Roentgenol* 1961, 85:663–679.

Atlas SW: *Magnetic Resonance Imaging of the Brain and Spine.* New York, Raven Press, 1991, pp 1–128.

Baierl P, Muhlsteffen A, Haustein J: Comparison of plain and Gd-DTPA–enhanced MR-imaging in children. *Pediatr Radiol* 1990; 20:515–519.

Balakrishnan V, Rice MS, Simpson DA: Spinal neuroblastomas: Diagnosis, treatment and prognosis. *J Neurosurg* 1974; 40:431–438.

Beltram J, Noto AM, Chakeres DW, et al: Tumors of the osseous spine: Staging with MRI imaging verous CT. *Radiology* 1987; 162:565–569.

Blews DE, Wang H, Jumbar AJ, et al: Intradural spinal metastases in pediatric patients with primary intracranial neoplasms: Gd-DTPA enhanced MR vs CT myelography. *J Comput Assist Tomogr* 1990; 14:730–735.

Cohen MD, Edwards MK: *Magnetic Resonance Imaging of Children.* Philadelphia, BC Decker, 1990, pp 1–55.

Dohrmann GJ, Farwell JR, Flannery JR: Ependymomas

and ependymoblastomas in children. *J Neurosurg* 1976; 45:273–280.

Edeu K: The dumb-bell tumors of the spine. *Br J Surg* 1941; 28:549–569.

Epstein BS: *The Spine. A Radiological Text and Atlas,* ed 4. Philadelphia, Lea & Febiger, 1976.

Epstein F, Epstein N: Surgical management of holocord spinal astrocytomas. *J Neurosurg* 1981; 54:829–832.

Farwell JR, Dohrman GJ: Intraspinal neoplasms in children. *Paraplegia* 1977; 15:262–273.

Herrman J. Sarcomatous transformation in multiple neurofibromatosis (von Recklinghausen's disease). *Ann Surg* 1950; 131:206–217.

Hughes JO: *Pathology of the Spinal Cord Tumors.* London, Lloyd-Luke, 1966, pp 160–180.

Izant RJ, Filston HC: Sacrococcygeal teratomas, analysis of forty-three circle. *Am J Surg* 1975; 130:617–620.

Kadonaga JN, Frieden IJ: Neurocutaneous melanosis: Definition and review of the literature. *Acad Dermatol* 1991; 24:747–755.

Kozlowski K, Beluffi G, Masel J, et al: Primary vertebral tumors in children. Report of 20 cases with brief review of the literature. *Pediatr Radiol* 1984; 14:129–139.

Lee C, Dean BL: Contrast-enhanced magnetic resonance imaging of the spine. *Top Magn Reson Imaging* 1991; 3:41–73.

Levy WJ, Bay J, Dohn D: Spinal cord meningioma. *J Neurosurg* 1982; 57:804–812.

Lewis TT, Kingsley DP: Magnetic resonance imaging of multiple spinal neurofibromata neurofibromatosis. *Neuroradiology* 1987; 29:562–564.

Masaryk TJ: Spine tumors, in Modic MT, Masaryk TJ (eds):

Magnetic Resonance Imaging of the Spine. St Louis, Mosby–Year Book, 1989, pp 183–213.

Rawlings CE, Giangaspero F, Burger PC, et al: Ependymomas: A clinicopathalogic study. *Surg Neurol* 1988; 29:271–281.

Reimer R, Onofrio BM: Astrocytomas of the spinal cord in children and adolescents. *J Neurosurg* 1985; 63:669–675.

Runge VM, Gelbum DY: The role of gadolinium-diethylenetriaminepentaacetic acid in the evaluation of the central nervous system. *Magn Reson Q* 1990; 6:85–107.

Schey WL, Shknolnik A, White H: Clinical and radiographic consideration of sacrococcygeal teratomas: An analysis

of 26 new cases and review of the literature. *Radiology* 1977; 125:189–195.

Sze G, Stimac GK, Bartlett C, et al: Multicenter study of gadopentetate dimeglumine as an MR contrast agent: Evaluation in patients with spinal tumors. *AJNR* 1990; 11:967–974.

Wiener MD, Boyko OB, Friedman HS, et al: False-positive spinal MR findings for subarachnoid spread of primary CNS tumor in postoperative pediatric patients. *AJNR* 1990; 11:1100–1103.

Zimmerman RA, Bilaniuk LT: Imaging of tumors of the spinal canal and cord. *Radiol Clin North Am* 1988; 26:965–1007.

SECTION 14

Miscellaneous Lesions

VASCULAR MALFORMATIONS

Vascular malformations of the spinal cord are rare. They may occur in any of the compartments of the spine (intramedullary, extramedullary, or intradural). However, the most common location is intramedullary with involvement of the dorsal aspect of the spi-

nal cord, usually in the thoracic region. Vascular malformations may bleed and produce an intramedullary hematoma or subarachnoid hemorrhage. If the vascular malformation is large, abnormally enlarged tortuous vessels may be demonstrated on CT, myelography, and MRI. The MR signal characteristics depend on the state of the hemorrhage. Subarachnoid hemor-

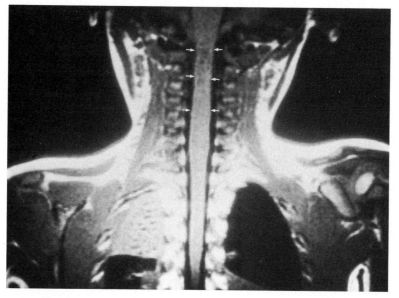

FIG 3–240.
FIG 3–Coronal T1-weighted image of the cervical spine showing ischemic infarction of the cervical cord with enlargement and hypointensity *(arrows).*

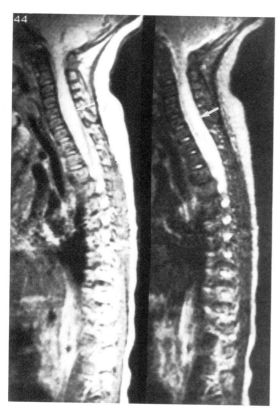

FIG 3–241.
Sagittal T2-weighted images of the cervical spine demonstrating hyperintensity *(arrows)* of the cervical cord with ischemic infarction.

rhage may be present, but is usually difficult to demonstrate radiologically. The late sequelae of chronic changes of vascular malformation of the spinal cord are atrophy with or without myelomalacia and, at times, syringomyelia. The best radiologic modality to demonstrate vascular malformations is spinal angiography. Certain spinal cord tumors, such as the highly malignant glioblastoma multiforme, may be highly vascularized and may simulate a vascular malformation of the spinal cord.

SPINAL CORD INFARCTION

Infarction in the spinal cord is usually secondary to compression of the vascular supply. The most common cause is trauma, with either compression of the anterior spinal artery or disruption of the intramedullary vessels. The early changes consist of edema with swelling, increased cord size, hypointensity and enlargement on CT, isointensity or hypointensity on T1-weighted MR images, and hyperintensity on T2-weighted MR images. If the child survives, later sequelae are atrophy with or without myelomalacia. On CT, the small cord is hypodense. On MR, the cord is small and hypointense or isointense on T1-weighted and isointense or hyperintense on T2-weighted images, depending on the degree of gliosis and scar formation (Figs 3–240 and 3–241).

REFERENCES

Spinal Cord Infarction

Atlas S: *Magnetic Resonance Imaging of the Brain and Spine.* New York, Raven Press, 1990.

Brown E, Virapongse C, Gregorios JB: MR imaging of cervical spine cord infarction. *J Comput Assist Tomogr* 1989; 13:920–922.

Cohen MD, Edwards MK: *Magnetic Resonance Imaging of Children.* Philadelphia, BC Decker, 1990.

Gebarski SS, Maynard FW, Gabrielsen TO, et al: Post traumatic progressive myelopathy. *Radiology* 1985; 157:379–385.

Hughes JT: Thrombosis of the posterior spinal artery. A complication of an intrathecal injection of phenol. *Neurology* 1970; 20:659–664.

Mawad ME, Rivera V, Crawforde S, et al: Spinal cord ischemia after resection of thoracoabdominal aortic aneurysms: MR findings in 24 patients. *Am J Neuroradiol* 1990; 11:987–991.

McArdle CB, Wright JW, Prevost WJ, et al: MR imaging of the acutely injured patient with cervical traction. *Radiology* 1986; 159:273–274.

Regenbogen VS, Rogers LF, Atlas SW, et al: Cervical spinal cord injuries in patients with cervical spondylosis. *Am J Roentgenol* 1986; 146:277–284.

PART II

The Neck and Respiratory System

JERALD P. KUHN

THOMAS L. SLOVIS

FREDERIC N. SILVERMAN

LAWRENCE R. KUHNS

4

Diagnostic Overview of Imaging Procedures in the Pediatric Neck and Thorax

DISORDERS OF SOFT TISSUES OF THE NECK

Imaging of the neck may be requested by a clinician to detect possible enlargement of normal anatomical structures, such as the adenoids; in other instances, the examining physician may feel a mass and require further information regarding its nature and extent. Retropharyngeal abscess is also a relatively common indication for imaging of the neck. The investigation usually begins with frontal and lateral plain films using conventional techniques (Table 4–1). This study provides information about normal anatomical structures, calcifications, bone destruction, and anomalies. It is important that the lateral radiograph be made in inspiration and with the head extended in order to satisfactorily evaluate the retropharyngeal soft tissues which may appear spuriously enlarged on technically poor films. If further information is required, the next step is selection of a cross-sectional imaging technique (Fig 4–1). Ultrasound is the least expensive and least invasive modality, and with the addition of color flow Doppler provides important information about the vascularity of the mass and its relationship to the great vessels. However, ultrasound is not as good as CT or MRI at clearly defining the anatomical space that the mass occupies nor in specifically identifying the nature of a mass. If the mass appears to be related to the thyroid gland, nuclear imaging with ^{99m}Tc pertechnetate will be the next diagnostic step. CT is superb at delineating the anatomical spaces in the neck and, with contrast enhancement, provides in-

formation regarding whether a mass is vascular in origin or has an enhancing rim, which would suggest an inflammatory origin. CT is also limited to the axial projection and, for complete examination, requires contrast injection. MRI is the most expensive procedure and often requires sedation, but it provides the most complete evaluation of the anatomical relationships of the normal and abnormal structures and has superior contrast resolution to CT. With the advent of gadolinium DTPA (diethylenetriamine pentaacetic acid), MRI provides equivalent or greater information than the contrast-enhanced CT scan and has the additional advantage of sagittal and coronal planes of view.

DISORDERS OF THE THORAX

Available Imaging Techniques

Chest radiography is the most frequent procedure done in most pediatric radiology departments, accounting for between one third and one half of the total volume of cases. The examination can be done either with the child supine using a cross-table technique for the lateral radiograph or with the uncooperative patient held erect in any one of a number of homemade or commercially available immobilization devices. A high proportion of inpatient examinations are done with portable techniques and a single anteroposterior (AP) supine view. Some departments are using digital radiography, which tends to reduce exposure errors. In neonates, a par-speed

TABLE 4–1.

Neck Imaging Techniques

Modality	Technique
Plain film (conventional)	Lateral, nonrotated, head extended, inspiratory phase of respiration
Ultrasound	Highest possible frequency transducer; color flow Doppler; orientation relative to great vessels
Computed tomography	5–10 mm without IV contrast medium; 5 mm with IV contrast medium; administer as a bolus (2 mL/kg); axial always, ?coronals if possible
Magnetic resonance	T1-weighted imaging in two or three planes; T2-weighted imaging in best plane; Gd enhancement in best plane
Nuclear medicine	^{99m}Tc pertechnetate first

film-screen combination is favored by many for greater detail, but in older children most departments use a higher speed system to reduce exposure time and radiation exposure. Tight collimation of the primary beam should be employed as well as supplementary lead shielding to diminish any scattered radiation to the gonads. It is important that the patient not be rotated (check the anterior rib ends), and be in a proper degree of inspiration (at least five anterior ribs above the diaphragm), and that the film be properly exposed (penetrated enough to see the vertebral body pedicles and light enough to see the peripheral vascular markings).

Familiarity with the normal appearances of the pediatric thorax is required to avoid errors of over-interpretation. Particular pitfalls include expiratory or rotated films and variations in the size and shape of the normal thymus. Correlation with the clinical history is important to avoid diagnostic errors. Signs of disease include generalized hyperinflation, which usually signifies small-airway disease caused by bronchiolitis, viral pneumonia, asthma, or cystic fibrosis. These diseases also frequently are associated with peribronchial thickening, which results from edema or inflammation in the perivascular space, a common connective tissue space containing a bronchus and its accompanying pulmonary arterial branch. Peribronchial thickening is seen radiologically as ring shadows when the bronchi are seen end-on and as "tram tracks" when they are visualized along their long axis. Subpleural edema manifested by widening of the fissures and thickening of interlobular septa is another sign of interstitial disease and is most common in pulmonary edema, which may be due to cardiac or renal causes, especially acute glomerulonephritis. Airspace consolidation is manifested by ill-defined nodular opacities, confluent shadows with air bronchograms, and the silhouette sign. Focal air trapping is seen if there is partial bronchial obstruction, which may be due to foreign body, inflammatory disease, or extrinsic mass lesions. Depending on the degree of obstruction, atelectasis may develop. Atelectasis is also commonly seen with infection and in postoperative states. The presence of an air bronchogram in an atelectatic lobe suggests that primary lung disease rather than bronchial obstruction is the cause of the volume loss.

Supplementary radiographic examination may be required in addition to routine frontal and lateral radiographs. *Lateral decubitus films* are used for detection of small amounts of pleural fluid, or even large amounts of subpulmonic fluid, which may masquerade as an apparently elevated hemidiaphragm. A small pneumothorax is best seen on a lateral decubitus film. These views are also useful for clarification of equivocal parenchymal opacities, especially near the right heart border, because in a left lateral decubitus view, the heart falls away from the right lung, which in turn is slightly hyperinflated because of its elevated position. This same principle of hyperinflation of the "up" lung and underinflation of the "down" lung is helpful in determining unilateral air trapping in cases of suspected intrabronchial foreign body. Another way of evaluating possible unilateral air trapping is to apply gentle hand pressure to the

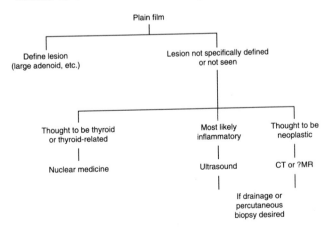

FIG 4–1.
Neck imaging algorithm.

baby's abdomen with a lead glove and produce a "forced" expiratory film.

Fluroscopy of the chest is used to evaluate dynamic abnormalities such as unilateral air trapping and mediastinal shift as well as to clarify questionable abnormalities seen on radiography. If there is a question of a mediastinal mass, an *esophogram* is a useful adjunct to the fluoroscopic examination, because the esophagus has a central position in the mediastinum and is often displaced by mediastinal masses or compressed by vascular rings. Rarely an esophageal perforation due to a chronic foreign body may actually be the cause of a mediastinal mass or airway symptoms. The esophagus and swallowing function have to be carefully studied in all cases of chronic, recurrent pneumonia to exclude aspiration, reflux, and, rarely, H-type tracheoesophageal fistula. If the baby does not swallow well, the esophagus can be filled by injecting barium through a feeding tube while slowly withdrawing the tube under fluoroscopic guidance.

A Thoraeus or copper filter on the table under the baby combined with a small focal spot allows the use of dynamic, (i.e., fluoroscopic) *high-kilovoltage magnification study* of the trachea. This is useful in cases of suspected subglottic stenosis as well as clarification of intrinsic or extrinsic abnormalities of the airway.

The need for *tracheobronchograms* has been reduced by the greater application of high-kilovoltage fluoroscopy techniques, and particularly by the more widespread availability of computed tomography (CT), but there are still a few cases when a positive contrast study of the tracheobronchial tree needs to be performed. The study is usually done with an endoscopist and with the patient anesthetized; it should be done under fluoroscopic control to optimally visualize the area of concern and to minimize the amount of contrast material needed. Many centers now use water-soluble, nonionic contrast media because they are less irritating than the oil-based contrast agents, although the water-soluble material does not coat as well.

Angiography is now used less than in the past because of the advent of the newer, less invasive modalities. Pulmonary arteriography remains the gold standard for detection of pulmonary embolism and is used in some congenital malformations for delineation of arterial and venous supply if this information cannot be obtained in other ways. Angiography is also used to localize and embolize bleeding vessels in the thorax, especially in children with cystic fibrosis and who have severe hemoptysis. Aortography is used in some cases of bronchopulmonary foregut

malformation if noninvasive studies have not established arterial supply.

Ultrasound is an attractive imaging modality for pediatric patients because it does not use ionizing radiation. Unfortunately, its application in thoracic diseases is less effective than in other parts of the body because of interference by the bony thorax and the fact that the air-containing lungs reflect the sound waves so that ultrasonic visualization is limited to portions of the heart and mediastinum. It can be used to evaluate the diaphragm and juxtadiaphragmatic masses. It can also be used to guide thoracentesis when pleural effusions are present and may be useful if a mass or consolidation contacts the thoracic wall without intervening lung. Ultrasound with color flow Doppler can sometimes visualize an abnormal vessel supplying a sequestration.

Nuclear medicine procedures are also used relatively infrequently. Technetium 99m pertechnetate or iodine-containing radioisotopes are used for evaluation of thyroid masses and functional abnormalities. Gallium 67 citrate is used in some lymphomas and can be helpful in differentiating fibrosis from residual tumor when soft-tissue masses persist in the mediastinum after therapy. It also is occasionally used to determine the activity of certain diffuse lung diseases, such as sarcoid. Bone scintigraphy is useful for evaluation of metastatic disease and detection of subtle rib fractures in cases of suspected child abuse. Ventilation-perfusion lung scanning is useful as an adjunct to pulmonary function tests and in diagnosis of suspected pulmonary embolism.

Computed tomography is the most important adjunctive imaging modality in the pediatric chest. For optimal examination, the child must be cooperative, restrained, or sedated. The child should be carefully centered in the gantry. The smallest field of view possible should be used to minimize pixel size and maximize spatial resolution. Usually, the shortest scan time available should be used and the images reconstructed using a high-spatial-frequency (bone- or edge-enhancing) algorithm if the pulmonary parenchyma is the area of interest, and a conventional algorithm for evaluation of mediastinal and mass lesions. Slice thickness and contiguity vary with the size of the patient and the reason for the examination. When searching for metastatic disease, contiguous slices should be used. For high-resolution CT (HRCT) studies, the thinnest slice available (1–3 mm) is required. Intravenous contrast enhancement is mandatory for evaluation of mediastinal pathologic changes and for differentiation of pleural from parenchymal processes. It is also required for analysis of the internal structure of mass lesions. The usual dose is 2 mL/kg administered as a bolus. Non-ionic contrast media should be used when possible, as there is less likelihood of vomiting or other side effects which could produce unwanted patient motion. Drawbacks to CT include cost, radiation exposure (0.5–2.0 rads per slice), and often, the need for sedation and contrast enhancement. Current applications of CT in the pediatric thorax are listed in Table 4–2. CT is usually limited to direct acquisition in only the axial plane, although in infants direct coronal and sagittal images can be made. Also, images can now be reformatted in any plane, and even in three dimensions. Ultrafast CT with scan times of 0.1 second can provide essentially motion-free images in any pediatric patient, and dynamic abnormalities can be studied using the cine mode of this scanner, which can produce up to 17 images per second. Spiral or helical scanning, now becoming more widely available on conventional CT scanners, will probably extend the applications of CT, particularly in the mediastinum, as up to 32 scans can now be obtained in 32 seconds, minimizing the amount of contrast media needed and also minimizing the deleterious effects of motion.

TABLE 4–2.

Indications for Computed Tomography in Diseases of the Pediatric Thorax

Evaluation of the bony thorax
  Mass
  Deformity
  Trauma
Mediastinal masses
  Location
  Extent
  Nature
Vascular rings
Airway
  Anomalies
  Stenosis
  Bronchiectasis
  Foreign body
Infection
  Evaluation of the opaque thorax
  Empyema vs. abscess
  Negative x-ray film with positive clinical findings
  Clarification of equivocal or confusing chest film
  ?Staging of early cystic fibrosis
Evaluation of bronchopulmonary anomalies
  Determination of parenchymal vascular and airway components
Trauma
  Detection of pneumothorax
  Pulmonary contusion, laceration
  Airway fracture
Neoplasm
  Determination of presence and extent of metastatic disease
  Primary evaluation of the mass: cystic, vascular, calcified, solid, fatty.

Magnetic resonance imaging (MRI) is also becoming a valuable addition to the armamentarium of the pediatric radiologist. It is expensive, not universally available, and nearly always requires sedation for children less than 5 years of age. However, since it does not involve ionizing radiation and usually does not necessitate the use of contrast media, it is inherently an attractive pediatric imaging technique. It has spatial resolution nearly equal to CT and superior contrast resolution; images can be acquired directly in any plane. Blood vessels are seen as areas of signal void. Currently, lung parenchyma is poorly visualized and calcifications are not usually seen. The techniques used vary with the clinical problem, but T1-weighted, cardiac-gated scans are usually obtained in at least two planes, followed by a T2-weighted scan in the plane that best reveals the abnormality. The technology is still evolving very rapidly and new applications will undoubtedly be found. The current, common uses for MRI are listed in Table 4–3. The relative advantages of CT and MRI are listed in Table 4–4.

CHEST WALL LESIONS

Chest wall lesions usually present with external deformities or palpable masses. The most common scenario is that of a small child in whom a frightened parent has just noticed a hard, palpable mass. Usually this turns out on the plain film to be nothing more sinister than a bifid rib which had escaped previous notice. A soft-tissue mass will usually not be well delineated on a plain radiograph, although the investigation should still begin with plain radiography. Plain films should be carefully scrutinized for the possibility of any involvement of the adjacent bony structures. Soft-tissue masses generally require further investigation by ultrasound, contrast-enhanced CT, or MRI. Investigation of traumatic lesions of the chest wall and thoracic structures is ini-

TABLE 4–3.

Applications for Magnetic Resonance Imaging in the Pediatric Thorax

Mediastinal masses
  Especially posterior where there is a question of spinal invasion
  Masses near the hilum
  Differentiation of vascular from nonvascular structures
Vascular rings
Vascular supply to sequestrations and other bronchopulmonary foregut malformations
Bone marrow imaging
Direct visualization of the diaphragm
Determination of intrathoracic vs. intra-abdominal location of disease

TABLE 4–4.

Relative Strengths of Computed Tomography vs. Magnetic Resonance Imaging

Characteristic	CT	MRI
Lower cost	✓	
No ionizing radiation		✓
Less need for sedation	✓	
Shorter examination time	✓	
Multiple planes of view		✓
Detection of calcification	✓	
Evaluation of lung parenchyma	✓	
Spinal invasion		✓
Hilar masses		✓
Spatial resolution	✓	
Contrast resolution		✓
Less requirement for contrast material		✓

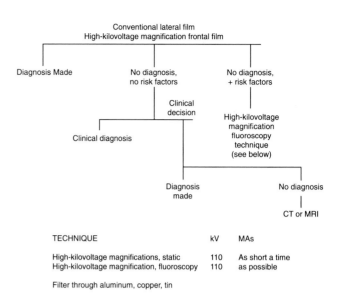

FIG 4–2.
Upper airway imaging algorithm.

TECHNIQUE	kV	MAs
High-kilovoltage magnifications, static	110	As short a time
High-kilovoltage magnification, fluoroscopy	110	as possible

Filter through aluminum, copper, tin

tiated with plain films. In most cases, detection of a subtle rib fracture is not clinically important; however, in cases of suspected child abuse, for purposes of documentation, radionuclide imaging is more sensitive to the detection of subtle fractures than is plain radiography. In cases of massive thoracic trauma, CT is helpful for evaluation of lung parenchymal abnormality and detection of mediastinal hemorrhage; however, if hemorrhage is detected or if great-vessel injury is strongly suspected clinically, angiography is still required.

AIRWAY LESIONS

Evaluation of the pediatric airway is performed because of clinical findings of airway obstruction which may present as stridor (croupy or noisy breathing) or hoarseness. Common clinical conditions include croup, epiglottitis, foreign body, or suspected mass lesion. If epiglottitis is suspected clinically, it is important to make an *upright* lateral film of the neck to exclude epiglottitis before placing the child in a supine position, a procedure which, if epiglottitis is present, may result in acute upper airway obstruction and death. After the conventional lateral film has been examined for evaluation of the supraglottic structures, a filtered high-kilovoltage frontal radiograph is obtained to clearly outline the structures of the upper airway, particularly the subglottic region (Fig 4–2). Some lesions, such as laryngomalacia or vocal cord abnormalities, are dynamic in nature and require real-time studies such as magnification high-kilovoltage fluoroscopy for further evaluation. Patients with risk factors as outlined in Table 4–5 may require additional investigation.

Diseases of the central or peripheral airways may present with wheezing (expiratory stridor), cough, recurrent infection, or the findings of focal or diffuse abnormalities of aeration discovered on chest radiography. In a child who is wheezing for the first time, the most likely diagnoses varies with the age of the patient. Under the age of 1 year, the most common diagnosis is bronchiolitis; radiography is indicated to exclude anomalies and foreign bodies, which are also common in children of this age. Initial evaluation of this group of children includes evaluation of the pulmonary parenchyma, which is achieved with a chest radiograph. If upper airway obstruction is suspected, a high-kilovoltage magnification airway film is indicated. If there is any suspicion of a foreign body, an expiratory film should be obtained, as the findings on the inspiratory film may be normal or extremely subtly abnormal. If a satisfactory expiratory radiograph cannot be obtained, either both lateral decubitus films or a "forced" expiration film should be obtained as described above. Thin-section CT is useful in problematic cases.

In the older child, the most common cause of wheezing is bronchospasm due to infection or an initial manifestation of asthma. However, because foreign bodies and anomalies may also present in this group, the older, first-time wheezing child should also be evaluated radiologically. Persistent

TABLE 4–5.

Risk Factors in Patients with Upper Airway Symptoms

Younger than 6 months of age
Prolonged stridor over 7 days
History of airway manipulation
History of foreign body
Recurrent symptoms

hyperinflation and mild peribronchial thickening are common radiographic manifestations of asthma, but these radiographic findings can also occur in cystic fibrosis, and this diagnosis should always be kept in mind and excluded clinically. In the known asthmatic patient, clinical evaluation and treatment are often indicated before resorting to radiography. Imaging of these children is reserved for clinically suspected complications such as major atelectasis, pneumothorax, or pneumomediastinum.

In selected cases of tracheobronchial anomalies, a bronchogram, thin-section CT, or MRI may be required to produce further information regarding the presence of an intrinsic or extrinsic lesion.

Investigation of a clinically suspected diaphragmatic abnormality is most often done by plain radiographs and fluoroscopy. Ultrasound can be used in the critically ill patient for bedside detection of diaphragmatic paralysis. The diaphragm is visible on CT, but since it is viewed in cross section it is often difficult to visualize the whole diaphragm. This can be done with MRI, but is rarely necessary. Evaluation of esophageal hiatal hernias is discussed in Chapter 25.

PULMONARY PARENCHYMAL ABNORMALITIES

Infection

Pneumonia and respiratory infection are the most frequent indications in childhood for chest radiography. The epidemiology of pneumonia suggests that viruses account for more than 90% of infections in children less than 2 years of age and 65% of pneumonias in childhood. *Mycoplasma* is the most common *single agent* producing pneumonia in childhood, and accounts for more than 65% of cases. Most of these are in children over 5 years of age. Bacteria account for only about 5% of pneumonias seen in childhood. The radiograph unfortunately cannot differentiate between the various causes of pneumonia; even in those instances in which lobar consolidation, pneumatoceles, or empyema are present, it is possible that more than a single agent is involved. Therefore, the indications for the radiograph are to detect the presence or complication of respiratory infection. The most frequent findings of viral pneumonia are hyperinflated lungs and peribronchial thickening. These findings are subjective and there is poor correlation from one observer to another. Acute complications of pneumonia include atelectasis, pneumatocele, lung abscess, and empyema; chronic effects of pneumonia may include bronchiectasis and oblitera-

tive bronchiolitis with resultant effects on the growth of the mature lung. Children with complicated pneumonia should have follow-up studies (Fig 4–3). It is important to remember that there may be a discrepancy between the radiographic clearing and the clinical response to therapy. In general, a follow-up radiograph is not necessary before 14 to 21 days, but is specifically indicated in extensive bacterial infection or in children with round pneumonias. If complications occur, follow-up must be individualized. Contrast-enhanced CT (CECT) is useful for differentiation of pleural from parenchymal abnormalities (Table 4–6). If there is a localized pulmonary opacity or an opaque hemithorax, it is often difficult from the plain radiograph to know if there is pleural or parenchymal disease, or if both are present. On rare occasions, an underlying neoplastic mass or pulmonary anomaly may be responsible for the radiographic findings.

Chronic recurrent pulmonary infection is a particularly difficult problem in childhood. Mechanical causes such as gastroesophageal reflux, aspiration, and H-type fistula necessitate careful radiographic evaluation of swallowing function and the esophagus. HRCT can be useful to exclude bronchiectasis, anatomical abnormality, and differentiation of interstitial and airspace disease. The chest radiograph may provide the first clue to systemic disease such as cystic fibrosis, acquired immunodeficiency syndrome (AIDS), altered immune function, and α_1 antitrypsin deficiency. The radiologist may be the first to suspect tuberculosis, which is a newly resurgent disease in the United States. Any child with hilar adenopathy deserves skin testing and evaluation for this eminently treatable disease.

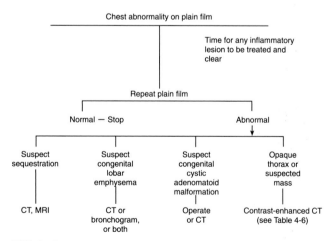

FIG 4–3.
Steps to take in investigation of the child with suspected pneumonia.

TABLE 4–6.

Computed Tomography Characteristics of the Opaque Thorax
or Large Thoracic Mass

Pleural fluid (empyema)
  Avascular
  Enhanced visceral or parietal pleura (split pleura sign)
  Lenticular-shaped
Parenchymal disease
  Pneumonia
    Air bronchograms
    Some enhancement
      Vessels may be visible in the opacified area
      May have localized areas of diminished enhancement
    Ill-defined border
  Abscesses
    Air-fluid level
    Thicker, irregular wall
    Acute angle with chest wall
  Neoplasms
    Moderate enhancement
    Center may be inhomogeneous
    Calcifications may or may not be visible
  Anomaly
    May be cystic, multicystic, or vascular
    No recognizable normal pulmonary structure
    May have an aberrant vessel
    Usually no normal bronchial supply
  Chest wall lesions
    May have associated bony or soft-tissue abnormality
    Obtuse angle with lung parenchyma
    May be inflammatory or neoplastic in origin
  Mediastinal mass
    Origin usually obvious on CT
    May be cystic, vascular, solid, calcified, or fatty

Pulmonary Circulatory Disorders

Abnormalities of the pulmonary arteries can be suspected on plain films and further evaluated when necessary by contrast-enhanced CT or MRI. The central pulmonary arteries are well visualized by echocardiography, although the peripheral vessels are usually not seen well utilizing this technique. The distinction of pulmonary edema from pneumonia is often difficult based on the radiographic findings alone; sometimes the conditions coexist. Pulmonary thromboembolic disease is difficult to diagnose in children because it occurs infrequently and thus is sometimes not even considered as a diagnostic possibility. Even when considered, it may be difficult to establish the diagnosis of thromboembolic disease. The possibility of pulmonary infarction should be considered in children with hypercoagulable states (nephrosis) and in sickle cell disease; in addition, other predisposing factors for thromboembolic disease include indwelling catheters, adolescents with pelvic inflammatory disease, and patients with

venous thrombosis of the lower extremity. Frequently, the chest film is normal or if abnormal is nonspecific. If pulmonary consolidation is present, radionuclide scanning will also be abnormal and therefore not usually helpful. If the chest film is normal, ventilation-perfusion lung scintigraphy is helpful. If the lung scan is negative or the chest film is abnormal but nondiagnostic, CECT may reveal the cause of the symptoms. The gold standard, however, remains pulmonary angiography.

Pulmonary Neoplasms

Evaluation for suspected pulmonary neoplasm can originate in one of two ways. Probably the most frequent circumstance is for a mass to be detected on a radiograph made for a suspected respiratory infection. The inexperienced may assume that the mass most likely represents a primary or metastatic neoplasm, because that would probably be true in an adult patient. In children, however, it is much more likely that the "mass" represents either a normal variant or an inflammatory mass such as "round pneumonia." Correlation with the clinical situation and follow-up radiography is all that usually needs to be done. It is relatively unusual, although not unheard of, for a malignancy to become manifest as an incidental finding on chest radiography. The second, less common, clinical situation exists when a patient has a known or strongly suspected malignancy. In this situation, CT of the lungs is indicated if detection of metastatic disease would change the staging or the therapy of the disease. Malignancies that are likely to spread to the lungs and mediastinum are listed in Table 13–1. Most of them will present as discrete nodules or masses, although in some lymphomas, and advanced cases of neuroblastoma and in rhabdomyosarcomas, an interstitial, lymphangitic pattern may be present. MRI has not proved as yet to be valuable in routine clinical use for evaluation of neoplastic pulmonary parenchymal abnormalities, although in suspected sequestrations and arteriovenous malformations it can demonstrate large-vessel abnormalities.

MEDIASTINAL DISORDERS

Evaluation of the pediatric mediastinum is most commonly performed for a suspected mediastinal mass. Again, the clinical history and the chest radiograph form the foundation upon which one begins to build the diagnostic exploration. CT and MRI have revolutionized our ability to visualize mediasti-

TABLE 4–7.

Imaging Characteristics of Common Pediatric Mediastinal Masses

Characteristic	CT*	MRI
Fatty masses (lipoma, lipoblastoma, teratoma)	Diminished attenuation (< −20 HU)	Bright on T1-weighted image; decreased intensity on T2-weighted image; chemical shift artifact
Cystic masses (bronchogenic enteric, and neurenteric cysts)	Usually near 0 HU although occasionally higher; no definable rim; no evidence of contrast enhancement	Low signal intensity on T1-weighted image; bright signal intensity on T2-weighted image; occasionally bright on T1-weighted image if containing mucoid material, protein, or blood
Solid masses (lymph nodes, neoplastic masses)	Near muscle attenuation on unenhanced scan; variable degree of enhancement; benign masses often show enhancement homogeneously and malignant ones often show enhancement heterogeneously; may or may not have a definable wall	Intermediate on T1-weighted image; bright on T2-weighted image; internal inhomogeneity occasionally present in malignant masses
Vascular masses (vascular malformations and aneurysms; vascular rings)	Marked enhancement	Flow void with no signal; if the vessel is large enough it will become bright on gradient-echo images
Calcified masses (granulomatous infections; rare germ cell tumors; neuroblastoma)	> 50 HU	No signal on T1- or T2-weighted images; calcifications may be missed unless very large; may have magnetic susceptibility on gradient-echo scans

*HU = Hounsfield unit.

nal structures. Chest fluoroscopy and the esophagogram are still useful tools, but often, regardless of what these studies reveal, CT or MRI is still required not only for more precise delineation of the extent of the mass, but also for more accurate assessment of its nature. The mediastinal masses usually occurring in children are listed according to their common locations and their CT characteristics in Chapter 14. It is not yet clear whether CT or MRI will have greater utility in exploring the pediatric mediastinum. The CT and MR imaging characteristics of common me-

diastinal masses are listed in Table 4–7. The relative advantages and drawbacks of these modalities are listed in Table 4–3. Our own current practice is to use MRI if preliminary studies reveal a paraspinal mass, to use CT if there is any possibility of pulmonary involvement (i.e., in a lymphoma), and to individualize the imaging protocol in most other instances. As MRI technology continues to improve, it is likely that it will probably replace CT for evaluation of the mediastinum, possibly even eventually for evaluation of the lung parenchyma.

5

Neck and Upper Airway

The cervical soft-tissue structures related to the upper airway are visible in roentgenograms by virtue of contrast with air in the pharynx, larynx, and trachea. Imaging of the neck is useful for identification and localization of foreign bodies, in the study of retropharyngeal and retroesophageal abscesses, and in the estimation of the size of the pharyngeal tonsils (adenoids). It is also used for evaluation of stridor, other neck masses, and various malformations. Accurate diagnosis can be made with available techniques in a high percentage of patients. Computed tomography (CT) maintains its efficacy in imaging soft-tissue structures and is particularly useful for identification of calcification that is not seen or poorly seen in conventional radiographs, as in the palatine tonsillar area, neoplasms, early fibrositis ossificans progressiva, etc. Magnetic resonance (MR) imaging is ideal for differentiation of soft tissues, including lymph nodes, muscles, vessels, thyroid, and tumors related to them. Ultrasound (US) and scintigraphy are excellent screening techniques, and may be sufficient for diagnosis in many instances. Scheible reported that high-resolution US is extremely helpful in the evaluation of neoplastic and inflammatory masses of the neck and in the identification of the position of thyroid nodules and even enlarged parathyroid glands. The sensitivity of thyroid tissue in infants and children to ionizing radiation should be considered in the choice of modality. For demonstration of the airways, the high-kilovoltage filtered-beam technique (Joseph et al.) is preferred to conventional radiography because of the fourfold reduction in radiation dose.

NORMAL ANATOMY

The major soft-tissue and skeletal structures seen in lateral projections of the neck are shown in Figures 5–1 and 5–2. During the first year—and particularly the first weeks—of life, the normal retropharyngeal tissues are abundant; in expiration, they thicken and sometimes cast a shadow not unlike that produced by a retropharyngeal abscess (Fig 5–3). Rivero and Young measured the thickness of the prevertebral soft tissues, as indicated in Figure 5–4, in films exposed *during inspiration* in 586 normal children. The maximal ratios of the soft tissues at the C2–3 level with the sagittal diameters of C2 at its lower border are shown in Table 5–1. In any equivocal examination, a repeat film exposed in inspiration usually resolves the matter.

In lateral projection, the superimposed normal shadow of the ear lobe can simulate an abnormal mass within the pharynx, as can normal large tonsils (Fig 5–5). The body and greater horns of the hyoid bone may be visible (Fig 5–6) in approximately 75% of term infants at the level of the second to third cervical vertebral body. The incidence of a visible hyoid center in the newborn period is greatly diminished in infants with the DiGeorge syndrome and in those with congenital heart disease, particularly those with interrupted aortic arch and with severe tetralogy of Fallot.

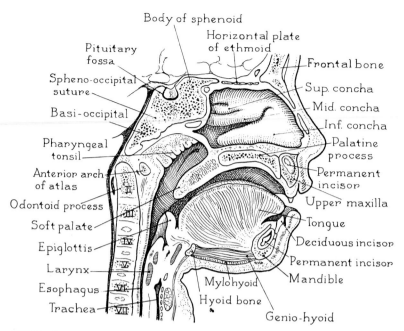

FIG 5–1.

Principal structures in a mesial sagittal section of the head of a boy 4 years of age.

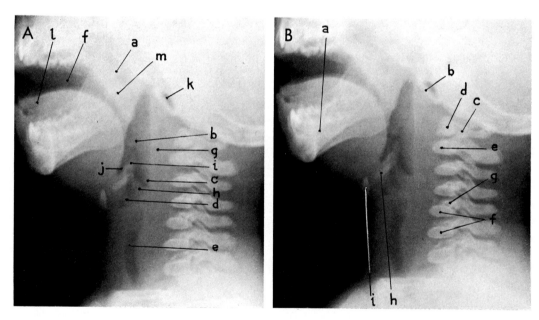

FIG 5–2.

A lateral projection of the neck of a patient 5 months of age shows the shadows of the normal structures. **A,** soft tissues: *a,* nasopharynx; *b,* oral pharynx; *c,* hypopharynx; *d,* larynx; *e,* trachea; *f,* oral cavity; *g,* prevertebral tissues; *h,* aryepiglottic fold; *i,* epiglottis; *j,* vallecula; *k,* external auditory canal; *l,* tongue; *m,* soft palate and uvula. **B,** skeletal tissues; *a,* mandible; *b,* ring of the tympanic bone; *c,* atlas; *d,* dens of the axis; *e,* body of the axis; *f,* body of cervical vertebra; *g,* lateral mass superimposed on the body of C5; *h,* greater wings of the hyoid; *i,* body of the hyoid.

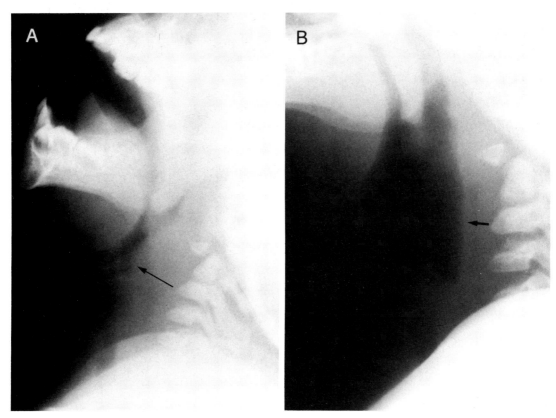

FIG 5–3.
Normal variation in the depth of the soft tissues of the retropharyngeal space *(arrows)* in expiration. **(A)** and inspiration **B.** This patient was a healthy 1-year-old.

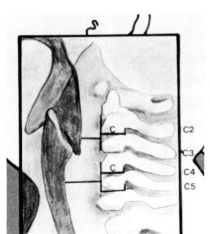

FIG 5–4.
Diagram for measurement of retropharyngeal and retrotracheal soft tissues according to Rivero and Young. The retropharyngeal soft tissues are measured from the posterior pharyngeal wall at the C2–3 interspace to the vertical line connecting the anterior margins of the bodies. The AP dimension of the body of C2 is measured at its caudal margin. Maximum ratios for retropharyngeal soft tissues in relation to the body of C2 at different ages are shown in Table 5–1. (From Rivero HJ, Young LW: Unpublished material, 1992.)

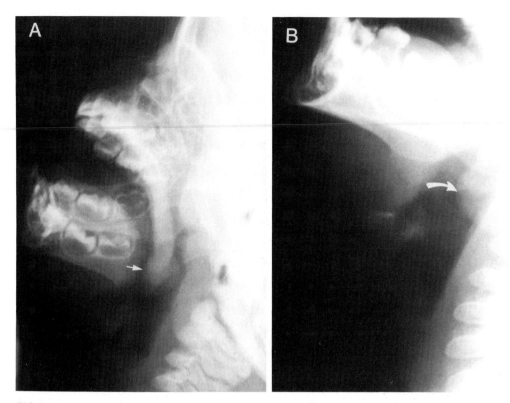

FIG 5–5.
Normal palatine tonsils **A,** *(small arrow)* and ear lobe **(B)** *(curved arrow)* seen projecting into the airway.

The styloid process and stylohyoid ligament vary considerably in size and mineralization (Fig 5–7); symptomatic elongation of the stylohyoid process in adults may produce obscure head and neck pain and is known as Eagle syndrome. Ossification occurs in the anterior arch of the atlas during the first postnatal year but may be present at birth. Calcification in the respiratory cartilages in children is pathologic; it occurs in chondrodysplasia punctata, the Keutel syndrome, and as an idiopathic phenomenon, occasionally in as-

sociation with stridor (Fig 5–8). It has been noted in children after prosthetic mitral valve replacement followed by lengthy periods of warfarin administration (Taybi and Capitanio).

The anatomy of the neck is well delineated by cross-section imaging and is conveniently divided into the suprahyoid neck and the infrahyoid region (Harnsberger). The reason for this distinction is that

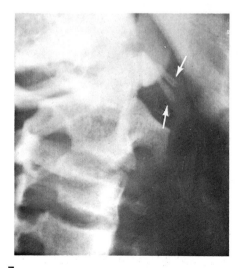

FIG 5–7.
The *arrows* indicate either calcification in the stylohyoid ligament, ossification in the styloid process, or both.

FIG 5–6.
The neck of an infant 2 days of age, lateral projection. The *white arrow* points to a large ossification center in the anterior arch of the atlas and the *black arrow,* to the mineralized body of the hyoid bone.

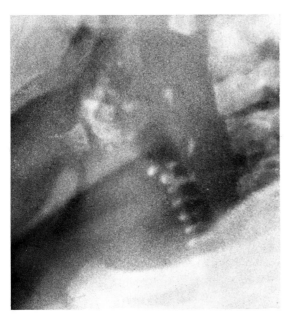

FIG 5–8.
Multiple calcifications of the tracheal and laryngeal cartilages of an infant 4½ months of age who had congenital stridor. (Courtesy of Drs. R.B. Goldbloom and J.S. Dunbar.)

TABLE 5–1.
Maximum Ratio of Retropharyngeal Soft Tissues to C2*

Age (yr)	Ratio
0–1	1.00
1–2	0.70
2–3	0.60
3–4	0.55
4–6	0.50
6–10	0.40

*Modified from Rivero HJ, Young LW: Unpublished material, 1992.

masses of the suprahyoid portion of the neck. It is a small fatty region immediately posterior and medial to the masticator space and directly anterior to the carotid space *(C)* and anterior and medial to the parotid space (Fig 5–9,B). Most important, it is anterior and lateral to the retropharyngeal space, where most inflammatory lesions occur in childhood. A mass in any of these spaces is defined by its effect on the PPS. Either contrast-enhanced CT at 3- to 5-mm intervals or MR imaging (MRI) can evaluate these spaces. CT is less prone to motion artifact, shows exquisite bone detail, and usually is faster to obtain. MRI (using 5-mm-thick T1- and T2-weighted slices) with its multiplanar approach is useful for planning therapy as well as for differentiating tumor(mass)-muscle interfaces.

The infrahyoid portion of the neck (Figs 5–10 and 5–11) is divided by fascia into circumferential

the three layers of the deep fascia that divide the suprahyoid portion of the neck merge on the hyoid bone (Fig 5–9,A). As in the adult, the parapharyngeal space *(PPS)* is the most important landmark in understanding the anatomy and, consequently,

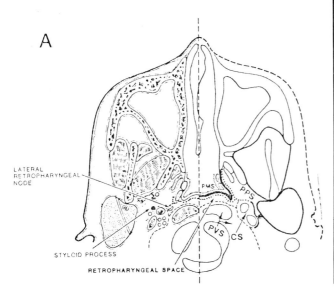

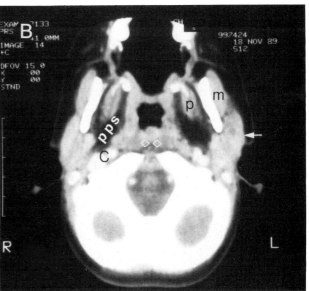

FIG 5–9.
Transaxial anatomy in the suprahyoid portion of the neck. **A,** section just below the nasopharynx reveals the parapharyngeal space *(PPS)* and the carotid space *(CS).* The pharyngeal mucosal space is indicated by *PMS,* and the prevertebral space by *PVS.* (From Harnsberger HR: *Handbook of Radiology: Head and Neck Imaging.* St Louis, Mosby– Year Book, 1990). **B,** axial CT scan demon-strating the anatomy at this level. *pps,* parapharyngeal space. *Arrow* is on the parotid gland denoting the parotid space; *m,* masseter muscle; *p,* pterygoid muscle; *p* and *m* define the masticator space; *C,* carotid space. The two diamonds are on the potential retropharyngeal space.

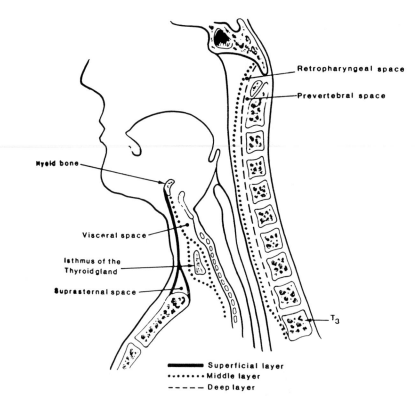

FIG 5–10.

Drawing showing the relations craniad and caudad of the retro-pharyngeal space to the prevertebral space. (From Harnsberger HR: *Handbook of Radiology: Head and Neck Imaging.* St Louis, Mosby– Year Book, 1990, p 151. Used by permission.)

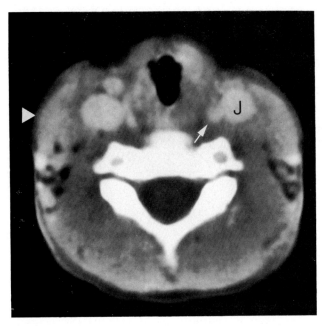

FIG 5–11.

Axial CT section through the high infrahyoid portion of the neck reveals the jugular vein *(J)* and the carotid artery *(arrow).* The sternocleidomastoid muscle is indicated by the *arrowhead.*

spaces. The superficial space extends from the hyoid downward to the sternum and upper margin of the clavicle and includes the sternocleidomastoid, trapezius, platysma, and inferior belly of the omohyoid muscles, as well as fat, blood vessels, cutaneous nerves, and lymph nodes. Immediately beneath the superficial space posteriorly is the posterior cervical space, formerly called the posterior triangle, and immediately deep to the superficial space anteriorly is the anterior cervical space. The middle or visceral space extends from the hyoid bone to the mediastinum and includes the thyroid and parathyroid glands, larynx, pharynx, trachea, esophagus, recurrent laryngeal nerves, infrahyoid strap muscles, and lymph nodes (Smoker). A third space is the deep or prevertebral space. It extends from the base of the skull to the coccyx and, in the neck, contains the prevertebral and scalene muscles, the brachial plexus, phrenic nerve, the vertebral vessels, and the vertebral body. In addition, the carotid and retropharyngeal spaces (including the "danger" space [Smoker]) are continuous from the suprahyoid portion of the neck to the mediastinum. The retropharyngeal space is a potential space anterior to the prevertebral space and normally contains only fat and lymph nodes.

CONGENITAL ABNORMALITIES

Torticollis (Wryneck)

Congenital wryneck is exceedingly rare and usually not associated with shortening of the sternocleidomastoid muscle or tumor formation within it. Instead, skeletal abnormalities such as Sprengel deformity, the Klippel-Feil syndrome, and multiple or single hemivertebrae are often the primary causes. Roentgen examination is essential for the satisfactory demonstration of these skeletal lesions. Muscular torticollis (fibromatosis colli), due to shortening of the sternocleidomastoid muscle, is a common lesion in infants. There are wide differences of opinion regarding the cause and causal mechanisms of both the muscular abnormality and the associated twist of the neck. The comprehensive monograph by Jones illustrates the uncertainties still remaining in a condition apparently recognized, and perhaps even treated, more than 2,000 years ago.

Included in the isolated muscular cases are patients with a sternomastoid "tumor" in infancy; those with diffuse fibrosis of the sternocleidomastoid muscle without a tumor, also presenting in infancy; and patients whose deformity was not appreciated until after the infant stage. The fibrotic changes in the sternocleidomastoid muscle are considered by some to be a form of juvenile fibromatosis. The muscular tumors became palpable between 1 and 15 weeks of age in 50 infants studied by MacDonald; one half of these were delivered by breech or forceps and one fourth were firstborn. Dunn found that the muscular swellings became palpable during the second postnatal week. In 12 of 61 infants with a tumor, discovery was made within the first week of life and primarily by the mother (Jones). Breech deliveries are very common in such

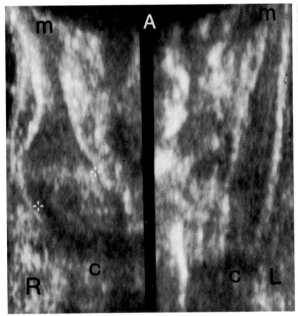

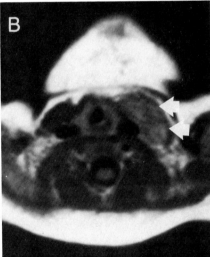

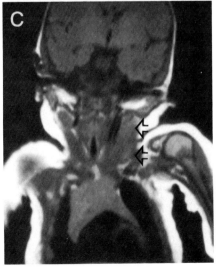

FIG 5–12.
A, composite coronal US views of the right and left neck region (*m,* mastoid region; *c,* clavicle) in a 5-week-old boy with torticollis, noted to have a hard 2- to 3-cm right neck swelling. On the left side *(L),* a lens-shaped section of normal sternocleidomastoid muscle is seen. On a comparable section of the right side *(R),* the muscle is expanded significantly in its lower half with patchy increased echogenicity centrally. These features are consistent with sternocleidomastoid muscle fibrosis. With massage and neck-stretching exercises, the swelling disappeared after several weeks. (Courtesy of Dr. R.G.K. McCauley, Boston.) **B,** axial and **C,** coronal T1-weighted MR images of another infant shows a mass *(arrows)* with intermediate signal intensity involving the sternocleidomastoid muscle.

patients. Transient torticollis and spontaneous recovery occurs in one fourth to one half of patients; this takes place within a few months after birth. About one third of the patients develop restriction of movement of the affected muscle after the tumor has disappeared, with some limitation of motion controlled by the muscle. Facial asymmetry and head tilt are mild or absent. In the remainder, progressive fibrosis of the muscle occurs and is associated with severe torticollis and early facial hemihypoplasia. The facial asymmetry may relate to mechanical flattening on the same side as the affected muscle. If the infant's sleeping position is largely prone, the face on the affected side is down and compressed; if the sleeping position is supine, the contralateral aspect of the cranium becomes plagiocephalic. These deformities occur in approximately 20% of cases. Thomsen and Koltai emphasize the resolution of mass or deformity with conservative management in the majority of patients. Wasting of the ipsilateral trapezius muscle may be associated.

Radiographic examination of the fibrotic sternocleidomastoid muscles and particularly of the lesion does not show any calcification. Lytic clavicular lesions have been reported in some cases at the site of the clavicular origins of the muscles. The chief value of x-ray examination lies in identification or exclusion of contributing skeletal abnormalities and the evaluation of alignment disturbances of which the progression or resolution may play a role in management. US reveals a hypoechoic, well-marginated mass within the surrounding normal muscle (Fig 5–12,A). It can be useful to differentiate the benign intramuscular tumor from cervical neuroblastoma, fibrosarcoma, and rhabdomyosarcoma. MRI has also been used (Fig 5–12,B and C), but in the typical clinical presentation these special procedures represent diagnostic overkill. In atypical cases, their contribution can be of value.

Wryneck may also occur in association with cervical lymphadenitis and retropharyngeal abscess as well as following upper pharyngeal surgery, as for tonsillectomy, and present as atlantoaxial rotatory subluxation. Localized inflammatory reaction is thought to promote lax capsular ligaments that permit excessive rotation and locking of the C1–2 articulating facets. It may also be a manifestation of posterior fossa and spinal tumors.

Hygromas (Cystic Lymphangiomas)

Hygromas are congenital abnormalities of the lymphatic system that are usually clinically evident at birth or may be diagnosed prenatally. Seventy per-

cent to 80% of hygromas occur in the neck, most commonly in the posterior cervical space (formerly called the posterior triangle). About 10% may extend into the mediastinum. They present as mass lesions, often quite large, but are soft and rarely cause airway obstruction. A primary mediastinal location without cervical involvement is rare but has been reported.

Most cystic hygromas occur in otherwise healthy children, but they have been diagnosed with prenatal sonography in fetuses with Turner syndrome (see Fig 44–27), Noonan syndrome, fetal alcohol syndrome, familial pterygium colli (Fryn syndrome), and several of the trisomy syndromes. Sonography reveals a multiloculated cystic mass with septa of variable thickness. Solid components may be seen to arise from cyst wall or from septa. Sonography is limited by its inability to fully define the extent of the lesion. On CT, the masses are avascular with attenuation values usually between 0 and 40 Hounsfield units (Fig 5–13). Smaller cysts are usually unilocular; larger ones may be septated. The fascial planes adjacent to the lesions are often poorly defined because cystic hygromas may infiltrate adjacent structures. On MRI, the lesions have a variable T1 time, probably because of varying amounts of protein content in the lymphatic fluid or because of hemorrhage; the T2 time is prolonged. CT or MRI may be useful to rule out mediastinal extension, thereby affecting the surgical approach.

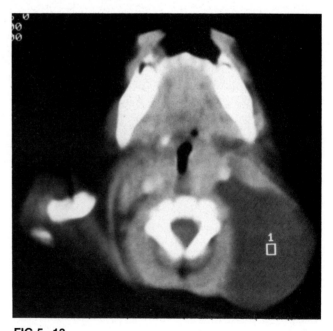

FIG 5–13.
Enhanced axial CT scan of a cystic hygroma shows a water attenuation mass in the lateral neck, posterior to the carotid space. The contents of a cystic hygroma may vary so that CT or MRI may show simple fluid, proteinaceous material, or fat.

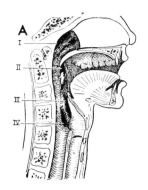
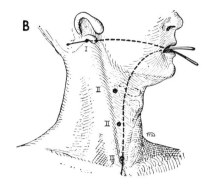

FIG 5–14.

A, sites of the cervical cysts and fistulas caused by persistence of the fetal pharyngeal pouches. **B,** sites of the cervical fistulas caused by persistence of the fetal branchial grooves. (From Arey LB: *Developmental Anatomy: A Textbook and Laboratory Manual of Embryology,* ed 3. Philadelphia, WB Saunders, 1937. Used by permission.)

Branchial Cleft Fistulas and Cysts

Cervical fistulas and cysts develop in the space immediately beneath the superficial spaces (i.e., the third branchial cyst develops in the posterior cervical space) from persistence of the branchial grooves or clefts externally and pharyngeal pouches internally, and from abnormal communications between them. The internal and external locations of the branchial fistulas and cysts are illustrated in Figure 5–14. The most common cystic mass results from the second branchial cleft along an embryologically defined line from the oropharyngeal tonsillar fossa to the supraclavicular region. These are found "wedged between the posterior submandibular space and carotid space presenting clinically as a mass at the angle of the jaw" (Vogelzand et al.) in older children or young adults. They displace the sternocleidomastoid muscles posteriorly or posterolaterally and displace the carotid-jugular complex posteriorly and medially. The cyst may occur alone or in conjunction with a sinus or fistula. On US, the mass is hypoechoic and unilocular. CT reveals an avascular mass with an enhancing rim that is thicker if the mass is chronically infected (Fig 5–15).

Thyroglossal Duct Cysts

Cysts that are derived from remnants of the thyroglossal duct are most often situated in the midline of the neck (Fig 5–16). Sixty-five percent occur below the level of the hyoid bone; in this location, they are characteristically embedded in the strap muscles. On US, these masses are usually cystic but may contain solid components or appear complex after hemorrhage. The characteristic CT appearance of a thyroglossal duct cyst is that of a well-circumscribed, low-density lesion with peripheral rim enhancement. Inflammation can alter the density of the cyst so that it

approaches or equals that of soft tissue. Septations are occasionally seen.

The absence of the normal "mass" anterior to the trachea (the thyroid gland) can be suggested by a ratio of measurements from the anterior border of the tracheal air column at the level of the cricoid cartilage constriction to the anterior fat–soft tissue interface and to the air-skin interface at the same level,

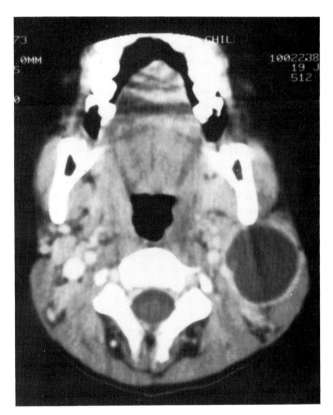

FIG 5–15.

Branchial cleft cyst. Axial contrast-enhanced CT scan of neck reveals a water-density mass with an enhancing rim posterior and lateral to the parapharyngeal space, behind the parotid space, and lateral to the carotid space.

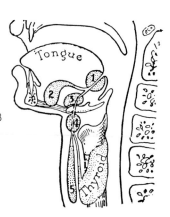

FIG 5–16.
Course of the thyroglossal duct and common sites *(1–5)* for cysts derived from it. (From Arey LB: *Developmental Anatomy: A Textbook and Laboratory Manual of Embryology,* ed 3. Philadelphia, WB Saunders, 1937. Used by permission.)

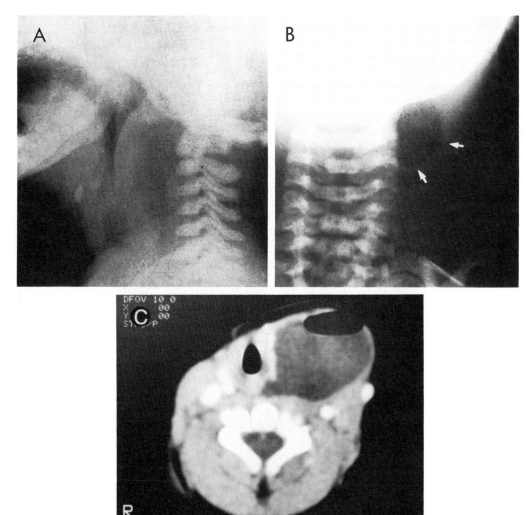

FIG 5–17.
A and **B,** pharyngeal diverticulum in newborn infant with neck swelling at 12 hours, increasing with first feeding. Progressive respiratory distress at 24 hours required excision and closure of communication. The cyst wall was lined with stratified squamous epithelium; there were mild acute and chronic inflammatory reaction and thyroid follicles, but no lymphoid aggregates were present. (Courtesy of Dr. J.B. Campbell, Denver, Colo.) **C,** pyriform sinus cyst that presented as an asymptomatic left cervical mass in a 1-week-old infant. US demonstrated a hypoechoic mass adjacent to the left lobe of the thyroid. CT demonstrates the anatomy in better detail. The intracystic gas apparently developed when the infant cried during placement of an intravenous needle prior to the CT examination. (Courtesy of Dr. Eric Effmann, Duke University, Durham, N.C., from Tyler D, Effmann E, Shorter NA: *J Pediatr Surg,* in press, 1991.)

according to Mahboubi et al. Normal subjects have a mean pretracheal ratio of 70 (range, 60–85) whereas hypothyroid patients without goiters and patients with ectopic thyroids have a mean ratio of 36 with a range of 25 to 50. The presence of a mass at the base of the tongue resembling an enlarged lingual tonsil in association with a low ratio suggests that this mass is a lingual thyroid. Confirmation of ectopic thyroid tissue in this position and others can be made with radionuclide scintigraphy.

Other Congenital Masses

A mass lesion may be produced by distention of a pharyngeal diverticulum with gas or fluid (Fig 5–17,A). It may compromise the upper airway in the newborn. Its communication with the lateral recess of the pharynx and the incorporation of thymic or thyroid tissue, or both, in its wall favor its origin from the branchial clefts. The cystic structure illustrated in Figure 5–17,B occurs when there is a fistula extending from the pyriform sinus to the thyroid gland. These are almost always on the left side and are associated with a cyst or abscess and, often, with recurrent suppurative thyroiditis. They can be identified by US or CT. Ranulas are uncommon cystic masses in the floor of the mouth in the newborn but have imaging characteristics similar to those occurring later. Other rare parenchymal cysts arising in the lower part of the neck are those of parathyroid, thyroid, or cervical thymic origin (Fig 5–18). An anterior cervical myelomeningocele is a rare malforma-

tion that may simulate a cystic hygroma on US. Pseudodiverticula of the pharynx acquired in the newborn period are described in Chapter 25.

INFLAMMATORY MASSES

Inflammatory masses in the superficial soft tissues are usually related to lymphadenitis or infection of a congenital cyst. A diagnosis of lymphadenitis is established clinically. US, CT, or MRI may be used to delineate the extent of the lesion and to try and differentiate cellulitis from an abscess (Fig 5–19). Any of the aforementioned parenchymal cysts may become infected; acute suppurative thyroiditis is a rare condition in childhood but, when present, occurs most often in the left lobe of the gland and is associated with a congenital fistula from the left pyriform sinus.

NEOPLASMS

Most neck masses in infants and children are of congenital or inflammatory origin. The incidence of inflammatory lesions is underestimated in most published series, as these infrequently come to histologic evaluation. In a recent article by Torsigliere et al., 55% of all lesions were congenital (branchial cleft cyst, 17%; thyroglossal duct cyst, 16%; dermoid cyst, 10%; lymphangioma, 8%; hemangioma, 2%). Inflammatory lesions represented 27% of the total with most being reactive lymphadenopathy. Malignant lesions represented 11% of the group with the most

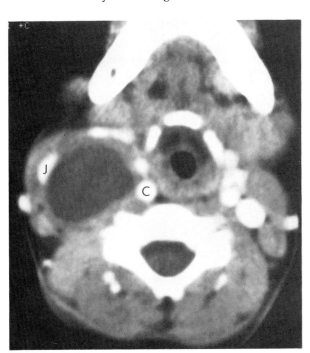

FIG 5–18.
Cervical thymic cyst. A contrast-enhanced CT scan of the neck of a 4-year-old girl reveals a water-density mass, apparently arising in the carotid sheath, that widely separates the jugular vein *(J)* and the carotid artery *(C)*. This location suggests a cervical thymic cyst, which was surgically proved.

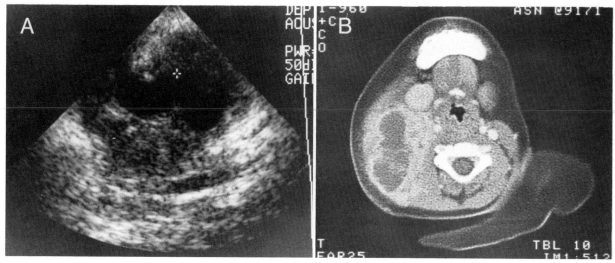

FIG 5–19.
Cervical abscess. **A,** US examination in a 1-year-old child reveals an irregular sonolucent mass surrounded by a hypoechoic area, which is consistent with an abscess with surrounding edema. **B,** a contrast-enhanced CT scan, same patient, reveals a well-defined, hypolucent area with an enhancing rim.

prevalent lesion being lymphoma (8%), thyroid carcinoma (1%), and a combination of rhabdomyosarcoma, neuroblastoma, histiocytosis, and fibrous histiocytoma accounting for 1% (Figs 5–20 and 5–21). In other studies (Cotton et al.), the incidence of rhabdomyosarcoma and neuroblastoma was somewhat greater. The location of the lesion gives a hint as to its origin, since those anterior to the sterno-cleidomastoid muscle in the submandibular space are more likely to be inflammatory or benign neoplastic lesions, while those more posteriorly located are more likely to be lymphoma or neuroblastoma (Table 5–2). The majority of thyroid lesions should be considered to be malignant until proved otherwise. The major cervical site of rhabdomyosarcoma is high in the posterior nasopharynx. Though rare, the overwhelming majority of pediatric salivary malignancies are located in the parotid gland (see Fig 5–20), and therefore focal parotid lesions should be examined histologically.

The age differential was interesting in the study of Torsiglieri et al. The lymphoma patients ranged in age from 4 to 21 years with an average of 11.7 years. In a large study of cervical neuroblastoma patients (Cushing et al.), none of the children at the time of diagnosis were over 2½ years old, and only two of the six were over 6 months old. Cervical neuroblastoma patients may present with a calcified (50%) cervical mass, inability to feed, Horner syndrome, or changes in color of the iris. Other neck masses that may calcify include hemangiomas, hematomas, teratomas, and chronic infections, especially granulomatous ones, such as those caused by atypical mycobacteria.

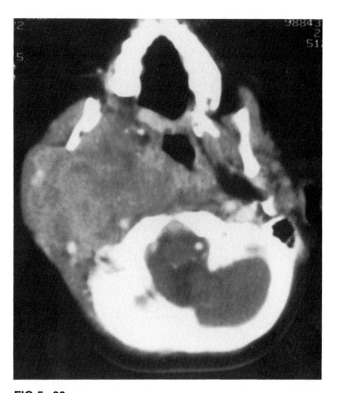

FIG 5–20.
Rhabdomyosarcoma of the parotid. Axial contrast-enhanced CT scan of a 6-year-old girl reveals obliteration of the right parapharyngeal space, separation of the vessels in the carotid sheath, involvement of the pterygoid muscles, and deviation of the hypopharynx. The mass enhances irregularly.

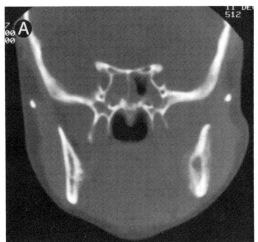
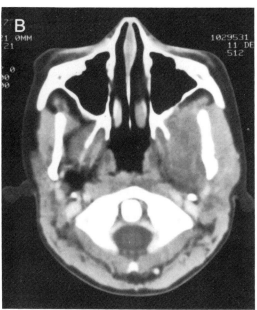

FIG 5–21.
Leukemic invasion of the masticator space. **A,** coronal CT scan shows permeation and destruction of the left mandible. **B,** axial contrast-enhanced CT scan reveals the left parapharyngeal space to be pushed medially and compressed. The pterygoid muscles are infiltrated and of low density with irregular enhancement.

The sonographic study of long-term survivors of Hodgkin's disease (Soberman et al., 1991) has added significant information to the pathophysiology of thyroid cancer. US detected abnormalities in 16 of 18 patients including diffuse atrophy (6), solitary nodules (4), multiple nodules (5), and gland heterogeneity with calcification (1). Of these 18 patients who had received radiation, with a mean of 6.4 years follow-up, one had multiple foci of papillary carcinoma.

The pediatric AIDS patient may present with a cervical mass. Most frequently, these are lymphoepithelial lesions occurring in lymph nodes and the parotid gland (Soberman et al.).

OROPHARYNX AND NASOPHARYNX

Most lesions of the tongue are obvious on direct visual inspection. Encroachment on the airway may result from either macroglossia (Beckwith-Wiedemann syndrome, hypothyroidism) or micrognathia (Pierre Robin syndrome or the cerebrocostomandibular syndrome). Hemangioma and lymphangioma may cause enlargement of the tongue. Other mass lesions include thyroglossal duct cyst, ectopic thyroid, and dermoid cyst. If further investigation beyond a lateral radiograph of the neck is necessary, the extent of these lesions is well demonstrated by MRI (Figs 5–22 and 5–23). Thyroid scintigraphy should be performed prior to surgical intervention to exclude the possibility that a mass represents ectopic thyroid tissue that is the only thyroid tissue in the body.

Ranulas (Latin diminutive of *rana,* frog) are cysts occurring in the floor of the mouth resulting from retention or extravasation of secretions from the sublingual gland; they are so named because the thin, flabby, cyst wall resembles the belly of a tadpole. They present clinically as a sublingual, submandibular, or upper cervical mass. The simple ranula, a retention cyst of salivary gland origin, has an intact wall; the "plunging" or "diving" ranula extends beyond the sublingual region where it originates into the deep fascial planes of the neck, usually because of extravasation. Both types are ideally identified by MRI but can be visualized also by CT (Figs 5–24 and 5–25). The differential diagnosis includes cystic hygroma, cervical adenitis, branchial cleft cyst, thyroglossal duct cyst, dermoid, and epidermoid cyst.

Tonsils and Adenoids

Normal adenoid tissue becomes visible in lateral radiographs of the nasopharynx at between 3 and 6 months of age. A lack of development suggests agammaglobulinemia. Grossly enlarged adenoids (Fig 5–26) can produce narrowing of the nasopharyngeal airway; enlarged palatine tonsils (Fig 5–27) can contribute, and the combination may result in hypercapnea, hypoxia, and cardiomegaly. The ob-

TABLE 5–2.

Differential Diagnostic Considerations in the More Common
Pediatric Neck Lesions by Anatomical Space Location

Suprahyoid Neck
  Masticator space
    Hemangioma
    Cystic hygroma-lymphangioma
    Mandibular osteomyelitis
    Lymphoma, leukemia
  Carotid space
    Neurofibroma
    Neural sheath tumors
  Parotid space
    Branchial cleft cyst
    Hemangioma
    Cystic hygroma-lymphangioma
    Parotid tumors
    Lymphoepithelial lesions of acquired immunodeficiency
      syndrome
    Reactive lymphadenopathy
  Retropharyngeal space
    Abscess
    Cellulitis
    Neuroblastoma (from prevertebral space)
    Hematoma

Infrahyoid neck
  Superficial space
    Rare muscle tumors
  Anterior and posterior cervical space
    Cystic hygroma-lymphangioma
    Branchial cleft cyst (3rd) in posterior cervical space
  Visceral space
    Thyroglossal duct cysts
    Aberrant thyroid tissue
    Esophageal duplication
    Lymphoma
    Abscess
    Cellulitis
  Carotid space
    Abscess
    Cellulitis
    Neural sheath tumor
  Retropharyngeal space (includes "danger" space)
    Abscess
    Cellulitis
    Lymphoma
    Hematoma

Transpatial lesions*
  Developmental
    Cystic hygroma-lymphangioma
    Hemangioma
    Thyroglossal duct cyst
    Branchial cleft cyst
  Infectious
    Abscess
    Cellulitis
  Neoplastic
    Lymphoma

*Modified from Vogelzang P, Harnsberger HR, Smoker WRK: *Semin Ultra-sound CT MR* 1991; 12:274–287.

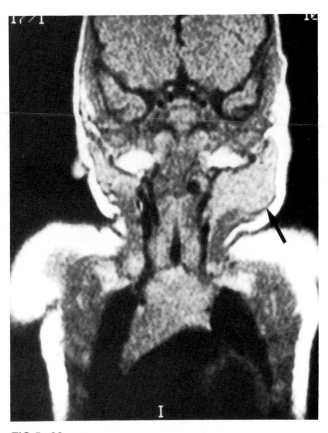

FIG 5–22.
Nondescent of the left thymic component. Coronal T1-weighted
MR image of a 4-month-old infant with a left neck mass *(arrow)*.
The intensity is equal to that of the normally positioned thymus.

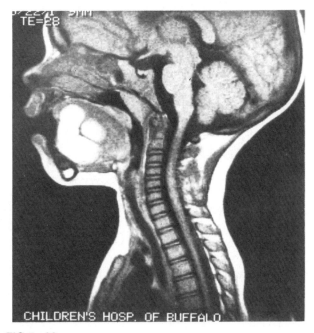

FIG 5–23.
Sublingual dermoid cyst. Sagittal T1-weighted MRI reveals a sep-tated mass that has a short T1 and is therefore bright. The mass
displaces the tongue superiorly and posteriorly.

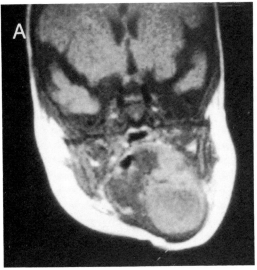
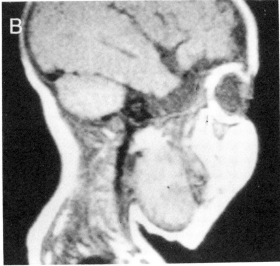

FIG 5–24.
Plunging ranula in a 2-month-old infant with a neck mass that had been enlarging for 2 weeks. Coronal and sagittal T2-weighted MR images (**A** and **B**) demonstrate a cystic mass in the floor of the mouth, in continuity with the left sublingual gland, displacing the base of the tongue posteriorly. Increased signal intensity in the floor of the mouth indicated inflammation. (From Matt BH, Crockett DM: *Otolaryngol Head Neck Surg* 1988; 99:330–333. Used by permission.)

struction causes alveolar hypoventilation and secondary pulmonary hypertension. Introduction of an airway and restoration of adequate ventilation reverses the pathophysiology.

Retropharyngeal and Parapharyngeal Tissues

Thickening of the retropharyngeal tissues may be simulated on a lateral film made with the patient in partial expiration or with the neck flexed. Repeat examination, with attention to exposure during inspiration, will usually establish the normality of the structures. The most common cause of true thickening of the retropharyngeal tissues is inflammation. A majority of retropharyngeal abscesses occur in children between 6 and 12 months of age. Retropharyngeal and retroesophageal abscesses produce convex thickening of the retropharyngeal-retroesophageal

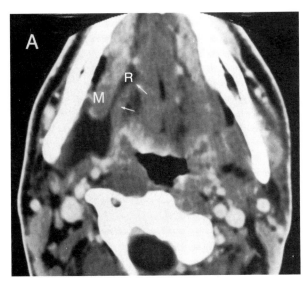
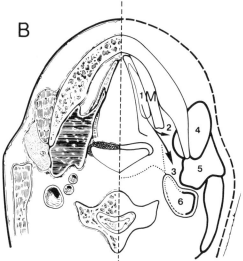

FIG 5–25.
A, plunging (or diving) ranula demonstrated by CT. The tail *(arrows)* of the ranula *(R)* is the clue to its origin and nature. The myelohyoid muscle *(M)* divides the floor of the mouth into the sublingual space and the submandibular space (*1* and *2* in **B**) that are continuous with the parapharyngeal space *(3)* and adjacent spaces. **B,** diagram of **A** and pertinent anatomy: *4,* masticator space; *5,* parotid space; *6,* carotid space. (From Coit WE, Harnsberger JR, Osborn AG, et al: *Radiology* 1987; 163:211–216. Used by permission.)

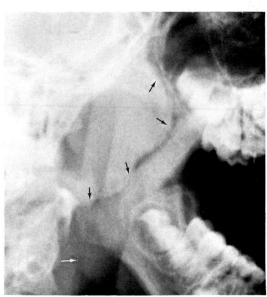

FIG 5–26.
Massive obstructive hypertrophy of the adenoids *(upper arrows)* with relatively small palatine tonsils *(lower arrows)* in a girl 5 years of age.

spaces (Fig 5–28), which displaces the parapharyngeal space anteriorly and laterally. The esophagus, larynx, and trachea are pushed forward. The normal cervical lordotic curve may be straightened or reversed owing to muscle spasm that, at times, may be so extreme as to suggest subluxation. Torticollis is often present. The malalignment, which affects the upper cervical vertebrae, disappears with resolution of the inflammatory process; the sequence of symptoms and signs has been called Grisel syndrome. Retropharyngeal calcific tendinitis affecting the longus colli muscle occurs primarily in adults, but rare instances are reported in childhood. The clinical features can be mistaken for those of retropharyngeal

or peritonsilar abscess, and the diagnosis is supported by the observation of amorphous calcification anterior to C1 or C2.

Plain radiography is limited in its ability to distinguish between retropharyngeal or parapharyngeal cellulitis and an abscess. CT cannot always be used to localize the abscess accurately and determine if there is drainable pus, but a low-density center surrounded by an enhancing rim, when present, is characteristic of an abscess (Fig 5–29). An abscess may extend into the neck up to the level of the ear or even down into the thorax (see Fig 5–28). Other conditions that cause thickening of the retropharyngeal tissues are uncommon but include hemorrhage,

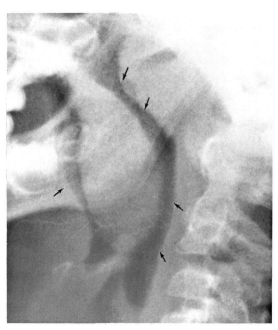

FIG 5–27.
Massive enlargement of the palatine tonsils in a lateral projection of the nasopharynx of a girl 3 years of age who had had recurrent cervical and submandibular hypertrophic lymphadenitis. Superimposition of the uvula produces spurious continuity of the tonsils with the palate.

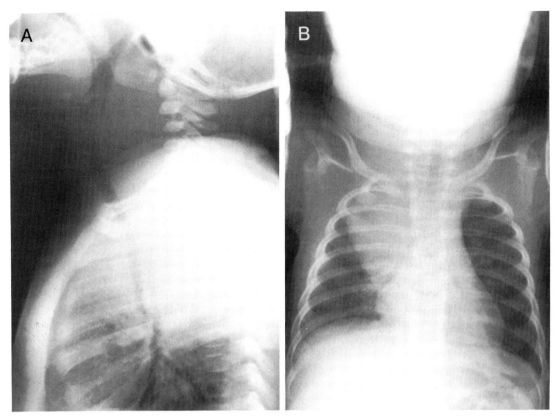

FIG 5–28.
Retropharyngeal abscess with extension into the posterior mediastinum. **A,** lateral view shows the marked increase of the retropharyngeal space, with anterior deviation of the trachea within both neck and thorax. **B,** frontal chest film shows the extension of this retropharyngeal abscess into the posterosuperior mediastinum on the right.

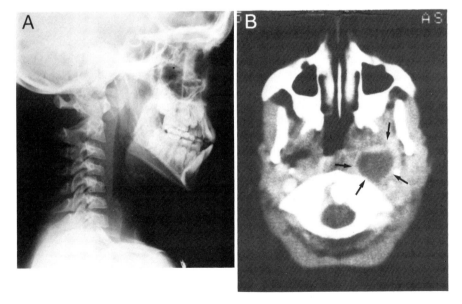

FIG 5–29.
Parapharyngeal abscess in a 12-year-old boy. **A,** a lateral radiograph of the neck shows slight straightening of the cervical lordotic curve, but no mass lesion is apparent. **B,** a contrast-enhanced CT scan, same patient, shows a well-defined low-density area with an enhancing rim *(arrows),* which is characteristic of an abscess.

especially in hemophilia; neuroblastoma; anterior myelomeningocele; and congenital hypothyroidism.

THYROID SCINTIGRAPHY IN PEDIATRICS*

The thyroid uptake of radioactive iodine may be quantitated. Scintigraphy for the study of thyroid function has continued to be a routine diagnostic tool even though more sophisticated procedures, such as the determination of thyroid hormone and thyroid-stimulating hormone (TSH) levels, are now available. The uptake test is based upon the fact that the administered radiopharmaceutical will be concentrated by the gland in a manner that reflects the thyroid's handling of dietary iodine and thereby reveals the functional status of the gland.

Technetium 99m pertechnetate is usually preferred over ^{123}I and ^{131}I because of the marked decrease in absorbed thyroid dose. There is a sevenfold reduction when ^{99m}Tc pertechnetate is used in comparison with ^{123}I, and ^{131}I has an even higher exposure. The major indications for the use of thyroid scintigraphy in pediatrics are:

1. Evaluation of neonatal hypothyroidism.
2. Evaluation of possible hyperthyroidism.
3. Evaluation of a thyroid nodule or a midline neck mass.

Neonatal thyroid screening reveals an incidence of elevated TSH of 1 in 4,254 to 1 in 5,200 births. The goal of imaging is to detect any functioning thyroid tissue, be it in normal position or ectopic position. ^{99m}Tc pertechnetate scintigraphy is very helpful in meeting these goals and is more reliable than US in detecting the ectopic gland. Detection of the ectopic gland is crucial, as it may support growth and development for a few months, after which it may fail, leading to defective brain development. A pitfall of using ^{99m}Tc pertechnetate in the neonate with a high TSH level is that a normal-appearing gland does not exclude an organification defect (conversion of iodide to iodine and binding to tyrosine in thyroglobulin). In these rare instances (elevated TSH and normal-appearing thyroid gland on scintigraphy), ^{123}I administration with perchlorate washout is required. If the iodide is trapped by the thyroid cells but not organified, it will be released when perchlorate is given.

In the evaluation of hyperthyroidism, the uptake of ^{123}I at 4 and 24 hours after administration is measured in conjunction with imaging to identify diffuse hyperthyroidism and differentiate it from a function-

ing autonomous nodule. The normal range for uptake in most of the United States is about 5% to 12% at 4 hours and 10% to 40% at 24 hours. If the uptake values are elevated and the patient is hyperthyroid, propylthiouracil may be administered and will often control the hyperthyroidism. Eventually, breakthrough or drug reaction may occur, necessitating subtotal thyroidectomy or ^{131}I ablation of the gland. In general, ^{131}I ablation is safer than surgery and results in fewer relapses. The risk of thyroid cancer is not increased by the ablation. In the usual case, the child will be rendered permanently hypothyroid and require lifetime thyroid replacement therapy. A functioning autonomous nodule may also be treated with ^{131}I or surgery.

The third indication for thyroid scintigraphy in pediatrics is evaluation of a thyroid nodule or neck mass. Most pertinent data on thyroid nodules come from evaluation of schoolchildren in the major atomic fallout area, and nonfallout areas, of Utah, Nevada, and Arizona. Of 5,179 children studied, 93 were found to have nodular thyroid glands. Thirty-four were nodular because of adolescent lobulation, a normal finding; 31 had thyroiditis. Only two of the 5,179 children had thyroid cancer, and neither of these thyroid cancers occurred in the fallout area of Utah-Nevada. This is the most carefully performed epidemiologic study of thyroid cancer to have been completed in the United States. It is likely that these two cancers might not have been discovered until adulthood if the screening program had not detected them.

The 1990 Biological Effects of Ionizing Radiation (BEIR) report on the health effects of ionizing radiation suggests the following generalizations with respect to which patients are at increased risk for thyroid carcinoma after therapeutic radiation to the neck:

1. Susceptibility is maximal in early childhood.
2. Females are two to three times more susceptible than males.
3. Radiogenic cancer is frequently associated with benign nodules; most cancers are papillary carcinomas; growth is increased by hormonal stimulation.

The Israel tinea study and the Rochester thymus irradiation study suggest that the relative risk after 1 Gy (100 rads) for ages 6 months to 15 years is 8.3 compared with that of the control population. The effect of lower exposures can only be extrapolated from the 1-Gy exposure range.

In children exposed to significant therapeutic radiation, the incidence of thyroid carcinoma is 7 per

---

*This section prepared by L.R. Kuhns, M.D.

100 in childhood, and the risk continues to rise in adulthood. In these patients, more careful follow-up by clinical examination and imaging is imperative.

In any patient, when a cold nodule is detected by ^{99m}Tc pertechnetate, several approaches are possible. US may be used to determine if the nodule is cystic or solid. Fourteen percent of cystic thyroid lesions were malignant in an adult series; no pediatric series is presently available. Needle aspiration requires expertise of both the operator and the cytopathologist. In many children's facilities, these experienced personnel are not available, so both cystic and solid cold nodules are often removed by the pediatric surgeon.

Any neck mass between the base of the tongue and the suprasternal notch may represent ectopic thyroid tissue. If the patient is euthyroid, removal of this thyroid tissue in an ectopic location can induce hypothyroidism. In such patients, a ^{99m}Tc pertechnetate scan is obtained preoperatively to determine if the mass is of thyroid origin and whether it is the only functioning thyroid tissue. Removal under these circumstances would be detrimental to the patient.

LARYNX AND CERVICAL TRACHEA

Anatomy

The larynx extends from the base of the tongue to the trachea. Its skeletal framework consists of three single cartilages (epiglottis, thyroid, and cricoid) and three smaller pairs of cartilages (arytenoid, cuneiform, and corniculate). The hyoid bone encircles the upper end of the epiglottis from the sides and in front; it may be ossified, even at birth. The epiglottis forms the anterior boundary of the supraglottic larynx. It is a thin, leaf-shaped cartilage that arches diagonally posteriorly and superiorly from the anterior portion of the thyroid cartilage to the root of the tongue. The aryepiglottic folds extend from the posterior surface of the epiglottis in a lateral inferior and posterior direction to the arytenoid cartilages. The aryepiglottic folds separate the central laryngeal vestibule from the paired lateral pyriform sinuses, which lie just medial to the thyroid cartilage. The pyriform sinuses increase in size with pharyngeal distention. On an anteroposterior (AP) radiograph, their inferior tip marks the level of the laryngeal ventricle. The thyroid cartilage is shield-shaped and formed of two laminae that meet in the midline anteriorly. Superior and inferior cornua are present posteriorly. In children, the thyroid cartilage usually

is not ossified. The interior of the larynx extends from its origin at the epiglottis to its lower limits at the inferior edge of the cricoid cartilage. It is generally divided into three portions. The supraglottic larynx contains the epiglottis, the aryepiglottic folds, and the false vocal cords. The glottic portion extends from the laryngeal ventricle below the false cords to the inferior margin of the true cords. The subglottic region extends from the inferior margin of the glottis to the lower edge of the cricoid cartilage. The cricoid cartilage itself is shaped like a signet ring and is normally the only complete ring in the airway.

Supraglottic Abnormalities

Larynx

Laryngomalacia is a common cause of inspiratory stridor in the first year of life. It is a self-limited condition that is thought to be related to inherent softness of the supraglottic structures. The diagnosis can be confirmed by endoscopy, by cross-table lateral fluoroscopy, or by cine-CT. Because of the symptoms of stridor, the much more frequent laryngomalacia is commonly confused with "tracheomalacia." Tracheomalacia refers to an abnormal tracheal collapse.

Epiglottitis

The most common lesion of the epiglottis, acute epiglottitis, is usually caused by *Haemophilus influenzae* infection and presents with symptoms of acute respiratory obstruction associated with high fever, dysphagia, and prostration. Its peak incidence is in children between 3 and 6 years of age. It is one of the most dangerous causes of acute upper airway obstruction. If there is any clinical question about the diagnosis, the patient should be accompanied to the radiology department by a physician prepared to introduce an airway. An upright, lateral radiograph of the lower part of the face and neck is then obtained to demonstrate the typical enlargement of the epiglottis and aryepiglottic folds (Fig 5–30). Approximately 25% of affected children will also have subglottic edema, as in croup. Although the epiglottis is enlarged, the accompanying edema of the aryepiglottic folds may be primarily responsible for the airway obstruction.

The major differential diagnoses are croup, foreign body, or retropharyngeal abscess. Other conditions associated with enlargement of the epiglottis include hereditary angioneurotic edema, aryepiglottic or epiglottic cysts, and hemophilia.

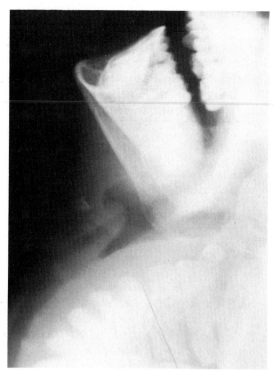

FIG 5–30.
Acute epiglottitis. Note the swollen epiglottis protruding into the posterior pharyngeal airspace and the marked extension of the neck and the dilated pharynx.

Glottic Abnormalities

Anomalies of the glottic portion of the larynx are rare in children. Vocal cord paralysis can be suspected at birth because of respiratory embarrassment unrelated to chest disease or inspiratory stridor with crying. Of the 149 infants and children described by Holinger et al., 82 had congenital lesions; in 42 (51%) of these, other congenital anomalies were present. Fifty-nine of the infants had secondary vocal cord paralysis related to meningomyelocele, Arnold-Chiari malformation, and hydrocephalus. In all of the congenitally affected infants, the vocal cords were in the abducted position, allowing for phonation but causing respiratory distress because of the narrow airway. In 8 of the 149 patients, the cause of the vocal cord paralysis could not be ascertained. The radiographic diagnosis of vocal cord paralysis is best determined on high-kilovoltage magnification films in the frontal projection on fluoroscopy (Fig 5–31).

Laryngotracheal-esophageal cleft occurs much less frequently than does tracheoesophageal fistula but probably is embryologically related. The most common form is a posterior laryngeal cleft or laryngeal fistula. Calcification of the cartilages of the lar-

ynx may occur in association with that of the trachea in chondrodystrophia punctata.

Multiple benign epithelial papillomas are the most common laryngeal tumors in infancy and childhood. Two thirds of affected children are less than 4 years of age at the time of the onset of symptoms. The diagnosis is made on endoscopy by identification of nodules on the vocal cords. The lesions may seed inferiorly into the tracheobronchial tree and lung as described in Chapter 13.

Subglottic Abnormalities

Croup

This very common cause of acute upper airway obstruction occurs in infants and young children, usually from 6 months to 3 years of age, and is most commonly caused by viral infection. The child typically presents with a short history of upper respiratory infection and a harsh, often brassy or barking cough followed by inspiratory stridor. Radiographic examination is not necessary in the classic case but is valuable to exclude other causes of respiratory distress, such as foreign body aspiration or epiglottitis. On high-kilovoltage AP projections of the neck, edema of the subglottic mucosa narrows the tracheal air column for about 5 to 10 mm or more below the level of the vocal cords, where the normal width of the column is resumed, resulting in an upward tapering appearance (Fig 5–32). Normally, the tracheal air column maintains an almost uniform width up to the vocal cord region, the level of which can be identified on a film exposed during inspiration by the inferior tips of the air-containing, pyriform sinuses. Subglottic and proximal tracheal stenosis, as well as radiolucent foreign body in the subglottic mucosa, may simulate the findings in croup; persistence of the swelling and the symptoms for 7 days or longer warrants endoscopic evaluation.

Membranous croup has similar radiographic findings, but an inflammatory membrane can be observed endoscopically in the subglottic area. Membranous croup is often more severe than the viral form and is associated with superimposed bacterial infection.

The radiographic features of subglottic stenosis (Fig 5–33) may resemble those of croup; in congenital cases, the onset of stridor is much earlier than in patients with the infectious disorder. The condition can be acquired in infants who have undergone prolonged tracheal intubation, or following tracheostomy. A variant of the congenital form is associated with an elliptic cricoid cartilage, in which case an

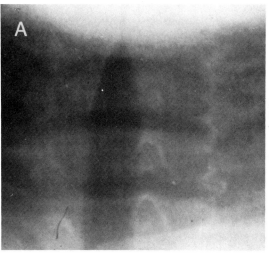

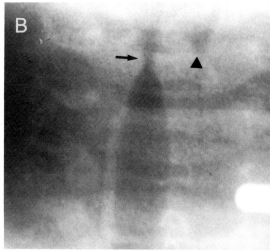

FIG 5–31.
Vocal cord paralysis in a 3-year-old. **A,** during phonation, the cords are medially positioned. **B,** during quiet respiration, the true cords *(arrow)* are in the paramedian position. Note the pyriform si-nus *(arrowhead)* indicating the level of the true cords. This is the widest the airway ever got at the level of the vocal cords.

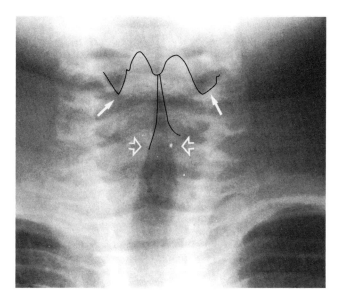

FIG 5–32.
AP view of the upper airway in a child with croup. The *upper arrows* indicate the level of the pyriform sinuses which are related to the level of the vocal cords. It is at this level that the normal trachea achieves almost its full subglottic diameter instead of tapering upward from the level of the *lower arrows* as a result of subglottic edema in croup.

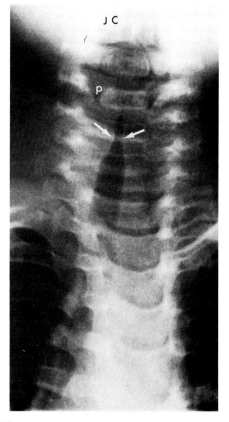

FIG 5–33.
Congenital subglottic stenosis. A long, relatively narrow, fixed area of stenosis extends from the vocal cords inferiorly *(arrows)*. The tip of the pyriform sinus *(p)* is at the level of the vocal cords.

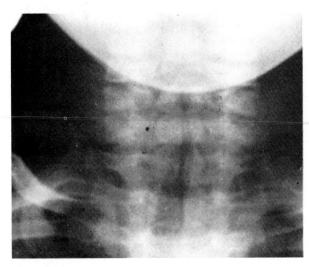

FIG 5–34.
AP projection of the upper portion of the trachea with subglottic hemangioma. Note the asymmetric narrowing of the lumen opposite the *black dot*. The narrowed lumen is superimposed on the still-open synchondroses of the neural arches of the cervical and upper thoracic vertebrae. The symmetric pyriform sinuses can be seen just below the curved edge of the mandible with the air-containing ventricle between them; this indicates a subglottic location of the obstruction.

hourglass constriction may be seen in the subglottic area.

Subglottic hemangioma is a rare cause of stridor in infants. Classic radiographic features are asymmetric narrowing of the subglottic trachea (Fig 5–34), but the narrowing may be symmetric. Affected infants usually develop stridulous breathing during the second half of the first year, at the time when cutaneous hemangiomas enlarge rapidly. Acquired subglottic cysts may present the same radiographic appearance according to Holinger et al., who recommend direct laryngoscopy for differential diagnosis. Rarely, dyspnea can result from cervical thymic tissue that is ectopic, or from an undescended thymic remnant in the submucosa of the airway (see Fig 5–18).

REFERENCES

Arey LB: *Developmental Anatomy: A Textbook and Laboratory Manual of Embryology,* ed 3. Philadelphia, WB Saunders, 1937.

Ben-Ami T, Yousefzadeh DK, Aramburo MJ: Presuppurative phase of retropharyngeal infection: Contribution of ultrasonography in the diagnosis and treatment. *Pediatr Radiol* 1990; 21:23–26.

Benanti JC, Gramling P, Bulat PI, et al: Retropharyngeal calcific tendinitis: Report of five cases and review of the literature. J *Emerg Med* 1986; 4:15–24.

Bistritzer T, et al: Severe dyspnea and dysphagia resulting from an aberrant cervical thymus. *Eur J Pediatr* 1985; 144:86–88.

Coit WE, Harnsberger HR, Osborn AG, et al: Ranulas and their mimics: CT evaluation. *Radiology* 1987; 163:211–216.

Cotton RT, Ballard ET, Going JA, et al: Tumors of the head and neck in children, in Thawley SE, Panje WR (eds): *Comprehensive Management of Head and Neck Tumors,* vol 2. Philadelphia, WB Saunders, 1987.

Cushing BA, Slovis TL, Philippart AI, et al: A rational approach to cervical neuroblastoma. *Cancer* 1982:50:785–787.

Dubousset J: Torticollis in children caused by congenital anomalies of the axis. *J Bone Joint Surg [Am]* 1986; 68:178–188.

Dunn PM: Congenital postural deformities: Further perinatal associations. *Proc R Soc Med* 1974; 67:1174–1178.

Fisher DA, Dussault JH, Foley TP Jr, et al: Screening for congenital hypothyroidism: Results of screening one million North American infants. *J Pediatr* 1979; 94:700–705.

Harnsberger HR: *Handbook of Radiology: Head and Neck Imaging.* St Louis, Mosby–Year Book, 1990.

Harnsberger HR (ed): The suprahyoid neck: A spatial approach. *Semin Ultrasound CT MR* 1990; 11:433–533.

Harnsberger HR, Osborn AG: Differential diagnosis of head and neck lesions on their space of origin. 1. The suprahyoid part of the neck. *Am J Roentgenol* 1991; 157:147–154.

Hensinger RN: Orthopedic problems of the shoulder and neck. *Pediatr Clin North Am* 1986; 33:1495–1509.

Holinger LD, Holinger PC, Holinger PH: Etiology of bilateral abductor vocal cord paralysis. A review of 389 cases *Ann Otol Rhinol Laryngol* 1976; 85:428–436.

Holinger PC, Holinger LD, Reichert TJ, et al: Respiratory obstruction and apnea in infants with bilateral abductor vocal cord paralysis, meningomyelocele, hydrocephalus, and Arnold-Chiari malformation. *J Pediatr* 1978; 82:368–373.

Holinger PH, Kutnick SL, Schild JA, et al: Subglottic stenosis in infants and children. *Ann Otol Rhinol Laryngol* 1976: 85:591–599.

Holinger LD, Toriumi DM, Anandappa EC: Subglottic cysts and asymmetrical subglottic narrowing on neck radiograph. *Pediatr Radiol* 1988; 18:306–308.

Jones PG: *Torticollis in Infancy and Childhood: Sternomastoid Fibrosis and the Sternomastoid "Tumor."* Springfield, Ill, Thomas, 1968.

Joseph PM, Berdon WE, Baker DH, et al: Upper airway obstruction in infants and small children: Improved radiographic diagnosis by combining filtration, high kilovoltage, and magnification. *Radiology* 1976; 121:143–148.

Kirshenbaum KJ, Hadimpalli SR, Friedman M, et al: Benign lymphoepithelial parotid tumors in AIDS patients: CT and MR findings in 9 cases. *AJNR* 1991; 12:271–274.

Kraus R, Han BK, Babcock DS, et al: Sonography of neck masses in children. *Am J Roentgenol* 1986; 146:609–613.

Lorman JG, et al: The Eagle syndrome. *Am J Roentgenol* 1983; 140:881–882.

Lucaya J, Berdon WE, Enriquez G, et al: Congenital pyriform sinus fistula: A cause of acute left-sided suppurative thyroiditis and neck abscess in children. *Pediatr Radiol* 1990; 21:27–29.

MacDonald D: Sternomastoid tumor and muscular torticollis. *J Bone Joint Surg [Br]* 1969; 51B:432–443.

Mahboubi S, Tenore A, Kirkpatrick JA: Diagnosis of ectopic thyroid: Value of pretracheal soft-tissue measurements. *Am J Roentgenol* 1981; 137:717–719.

Matt BH, Crockett DM: Plunging ranula in an infant. *Otolaryngol Head Neck Surg* 1988; 99:330–333.

McHenry C, Smith M, Lawrence AM, et al: Nodular thyroid disease in children and adolescents: A high incidence of carcinoma. *Am Surg* 1988; 54:444–447.

Mlnarski FG, Parnes SM, Polanski S: Congenital calcifications of the larynx and trachea. *Otolaryngol Head Neck Surg* 1985; 93:99–101.

Muir A, Daneman MB, Daneman A, et al: Thyroid scanning, ultrasound, and serum thyroglobulin in determining the origin of congenital hypothyroidism. *Am J Dis Child* 1988; 142:214–216.

Parke WW, Rothman RH, Brown MD: The pharyngovertebral veins: An anatomical rationale for Grisel's syndrome. *J Bone Joint Surg [Am]* 1984; 66:568–574.

Reede DL, Bergeron RT, Som PM: CT of thyroglossal duct cysts. *Radiology* 1985; 157:121–125.

Rivero, Young: In press, 1992.

Sartoris DJ, Mochizuki RM, Parker BR: Lytic clavicular lesions in fibromatosis colli. *Skeletal Radiol* 1983; 10:34–36.

Scheible W: Recent advances in ultrasound: High-resolution imaging of superficial structures. *Head Neck Surg* 1981; 4:58–63.

Slovis TL: Noninvasive evaluation of the pediatric airway: A recent advance. *Pediatrics* 1977; 59:872–880.

Smoker WRK: *Semin Ultrasound CT MR* 1991; 12:192–203.

Smoker WRK, Harnsberger HR: Differential diagnosis of head and neck lesions based on their space of origin. 2. The infrahyoid portion of the neck. *Am J Roentgenol* 1991; 157:155–159.

Soberman N, Leonidas JC, Berdon WE, et al: Sonographic observations of parotid enlargement in 10 HIV positive children. *Am J Roentgenol* 1991; 157:553–556.

Soberman N, Leonidas JC, Cherrick I, et al: Sonographic abnormalities of the thyroid gland in longterm survivors of Hodgkin disease. *Pediatr Radiol* 1991; 21:250–253.

Som PM, Bergeron RT: *Head and Neck Imaging,* ed 2. St Louis, Mosby–Year Book, 1991.

Taybi H, Capitanio MA: Tracheobronchial calcification: An observation in three children after mitral valve replacement and warfarin sodium therapy. *Radiology* 1990; 176:728–730.

Thomsen JR, Koltai PJ: Sternomastoid tumor of infancy. *Ann Otol Rhinol Laryngol* 1989; 98:955–959.

Tom LWC, Rossiter JL, Sutton LN, et al: Torticollis in children. *Otolaryngol Head Neck Surg* 1991; 105:1.

Torsiglieri AJ Jr, Tom LWC, Ross AJ III, et al: Pediatric neck masses: Guidelines for evaluation. *Int J Pediatr Otorhinolaryngol* 1988; 16:199–210.

Tyler D, Effman E, Shorter N: Pyriform sinus cyst and fistula in the newborn: The value of endoscopic cannulation. *J Pediatr Surg,* in press.

Vogelzand P, Harnsberger HR, Smoker WRK: Multispatial and transpatial diseases of the extracranial head and neck. *Semin Ultrasound CT MR* 1991; 12:274–287.

Watts FB Jr, Slovis TH: The enlarged epiglottis. *Pediatr Radiol* 1977; 5:133–136.

Wells RG, Sty JR, Duck SC: Technetium 99m pertechnetate thyroid scintigraphy: Congenital hypothyroid screening. *Pediatr Radiol* 1986; 16: 368–373.

Wells TR, Gilsanz V, Senac MO Jr, et al: Ossification centre of the hyoid bone in DiGeorge syndrome and tetralogy of Fallot. *Br J Radiol* 1986; 59:1065–1068.

6

Chest Wall, Diaphragm, and Pleura

External deformities of the thoracic walls, except those involving the vertebral column, may often be satisfactorily evaluated without roentgenographic examination; such examination is helpful, however, to demonstrate details of skeletal features, to show associated anomalies, and to determine the exact positions of the intrathoracic structures. Computed tomography (CT) and magnetic resonance imaging (MRI) provide important additional information and should be considered whenever detailed anatomical evaluation is indicated. Fetal ultrasound (US) has been found useful for evaluation of thoracic circumference and length, and standard measurements have been described in relation to fetal age. In addition to predictive value with respect to pulmonary hypoplasia, the measurements may provide an additional or alternative parameter for evaluation of fetal growth. Their relations to abdominal circumference and humeral length are said to be constant in normal pregnancies.

SECTION 1

Soft Tissues

During the first years of life the thoracic walls are relatively thin; the apices of the lungs occasionally protrude through the superior thoracic inlet well above the first ribs (Fig 6–1), but such changes have no clinical significance. Jones described a boy 9 years of age who had permanent but intermittent bulging of the neck, above the clavicles medially, which met in the suprasternal regions. The bulging could be reduced by palpation and could be prevented by finger pressure. During the Valsalva maneuver the api-

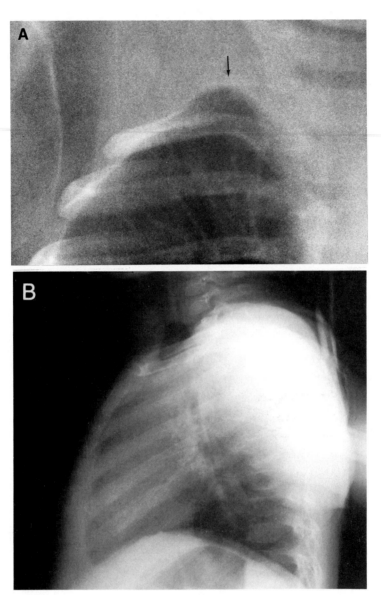

FIG 6–1.
A, protrusion of the apex *(arrow)* of the right lung above the first rib of a healthy girl 3 years of age. This change is sometimes bilateral and is asymptomatic. **B,** lateral projection in another child.

ces of the lungs extended to the midlevel of C6 on the right and C7 on the left. He found 61 reported cases of similar protrusions that he considered cervical hernias of the lung. The occurrence of a cervical hernia in the daughter of a woman with a Morgagni hernia of the diaphragm raised the question of a hereditary defect of the cervical mesenchyme (Catalona et al.).

Air in the suprasternal fossa is superimposed on the trachea and esophagram and may cast fictitious images of air-fluid levels in them in posteroanterior projections (Ominsky and Berinson). The structural changes responsible for the gas-filled depressions

are shown in Figures 6–2 and 6–3. At any age, the apices of the lungs may be obscured by thickening of the overlying tissues such as the folds of skin over the clavicles, the heavy subcostal muscles on the posterior arcs of the first and second ribs, and the subclavian artery (Fig 6–4). The internal surface of the posterior segment of the thoracic wall is to a great extent covered by thick subcostal muscles and other muscular bundles that form a fleshy lining interposed between the internal surface of the ribs and the parietal layer of the pleura (Fig 6–5). The companion shadows of the first three ribs are cast by the heavy subcostal muscles in these levels and the con-

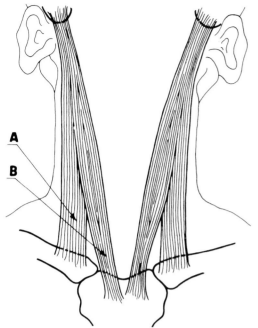

FIG 6–2.
Drawing of the clavicular *(A)* and sternal *(B)* insertions of the sternocleidomastoid muscles that form the edges of the suprasternal fossae. (From Ominsky S, Berinson HS: *Radiology* 1977; 122: 311–313. Used by permission.)

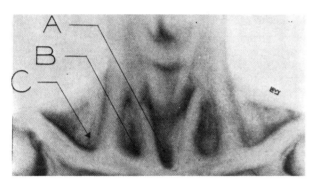

FIG 6–3.
Drawing of the fossae (outlined by skin and elements of the sternocleidomastoid muscles and the clavicles). *A,* suprasternal fossa; *B,* lesser supraclavicular fossa; *C,* greater supraclavicular fossa. (From Ominsky S, Berinson HS: *Radiology* 1977; 122:311–313. Used by permission.)

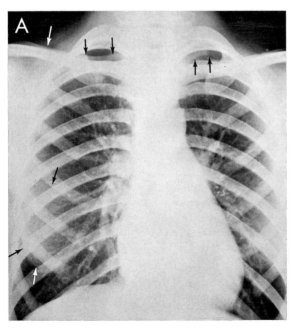

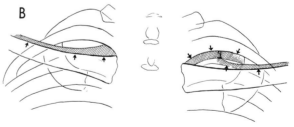

FIG 6–4.
A, some shadows of the soft tissues in the thoracic wall. The companion shadow of the right clavicle *(arrows)* is cast by a heavy fold of skin. The companion shadow of the left second rib obscures the left pulmonary apex *(arrows);* it is cast either by the thick subcostal muscles on the internal aspects of the left second rib, by the left subclavian artery, or by both. The adolescent mammary glands are responsible for the haze over the lower part of the lungs *(lower arrows).* **B,** schematic drawing of **A.**

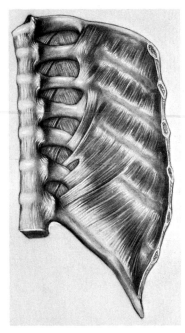

FIG 6–5.
Normal posterior thoracic wall viewed from the front to show the subcostal muscles, which are interposed between the ribs and the parietal layer of the pleura. (Redrawn from Knuttson F: *Acta Radiol* 1932; 13:638–677.

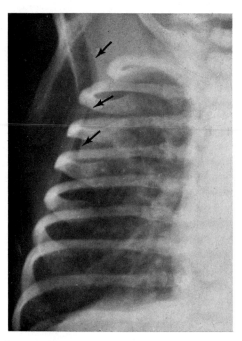

FIG 6–6.
Heavy anterior axillary fold superimposed on the right hemithorax in a fashion that simulates pleural thickening with pneumothorax. The edge of the shadow superimposed on the lungs *(arrows)* is directly continuous with the axillary shadow above and lateral to the lung. The patient was a malnourished infant 28 days old.

nective tissue sheath interposed between the medial segments of the ribs and the dome of the pleura. This posterior muscular layer also can be visualized in oblique projections as a shadow of water density that tapers off inferiorly because the lateral extent of the subcostal muscles diminishes from the level of the third rib downward; despite the downward tapering, it is often confused with a pleural effusion.

Often the lateral margins of the lungs are covered by the shadows of the axillary folds, which may resemble pleural exudates and sometimes have the appearance of pneumothorax. Longitudinal folds of skin of marasmic infants, and the lateral borders of breast shadows may cause similar diagnostic confusion (Fig 6–6). Normal and abnormal soft-tissue masses on the thoracic wall may produce ill-defined increases in density that simulate intrathoracic pathologic change. The medial border of the soft tissues of the arm, when superimposed on the lateral chest wall, may cause confusing linear densities, particularly when collimation of the x-ray beam has eliminated the bony humerus for orientation. Absence or loss of soft tissues in the thoracic wall produces fictitious extra radiolucencies of the underlying lungs. The false hyperaeration of the right lung in Figure 6–7 is due to congenital hypoplasia of the right thoracic wall; and as seen in Figure 6–8, to congenital

absence of the pectoralis major muscle. This is a common associated malformation in the Poland syndrome, in which rib defects may also be present. Thoracic muscular atrophy and hypoplasia in acquired disease produce similar false hyperradiolucencies of the underlying lung (Fig 6–9). Adjacent edges of images of soft tissue and partially superimposed skeletal structures may produce spurious "radiolucent" zones or lines simulating abnormal gas collections (Fig 6–10).

Inflammatory, hemorrhagic, and neoplastic thickenings of the thoracic wall produce areas of increased radiodensity and may simulate intrathoracic pathologic change (Fig 6–11). The shadows of enlarged lymph nodes in the axilla and supraclavicular regions are frequently visible; calcifications in supraclavicular nodes are sometimes superimposed on a pulmonary apex and may be mistaken for apical pulmonary tuberculous foci. Calcification in the thoracic wall in angiomas and in myositis ossificans, and superimposition of long hair may also cast factitious dense shadows. Pockets of gas in the thoracic wall (Fig 6–12) superimposed on the lung may resemble gas-containing cavities. Deep defects in the thoracic wall that are sequelae of previous surgery may be similarly confusing.

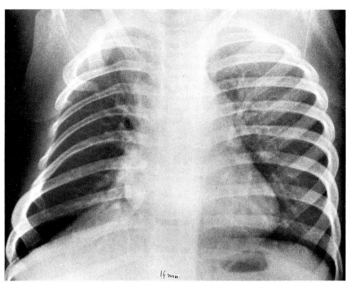

FIG 6–7.
Increased radiolucency of the right hemithorax suggests overaeration of the right lung but is really due to thinness of its overlying right thoracic wall, which was congenitally hypoplastic. There may also be a contribution from an overexpanded, congenitally hypoplastic right lung. The patient, a girl, was 19 months of age. Many of the ribs are also hypoplastic.

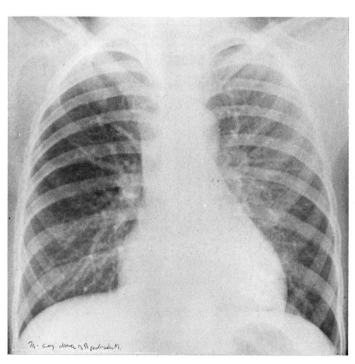

FIG 6–8.
Factitious overaeration of the upper part of the right lung due to a congenital absence of the right pectoralis major muscle. The increased radiolucency is due to a regional deficiency of the anterior thoracic wall. The patient was a boy 7 years of age. This phenomenon is common in the Poland syndrome.

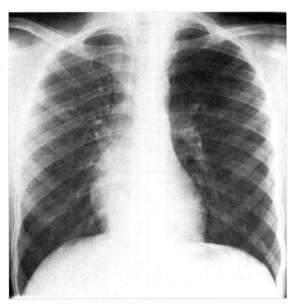

FIG 6–9.
Factitious overaeration of the left lung due to atrophy of the left thoracic wall, including the left pectoralis major muscle, following disarticulation of the left humerus at the shoulder in treatment of malignancy of the left humerus. The entire left hemithorax is more radiolucent than the right owing to the greater penetration of the photons through the thinner-walled left hemithorax. Slight rotation of the chest to the right has produced factitious displacement of the heart and mediastinum to the right. This patient was a boy 10 years of age.

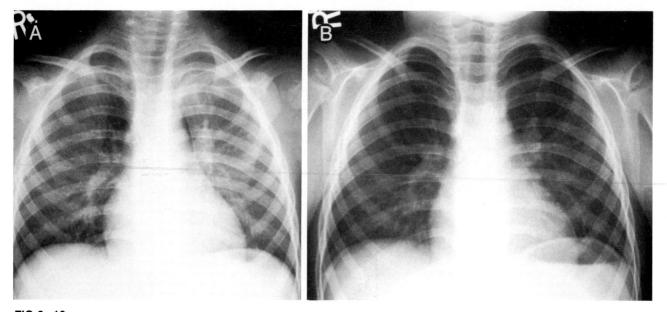

FIG 6–10.
A, frontal chest film reveals a sharp black line adjacent to the aortic arch on the left. This might be mistaken for free air. **B,** the position of the shoulder girdle is changed, and a repeat examination shows a normal chest.

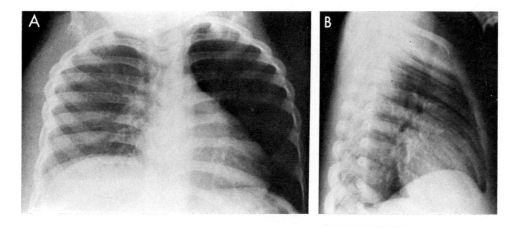

FIG 6–11.
Traumatic hematoma of the right thoracic wall that overlaps on the right lung in both frontal **(A)** and lateral **(B)** projections to produce a generalized haziness of the right hemithorax. In contrast, the left lung is more radiolucent owing to the relative thinness of its wall and the compensatory overbreathing. Note the clarity of the elevated right diaphragm in the lateral projection.

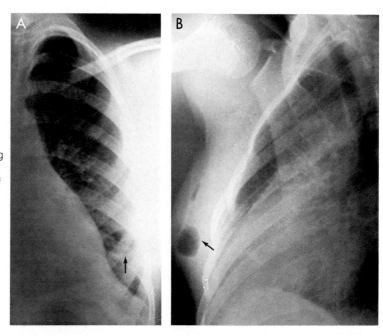

FIG 6–12.
Pockets of gas *(arrows)* in the left thoracic wall following thoracotomy that simulate a pneumatocele in the frontal projection **(A)** but are clearly confined to the swelling of the thoracic wall in the tangential projection **(B).**

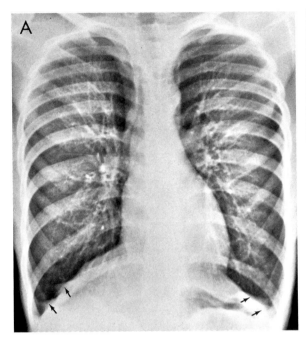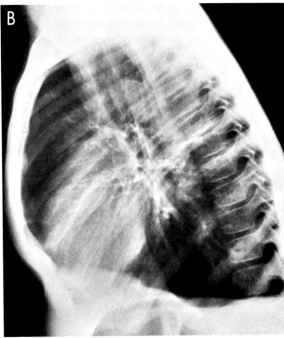

FIG 6–13.

Bilateral severe pulmonary emphysema secondary to severe long-standing atopic asthma that has dilated the thoracic cage and stretched and narrowed the mediastinum and heart longitudinally. **A,** frontal, and **B,** lateral projections. The upper portions of both sides of the thorax are widened and the lower intercostal spaces deepened. The leaves of the diaphragm are depressed, and costal attachments *(arrows)* are conspicuous because of stretching

due to the low position of the diaphragm. The wide radiolucent marginal strips on both sides of the mediastinum could be caused by medial pneumothorax or by overdistended gas-filled alveoli in the periphery of both lungs where the blood vessel content is minimal. In **B,** the thorax is deepened at all levels, and the volume of the radiolucent lung between the sternum and great vessels is markedly increased.

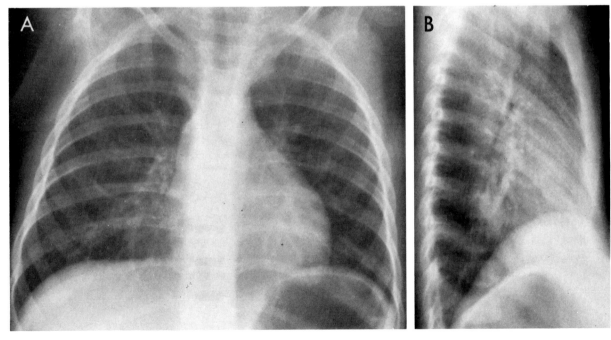

FIG 6–14.

Idiopathic flat, shallow chest in a boy 15 months of age. The thorax is wide at all levels **(A)** but is shallow ventrodorsally at all levels

(B). The sternum is not depressed. The spine is straight; the shallow kyphosis characteristic of this early age is reduced.

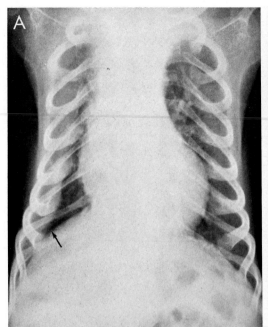
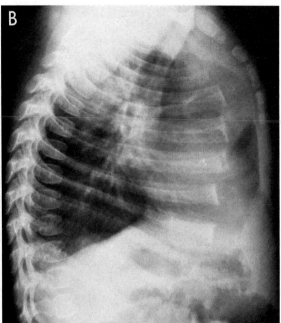

FIG 6–15.
Paralytic thorax in a boy 4 months of age with amyotonia congenita. In **A,** a frontal projection, the long, narrow thorax is constricted in the middle and bulges laterad below. The normal caudal pitch of the ribs is increased. The cardiac shadow, although normal in size, is disproportionately large in relation to the stenosed thorax. In **B,** a lateral projection, the thorax is surprisingly deep ventrodorsad. In both films, the muscular masses are hypoplastic, and the bones of the thoracic cage are osteoporotic.

EXTERNAL CONTOUR

Under normal circumstances, the bony thorax is bilaterally symmetric and narrower in its upper portion than in the lower three fourths. When the thorax is deformed and asymmetric, the densities of the two sides may be unequal owing to differences in the volume of each lung and to differences in the thickness of the thoracic wall on the two sides rather than to intrathoracic disease. The shoulder girdle—composed of the scapulae, clavicles, and manubrium sterni—is supported above the narrowest portion of the thoracic cage and, together with the upper limbs, accounts for the variable inverted triangular shape of the chest.

In patients with long-standing emphysema, the chest expands in all axes. The pattern is particularly prominent in lateral projections. This is the case in children with asthma (Fig 6–13) and in cystic fibrosis of the pancreas. In what Caffey called idiopathic flat chest (Fig 6–14), a flat, wide thorax is noted, probably as an anatomical variation. The normal thoracic kyphosis is reduced and the heart is displaced slightly to the left, but there are no cardiac murmurs. The sternum is not deformed. This pattern may be a variant of the straight back syndrome.

In neuromuscular abnormalities, such as amyotonia congenita (Oppenheim disease) and in cord injuries in the cervical spine, the thoracic cage may assume an hourglass or truncated cone configuration caused by weakness and paralysis of the external muscles of respiration (Fig 6–15). In frontal projection, the thorax is elongated and stenosed, with the greatest narrowing near the middle. The lower segments bulge externally, owing to the enlarged abdomen. A similar configuration is common in premature infants who have been treated with muscle relaxants to facilitate mechanical ventilation. The caudal pitch of the ribs is increased. Respiration is almost exclusively diaphragmatic and is paradoxical; the thorax elongates and narrows during inspiration while the abdomen balloons outward.

REFERENCES

Catalona WJ, Crowder WL, Cretien PB: Occurrence of hernia of Morgagni with filial cervical lung hernia: A hereditary defect of the cervical mesenchyme? *Chest* 1972; 62:340–342.

Collins JP, Pagani JJ: Extrathoracic musculature mimicking pleural lesions. *Radiology* 1978; 120:21–22.

Jones JG: Cervical hernia of the lung. *J Pediatr* 1970; 76:122–125.

Lightwood RG, Cleland WP: Cervical lung hernia. *Thorax* 1974; 29:349–351.

Ominsky S, Berinson HS: The suprasternal fossa. *Radiology* 1977; 122:311–313.

SECTION 2

Bones

In generalized skeletal disease, the changes in the bones of the thoracic walls resemble those in other parts of the skeleton. Lesions caused by trauma, infection, and anomalous growth have the same roentgenographic characteristics as those in extrathoracic bones. Heavy shadows of intrathoracic disease may obscure slight, and sometimes even marked, changes in the overlying portions of the thoracic skeleton.

CONGENITAL DEFORMITIES

Pectus Excavatum (Funnel Chest)

Pectus excavatum is characterized by an internal depression of the lower portion of the sternum and its attached costal cartilages (Figs 6–16 and 6–17). The depression varies from a shallow cup to a deep funnel, and the sternum is usually partially rotated to the right as well as depressed. In the most severe cases, the entire thorax may be flattened ventrodorsally and widened laterally. The pectus is caused by an overgrowth of costal cartilages, although some attribute it to an abnormal growth in the length of the

ribs. The cause of the condition is unknown but its incidence is 1 in 300 births. It occurs frequently in families; McKusick lists it among autosomal dominant traits. The disease is commonly seen in Marfan syndrome and has been associated with Hurler syndrome. There is an increased incidence (21%) of scoliosis in patients with anterior chest wall deformities; it is mild in most, although approximately one fifth of those with scoliosis require some therapeutic intervention.

The plain film (Fig 6–18) shows the body of the sternum forming the floor of the depression. In cases of slight sternal depression, there are no cardiac changes; with deep depressions, the heart, lung, diaphragm, and esophagus may all be compressed. In moderate and severe cases, the heart is displaced to the left. The soft tissues and cartilages of the right wall of the depression are sufficiently tangential to the x-ray beam to obliterate the lower right cardiac border (see Fig 6–18,A and B), simulating middle lobe disease. Compression atelectasis may contribute to the obliteration. Rarely, the cardiac shadow is displaced to the right and its left border is obliterated (Shevland and Abu-Yousef). Fol-

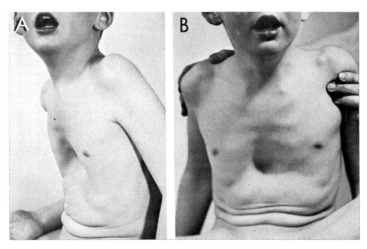

FIG 6–16.
A boy 4 years of age with a deep funnel chest. **A,** lateral, and **B,** frontal views.

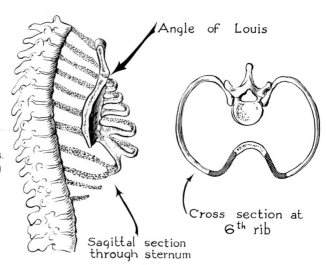

FIG 6–17.
Schematic drawing of a funnel chest that shows the depression of the sternum. The manubrium is not affected, and the angle of Louis is prominent. The body (gladiolus) is depressed internally, and the costal cartilages at the same levels are all bent inward on both sides. (From Bill AH Jr: *Pediatrics* 1953; 11:582–587. Used by permission.)

lowing surgical elevation of the sternum and costal cartilages, the dead space may fill with fluid and simulate pulmonary consolidation or atelectasis.

There has been significant new information recently concerning cardiac and respiratory function in adolescents with pectus excavatum (Ghory et al.; Derveaux et al.; Wynn et al.). Though it is difficult to obtain a consensus, it appears that lung capacity is somewhat reduced prior to any operation, in both the control group and those who eventually receive surgery, and the abnormalities do not change after operation. Most feel that the decrease in total lung capacity is specifically due to the decreased vital ca-

pacity. Evaluation of cardiac function by many techniques, including radionuclide procedures, found no apparent abnormalities of cardiac output and stoke volume during exercise before and after operation.

Some clinicians feel that CT is the best modality for evaluation of the severity of pectus excavatum. A ratio of the transverse diameter of the chest to the narrowest anteroposterior (AP) diameter of the chest on CT seems to provide important information for discrimination between those with mild and those with moderate to severe defects. A ratio greater than 3.25 defines the moderate to severe group (Haller et al.).

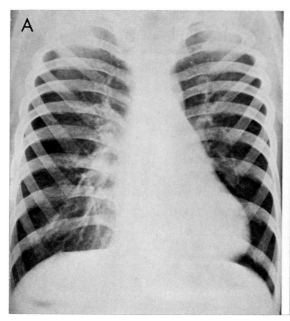

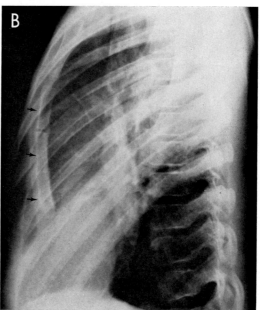

FIG 6–18.
Funnel chest in a boy 7 years of age. **A,** frontal, and **B,** lateral projections. The cardiac shadow is displaced to the left, and as a result the right hilum and bronchovascular markings below it are un-

usually conspicuous. In **B,** the lower portion of the sternum is displaced dorsad several centimeters *(arrows)*, and the fourth sternal ossification center is not yet mineralized.

Surgical correction of the deformity is used in moderate to severe deformities for cosmetic reasons. A conservative surgical point of view was supported by Humphreys and Jaretzki. They reviewed the records of 334 patients with funnel chest deformity; 166 had been operated on at least once and 168 had not had surgery. Eighteen percent of the entire group died of associated anomalies. The deformity improved or disappeared in 50% of the surviving infants not operated on and in some children up to 6 years of age. After that age, the condition worsened or did not change. Mild deformity was compatible with long life without symptoms, whereas severe deformity could lead to chronic disability. The authors believed that operation was justified in appropriate cases but was seldom indicated in children under 3 years of age; the best results were obtained in children 3 to 6 years of age in whom better results were obtained with the more radical types of surgery.

A few reports have appeared of acquired pectus excavatum from chronic airway obstruction due to hypertrophied adenoids and tonsils and of improvement in cardiorespiratory status together with improvement in the degree of pectus deformity after removal of the obstruction. In view of the high rate of spontaneous improvement of the deformity noted above, a cause-and-effect relation can be questioned even if relief of the obstruction is a valid reason for surgical management.

Other Deformities

Congenital chondrosternal prominence (pigeon breast, pectus carinatum), the converse of funnel chest, is characterized by ventrad protrusion of the upper portion of the sternum and its costal cartilages, with bilateral flattening of the sides of the chest. Usually, deep Harrison grooves furrow both lateral thoracic walls in the lower levels. This deformity, formerly attributed to rickets, is usually a congenital malformation that is secondary to congenital hypoplasia and weakness in the ventral (chondrosternal) segment of the diaphragm (Brodkin). The muscles in the lateral and posterior segments of the diaphragm are, in contrast, thick and long. It is a common feature in Marfan syndrome (Fig 6–19) and occurs also in other dysmorphic syndromes. As in the case of pectus excavatum, children with pectus carinatum may have scoliosis of a degree requiring orthopedic management.

The rachitic chest exhibits multiple deformities owing to the softening of the bony cage; the chest wall gives way at sites of greatest weakness and

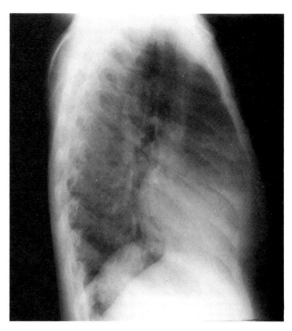

FIG 6–19.
Lateral chest film of a patient with Marfan syndrome and pectus caranatum. The ribs are elongated and the long sternum extends downward and forward with no intrinsic anterior curve. Clinically, the projecting lower end of the straight sternum resulted in a silhouette similar to that illustrated in Figure 43–17. (Courtesy of Dr. Janet Strife, Cincinnati.)

greatest stress and the total volume of the thorax is reduced. At the costochondral junctions, the ends of the softened ribs are displaced inward, flattening the anterolateral aspects of the chest wall and producing symmetric, obliquely oriented, longitudinal grooves (Fig 6–20). The costochondral junctions are swollen; the sternal ends of the ribs are expanded and cupped. Bilateral Harrison grooves may appear in the lower thoracic levels as a result of the drag of the diaphragm on the softened ribs. Caudal to these grooves, the thoracic wall is everted by the underlying distended alimentary tract and the ptotic liver and spleen. Rachitic deformities are usually more conspicuous on the right side because the heart buttresses the left.

Defects of the anterior ribs of the upper thorax are commonly present in the Poland syndrome (see Fig 6–8). Defects also occur in association with hemivertebra malformations and may be of sufficient size to affect respiratory function. Both deformities may reflect the effect of a congenital anomaly in one system on another closely associated one or simultaneous response of two spatially related tissues to a common noxious influence. The absence of pectoral muscle may adversely affect adjacent rib development in the Poland syndrome. In the hemivertebra anomaly, there may be a concomitant absence

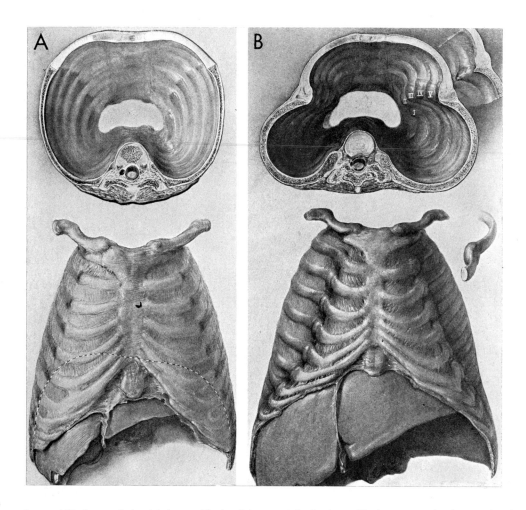

FIG 6–20.
Morbid changes in a rachitic thorax. **A,** frontal view and horizontal section of the normal thorax at the level of the sixth vertebral segment; the latter is viewed from below. **B,** similar views of a deformed rachitic thorax. In the section, it is evident that the thoracic cavity is partially divided into three chambers by the inward projection of the swollen costochondral junctions (rachitic rosary) and vertebral column. The heart occupies the anterior chamber. All deformities seen here are exaggerated during inspiration. A detail drawing of the costochondral deformity is appended to the left side of the thorax in both views. (From Park EA, Howland J: *Bull Johns Hopkins Hosp* 1921; 32:101–109. Used by permission.)

of a rib since, in early embryonic development, the transverse process has continuity with the rib.

The bones of the thoracic cage participate in generalized skeletal dysplasias. In achondroplasia, owing to undergrowth of the ribs and sternum, the thorax is reduced in girth and depth and its anterior wall is shortened. In contrast, the clavicles are overlong and the scapulae and shoulders are widely spaced in relation to the thoracic wall. These features are exaggerated in thanatophoric dysplasia, Jeune syndrome, and rib-polydactyly syndromes. The thoracic cage is short and wide in the Kniest syndrome and may have an outward, rounded configuration in the Cornelia de Lange syndrome (see Chapter 43). A wide variety of congenital thoracic malformations is associated with multiple hemivertebrae; severe deformities arise from abnormalities affecting the ribs.

BLUNT TRAUMA

Practically any intrathoracic structure can be damaged during blunt injury to the chest without definite evidence of skeletal injury because of the extremely pliant thoracic cage in children. Serious or even potentially fatal mechanical injuries may not be visible on standard films, and CT is the examination of choice, for evaluation of intrathoracic injuries. Identification of bony injuries is important to convey information on the extent of the trauma and may indicate specific associated conditions (Fig 6–21). Fractures of the first three ribs are often associated with serious injury to the mediastinal blood vessels, airways, and bronchi; fractures of the lower ribs are commonly associated with lacerations of the liver, spleen, and diaphragm. Rib fractures in various stages of healing warrant consideration of child

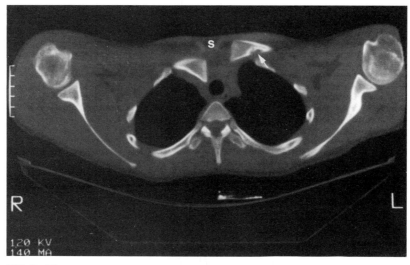

FIG 6–21.
CT scan of a disrupted sternoclavicular joint reveals posterior dislocation of the right clavicle. *S*, sternum. Note the rhomboid fossa on the left *(arrow).*

abuse. Traumatic pneumothorax, hemothorax, and diaphragmatic hernia do not differ radiographically from their nontraumatic counterparts. Traumatic chylothorax commonly causes enlargement of the mediastinum before the pleural space is filled with chyle. Diagnosis depends, however, on the nature of the fluid removed by thoracentesis. Blunt trauma to the chest wall may cause pulmonary hematomas from lacerations. Intercostal pulmonary hernia may develop following penetrating chest wall trauma. Smith and Stempel reported an instance in which such a hernia appeared at the site of a hematoma following a nonpenetrating injury. The mass appeared during expiration but disappeared on inspiration and was accentuated by the Valsalva maneuver. Spontaneous healing occurred within a few weeks.

Thoracic trauma is discussed in greater detail in Chapter 12.

STERNUM

In frontal projection, the shadow of the sternum is superimposed on the spine and is invisible except for the margin of the manubrium, which sometimes projects laterad beyond the paravertebral lines. On oblique and lateral projections, the entire sternum can be satisfactorily visualized. The number of sternal ossification centers and their pattern of appearance vary greatly. The first center usually appears in the manubrium during the sixth fetal month, and subsequently centers appear in the body of the sternum at approximately 1-month intervals, progressing from above downward (Fig 6–22; see also Fig

6–25). Initially, there are two foci of ossification in each center which later fuse. The initial foci may be at alternate horizontal levels and tend to occur between sites of junction of the rib cartilages with the sternum. The segmental centers then fuse with one another from below upward. The manubrium, gladiolus, and ensiform cartilage remain separate throughout childhood except in some infants and children with congenital heart disease in whom manubrial-gladiolar fusion is common. Fusion of the gladiolar centers occurs early in the same group of children and is often associated with pectus carinatum. The frequency of these fusions increases with age and is greatest in cyanotic females. Ossification of persistent episternal cartilage is responsible for the small accessory suprasternal bones occasionally found on the superior margins of the manubrium (Fig 6–23). These can be shown by CT and must be differentiated from fracture fragments, sequestra, foreign bodies, or calcified lymph nodes in the appropriate clinical setting. Separate superior and inferior manubrial centers are common in infants with Down syndrome, occurring approximately four times as frequently as in unaffected infants.

The most important lesion of the sternum, pectus excavatum, has already been described. Cleft and notched sternums (Fig 6–24) result from failure of fusion of paired embryonal components (Fig 6–25). The sternal defect is not visible in conventional radiography but can be inferred from marked lateral displacement of the medial ends of the clavicles. Ravitch classified sternal clefts into four major and ten minor categories. The sternal aperture illustrated in Figure 6–26 probably is a minor form of

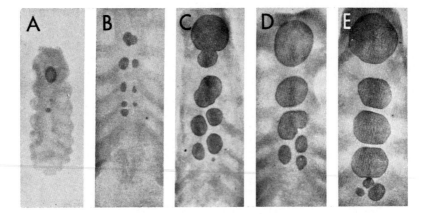

FIG 6–22.
Roentgenograms of specimens of the sternum that show ossification patterns at different ages. **A,** at the sixth fetal month, there are single tiny centers in the manubrium and body. **B,** at the age of 18 days, the paired manubrial centers are partially fused; in contrast, the first three centers in the body are paired but not fused, and the single fourth center is unpaired. **C,** at 8 months. **D,** at 10 months. **E,** at 15 months. (From Diwami M: *Arch Dis Child* 1940; 15:159–1970. Used by permission.)

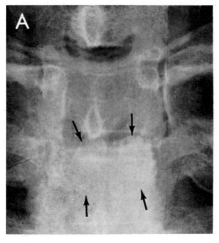
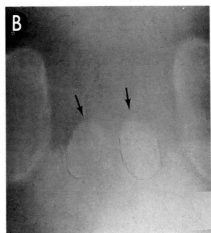

FIG 6–23.
Suprasternal bones in an adult. **A,** frontal projection with standard technique. Indefinite shadows of increased density are seen in the suprasternal region *(arrows),* but contrast is poor owing to the heavier shadow of the spine. **B,** frontal projection, tomogram of ventral thoracic wall at depth of 1 cm. Well-defined, paired oval ossicles are clearly visible in the suprasternal regions, each just lateral to the midsagittal thoracic plane.

FIG 6–24.
Congenital cleft of the sternum in an infant 4 months of age (proved at surgical exploration). The sternum itself cannot be seen; the diagnosis is indicated by displacement laterad of the medial ends of both clavicles. During expiration, a large mass of tissue bulged forward above the defective sternum and between the laterally displaced clavicles.

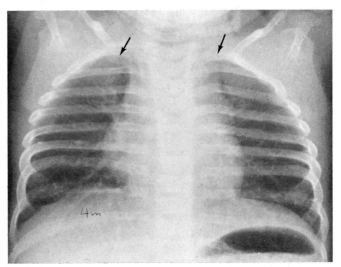

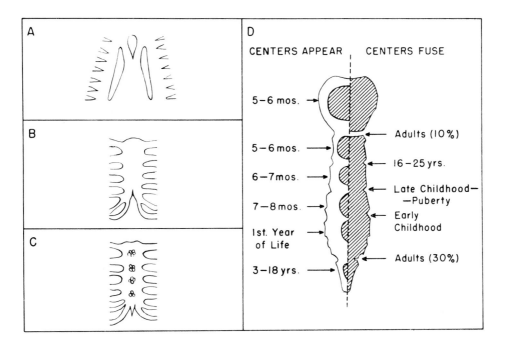

FIG 6–25.
Diagrammatic resume of the development of the sternum. **A,** the mesoblastic primordia (two lateral bands and a median rudiment). **B,** plate of hyaline cartilage originating from the chondrification and midline fusion of the primordia. **C,** appearance of islands of hypertrophied chondroblasts—the future ossification centers. **D,** ossification and fusion of the various sternebrae (infant and adult sternum). (From Currarino G, Silverman FN: *Radiology* 1958; 70:532–540. Used by permission.)

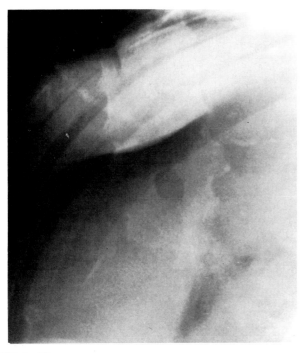

FIG 6–26.
Sternal aperture found incidental to oblique projections of the chest for unrelated complaint.

this embryologic defect. A defect occurs in the lower part of the sternum in association with a high omphalocele that is accompanied by a pericardial and diaphragmatic defect and, not infrequently, a ventral diverticulum of the left ventricle. The last may present as a pulsating mass extending as far down as the umbilicus. The association is known as the 'Cantrell syndrome.' The most severe form of sternal cleft is that associated with ectopia cordis. Sternal defects characterized by incomplete fusion of the lateral sternal bands may be associated with craniofacial hemangiomas as well as with similar internal vascular lesions that may be large and life-threatening. Often, cutaneous scars occur over the region of the bony defect. The condition does not appear to be hereditary.

Fractures of the sternum are not common; in young infants, they warrant consideration of child abuse (Kleinman). A spontaneous sternal fracture has been reported during exercise in a teen-age boy with cystic fibrosis of the pancreas. It was believed to result from bone demineralization secondary to the disease and its complications. It is also possible that excessive respiratory efforts caused a minor stress fracture that became complete under appropriate force. Median sternotomy wound infections have occurred with diagnosis between 5 to 30 days postoperatively in most patients, and after 4 years in an instance of chronic sternal osteomyelitis. Mediastinal involvement may occur. Neoplasms are rare and are generally metastatic.

CLAVICLES

The inferior surface of the clavicle near its sternal end is often marked by a depression that is visible roentgenographically (Fig 6–27). This depression, the rhomboid fossa, has a roughened floor that serves to attach the costoclavicular ligament, which originates on the cartilage of the first rib. The fossa may be unilateral or bilateral. The foramen of the canal for the midclavicular nerve may be visible at times because of angles of projection despite its usual oblique orientation (Fig 6–28). Ossification centers in epiphyseal cartilage at the medial end of the clavicles may be visible in teen-agers and simulate fracture fragments (Fig 6–29).

The common types of clavicular defects include complete or partial aplasias, which are sometimes associated with the other lesions of cleidocranial dysplasia (see Fig 43–63). Fibrosis of the clavicles in progeria may cause gradual rarefaction and finally disappearance of both clavicles. Congenital pseudarthroses of the clavicle, both unilateral and bilateral, have been described in a number of cases. At birth a swelling is noted just lateral to the middle of the clavicle. Radiographically, a middle segment is missing, but the terminal segments are enlarged. The larger medial segment always lies in front of and above the smaller lateral segment. At the site of the central defect the tissues are movable, as are the terminal segments, without inducing pain. Swelling and mobility increase with advancing age; spontaneous union does not occur. Behringer and Wilson ac-

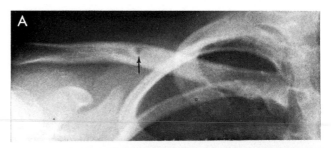

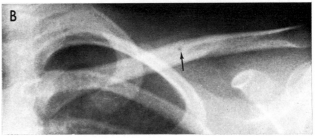

FIG 6–28.
Foramina of the normal canals for the midclavicular nerve in the right **(A)** and left **(B)** clavicles of a healthy boy 11 years of age.

cepted 18 cases from the literature as "documented" and added another; 57 reports of what they termed anecdotal cases were also found. Like previous authors, they comment on the practically universal involvement of the right clavicle. Sclerotic, opposing ends of bone at the site of the defect are generally separated by fibrous tissue in which fluid is occasionally found, although Alldred reported articular cartilage covering the bone ends with a joint cavity

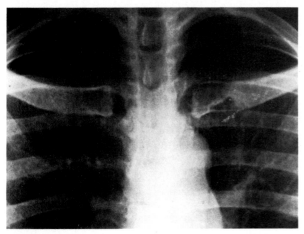

FIG 6–27.
Young man with unilateral rhomboid fossa of the clavicle.

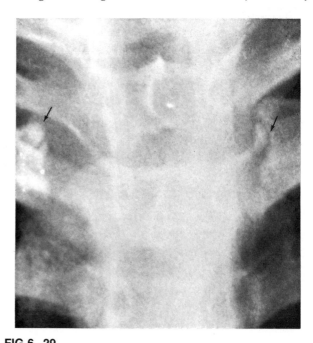

FIG 6–29.
Normal ossification centers in the medial epiphyseal cartilages of the clavicles of a healthy boy 17 years of age.

between them. Neurofibromatosis has not been established in any of the definite cases. Many excellent results have been obtained after excision and bone grafting or internal fixation.

The cause of pseudarthrosis of the clavicle remains a mystery; the differential diagnosis is considered to lie between cleidocranial dysplasia and a birth fracture. No definite genetic patterns have been found. Behringer and Wilson favor a birth fracture related to the common left occiput posterior presentation in which the right shoulder is behind the pubis. They postulate that traction upon the head, employed to deliver the posterior shoulder, might fracture the right clavicle, and point out that fracture of the clavicle is the most common birth fracture. Lloyd-Roberts and associates believe that, in many cases, congenital pseudarthrosis is due to habitual pressure on the growing clavicle during fetal life. They have found a high correlation of pseudarthrosis of the clavicle with ipsilateral cervical ribs and highly placed first right ribs. In arteriograms, they demonstrated the close anatomical relation between the pseudarthroses of the clavicle and the apex of a highly placed angulated subclavian artery.

A primitive, supernumerary clavicle was found below a normal left clavicle in a patient described by Goldthamer (Fig 6–30); this little bone was fixed laterally to the coracoid process, but its medial end was freely movable in the soft tissue of the thoracic wall.

In anterior sternoclavicular dislocations, which are rare in infants and children, the medial end of the clavicle is displaced upward and outward. The swollen deformity above the sternum is usually obvious both clinically and radiographically. Posterior sternoclavicular dislocations are uncommon, and are

generally associated with significant vectors of force (Fig 6–31; see also Fig 6–21). The displaced clavicle may compress vital structures in the mediastinum and cause serious disability, even death (Lee and Gwinn).

Fractures of the clavicle are common; during the neonatal period clavicular fractures are more frequent than all other fractures combined. The lateral half of the clavicle is almost always affected; the site of the fractures is usually near the junction of the lateral and middle thirds of the shaft. In breech presentations, direct traction of the obstetrician's finger in the attempt to depress the shoulders and to free the arms in the delivery of the head is responsible for clavicular injury. Callus formation is usually evident roentgenographically in 8 or 9 days. Healing occurs usually without significant deformity, despite marked initial overriding of the fragments and even without corrective therapy. Fresh fractures of the medial third of the clavicle are often invisible or difficult to see in standard projections but become clearly visible in lordotic projections (Fig 6–32). The medial fragment is usually flexed cephalad by the pull of the sternocleidomastoid muscle while the lateral fragment is anchored at the intact acromioclavicular joint (Fig 6–33). The lateral end of the clavicle may be broken following a fall directly on the shoulder or other axial impact to the lateral end of the clavicle (Fig 6–34).

Focal lesions of the clavicle are uncommon (Fig 6–35). Osteomyelitis, osteoid osteomas, Ewing sar-

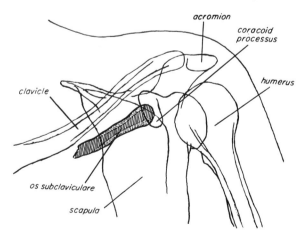

FIG 6–30.
Supernumerary left clavicle in a man 34 years of age. Drawing of a radiograph in which a primitive small clavicle lies below the normal clavicle. (From Goldthamer CR: *Radiology* 1957; 68:576–578. Used by permission.)

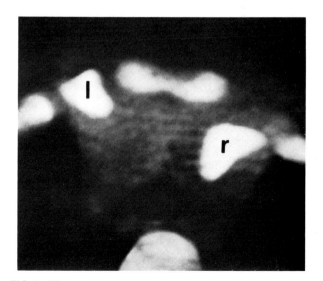

FIG 6–31.
CT demonstration of right posterior sternoclavicular dislocation. The discrepancy in position of the medial ends of the left *(l)* and right *(r)* clavicles is clearly shown, and the proximity of the displaced clavicle to mediastinal structures is obvious. (Courtesy of Dr. R. Jaffe, Salt Lake City.)

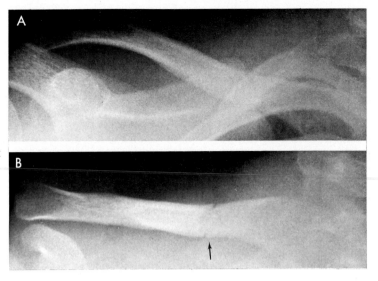

FIG 6–32.
Transverse fracture of the clavicle in its medial third is invisible in a standard projection **(A)** but clearly visible in the lordotic projection **(B).** The latter projection should be considered when the findings are normal in the standard position but the history and clinical signs strongly support injury in this area. This patient, a boy 10½ years of age, had fallen on his shoulder, and his point of tenderness *(arrow)* was over the medial third of the clavicle.

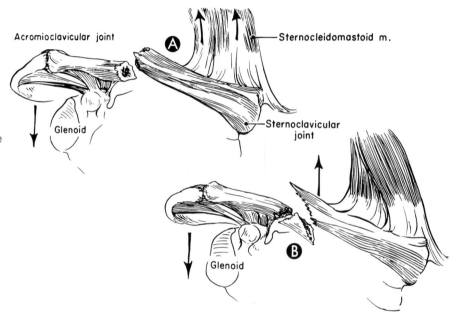

FIG 6–33.
Fractures of the clavicle. Typical flexion cephalad of the medial fragment by the pull of the sternocleidomastoid muscle with the medial fragment anchored at the sternoclavicular joint. **A,** simple transverse fracture; **B,** comminuted fracture with medial, middle, and lateral fragments. (From Cave EF: *Fractures and Other Injuries.* St Louis, Mosby–Year Book, 1958, p 258. Used by permission.)

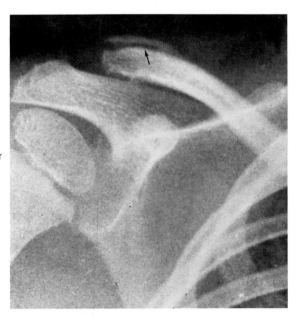

FIG 6–34.
This boy, 15 years of age, fell out of bed directly onto his right shoulder and broke off a superficial layer of the superior cortical wall of the right clavicle at its very lateral end.

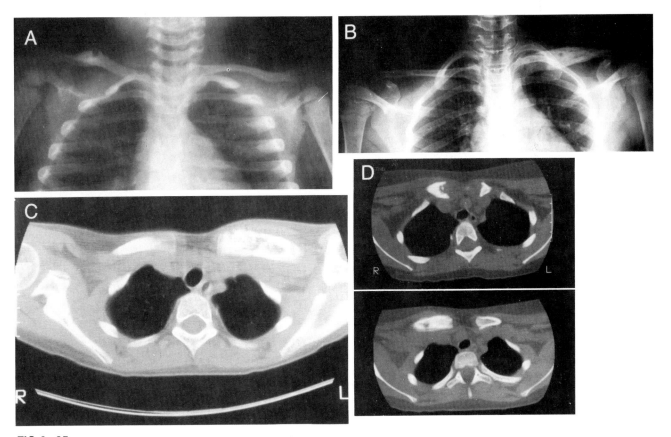

FIG 6–35.

Lesions of the clavicle. **A,** sclerotic midportion of the right clavicle with a lytic superior margin. This was osteomyelitis. **B,** enlarged, primarily sclerotic lesion of the left proximal clavicle. There is periosteal reaction about, and some lucencies within the lesion. **C,** CT scan of the same patient as in **B** reveals some soft-tissue swelling but little mass. The bone is expanded and permeated. This was

osteomyelitis. **D,** two sections of a CT scan on a 15-year-old patient with pain in the right clavicle at the sternoclavicular junction. The upper section shows the nidus and soft tissue about the nidus. The lower section reveals expanded sclerotic bone. This was an osteoid osteoma.

coma, and aneurysmal bone cyst all have been described. Cross-sectional imaging is important to discern soft-tissue mass, extent of involvement of the marrow cavity, and, in general, to further define the lesion.

Fibrous cortical defects are extremely rare in the clavicle. Gardiner reported one in the tender, swollen, medial end of the clavicle of a boy 10 years of age. Microscopic examination disclosed that the radiolucent tissue was made up of whorls of spindle-shaped cells and scattered multinucleated giant cells characteristic of benign cortical defect. Inflammatory changes in the clavicle are no different from inflammatory changes in other tubular bones. Periosteal reaction in the clavicle has been described following percutaneous subclavian venous catheterization. The subperiosteal bone formation was observed 1 week following catheterization and resolved in 1 month. It was believed to represent a subperiosteal hematoma following injury to the periosteum by the

needle, and can be confused with osteomyelitis. Regional demineralization of the acromial ends of both clavicles is a common and important diagnostic finding in primary and secondary hyperparathyroidism and in renal osteodystrophy. Teplick and associates found similar erosive changes at the sternal ends in the same diseases. Similar changes may be observed in severe rheumatoid arthritis.

The clavicles are frequently affected in infantile cortical hyperostosis. Roentgenographic examination discloses irregular thickening and sclerosis of one or both clavicles (Fig 6–36; also see Fig 47–35). Focal thickenings of the inferior edge of the clavicle may develop in long-standing, severe cases of rheumatoid arthritis (Fig 6–37). Similar bony projections may be present in association with a true coracoclavicular joint (Moore and Renner). Figure 6–38 had been presented earlier as an example of calcification in coracoclavicular ligaments in a 4-year-old boy; in view of his age, the clavicular excrescences more

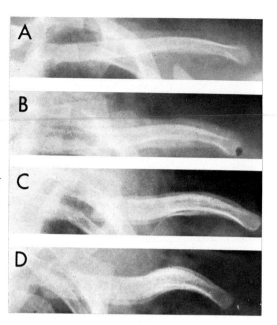

FIG 6–36.
Infantile cortical hyperostosis exemplified by serial early changes in the clavicle of an infant 5½ months of age whose face and jaws had been swollen for several days. **A,** early even external thickening directly from the original cortex; there is no independent thin shell of peripheral bone. **B,** 7 days after **A,** cortical thickening is deeper and more sclerotic, but still there is no independent peripheral shell of bone. **C,** 30 days after **A,** the hyperostosis is shrinking but for the first time is capped by a thin peripheral shell. **D,** 43 days after **A,** the peripheral cortical cap is still clearly visible. This sequence could be produced by a healing nondisplaced fracture.

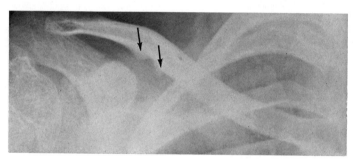

FIG 6–37.
Bony spurs *(arrows)* on the clavicle at the site of attachment of a coracoclavicular ligament (conoid) in a girl 9 years of age who had had severe rheumatoid disease for 4 years. There were similar spurs at the same site on the other clavicle.

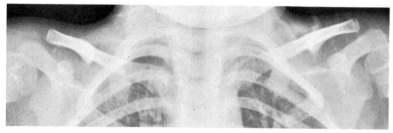

FIG 6–38.
Probable early appearance of coracoclavicular joints in an asymptomatic 4-year-old boy.

likely represent early features of development of a coracoclavicular joint, and resemble closely those illustrated in the literature as reviewed by Cockshott.

In Friedrich disease tomographic examination of painful swelling in the region of the sternoclavicular joints has demonstrated focal destruction in the adjacent clavicle with some bony sclerosis. Biopsy to exclude osteomyelitis or tumor demonstrates only necrotic bone. There are no systemic signs of disease and no history of trauma. The condition is thought to be an aseptic necrosis of the epiphyseal bone in this region. It may be similar to Tietze syndrome (see under Ribs below). The condition is quite different from sternocostoclavicular hyperostosis described by Köehler and associates in adults. In this condition, painful swelling of the sternum, clavicles, and upper ribs occurs and is associated with hyperostotic periostitis and end-stage spongy hyperostosis. Bilateral subclavian vein occlusion has been demonstrated on phlebography.

SCAPULAE

All of the postnatal ossification centers, except for the one for the coracoid process, make their appearance in the pubertal and postpubertal periods. The coracoid center usually appears by 4 months of age but can be present at birth. Two centers may appear in the acromial process between 12 and 15 years of age, and a secondary coracoid center may appear between 13 and 16 years. Multiple centers occur in the cartilaginous vertebral border of the scapula and in its continuation into the inferior angle, as well as in the rim of the glenoid cavity at a slightly later age. Most of these centers fuse with the main body of the bone beginning about 17 years of age but they can remain separate until the middle of the third decade. The above appearance times apply primarily to boys; girls are advanced by 1 or 2 years in the later-ap-

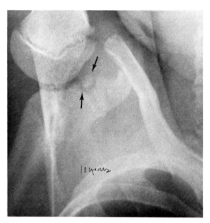

FIG 6–39.
Accessory ossification center in the base of the coracoid process in a healthy boy 10 years of age with no local clinical signs.

pearing centers. Examples are shown in Figures 6–39 and 6–40. Ogden and Phillips found that the glenoid cavity in cadavers, ranging from newborn to 14 years of age, was always concave, although the osseous subchondral contour was often flat or slightly convex in radiographs.

Anomalies of the scapula include ossification of structures normally ligamentous, absence of ossification centers usually present, or the presence of abnormal or accessory centers that may persist without union. Deep marginal radiolucent notches (Fig 6–41) have been observed in the caudal border of the scapula in a few cases (Khoo and Kuo). When neighboring bones are injured, the normal ossification centers in the cartilaginous portions of the scapula may be mistaken for fracture fragments (Fig 6–42). Gross irregular and incomplete ossification of the acromial processes in both scapulae was observed by Caffey in a 14-week-old girl (Fig 6–43). These defects may possibly represent unfused acromial processes, which are occasionally seen in older children and adults and are twice as frequent unilaterally as bilaterally (Köhler).

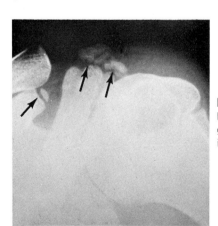

FIG 6–40.
Normal secondary ossification centers in the acromial and coracoid processes of a healthy girl 12 years of age. The acromial center is developing from three centers that are irregular in density and margin. These should not be mistaken for fractures or osteochondroses.

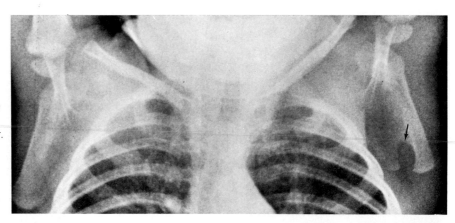

FIG 6–41.
Deep radiolucent notches in the left scapula *(arrow)* of an asymptomatic boy 8 months of age. The scapula is also highly placed and small. (Courtesy of Dr. Virgil Condon, Salt Lake City.)

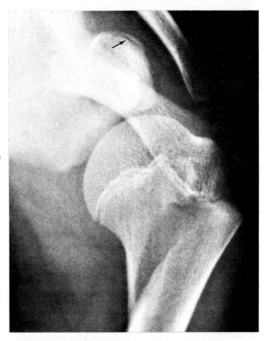

FIG 6–42.
Oblique fracture of the proximal end of the left humerus of a girl 12 years of age who fell off a bannister. The *arrow* points to the scale ossification center in the apophyseal cartilage of the uninjured coracoid process of the scapula.

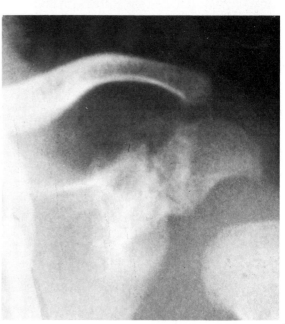

FIG 6–43.
Irregular, incomplete ossification at the base of the acromial process of the left scapula in an asymptomatic girl 14 weeks of age. Both gestation and parturition were normal, with no evidence of trauma to the shoulder at birth and no history or clinical signs of trauma after birth. Similar, practically identical changes were present in the right acromial process. (Courtesy of Dr. James R. Marquis, Newark, NJ.)

When one of the acromial ossification centers fails to unite with the rest of the bone, and an articulation is formed with a synovial lining, the ununited portion is called the os acromiale. We have had occasion to see a "hook-shaped" scapula (Fig 6–44) in which the inferior angle bent outward. The patient had several features consistent with pseudopseudohypoparathyroidism but also had hearing difficulties, a high arched palate, mild skeletal dysmorphism, and restricted extension of the elbows. An identical scapular "hook" was present in a patient with the Pierre Robin syndrome and clubfoot reported by Bezirdjian and Szucs.

The most important congenital anomaly is congenital failure of descent, or Sprengel deformity (Figs 6–45 and 6–46), resulting in an elevated scapula on one or both sides. In some patients, the elevated scapula is anchored to the spine by an anomalous omovertebral bone that articulates laterally with the medial border of the scapula and medially with one or more of the cervical vertebrae. Sometimes this union is made by fibrous tissue. The origin of the omovertebral bone is unknown. The fixation is frequently responsible for the medial position of the scapula in addition to its elevation. Removal of the omovertebral bone ameliorates the deformity of the scapula and permits an increase in the range of motion, especially abduction, at the affected shoulder.

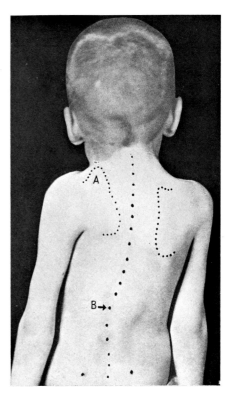

FIG 6–45.
Congenital failure of descent of the left scapula (Sprengel deformity) in a boy 6 years of age. *A* indicates the high position of the left scapula and *B*, thoracolumbar scoliosis. (From Rotch TM: *Living Anatomy and Pathology: The Diagnosis of Diseases in Early Life by the Roentgen Method. [The Roentgen Ray in Pediatrics.]* Philadelphia, JB Lippincott, 1910, p 75.)

Scoliosis is a common associated feature, and in one third of these cases, renal anomalies occur. A Klippel-Feil deformity (congenital failure of segmentation) of the cervical vertebral column may accompany Sprengel deformity, and other vertebral anomalies are frequent (see Fig 6–46,B).

The scapula may participate in generalized disorders of the skeleton. Large and small scapular defects are present in some cases of reticuloendotheliosis. In the more severe cases of multiple cartilaginous exostoses (Fig 6–47), bony tumors may project from the scapular margins, usually the vertebral. Exostoses of the internal edge of the scapula or on the subscapular ribs may displace the scapula, impinge on the thoracic cage or the scapula, respectively, and generate grating and snapping sounds on movement of the scapula on the ribs (the "snapping scapula," according to Parsons). Both frontal and oblique projections of the thorax are essential for optimal radiographic visualization of these lesions. External scapular exostoses cause localized swellings (Fig 6–48). Similar features can be observed with exostoses following radiation therapy in the region.

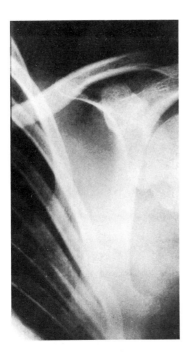

FIG 6–44.
Hook-shaped protrusion at the inferior tip of the scapular blade in a patient with some features of pseudopseudohypoparathyroidism. See text.

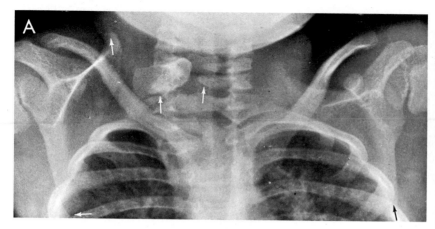

FIG 6–46.
Failure of descent of the right scapula (Sprengel deformity). The scapula is also rotated and clinically "winged." **A,** a large omovertebral bone is superimposed on the right side of the cervical spine, probably connected by membranous tissue or cartilage to the abnormally positioned scapula. The superior medial angle of the scapula is prominent, possibly because of projection. The right clavicle is small in caliber, and its normal curves are diminished. Hemivertebra deformities are present in the sixth and seventh cervical segments. **B,** in the lower thoracic and lumbar levels, variations in the pedicles *(arrows)* are related to deletions of portions of the neural arches and compensatory hypertrophy.

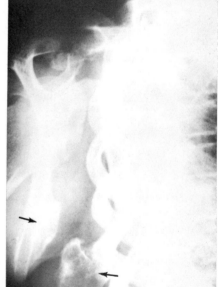

FIG 6–47.
Two large cartilaginous exostoses *(arrows),* one extending laterad off a rib and the other mediad off the inner edge of the scapular plate, in a 14-year-old boy.

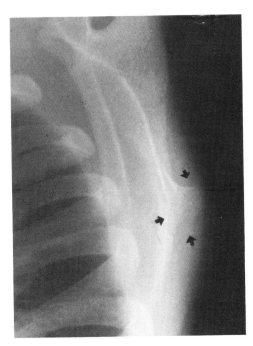

FIG 6–48.
A large cartilaginous exostosis *(arrows)* that extends outward from the external edge of the left scapula caused a visible and palpable soft-tissue swelling in this boy of 12 years.

In skeletal dysplasias with altered longitudinal growth, the scapular dimensions are similarly affected, particularly in their height. Dysplasia epiphysealis hemimelica has been described in the scapula (Bigliani et al). Aneurysmal bone cysts of great size may destroy large segments of the scapula and, like other tumors (Fig 6–49), tend to maintain their usually diagnostic features. One of the most striking of all the scapular lesions is seen in infantile cortical hyperostosis (Fig 6–50). Scapular swelling may appear as early as the third week of life and has been confused with neoplastic disease. Roentgenographic evidence of changes persist for months after the active clinical manifestations have completely subsided.

Fractures and infections of the scapula are rare in children. Forceful lateral traction of the arm or direct impaction stresses on the scapula itself may drive the inferior angle of the scapula between the fourth and fifth ribs and lock it there, according to Nettrour and associates. This is a rare displacement because, in most cases of this type of violence, the involved soft tissues tear and prevent the scapular displacement. Scapular fractures, particularly acromion fractures, in young children should be considered pathognomonic of child abuse according to Kleinman. They may be the initial clue in a battered child who presents with irritability and may be discovered only serendipitously on the chest film (Fig 6–51).

RIBS

During the ninth fetal week the primary ossification centers appear near the angles of the ribs prior to the beginning of ossification in the corresponding vertebrae. From the angles, ossification extends rap-

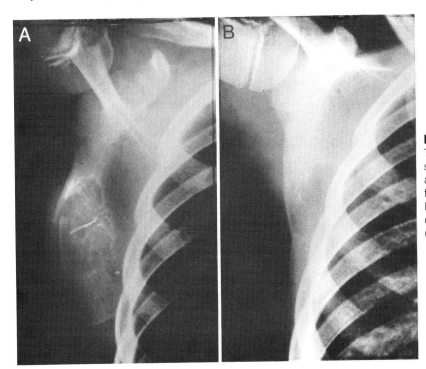

FIG 6–49.
Typical unicameral bone cyst affecting the scapula. **A,** pathologic fracture of a previously asymptomatic lesion. Note the intracystic fragment of wall in addition to the fracture of the lateral wall. **B,** spontaneous healing after conservative management 10 months later. (Courtesy of Dr. J. Gamble, Stanford, Calif.)

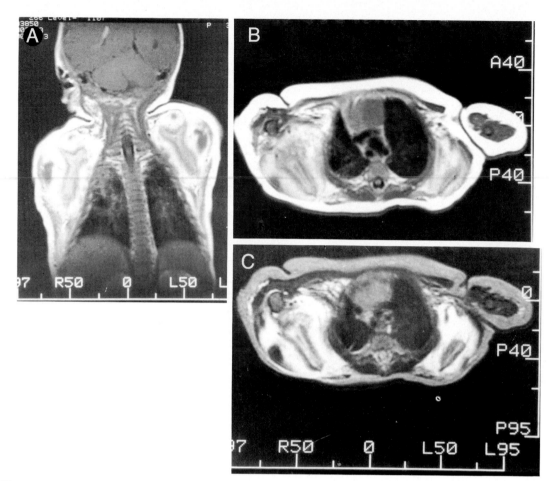

FIG 6–50.
Infantile cortical hyperostosis demonstrated on MRI scan. This 7-week-old infant was referred for neurologic evaluation because of bilateral Erb palsy and posterior shoulder masses. MRI demonstrates regions of increased signal intensity completely surrounding both scapulae with thickening of cortical bone. **A,** Coronal T1-weighted (TR/TE = 750/20) scan. **B,** axial T1-weighted (TR/TE = 800/20) scan. **C,** axial T2-weighted (TR/TE = 2,000/80) scan. (Courtesy of Dr. Bruce Parker, Stanford, Calif.)

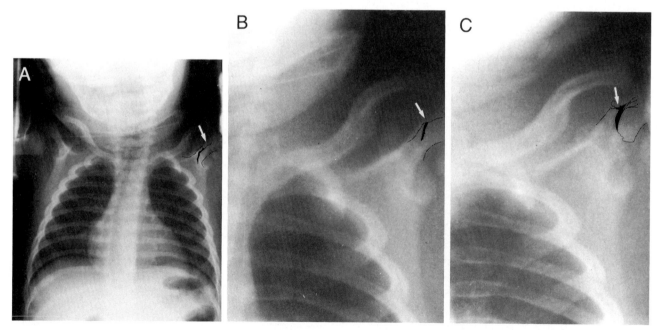

FIG 6–51.
Acromial fracture in child abuse. **A,** chest film in a 3-month-old infant. The left acromial fracture was seen and led to the confirmation of child abuse. **B,** close-up of the fracture. **C,** close-up of the healing fracture 1 month later.

idly forward so that the shafts are ossified and surround the greater part of the thoracic wall as thin bony strips at the end of the fourth fetal month. The anterior extremities of the ribs remain cartilaginous in the form of costal cartilages; the final relative length of the bony and cartilaginous segments is said to be established before birth. Because of observations of defective rib ossification in the cerebrocostovertebral syndrome (see below), questions have been raised concerning the adequacy of theories on the origin of ribs and their subsequent ossification. During adolescence, secondary ossification centers appear in the tubercle and in the head of each rib except the 10th, 11th, and 12th; these secondary centers fuse with the shaft early in the third decade. Occasionally a supernumerary center appears in the anterior end of the 12th ribs; this small opaque shadow, superimposed on the kidney, may resemble a renal stone. Physiologic calcification of the costal cartilages apparently never begins prior to adolescence, even in cases of markedly accelerated development in other structures; it is much more prominent in females than in males.

Congenital anomalies of the ribs are common; they constitute about 2% of all malformations ac-

cording to Coury and Delaporte. Supernumerary ribs are the most common abnormality, approximating 30% of the group. Agenesis and aplasia are next in frequency (about 26%), and errors of segmentation, including synostoses, follow at 20%. The last are often associated with vertebral anomalies. Synostoses occur as isolated events, most frequently in the first and second ribs. Forked rib deformity in the sternal ends of the ribs has no clinical significance in most cases, but in the upper three or four ribs may be a clue to the diagnosis of multiple basal cell syndrome. In more than three fourths of the cases, rib anomalies are asymptomatic; they usually are incidental findings in chest radiographs or are discovered by the observation of a palpable bony protrusion. A rare malformation is an intrathoracic rib that extends obliquely downward within the thoracic cage from its origin in an upper vertebral body (Fig 6–52).

Infections of the chest wall are rare but potentially serious disorders. Recognition of these disorders can be difficult as patients may present with fever, pain, and only minor skin changes. Physical examination underestimates the extent of deep-tissue involvement. Cross-sectional imaging with CT and

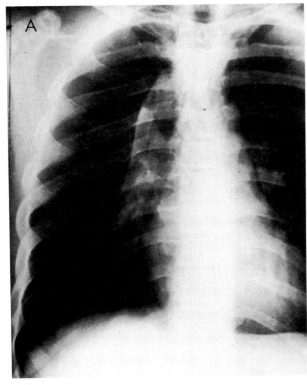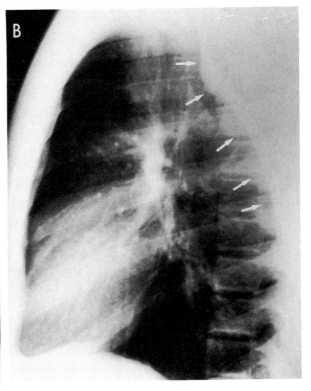

FIG 6–52.
Frontal **(A)** and lateral **(B)** views of intrathoracic rib that was an incidental finding in the course of evaluation for unrelated complaints. The accessory rib takes its origin from the fourth thoracic vertebral body, apparently more ventrad than the normal rib, and courses downward and backward within the right hemithorax.

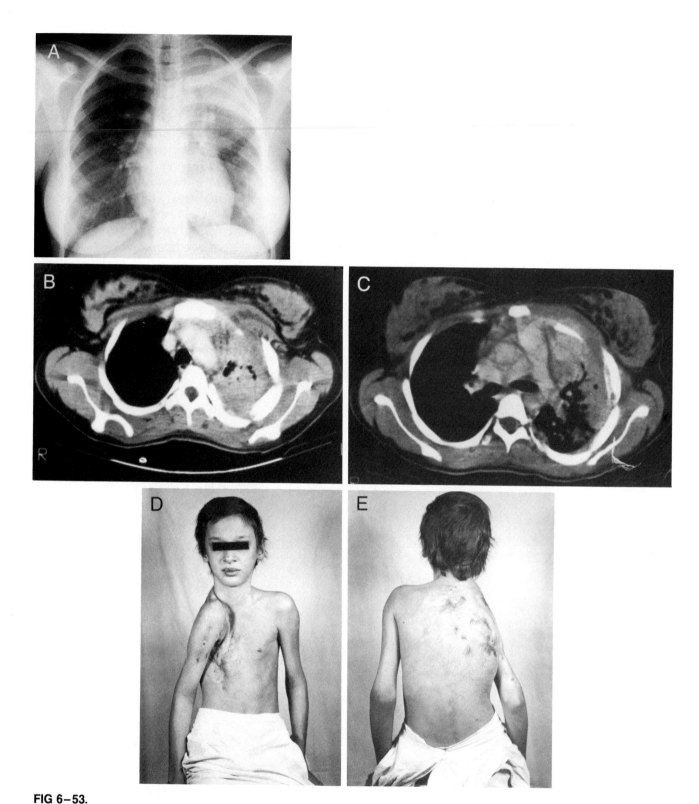

FIG 6–53.
Actinomycosis. **A,** chest film of a 13-year-old girl with cough and chest pain. Diffuse density is seen in the left upper thorax. There are permeative changes of the lateral aspect of the third left rib. **B,** enhanced axial CT scan at the level of the arch reveals the exten-sive chest wall involvement as well as the parenchymal disease. **C,** bone windows on a CT section at the level of the carina demon-strate the rib involvement. **D** and **E,** residual deformity in another patient following recovery from the infection.

MR provides the most information about the nature and extent of these infections (see Fig 40–4). An unusual chest wall infection in children is caused by actinomycosis (Fig 6–53). Thoracic actinomycosis accounts for only 15% of all systemic actinomycoses (craniofacial represents 63% and abdominal, 22%). The disease is usually spread after dental extraction. The triad of lower lobe pulmonary consolidation, empyema, and "wavy" periostitis is typical for this disease. Occasionally, there is vertebral body involvement by direct extension. It is important to diagnose this disease quickly, as it is easily treatable with antibiotics (Golden et al.).

Costochondral involvement has been reported in heroin addicts with systemic candidiasis. Although addiction is not ordinarily a pediatric problem, several of the patients were adolescents. It is believed that the infection was acquired through contamination of lemons used to dissolve "brown" heroin by strains of *Candida* from oropharyngeal or cutaneous areas. The condition presents clinically as a noninflammatory mass in a costochondral site. In all 12 of 26 affected drug abusers who had biopsies, perichondritis was observed; myositis and secondary involvement of bone and cartilage were less frequent. Those with osteitis had positive gallium scintiscans; radiographic studies generally do not reveal bone lesions in affected ribs.

Rib fractures may occur as a result of vigorous efforts during respiratory therapy; they have also been damaged in vigorous play in which parents toss infants into the air and catch them. Healing fractures are observed frequently in children who have been subjected to physical abuse. The characteristic fracture in child abuse is a paravertebral rib fracture which may result either from fixation against the transverse processes or from a direct blow. When forcible direct pressure is applied to the anterior chest wall producing rib fractures, their location is usually more lateral.

Residual traumatic lesions in the ribs may persist for weeks and months after rib resection and intercostal drainage. Diffuse periosteal new bone formation has been noted in the ribs of an infant in an intensive care unit who was receiving physiotherapy to the chest performed with a vibrator. Infants receiving prostaglandin E_1 to maintain patency of the ductus arteriosus may develop periosteal reactions about the ribs and clavicles, and very rarely, the mandible.

The ribs are heir to practically all of the localized lesions found in the long tubular bones of the extremities. They are often affected by enchondromas and multiple or solitary eosinophilic granulomas. In primary or secondary hyperparathyroidism, cystic rarefaction may be found in one or several ribs. This is also true in fibrous dysplasia. Cartilaginous exostoses may grow from the ribs, usually from the sternal ends (Figs 6–54 and 6–55), and enchondromas are not infrequent.

Chest wall tumors are infrequent in infants and children. The most frequent lesions are small round cell tumors (Askin tumor and Ewing sarcoma). Other lesions include undifferentiated spindle cell sarcoma, osteogenic sarcoma, large cell lymphoma, and synovial sarcoma, as well as osteoid osteoma and hamartoma. Ewing tumor has the same characteristics as when it occurs in other flat bones. Osteoid osteoma has been associated with scoliosis in some cases. Hamartomas, also known as mesenchymomas (an improper term according to McLeod and Dahlin), are usually present at birth, frequently in-

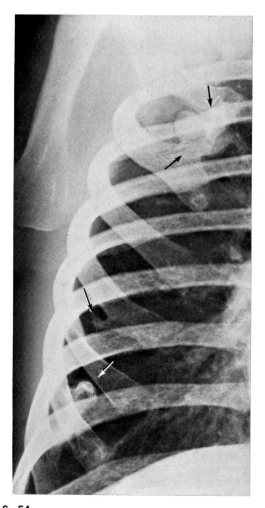

FIG 6–54.
Multiple cartilaginous exostoses *(arrows)* near the sternal ends of the ribs in a patient who had similar bony overgrowths attached to the ends of the shafts of several bones in the limbs. Several members of the family had multiple cartilaginous exostoses.

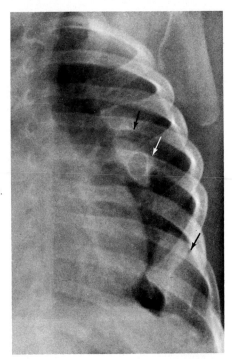

FIG 6–55.
Cartilaginous exostoses *(arrows)* at the sternal ends of the ribs, which could be mistaken for intrapulmonary lesions in an otherwise healthy girl 3½ years of age.

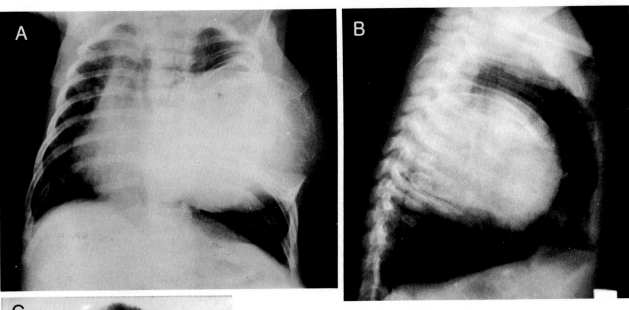

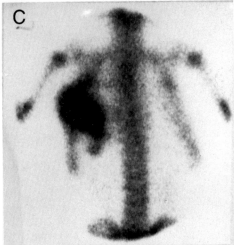

FIG 6–56.
Benign mesenchymoma of the chest wall in a 6-week-old boy. AP and lateral projections (**A** and **B**), and posterior bone scan **(C).** A large left chest wall mass arises from the fifth and sixth ribs, and displaces the mediastinum to the right. The affected ribs are partially destroyed in their midportions and the adjacent ribs are displaced and eroded. Some irregular calcification is present within the mass. A second, smaller mass (also containing calcification) is arising from the inferior border of the ninth rib causing pressure erosion on the tenth rib. The high uptake of radionuclide in the tumor indicates the large amount of cartilage calcification and bone within it. (From Oakley RH, Carty H, Cudmore E: *Pediatr Radiol* 1985; 15:58–60. Used by permission.)

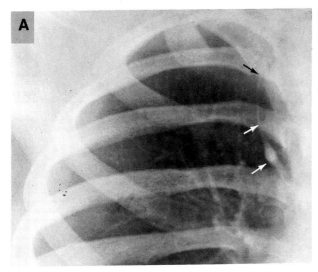

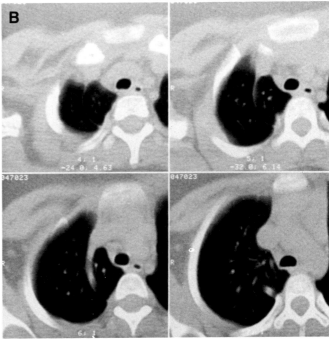

FIG 6–74.
A, normal azygos lobe. The azygos lobe is delineated by the inverted "shadow" *(arrows)* of the azygos fissure and azygos vein. **B,** four contiguous CT images in a patient with an azygos lobe.

Note the lateral and posterior displacement of the azygos vein. There is aerated lung between the azygos vein and the trachea *(T)*.

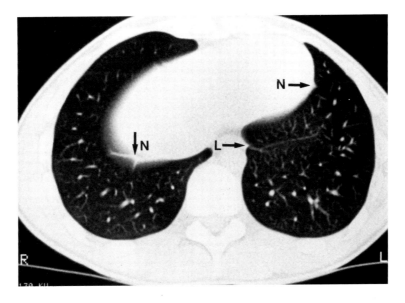

FIG 6–75.
CT demonstration of normal pulmonary ligament and phrenic nerves. A 6 mm CT scan through the lung base in a normal teenage patient reveals the origin of the left pulmonary ligament (L) seen as a branching structure originating from the esophagus medially and extending laterally. This structure can sometimes be seen to branch as it inserts on the diaphragm. The branching structure visualized on the right side (N) is the right phrenic nerve, which on other images was seen to lie adjacent to the inferior vena cava, which differentiates it from the right pulmonary ligament which also is connected to the esophagus. A tiny bump representing the left phrenic nerve (N) is seen adjacent to the pericardium.

TABLE 6–1.

Laboratory Characteristics of an Exudate*

Pleural fluid to serum protein ratio >0.5
Pleural fluid to serum protein ratio for lactic dehydrogenase (LDH) >0.6
Pleural fluid LDH >200 IU
Pleural fluid protein > 3.0 g/dL
pH <7.2
Glucose < 50–60 mg/dL
Positive Gram stain

*Modified from Light RW: *Pleural Diseases.* Philadelphia, Lea & Febiger, 1983.

TABLE 6–2.

Causes of Pleural Effusion

Congenital
  Chylothorax
  Lymphangiectasia
Cardiac
  Congestive heart failure
Renal
  Acute glomerulonephritis (AGN)
  Nephrotic syndrome
  Renal failure
Inflammatory
  Infection
    Staphylococcal, *Haemophilus influenzae*, pneumococcal, tuberculosis, *Mycoplasma*
  Subphrenic abscess
Traumatic
  Hemothorax
  Malpositioned intravascular catheter
  Surgical sequelae
    Thoracotomy
    Postpneumonectomy
    Esophageal rupture
    Chylothorax
  Esophageal rupture
Neoplastic
  Mediastinal mass (especially lymphoma)
  Malignant effusion
    Chest wall sarcoma, metastatic disease
  Hemangiomatosis
  Leukemia
Other
  Ascites
  Collagen-vascular disease
  Hypoproteinemia of any cause
  Fluid overload
  Ventriculopleural shunt

Causes

Pleural effusion has many causes in children. The nature of the effusion, whether transudate, exudate, hemorrhagic effusion, or even chylothorax, can, of course, be determined only by microscopic and laboratory examination. Common causes of pleural effusion seen in childhood are listed in Table 6–2.

In congestive heart failure, pleural fluid accumulation may be bilateral or unilateral; thickening of the fissures, Kerley lines, and pulmonary vascular congestion are commonly seen.

Pleural effusion occurs commonly in association with pneumonia; the incidence is probably greatest with *Staphylococcus* and *Haemophilus influenzae*. Effusions are seen infrequently in viral pneumonia. Once thought to be uncommon, small effusions are now known to be present in up to 25% of cases of mycoplasma pneumonia. Effusions that are usually sterile are also seen as a complication of tuberculosis.

Pleural effusion is usually present in both the nephrotic syndrome and in acute glomerulonephritis (AGN). The amount tends to be greater in those with the nephrotic syndrome. Heart size tends to be normal to small in nephrosis and slightly large in AGN. Recurrent effusion is sometimes the presenting sign of collagen-vascular disease, most commonly systemic lupus erythematosus or rheumatoid arthritis. Interstitial lung disease may be associated later in the disease.

Pleural effusion can occur in patients with ascites, either spreading through existing channels of communication (esophageal and aortic hiatus) or through transdiaphragmatic lymphatic connections.

Hydrothorax is a complication of hyperalimentation when the catheter is placed in a small peripheral vein rather than in the superior vena cava. Hydrothorax occurs due to gradual erosion of the thin-walled, peripheral, intrathoracic vein by the stiff catheter tip.

Chylothorax usually is secondary to trauma to the thoracic duct, most commonly after cardiac surgery. Lethal chylothorax has been reported as a complication of superior vena caval thrombosis secondary to prolonged central line placement. Chylothorax is a relatively common cause of pleural effusion in neonates. This can be diagnosed by thoracentesis although the effusion may not become chylous until after the infant has been fed. Lymphangiomas of the lung or mediastinum can be complicated by chylothorax.

Radiologic Detection

Pleural fluid is typically seen on erect chest films as areas of homogeneous opacity causing rounding of the costophrenic angles. The water-density shadows extend laterally, posteriorly, and anteriorly up the chest wall with concave medial margins and taper smoothly superiorly (Fig 6–76). The fluid layers in a dependent position on decubitus radiographs.

Distribution of fluid in the pleural cavity is determined primarily by gravity and secondarily by the elastic recoil of the lung. Normal, healthy lung tends to retract toward the hilum but maintains its shape, although its volume is diminished. Atypical arrangements of pleural effusion are thought to be explained by varying combinations of the above two factors and have been beautifully explained in Fleischner's classic article.

In the *upright* position, pleural fluid accumulates first in the subpulmonic space between the inferior surface of the lung and the hemidiaphragm. A small amount of fluid in this location will be detected only if a lateral decubitus view is obtained. As the amount of subpulmonary fluid increases, it spills first into the posterior and then the lateral costophrenic sinuses and blunts them. By the time this occurs in adults, about 200 mL of free fluid is present. Occasionally, much larger amounts of fluid may be confined to the subpulmonary space without spilling into the costophrenic sulcus. Radiographic findings suggesting subpulmonary effusion include the following (Fig 6–77): apparent elevation of one or both diaphragms, a shallow costophrenic sinus, lateral displacement of the uppermost portion of what appears to be the diaphragm, widening of the space between the stomach bubble and the apparent diaphragm, minimal thickening of the interlobar fissures, and fluid extending in a spurlike fashion into the fissure at the lung base. Surprisingly large

amounts of fluid can accumulate in the subpulmonary space without blunting of the costophrenic angle, particularly in children with nephrosis. Frequently, when patients have a pleural effusion, subpleural edema is also present and is manifested by thickening of the interlobar fissures. Awareness of this finding should suggest an effusion, which can then be confirmed by decubitus views.

In the *supine* position, fluid accumulates first in the most dependent portion of the lung posteriorly and medially and extends superiorly behind the lung to produce a generalized haziness of the lung before fluid can be detected extending laterally between the lung and the chest wall (Fig 6–78). As the size of the effusion increases, an opaque meniscus develops laterally, followed by formation of an apical "cap."

A large pleural effusion usually produces a shift of the mediastinum toward the contralateral side. The ipsilateral lung collapses concentrically, much as it does with a large pneumothorax (Fig 6–79).

Larger amounts of pleural effusion, while not difficult to detect radiographically, may simulate other abnormalities or obscure underlying pulmonary disease. Views of the chest after thoracentesis or with the child in the lateral decubitus position may be of benefit in visualizing the lung. CT is the most accurate method to separate pleural processes from parenchymal or mediastinal abnormalities although US of the chest can be used to document the fluid nature of the radiographic opacity and may give information about underlying parenchymal abnormalities. Lesions arising in the pulmonary parenchyma or chest wall may simulate loculated effusion as discussed and illustrated later in this chapter. Pleural fluid may be simulated by an atypical form

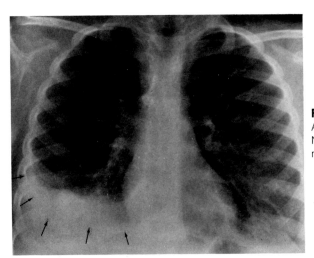

FIG 6–76.
Appearance of free pleural effusion on an upright chest radiograph. Note the right pleural effusion *(arrows)* in a 7-year-old with nephrosis. A meniscus sign is seen both medially and laterally.

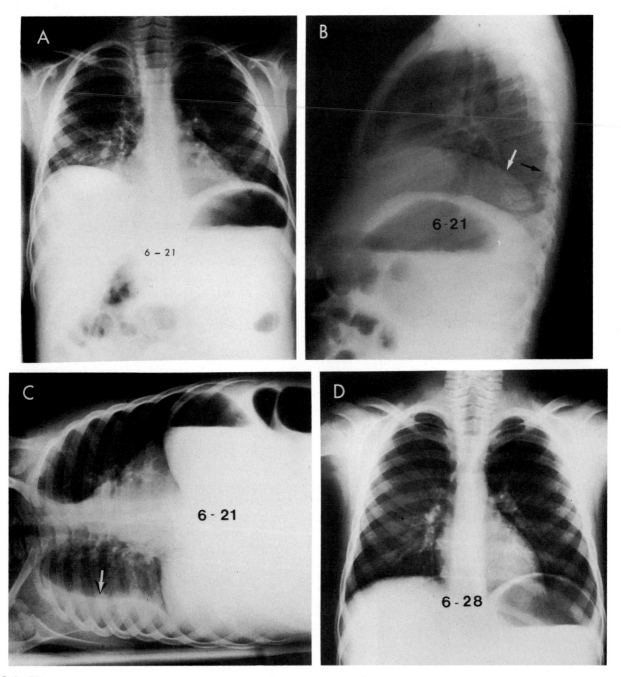

FIG 6–77.
Subpulmonary effusion on an erect film simulating high dia-phragms. A 6-year-old child presented with dyspnea. **A,** frontal ra-diograph shows elevation of both hemidiaphragms but especially the right. Note that the apex of the diaphragm is slightly farther lat-erad than usual. Also, on the left side there is some apparent thick-ening of the space between the upper portion of the gastric bub-ble and what appears to be the bottom of the lung. **B,** the lateral film also shows an "elevation" of the right hemidiaphragm. Note that the posterior costophrenic angle is sharply preserved al-though there is a soft-tissue opacity extending superiorly *(arrows).* **C,** right lateral decubitus radiograph made because of suspicion of pleural effusion based on the appearance of the frontal and lat-eral x-ray films shows a surprisingly large effusion in the right hemithorax *(arrow).* A much smaller effusion was also present on the left side. **D,** 1 week later the bilateral effusions have cleared. Compare the appearance of the diaphragms in this normal radio-graph with **A,** when bilateral subpulmonary effusions were present.

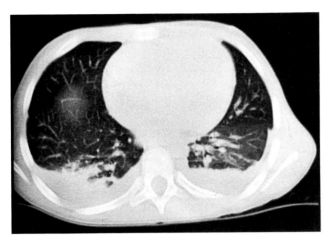

FIG 6–78.
Free pleural effusion on CT scan. This nonenhanced CT image shows bilateral pleural effusions that layer posteriorly, a normal distribution in the recumbent patient. Note the relatively large amount of fluid present. On the right side no fluid has extended laterally, where it would be tangential to the beam on a frontal supine radiograph. On the left slight lateral extension into the major fissure is noted. On a supine radiograph of the chest the right lung appeared slightly hazy, but no free fluid was detected. Only a small amount of fluid was suspected on the left side on the basis of supine radiographic findings (not shown).

of peripheral upper lobe atelectasis (Franken and Klatte) (Fig 6–80).

Appearance of Pleural Fluid on CT and US Scans

US and CT are helpful in evaluating pleural effusion. On US images, the diaphragm is seen as a curvilinear echogenic structure, the movement of which can be assessed with real-time techniques. Effusions are seen as sonolucent areas in the supradiaphragmatic region (Fig 6–81). On CT, fluid is distributed in a gravity-dependent position and therefore is usually posterior. Its attenuation values are in the range of water or higher, but measurement of Hounsfield units (HU) has not been helpful in identifying the nature of the effusion. On images near the lung base, it can be difficult to determine if effusion, ascites, or both are present. The key to correct localization of the fluid collection is to accurately identify the hemidiaphragm. A common error is to mistake thickening of the parietal pleura for the diaphragmatic crus. The signs that are useful in localization include: (1) is the fluid anterior or posterior to the diaphragm? (pleural fluid is posterior). (2) Is the crus displaced anteriorly? (effusion). (3) Is the interface with the liver fuzzy (effusion) or sharp? (ascites). (4) Is fluid seen medial to the bare area of the liver? (effusion) (Fig 6–82).

Loculated Pleural Fluid, Parapneumonic Effusions, and Empyema

Loculation of pleural fluid usually indicates a purulent pleural exudate. Occasionally, interlobar loculations may occur without associated infection. Classification of pleural fluid as a transudate or exudate requires thoracentesis and laboratory analysis, as described previously. Light further subdivides exudates into simple and complicated (parapneumonic) effusions based on decreased pH and glucose levels

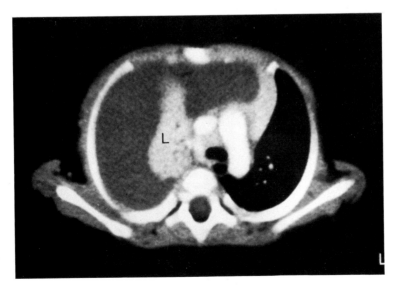

FIG 6–79.
Compression atelectasis due to large pleural effusion. Contrast-enhanced CT (CECT) image of a 9-month-old boy with pneumococcal pneumonia and a huge pleural effusion shows the lung (L) to be markedly compressed by the effusion and the mediastinum dramatically shifted to the left side.

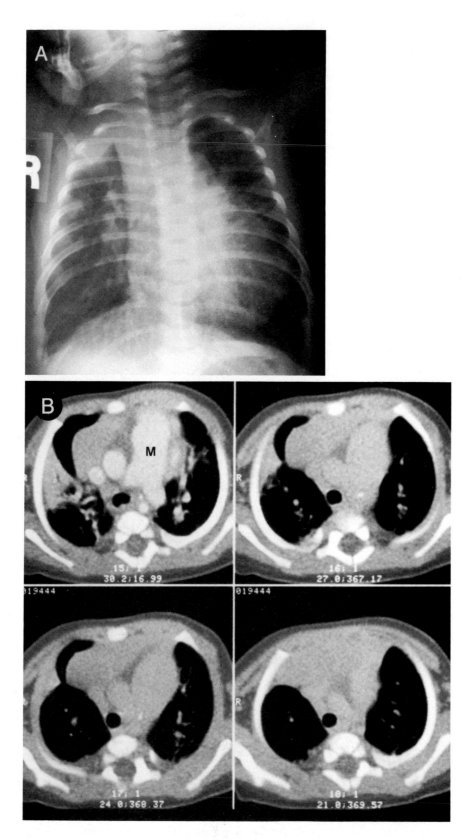

FIG 6–80.
Peripheral atelectasis simulating pleural effusion. **A,** frontal supine radiograph in a 4-month-old infant reveals cardiomegaly, increased pulmonary vascularity, and a peripheral opacity in the right upper lobe which was thought to represent a pleural effusion. **B,** a series of 0.1-second ultrafast CT (UFCT) images from inferior to superior at 3-mm increments reveals no evidence of pleural effusion. Instead there is segmental peripheral atelectasis of the anterior subsegment of the right upper lobe. Note the enlargement of the main pulmonary artery *(M)* as a result of this infant's large ventricular septal defect.

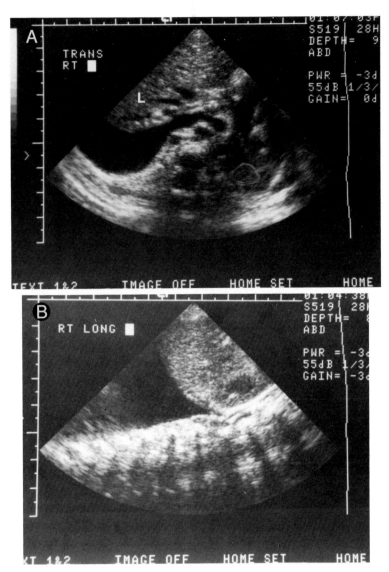

FIG 6–81.
Ultrasound appearance of pleural effusion. **A,** transverse US section shows a sonolucent collection posterior to the liver *(L)*. **B,** longitudinal section in the same patient shows fluid in the posterior costophrenic sulcus. (Courtesy of Dr. Thomas L. Slovis, Children's Hospital of Michigan.)

and an increased lactic dehydrogenase level. Empyema is diagnosed when frank pus is found.

Empyema most commonly follows bacterial pneumonia. *Staphylococcus aureus, Streptococcus pneumoniae,* and *H. influenzae* type b are the most frequent offenders. It may also occur secondary to septic pulmonary emboli, lung abscess, or spread of infection from the rib, spine, liver, or the subphrenic or retropharyngeal regions. Regardless of the cause, the natural history of empyema is similar and has been classified by the American Thoracic Society into three stages: exudative, fibrinopurulent, and organized.

In the exudative stage, the pneumonic process causes inflammation of the visceral pleura and accumulation of watery, uninfected pleural fluid. The radiographic separation of pneumonia from effusion can be difficult unless decubitus positioning is employed. The empyema may resolve without drainage if the primary infection is rapidly and effectively treated, but the amount of fluid can increase very quickly, sometimes in 24 hours, and can become fibrinopurulent and loculated. Therapy at this second stage often requires closed chest tube drainage. The fluid is usually infected unless antibiotics have been given. The radiographic appearance depends on the site and amount of loculations. Loculation is suggested on the chest film when the meniscus is unusually large or extends further cephalad than would be expected for the visible amount of pleural

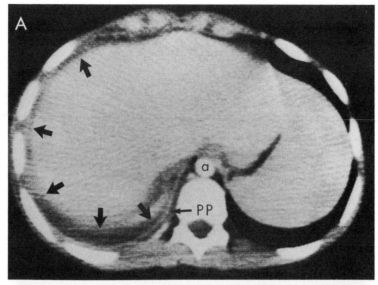

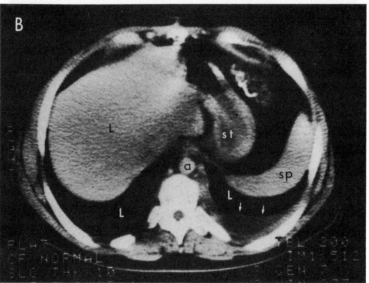

FIG 6–82.
CT appearance of pleural effusion and peritoneal fluid. **A,** CT scan at the level of the hemidiaphragm. The patient has a small pleural effusion *(arrows)* which is seen as a low-attenuation collection peripheral to the liver. This could be mistaken for ascites were the parietal pleura *(arrow, PP)* mistaken for the crus of the diaphragm. Peritoneal fluid occurs anterior to the crus and pleural effusion posterior to it. *a,* aorta. **B,** CT of a different patient with peritoneal fluid secondary to splenic trauma. Note the sharp interface with the liver, the position of the diaphragm, and the lack of fluid over the bare area of the liver.

fluid (Fig 6–83). Failure of the fluid to move on decubitus views confirms the loculation.

In the organizing stage (stage 3), there is ingrowth of fibroblasts along fibrin sheets lining the visceral and parietal pleurae that results in pleural fibrosis, the development of which may necessitate open pleural drainage (Fig 6–84,A and B).

When empyema loculates, large or small areas of any segment of the pleural space may be affected in single or multiple loci (Fig 6–84,C). Purulent fluid encapsulations usually have smooth, rounded, external contours on plain films. US examination

shows them to be sonolucent in the exudative stage with septations and echogenic foci common in the fibrinopurulent and organized stages.

Interlobar loculations of effusions, confined to the major fissures, cast poorly defined, broad shadows in frontal projections owing to the oblique planes of their projection. In lateral views, the shadows are sharply defined, typically with biconvex borders and tapered margins. Contrast-enhanced CT (CECT) reveals a rounded mass with an enhancing rim and a low-attenuation center (Fig 6–85).

Fluid in the minor fissure on the right side is

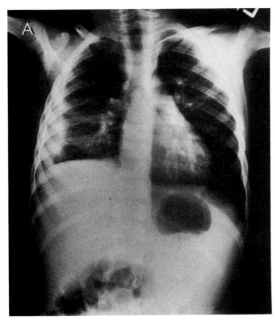

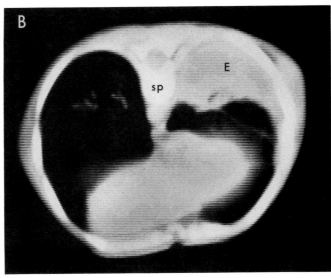

FIG 6–83.
Loculated pleural fluid. **A,** chest radiograph shows a peripheral opacity which appears primarily lateral. It has tapered margins both inferiorly and superiorly. **B,** unenhanced prone CT scan re- veals that most of the exudate *(E)* is actually posterior in location. *sp,* spine.

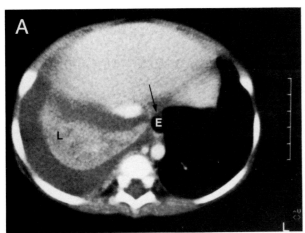

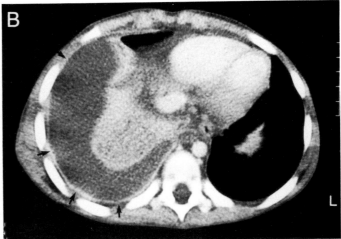

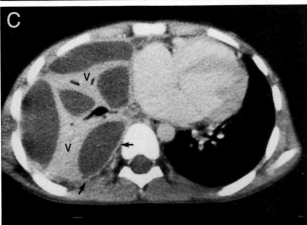

FIG 6–84.
CT appearance of various stages of empyema. **A,** a 9-month-old infant with parapneumonic effusion which was serosanguinous at thoracentesis. CECT reveals compressive atelectasis of the lung *(L)* which is tethered to the esophagus *(arrow, E)* at the level of the pulmonary ligament. No enhancement of the pleural surfaces is noted. **B,** CECT scan in an 8-year-old child with pneumococcal pneumonia. There is compressive atelectasis of the right lower lobe, and rather marked enhancement *(arrows)* of the parietal pleura. Cloudy, infected fluid was withdrawn at thoracentesis. **C,** CECT on an 11-year-old child reveals marked loculation of fluid collections with enhancement of the visceral pleura *(arrows)* V indicates lung tissue. Grossly infected fluid was removed at thoracentesis. Note the marked compression of the intervening normal lung, which shows moderate contrast enhancement

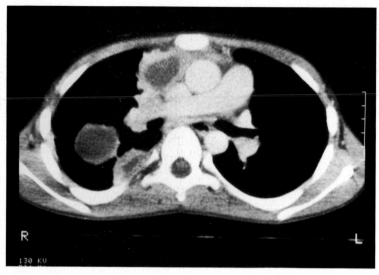

FIG 6–85.
Empyema loculated in the right major fissure. Note the enhanced rim of the visceral pleura. Loculations are also present posteriorly and in the mediastinal pleura anteriorly.

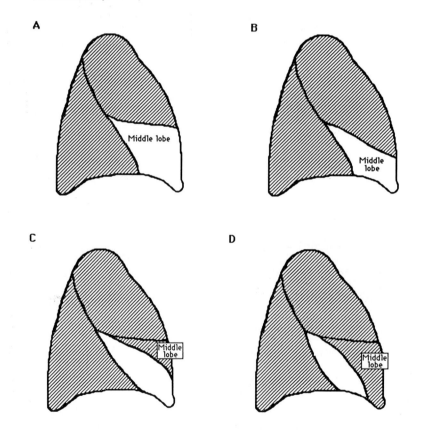

FIG 6–86.
Diagrams illustrating the similarity of consolidations in the right middle lobe and loculated pleural exudates in the inferior portion of the major fissure. **A,** consolidation in a large right middle lobe. **B,** consolidation in a small right middle lobe. **C,** large interlobar loculation between the right middle and lower lobes. **D,** small interlobar loculation in the same position as **C.** (Redrawn by Jonas C from Schoenfield H: Die Pleura und ihre Erkrankungen, in Engel S, Schall L (eds): *Handbuch der Roentgendiagnostik und Therapie im Kindesalter.* Leipzig, Georg Thieme Verlag, 1933.)

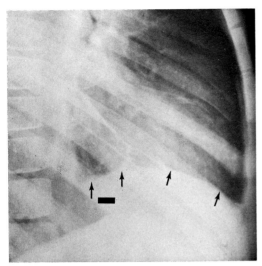

FIG 6–87.
"Overlap" shadow of the right hemidiaphragm simulating consolidation in the right middle lobe produced by the superimposed shadows of the base of the heart and the dome of the right diaphragm *(arrows)*. Right lower lobe consolidation silhouettes the right diaphragm posteriorly.

sharply defined in both lateral and frontal views. Differentiation between fluid in the base of the major fissure and consolidations in the right middle lobe directly anterior to the fissure is difficult and, at times, impossible unless CT is utilized. Difficulties in distinguishing between these two lesions are due to the great variation in size and shape of the middle lobe and in the position of the interlobar fissures (Fig 6–86). Further confusion may arise because an "overlap" shadow may simulate a supradiaphragmatic fluid collection (Fig 6–87).

CT is useful in evaluation of parapneumonic effusions and empyema by accurately localizing the site and extent of the fluid collections, determining the adequacy of chest tube drainage, and aiding in the differentiation of pleural from parenchymal pro-

cesses. In the exudative stage, CT reveals free pleural effusion indistinguishable from any transudative pleural fluid collection. Contrast enhancement is extremely useful in evaluation of pleural abnormalities. If pleural inflammation or irritation is present, the pleura usually shows enhancement (see Fig 6–84). As the fibrinopurulent phase progresses, the pleural enhancement becomes more marked; the enhancement of both the visceral and parietal layers results in the "split pleura" sign, diagnostic of a pleural process (Fig 6–88). Similar findings are present on T1-weighted gadolinium-enhanced MR studies (Fig 6–89). Fluid may be loculated in one or more locations in the thorax. The adjacent extrathoracic soft tissues may be inflamed. Chronic, organized empyema is now infrequently seen in chil-

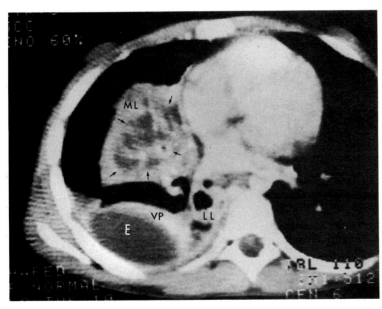

FIG 6–88.
Loculated pleural collection. CT scan of a 12-year-old boy with acute streptococcal pneumonia demonstrates pneumonic consolidation of the right middle lobe *(arrows, ML)*. The right lower lobe *(LL)* is collapsed posteriorly. A large loculated empyema *(E)* is outlined by contrast-enhanced parietal pleura posteriorly and thickened visceral pleura anteriorly *(VP)*.

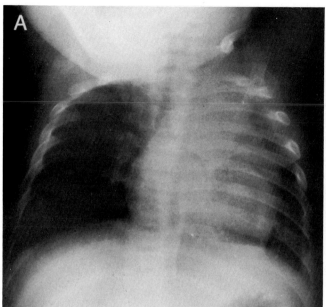
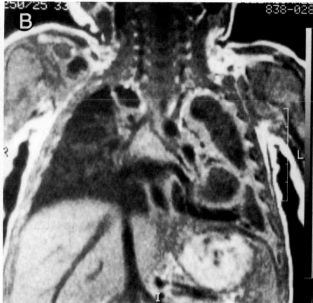

FIG 6–89.
MR appearance of loculated empyema. **A,** supine chest radiograph of a 6-month-old infant thought clinically to have a neuroblastoma. Radiograph reveals opacity in the left superior mediastinum as well as slight paravertebral widening and pleural thickening *(arrows).* **B,** coronal gadolinium DTPA–enhanced T1-weighted MR image reveals three fluid-filled loculations with thick enhancing rims consistent with loculated empyema. This was confirmed by thoracentesis.

dren, but its hallmarks are progressive pleural thickening showing marked contrast enhancement and associated with compression of the adjacent lung.

In addition to antibiotics, therapy of empyema usually includes repeated thoracentesis or closed chest tube drainage. More recently, radiologically guided percutaneous catheter drainage has been shown to be safe and effective. CT can be used to assure adequacy of the drainage procedures and to recognize chest tubes inadvertently placed in the fissures or actually through the lungs themselves. Some studies have shown no significant difference in the long-term outcome of empyema regardless of the method of therapy employed. Decortication of a chronic, organized empyema is necessary in well under 10% of children.

While the plain film separation of pleural from parenchymal abnormalities is difficult or impossible, CT in most cases can not only make this distinction, but can also characterize the parenchymal abnormality. Pleural disease is recognized, following contrast enhancement, by the findings of enhancement, usually of both the visceral and parietal pleural layers enclosing an avascular collection which is usually thin-walled with smooth margins, of lenticular shape, and forming obtuse angles with the chest walls (see Fig 6–88).

Characterization of the underlying parenchymal

abnormality is also aided by CECT. Neoplasms are fortunately rare in children, but mediastinal masses such as lymphoma can be associated with pleural effusion. These conditions are more fully described in Chapter 14, but typically present as masses in the anterior or middle mediastinum and are associated with hilar adenopathy. The mediastinal mass itself usually shows inhomogeneous enhancement with areas of necrosis (Fig 6–90). Chest wall neoplasms can also simulate empyema (Fig 6–91). Uncomplicated bacterial pneumonia typically appears on CT as poorly marginated airspace disease with air bronchograms and relatively uniform enhancement. Major atelectasis shows a lobar or segmental configuration, usually an air bronchogram, and relatively marked enhancement. We have seen several cases of *S. pneumoniae* and *S. aureus* pneumonia in which the area of lobar consolidation was inhomogeneous and marked by poorly marginated areas of low attenuation without enhancing rims, probably representing areas of incipient necrosis (Fig 6–92). Air-containing spaces, presumably pneumatoceles or areas of actual pulmonary breakdown, have been noted in some such cases (Fig 6–92). Gas in an empyema suggests a bronchopleural fistula and, when air-fluid levels are present, confusion with a lung abscess may occur (Fig 6–93). The criteria listed in Table 6–3 usually allow differentiation of abscess from empyema;

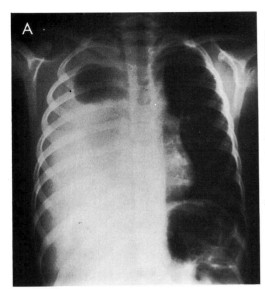

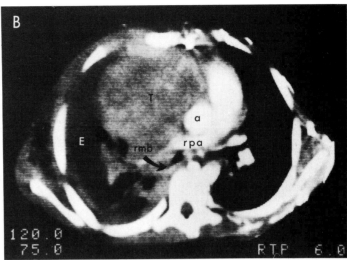

FIG 6–90.
Utility of CT evaluation of opaque hemithorax. **A,** chest radiograph in a patient thought clinically to have pneumonia and empyema. **B,** CECT made because of rapid recurrence of fluid after thoracentesis reveals a large effusion *(E)* and a large mediastinal mass *(T),* which compresses the right mainstem bronchus *(rmb)* and displaces the right pulmonary artery *(rpa)* posteriorly. Diagnosis: non-Hodgkin lymphoma. *a,* aorta.

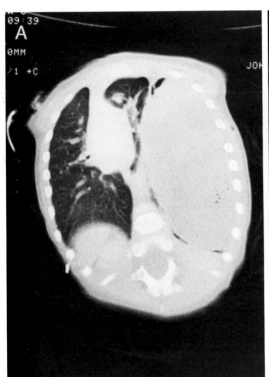

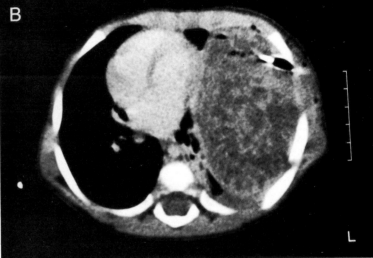

FIG 6–91.
Chest wall mass simulating empyema. This 1-year-old child was thought to have empyema on the basis of a radiographic examination. A thoracostomy tube was placed and only a small amount of serosanguinous fluid was obtained. The patient was referred for CT. **A,** oblique direct coronal scan with the patient sitting upright in the gantry of the scanner reveals a large extrapleural mass occupying the left hemithorax. Note the small rim of lung inferiorly separating the mass from the diaphragm. **B,** transaxial contrast-enhanced 3-mm CT image reveals the chest tube entering the mass. The mass has a thin enhancing capsule and a heterogeneous internal architecture. At surgery a primitive neuroectodermal tumor arising from the chest wall was partially removed.

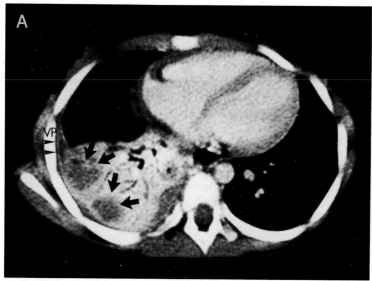

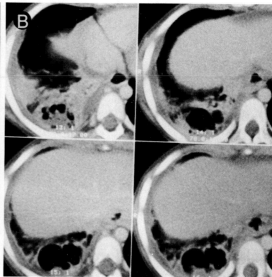

FIG 6−92.

Combined pleural and parenchymal disease caused by pneumonia, pneumatoceles, and parapneumonic effusion. The patient was a 3-year-old child with pneumococcal pneumonia. **A,** contrast-enhanced UFCT scan reveals right lower lobe consolidation. Air bronchogram and enhancement of the affected lobe is noted, as are two large, round, low-attenuation areas in the lower lobe *(ar-*

rows). Slight thickening *(arrowheads)* of the visceral pleura *(VP)* is also evident. The low-attenuation lesions are thought to represent areas of pulmonary necrosis that may or may not go on to become pneumatoceles. **B,** contiguous serial 3-mm sections *1* through *4* inferior to **A** reveal multiple air-containing cavities in the inferior portion of the right lower lobe representing pneumatoceles.

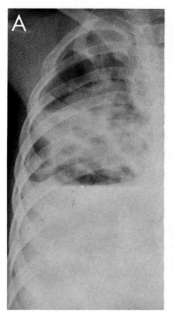

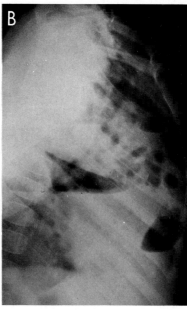

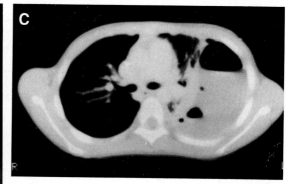

FIG 6−93.

Pyopneumothorax. Multiloculated pyopneumothorax presenting with numerous separate gas spaces in the right pleural space, some of which have gas-fluid levels. **A,** frontal and **B,** lateral projections. **C,** CT scan in a different patient who also had pyopneu-

mothorax. Note the multiple gas-fluid levels in the left pleural space with marked compression atelectasis of the left lung. Without the use of CT it is often impossible to be certain if the gas collections are in the lung, the pleural space, or both.

TABLE 6–3.
Computed Tomography (CT) Findings in the Differentiations of Lung Abscess and Empyema*

CT Findings	Abscess (%)	Empyema (%)
Wall characteristics		
Thick	88	6
Thin	12	94
Uniform width	0	93
Smooth internal margin	14	91
Smooth external margin	17	91
Split pleural sign	0	68
Angle with chest wall		
Acute	83	14
Obtuse	0	70
Shape		
Round	67	11
Lenticular	0	63

*Modified from Stark DP, Federle MP, Goodman PC, et al: *Am J Roentgenol* 1983; 141:163.

at times, however, the differentiation of abscess from empyema may be difficult, and they may even coexist.

PLEURAL NEOPLASMS

Neoplasms of the pleura are rare in children. Benign, malignant, and inflammatory chest wall masses, discussed earlier in this chapter, can breach the pleura or simulate pleural masses. Pulmonary metastatic disease is often peripheral and may be pleural-based. Both Wilms tumor and neuroblastoma (Fig 6–94) may involve the pleura, as can metastatic sarcomas. Pleural lipomas are diagnosed by findings of an ovoid, extrapleural mass with imaging characteristics on CT or MR consistent with a homogeneous fatty mass (Fig 6–95). They are differentiated from liposarcomas because the latter are rarely intrathoracic, but tend to be symptomatic, infiltrative, heterogeneous, and usually have attenuation coefficients greater than −50 HU. Mesothelioma, the commonest adult pleural malignancy, is very rare in children but has been reported to be associated with prior radiation therapy, usually for Wilms tumor.

PNEUMOTHORAX

Air may enter the pleural space by way of the parietal or the visceral pleura. Many causes of pneumothorax are known: exploratory needle punctures, therapeutic introduction of air, tracheotomy, traumatic lacerations of the lung, and penetrating foreign bodies in the lung, bronchial tree, and occasionally the esophagus. Pneumothorax has also been reported in association with many pediatric pulmonary diseases, including asthma, cystic fibrosis, histiocytosis X, Marfan syndrome, metastatic neoplasms (especially osteogenic sarcoma), lymphangiomatosis, cystic adenomatoid malformation of the lung, bronchogenic cyst, and, rarely, endometriosis. Many cases of pneumothorax in children, especially in teen-agers, are "spontaneous" and may result from rupture of apical subpleural blebs.

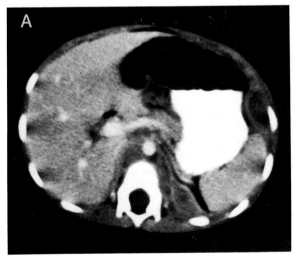
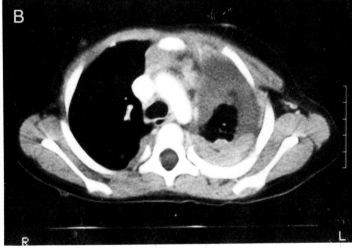

FIG 6–94.
Metastatic neuroblastoma with pleural effusion in a 4-year-old child. **A,** CECT 6-mm slice through the upper abdomen reveals displacement of the diaphragmatic crus on the left side by a solid tumor mass demonstrating irregular enhancement. A loculated fluid collection is noted laterally with enhancement of the visceral pleura. **B,** a more superior section at the level of the aortic arch in the same patient reveals a large pleural effusion, a compressed air containing lung, enhancement of the solid tumor mass posteriorly, and mediastinal metastases.

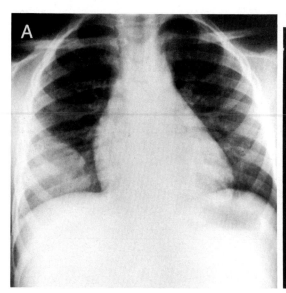

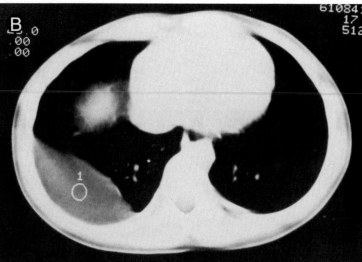

FIG 6–95.
Pleural lipoma. **A,** chest radiograph reveals an extrapleural opacity at the right lung base which is of relatively low attenuation. **B,** unenhanced CT scan reveals a low-attenuation pleural mass. Hounsfield units confirmed its fatty nature. (Courtesy of L. Das Narla, Richmond, Va.)

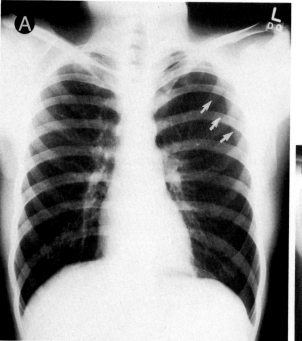

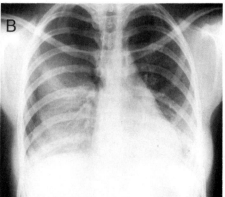

FIG 6–96.
Pneumothorax. **A,** posteroanterior inspiration radiograph reveals a small apical left pneumothorax diagnosed by seeing a faint pleural line *(arrows)* and lack of pulmonary vascular markings peripheral to the pleural line. **B,** expiratory film in a different patient shows accentuation of a small pneumothorax on the right side. The total volume of air in the pleural space does not increase, but the lung volume decreases on expiration, increasing the opacity of the lung and making the relative amount of air larger and the findings more obvious.

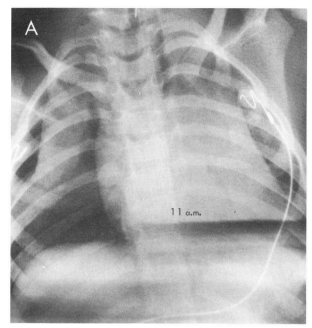

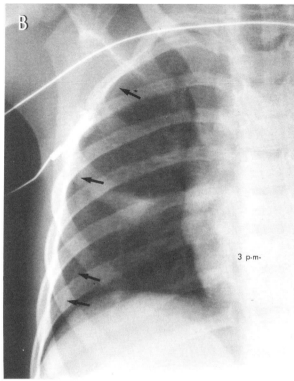

FIG 6–97.
"Loculated" pneumothorax. This portable chest radiograph was made following nephrectomy because the surgeon thought he had inadvertently entered the pleural space. **A,** radiograph shows a loculated pneumothorax superiorly and laterally on the right side. There is partial loss of volume in the right upper lobe which has caused "loculation" of the pneumothorax adjacent to the atelectatic lobe. **B,** repeat portable radiograph 4 hours later. The right upper lobe is now reexpanded and is of the same density as the rest of the lung. The pneumothorax now assumes a more typical peripheral location *(arrows).*

In the erect position, the radiographic appearance of pneumothorax depends on the amount of gas in the pleural space, the degree of collapse of the lung, and the presence or absence of underlying lung disease. A constant finding, however, is that the outer margin of the lung (visceral pleura) is separated from the chest wall (parietal pleura) by a radiolucent space devoid of any pulmonary vascular markings (Fig 6–96). In equivocal cases, the findings may be made more obvious by obtaining either a lateral decubitus film or one exposed in expiration. The volume of gas in the pleural space stays the same while the overall volume of the thorax decreases, which allows the extrapulmonary gas to occupy a relatively greater volume. In supine patients the lung collapses more posteriorly, and gas layers anteriorly and medially to produce a "hyperlucent" lung or medial radiolucency simulating a pneumomediastinum. An unusually prominent costophrenic sulcus is an additional sign of pneumothorax on an AP supine radiograph, as is visualization of the anterior junction line in neonates.

An unusual form of localized pneumothorax pe-

ripheral to a collapsed lobe was described by Lipinski and Goodman. Berdon et al. reported three similar cases and theorized that the lucency was not a true pneumothorax but in fact was the result of gas filling the space between parietal and visceral pleurae in a manner analogous to the so-called vacuum phenomenon in joints. This form of "pneumothorax" is associated with lobar bronchial obstruction, and relief of the bronchial obstruction causes rapid disappearance of the gas collection. An alternative explanation for this atypical localization of gas is that gas, free in the pleural space, may be attracted by the increased elastic recoil of a collapsing lung in much the same way that atypical fluid loculations are thought to occur. Relief of the atelectasis then allows "typical" distribution of pneumothorax (Fig 6–97). Occasionally, the upper lobe will collapse completely and may even undergo torsion with the ptotic, consolidated lobe, simulating a mediastinal or hilar mass (Fig 6–98).

An accurate estimation of the size of a pneumothorax is difficult. In an adult sized patient, a pneumothorax that occupies the peripheral inch of the

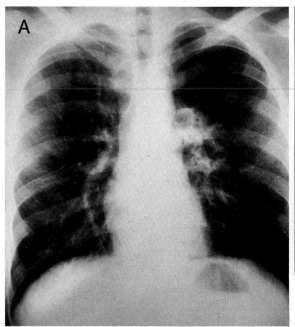

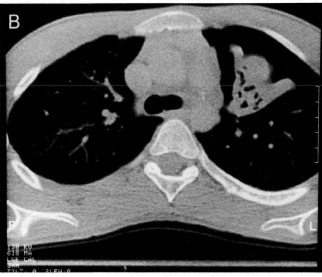

FIG 6–98.
Pneumothorax with left upper lobe collapse simulating a hilar mass. **A,** chest radiograph in a 15-year-old boy presenting with chest pain and shortness of breath. The child was referred for CT because of an apparent left hilar mass. A subtle pneumothorax was visible on the chest radiograph only in retrospect. **B,** unenhanced CT section reveals tight atelectasis of the left upper lobe which is surrounded by a "loculated" pneumothorax. The left lower lobe is fully expanded and appears normal.

thorax amounts to about 30% of total lung volume. One must be careful to differentiate pneumothorax from soft-tissue artifacts, especially skin folds, to avoid overdiagnosis. Usually, a skin fold looks like a boundary with a fine, dark line (a Mach line) along its lateral margin. A pneumothorax shows the visceral pleura, which appears as a fine, white line. A rotated lateral chest film may also erroneously suggest a pneumothorax (Fig 6–99).

A large cystic lesion, either congenital or acquired, can simulate a tension pneumothorax. The diagnosis is usually not considered until the presumed pneumothorax has failed to respond to chest tube placement. CT examination may be done to verify tube placement and will discover septations in the cystic lesion, differentiating it from a tension pneumothorax (Fig 6–100).

Tension Pneumothorax

The most common manifestations of tension pneumothorax are mediastinal shift, diaphragmatic depression, and rib cage expansion. True tension pneumothorax is uncommon. The degree of lung collapse can neither confirm nor rule out tension. Underlying lung disease may prevent total collapse even if tension is present. With any large pneumothorax, there is a shift of the mediastinum away

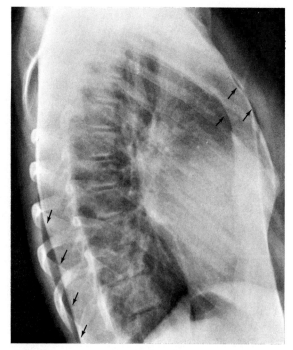

FIG 6–99.
A slightly obliqued lateral radiograph simulating a pneumothorax. On a slightly oblique lateral projection, radiolucent strips of intrapulmonary air both fore and aft may simulate pneumothorax or subcutaneous emphysema *(arrows).* This boy was 13 years old.

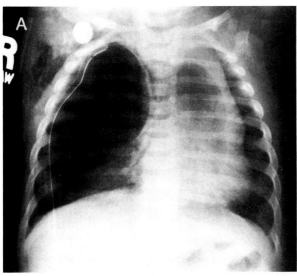
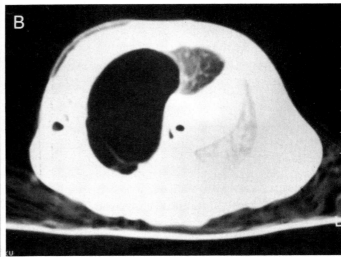

FIG 6–100.
Congenital cystic disease of the lung simulating a pneumothorax. **A,** a 1-year-old infant was referred from an outside hospital after placement of a right chest tube for a pneumothorax with failure of therapeutic response. This supine frontal radiograph reveals a right chest tube in place. There is a large air collection in the right thorax, herniation of air across the midline, and compressive atelectasis of the right lower lobe. **B,** unenhanced CT scan in this patient reveals septa in the large air collection indicating that this is a cystic lesion rather than a true pneumothorax. At surgery a cystic adenomatoid malformation was removed.

from the pneumothorax, since pressure on the normal side is lower (more negative) than on the affected side. The diagnosis can be established on fluoroscopy, where it will be seen that there is minimal, if any, shift toward the side of the pneumothorax on inspiration and that there is limited diaphragmatic excursion.

Hydropneumothorax

Hydropneumothorax is diagnosed when there are solitary or multiple air-fluid levels in the pleural space. The fluid may be serous, bloody, or infected. Lung abscess or infected pneumatoceles may produce a similar radiographic appearance, as described above. CT is often required to differentiate these conditions. If the fluid or air crosses a fissure, pleural origin can be presumed. Unless the gas has been introduced by thoracentesis, communication with the lung is presumed since gas-forming infections are uncommon in children.

REFERENCES

Anatomy, Normal Radiographic Appearance

Berkmen YM, Auh YH, Davis SD, et al: Anatomy of the minor fissure: Evaluation with thin-section CT. *Radiology* 1989a; 170:647-651.

Berkmen YM, Davis SD, Kazam E, et al: Right phrenic nerve: Anatomy, CT appearance, and differentiation from the pulmonary ligament. *Radiology* 1989b; 173:43-46.

Chasen MH, McCarthy MJ, Gilliland JD, et al: Concepts in computed tomography of the thorax. *Radiographics* 1986; 6:793-832.

Friedman E: Further observations on the vertical fissure line. *Am J Roentgenol* 1966; 97:171.

Glazer HS, Anderson DJ, DiCroce JJ et al: Anatomy of the major fissure: Elevation with standard and thin-section CT. *Radiology* 1991; 180:839.

Godwin JD, Vock P, Osborne DR: CT of the pulmonary ligament. *Am J Roentgenol* 1983; 141:231

Im JG, Webb WR, Rosen AW, et al: Costal pleura: Appearances at high-resolution CT. *Radiology* 1989; 171:125.

Naidich D, Zerhouni EA, Siegelman SS (eds): *Computed Tomography and Magnetic Resonance of the Thorax,* ed 2. New York, Raven Press, 1991, p 411.

Rabinowitz JG, Wolf BS: Roentgen significance of the pulmonary ligament. *Radiology* 1966; 87:1013.

Rost RC Jr, Proto AV: Inferior pulmonary ligament: Computed tomographic appearance. *Radiology* 1983; 148:479.

Spackman JM, et al: Alterations in CT mediastinal anatomy produced by an azygos lobe. *Am J Roentgenol* 1981; 137:47-50.

Pleural Effusion

Broaddus C, Staub NC: Pleural liquid and protein turnover in health and disease. *Semin Respir Med* 1987; 9:7–12.

Eklof O, Torngren A: Pleural fluid in healthy children. *Acta Radiol* 1971; 11:346.

Fleischner FG: Atypical arrangement of free pleural effusion. *Radiol Clin North Am* 1963; 1:347.

Franken EA, Klatte EC: Atypical (peripheral) upper lobe collapse. *Ann Radiol (Paris)* 1977; 28:87.

Griffen DJ, Gross BH, McCracken S, et al: Observations on CT differentiation of pleural and peritoneal fluid. *J Comput Assist Tomogr* 1984; 8:24.

Halvorsen RA, Fedyshin PJ, Korobkin M, et al: Ascites or pleural effusion? CT differentiation: Four useful criteria. *Radiographics* 1986; 6:135.

Henschke CI, Yankelevitz DF, Davis SD: Pleural diseases: Multimodality imaging and clinical management. *Curr Probl Diagn Radiol* 1991; 20(5):155.

Light RW: *Pleural Diseases.* Philadelphia, Lea & Febiger, 1983.

McLoud TC, Flower CDR: Imaging the pleura: Sonography, CT and MR imaging. *Am J Roentgenol* 1991; 156:1145.

Miserocchi G: Pleural pressures and fluid transport, in crystal RG (ed): The Lung: Scientific Foundations. New York, Raven Press, 1991, pp 885–893.

Moskowitz H, Platt RT, Schachar R, et al: Roentgen visualization of minute pleural effusion. *Radiology* 1973; 109:33.

Naidich DP, Megibow AJ, Hilton S, et al: Computed tomography of the diaphragm: Peridiaphragmatic fluid localization. *J Comput Assist Tomogr* 1983; 7:641.

Pecorari A, Weisbrod GL: Computed tomography of pseudotumoral pleural fluid collections in the azygoesophageal recess. *J Comput Assist Tomogr* 1989; 13:803.

Vix VA: Roentgenographic manifestations of pleural disease. *Semin Roentgenol* 1977; 12:277.

Empyema

Andrews NC, et al: Management of nontuberculous empyema. *Am Rev Respir Dis* 1962; 85:935.

Bressler EL, Francis IR, Glazer GM, et al: Bolus contrast medium enhancement for distinguishing pleural from parenchymal lung disease: CT features. *J Comput Assist Tomogr* 1987; 11:436.

Cleveland RH, Foglia RP: CT in the evaluation of pleural versus pulmonary disease in children. *Pediatr Radiol* 1988; 18:14–19.

Freij BJ, Kusmiesz H, Nelson JD, et al: Parapneumonic effusions and empyema in hospitalized children: A retrospective review of 227 cases. *Pediatr Infect Dis* 1984; 3:578–591.

Redding GJ, Walund L, Walund D, et al: Lung function in children following empyema. *Am J Dis Child* 1990; 144:1337.

Stark DP, Federle MP, Goodman PC, et al: Differentiating lung abscess and empyema: Radiography and computed tomography. *Am J Roentgenol* 1983; 141:163.

Wise MB, Beaudry PH, Bates DV: Long-term follow-up of staphylococcal pneumonia. *Pediatrics* 1966; 38:398–401.

Neoplasms

Anderson KA, Hurley WC, Hurley BT, et al: Malignant pleural mesothelioma following radiotherapy in a 16-year-old boy. *Cancer* 1985; 56:273.

Antman KH, Ruxer RL Jr, Aisner J, et al: Mesothelioma following Wilms' tumor in childhood. *Cancer* 1984; 54:367.

Kawashima A, Libshitz HI: Malignant pleural mesothelioma: CT manifestations in 50 cases. *Am J Roentgenol* 1990; 155:965.

Lorigan JG, Libshitz HI: MR imaging of malignant pleural mesothelioma. *J Comput Assist Tomogr* 1989; 13:617.

Storey TF, Narla LD: Pleural lipoma in a child—CT evaluation. *Pediatr Radiol* 1991; 21:141-142.

Pneumothorax

Beg MH, Reyazuddin, Faridi MMA, et al: Spontaneous pneumothorax in children. A review of 95 cases. *Ann Trop Paediatr* 1988; 8:18.

Berdon WE, Dee GJ, Abramson SJ, et al: Localized pneumothorax adjacent to a collapsed lobe: A sign of bronchial obstruction. *Radiology* 1984; 150:691.

Berkmen YM, Yankelevit D, Davis SD, et al: Torsion of the upper lobe in pneumothorax. *Radiology* 1989c; 173–447.

Goodman LR, Foley WD, Wilson CR, et al: Pneumothorax and other lung diseases: Effect of altered resolution and edge enhancement on diagnosis with digitized radiographs. *Radiology* 1988; 167:83.

Lipinski JK, Goodman A: Pneumothorax complicating bronchiolitis in an infant. *Pediatr Radiol* 1980; 9:244.

Markowitz RI: The anterior junction line: A radiographic sign of bilateral pneumothorax in neonates. *Pediatr Radiol* 1988; 167:717.

Normal Lung and Anomalies

NORMAL LUNG

The lungs develop as a primitive bud from the foregut; during the fifth week of fetal life the lung bud normally separates completely from the esophagus, which also is of foregut origin. A failure to completely separate leads to anomalies along the spectrum of tracheoesophageal fistula. Abnormal budding of the primordial foregut results in bronchogenic and neurenteric cysts as well as sequestrations. Insults occurring after the 26th day of fetal life interfere with the growth and development of the terminal air sac. At birth, there are approximately 24 million alveoli present; they grow in number and size until they reach the adult number of some 300 million by the time the child reaches 8 years of age.

The radiologic anatomy of the normal tracheobronchial tree and lung is not significantly different in the pediatric patient from that seen in the adult. The left lung has two lobes and the right, three lobes (Fig 7–1). The pleural fissures separating the lobes of the lungs are often anatomically incomplete. Portions of the fissures are occasionally visualized in healthy infants as hairlike lines. The lungs are further subdivided into eight segments on the left and ten on the right, each served by a segmental bronchus (Fig 7–2). Collateral ventilation can occur across pulmonary segments since there is no pleura separating them. Fraser and Paré describe three routes of collateral ventilation: (1) pores of Kohn (circular discontinuities in alveolar walls); (2) canals of Lambert (epithelial-lined tubules between preterminal bronchioles and alveoli surrounding them); and (3) direct airway anastomosis.

From a structural and functional point of view, the lung is divided into two major components: (1) the airways and the vasculature, and (2) their interstitial supporting structures. The airways are further subdivided into pure conducting, partially conducting, and gas-exchanging zones (Fig 7–3).

The trachea, the largest of the conducting airways, is a fibromuscular tube lined by a mucous membrane and supported by 16 to 20 cartilaginous rings, which are incomplete posteriorly, where the tracheal wall is comprised of fibrous, muscular, and elastic tissue. The trachea extends from the cricoid cartilage at C4 to the carina at about T4 at birth, but by about 2 years of age it is at T5 (Noback). The right main bronchus originates from the trachea at an angle of 32 ± 5.5 degrees and the left at an angle of 51 ± 9.5 degrees from birth to 2 years of age.

The *bronchi* are also conducting airways which consist of the first 11 branching generations after the carina. The first four bronchial generations (through the segmental branches) are strongly supported by cartilaginous plates that aid in keeping the bronchi patent. The smaller cartilaginous bronchial branches, from the 5th to the 11th generation, dou-

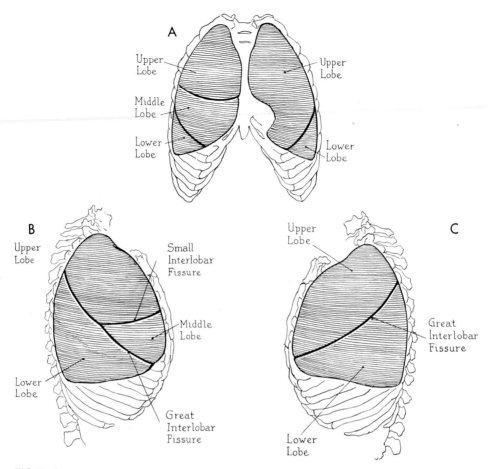

FIG 7–1.
Lobes and fissures of normal lungs. **A,** frontal aspect of both lungs. **B,** lateral aspect of the right lung. **C,** lateral aspect of the left lung.

ble in number with each branching generation and decrease in size down to about 1 mm in diameter. They are in a common fibrous sheath with a pulmonary arterial branch. The bronchioles are the conducting airways which extend to the 16th generation and are distinguished by a lack of cartilage in their walls. They are dependent for their patency on the support of the surrounding lung parenchyma. As the lung expands, the bronchioles dilate. The last conducting branch of the airway is the *terminal bronchiole*, which gives rise to transitional structures, the *respiratory bronchioles*, of which there are three generations, each giving rise to progressively greater numbers of alveoli. The alveoli, and the alveolar ducts and sacs which give rise to them, constitute the pure gas-exchange portion of the airways.

The alveolus, 200μm in diameter, is obviously too small to visualize radiologically. Controversy exists about what actually is being seen radiologically in "airspace" consolidation, but many now believe that the acinus is the pulmonary unit actually being visualized. The acinus is the unit of lung served by

the terminal bronchiole; it consists of three generations of respiratory bronchioles and about 400 alveoli. In the adult it measures about 7.5 mm in diameter; the size of the acinus, about 1 mm in infants, has been shown to increase throughout childhood.

The *secondary pulmonary lobule* is a cluster of about three to four dozen primary lobules that are separated from other primary lobules by intralobular septa of fibrous tissue. The secondary lobules and their septa are much better developed in the periphery of the lung than in the center (Fig 7–4). Heitzman has suggested that the lung is made up of a peripheral cortex of well-developed lobules and a medullary portion of lung in which the interlobular septa are poorly developed. The pulmonary veins and lymphatics course through the interlobular septa, the core structures of which are the pulmonary arteries and the terminal bronchioles. Thickened septa are visible in radiographs as Kerley B lines. Although the walls of the secondary pulmonary lobule are rarely visible in radiographs, several pulmonary lesions actually represent disease limited to the sec-

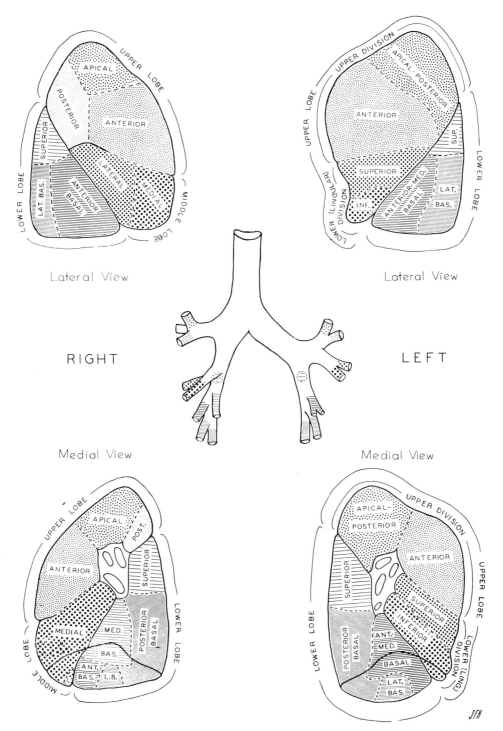

FIG 7–2.
Tracheobronchial anatomy. Tracheobronchial branches according to the pulmonary segments in which they ramify; each bronchial branch is named after its corresponding segment of lung. (The names used are those suggested by Jackson, Huber: *Dis Chest* 1943; 9:1.)

ondary lobule or clusters of them, according to Heitzman.

The lung has both a systemic and pulmonary arterial supply. The main pulmonary artery arises from the right ventricle distal to the pulmonic valve and forms a segment of the left heart border before it bifurcates at the level of the carina. The left pulmonary artery curves superiorly and posteriorly to the left hilum anterior to the left main bronchus where it divides into two branches. The lower

FIG 7–3.

Bronchial generations. The bronchi and airways from the 1st generation, the trachea, to the last generation, the alveolar sacs, are represented. Bronchi, which contain cartilage within their walls, measure between 10 and 3 mm in diameter and extend to the 4th generation, i.e., the subsegmental branches. They are easily visible by high-resolution computed tomography *(HRCT).* Bronchioles, which do not contain cartilage but rather an extensive network of fibers within their walls, are only seen to the 8th generation, which corresponds to a diameter of about 1.5 mm. Beyond the 8th generation, the bronchiolar walls are not resolvable by HRCT unless abnormal. The terminal bronchioles are the 16th-generation bronchioles and conduct air into the lobules. Beyond the terminal bronchioles, four to eight respiratory bronchioles lead to the formation of acini. Respiratory bronchioles are characterized by the presence of outpouchings representing alveolar structures. Each respiratory bronchiole leads to a series of alveolar ducts and terminal groupings of alveolar sacs. (From Naidich DP, Zerhouni EA, Siegelman SS (eds): *Computed Tomography and Magnetic Resonance of the Thorax,* ed 2. New York, Raven Press, 1991, p 349. Used by permission.)

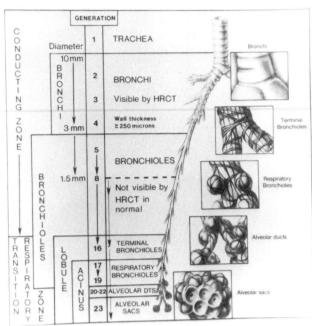

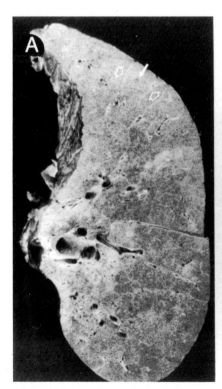

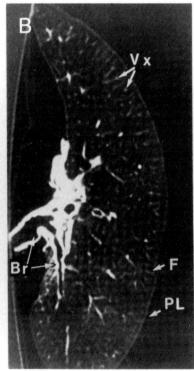

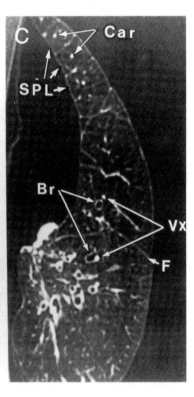

FIG 7–4.

Secondary pulmonary lobular anatomy. **A,** inflated fixed lung section shows characteristic appearance of a subpleural secondary pulmonary lobule when oriented perpendicular to the plane of section. The secondary pulmonary lobule is defined as that portion of the lung subtended by three to five terminal bronchioles, and typically ranges from 1.0 to 2.5 cm in size. Peripherally, lobules are bordered by interlobular septa *(open arrows)* within which pulmonary veins and lymphatics are located; centrally, the lobule is defined by core structures, including bronchioles and accompanying branches of the pulmonary artery *(white arrow).* Note that in this section only a few well-defined peripheral and occasional central lobules can actually be identified. **B,** and **C,** in vitro CT evaluation: 2-mm-thick CT sections through the periphery of an inflated fixed lung specimen. A number of secondary lobules *(SPL)* can be identified, within which characteristic central arteries *(Car)* can be seen. *F,* fissure; *PL,* pleura; *Br,* central bronchi; *Vx,* vessels accompanying bronchi, presumably pulmonary artery branches. Note that within definable lobules, core or central bronchioles are too small to be visualized. (In Naidich DP, Zerhouni EA, Siegelman SS (eds): *Computed Tomography and Magnetic Resonance of the Thorax,* ed 2. New York, Raven Press, 1991, p 351. Used by permission.)

branch is directed posteriorly and crosses over the left upper lobe bronchus, descending parallel with but lateral to the left lower lobe bronchus. This vessel gives branches to the lingula and to the superior segment of the lower lobe as well as to the basilar segments. The smaller superior branch divides, and its branches parallel the bronchial divisions to the upper lobe. The right pulmonary artery is almost horizontal and divides into its two major branches while still within the pericardium. It lies posterior to the aorta and superior vena cava and anterior to the right main bronchus. The main upper lobe branch, the truncus anterior ascends anterior to the right upper lobe bronchus and subdivides into three branches which parallel the three segmental bronchi to the right upper lobe. The largest branch of the right pulmonary artery is the interlobar artery, which passes anteriorly to the bronchus intermedius and descends laterally to it, giving branches, in order, to the middle lobe, the superior segment of the lower lobe, and four branches to the basilar segments of the lower lobe.

In the lung parenchyma, the pulmonary arterial branches travel and divide with the bronchial branches, although they give off some branches which are not accompanied by bronchial branches. There are approximately 23 divisions of the airway and approximately 28 divisions of pulmonary arterial branching; these vessels can be visualized on high-resolution computed tomography (HRCT) to about the level of the 16th generation, which is a few millimeters from the pleural surface and corresponds to the level of the terminal bronchioles, allowing identification of the secondary pulmonary lobule (the parenchyma supplied by three to five terminal bronchioles). The arterioles continue to divide until they form a dense capillary network surrounding the alveolus that Wiebel has calculated to be a total number of 280 billion capillary segments with a total blood volume of 140 mL, which can be nearly doubled during exercise.

The primary role of the pulmonary circulation is to transport deoxygenated blood from the heart to the alveolar capillaries where oxygenation occurs, and then through the pulmonary veins back to the left atrium. The pressure in the pulmonary circuit is about one sixth that of the systemic circuit; total pulmonary blood flow is determined primarily by cardiac output, although the control of pulmonary blood flow is complex and also depends on the relative systemic and pulmonary pressures as well as gravity and local pulmonary factors. There are large numbers of capillaries which normally are only minimally perfused; therefore the lung has a large capacity for arterial flow to increase or shift significantly without increasing the pulmonary arterial pressure. Gravity is an important determinant of regional pulmonary blood flow, with the more dependent regions receiving a greater volume of blood. The smaller, muscular, pulmonary arterial branches vasoconstrict under conditions of hypoxia in an attempt to maintain the ventilation-perfusion balance. When lung disease becomes severe enough, this protective mechanism is overwhelmed and poorly ventilated alveoli are perfused, which results in systemic deoxygenation. Right-to-left shunts occur as poorly oxygenated blood flows past atelectatic alveoli and returns, still poorly oxygenated, to the heart. Hypoxemia and accompanying acidosis increase pulmonary vascular resistance which leads to right ventricular hypertrophy and eventually to cor pulmonale. The vast pulmonary capillary bed serves the function of gas exchange. The endothelial lining is quite sensitive to toxins, including high oxygen concentrations, and when damaged, results in permeability-type pulmonary edema.

The pulmonary venous radicles arise distal to the capillary mesh and travel in the interlobular septa, which form the walls of the secondary pulmonary lobules; the veins thus do not travel with the pulmonary artery and bronchial branches. They drain toward the hilum and gradually increase in size. There usually are two large veins on each side. The upper lobe veins are more vertical in orientation and the lower ones more horizontal before they enter the left atrium. The right superior vein is posterior to the superior vena cava and anterior to the right inferior pulmonary artery. The left superior pulmonary vein is anterior to the left main pulmonary artery and is also just anterior to the left upper lobe bronchus. The right inferior branch enters the left atrium anterior to the right lower lobe bronchus, and the left inferior pulmonary vein enters the left atrium at a point just anterior to the descending aorta and posterior to the left lower lobe bronchus.

The systemic circulation to the lung is via bronchial arteries that are branches of the thoracic aorta. These vessels provide nourishment to the structures of the lung and mediastinum. In the presence of pulmonary artery obstruction, collateral circulation to the pulmonary capillaries can develop through precapillary anastomotic channels.

ANOMALIES OF THE LUNG

There is no widely accepted embryologic basis for lung anomalies. For this reason many theories have been presented to show that the major anomalies

TABLE 7–1.

Anomalies of the Trachea and Lungs*

Anomaly	Origin of Defect	First Appearance (of Other Diagnostic Clues)	Sex Chiefly Affected	Relative Frequency	Remarks
Tracheal atresia	3rd to 4th week	At birth	?	Very rare	Fatal at birth
Bilateral agenesis of the lung	4th week	At birth	?	Very rare	Fatal at birth
Congenital tracheal stenosis	3rd to 4th week	At birth	?	Rare	Usually fatal soon after birth
Tracheobronchomegaly	5th month?	Late childhood or later	?	Rare	
Unilateral agenesis and hypoplasia of the lungs	Late 4th week	Infancy and childhood	Female	Uncommon	50% die in first 5 years
Anomalies of lobulation	10th week	None	Male?	Common	Asymptomatic
Pulmonary isomerism	Unknown	None	?	Uncommon	Associated with heterotaxy, asplenia, and anomalous pulmonary veins
Congenital cysts of respiratory tract					
Bronchogenic cysts	6th to 7th week	Infancy, if at all	?	Uncommon	Compression of trachea may be fatal
Pulmonary cysts	24th week	Infancy and childhood	Male	Uncommon	Eventually fatal if untreated

*From Gray SW, Skandalakis JE: *Embryology for Surgeons.* Philadelphia, WB Saunders, 1972. Used by permission.

are a continuum of developmental defects based to a large extent on the timing of the insult (Table 7–1). The major exception to these theories is agenesis of the lung. It is accepted that either a simple arrest of development occurs (bilateral agenesis) or there is a "failure to maintain the developmental balance of the two lung buds" (Gray and Skandalakis). Many

of the pulmonary malformations have a high incidence of associated anomalies (Table 7–2).

Pulmonary Agenesis and Aplasia

Pulmonary agenesis is defined as a total absence of the lung parenchyma, its vasculature, and its bron-

TABLE 7–2.

Anomalies Associated with or Part of Bronchopulmonary Foregut Malformations

Disease	Incidence of Anomalies	Association
Pulmonary agenesis	50%	Cardiovascular (patent ductus arteriosus) Gastrointestinal (tracheoesophageal fistula) Genitourinary Skeletal (limbs, vertebrae)
Congenital lobar emphysema	14%	Congenital heart disease
Hypogenetic lung syndrome	Frequent	Congenital heart disease Vertebral anomalies Horseshoe lung
Congenital cystic adenomatoid malfunction	Approximately 30% in type II	Renal Gastrointestinal Cardiac Osseous
Sequestration		
Intralobular	Rare	—
Extralobular	Frequent	Diaphragmatic hernia Pulmonary vascular anomalies Congenital heart disease

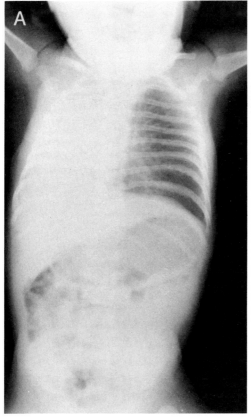

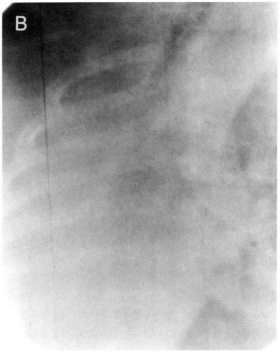

FIG 7–5.
Pulmonary atresia. **A,** frontal radiograph of this 2-month-old infant reveals an opacification of the right hemithorax with a shift of the mediastinum to the right. **B,** high-kilovoltage frontal examination shows the trachea and left mainstem bronchus. There is no evidence of any right mainstem bronchus. This patient also had another congenital anomaly—an atrial septal defect.

chus beyond the bifurcation (Fig 7–5). Pulmonary aplasia is similar except that a blind-ending rudimentary bronchus is present (Fig 7–6). The sex incidence of the lesion is equal, and it occurs as often on the right side as on the left. Anomalies accompanying pulmonary agenesis often involve the cardiovascular (patent ductus arteriosus), gastrointestinal (tracheoesophageal fistula), and genitourinary systems. Hemivertebra and ipsilateral skeletal anomalies are frequent.

Radiologic Findings

There is a marked shift of the heart and mediastinal structures to the affected side, which is mostly opaque except for some lucency superiorly resulting from displacement of the contralateral, emphysematous, and hyperplastic lung, which herniates across the midline. A clue to the diagnosis of pulmonary agenesis is found by careful investigation of the "carina" as there is absence of the bronchus on the affected side (see Figs 7–5 and 7–6).

Pulmonary Hypoplasia

Pulmonary hypoplasia can be due to a decreased number of branching generations in the airway with a consequently decreased number of acini, decreased alveolar size, or a combination of the two. It may be unilateral or bilateral. In bilateral cases, the radiographic recognition of small lungs is difficult. Pneumothoraces and neonatal respiratory distress are common. Neonatal pulmonary hypoplasia is associated with the oligohydramnios syndrome, especially when due to renal agenesis. Diaphragmatic hernia is associated with pulmonary hypoplasia. Other intrauterine abnormalities encroaching on the intrathoracic space and associated with pulmonary hypoplasia include large fetal pleural effusions, thoracic spinal deformities, malformation syndromes associated with small bony thoraces, and intrathoracic masses such as cystic hygroma and congenital cystic adenomatoid malformation (CCAM).

Pulmonary hypoplasia can be acquired following infection (Swyer-James syndrome), radiation ther-

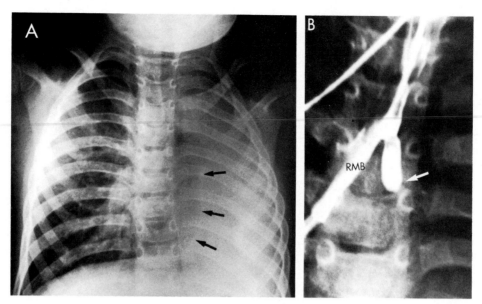

FIG 7–6.
Pulmonary aplasia. **A,** a chest radiograph in an asymptomatic 6-year-old boy shows complete opacification of the left hemithorax with some crowding of the ribs superiorly. The heart and mediastinal structures are shifted to the left, and a portion of the right lung is herniated across the midline *(arrows)*. **B,** a bronchogram shows a rudimentary left mainstem bronchus *(arrow)*. *RMB,* right mainstem bronchus.

apy, aspiration of toxic substances, and scoliosis. Fletcher and associates reported two infants in whom the lung volume diminished after postsurgical occlusion of the right pulmonary artery.

Unilateral pulmonary hypoplasia is usually associated with a small or atretic pulmonary artery. If the pulmonary artery is not clearly seen on chest films, it can be noninvasively visualized by computed tomography (CT) or magnetic resonance imaging (MRI) to exclude unilateral pulmonary artery agenesis. The absent pulmonary artery is usually on the side opposite the aortic arch (Fig 7–7). Characteristic radiographic features include volume loss in the affected hemithorax, which is manifested by a mediastinal shift toward the affected side, and a small hilar shadow (Fig 7–8). The lung is often hyperlucent. The differential diagnosis includes the Swyer-James syndrome. It can be excluded if the ventilation lung scan shows no evidence of expiratory obstruction. Vertebral abnormalities (Fig 7–9), congenital heart

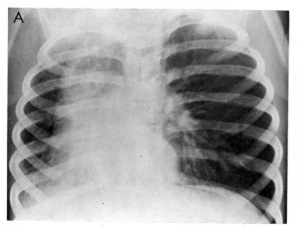
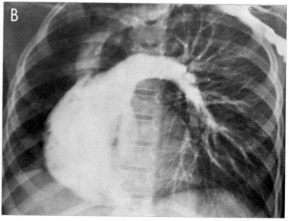

FIG 7–7.
Congenital hypoplasia of the right lung with congenital absence of the right pulmonary artery in a boy 9 years of age. **A,** in a standard frontal projection, the entire right hemithorax is small, but all of the mediastinal structures are shifted to the right side. **B,** a frontal an- giocardiogram 2.5 seconds after the intravenous injection of contrast agent shows opacification of the right chambers of the heart and the main pulmonary artery and its left branch. The right pulmonary artery is absent.

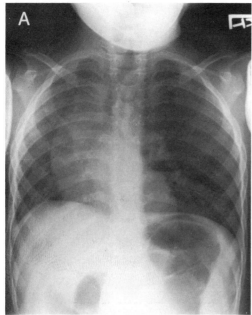

FIG 7–8.
Pulmonary hypoplasia. **A,** frontal radiograph in an 8-month-old infant shows marked differential volume between the right and left side. The left side is much more lucent and there is prominence of the left pulmonary artery. **B,** CT scan with bone windows reveals smaller arterial supply to the defect on the right. **C,** mediastinal settings reveal the clear difference in volume between the two sides. This patient was a premature baby without any problems who had the chest film for a respiratory infection.

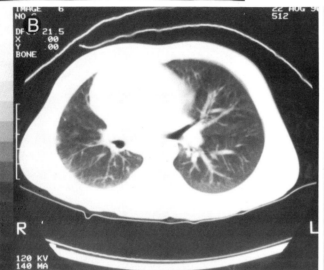

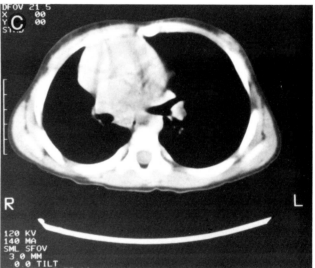

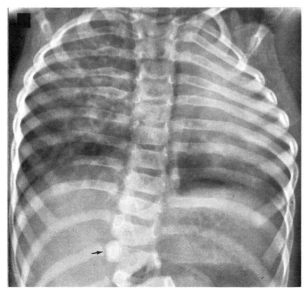

FIG 7–9.
Anomalies and pulmonary hypoplasia. Congenital hypoplasia of the left lung with scoliosis and hemivertebra *(arrow)* at the 11th thoracic segment. The left hemithorax is small and its lateral wall is flat. The left intercostal spaces are all narrow. The heart is displaced into the opaque left hemithorax. The left leaf of the diaphragm is not elevated. A substantial segment of the gas-containing right lung has protruded into the left hemithorax in this boy 5 years of age.

disease, and often the tetralogy of Fallot are found in many patients. Pulmonary hypoplasia is also present as part of many of the more complex bronchopulmonary anomalies discussed in the following section.

The Continuum of Bronchopulmonary Foregut Malformations (Sequestration Spectrum)

The most common pulmonary anomalies are lobar emphysema, bronchogenic cyst, cystic adenonatal malfunction, sequestration, hypogenetic lung, and pulmonary arteriovenous malformation. Each will be considered separately, but several anomalies occur in the same patient, and sometimes separation of one from the other, even histologically, is impossible. Heothoff et al. have proposed lumping these complex anomalies under the name "sequestration spectrum," which they define as:

> A collection of anomalies of the lung parenchyma and of its blood supply, including sequestrations, with associated anomalies of the gastrointestinal tract and diaphragm—at one end of the spectrum is abnormal pulmonary tissue similar to that found in sequestration but without anomalous vascular supply, namely, bronchopulmonary cyst. Between these two extremes lie the variants of sequestration.

Congenital Lobar Emphysema (Neonatal Lobar Hyperinflation)

Congenital lobar emphysema is a condition in which one or occasionally two lung lobes are overdis-

tended, causing compression of normal lung tissue. It has multiple causes such as focal bronchial obstruction (intrinsic or extrinsic) in 40% to 60% of cases, primary abnormalities in alveolar number (polyalveolar lobe or too many alveoli, and congenital hypoplastic emphysema or too few alveoli), and primary abnormalities in alveolar structure (alveolar fibrosis). Since this condition usually presents in the neonate, it is discussed in Chapter 51. It should be noted, however, that if there is little mediastinal compression or obstructive component, congenital lobar emphysema may not present in the neonatal period but will become symptomatic in infants and children. These patients present with pulmonary infection or wheezing, and the radiograph reveals the hyperlucent lobe—usually the left upper (40%), right middle (34%), or right upper lobe (21%) (Table 7–3). The major clinical consideration is a bronchial obstruction. A CT scan or bronchogram will help resolve this problem. Panicek et al. consider this condition, in which the lung is abnormal but its vascularity is normal, to be part of the sequestration spectrum.

Bronchogenic Cyst

A bronchogenic cyst may represent the most common type of congenital lung cyst. It is a developmental anomaly which probably results from defective growth of the lung bud or the mesenchymal cells growing near the lung bud. A bronchogenic cyst may either be intrapulmonary or mediastinal; the latter is discussed in Chapter 14. An intrapulmo-

TABLE 7–3.

Common Characteristics of Bronchopulmonary Foregut Malformations*

Malformation	Location	Differential Diagnosis
Lobar emphysema	LUL (41%)	Lung cyst
	RML (34%)	Pneumothorax
	RUL (21%)	CCAM
Bronchogenic cyst	Mediastinal (85%)	Round pneumonia
	Intrapulmonary (15%)	Metatastic neoplasm
	Two thirds are lower lobes	Interlobar effusion
		Plasma cell granuloma
		Cavitated abscess
Congenital cysts	Equal in lobes (middle rare)	Lobar emphysema
Adenomatoid malfunction	One third have more than	Bronchogenic cyst
	1 lobe involved	Diaphragmatic hernia
		Pulmonary interstitial
		emphysema
Sequestration		
Intralobar	60% left, basal segment	Pneumonia
Extralobar	80% left at or below	"Abdominal" mass
	diaphragm	

*LUL = left upper lobe; RML = right middle lobe; RUL = right upper lobe; CCAM = congenital cystic adenomatoid malformation.

nary bronchogenic cyst probably results from an earlier embryologic error than does a mediastinal cyst. Intrapulmonary bronchogenic cysts often communicate with the bronchial tree, and about two thirds are aerated. They are lined with respiratory epithelium and may be filled with clear or mucoid material.

Radiographs show a round or oval, either fluid- or air-filled cyst with a wide range of sizes (Fig 7–10). If air-filled, the cyst wall is thin and smooth. The cyst is unilocular and about two thirds of the time occurs in the lower lobes. The differential diagnosis of a fluid-filled intrapulmonary bronchogenic cyst includes round pneumonia, primary or metastatic pulmonary neoplasm, interlobar effusion, and plasma cell granuloma. Air- or air and fluid–filled cysts must be differentiated from small CCAMs, pneumatocele, pulmonary abscess, and cavitating laryngeal papilloma.

Congenital Cystic Adenomatoid Malformation (CCAM)

CCAM may be defined as a multicystic mass of pulmonary tissue in which there is a proliferation of bronchial structures at the expense of alveolar development. Pathologically, the affected lobe is increased in volume and weight. It is composed of a cystic lesion with an overgrowth (adenomatoid increase) of the terminal portion of the bronchial tree. The bronchial structures are disorganized, but some bronchial communication may be present; the blood supply is usually from the pulmonary circulation. In

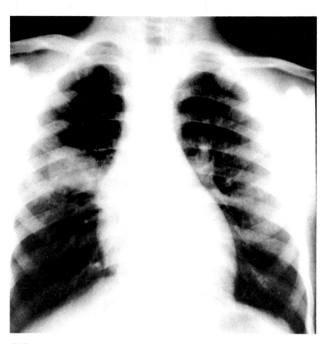

FIG 7–10.
Bronchogenic cyst. Frontal radiograph in this 3-year-old girl revealed an oval density in the right midlung field. This did not communicate with the bronchus. The child had been asymptomatic and the lesion was found at the time of the chest film for upper respiratory infection.

some cases there is communication with the gastrointestinal tract. Three types of CCAM have been described: (1) type I (most common), with multiple, varying-sized large cysts that radiologically resemble congenital lobar emphysema; (2) type II (40% of

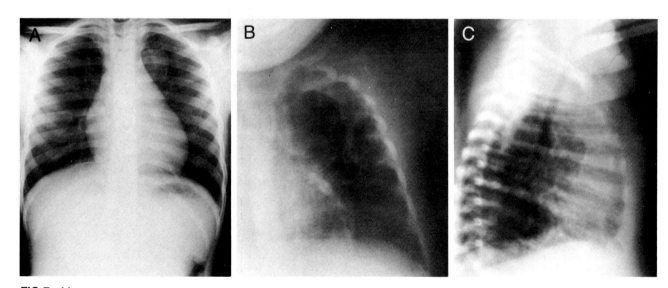

FIG 7–11.
Congenital adenomatoid malformation. **A,** frontal film of a 7-year-old asymptomatic girl with a mixed solid and air-filled lesion in the left upper lobe. At surgery this was shown to be an adenomatoid malformation. **B,** and **C,** newborn with cystic congenital adenomatoid malformation in the left upper lobe There is little solid component.

cases), with multiple thin-walled, even-sized (1–2 cm in diameter) cysts with associated congenital malformations and common early death (Fig 7–11); and (3) type III (rarest), with a bulky, firm mass and multiple tiny cysts that may appear solid to the naked eye.

The lesion has been found in stillborn infants; we have identified it in utero. The triad of findings includes maternal hydramnios, fetal anasarca, and a cystic or solid mass in the fetal chest. The anasarca is probably related to venous obstruction secondary to the expanding intrathoracic mass.

The lesion occurs with equal frequency in both lungs, but there is a slight tendency for upper lobe predominance (Fig 7–12). Radiographic examination shows a mass lesion with signs of an associated shift. The mass is often lobulated and contains both fluid and air. In the older child, more air-filled cysts tend to be evident. Air gets into the lesion not through normal bronchial connections but from the neighboring well-ventilated lung diffusing through the pores of Kohn. The differential diagnosis includes diaphragmatic hernia, particularly if the patient is seen at birth. Congenital lobar emphysema can also be confused with CCAM. If the clinical question persists, CT shows multiple cysts in CCAM in contrast with an emphysematous, but otherwise normal lung in lobar emphysema. Severe staphylococcal pneumonia with pneumatocele formation may be confused radiographically with CCAM. Pulmonary interstitial emphysema confined to a lobe could be confused with CCAM but air-fluid levels are lacking in pulmonary interstitial emphysema, and the history is usually helpful (Fig 7–13). If

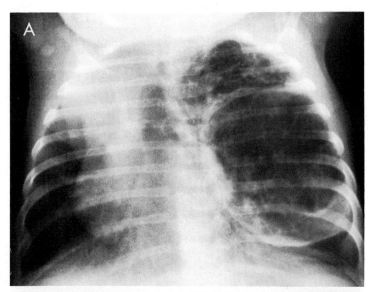

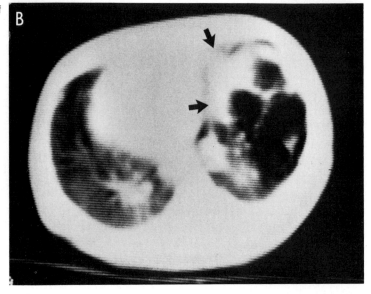

FIG 7–12.
Adenomatoid malfunction. Chest radiograph **(A)** and CT scan **(B)** in a 1-year-old child with type I cystic adenomatoid malformation. Note the many large cysts of varying sizes, some of which have relatively thick walls *(arrows)*.

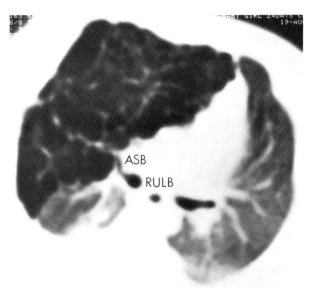

FIG 7–13.
Pulmonary interstitial emphysema in a neonate with an expansile cystic right upper lobe who was thought possibly to have cystic adenomatoid malformation. An ultrafast CT scan revealed that the hyperinflated lobe was being supplied by the anterior segmental branch *(ASB)* of the right upper lobe bronchus *(RULB)*. No air-fluid levels or solid tissue are present, and the multiple hyperexpanded areas of lung are consistent with pulmonary interstitial emphysema, which was subsequently proved as the lesions spontaneously returned to normal.

CCAM occurs in the lower lobes, its radiologic appearance can simulate sequestration of the lung.

Bronchopulmonary Sequestration

Bronchopulmonary sequestration is a congenital mass of nonfunctioning pulmonary tissue that has no normal connection with the bronchial tree or the pulmonary arteries. Its arterial supply arises from a systemic vessel, usually a branch of the abdominal aorta. Its venous drainage may be via the pulmonary veins, the inferior vena cava, or the azygos system. At least 40 hypotheses have been proposed to explain the development of this anomaly, but none is completely satisfactory. Many authors distinguish between intralobar sequestration and extralobar sequestration because they may present in different ways, i.e., intralobar as a pulmonary mass with or without infection, whereas extralobar is most often an incidental finding of an asymptomatic mass at or below the diaphragm. Additionally, extralobar sequestration is frequently associated with other congenital anomalies (see Table 7–2). Intralobar sequestration is contiguous to normal lung parenchyma and within the pleural covering of the normal lung. Extralobar sequestration is separate from the normal lung parenchyma and has its own pleural covering. Further differentiation via arterial supply and pul-

monary venous drainage, however, is not helpful because there is so much variability in each type of sequestration. In some cases of either type, there is communication with the gastrointestinal tract.

Intralobar Sequestration

Intralobar sequestrations occur in the left paravertebral gutter in approximately two thirds of cases and in the right paravertebral region in most of the remainder. Upper lobe involvement and bilateral cases have been reported but are very rare.

This lesion is usually recognized because of secondary infection or, occasionally, as an incidental finding on a routine chest radiograph (Fig 7–14). The sequestered segment communicates with the surrounding lung primarily as a result of infection, although some authors have reported that cystic spaces in the lesion may communicate directly with the normal bronchial tree without any evidence of supervening infection. Hemoptysis can be noted if communication with the bronchial tree occurs; some younger patients have presented with congestive heart failure due to a right-to-left shunt through the sequestered segment.

The radiographic appearance depends on the degree of aeration and the presence or absence of superimposed infection. Emphysematous lung tissue (in the "normal" lung) may be seen surrounding the sequestration and is thought to be due to collateral ventilation. Intralobar sequestration can be present without any obvious abnormality in the lung parenchyma. The lesion may appear as a water-density mass that is oval, spherical, or triangular (Fig 7–15,A). It may be mistaken for pneumonia, atelectasis, bronchogenic cyst, or neoplasm. More commonly, it may be an air-containing cystic mass, often containing multiple cysts of varying sizes, and may simulate a CCAM. On bronchography, the normal bronchial tree is draped around the mass, although rarely the lesion can fill on a bronchogram. Should this happen, an erroneous diagnosis of bronchiectasis may be made. An upper gastrointestinal series is indicated to exclude communication with the stomach or esophagus. It is important to try to demonstrate the anomalous feeding vessel, not only for diagnostic purposes but also to help avoid potential hemorrhage if surgery is contemplated. The abnormal vessel is best seen by angiography but can often be satisfactorily visualized on MRI (Fig 7–15,B and C).

Extralobar Sequestration

Extralobar sequestration, or accessory lung, occurs in contiguity with the left hemidiaphragm in 90% of

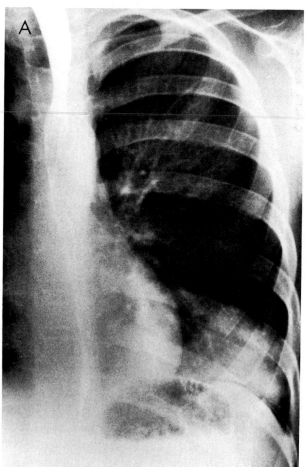

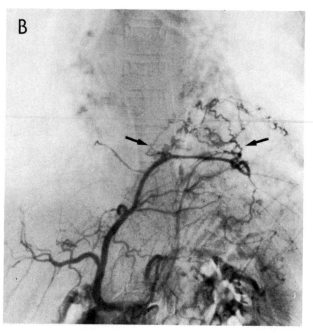

FIG 7–14.
Intralobar sequestration. **A,** a 10-year-old girl with a persistent left lower lobe "infiltrate." **B,** a selective angiogram reveals an anomalous supply from the left hepatic artery. An intralobar pulmonary sequestration was found at surgery.

cases. It is usually unilateral (Fig 7–16). Rarely, a hemodynamically significant left-to-right shunt may develop. There is a 30% incidence of associated diaphragmatic hernia. In lesions close to the diaphragm, CT can aid in determining whether there is any intra-abdominal extension. Because this type of sequestration is more completely separated from the lung than is the intralobar type, there is less chance of secondary infection. Most cases present as a basilar soft-tissue density, although aeration sometimes occurs.

Recently, the association of extralobar sequestration and tension hydrothorax has been described (Hernanz-Schulman et al.). Prior to this report, the tension hydrothorax and subsequent hydrops has always been fatal. However, the authors report the use of color flow Doppler to diagnose the systemic blood supply to the sequestration, and at surgery there was torsion of the sequestration. The torsion most likely occludes "efferent venous and lymphatic channels, initiating the accumulation of pleural fluid" (Hernanz-Schulman et al). Two of the authors' three patients survived.

Bronchopulmonary Foregut Malformation

Gerle et al., Heithoff et al., and Leithiser et al. have suggested that, since connection with the foregut is seen in some cases of bronchopulmonary sequestration, the general term *bronchopulmonary foregut malformation* is more accurate (Figs 7–17 and 7–18). These authors suggest that sequestration occurs when a supernumerary lung bud develops caudad to the normal lung bud. If arrest occurs early in development, it may stay in communication with the foregut and share its blood supply. Should arrest occur later, a fibrous strand may be all that is left connecting the sequestered segment to the foregut. The location of the sequestered segment may reflect the time at which the outpouching occurs. If it occurs early, and therefore closer to the normal lung bud, the sequestration will be intralobar; if it occurs later in embryonic life, an extralobar sequestration will result.

Esophageal Lung

This anomaly may result from an ectopic supernumerary lung bud that retains its primitive connection

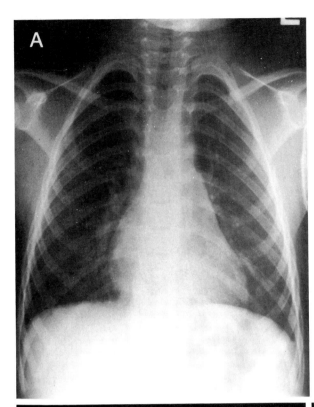

FIG 7–15.
Intralobar sequestration. **A,** frontal chest radiograph in this 5-year-old child reveals a persistent density in the left lower lobe. **B,** and **C,** MRI (coronal T1-weighted gated images) reveals the vascular supply coming from the aorta and feeding the left lower lobe sequestration.

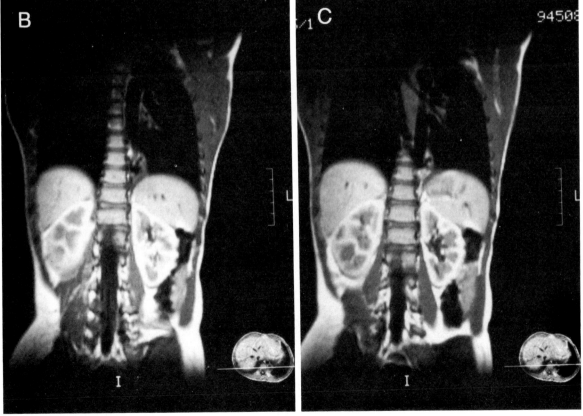

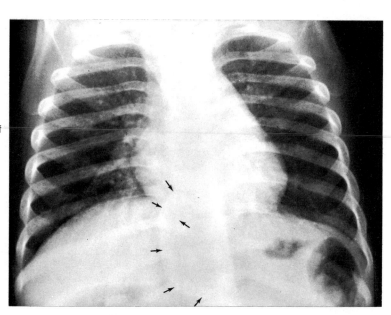

FIG 7–16.
Extralobar congenital pulmonary sequestration (accessory lobe) in an asymptomatic boy 18 months of age. The smooth mass of water density *(arrows)* extends along the right vertebral edge from ribs 8 to 12. Contiguous bones are normal. A neurogenic tumor was suspected from these radiographic changes. At surgical exploration an accessory pulmonary lobe was found with its own blood supply directly from the descending aorta below the diaphragm.

to the gastrointestinal tract. It can be considered as part of the bronchopulmonary foregut spectrum. An anomalous lobe of one lung communicates directly with the esophagus through a bronchus or bronchus-like structure. Most often, this anomaly involves a lower lobe, but an entire lung may be supplied by the esophageal bronchus. The clinical and radiologic findings vary with the anatomical defect.

If only a lobe or segment is anomalously supplied, it may remain normal until infection supervenes. The diagnosis is usually established by a barium esophagogram demonstrating the fistula to the lung.

Systemic Arterial Supply to Normal Lung
Also considered to be part of the sequestration spectrum is the relatively rare condition in which normal

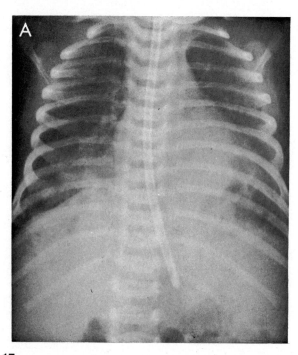

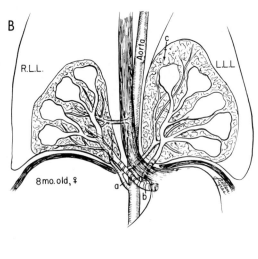

FIG 7–17.
Bilateral bronchopulmonary foregut congenital malformation that casts images of increased density in the bases of both lungs. **A,** in the radiograph, the patches of increased density intermingle with radiolucent patches that suggest cysts. **B,** schematic drawing of

A: *R.L.L.,* right lower lobe; *L.L.L.,* left lower lobe; *a,* blood supply from the aorta; *b,* patent foregut communication; *c,* accessory pulmonary tissue. (From Gerle RD, Jaretzki A III, Ashley CA, et al: *N Eng J Med* 1968; 278:1413. Used by permission.)

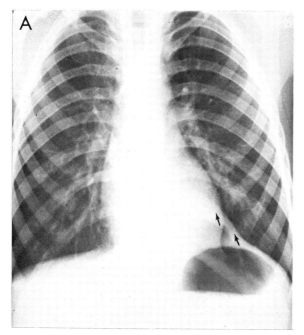

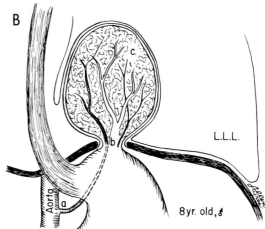

FIG 7–18.
Unilateral congenital bronchopulmonary communication with a left-sided diaphragmatic hernia. **A,** in the radiograph, an extra density is superimposed on the cardiac image *(arrows).* **B,** schematic drawing of **A:** *a,* main arterial supply from the aorta; *b,* communi-cation with the stomach; *c,* accessory pulmonary tissue. (From Gerle RD, Jaretzi A III, Ashley CA, et al: *N Engl J Med* 1968; 278:1413. Used by permission.)

lung, usually the lower lobe, is supplied by an abnormal vessel of systemic origin. Venous drainage is usually via the pulmonary veins. Patients may present with findings secondary to a left-to-right shunt, including heart murmur or congestive failure, or the lesion may be diagnosed incidentally on routine radiographic examination. The area of increased vascularity may be mistaken radiographically for pneumonia. Typically, the large abnormal vessel arises from the aorta. Its presence may be diagnosed noninvasively by CT or MRI or directly by angiography (Fig 7–19). Differentiation from bronchopulmonary sequestration is established by the fact that the lung itself appears normal on CT except for increased vascularity; typically, no cysts, abnormalities of aeration, or mass lesions are present. The affected portion of lung has a normal bronchial supply which may be demonstrated either by CT or by bronchography.

"Acquired" Sequestration
In cases of severe chronic inflammation and bronchiectasis, dilated large abnormal vessels may arise from the descending aorta supplying the area of chronic inflammation and mimicking the findings of sequestration (Fig 7–20). Differentiation from sequestration is made by demonstrating broncho-graphically that the dilated bronchi are branches of normal lobar and segmental bronchi.

Hypogenetic Lung Syndrome (Pulmonary Venolobar Syndrome, Scimitar Syndrome), Horseshoe Lung

Hypogenetic lung syndrome nearly always affects the right lung; its lower portion is drained by an anomalous vein which characteristically extends below the diaphragm and empties into the inferior vena cava, portal vein, or hepatic vein. Arterial supply to the hypoplastic lung is usually from a small pulmonary artery, but systemic arterial supply may also be present. Other anomalies are frequent including errors in pulmonary lobation, hemivertebra, scoliosis, and congenital heart disease. The affected lung is supplied by bronchi but anomalies of branching are frequent. Radiographs typically show dextroposition of the heart, a small right lung, and the scimitar sign of the anomalous vein extending inferiorly (Fig 7–21). There is usually a prominent retrosternal soft-tissue density present in the lateral radiograph which has been thought to be due to retrosternal areolar connective tissue. However, CT in several cases has demonstrated that the density is due to mediastinal shift and rotation secondary to

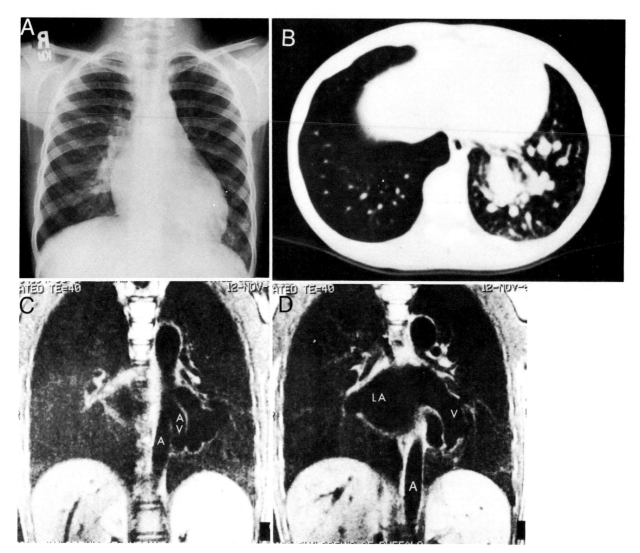

FIG 7–19.
Systemic arterial supply to a normal lung in a 6-year-old child with "chronic left lower lobe pneumonia." **A,** a chest radiograph reveals increased opacity in the left lower lobe, cardiomegaly, and prominent vessels. **B,** a contrast-enhanced CT scan reveals large vessels in the left lower lobe with no evidence of cystic malformation of the lung. **C,** a coronal MRI reveals a large vessel *(AV)* arising from the aorta *(A)*. **D,** coronal MRI, 1 cm anterior to **C,** reveals a huge draining vein *(V)* inserting into the left atrium *(LA)*. At surgery, a normal left lower lobe supplied by an anomalous vessel arising from the aorta was removed. *A,* aorta.

the loss of normal pulmonary volume. CT is also valuable for demonstration of hypoplasia of the pulmonary artery, anomalies of pulmonary venous return, and bronchial abnormalities. Although there is a left-to-right shunt present, it usually is not hemodynamically significant. Related disorders include horseshoe lung and the accessory diaphragm syndrome.

Horseshoe lung is a malformation in which the lungs are joined posteriorly. Dextroversion of the heart is present, as is hypoplasia of the right lung. Vascular anomalies include partial anomalous pulmonary venous return (PAPVR) to the inferior vena cava and aberrant systemic arterial supply to the af-

fected lung. Radiologic findings are similar to those in the scimitar syndrome except that one may see a small area of hyperlucent lung in the left cardiothoracic sulcus which represents the isthmus of the horseshoe. Pulmonary angiograms show arterial branches extending inferiorly and crossing the midline behind the heart. HRCT is required to determine whether the two lungs are truly fused or whether there is pleura separating the herniated lung from the hypoplastic one.

In *accessory diaphragm syndrome,* hypoplasia of the lung, usually the right, is also present (see Figs 6–65 and 6–66). Associated anomalies include anomalous pulmonary venous return, congenital

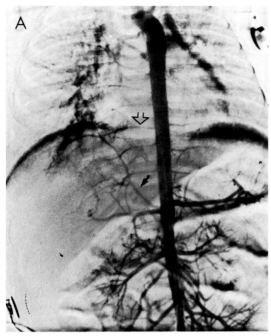

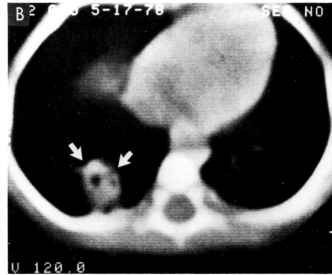

FIG 7–20.
Acquired sequestration. **A,** persistent right lower lobe infiltrate and recurrent hemoptysis led to an abdominal aortogram. In this 2-year-old child, hypertrophied phrenic artery branches *(black arrow)* and intercostal vessels *(open arrow)* supply the area of the infiltrate. **B,** a CT scan in the same patient shows a well-defined pleural-based mass density posteriorly *(arrows)*. Air-filled structures not clearly identifiable as bronchi are seen centrally. The location is, however, atypical for sequestration. At surgery, an area of chronic bronchiectasis distal to an intrabronchial foreign body (pine needle) was found.

heart disease, diaphragmatic hernia, and occasional vertebral anomalies. This syndrome cannot be separated radiologically from hypoplastic right lung of other causes; surgery is required for diagnosis.

Pulmonary arteriovenous malformation is discussed in Chapter 11.

Pulmonary Lymphangiectasia

Developmental lymphatic disorders are rare and are divided into four types by Scalzetti et al. These categories are[11] (1) lymphangiectasis, characterized by congenital anomalous dilatation of pulmonary lymph vessels; (2) localized lymphangioma, a rare and benign, usually cystic, lesion characterized by masslike proliferation of lymph vessels; (3) diffuse lymphangioma, a proliferation of vascular, mainly lymphatic, spaces in which visceral and skeletal involvement is common; and (4) lymphangioleiomyoma, which involves a haphazard proliferation of smooth muscle in the lungs and dilatation of lymphatic spaces" (Scalzetti et al.).

Pulmonary lymphangiectasia can involve both lungs diffusely, is frequently seen in stillborn infants, and may accompany congenital heart disease (usually total anomalous pulmonary venous return or hypoplastic left heart syndrome). It is seen in Noonan syndrome. Radiographic findings are those of lymphatic engorgement with prominent diffuse interstitial lung markings. Noonan, in a review of 48 cases, divided pulmonary lymphangiectasia into the following types: (1) those occurring as a part of generalized lymphangiectasia; (2) those secondary to pulmonary venous obstruction; and (3) a primary developmental abnormality in the lung. About one third of the reported cases of pulmonary lymphangiectasia appear to be secondary to cardiac defects associated with pulmonary venous obstruction.

In those children with noncardiac pulmonary lymphangiectasia, there appear to be two groups. In one, symptoms develop at, or shortly after, birth and most of the affected infants die in the first 24 hours of life. In the late-onset group, initial radiographs are said to be normal, but when symptoms develop, radiographic findings consist of diffuse parenchymal changes with or without Kerley B lines. It is not known whether pulmonary lymphangiectasia in these patients represents the same disease as that seen in those who die early.

Gorham syndrome is lymphangioma of the skeleton (osteolytic lesions, vanishing bone disease) and chylothorax. The latter may be secondary to a pleural component. Tuberous sclerosis rarely has pulmonary changes of lymphangioleiomyomatosis.

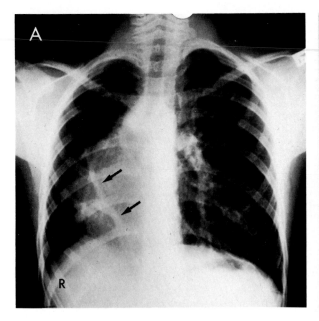

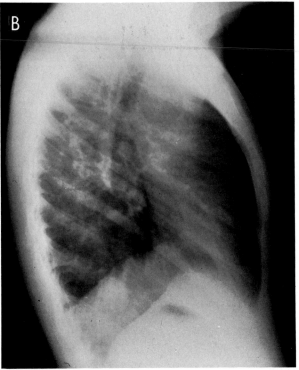

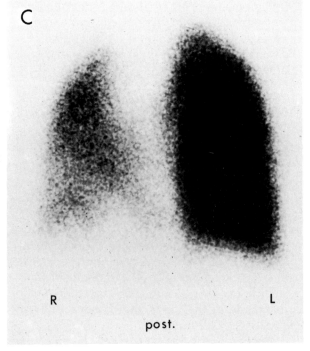

FIG 7–21.

Hypogenetic lung syndrome. **A,** a 10-year-old girl with a history of recurrent respiratory infections. A frontal radiograph shows dextroposition of the heart, a small hypovascular right lung, and a linear branching shadow *(arrows),* which on cardiac catheterization was shown to be an anomalous vein draining into the inferior vena cava. **B,** a lateral chest film reveals increased soft-tissue density anteriorly and elevation of the right hemidiaphragm, signs consistent with pulmonary hypoplasia on the right. **C,** a radionuclide perfusion scan shows a marked difference in perfusion in the two lungs.

REFERENCES

Ellis K: Developmental abnormalities in the systemic blood supply to the lungs. *Am J Roentgenol* 1991; 156:669.

Fraser R, Paré J; *Diagnosis of Diseases of the Chest,* vol 1. Philadelphia, WB Saunders, 1977.

Gray SW, Skandalakis JE: *Embryology for Surgeons.* Philadelphia, WB Saunders, 1972.

Heitzman RE: *The Lung,* ed 2. St Louis, Mosby–Year Book, 1984.

Keslar P, Newman B, Oh KS: Radiographic manifestations of anomalies of the lung. *Radiol Clin North Am* 1991; 29:255.

Mata JM, Caceres J, Lucaya J, et al: CT of congenital malformations of the lung. *Radiographics* 1990; 10:651–674.

Naidich DP, McCauley DI, Siegelman SS: Computed tomography of bronchial adenomas. *J Comput Assist Tomogr* 1982; 6:725.

Naidich DP, Zerhouni EA, Siegelman SS (eds): *Computed Tomography and Magnetic Resonance of the Thorax,* ed 2. New York, Raven Press, 1991.

Noback GJ: The developmental topography of the larynx, trachea and lungs in the fetus, newborn, infant and child. *Am J Dis Child* 1923; 26:515.

Panicek DM, Heitzman ER, Randall PA, et al: The continuum of pulmonary developmental anomalies. *Radiographics* 1987; 7:747–772.

Sane SM, Girdany BR: Cysts and neoplasms in the infant lung. *Semin Roentgenol* 1972; 7:122.

Spencer R: *Pathology of the Lung,* ed 4. Oxford, England, Pergamon Press, 1984.

Stocker JT, Drake RM, Madewell JE: Cystic and congenital lung disease in the newborn. *Perspect Pediatr Pathol* 1978; 4:93.

Weibel ER: *Morphometry of the Human Lung.* New York, Academic Press, 1963.

Wellons HA, Eggleston P, Golden GT, et al: Bronchial adenoma in childhood: Two case reports and review of the literature. *Am J Dis Child* 1976; 130:301.

Wolson AH: Pulmonary findings in Gaucher's disease. *Am J Roentgenol* 1973; 123:712.

Pulmonary Agenesis, Hypoplasia

Currarino G, Williams B: Causes of congenital unilateral pulmonary hypoplasia: A study of 33 cases. *Pediatr Radiol* 1985; 15:15–24.

Felson B: Pulmonary agenesis and related anomalies. *Semin Roentgenol* 1972; 7:17.

Fletcher BD, Garcia EJ, Colenda C: Reduced lung volume associated with acquired pulmonary artery obstruction in children. *Am J Roentgenol* 1979; 133:47.

Swischuk LE, Richardson CJ, Nichols MM, et al: Primary pulmonary hypoplasia in the neonate. *J Pediatr* 1979; 95:573.

Congenital Lobar Emphysema (Neonatal Lobar Hyperinflation)

Gordon I, Dempsey JE: Infantile lobar emphysema in association with congenital heart disease. *Clin Radiol* 1990; 41:48.

Kennedy CD, Habibi P, Matthew DJ, et al: Lobar emphysema: Long-term imaging follow-up. *Radiology* 1991; 180:189–193.

Bronchogenic Cyst, Congenital Cystic Adenomatoid Malformation (CCAM)

Diwan RV, Brennan JN, Philipson EH, et al: Ultrasonic prenatal diagnosis of type III congenital cystic adenomatoid malformation of the lung. *J Clin Ultrasound* 1983; 11:218.

Madewell JE, Stocker JT, Korsower JM: Cystic adenomatoid malformation of the lung: Morphologic analysis. *Am J Roentgenol* 1975; 124:436.

Miller RK, Sieber WK, Eunace EJ: Congenital adenomatoid malformation of the lung: Report of 17 cases and review of the literature. *Pathol Annu* 1980; 5:387–402.

Rogers LF, Osmer JC: Bronchogenic cyst: A review of 46 cases. *Am J Roentgenol* 1964; 91:273–283.

Rosado-de-Christenson ML, Stocker JT: Congenital cystic adenomatoid malformation. *Radiographics* 1991; 11:865–886.

Shackelford GD, Siegel MJ: The appearance of cystic adenomatoid malformation. *J Compu Assist Tomogr* 1989; 31:612–616.

Stocker JT, Madewell JE, Drake RM: Congenital cystic adenomatoid malformation of the lung: Classification and morphologic spectrum. *Hum Pathol* 1977; 8:155–171.

Hypogenetic Lung Syndrome (Pulmonary Venolobar Syndrome, Scimitar Syndrome), Horseshoe Lung

Ang JG, Proto AV: CT demonstration of congenital pulmonary venolobar syndrome. *J Comput Assist Tomogr* 1984; 8:753–757.

Davis WA , Allen RP: Accessory diaphragm: Duplication of the diaphragm. *Radiol Clin North Am* 1968; 6:153.

Godwin JD, Tarver RD: Scimitar syndrome: Four new cases examined with CT. *Radiology* 1986; 159:15–20.

Greene R, Miller SW: Cross-sectional imaging of silent pulmonary venous anomalies. *Radiology* 1986; 159:279–281.

Hawass ND, Badawi MG, Muzrakchi AM, et al: Horseshoe lung: Differential diagnosis. *Pediatr Radiol* 1990; 20:580.

Takeda K, Kato N, Nakagawa T, et al: Horseshoe lung without respiratory distress. *Pediatr Radiol* 1990; 20:604.

Sequestration Spectrum

Choplin RH, Siegel MJ: Pulmonary sequestration: Six unusual presentations. *Am J Roentgenol* 1980; 134:695.

Felson B: Pulmonary equestration evisited. *Medical Radiography and Photography* 1988; 64:1–27.

Gerle RD, Jaretzki A III, Ashley CA, et al: Congenital bronchopulmonary foregut malformation: Pulmonary sequestration communicating with the intestinal tract. *N Engl J Med* 1968; 278:1413.

Heithoff KB, Sane SM, Williams HJ, et al: Bronchopulmonary foregut malformations: A unifying etiological concept. *Am J Roentgenol* 1975; 126:46.

Hernanz-Schulman M, Stein SM, Neblett WW, et al: Pulmonary sequestration: Diagnosis with color Doppler sonography and a new theory of associated hydrothorax. *Radiology* 1991; 180:817–821.

Ikezoe J, Murayama S, Godwin JD, et al: Bronchopulmonary sequestration: CT assessment. *Radiology* 1990; 176:375–379.

Leithiser RE Jr, Capitanio MA, Macpherson RI, et al: "Communicating" bronchopulmonary foregut malformations. *Am J Roentgenol* 1986; 146:227–231.

Maulik D, Robinson L, Dailey DK, et al: Prenatal sonographic depiction of intralobar pulmonary sequestration. *J Ultrasound Med* 1987; 6:703–706.

Naidich DP, Rumancik WM, Lefleur RS, et al: Intralobar pulmonary sequestration: MR evaluation. *J Comput Assist Tomogr* 1987; 11:531–533.

Panicek DM, Heitzman ER, Randall PA, et al: The continuum of pulmonary developmental anomalies. *Radiographics* 1987; 7:747–772.

Sade RM, Clouse M, Ellis FH Jr: The spectrum of pulmonary sequestration. *Ann Thorac Surg* 1974; 18:644–658.

Stern EJ, Webb WR, Warnock ML, et al: Bronchopulmonary sequestration: Dynamic, ultrafast, high-resolution CT evidence of air trapping. *Am J Roentgenol* 1991; 157:947–949.

Pulmonary Lymphangiectasia

Bentur L, Canny G, Thorner P, et al: Spontaneous pneumthorax in cystic adenomatoid malformation. *Chest* 1991; 99:1292–93.

Galvin JR, Mori M, Stanford W: High-resolution computed tomography and diffuse lung disease. *Curr Probl Diagn Radiol* 1992; 2:1–74.

Glazer HS, Anderson, DiCroce JJ, et al: Anatomy of the major fissure: Evaluation with standard and thin-section CT. *Radiology* 1991; 180:839–844.

Noonan JA: Congenital pulmonary lymphangiectasia. *Am J Dis Child* 1970; 120:314–315.

Scalzetti EM, Heitzman ER, Groskin SA, et al: Developmental lymphatic disorders of the thorax. *Radiographics* 1991; 11:1069–1085.

Zwirewich CV, Mayo JR, Müller NL: Low-dose high-resolution CT of lung parenchyma. *Radiology* 1991; 180:413–417.

8

Diseases of the Airways and Abnormalities of Pulmonary Aeration

CENTRAL AIRWAYS—TRACHEA AND BRONCHI

Radiographic Appearance

On frontal chest radiographs the trachea usually lies in the midline or slightly to the right of it; on an expiratory film, especially in infants, the trachea may buckle anteriorly and to the right, sometimes so markedly as to suggest a mediastinal mass to the inexperienced observer (Fig 8–1). Deviation to the left suggests a right aortic arch or other mass lesion.

On lateral views, the trachea inclines gently posteriorly relatively parallel to the spine, normally maintaining an even caliber until the bifurcation (Fig 8–2). After the neonatal period, the normal trachea shows little, if any, change in caliber during quiet breathing unless peripheral airway obstruction is present; then the trachea can collapse by about 50% on expiration. Collapse of a greater extent suggests tracheomalacia rather than normal tracheal response to increased intrathoracic pressure. Cine computed tomography (CT) can precisely demonstrate changes in tracheal diameter with respiration. Normal age-related CT values for tracheal dimensions have been published by Griscom. Both the length and cross-sectional areas of the trachea increase with age and correlate well with body height.

The tracheobronchial tree is optimally visualized

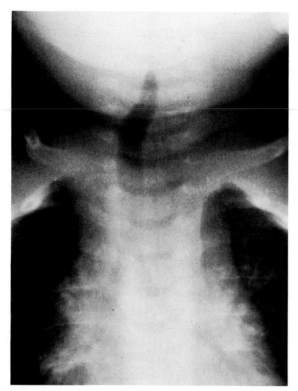

FIG 8–1.
Normal high-kilovoltage film of the trachea in an infant. Note the normal slight buckling to the right side just above the thoracic inlet.

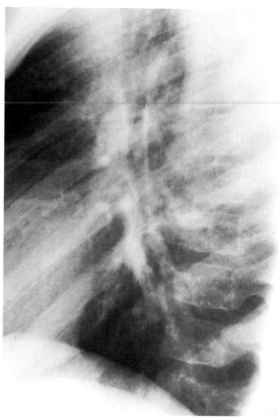

FIG 8–2.
Normal lateral radiograph of the trachea. The trachea narrows at the bifurcation. The origin of the right upper lobe bronchus is a faintly visible, rounded radiolucency.

by the use of filtered, high-kilovoltage magnification film or fluoroscopic techniques. If further information is required, CT provides superb visualization of the trachea and major bronchi. The normal trachea is nearly circular on axial CT examination. Direct coronal CT can be applied in younger children. Positive contrast tracheobronchograms are rarely necessary but if needed, should be performed with water-soluble nonionic contrast agents. Magnetic resonance imaging (MRI) can provide excellent visualization of the trachea and proximal bronchi in multiple planes.

The anatomy of the major bronchi is depicted in Figure 7–2. Knowledge of CT anatomy is important as this modality is becoming widely used in evaluation of the tracheobronchial tree. CT anatomy at five levels is shown in Figure 8–3. On the right side, the anterior and posterior segmental right upper lobe branches are usually clearly seen on CT as they are parallel to the plane of section. The apical branch is visualized in cross section and can be difficult to identify unless its wall is thickened. The medial and lateral segmental branches of the right middle lobe bronchi are visualized just inferior to the bronchus intermedius in nearly all patients. Usually the superior segmental branch of the right lower lobe bronchus can be seen at the level of the right middle lobe

bronchus, and then just distal to this, one can see the other segmental bronchi of the right lower lobe.

On the left side, the left upper lobe bronchus originates at a level inferior to the right upper lobe bronchus, usually at the level of the bronchus intermedius. At this point, the apicoposterior branch arises. The lingular bronchus extends laterally, obliquely, and inferiorly at or just before the division into the lower left bronchus. The anterior segmental bronchus is identified easily as it is the only left upper lobe bronchus which courses anteriorly and is horizontal. Its origin is variable, but most commonly it originates as a branch of the apical posterior segmental bronchus. The lower lobe segmental bronchi are often visualized as a trifurcation. Greater detail of normal CT anatomy is presented in the textbook of Naidich and associates.

Congenital Anomalies of the Tracheobronchial Tree

Tracheal Development

The pulmonary system arises as a midline ventral diverticulum from the foregut during the 21st to 24th

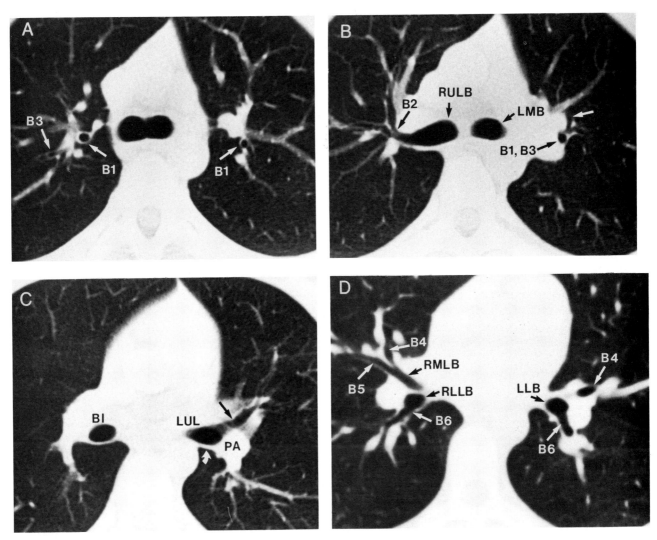

FIG 8–3.

A, normal bronchial anatomy as seen on CT using contiguous 6-mm slices. CT scan image at the level of the carina reveals the origin of both main stem bronchi. The apical bronchus (B1) of the right upper lobe is visualized in cross section. Subsegmental branches of the posterior segmental branch (B3) are seen coursing horizontally just lateral and posterior to the B1 bronchus (arrows). On the left side the posterior segment of the apical posterior bronchus is sectioned transversely. **B,** just inferior to the carina the origin of the right upper lobe (RULB) and the left main stem (LMB) bronchi are visualized. On the left side the apical posterior segmental bronchus (B1, B3) is sectioned transversely. The origin of the anterior segmental bronchus to the left upper lobe is seen coursing horizontally (arrow). **C,** section through the bronchus intermedius (BI) on the right side. At this level on the left side the superior division of left upper lobe (LUL) bronchus is seen, as is the origin of the apical posterior segmental bronchus (straight black arrow). The left inferior pulmonary artery (PA) is seen, as is the left retrobronchial stripe (curved white arrow). **D,** just below the origin of the right middle lobe bronchus it is seen dividing into medial (B4) and lateral (B5) segments. The origin of the right lower lobe bronchus and its first segmental branch (B6), the superior segment, are also easily identified. On the left side, the section is just below the origin of the lingular bronchus (B4). There is also visualization of the left lower lobe bronchus (LLB) and its superior segmental branch (B6). RMLB, right middle lobe bronchus; RLLB, right lower lobe bronchus. **E,** this series of four contiguous images extends from the previous level inferiorly through the truncus basalis on both sides inferiorly toward the trifurcation of the basilar segmental bronchi. **F,** just inferior to **E,** the inferior pulmonary veins are visualized entering the left atrium bilaterally. On the left side, the anterior and medial basilar segments have a common origin (B7 and B8); the lateral and posterior segments of the bronchi (B8 and B10) are also well visualized. On the right side, the medial (B7), lateral (B9), and posterior (B10) basilar bronchi are seen near their point of origin.

(Continued.)

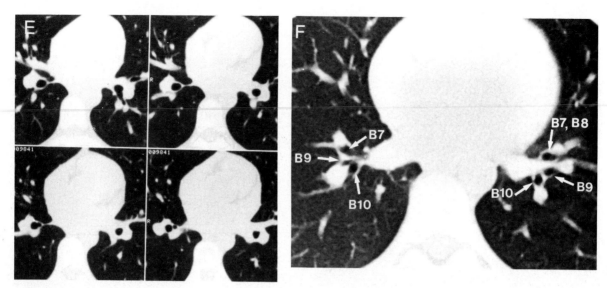

FIG 8–3 (cont.)

day of embryonic development. As this occurs, a longitudinal laryngeal tracheal groove forms. At approximately 24 to 27 days, development of the tracheoesophageal septum begins. The process of division of the respiratory from the digestive system begins caudally, extends cranially, and is nearly complete by the 32nd to 34th day (Smith) (Fig 8–4). Abnormal development of this septum results in anomalies such as tracheal or esophageal atresia and tracheoesophageal fistula.

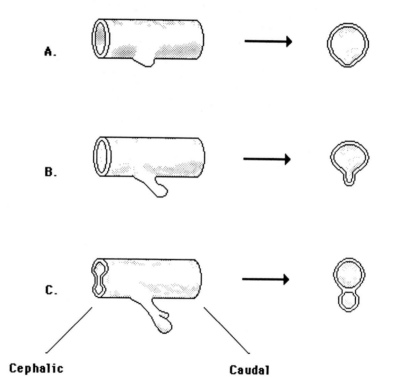

FIG 8–4.
Differentiation of foregut into esophagus and trachea: schematic representation of the separation of the trachea and esophagus in normal embryogenesis. **A,** development of the laryngotracheal groove on the ventral aspect of the foregut. **B,** evolution into a lung bud and beginning formation of the tracheoesophageal septum. **C,** bifurcation of the single lung bud into main bronchi and partial construction of the tracheoesophageal septum. (From Effmann EI, Spackman TJ, Berdon WE, et al: *AJR* 1975; 125:767. Used by permission.)

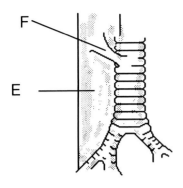
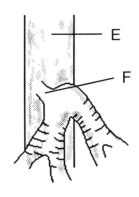
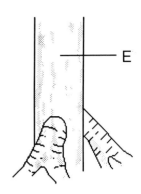

Type I   **Type II**   **Type III**

FIG 8–5.
Three types of tracheal agenesis. Type II, with absence of the trachea to the level of the carina, is the most common. E = esophagus, F = fistula. (From Effmann EI, Spackman TJ, Berdon WE, et al. *AJR* 1975; 125:767. Used by permission.)

Tracheal Atresia

Tracheal atresia is a rare lethal anomaly, producing severe neonatal respiratory distress. The entire trachea is usually absent. Three anatomical types are recognized (Fig 8–5). What little pulmonary aeration there is occurs through a distal trachea or broncho-esophageal fistula. The diagnosis should be suspected in any infant in whom improved ventilation is obtained despite difficult intubation and an apparent abnormal placement of the endotracheal tube in the esophagus. The diagnosis can be confirmed by CT (Fig 8–6).

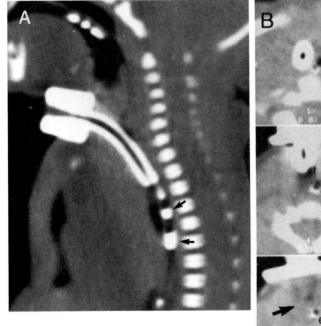
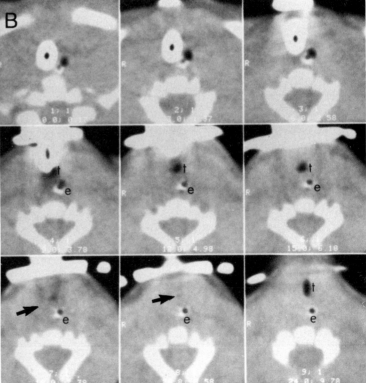

FIG 8–6.
CT of focal proximal tracheal atresia. This infant was born with respiratory distress and could not be intubated. Tracheostomy was performed. **A,** direct sagittal CT scan reveals the tracheostomy tube in the distal trachea. A nasogastric tube *(arrows)* is noted in the esophagus. No proximal tracheal airway is visualized. **B,** contiguous 3-mm transaxial CT images from inferior *(top left)* to superior *(bottom right)* reveal complete absence of the tracheal air column *(arrows)* at levels 7 and 8. *t*, trachea; *e*, esophagus.

Bronchial Atresia

Bronchial atresia may result from a developmental abnormality during the fifth fetal week when the segmental airways develop, or it could result from a later intrauterine interruption of the bronchial artery blood supply. The affected bronchus does not communicate proximally; its distal portion usually dilates and fills with mucus causing a small mass shadow in the hilar region. The bronchus serving the apical posterior segment of the left upper lobe is most commonly affected. In the newborn, this anomaly typically presents as a localized pulmonary opacity in the region served by the affected bronchus because there is a delay in the clearing of fetal lung liquid behind the atretic bronchus (Fig 8–7). This opacity is gradually replaced by hyperinflation

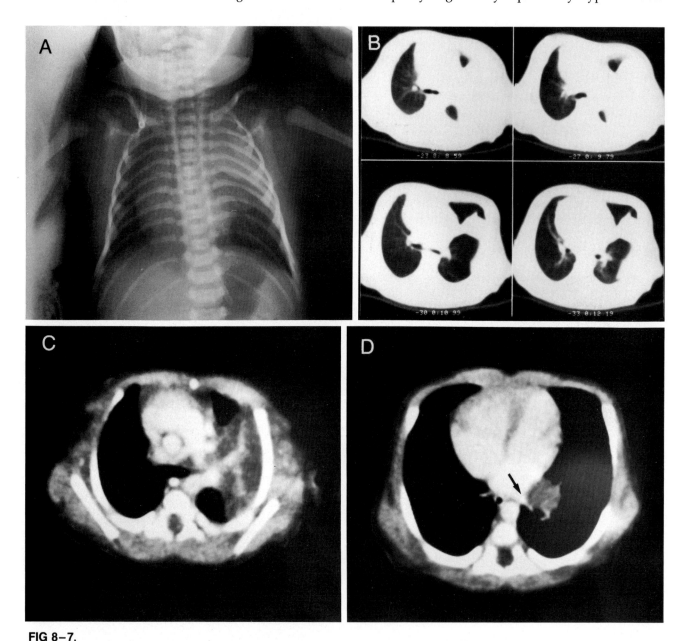

FIG 8–7.
Atresia of the apical posterior segmental bronchus of the left upper lobe. **A,** AP supine chest radiograph reveals left upper lobe opacity without an air bronchogram. There was a question of a left hilar mass as well. **B,** contiguous 3-mm ultrafast CT (UFCT) images reveal the superior division of the left upper lobe bronchus to be missing. **C,** contrast-enhanced 3-mm section at the level of the carina reveals the left upper lobe opacity to be vascularized, a find-ing consistent with normal lung parenchyma. *D,* ductus; *A,* aorta; *P,* pulmonary artery. **D,** CT section 2 cm inferior to **C,** reveals a 2-cm cystic avascular mass anterior to the left inferior pulmonary vein *(arrow).* At surgery this was a bronchogenic cyst which shared a common wall with the inferior portion of the lingular bronchus. The superior division of the left upper lobe bronchus was atretic.

resulting from collateral ventilation through the pores of Kohn. Localized hyperlucency is thus the usual appearance in the older child and adult. The affected bronchus may dilate distally, fill with fluid, and simulate a mass or mucoid bronchial impaction (Fig 8–8).

The occurrence of bronchial atresia with other malformations including bronchogenic cyst, intralobar sequestration, and adenomatoid malformation suggests a unifying embryologic theory for their concurrent development (Remy and Remy). There have been at least five cases of concurrent presence of bronchogenic cyst and bronchial atresia, suggesting that bronchial atresia may more likely develop from an early budding anomaly at the time of the development of the bronchogenic cyst (at 4–5 weeks) rather than being due to a later vascular accident.

Tracheal Fistula

In about 70% of patients with esophageal atresia, an associated tracheoesophageal fistula is present.

This topic is discussed in detail in Chapters 25 and 52.

Bronchobiliary Fistula

Bronchobiliary fistula is a very rare anomaly which is suggested by the coughing up of green mucoid material and the radiographic finding of gas in the gallbladder. Chronic recurrent pneumonia is usually present. The fistula usually arises from the proximal portion of the right main stem bronchus just below the carina and extends to the extrahepatic ductal system; its presence can be confirmed by bronchography.

Tracheal Bronchus

Although the right upper lobe bronchus normally arises directly from the trachea in swine and many other cloven-hoofed animals, this occurrence is unusual in man. The incidence in humans, gleaned from bronchographic studies, is thought to be about 1% on the right side. A left-sided tracheal bronchus

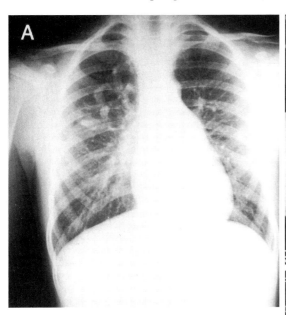

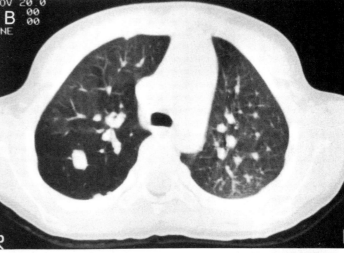

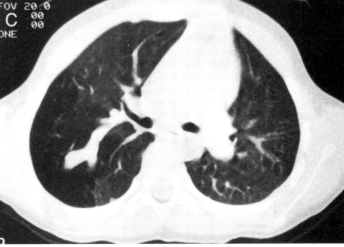

FIG 8–8.
Right upper lobe bronchial atresia in an 8-year-old child. **A,** chest radiograph reveals slight hyperlucency of the right upper lobe and branching opacities. **B** and **C,** transaxial CT images reveal a branching nonvascular opacity which can be followed down to the origin at the level of the posterior segmental bronchus of the right upper lobe. Note the peribronchial hyperinflation.

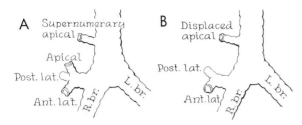

FIG 8–9.
The two common types of tracheal bronchus: **A,** supernumerary apical bronchus. **B,** displaced apical bronchus. (From McLaughlin FJ, et al: *J Pediatr* 1985; 106:751.)

is estimated to occur from 2.5 to 7 times less frequently (Remy et al., Ritsema).

The bronchus is either supernumerary if the right lobe has a normal trifurcating bronchus or, more commonly, is merely ectopic, with the missing segmental branch arising from the trachea or the main stem bronchus and usually supplying the apical segment of the lung (Figs 8–9 and 8–10). A double right tracheal bronchus has been observed (Iannacone et al.), as has duplication of the right upper lobe bronchus (Fig 8–11). The latter anomaly reportedly occurred 11 times in 1,200 bronchograms studied by Atwell. Remy and associates reported seven

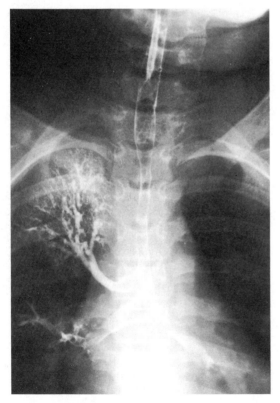

FIG 8–10.
Bronchogram of tracheal bronchus associated with tracheal stenosis of the segmental type.

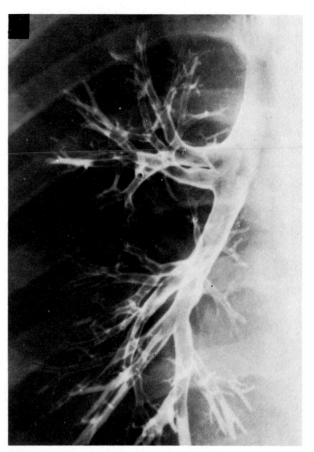

FIG 8–11.
Duplication of the right upper lobe bronchus. (Courtesy of Dr. Jack Sty, Milwaukee.)

cases of left tracheal bronchi, most of which involved the apical posterior segmental bronchus, which actually arose not from the trachea but from the left main stem bronchus. Four of the cases reported by Remy et al. had left upper lobe emphysema, as did seven similar cases described in the literature, suggesting that left-sided tracheal bronchus may be frequently associated with this radiographic abnormality. The emphysema could be due to pressure on the ectopic bronchus by the left pulmonary artery.

While many cases of tracheal bronchus are asymptomatic, some are associated with bronchiectasis and recurrent infection (Ritsema). In addition to the cases of left upper lobe emphysema referred to above, Siegel et al. and Holinger also reported cases in which there was cystlike hyperexpansion in the right upper lobe. Additionally, both cases presented by Siegel et al., as well as several others in the literature, have been associated with tracheal stenosis (Fig 8–12).

Tracheal bronchus should therefore be excluded in cases of tracheal stenosis or persistent upper lobe

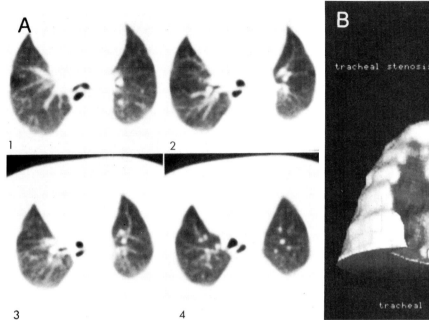

FIG 8–12.
Tracheal bronchus associated with tracheal stenosis. **A,** contiguous serial 3-mm images from the carina cephalad. Image *1* reveals the carina. The right main stem bronchus is slightly flattened. Image *2* reveals a branching bronchial structure superior to the level of the carina. Image *3* shows it nearing the trachea. Image *4* reveals the origin of the tracheal bronchus from the posterolateral wall of the trachea. *E,* esophagus. **B,** three-dimensional reconstruction of the transaxial images reveals the origin of the tracheal bronchus, the tracheal stenosis, and a carinal configuration suggestive of a bridging bronchus anomaly. (See also Fig 8-13.)

abnormalities, such as recurrent pneumonia or persistent, unexplained air trapping. This is especially true in children with Down syndrome or in those with anomalies of the upper ribs. The aberrant bronchus may be seen on plain film, CT examination, or tracheogram.

Bridging Bronchus
Bridging bronchus is a rare branching anomaly in which the middle and the lower lobes of the right lung are supplied by a bronchus which arises from the medial aspect of the left main bronchus and bridges the mediastinum in its course to the right lung. Radiologically, the bridging bronchus can be seen to branch from the left main bronchus at a lower level (T5–6) than the normal carina (Fig 8–13,A and B). Wells et al. suggest that in patients with pulmonary artery sling, the junction of the bridging bronchus and the left main bronchus has often been misinterpreted as a low-lying, inverted T-shaped carina, and that the right main bronchus, which supplies only the right upper lobe, has been misinterpreted as a tracheal or preeparterial bronchus. This anomaly occurs in about 80% of the reported cases of left pulmonary artery sling; this group of patients also frequently has tracheal stenosis due to complete cartilage rings as well as an in-

creased incidence of imperforate anus and absence of the gallbladder. It is not clear how many cases of "tracheal bronchus" really are the bridging bronchus anomaly, but if there is a "tracheal bronchus" and a low-lying carina with an increased subcarinal angle and tracheal stenosis, bridging bronchus should be strongly considered.

Other Branching Anomalies
Minor variations in normal branching of the tracheobronchial tree occur relatively frequently, but most are of little clinical significance and are described elsewhere for the interested reader (Atwell).

Landing and Wells have emphasized abnormal branching patterns associated with abnormalities of visceral and atrial situs. In patients with asplenia syndrome, the lungs are bilaterally "right-sided," and bilateral eparterial bronchi (first bronchial branch superior to the pulmonary artery) are present; in polysplenia, a less severe anomaly, bilateral left-sidedness is noted, and bilateral hyparterial bronchi (first bronchial branch inferior to the pulmonary artery) are present.

Congenital Tracheal Stenosis
Approximately 50% of cases of tracheal stenosis are of the focal or segmental variety, 30% of the "gener-

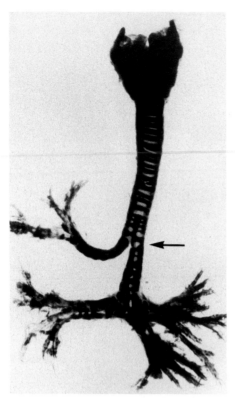

FIG 8–13.
Dissected, stained, and cleared specimen of a 2-day-old infant with classic "bridging bronchus." The *arrow* shows the level of tracheal bifurcation. The lower bifurcation (the pseudocarina) shows the inverted "T" pattern. (From Wells TR, Gwinn JL, Landing BH, et al. *J Pediatr Surg* 1988; 23:892. Used by permission.)

alized hypoplasia" type, and 20% are of the carrot- or funnel-like stenosis often associated with the pulmonary sling anomaly and "napkin-ring cartilages" (Landing and Wells) (Fig 8–14).

Many cases of tracheal stenosis occur in association with extrinsic pressure by anomalous vessels and are due to abnormalities of the adjacent tracheal cartilages. The airway deformity persists even after relief of the vascular compression. The most striking example of this occurs in the pulmonary sling anomaly, which is associated with abnormal complete circumferential tracheal cartilage rings which may be either focal or generalized. As discussed above, tracheal bronchus and bridging bronchus are commonly found with pulmonary sling and are associated with tracheal stenosis. In a report by Capitanio et al., compression of the trachea by the aorta was seen in four children with congenital heart disease. In each instance, the aorta was dilated, as it was the major or only conduit through which blood could leave the heart. The trachea was displaced posteriorly and had an anterior compression defect. Of significance were intrinsic anomalies of the trachea and

bronchi, including tracheostenosis, tracheomalacia, and bronchomalacia due to abnormalities of the cartilage rings.

Benjamin et al. reported on 21 children with congenital tracheal stenosis; all but two presented in the first year of life. Nonspecific signs of upper airway obstruction were present in all patients. Tracheal stenosis was associated with other congenital anomalies in all but two patients. Four patients had tracheal bronchus, five had hypoplasia of one or both lungs, and three had an H-type tracheoesophageal fistula. Skeletal and cardiovascular anomalies were also frequent. LaCrosse et al. reported an unusual form of tracheal stenosis, in which esophageal tissue was sequestered in the tracheal wall. This most likely results when the trachea fails to separate normally from the esophagus early in embryogenesis.

Tracheal abnormalities occurring in malformation syndromes have been studied by Landing and Wells, and the interested reader is referred to their comprehensive review. Conditions associated with the dysplasias include tracheal flattening, tracheal cartilage abnormalities, short trachea, abnormal bronchial branch pattern, and combinations thereof. Among the syndromes implicated are camptomelic syndrome, diastrophic dwarfism, thanatophoric dwarfism with cloverleaf skull, and Ellis–van Creveld syndrome. Also mentioned in the review article are the asplenia syndromes, Saldino-Noonan syndrome, partial chromosome 19 trisomy, and rib-gap syndrome. Of course, the most frequent tracheal abnormalities are found in association with esophageal atresia and the VATER and VACTERL syndromes (Landing and Wells).*

Diffuse tracheal narrowing has also been observed in 16% of patients with mucopolysaccharidoses (Peters et al.). In one autopsied case, it was demonstrated that the tracheal narrowing was due to mucopolysaccharide deposition. This can occur in the larynx and supraglottic portion of the airway, leading to respiratory obstruction and death. MRI is particularly useful to show the abnormal deposits.

Tracheal calcifications can be associated with tracheal narrowing and stridor. Most commonly, they occur in chondrodysplasia punctata, Keitel syndrome, and warfarin embryopathy, but also can be idiopathic (see Fig 5–8). Tracheal calcifications have been noted to develop following cardiac surgery, particularly in children who have been treated with

*VATER, an acronym for *v*ertebral defects, imperforate *a*nus, *t*racheo*e*sophogeal fistula, and *r*adial and *r*enal dysplasia; VACTERL, *v*ertebral, *a*nal, *c*ardiac, *t*racheal, *e*sophageal, *r*enal, and *l*imb.

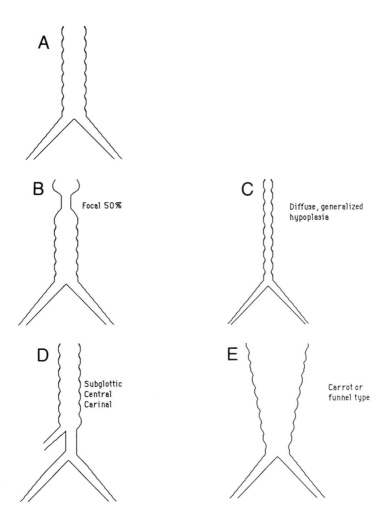

FIG 8–14.
Types of tracheal stenosis. **A,** normal tracheal bronchial tree. **B,** focal or segmental (50%). **C,** diffuse generalized hypoplasia (30%). **D,** focal tracheal stenosis may occur in the subglottic, central, or the carinal region. The focal type is often associated with the tracheal bronchus anomaly (see Fig 8–10). **E,** carrot or funnel type (20%). (Drawn by C. Jonas.)

warfarin sodium, suggesting a possible relationship to the calcifications which have been seen in warfarin embryopathy.

Tracheobronchomegaly

Tracheobronchomegaly, or Mounier-Kuhn syndrome, is a disorder of unknown etiology characterized by prominent dilation of the trachea and mainstem bronchi, probably due to a defect in the elastic and muscular tissues of these structures. Marked tracheal enlargement occurs on inspiration, and an abnormal degree of collapse is seen on expiration. Tracheograms can be used to confirm the diagnosis and may show "tracheal diverticuli" (Fig 8–15). The condition occurs only rarely in childhood, although it has been reported in an 18-month-old boy (Hunter et al.). Tracheobronchomegaly was associated with acquired cutis laxa in a boy 14 years of age described by Wanderer and associates. Their studies disclosed abnormal elastic fibers in the skin and abnormal recoil of the lungs. These findings suggest that tracheobronchomegaly may be due to a basic defect in elastic tissue at several sites. Landing (1979) thinks that some cases suggest an autosomal recessive inheritance.

Tracheomegaly, an increase in tracheal dimensions greater than 2 SD above the normal, has been increasingly observed in children who have either a history of prolonged ventilatory support or chronic pulmonary infection, including cystic fibrosis. Why most children with similar histories do not develop tracheomegaly is as yet unknown.

Tracheomalacia

Tracheomalacia is often suspected clinically when an infant has noisy or stridulous breathing. Most often, the symptoms are due to the self-limited "laryngomalacia" or, as it is more accurately called, the "supraglottic hypermobility syndrome" (see Chapter 5).

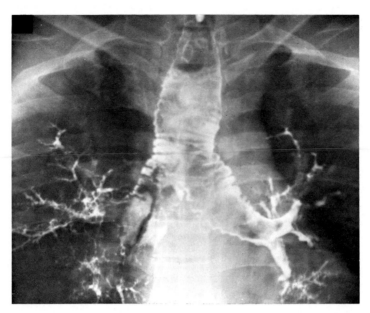

FIG 8–15.
Tracheogram reveals marked dilatation of the trachea and larger bronchi and indentations of the tracheal wall between the cartilag- inous rings. (From Katz I, LeVine M, Herman P: *Am J Roentgenol* 1962; 88:1084. Used by permission.)

The condition is usually self-limited. Tracheomalacia is interpreted to mean abnormal tracheal collapse (Fig 8–16). Most cases of what appear to be tracheomalacia actually represent normal tracheal response to abnormal airway pressures. Wittenberg et al. showed that the normal trachea could collapse by as much as 50%. Inspiratory collapse in the extrathoracic trachea can occur normally when upper airway obstruction (croup or epiglottitis) is present. Expiratory collapse of a long intrathoracic tracheal segment was associated with small airway obstruction, as occurs in bronchiolitis.

Benjamin et al. have suggested that true tracheomalacia be divided into primary and secondary types. *Primary tracheomalacia* is seen in a variety of syndromes and systemic diseases affecting cartilage such as Larsen syndrome and relapsing polychondritis. It may also be seen occasionally in premature infants as well as in otherwise apparently normal infants. *Secondary tracheomalacia* is seen in patients with tracheoesophageal fistula, extrinsic pressure by vessels and mediastinal masses, and also arises secondary to tracheal injury, most commonly, intubation. Tracheomalacia occurs in up to 50% of patients with tracheoesophageal fistula. According to Kao et al., in a study using cine-CT, the level of the tracheomalacia does not appear to correlate with the level of the fistula nor with the size of the adjacent dilated esophagus, the length of the atretic esophageal segment, or the site of surgery. Tracheomalacia may be either focal or diffuse and often persists and causes

stridor even after decompression of the dilated pouch and repair of the fistula.

Tracheomalacia also occurs in association with extrinsic pressure by mediastinal masses and abnormal vessels such as vascular rings and the innominate artery syndrome. The latter condition, discussed below, remains controversial.

Extrinsic Compression of the Tracheobronchial Tree

Anterior tracheal compression at the thoracic inlet was seen in 30% of children under 2 years of age in a study of randomly selected lateral chest films. Strife et al. (1981) in a review of pediatric angiograms, reported that the innominate artery arises to the left of the trachea and crosses in front of it, and is responsible for the tracheal indentation. Anterior tracheal compression is most often present in asymptomatic children but can occur in a much smaller group of children who have severe stridor and apnea. In some cases of the innominate artery syndrome, symptoms may be severe enough to warrant surgery.

Fletcher and Cohn, using MRI, studied normal infants and infants with anterior tracheal compression, and found that in both groups the normal innominate artery indeed was situated anterior and to the left of the trachea but that there was no apparent difference in the anatomical relationships in the two groups. Moreover, there was no evidence of excessive mediastinal crowding. These investigators con-

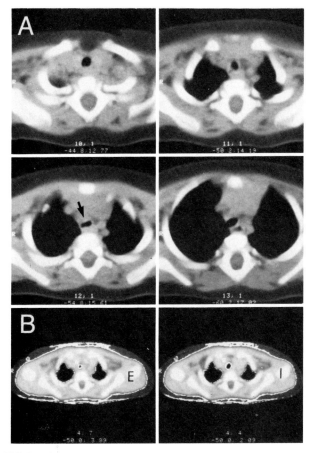

FIG 8–16.
Tracheomalacia. **A,** contiguous, transaxial 3-mm, 0.1-second UFCT images reveal narrowing of the trachea (arrow) at the level of the manubrium. **B,** same patient; UFCT in the cine mode reveals a 72% change in the caliber of the trachea between inspiration (I) on the right and expiration (E) on the left. At endoscopy, tracheomalacia was noted to be present.

cluded that the anterior tracheal narrowing was due to an intrinsic deficiency of the tracheal cartilage itself rather than to an aberrant position of the innominate artery.

The normal thymus, no matter how large, rarely compresses or displaces the trachea. A cause other than the thymus should be considered if tracheal displacement or compression is noted, although there is some evidence that a posterior or ectopic thymus may cause airway compression in rare instances.

The commonest pathologic cause of tracheal compression or displacement is a vascular ring. These malformations are discussed in greater detail in Chapter 17. The two commonest types are double aortic arch and right aortic arch with an aberrant left subclavian artery and a ligamentum arteriosum. The trachea is bowed forward on the lateral chest film and deviates to the left on the frontal film, some-

times enough to suggest a mediastinal mass. An esophagogram and high-kilovoltage films of the airway usually suffice for diagnosis. Vascular anatomy may be directly visualized with MRI or CT scanning (Fig 8–17). Angiography is rarely necessary.

Pulmonary artery sling (aberrant left pulmonary artery) often causes unilateral air trapping. Aneurysmal dilation of the pulmonary artery can also cause airway obstruction. Enlargement of the left atrium and left ventricle, as seen in patients with large ventricular septal defects of the myocardiopathies, may obstruct the left lower lobe bronchus or, occasionally, the entire left main bronchus, causing left lower lobe atelectasis.

In the newborn, a bronchogenic cyst is the most common mass to compress the tracheobronchial tree, but many mediastinal masses can cause extrinsic pressure on the airway (Fig 8–18). In the older child, lymphoma is the commonest mass to displace or obstruct the airway. Less commonly, inflammatory lymphadenopathy, especially tuberculosis, can produce similar findings. We have seen two patients with neurofibromatosis in whom extrinsic pressure in the upper trachea was caused by neurofibromatous masses. These conditions are discussed at greater length in Chapter 14.

Acquired Tracheobronchial Abnormalities and Focal Disturbances in Aeration

Focal Disturbances in Aeration

Tracheal lesions may cause bilateral increased or decreased inflation and often escape detection. Bronchial lesions are more easily diagnosed because they produce focal changes in aeration.

Compensatory Hyperinflation. When a lung, or a significant portion of it, undergoes volume loss, the remaining normal pulmonary tissue compensates by overexpansion due to alveolar enlargement. The characteristic radiographic finding is increased radiolucency due to increased tidal air; increased residual air may or may not be present. Ventilation and perfusion are normal on radionuclide examination.

Obstructive Hyperinflation. Obstructive hyperinflation occurs as a result of partial bronchial obstruction, either intrinsic or extrinsic. Intrinsic bronchial obstruction is caused by inflammatory disease, foreign bodies, mucous plugs and secretions, neoplasm, or bronchial stenosis. The most frequent cause of partial bronchial obstruction in our experience is edema and mucous plugging associated with inflammatory disease; foreign bodies are a more spectacular but less frequent cause of bronchial ob-

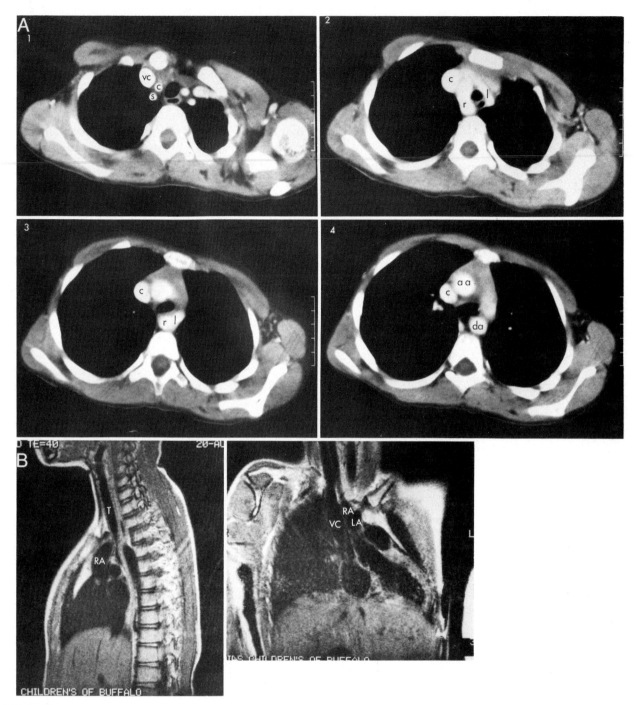

FIG 8–17.
A, CT and MRI of double aortic arch in a 5-year-old girl. Contiguous 6-mm UFCT images in level *1* reveal that each arch gives rise to a carotid and subclavian vessel, the so-called four-dot sign. *VC,* vena cava; *S,* subclavian; *C,* carotid). Level *2* shows a larger right and smaller left aortic arch circling the trachea. Level *3* shows the junction of the two arches into a midline descending thoracic aorta

that is displacing the trachea slightly anteriorly. Level *4* shows the now slightly left descending aorta *(da),* which is displacing the carina *(c)* and left main stem bronchus anteriorly. **B,** sagittal and coronal MR images, same patient. The sagittal image reveals tracheal *(T)* compression, and the coronal image reveals the branching of the left *(LA)* and right *(RA)* aortic arches.

struction. Extrinsic obstruction is due to pressure from congenital cystic masses, nodes, neoplasms, and vascular anomalies. These specific conditions are discussed elsewhere.

Whatever the cause of bronchial narrowing,

there are three possible effects on pulmonary aeration depending on the degree of obstruction. If the air flows freely through the narrow bronchial lumen, aeration of the lung is not disturbed. If, however, the ingress of air during inspiration exceeds the

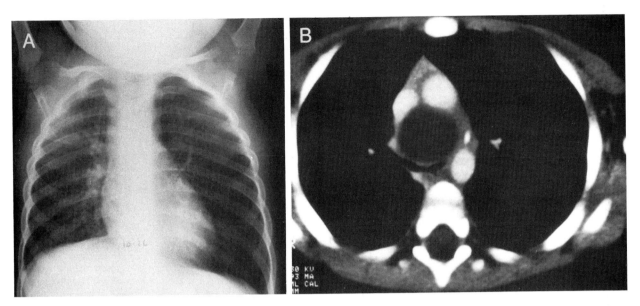

FIG 8–18.
Subcarinal bronchogenic cyst presenting as airway obstruction. This 2-year-old child presented with recent onset of wheezing. **A,** frontal radiograph shows air trapping in the left lung. An intrabronchial foreign body was suspected but none was found at bronchoscopy. There was a suggestion of a subcarinal mass noted at the bronchoscopic examination. **B,** contrast-enhanced CT examination, 0.1 second, reveals an avascular subcarinal mass extending up to the level of the aortic pulmonary window. The carina is displaced posteriorly. Incidental note is made of calcification in the ligamentum arteriosum. This subcarinal mass was completely missed on the radiographic examination even in retrospect. At surgery, a bronchogenic cyst was removed.

egress during expiration, as in the "ball-valve" type, the alveoli become overinflated and air trapping results. If both ingress and egress of air are blocked completely or if the egress exceeds the ingress, obstructive atelectasis develops (Fig 8–19). Rapidly shifting bronchial obstructions are seen, particularly in acute infections and bronchial asthma when, especially during coughing, obstructing plugs of exudate may be dislodged from some bronchi and sucked into others.

Postintubation Stenosis. Endotracheal intubation is now the commonest cause of tracheal stenosis

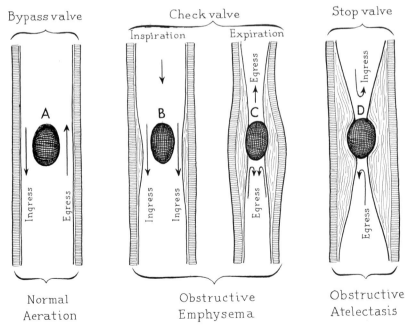

FIG 8–19.
The causal mechanism of obstructive atelectasis and emphysema. (Redrawn from Stoloff after Jackson.)

and granuloma. Granulation tissue and fibrosis develop following either endotracheal or tracheostomy tube placement, and can occur at the stoma, at the tip of the tube, or at the site of the cuff. Scott and Kramer reported tracheostomy-related complications in 26% of their pediatric patients.

The duration of intubation plays an important role in the incidence and severity of complications. Microscopic lesions occur after approximately 48 hours of intubation. Epithelial metaplasia is seen in children intubated for longer than 7 days, although occasionally granuloma may develop even after very brief periods of intubation. Stenosis may be weblike, fusiform, or irregular in shape (Fig 8–20). Diagnosis can usually be made by high-kilovoltage films but CT is useful to accurately measure cross-sectional areas (Fig 8–21) and may demonstrate intratracheal webs and granulomas. Fluoroscopy or cine-CT may be necessary to differentiate between a fixed tracheal stenosis and focal tracheomalacia; in some patients, both conditions may be present.

Airway Foreign Bodies. Aspiration of a foreign body into the tracheobronchial airway is a common cause of respiratory distress in children between the ages of 6 months and 3 years. In many cases, there

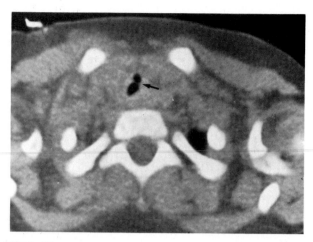

FIG 8–21.
A 2-year-old child with postintubation tracheal stenosis demonstrated on UFCT with a 0.1-second scan time. The normal trachea at this level should be round. The trachea in this patient is narrowed from side to side and has a weblike band *(arrow)* crossing its lumen.

is no clear-cut history of foreign body aspiration, and most foreign bodies are nonopaque. History of a choking episode, volunteered or elicited, carries a high index of suspicion. Clinical features may include stridor, wheezing, cough, recurrent pneumonia, or hemoptysis.

Radiographic features depend on the size, location, duration, and nature of the foreign body. Careful inspection of the tracheobronchial tree with high-kilovoltage films or fluoroscopy may reveal a barely visible opacity interrupting the air column. Most nonopaque foreign bodies are vegetable or food matter, but products of our society, such as aluminum pull tabs on beverage cans and pieces of plastic toys, also are found occasionally. If the foreign object is in the trachea, the chest radiograph may be normal, or may show bilateral under- or overinflation. Many intratracheal foreign bodies escape detection without the use of CT.

More commonly, however, the foreign body lodges in the bronchial tree, more often in the right than the left. The chest radiograph may reveal a variety of findings, the commonest of which is a unilateral hyperlucent lung. A film made at full inspiration may appear normal; close inspection may reveal relatively increased volume on the normal side with slight mediastinal shift toward the partially obstructed side. If a foreign body is suspected clinically, expiration films should always be obtained (Fig 8–22). The use of a gloved hand against the abdomen can aid in getting a film in good expiration. Lateral decubitus films have been suggested as an alternative if satisfactory inspiration-expiration stud-

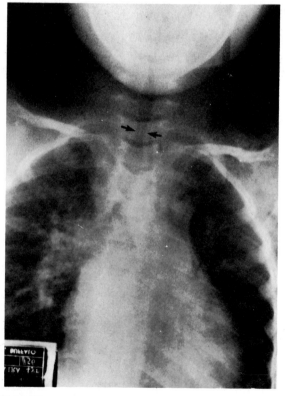

FIG 8–20.
Segmental tracheal stenosis following prolonged endotracheal intubation in a 4-year-old girl.

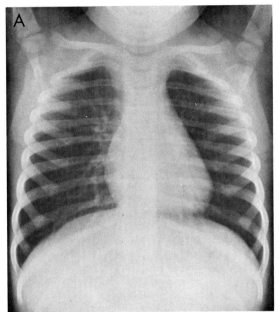 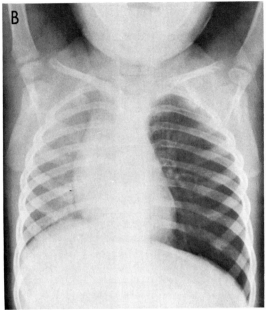

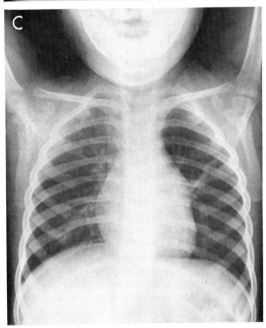

FIG 8–22.
The value of inspiratory and expiratory films in the diagnosis of obstructive emphysema in a child 30 months of age. **A,** chest radiograph exposed near the peak of a deep inspiration. Both lungs are about equally aerated and the mediastinal structures are in midline. The less prominent markings in the left lung suggest it may be emphysematous but the findings are subtle. In **B,** made at deep expiration, the right lung has deaerated normally but the left lung has failed to empty and remains hyperlucent. The mediastinal structures have shifted to the right, away from the side of the foreign body. This maneuver clearly shows the high residual air and low tidal air characteristic of obstructive emphysema. At bronchoscopy, a peanut was removed from the left main bronchus. In **C,** made 24 hours later in mid-inspiration, the left lung is still slightly hyperlucent and an opaque strip extends from the left hilum. Residual changes of this kind often persist after complete removal of a foreign body owing to localized chemical obstructive bronchitis from the peanut or edema to the bronchial walls resulting from the bronchoscopy. A second foreign body may also be responsible in some cases. (Courtesy of Dr. R. Parker Allen, Denver.)

ies cannot be obtained. When air trapping is present in a dependent lung on the decubitus view, the affected lobe or segment tends to remain hyperlucent rather than deflating, as would normally occur. Fluoroscopic examination of the chest is also valuable to detect air trapping. The examination shows inspiratory mediastinal shift toward the affected side and restricted diaphragmatic excursion on the affected side. Pneumomediastinum has been reported to occur in an otherwise unsuspected foreign body aspiration. The sensitivity and specificity of plain film technique recently have been questioned (Svedstrom et al.).

CT is the most sensitive diagnostic technique but is reserved for use in elusive cases of foreign body. It not only can demonstrate the relatively non-opaque foreign body in the bronchial tree in many instances, but also is a very sensitive means to detect differences in density in the lung parenchyma. Our experience suggests that if one uses contiguous thin (3 mm) slices, the foreign body can nearly always be directly visualized (Fig 8–23,A and B).

If the bronchial obstruction becomes more complete, atelectasis, pneumonia, or bronchiectasis may develop. Foreign body should be suspected clinically in all such unexplained cases. Timothy grass and

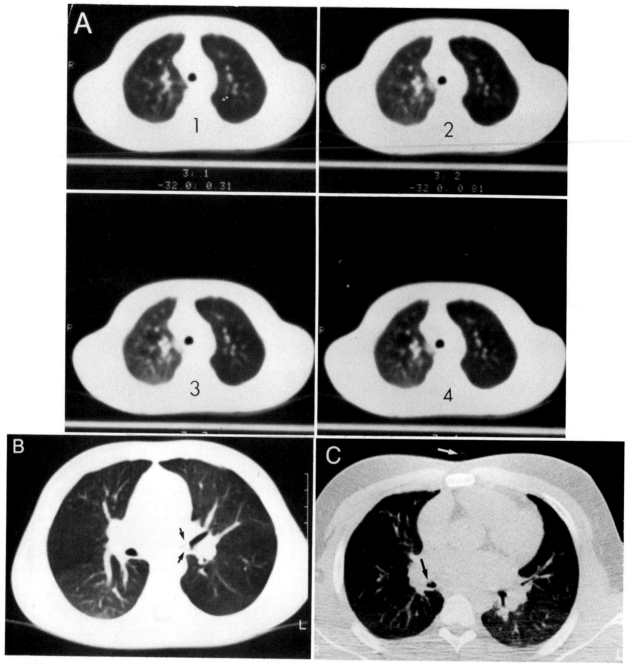

FIG 8–23.
CT demonstration of intrabronchial foreign bodies and normal radiographs. Foreign body in the left main stem bronchus of a 2-year-old child. Expiration films and fluoroscopy were equivocal. **A,** four frames from cine-CT performed at the same level, 0.05-second scan time at 0.7-second intervals, reveal relative hyperlucency of the left lung that is most marked on expiration. In frame 3, note the mediastinal shift toward the normal side on expiration. This subtle finding was not appreciated on conventional fluoroscopy. **B,** a high-resolution 0.1-second UFCT image reveals a 3-mm foreign body in the left main stem bronchus (arrows). At endoscopy, a small fragment of apple core was removed. **C,** 16-year-old boy with a barely opaque plastic foreign body in the right lower lobe bronchus (black arrow). A similar object (the end of a ballpoint pen) was taped to the patient's chest wall and is also only faintly visible (white arrow). A conventional expiration chest radiograph was normal.

certain weeds are particularly prone to produce complications of this type because the structure of the grass heads allows them to migrate distally down the bronchial tree into the pulmonary parenchyma. Hemoptysis associated with a chronic infiltrate should suggest foreign body. CT is less reliable if the lung is consolidated and the foreign body may escape detection unless it is calcified or opaque.

Esophageal foreign bodies can cause respiratory distress by inducing tracheospasm or by causing sec-

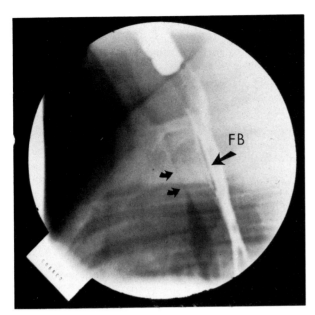

FIG 8–24.
Esophageal foreign body presenting with stridor. Lateral spot film from a 1-year-old patient shows a toothpick *(FB, large arrow)* in the barium-filled esophagus. Perforation had occurred and an abscess had developed causing marked narrowing of the trachea *(curved arrows).*

ondary tracheal compression (Fig 8–24). Foreign bodies tend to lodge in the coronal plane in the esophagus and in the sagittal plane in the trachea. Diagnosis of nonopaque foreign bodies requires an esophagogram.

Unilateral Hyperlucent Lung (Swyer-James-Macleod Syndrome). In 1953, Swyer and James described the constellation of radiographic findings of a small hyperlucent lung with ipsilateral small hi-

lum, diminished pulmonary vascularity, air trapping, and a lack of peripheral filling on bronchography in a 6-year-old patient. The pathology specimen revealed varying stages of bronchitis and bronchiolitis. Subsequently, numerous other reports concluded that the syndrome was due to an infectious insult to the bronchial tree in childhood, most commonly from adenoviral pneumonia, although several other types of pneumonia have been reported, including measles, tuberculosis, pertussis, and *Mycoplasma* pneumonia.

It is thought that the reduced number of alveoli, the emphysematous alveoli, the hypoplasia of the pulmonary arteries, and the decreased number of capillaries all result from an insult causing bronchiolitis obliterans occurring before the age of 8 years, before a full complement of alveoli would have developed.

The radiographic manifestations are easily recognized and virtually pathognomonic (Fig 8–25). The focal hyperlucency, whether it involves a lobe or the entire lung, is not caused by a relative increase in air in the affected lung but by decreased perfusion. The ipsilateral hilum is small but present, differentiating Swyer-James-Macleod syndrome from pulmonary artery agenesis. The volume of the affected lung or lobe is comparable to or smaller than that of the normal contralateral lung or may be reduced, but volume is seldom increased. A characteristic feature is air trapping on expiration, which indicates airway obstruction and differentiates Swyer-James syndrome from other conditions that may cause unilateral translucency. Pulmonary arteriography, seldom indicated in these patients, shows markedly dimin-

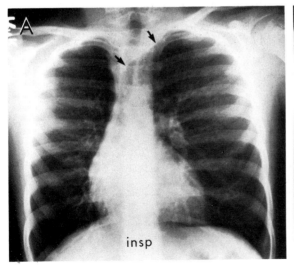
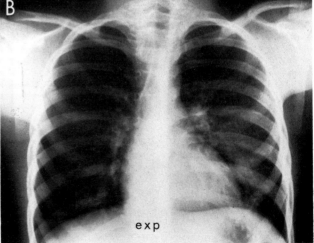

FIG 8–25.
Bronchiolitis obliterans (Swyer-James-Macleod syndrome) affecting the right lung. **A,** inspiration film shows hyperinflation on the left side with herniation of the left upper lobe across the midline ante- riorly *(arrows).* **B,** expiration film shows little change in position of the right hemidiaphragm. The right lung is hyperlucent and the mediastinum has shifted back toward the normal left side.

ished perfusion, a finding more easily demonstrated on radionuclide lung scanning or CT. Bronchography is usually not necessary but, if performed, shows a characteristic deformity of the bronchial tree. The segmental bronchi are irregularly dilated and end abruptly in squared or tapered terminations in fifth or sixth branches. Filling of peripheral bronchioles or radicles is notable by its absence.

CT has shown that despite the apparent unilateral involvement on the chest film, the abnormalities may be bilateral and are asymmetric. Features include patency of the central bronchi, small pulmonary vessels, bronchiectasis, usually cylindric, and a mosaic pattern of uneven ventilation and perfusion (Fig 8–26).

Differential diagnosis of unilateral hyperlucent lung syndrome is outlined in Table 8–1.

Tracheobronchial Neoplasms.—*Tracheal Neoplasms.* Tracheal neoplasms are rare in children. Laryngeal papillomas, discussed earlier, may seed into the trachea and, on occasion, into the lung parenchyma. Adenomas usually arise in the main stem bronchi and are discussed below. Granular cell myoblastoma or schwannoma can occur in the trachea. Hicks reported two cases which presented as obstructive lung disease in teenagers. Ectopic thymic and thyroid tissue have both reported to occur in the trachea.

Bronchial Adenomas. Bronchial adenomas are actually not adenomas but low-grade malignancies

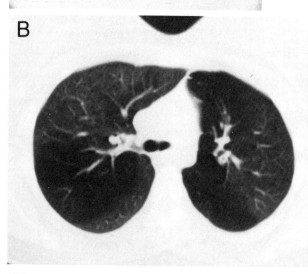

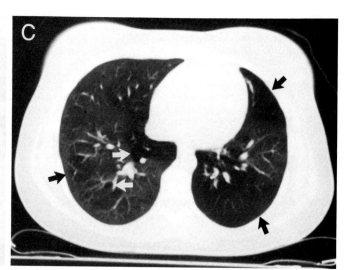

FIG 8–26.
CT findings in Swyer-James syndrome. **A,** frontal chest radiograph in a 14-year-old patient with previously documented left-sided bronchiolitis obliterans secondary to adenoviral pneumonia reveals the left lung to be small and hyperlucent with the left pulmonary artery inconspicuous. **B,** 6-mm CT scan at the level of the carina shows segmental hypoperfusion both anteriorly and posteriorly in the left upper lobe with a relatively normal segment noted laterally.

Of interest is a similar area of abnormality in the posterior segment of the right upper lobe. **C,** 6-mm CT scan through the lower portion of the left lung reveals cylindric bronchiectasis in the left lower lobe associated with marked diminution in the size of the vessels. There is again a relatively normal-appearing segment of left lung laterally. The right lower lobe shows scattered subsegmental areas of hypoperfusion *(arrows).*

TABLE 8–1.

Causes of Unilateral Hyperlucent Lung in Childhood

I. Technical factors
    A. Uneven film development
    B. Poor centering
    C. Patient rotation
II. Chest wall abnormalities
    A. Scoliosis
    B. Absent pectoralis muscle, with or without Poland syndactyly, and postoperative
       Blalock-Taussig shunt with mammary hypoplasia
III. Pleural disease
    A. Pneumothorax
    B. Pneumomediastinum
    C. Contralateral pleural effusion
IV. Idiopathic "congenital lobar emphysema"
V. Air trapping secondary to bronchial obstruction
    A. Extrinsic lesions
       1. Vascular
          a. Pulmonary artery sling
          b. Tetralogy of Fallot with absent pulmonary valve
       2. Mediastinal masses (e.g., bronchogenic cysts)
       3. Peribronchial adenopathy
    B. Intrinsic lesions
       1. Foreign body
       2. Mucous plug
       3. Bronchial stenosis
       4. Congenital bronchial atresia
       5. Bronchial adenoma
VI. Pulmonary vascular abnormalities
    A. Absent pulmonary artery on left, usually associated with tetralogy of Fallot
    B. Scimitar syndrome with pulmonary hypoplasia
    C. Hypoplastic pulmonary artery
    D. Patent ductus arteriosus
VII. Parenchymal disease
    A. Swyer-James-Macleod syndrome
    B. Congenital lung cysts
    C. Hypoplasia of lung
       1. Primary congenital
       2. Secondary to diaphragmatic hernia
       3. Vascular occlusion
       4. Injury from physical or chemical agents

of the tracheobronchial tree. In adults, they account for 6% of all primary bronchial neoplasms but are uncommon in children. Nonetheless, over 50 cases have been reported. They are of two types: (1) carcinoid, and (2) salivary gland types—the cylindromas and mucoepidermoid tumors. The carcinoid type accounts for up to 90% of all bronchial adenomas reported. The intrabronchial lesions present with hemoptysis, cough, and wheezing. The carcinoid syndrome that occurs in adults is rare in children. Carcinoid tumors are found most commonly in the tracheobronchial tree, but one third present as peripheral nodules. Cylindromas (adenoid cystic carcinoma) constitute approximately 10% of all bronchial adenomas. These lesions are the most aggressive type of bronchial adenoma and may penetrate diffusely into the bronchial wall. Mucoepidermoid tumors are the rarest type, accounting for less than 2% of bronchial adenomas. They tend to occur in the main stem bronchus.

Radiographic Findings. When the adenoma is intrabronchial, depending on the size and location of the lesion, the chest film may be normal. Most patients, however, have radiographic findings of partial or complete bronchial obstruction. Segmental, lobar, or total lung collapse may be present, or unilateral air trapping may be seen. CT is of value in the diagnosis of both the intrabronchial and extrabronchial extent of the tumor, which is also demonstrable by MRI (Fig 8–27).

Focal Diminished Aeration

Atelectasis. Atelectasis, a decrease in lung volume or collapse of part or all of the lung, may be

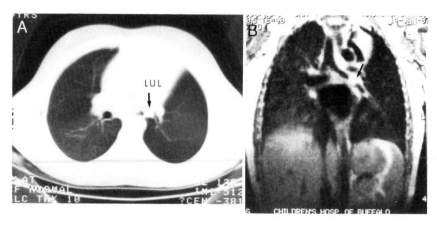

FIG 8–27.
Bronchial adenoma in a 10-year-old girl with left upper lobe atelectasis. **A,** CT scan revealed a soft-tissue density *(arrow)* in the left main stem bronchus. The left upper lobe *(LUL)* is atelectatic, and the left lower lobe is hyperinflated. **B,** T1-weighted MRI reveals an area of shortened T1 in the left main stem bronchus. At surgery, a bronchial adenoma was found.

classified as obstructive (resorptive), adhesive, compressive (passive), or cicatrizing.

In *obstructive* or *resorptive atelectasis,* the bronchial obstruction does not allow enough air to reach the distal airspaces to maintain their volume. As collapse ensues, a water-density shadow develops, usually without an air bronchogram. *Adhesive atelectasis* occurs in the presence of a patent airway and may be due to a surfactant deficiency. Hyaline membrane disease is the most common example, although this type of atelectasis commonly occurs in infection and postoperative states. Air bronchograms are common. *Compressive* or *passive atelectasis* occurs because of extrinsic pressure on the lung. The collapsed, airless segment casts a water-density shadow, but the bronchial tree is patent and an air bronchogram is usually seen. This type of atelectasis occurs with pneumothorax, large pleural effusion, or compression of the lung by a mass lesion. *Cicatrizing atelectasis* is volume loss resulting from local or generalized pulmonary fibrosis; bronchiectasis is often present.

The radiographic diagnosis of lobar atelectasis has been described in detail and is only summarized here. General signs of atelectasis relate to volume loss. The most direct and reliable sign is the displacement of an interlobar fissure. Other signs of volume loss, such as elevation of the hemidiaphragm and mediastinal shift, are maximal nearest the point of volume loss. Hilar shadows may be displaced toward the atelectatic lobe, and the ribs may be crowded. Compensatory overinflation of the remaining aerated segments in the affected lobe is present, and the collapsed portion of the lung is of increased opacity and often triangular in at least one projection.

Total unilateral pulmonary collapse, less common than collapse of a lobe or segment, may be due to a misplaced endotracheal tube or other bronchial obstruction of less obvious cause. A marked shift of the mediastinum occurs ipsilaterally and posteriorly (Fig 8–28). When atelectasis of the left lung occurs, the right lung may herniate anteriorly or posteriorly at the azygoesophageal recess.

Right Upper Lobe Atelectasis. Right upper lobe atelectasis (Figs 8–28 and 8–29) is usually relatively easy to diagnose, whether the collapsed segment is partially or totally airless, because the right minor fissure is elevated. The right hilum may be elevated, although there is usually little mediastinal shift. At the end stage of right upper lobe atelectasis, the lobe is pancaked against the lung apex or the mediasti-

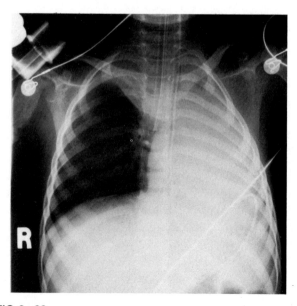

FIG 8–28.
Malpositioned endotracheal tube causing atelectasis of the right upper lobe and the entire left lung.

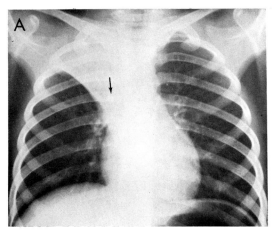

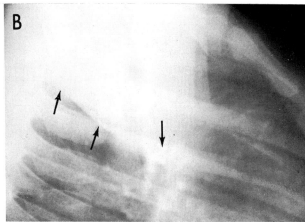

FIG 8–29.
Complete obstructive atelectasis of the right upper lobe due to a foreign body *(tooth; arrow)* in the right upper lobe bronchus of a 7-year-old girl. **A,** frontal, and **B,** lateral radiographs reveal that the right upper lobe is opaque and reduced in volume and its lower margin is concave *(arrows).* There is no shift of the heart and mediastinum and only minimal elevation of the hemidiaphragm because there has been compensatory expansion of the right lower lobe.

num, so it may be confused on the posteroanterior (PA) view with apical pleural thickening or mediastinal widening (Figs 8–30 and 8–31). When this severe degree of atelectasis is present, the middle and lower lobes may be overinflated and may be misconstrued as being the radiographic abnormality, while the true abnormality, collapse of the upper lobe, may go unrecognized. A compensatorily overin-

flated lung, however, should reduce in volume on ever, should reduce in volume on expiration, while hyperexpansion from air trapping remains unchanged on the expiratory view.

Left Upper Lobe Atelectasis. When the left upper lobe collapses, it moves anterosuperiorly rather than directly superiorly, as with right upper lobe collapse. Thus, a completely collapsed left upper

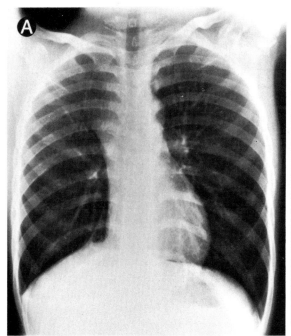

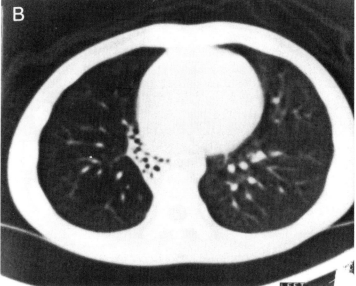

FIG 8–30.
Right upper lobe atelectasis simulating a mediastinal mass. **A,** frontal radiograph shows widening of the superior mediastinum on the right side with an indistinct superior border. **B,** unenhanced CT image reveals a tightly atelectatic right upper lobe which is pan-caked against the mediastinum. Cylindric bronchiectasis is present in the atelectatic lobe. Vascularity in the right lung is diminished. (Courtesy of Dr. John P. Dorst, Baltimore.)

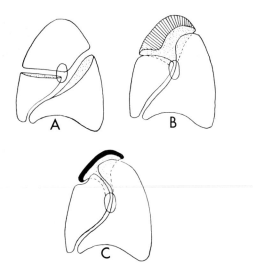

FIG 8–31.
Schematic representation of the progressive collapse of the right upper lobe as viewed in a lateral projection, mediastinal aspect. **A,** at the beginning of collapse. **B,** further collapse with upward displacement of the shrunken right upper lobe and compensatory expansion upward of the right middle and lower lobes. Crosshatching marks the segment of atelectatic lobe still in contact with the lateral thoracic wall; the *dotted area* represents extension of the atelectatic lobe from the chest wall to the hilum. **C,** further collapse. The segment against the chest wall (marked in *black*) is smaller, as is the hilar extension *(dotted area)*. The right middle and lower lobes are further expanded to fill in the space previously occupied by the strunken right upper lobe. Compare with the CT scan in Figure 8–30.

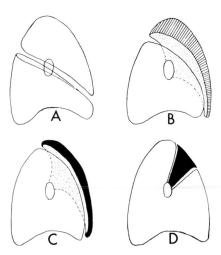

FIG 8–32.
Schematic representation of the progressive collapse of the left upper lobe as viewed in the lateral projection, mediastinal aspect. **A,** at beginning of collapse. **B,** further collapse. The interlobar septum is displaced forward as the upper lobe shrinks forward and flattens on the chest wall, and the lower lobe expands ventrad in compensation. *Crosshatching* marks the segment of shrunken lobe still in contact with the lateral and ventral chest walls; the extension of the shrunken lobe to the hilum is *dotted*. **C,** further collapse. The segment of collapsed lobe still in contact with the chest wall *(black)* is smaller than in **B,** and the left lower lobe is still expanding upward and forward. **D,** a nearly complete collapse shows only a black wedge with its base on the chest wall and its apex at the hilum; the lower lobe, distended by compensatory emphysema, occupies the rest of the left hemithorax.

lobe demonstrates its opacity on the PA view in the suprahilar position rather than paramediastinally, as with the completely collapsed right upper lobe (Fig 8–32). The lobe thins as it moves anteriorly. The typical appearance on the frontal radiograph is that of a hazy opacity distributed about the hilar area, fading superiorly, laterally, and inferiorly, and associated with a partially obscured cardiac margin. On the lateral view, there may be a sharply marginated interface anteriorly (Fig 8–33,A and B). A type of collapse, similar to the peripheral form of right upper lobe collapse described by Franken and Klatte, has been seen also in the left upper lobe. This occurs most often in children with cardiomegaly. The enlarged heart displaces the left upper lobe laterally so that the lung is compressed between the heart and the chest wall; the collapsed lobe may simulate pleural effusion.

Lower Lobe Collapse. Collapse of the lower lobes may be considered together since the radiographic pattern of atelectasis is similar regardless of the side involved. As collapse occurs, the lateral portion of the major fissure moves posteriorly toward the costophrenic angle. This abnormality is well delineated on the lateral view (Fig 8–34). On the fron-

tal view, the lateral margin of the lobe may be either well defined or ill defined, depending on whether or not the adjacent hyperexpanded lung has made the lower lobe fissures tangential to the x-ray beam. If the lateral margin is well defined, the lobe assumes a typical triangular shape, with the apex in the hilar area. A right lower lobe collapse obscures the silhouette of the right hemidiaphragm. A left lower lobe collapse can be more difficult to see if the radiograph is underpenetrated and the retrocardiac area is not clearly visible. Again, however, obliteration of the left hemidiaphragmatic silhouette should be noted. One should also note downward shift of the hilum and a decrease in hilar size.

Right Middle Lobe Collapse. As the middle lobe loses volume, the major and minor fissures move toward each other in superomedial and inferomedial directions, respectively. The middle lobe thus assumes an oblique orientation and does not appear sharply marginated on the PA view, although the right cardiac border may be ill defined. On the lateral view, however, the typical triangular opacity of right middle lobe collapse can be readily recognized. Distinction between complete and segmental volume loss in the right middle lobe may be

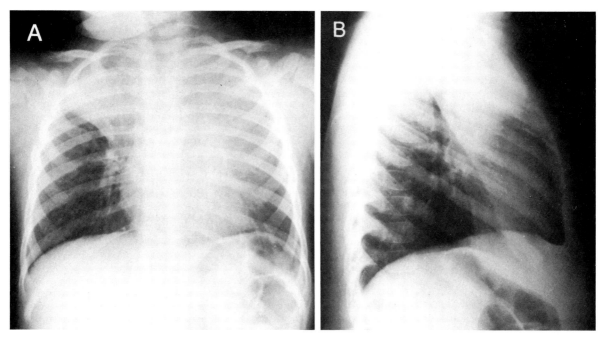

FIG 8–33.
Bilateral upper atelectasis in a 3-year-old child with asthma. **A,** Frontal radiograph reveals typical findings of right upper lobe atelectasis with consolidation and superior displacement of the right minor fissure. On the left side the more subtle changes of left upper lobe atelectasis are manifest by diffuse haziness and poor definition of the upper two thirds of the cardiac margin. **B,** lateral radiograph reveals anterior displacement of the major fissure and increased opacity of both upper lobes. The displaced major fissure appears to be the left fissure as it extends below the plain of the left hemidiaphragm. The patient was asthmatic and a follow-up radiograph 3 days later (not shown) was normal.

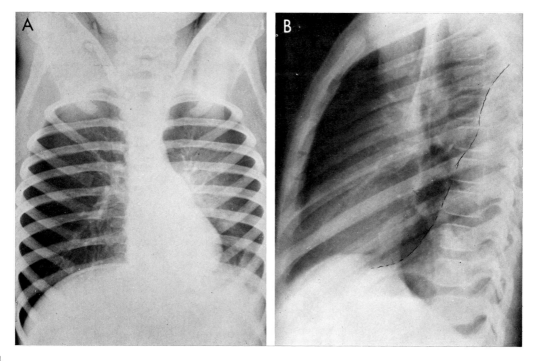

FIG 8–34.
Massive obstructive atelectasis of the left lower lobe, **A,** dorsoventral, and **B,** left lateral projections. The shrunken left lower lobe is opaque; the concavity of its anterior border is noteworthy. The heart is shifted toward the left. The decrease in volume of the atelectatic left lower lobe is largely compensated for by expansion of the left upper lobe, which appears to occupy approximately four fifths of the left hemithorax.

difficult. The right heart border may be obliterated by either. Typically, however, atelectasis of only the lateral segment does not obliterate the right heart border.

Right middle lobe collapse is relatively common in children and has been the source of considerable interest in the literature since first described by Brock and associates in 1937. They believed that the anatomical characteristics of the right middle lobe made it peculiarly susceptible to compression and stenosis by peribronchial lymphadenopathy. "Middle lobe syndrome" refers to a complex of recurrent atelectasis, pneumonia, and bronchiectasis. Culiner suggested that the importance of bronchial obstruction had been overemphasized in the etiology of this syndrome. In his view, impaired collateral ventilation caused difficulty in clearing secretions following pneumonia and this resulted in protracted atelectasis and recurrent infections (Fig 8–35). In most published series of "right middle lobe syndrome" in children, persistent middle lobe collapse has been found to be due to both mechanisms. Asthma is the most frequently associated condition. In our experience, using CT, the middle lobe bronchi nearly always are patent in cases of chronic right middle lobe collapse.

Radiographic Appearances Simulating Pulmonary Collapse. Pleural space diseases, particularly collections of fluid, may simulate areas of atelectasis just as atelectasis may simulate pleural effusions.

Consolidation due to inflammatory processes (pneumonia) and consolidation due to volume loss cannot always be distinguished; air bronchograms may be present in either condition.

Congenital pulmonary venolobar syndrome (scimitar syndrome) and other causes of pulmonary hypoplasia may mimic atelectasis, especially on the lateral view. The normally aerated lung sharply outlines a soft-tissue opacity that fills in the space normally occupied by the missing lobe or lobes. Anterior displacement of the major fissure is simulated on the lateral view. However, in hypogenetic lung syndrome, the anterior soft-tissue opacity extends inferiorly to the diaphragms, as opposed to right upper lobe atelectasis, which has a more wedge-shaped appearance and does not extend to the diaphragms. CT examination in hypogenetic lung syndrome suggests that the anterior soft-tissue density is due to mediastinal rotation and shift. Pulmonary agenesis radiologically resembles atelectasis of the entire lung, although associated anomalies or the history may aid in proper diagnosis.

Bronchiectasis

Bronchiectasis may be defined as localized (usually) irreversible dilation of the bronchial tree. *Irreversible* is included in the definition so as to exclude the localized but transient airway dilation associated with pneumonia and atelectasis. It may require a trial of therapy to distinguish these two conditions. Bron-

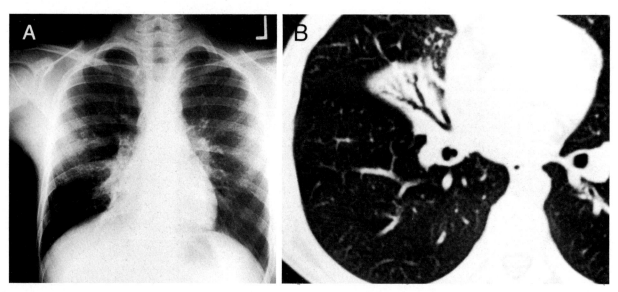

FIG 8–35.
Chronic right middle lobe atelectasis. **A,** frontal radiograph reveals increased opacity and the silhouette sign involving the right heart border indicating right middle lobe atelectasis. **B,** 6-mm CT scan reveals the lateral segment of the right middle lobe to be completely atelectatic, and patchy consolidation is noted in the medial segment. There is mild cylindric bronchiectasis associated. No evidence of bronchial obstruction is seen on the CT scan and at bronchoscopy the bronchus was patent as well. Recurrent atelectasis and pneumonia had been present since shortly after birth.

chiectasis is seen much less frequently since the advent of effective antibiotic therapy, and vaccines effective against measles and pertussis, but its precise current incidence is unknown because bronchography or surgery is required for definitive diagnosis. It has been referred to in a recent review (Barker and Bardona) as an "orphan disease." Persistent infection seems to be the most important etiologic factor causing destruction of the elastic tissue and musculature of the bronchial walls. A previous history of pneumonia, either bacterial, measles, pertussis, or adenoviral, is present in many cases. Bronchiectasis also occurs in chronically obstructed bronchi, but associated infection is usually also present.

Reid, in 1950, classified the disease into three groups using the criteria of severity of bronchial dilation and the degree of bronchial and bronchiolar obliteration.

Group 1: Cylindrical bronchiectasis is the least severe form. The bronchi retain their regular outline but are mildly dilated and fail to taper distally, instead terminating abruptly with squared-off ends. The most distal bronchi and bronchioles are plugged with secretions, but pathologically the number of bronchial subdivisions is normal.

Group 2: Varicose bronchiectasis is marked by a greater degree of dilation and accompanied by local ballooning of the airway. The bronchi have an irregular, beaded outline, and have a typical bulbous termination. The number of patent airway divisions is

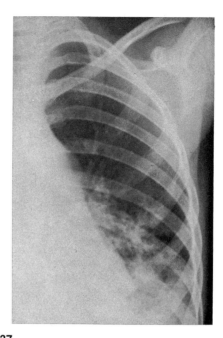

FIG 8–37.
The honeycomb lung of bronchiectasis. The irregular density in the base of the left lung was suggestive of the diagnosis; saccular bronchial dilatations were demonstrated in bronchograms a few days later. The honeycomb pattern is found only in advanced cases.

reduced from the normal of up to 20 to about 6 or 7 (Fig 8–36).

Group 3: Cystic or saccular bronchiectasis is the most severe form. Bronchial dilatation increases progressively toward the lung periphery. The bronchi have balloonlike dilation and only four to five branching generations can be counted and the distal branches are occluded (bronchiolitis obliterans).

Radiographic Findings. The chest film, although nonspecific, is usually abnormal in bronchiectasis (Fig 8–37). Gudjberg found normal chest radiographs in only 7.1% of proven cases (Fig 8–38,A and B). Radiographic findings vary with the severity of the disease and range from normal to a severe honeycomb lung appearance with obvious cysts and air-fluid levels in cases of advanced cystic bronchiectasis. Bronchial wall thickening, manifest as ring and tramline shadows, can be seen and should mucoid impaction supervene, the dilated airways may appear as rounded or oval nodular opacities when seen end-on, or as a combination of V- or Y-shaped branching bandlike shadows.

Vandevivre and associates have suggested that technetium 99m perfusion lung scanning may aid in detection. A normal chest film and a normal perfusion scan essentially rule out bronchiectasis. Ventilation scanning with krypton 81m also appears to be an accurate method to exclude this disease.

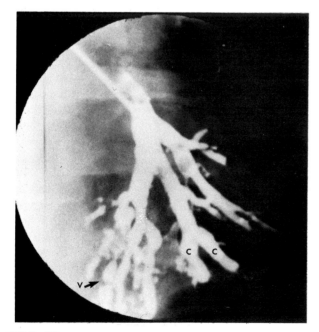

FIG 8–36.
Cylindric *(c)* and varicose *(v)* bronchiectasis demonstrated on a single spot radiograph from a bronchogram.

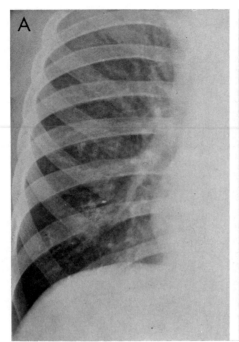
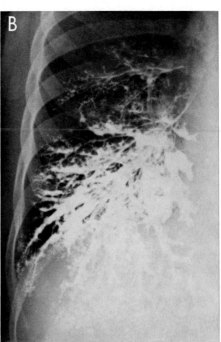

FIG 8–38.
Unusual finding of a normal plain radiograph and documented bronchiectasis. **A,** plain radiograph shows no abnormality in the right lower lobe. **B,** bronchogram 24 hours later reveals varicose bronchiectasis.

CT has become widely used for the diagnosis of bronchiectasis. There is still some controversy as to the optimal technique (Fig 8–39,A–D), but most authors favor the use of thin or medium (1.5–5.0 mm.) slices and image reconstruction using an edge-enhancing (bone) algorithm. Gantry angulation shows the middle lobe and lingular branches more consistently. Sensitivity and specificity ranges between 90% and 95% in most adult series. Kuhn (in Naidich, Zerhouni, et al.) demonstrated sensitivity and specificity exceeding 90% in a series studying pediatric bronchiectasis. When seen parallel to the plane of section, cylindric bronchiectasis is characterized by dilated, thick-walled bronchi visible farther toward the lung periphery than usual. On axial section the dilated bronchus is accompanied by a pulmonary arterial branch producing a signet-ring appearance. The CT appearance of varicose bronchiectasis is similar except that the bronchial walls appear somewhat beaded when the bronchi lie parallel to the plane of the cut. Cystic bronchiectasis is characterized by marked bronchial dilation with strings or clusters of cysts, some of which may contain fluid.

If plain films, CT, and radionuclide scans are normal, positive contrast bronchography is rarely indicated since it is unlikely that significant disease is present. If surgery is contemplated when other examinations have positive findings, bronchography may be helpful to determine the extent of disease.

Either oily diosonil or nonionic water-soluble contrast agents are now used for positive contrast bronchography. On the positive contrast bronchogram, bronchiectasis may be cylindric, varicose, or saccular, as described by Reid's pathologic classification. Differentiation between cylindric bronchiectasis and reversible bronchial dilation seen following pneumonia or atelectasis is difficult (Fig 8–40). The bronchi show tubular dilatation with a smooth outline. Pathologic changes may be noted as long as 3 to 4 months following an initial insult. The appearance of varicose bronchiectasis (dilation and distortion by constriction) and saccular bronchiectasis (dilation with ballooned termination) corresponds to the aforementioned pathologic descriptions.

Diseases Associated With Bronchiectasis. *Williams-Campbell Syndrome.* In 1960, Williams and Campbell described five patients with the onset of bronchiectasis in infancy. Autopsy showed near-total absence of cartilage in the segmental and subsegmental bronchi. Additional cases have since been described, including a series of 11 by Williams et al. The disease has also been reported in siblings. In patients who have superimposed infection, it may be impossible to state with certainty that the disease was congenital and not acquired (Fig 8–41).

Primary Ciliary Dyskinesia (Immotile Cilia Syndrome). Situs inversus, sinusitis, and bronchiecta-

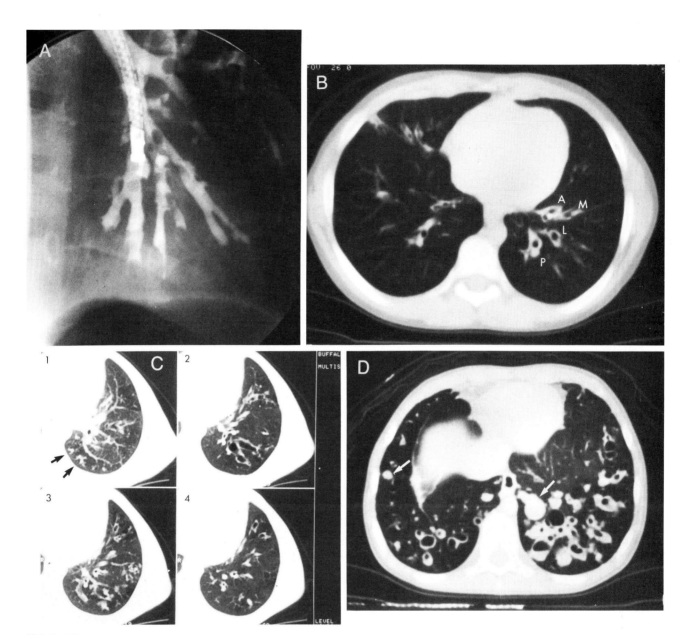

FIG 8–39.
Correlation of bronchography and CT in the diagnosis of bronchiectasis. **A,** fiberoptically guided bronchogram in a 10-year-old boy with asthma. Mild cylindric bronchiectasis is noted in the posterior and lateral basilar segments. **B,** 6-mm CT image in the same patient reveals a signet-ring sign in the posterior basilar segment *(P)* with mild peribronchial thickening and slight dilation of the segmental bronchus so that it is larger than its accompanying artery—findings of cylindric bronchiectasis. Mild cylindric bronchiectasis is also noted in the lateral segmental bronchus *(L);* the anterior *(A)* and medial *(M)* segmental bronchi show peribronchial thickening and minimal dilatation. Also noted on the CT scan and not observed on the localized bronchogram is cylindric bronchiectasis in the posterior basilar segment of the right lower lobe as well as in

the inferior portion of the right middle lobe. **C,** cylindric and varicose bronchiectasis in a teenage boy with lung disease of unknown cause. Level *1* reveals peripheral mucoid impaction *(arrows)*. Level *2* reveals both cylindric bronchiectasis with a signet-ring sign as well as varicose bronchiectasis where segmental basilar branches in the left lower lobe are imaged along their long axis. Level *3* reveals further areas of peripheral mucoid impaction and cylindric bronchiectasis. Level *4* reveals cylindric bronchiectasis peripherally in the anterior segment of the left lower lobe. **D,** cystic bronchiectasis in a teenage patient with cystic fibrosis. Multiple 1.5- to 2-cm areas of cystic bronchiectasis are noted in both lungs. Most contain air-fluid levels, although some dilated bronchi *(arrows)* are completely fluid-filled.

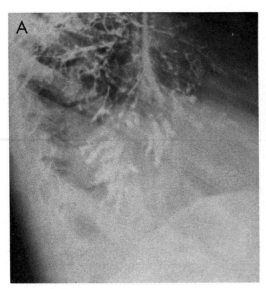

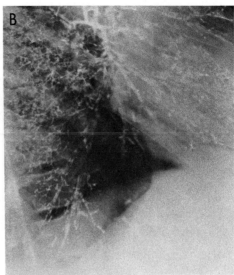

FIG 8–40.
Transient cylindric bronchiectasis due to chronic atelectasis in a girl 10 years of age. A previous film (not shown) disclosed massive atelectasis of the right lower lobe. **A,** bronchogram 2 weeks later shows extensive cylindric bronchiectasis in the right lower lobe associated with atelectasis of this lobe. Six months later this patient was asymptomatic. **B,** bronchogram performed 2 years after **A** shows the right lower lobe bronchi to be normal.

sis (Kartagener syndrome) occur in 1 in 40,000 whites. These patients have a deficiency in the dynein arms of the cilia in the epithelial cells lining the respiratory tract. The affected cilia are immotile or dysmotile, resulting in impaired ability to clear secretions and, presumably, causing increased susceptibility to infection, bronchiectasis, and sinusitis.

The primary ciliary dyskinesia syndrome is associated with chronic recurrent respiratory infection in patients with or without situs inversus (Fig 8–42).

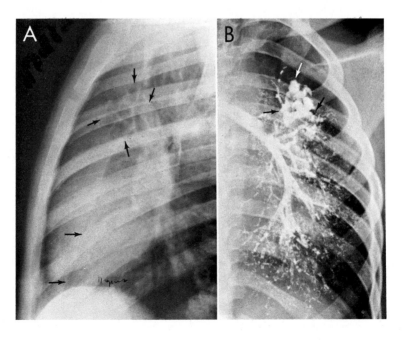

FIG 8–41.
Congenital segmental bronchiectasis and hypoplasia of the left upper lobe in a boy 11 years of age. **A,** in plain films, and best seen in lateral projection, there were several cavities ventrad and cephalad to the left hilum *(arrows).* **B,** bronchograms showed limited saccular dilatation of all the branches of the left upper lobe. In the excised specimen, the left upper lobe was markedly hypoplastic, being about the size of a thumb, with no evidence of inflammation but marked dilation of the hypoplastic bronchi.

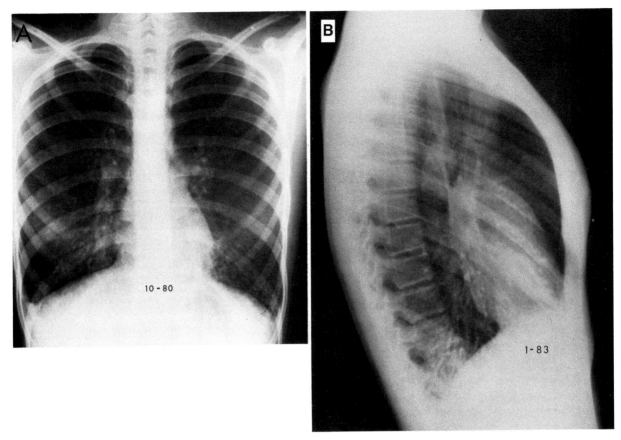

FIG 8–42.
Immotile cilia syndrome with bronchiectasis in one of two affected sisters. **A,** chest radiograph at 13 years of age shows linear basilar opacities consistent with bronchiectasis. **B,** lateral chest radio-graph shows "tram tracking" in the posterior aspect of both lower lobes. A lung scan, not shown, showed poor perfusion in both lower lobes, findings consistent with bronchiectasis.

Ciliary activity is required for normal rotation of the fetal gut. In its absence there is an equal likelihood of situs inversus and situs solitus. Kartagener syndrome is but one point on the spectrum of diseases with ciliary dyskinesia. In addition to sinorespiratory ailments, defective ciliary motility also contributes to deafness and infertility. Abnormalities of mucociliary clearance can be acquired, particularly in cases of chronic recurrent infection, perhaps accounting for the impaired mucociliary clearance seen in cystic fibrosis as well as in asthma.

Chronic Recurrent Infection. Bronchiectasis occurs in children with immunodeficiency syndromes such as hypogammaglobulinemia, agammaglobulinemia, and Wiskott-Aldrich syndrome, presumably because of their susceptibility to chronic, recurrent infections. Other pulmonary infections, particularly measles, pertussis, and tuberculosis, can damage bronchi and make them susceptible to secondary infection and bronchiectasis (Fig 8–43). There is also evidence that adenoviral infections may produce not only bronchiectasis but also obliterative bronchioli-tis. Eskimo and Polynesian children may be particularly susceptible.

Cystic Fibrosis of the Pancreas (Mucoviscidosis)
Cystic fibrosis is the commonest lethal, genetically transmitted syndrome affecting white children. Its transmission is autosomal recessive. The gene responsible for cystic fibrosis has been identified on the long arm of chromosome 7. Multiple different mutations of the gene exist, probably explaining the marked variability of the disease. The estimated incidence is 1 in 1,600 white live births but only 1 in 17,000 black live births. It is even less common in Oriental children.

About 10% of cases are discovered in infancy when they present as meconium ileus syndrome. Most of the rest present in early childhood with symptoms that may include failure to thrive, malabsorption syndrome, chronic recurrent respiratory infections, a salty taste to the skin, wheezing, nasal polyposis, or rectal prolapse. Nearly all patients develop pulmonary symptoms that ultimately prove

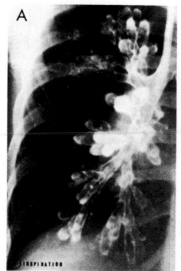

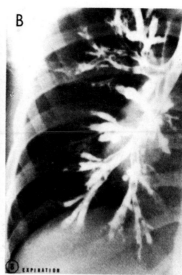

FIG 8–43.
Obliterative bronchiectasis following measles and pneumonia in a boy 5 years of age. **A,** chest radiograph made during inspiration shows dilatation of the bronchi. Note the lack of peripheral filling. **B,** chest radiograph made during expiration reveals that some of the peripheral bronchi have narrowed in caliber; others remain dilated. (From Capitanio M: *Pediatrics* 1975; 87:230. Used by permission.)

fatal, although survival into the late teens and early adulthood is increasingly common with most patients surviving beyond 18 years of age and some large cystic fibrosis centers projecting median survival to age 30.

The cause remains unknown, although the key dysfunction occurs in those organs which have exocrine-secreting glands. The mucus-containing liquids of the airways are secreted in excessive amounts and are poorly cleared, obstructing the lumen of the organs into which they are secreted. The respiratory tract, the gastrointestinal system, and the reproductive systems are the most severely involved. There may be extensive gastrointestinal involvement, including meconium ileus, pancreatic insufficiency, malabsorption, gallbladder disease, portal hypertension, splenomegaly, biliary cirrhosis, and esophageal varices. These abnormalities are discussed in detail in Part IV.

Involvement of the pulmonary system is the major cause of morbidity and mortality in affected children. Pulmonary abnormalities are invariable, except in infants dying of meconium ileus. There are histologic changes of hyperplasia and obstruction of the submucosal glands of the trachea and major bronchi. Lung disease begins in the bronchioles. The pathophysiology is still incompletely understood but has been recently reviewed by Zach. The basic defect in the respiratory mucosa seems to be decreased chloride ion permeability. This defect, coupled with some unknown combination of factors, perhaps including a viral infection, leads to increased bacterial adherence. The first bacterial infection is often with *Staphylococcus aureus* which may further damage the respiratory epithelium which then becomes chronically colonized with *Pseudomonas aeruginosa*, often the mucoid strain. As the infection persists, mucociliary clearance is damaged, secretions increase, and more obstruction and infection result. There is evidence that interaction between the *Pseudomonas* and activated B lymphocytes may result in immune complexes being formed, which, via complement activation, ultimately lead to the release of lysosomal enzymes and oxygen radicals from the neutrophils that have been mobilized to the area, thus causing further tissue damage, perhaps ultimately leading to destruction of the connective tissue walls of the bronchi. Dilatation of the bronchial airways occurs at the expense of the lung parenchyma. In the dissections of Esterle and Oppenheimer, bronchitis and bronchiolitis were found in nearly every infant over 1 month of age, and bronchiectasis had developed in all patients 6 months or older. Focal areas of overinflation occur distal to segmentally obstructed bronchi. True emphysema (alveolar destruction), however, is uncommon, although the lungs are severely hyperaerated as a result of small-airway obstruction. Multiple bronchiectatic cavities and lung abscesses of varying sizes are common complications of the pneumonia as the disease progresses. Despite severe extensive involvement of the lungs, pleural effusion is unusual. The extensive pulmonary abnormalities increase pulmonary vascular resistance, eventually resulting in cor pulmonale. Right heart

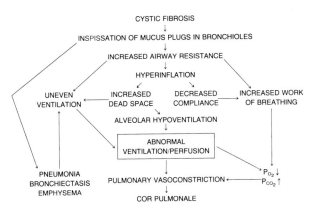

```
                    CYSTIC FIBROSIS
                          ↓
    INSPISSATION OF MUCUS PLUGS IN BRONCHIOLES
                          ↓
              INCREASED AIRWAY RESISTANCE
                          ↓
                    HYPERINFLATION
    UNEVEN      INCREASED    DECREASED    INCREASED WORK
  VENTILATION   DEAD SPACE   COMPLIANCE   OF BREATHING
                ALVEOLAR HYPOVENTILATION
                  ┌─────────────────┐
                  │    ABNORMAL     │
                  │ VENTILATION/PERFUSION │
                  └─────────────────┘
                                          PO₂ ↓
PNEUMONIA                                 PCO₂ ↑
BRONCHIECTASIS  PULMONARY VASOCONSTRICTION ←
EMPHYSEMA
                    COR PULMONALE
```

FIG 8–44.
Pulmonary manifestations of cystic fibrosis. Correlation of radiologic changes with pulmonary function. P_{O_2}, partial pressure of oxygen; P_{CO_2}, partial pressure of carbon dioxide. (From Reilly BJ, Featherby EA, Weng T, et al: *Radiology* 1971; 98:281. Used by permission.)

failure is a common cause of death. The proposed pathophysiology of the pulmonary manifestations of cystic fibrosis has been summarized by Reilly et al. (Fig 8–44).

The diagnosis of cystic fibrosis may be suggested by the family history or radiographic findings. Confirmation requires a positive sweat test. The test should be done in a center with personnel experienced in the technique because false-positive results are common otherwise. The only method accepted by the Cystic Fibrosis Foundation is the pilocarpine iontophoresis sweat collection test with chemical analysis of the chloride concentration which, in abnormal cases, will be greater than 60 mEq/L.

The radiographic findings vary with the age of the patient and the severity of the disease. They reflect extensive airway (rather than airspace) involvement. In infancy, the chest film may be normal, and, uncommonly, even in older children with mild pulmonary involvement, a normal chest film may be seen.

The first radiographic manifestation of the disease in the lungs is usually hyperinflation, which results from the obstruction of the small airways (terminal and respiratory bronchioles). The chest radiograph at this stage usually appears otherwise normal, although right upper or middle lobe atelectasis is likely to occur, even in infancy (Fig 8–45). A thickened right upper lobe bronchus, best detected on the lateral film, can be an early finding of peribronchial involvement, and is much more common in cystic fibrosis than in other airway diseases. Signs of growth failure, such as humeral metaphyseal bands and other signs of poor nutrition, may also be noted. Rarely, a fatty liver may be suspected on plain films. Bulky stool, visible in the colon, is another finding that suggests the diagnosis. Paranasal sinuses are nearly always opacified.

The radiologic differential diagnosis in the early stages of disease includes bronchiolitis, bronchial asthma, viral bronchopneumonia, and other causes of recurrent pneumonia in childhood. Airway involvement is the hallmark of this disease and it is increasing involvement of the airways that provides radiologic insight into the progression of the disease. Bronchial wall thickening becomes more widespread, producing an overall increase in ring and tramlines. This is the result of peribronchial inflammation which is also manifested by the presence of small nodular opacities measuring from 1 to 3 cm, best seen in the lung periphery. These findings wax and wane to some extent with the onset and resultant therapy of superimposed acute infections (Fig 8–46). Lobar pneumonia is surprisingly uncommon.

Bronchiectasis accompanies the chronic inflam-

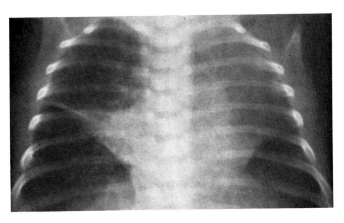

FIG 8–45.
Pulmonary changes of cystic fibrosis in an infant 6 weeks of age who had been dyspneic since the first week of life. The lungs are markedly hyperinflated. There is right middle lobe atelectasis and partial left upper lobe atelectasis. Incidental note is made of a healing rib fracture on the left.

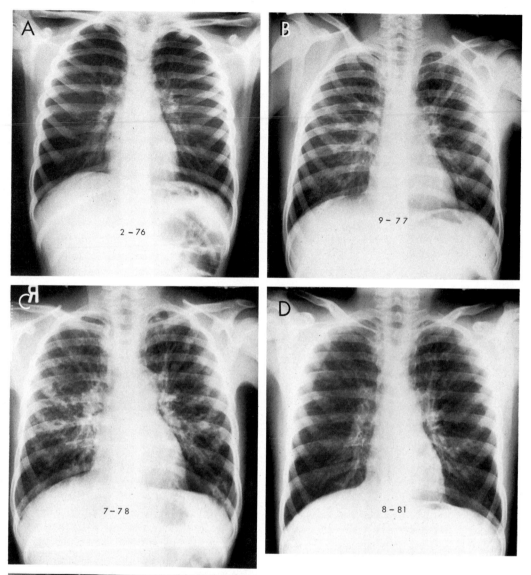

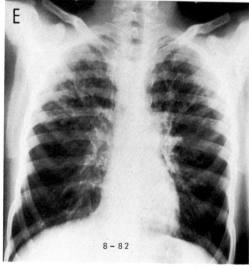

FIG 8–46.

A, serial radiographs in a 9-year-old boy show the changing appearance of cystic fibrosis over 6 years. At age 9 years the frontal radiograph shows minimal peribronchial thickening and hyperaerated lungs indistinguishable from asthma. **B,** 19 months later, the radiographic picture has worsened considerably. Extensive peribronchial thickening is now noted. Mucoid impaction of the bronchus is seen in the left upper lobe, and hilar shadows have become abnormally prominent. **C,** 10 months later, further deterioration is obvious. Widespread typical changes of cystic fibrosis are noted throughout both lungs. The patient was acutely ill at this time; follow-up studies **(D)** showed considerable improvement, which suggested that some of the changes evident on **C** were due to superimposed infection. **E,** 1 year after **D.** Note the progressive changes of cystic fibrosis—most severe in the upper lobes bilaterally.

mation and can be recognized, as the bronchus, whether seen end-on or en face, becomes larger than its accompanying pulmonary artery. These changes are better appreciated on CT but can, with experience or when severe, be recognized on plain film examinations. Bronchiectasis tends to be more severe in the upper lobes, especially the right (Fig 8–47). The reason for this is not known with certainty but it has been theorized that the decreased ventilatory excursions in the upper lobes may contribute to the already impaired drainage of secretions.

Mucoid impaction of the bronchi is almost invariable in advanced cases, and may be seen on plain films as branching tubular opacities; however, surprisingly large impactions may be revealed only by CT (Fig 8–48). Allergic bronchopulmonary aspergillosis (ABPA) develops in up to 10% of patients, and is manifest by central bronchiectasis and gloved-finger opacities.

In spite of the amount and degree of chronic bronchial obstructions, pneumatoceles are rare. Large cystic spaces probably representing severe cystic bronchiectasis are seen in older children and adults. Pneumothorax occurs occasionally, particularly in the older child, and may be quite refractory to therapy. Tomashefski has demonstrated that while interstitial air, subpleural blebs, and cystic bronchiectasis are present on pathologic examination, only areas of cystic bronchiectasis are large enough to be recognized, usually in the upper lobes, on x-ray films of the chest. Tracheomegaly and abnormal tracheal flaccidity are common in older patients.

The hilar shadows are usually enlarged and often show progressive enlargement (Fig 8–49), but without CT or MRI it is difficult to distinguish between lymphadenopathy, pulmonary arterial dilatation and perihilar pneumonia as the cause. All may be present, with lymphadenopathy most common. Cor pulmonale, with right ventricular hypertrophy secondary to lung disease, develops terminally in many cases and, when recognized, heralds a grave prognosis. It is diagnosed radiologically when right ventricular dilatation and the vascular changes of pulmonary hypertension are recognized. Hemoptysis, often massive and life-threatening, is seen with increasing length of survival. The site of bleeding may be localized by fiberoptic bronchoscopy, by bronchial arteriography, or with radionuclide techniques. It may be controlled with bronchial artery embolization.

Several authors have proposed grading systems to judge the severity of the radiologic findings. The Brasfield system, for example, assigns scores from 0 (absent) to 5 (most severe) for findings of air trap-

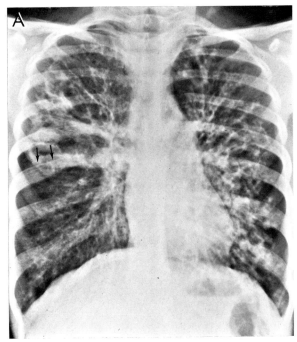
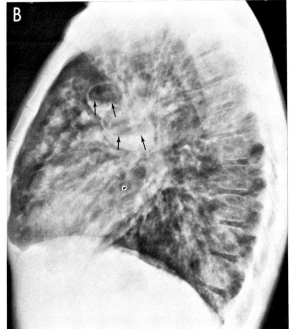

FIG 8–47.
Advanced cystic fibrosis with cystic bronchiectasis. Two large cavities with gas-fluid levels are seen in the right upper lobe of a girl 11 years of age who had severe cystic fibrosis. **A,** frontal, and **B,** lateral projections. These large cavities probably represent cystic bronchiectasis although pneumatoceles or lung abscess filled with gas and fluid have a similar appearance.

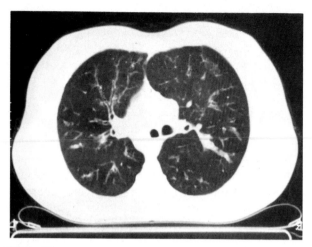

FIG 8–48.
Cylindric bronchiectasis and mucoid impaction of the bronchus are demonstrated in this 15-year-old patient with cystic fibrosis. Anterior segmental bronchi in the left upper lobe are affected with cylindric bronchiectasis, and the superior segmental bronchus of the right lower lobe is seen to be filled with mucus and dilated. The mucoid bronchial impaction was not detected on plain radiographic examination.

ping, linear markings (bronchial shadows), nodular cystic lesions, large lesions, and general severity. CT grading systems, based primarily on the severity of bronchiectasis, have also been proposed (Fig 8–50).

Differential Diagnosis in the Older Child. In the vast majority of cases the diagnosis is well established, and the radiograph is used to evaluate the progression of disease. The typical patterns just de-

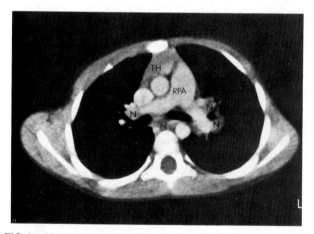

FIG 8–49.
Hilar and subcarinal adenopathy in a 5-year-old patient with cystic fibrosis. Plain film revealed prominent hilar shadows bilaterally. Contrast-enhanced CT (CECT) scan reveals the right pulmonary artery (RPA) to be of normal caliber. Low-density nodes (N) surround the main stem bronchus and are seen in the subcarinal area and posterior to the right pulmonary artery. In our experience, hilar and some carinal adenopathy has been a nearly universal finding on CECT examinations in children with cystic fibrosis.

scribed are virtually pathognomonic; other entities to be considered in atypical or early cases include other causes of severe chronic airway infection such as severe asthma, primary cilia dyskinesia, and immunodeficiency syndromes.

The radiologist should be familiar with the complications of cystic fibrosis of the pancreas, many of which are diagnostically important. In almost all males, sterility develops due to aspermia and structural defects in the epididymis, seminal vesicles, and vas deferens. The adult female with cystic fibrosis may be infertile. Patients with cystic fibrosis of the pancreas are highly sensitive to heat unless treated effectively with salt and water replacement. In the respiratory tract, atelectasis, bronchiectasis, pulmonary abscesses, recurrent pneumothorax, and hemoptysis are all common. Empyema is relatively rare. The paranasal sinuses are opaque radiographically in almost all patients older than 2 years but without clinical signs of sinusitis. The opacification is probably due to hypertrophied mucosa rather than to inflammation. Nasal polyps may cause severe deformities of the face in older patients. Hearing impairment has been found in more than 50% of patients.

In the alimentary tract, complications include fecal impaction, small bowel obstruction (meconium ileus equivalent), rectal prolapse, intussusception, pneumatosis intestinalis, duodenal ulcers, biliary cirrhosis with portal hypertension with resultant hypersplenism, cholelithiasis, and pancytopenia.

In a single patient, Wood found pneumatosis coli and prolapse of the rectum associated with cystic fibrosis of the pancreas. The proximal half of the colonic mucosa was "stretched over a solid mass of air-filled blebs." These blebs became less numerous in the distal portion of the colon but were also present in the rectum and at the anorectal junction.

Of 22 patients, Sauvegrain and Feigelson found microgallbladder in 7; only 1 patient had hepatic disease. All of 29 sialograms obtained by Leake and others were normal in children suffering from cystic fibrosis.

Older children may develop glycosuria and hyperglycemia which appears not to be true diabetes mellitus but rather due to structural disorganization and fibrosis of the islands of Langerhans. These patients also do not suffer from the usual complications of diabetes mellitus, nor are their family histories characteristic of diabetes mellitus. Small to moderate amounts of insulin readily control the hyperglycemia.

Both vascular and perivascular calcifications were present in two patients with cystic fibrosis

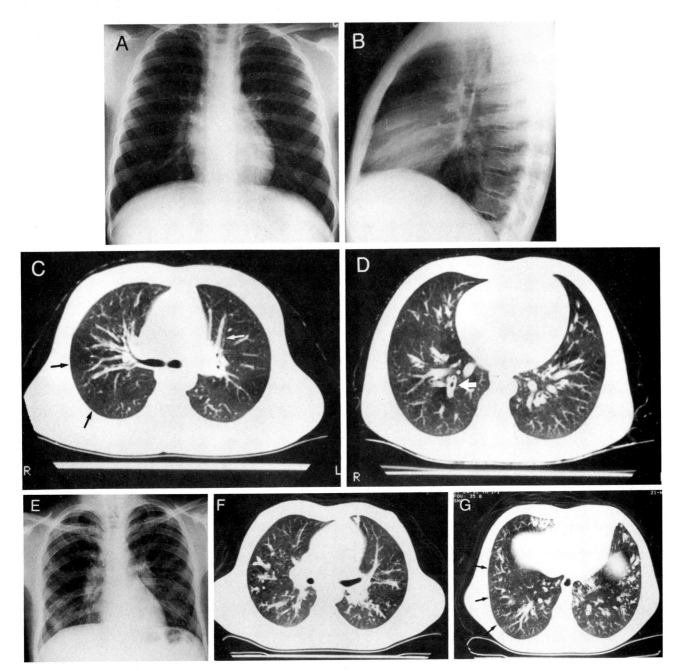

FIG 8–50.

Radiographic and CT findings in cystic fibrosis. **A,** frontal, and **B,** lateral chest radiographs in an 11-year-old boy. The radiographs prospectively were interpreted as being normal, although there is mild peribronchial thickening in the anterior segmental bronchus of the left upper lobe and on the lateral radiograph **(B)** the lungs appear hyperinflated. **C,** 6-mm CT scan at the level of the origin of the anterior and posterior segmental bronchi of the right upper lobe reveals marked peribronchial thickening on the right, especially centrally, which results in delineation of the bronchial wall into the outer third of the right upper lobe. Although the bronchus is not dilated, focal subsegmental areas of hyperinflation are present in the right upper lobe laterally. On the left side, central peribronchial thickening is noted as well as bronchial wall thickening along the anterior segmental bronchus *(arrows).* **D,** 6-mm CT scan through the lung base in the same patient reveals marked disturbance of perfusion in the right lower lobe. Marked peribronchial thickening is noted in the basilar segments of the right lower lobe, especially the medial basilar segment *(arrow).* Marked peribronchial thickening is also present in the segmental bronchi of the

left lower lobe. There are also a few small areas of mucoid impaction noted in the anterior segment of the left lower lobe. **E,** moderately severe cystic fibrosis in a 14-year-old boy. Radiograph shows bilateral hilar adenopathy and ill-defined patchy linear opacities peripherally, somewhat worse on the right than on the left side. Some tramlines and ring shadows are visible centrally. **F,** 6-mm CT scan through the level of the bronchus intermedius reveals multiple areas of mucoid impaction peripherally in the right upper lobe laterally and posteriorly with relative sparing of the anterior segment. A few areas of mucoid impaction are present in the left upper lobe. The segmental bronchi of the left upper lobe show bronchial wall thickening and are visible abnormally far into the periphery of the lung parenchyma. An area of relative hypoperfusion is noted just posterior to this thickened bronchus. **G,** 6-mm CT scan through the lung base reveals the lungs to be of large volume. Multiple areas of mucoid impaction and dilated bronchi are noted, especially anteriorly in both lower lobes. Many of the secondary pulmonary lobules *(arrows)* are underperfused owing to focal air trapping.

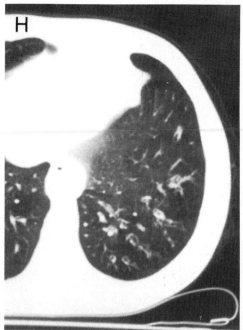

FIG 8–50 (cont.).
H, cylindric bronchiectasis without mucoid impaction is noted in the periphery of the left lower lobe in another patient with cystic fibrosis. Compare the appearance in this patient with the mucoid impaction seen in **F** and **G. I,** chest radiograph in a young adult with advanced cystic fibrosis and loss of lung volume in the left up per lobe with some cystic airspaces visible on the plain radiograph. **J,** 6-mm CT scan image through the upper lobes in this patient reveals complete destruction of the left upper lobe with marked cystic bronchiectasis. Cylindric bronchiectasis involving the superior segment of the left lower lobe is visible posteriorly. Extensive cylindric bronchiectasis peribronchial thickening, and areas of cystic bronchiectasis also are obvious in the right upper lobe.

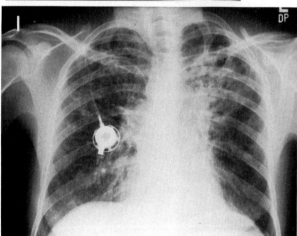

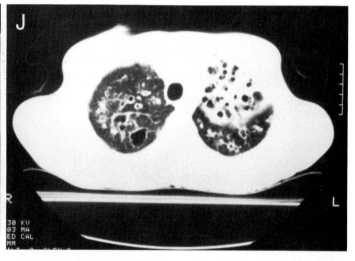

studied by Kuhn and associates at necropsy. One was a girl 14 years of age and one an infant 5 months of age.

Myocardial fibrosis with coarse scarring of the left ventricle and atrium and fibroelastic thickening of the endocardium has been observed in a few cases. The cause of the myocardial fibrosis is not known; a secondary nutritional deficiency is a possible cause.

DISORDERS OF THE PERIPHERAL AIRWAYS AND DISEASES ASSOCIATED WITH DIFFUSE HYPERINFLATION

Although the smaller airways, the bronchioles, are invisible radiologically, diseases which affect them produce disturbances in pulmonary aeration, usually resulting in diffuse air trapping because of ventilatory obstruction. When complications of inflammation and atelectasis ensue, pulmonary parenchymal opacities may develop.

Diseases Causing Generalized Hyperinflation (Air Trapping)

Generalized air trapping is commonly seen in bronchiolitis, asthma, cystic fibrosis, and viral lower respiratory infection—diseases that affect the smaller airways. Patients with large left-to-right shunts often exhibit marked pulmonary hyperaeration. This may be due to decreased pulmonary compliance or increased pulmonary arterial pressure. Other mechanisms such as increased pulmonary airway resistance due to peribronchial edema may also play a role. Pulmonary hyperinflation can also occur in diabetic acidosis, aspirin intoxication, and other causes of metabolic acidosis. Radiographic diagnosis of hyperinflated lungs is subjective, but the findings of increased lung volume are readily recognized in more severe cases (Fig 8–51). One looks for flattening of the diaphragmatic domes, especially on the lateral view, and increased anteroposterior (AP) diameter of the chest; increased retrosternal and posterior cardiac air spaces; abnormally radiolucent lungs; horizontal ribs; elongated, vertical heart; and outward bowing of the upper part of the sternum. However, experience is probably the best teacher when estimating the presence and degree of air trapping.

Bronchiolitis

The subject of viral pneumonia is considered in Chapter 9; bronchiolitis could be considered there as well, since the dividing line between bronchiolitis, bronchitis, and viral bronchopneumonia is, in many cases, indistinct. However, since the radiographic hallmark of bronchiolitis is pulmonary hyperaeration, it is appropriate to discuss bronchiolitis here.

Bronchiolitis is a common lower respiratory tract infection which usually occurs in infants under the age of 1 year. It is nearly always of viral origin, with respiratory syncytial virus and, less commonly, parainfluenza virus the leading pathogens. The viral antigen can now be rapidly identified using immunofluorescent techniques on nasal secretions. There is a strong seasonal incidence; most cases occur in winter and spring. Epidemic occurrence is common. Clinically, bronchiolitis begins as coryza with a progressive cough and the development of wheezing, tachypnea, tachycardia, and retractions. In some cases, wheezing is the only symptom, but respiratory distress can be severe and, in rare instances, death can result.

Typically, the chest film shows generalized hyperinflation (Fig 8–52). Mild degrees of peribronchial inflammatory edema may be seen as bronchial "cuffing." If infiltrates or areas of atelectasis are present, differentiation from viral bronchopneumonia becomes difficult. Most infants with bronchiolitis improve within 3 to 4 days and recover within 2 weeks, but there are some for whom the first bout of wheezing is the harbinger of recurrent symptoms. In these children, where "bronchiolitis" ends and "asthma" begins is unclear. Whether these children have "reactive airways" that predispose them first to bronchiolitis and then to asthma, or whether the initial bout of bronchiolitis may cause permanent dam-

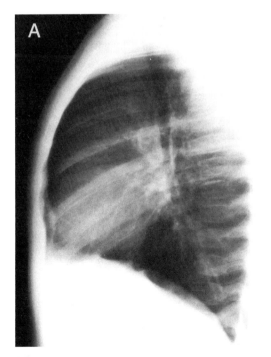

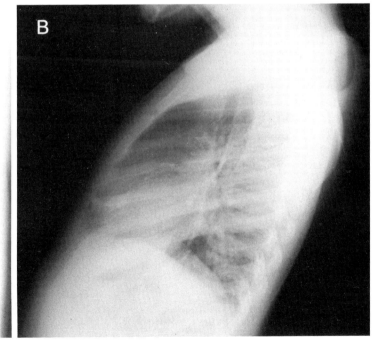

FIG 8–51.
Hyperinflation of the lungs during an acute asthmatic attack. **A,** lateral radiograph of a 2-year-old child with asthma shows severe pulmonary hyperaeration with flattening of the hemidiaphragms and an increase in the retrosternal and retrocardial air spaces. **B,** 5 days later, the lungs are normally aerated.

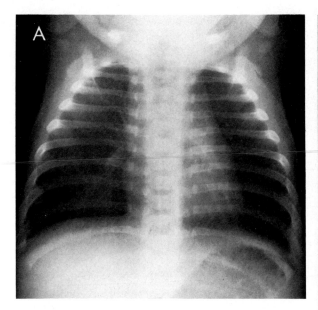

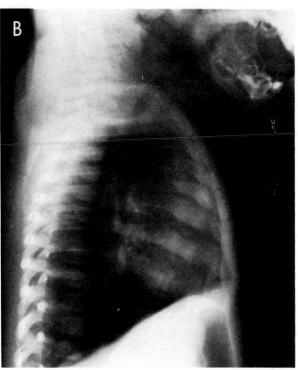

FIG 8–52.
Bronchiolitis in a 4-month-old infant. Note the pulmonary hyperaeration but generally clear lungs.

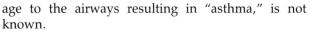

age to the airways resulting in "asthma," is not known.

The relation between bronchiolitis and asthma is not clear, but it seems likely that the conditions are related. In any case, since viral bronchiolitis rarely recurs, infants having three or more attacks should be considered to have asthma.

Bronchial Asthma

Bronchial asthma is a common, recurrent, pulmonary disease characterized by wheezing, cough, and dyspnea due to increased resistance to airflow in intrapulmonary airways. Reversible bronchospasm can begin in infancy, in association with respiratory infections, later in childhood, or even in adulthood. It may be precipitated by exposure to allergens, irritants such as smoke, or infections, but in many cases no obvious external stimulus is apparent. It is a type I or IgE-mediated immune response (see Chapter 10). Areas of controversy include the roles of allergy, gastroesophageal reflux, adenoid enlargement, and chronic sinusitis in causation and exacerbation of the disorder.

Pathology. At autopsy, the lungs of asthmatic patients reveal hyperinflation with smooth muscular hyperplasia of bronchial and bronchiolar walls, markedly thickened basement membrane, mucous plugging, and various degrees of mucosal edema and epithelial damage. The last-named findings are thought to contribute to abnormal mucociliary clearance. Destructive emphysema and bronchiectasis are rare except in those few patients who have allergic bronchopulmonary aspergillosis.

Airflow obstruction in asthma is multifactorial. Bronchospasm, mucosal edema, and mucous plugging occur in varying combinations. In most patients with asthma, both larger and smaller airways are involved. Because of the increased resistance to airflow, hyperinflation develops leading to increased residual volume and decreased vital capacity. Ventilation-perfusion imbalances result from the uneven distribution of inspired air. Hypoxemia is common, although carbon dioxide retention may not be present.

Radiology. Radiographic findings vary with severity of the disease. Most children with intermittent bouts of asthma have normal radiographic findings when they are not ill. In children with asthma who require steroids or bronchodilators to maintain a normal daily life, there is a slightly greater than 20% likelihood that radiographic abnormalities will be present. Findings of uncomplicated asthma, in addition to hyperinflation, are hilar vessels that are relatively large for the size of the intrapulmonary vessels, suggesting pulmonary hypertension, and a mild degree of bronchial wall thickening, especially in the hilar regions (Fig 8–53).

Patchy, irregular areas of opacity may occur and

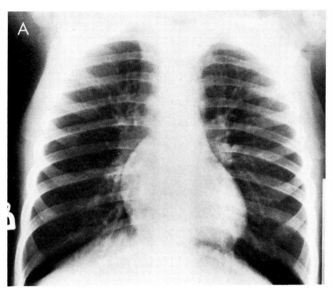

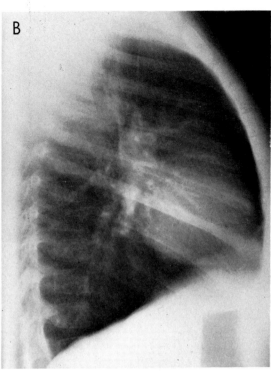

FIG 8–53.
A 4-year-old boy with asthma. Frontal **(A)** and lateral **(B)** radiographs show pulmonary hyperaeration and minimal peribronchial thickening. No asthmatic complication is apparent.

be due to either subsegmental atelectasis or to infection; viral infection is common and difficult to exclude. Atelectasis may be severe and involve a lobe or even an entire lung. Spontaneous remission is the rule, but occasionally a collapsed lobe, especially the right middle or the left lower lobe, will not reexpand. In the series of Eggleston et al. of 479 hospitalized children with asthma, 22% had radiographic abnormalities in addition to the usual hyperinflation and bronchial wall thickening.

In another series of 128 radiographic examinations in children hospitalized for asthma, one third had normal chest films and one third had hyperinflated lungs. In addition to hyperinflation, findings in the abnormal group included peribronchial thickening in 43%, subsegmental atelectasis in 20%, and either pneumonia or segmental atelectasis in 10%.

Allergic bronchopulmonary aspergillosis (ABPA) may occur in cases of long-standing asthma. Pneumomediastinum occurs in about 5% of asthmatic children; they may be asymptomatic or present with substernal chest pain or dysphagia. Pneumothorax is surprisingly uncommon but may rarely be responsible for sudden death.

Although many asthmatic children have radiographic abnormalities, the chest film is not used to establish a diagnosis of asthma but rather to exclude complications and to eliminate other causes of wheezing. Zieverink et al. studied the efficacy of 464 chest radiographs in 188 children treated in the emergency department for acute asthmatic attack. Radiographic abnormalities were found in 13%. The radiographic examination was most likely to be abnormal in children who had rales or rhonchi in addition to wheezing.

All children with wheezing do not have asthma, and the chest x-ray examination is helpful to reach a correct diagnosis in some problem cases. Vascular rings cause inspiratory stridor and certainly have been mistaken for asthma, as have intratracheal foreign bodies and tumors. A nonopaque, esophageal foreign body can be an elusive cause of respiratory distress that simulates asthma. Extrinsic tracheobronchial compression by lymphadenopathy, bronchogenic cysts, or other mediastinal masses can also cause wheezing. Congenital cardiac disorders, especially those with left atrial enlargement, and pulmonary diseases such as bronchiolitis, cystic fibrosis, and pneumonia may simulate asthma, both clinically and radiologically. Many centers thus obtain radiographs in children with a first bout of wheezing but do not obtain radiographs in known asthmatic children unless they are very ill or a complication is suspected. ABPA is a complication of both asthma and cystic fibrosis. Primary criteria for the diagnosis of the disease, according to Mintzer and associates, are as follows:

1. Asthma.
2. Blood eosinophilia.

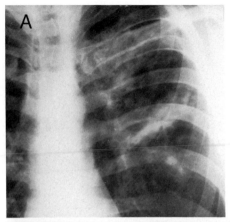

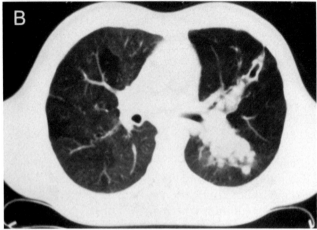

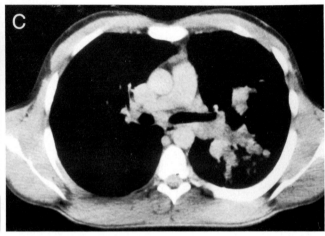

FIG 8–54.
Radiographic and CT findings in allergic bronchopulmonary aspergillosis. This 20-year-old patient had a long history of asthma.
A, close-up view of the left upper lobe shows ill-defined, question-
ably branching opacities. **B,** unenhanced CT scan reveals subsegmental mosaic areas of air trapping in the right lung. On the more
affected left side, there is severe central bronchiectasis with a lobulated mass in the posterior segment of the left upper lobe. **C,**
CECT reveals the mass to be avascular, which suggests that it is
fluid in a dilated bronchial tree. A diagnosis of allergic bronchopulmonary aspergillosis was established clinically.

3. Immediate skin reactivity to *Aspergillus.*
4. Precipitating antibodies against *Aspergillus.*
5. Elevated serum IgE levels.
6. Central bronchiectasis (plain films or bronchographic evidence).

   In ABPA, there is an endobronchial allergic reaction to *Aspergillus* that contributes to the formation
of thick intrabronchial mucous plugs. Collateral air
drift occurs around these plugs, allowing visualization of the typical "toothpaste" or "gloved-finger"
signs. Early diagnosis is important because steroid
therapy appears to be effective in preventing permanent bronchial damage. The classic radiographic
findings include patchy infiltrates, massive homogeneous consolidations, tramline shadows, ring shadows, and other signs of mucoid bronchial impaction
as well as perihilar infiltrates simulating adenopathy. CT reveals a high incidence of bronchiectasis
which often is central and associated with mucoid
impaction (Fig 8–54).

REFERENCES

Congenital Anomalies of the Tracheobronchial Tree
Atwell SW: Major anomalies of the tracheobronchial tree
with a list of minor anomalies. *Dis Chest* 1967; 52:611.
Auringer ST, Bissett GS III, Myer CM III: Magnetic resonance imaging of the pediatric airway: Compared with
findings at surgery and/or endoscopy. *Pediatr Radiol*
1991; 21:329.
Bar-Ziv J, Solomon A: Direct coronal CT scanning of
tracheo-bronchial, pulmonary and thoraco-abdominal lesions in children. *Pediatr Radiol* 1990; 20:245.
Benjamin B, Pitkin J, Cohen D: Congenital tracheal stenosis. *Ann Otol Rhinol Laryngol* 1981; 90:364.

Brasch RC, Gould RG, Gooding CA, et al: Upper airway obstruction in infants and children: Evaluation with ultrafast CT. *Radiology* 1987; 165:459.

Brody AS, Kuhn JP, Seidel FG, et al: Airway evaluation in children with use of ultrafast CT: Pitfalls and recommendations. *Radiology* 1991; 178:181.

Brown SB, Hedlung GL, Glasier CM, et al: Tracheobronchial stenosis in infants: Successful balloon dilatation therapy. *Radiology* 1987; 164:475.

Capitanio M, et al: Obstruction of the airway by the aorta: An observation in infants with congenital heart disease. *Am J Roentgenol* 1983; 140:675.

Carpenter BLM, Merten DV: Radiographic manifestations of congenital anomalies affecting the airway. *Radiol Clin North Am* 1991; 29:219.

Effmann EL, Spackman TJ, Berdon WE, et al: Tracheal agenesis. *Am J Roentgenol* 1975; 125:767.

Ell SR, Jolles H, Galvin JR: Cine CT demonstration of non-fixed upper airway obstruction. *Am J Roentgenol* 1986; 146:669.

Ell SR, Jolles H Keyes WD, et al: Cine CT technique for dynamic airway studies. *Am J Roentgenol* 1985; 145:35.

Evans JA: Aberrant bronchi and cardiovascular anomalies. *Am J Med Genet* 1990; 35:46.

Fletcher BD, Cohn RC: Tracheal compression and the innominate artery: MR evaluation in infants. *Radiology* 1989; 170:103.

Godfrey S: Association between pectus excavatum and segmental bronchomalacia. *J Pediatr* 1980; 96:649.

Goldbloom RB, Dunbar JS: Calcification of the cartilage in the trachea and larynx in infancy associated with congenital stridor. *Pediatrics* 1960; 26:699.

Griscom NT: Computed tomographic determination of tracheal dimensions in children and adolescents. *Radiology* 1982; 145:361.

Griscom NT: CT measurement of the tracheal lumen in children and adolescents. *Am J Roentgenol* 1991; 156:371.

Griscom NT, Martin TR: The trachea and esophagus after repair of esophageal atresia and distal fistula: Computed tomographic observations. *Pediatr Radiol* 1990; 20:447.

Holinger PH, et al: Congenital malformations of the trachea, bronchi and lung. *Ann Otol Rhinol Laryngol* 1952; 61:1159.

Hunter TB, Kuhns LR, Roloff MA, et al: Tracheobronchomegaly in an 18-month-old child. *Am J Roentgenol* 1975; 123:687.

Iannacone G, Capocaccia P, Colloridi V, et al: Double right tracheal bronchus: A case report in an infant. *Pediatr Radiol* 1983; 13:156.

Kao SCS, Smith WL, Sato Y, et al: Ultrafast CT of laryngeal and tracheobronchial obstruction in symptomatic postoperative infants with esophageal atresia and tracheoesophageal fistula. *Am J Roentgenol* 1990; 154:345.

Karsh S, Mahboubi S: Tracheomegaly in children. *Clin Imaging* 1989; 13:77.

Katz I, LeVine M, Herman P: Tracheobronchomegaly: The Mounier-Kuhn syndrome. *Am J Roentgenol* 1962; 88:1084.

Kirks DR, Fram EK, Vock P, et al: Tracheal compression by mediastinal masses in children: CT evaluation. *Am J Roentgenol* 1983; 141:647.

Lacasse JE, Reilly BJ, Mancer K: Segmental esophageal trachea: A potentially fatal type of tracheal stenosis. *Am J Roentgenol* 1980; 134:829.

LaCrosse JE, Reilly BJ, Mancer K: Segmental esophageal trachea: A potentially fatal type of tracheal stenosis. *Am J Roentgenol* 1980; 134:829.

Landing B: Congenital malformations and genetic disorders of the respiratory tract (larynx, trachea, bronchi and lungs). *Am Rev Respir Dis* 1979; 20:151.

Landing BH: Syndromes of congenital heart disease with tracheobronchial anomalies. *Am J Roentgenol* 1975; 123:679.

Landing BH, Wells TR: Tracheobronchial anomalies in children. *Perspect Pediatr Pathol* 1973; 1:1.

Lee KS, Bae WK, Lee BH, et al: Bronchovascular anatomy of the upper lobes: Evaluation with thin-section CT. *Radiology* 1991; 181:765-772.

MacMahon HE, Ruggieri J: Congenital segmental bronchomalacia. *Am J Dis Child* 1969; 118:923.

McLaughlin FJ, Strieder DJ, Harris GBC, et al: Tracheal bronchus: Association with respiratory morbidity in childhood. *J Pediatr* 1985; 106:751.

Newth CJL, Lipton MJ, Gould RG, et al: Varying tracheal cross-sectional area during respiration in infants and children with suspected upper airway obstruction by computed cinetomography scanning. *Pediatr Pulmonol* 1990; 9:224.

Peters ME, Arya S, Langer LO, et al: Narrow trachea in mucopolysaccharidoses. *Pediatr Radiol* 1985; 15:225.

Remy J, Smith M, Marache P, et al: Le bronche "trachéale" gauche pathogène: Revue de la littérature à propos de 4 observations. *J Radiol Electrol Med Nucl* 1977; 58:621.

Ritsema GH: Ectopic right bronchus: Indication for bronchography. *Am J Roentgenol* 1983; 140:671.

Sane SM, Sieber WK, Girdany BR: Congenital bronchobiliary fistula. *Surgery* 1971; 69:599.

Santos JMG: Laryngotracheobronchial cartilage calcification in children: A case report and review of the literature. *Pediatr Radiol* 1991; 21:377.

Siegel MJ, et al: Tracheal bronchus. *Radiology* 1979; 130:353.

Smith EI: Early development of the trachea and esophagus in relation to atresia of the esophagus and tracheoesophageal fistula. *Contrib Embryol Carnegie Inst* 1957; 36:41.

Strife JL: Upper airway and tracheal obstruction in infants and children. *Radiol Clin North Am* 1988; 26:309.

Strife JL, Towbin RB, Francis P, et al: Retained fetal lung fluid in two neonates with congenital absence of the pulmonary valve and tetralogy of Fallot. *Radiology* 1981; 141:675.

Strife JL, Baumel AS, Dunbar JS: Tracheal compression by the innominate artery in infancy and childhood. *Radiology* 1981; 139:73.

Strife JL, Matsumoto J, Bissett GS III, et al: The position of the trachea in infants and children with right aortic arch. *Pediatr Radiol* 1989; 19:226.

Taybi H, Capitanio MA: Tracheobronchial calcification: An observation in three children after mitral valve replacement and warfarin sodium therapy. *Radiology* 1990; 176:728.

Vogl T, Wilimzig C, Hofmann U, et al: MRI in tracheal stenosis by innominate artery in children. *Pediatr Radiol* 1991; 21:89.

Wanderer AA, Ellis EF. Goltz RW, et al: Tracheobronchomegaly and acquired cutis laxa in a child. Pediatrics 1969; 44:709

Wells TR, Gwinn JL, Landing BH, et al: Reconsideration of the anatomy of sling left pulmonary artery: The association of one form with bridging bronchus and imperforate anus. Anatomic and diagnostic aspects. *J Pediatr Surg* 1988; 23:892.

Wells TR, Stanley P, Padua EM, et al: Serial sectioreconstruction of anomalous tracheobronchial branching patterns from CT scan images: Bridging bronchus associated with sling left pulmonary artery. *Pediatr Radiol* 1990; 20:444.

Wittenberg MH, Gyepes Gypes MT, Crocker D: Tracheal dynamics in infants with respiratory distress, stridor and collapsing trachea. *Radiology* 1967; 88:653.

Woodring JH, Barrett PA, Rehm SR, et al: Acquired tracheomegaly in adults as a complication of diffuse pulmonary fibrosis. *Am J Roentgenol* 1989; 152:743.

Woodring JH, Howard RS II, Rehm SR.: Congenital tracheobronchomegaly (Mounier-Kuhn syndrome): A report of 10 cases and review of the literature. *J Thorac Imaging* 1991; 6:1.

Acquired Abnormalities of the Tracheobronchial Tree

Brock RC, Carn RJ, Dickinson J: Tuberculous mediastinal lymphadenitis in childhood: Secondary effects on the lung. *Guy Hosp* Rep 1937; 7:195.

Cohen SR, Seltzer H, Geller KA, et al: Papilloma of the larynx and tracheobronchial tree in children: A retrospective study. *Ann Otol Rhinol Laryngol* 1980; 89:497.

Faw K, Muntz H, Siegel M: Computed tomography in the evaluation of acquired stenosis in the neonate. *Laryngoscope* 1982; 92:100.

Gold R, Wilt JC, Adhihari PK, et al: Adenoviral pneumonia and its complications in infancy and childhood. *J Can Assoc Radiol* 1969; 20:218.

Kramer SS, Wehunt WD, Stocker JT, et al: Pulmonary manifestations of juvenile laryngotracheal papillomatosis. Am J Roentgenol 1985; 144:687.

Lack EE, Harris GBC, Eraklis AJ, et al: Primary bronchial tumors in childhood: A clinicopathologic study of six cases. *Cancer* 1983; 51:492.

Lynch DA, Brasch RC, Hardy KA, et al: Pediatric pulmonary disease: Assessment with high-resolution ultrafast CT. *Radiology* 1990; 176:243.

Macleod WM: Abnormal transradiancy of one lung. *Thorax* 1954; 9:147.

MacPherson RI, Cummings GR, Chernik V: Unilateral hyperlucent lung. A complication of viral pneumonia. *J Can Assoc Radiol* 1969; 20:225.

Marti-Bonmati L, Perales FR, Catala F, et al: CT findings in Swyer-James syndrome. *Radiology* 1989; 172:477

Mu L, Sun D, He P: Radiological diagnosis of aspirated foreign bodies in children: Review of 343 cases. *J Laryngol Otol* 1990; 104:778.

Naidich DP, McCauley DI, Seigelman SS: Computed tomography of bronchial adenomas. *J Comput Assist Tomogr* 1982; 6:725.

Othersen HB: Intubation injuries of the trachea in children. *J Pediatr Surg* 1979; 189:601.

Reed L, Simon G: Unilateral lung transradiancy. *Thorax* 1962; 17:230.

Reed MH: Radiology of airway foreign bodies in children. *J Can Assoc Radiol* 1977; 28:111.

Scott JR, Kramer SS: Pediatric tracheostomy. II. Radiographic features of difficult decannulations. *Am J Roentgenol* 1978; 130:893.

Svedstrom E, Puhakka H, Kero P: How accurate is chest radiography in the diagnosis of tracheobronchial foreign bodies in children? *Pediatr Radiol* 1989; 19:520.

Swyer PR, James GCW: A case of unilateral pulmonary emphysema. *Thorax* 1953; 8:133.

Van Duc T, Tsan Vinh L. Huault G, et al: Laryngotracheal lesions induced by endotracheal intubation in children: Anatomic study of 53 cases. *Nouv Presse Med* 1974; 3:365.

Watterson KG, Wisheart JD: Tracheobronchial mucoepidermoid carcinoma in childhood with a ten year follow-up. *Eur J Cardiothorac Surg* 1990; 4:112.

Weber AL: Tracheal stenosis: Analysis of 150 cases. *Radiol Clin North Am* 1978; 16:291.

Atelectasis

Culiner MM: Right middle lobe syndrome: A nonobstructive complex. *Chest* 1966; 50:57.

Felman H: Lingular and upper lobe atelectasis and cardiomegaly: An usual pattern simulating pleural effusion. *Br J Radiol* 1972; 45:299.

Frankenen E, Klatte EC: Atypical (peripheral) upper lobe collapse. *Ann Radiol (Paris)* 1977; 28:87.

Livingston GL, Holinger LD, Luck SR: Right middle lobe syndrome in children. *Int J Pediatr Otorhinolaryngol* 1987; 13:11-23.

Lubert M, Kraus GR: Patterns of lobar collapse as observed radiogaphically. *Radiology* 1951; 56:165.

Proto AV, Tocino I: Radiographic manifestations of lobar collapse. *Semin Roentgenol* 1980: 15:117.

Bronchiectasis

Avery ME: Bronchography: Outmoded procedure? *Pediatrics* 1970; 46:333.

Barker AF, Bardana EJ Jr: Bronchiectasis: Update of an orphan disease. *Am Rev Respir Dis* 1988; 137:969-978.

Capitanio M: Congenital bronchiectasis due to deficiency of bronchial cartilage (Williams-Campbell syndrome). *Pediatrics* 1975; 87:230.

Gudjberg CE: Bronchiectasis: Radiological diagnosis and prognosis after operative treatment. *Acta Radiol Suppl* (Stockh) 1957;143.

Naidich DP, McCauley DI, Khouri NF, et al: Computed tomography of bronchiectasis. *J Comput Tomogr* 1982; 6:437.

Naidich DP, Zerhouni EA, Siegelman SS (eds): *Computed Tomography and Magnetic Resonance of the Thorax,* ed 2. New York, Raven Press, 1991.

Neels DA, Goodman LR, Gurney JW, et al: Computed tomography in the evaluation of allergic bronchopulmonary aspergillosis. *Am Rev Respir Dis* 1990; 142:1200.

Reid L: Reduction in bronchial subdivision in bronchiectasis. *Thorax* 1950; 5:233.

Remy-Jardin M, Remy J: Comparison of vertical and oblique CT in evaluation of bronchial tree. *J Comput Assist Tomogr* 1988; 12:956.

Sturgess JM, Chao J, Wong J, et al: Cilia defective radial spokes: A cause of human respiratory disease. *N Engl J Med* 1979; 300:53.

Vandevivre J, Spehl M, Dab I, et al: Bronchiectasis in childhood: Comparison of chest roentgenograms, bronchograms, and lung scintigraphy.*Pediatr Radiol* 1980; 9:193.

Wayne KS, Taussig LM: Probable familial congenital bronchiectasis due to cartilage deficiency (Williams-Campbell syndrome). *Am Rev Respir Dis* 1976; 114:15.

Cystic Fibrosis

Amodio JB, Berdon WE, Abramson S, et al: Cystic fibrosis in childhood: Pulmonary paranasal sinus and skeletal manifestations. *Semin Roentgenol* 1987; 22:1125

Bhalla M, Turcios N, Aponte V, et al: Cystic Fibrosis: Scoring system with thin-section CT. *Radiology* 1991:179: 783.

Brasfield D, Hicks G, Soong S, et al: The chest roentgenogram in cystic fibrosis: A new scoring system. *Pediatrics* 1979; 63:24.

Esterle JR, Oppenheimer EH: Observations in cystic fibrosis of the pancreas. 3: Pulmonary lesions. *Johns Hopkins Med J* 1968; 122:94.

Friedman PJ: Chest radiographic findings in the adult with cystic fibrosis. *Semin Roentgenol* 1987: 32:114-124.

Griscom NT, Capitanio MA, Wagner ML, et al: Visible fatty liver. *Radiology* 1975; 117:385.

Griscom NT, Vawter GF, Stigol LC: Radiologic and pathologic abnormalities of the trachea in older patients with cystic fibrosis. *Am J Roentgenol* 1987; 148:691.

Hardy KA, Lynch DA, Brasch RC, et al: Usefulness of high resolution computed tomography in infants and young children with cystic fibrosis: A comparison with chest radiography. *Pediatr Pulmonol* 1989; 4(suppl):141.

Kuhn JP, et al: Metastatic calcification in cystic fibrosis: Report of two cases. *Radiology* 1970; 97:59.

Maclusky I, Levinson H: Cystic fibrosis, in Chernick V (ed): *Kendig's Disorders of the Respiratory Tract in Children,* ed 5. Philadelphia, WB Saunders, pp 692-730.

Nathanson I, Conboy K, Murphy S, Afshani E, Kuhn JP: Ultrafast computerized tomography of the chest in cystic fibrosis: A new scoring system. *Pediatr Pulmonol* 1991; 11:81.

Reilly BJ, Featherbee EA, Weng TR: The correlation of radiological changes with pulmonary function in cystic fibrosis. *Radiology* 1971; 98:281.

Riordan JR, et al: Identification of the cystic fibrosis gene: Cloning and characterization of complementary DNA. *Science* 1989; 245:1066.

Sauvegrain J, Feigelson J: Cholecystography in mucoviscidosis. *Ann Radiol* 1970; 13:311.

Taussig LM (ed): Cystic fibrosis. New York, Thieme-Stratton, 1984.

Tizzano EF, Buchwald M: Cystic fibrosis: Beyond the gene to therapy. *J Pediatr* 1992; 120:337.

Tomashefski JP Jr, Bruce M, Stern RC, et al: Pulmonary air cysts in cystic fibrosis: Relation of pathologic features to radiologic findings and history of pneumothorax. *Human Pathol* 1985; 16:253-261.

van der Put JM, Meradji M, Danoesastro D, et al: Chest radiographs in cystic fibrosis. A follow-up study with application of a quantative scoring system. *Pediatr Radiol* 1982; 12:57.

Wood B, Boat TF, Dorschuk CF: Cystic fibrosis. *Am Rev Respir Dis* 1976; 113:833.

Wood RE: *Pneumatosis coli* in cystic fibrosis: Clinical, radiological and pathological features. *Am J Dis Child* 1975; 129:246.

Zach MS: Lung disease in cystic fibrosis - an updated concept. *Pediatr Pulmonol* 1990; 8:188.

Peripheral Airway Disorders

Blair DN, Coppage L, Shaw C: Medical imaging in asthma. *J Thorac Imaging* 1986; 1:23.

Brooks LJ, Cloutier MM, Afshani E: Significance of roentgenographic abnormalities in children hospitalized for asthma. *Chest* 1982; 82:315.

Coblentz CL, Babcook CJ, Alton D, et al: Observer variation in detecting the radiologic features associated with bronchiolitis. *Invest Radiol* 1991; 26:115.

Eggleston PA, Ward BH, Pierson WE, et al: Radiographic abnormalities in acute asthma in children. *Pediatrics* 1974; 54:442.

Friedman PJ: Radiology of the airways with emphasis on the small airway. *J Thorac Imaging* 1986; 1:7-22.

Hicks GM: Two cases of tracheal abnormality in teenagers presenting as obstructive lung disease. *Ann Radiol* 1976; 19:7781.

Hodson CJ, Trickey SE: Bronchial wall thickening in asthma. *Clin Radiol* 1960; 11:183.

Markowitz RI, Johnson KM, Weinstein EM: Hyperinflation of the lungs in infants with large left-to-right shunts. *Invest Radiol* 1988; 23:354.

Martinez FD, Cline M, Burrows B: Increased incidence of asthma in children of smoking mothers. *Pediatrics* 1992; 89:21.

Mintzer RA, et al: The spectrum of radiologic findings in allergic bronchopulmonary aspergillosis. *Radiology* 1978; 127:301.

Morrish WF, Herman SJ, Weisbrod GL, et al: Bronchiolitis obliterans after lung transplantation: Findings at chest radiography and high-resolution CT. *Radiology* 1991; 179:487.

Simon G, Connolly N, Littlejohns D, et al: Radiological abnormalities in children with asthma and their relation to the clinical findings and some respiratory function tests. *Thorax* 1973; 28:115.

Simon G: Type I immunologic reaction in the lungs. *Semin Roentgenol* 1975; 10:21.

Tabachnik E, Levinson H: Infantile bronchial asthma. *J Allergy Clin Immunol* 1981; 67:339.

Wyatt SE, Nunn P, Hows JM, et al: Airways obstruction associated with graft versus host disease after bone marrow transplantation. *Thorax* 1984; 39:887.

Zieverink SE, Harper AP, Holden RW, et al: Emergency room radiography of asthma: An efficacy study. *Radiology* 1982; 145:27.

9

Pulmonary Infection

TECHNIQUES AND DIFFERENTIAL DIAGNOSIS

The diagnosis of pneumonia is one of the most common challenges facing a radiologist interpreting children's chest films. It must be determined whether pneumonia is present, and if it is, the physician must localize it, characterize its pathologic nature, evaluate its possible cause, and look for complications. Knowledge of the clinical history, the age of the child, the duration and severity of symptoms, the white blood cell count, and the presence or absence of fever all help to narrow the differential diagnosis. High-quality chest radiographs, made with a short exposure time to minimize respiratory

511

motion, are essential for an accurate diagnosis. Films must be made in an adequate degree of inspiration to avoid errors of overinterpretation due to physiologic underaeration. Detailed consideration of the radiographic technique is beyond the scope of this discussion and is covered well elsewhere.

It is possible to obtain frontal and lateral films of good quality in younger or uncooperative children either erect or supine. Films are best exposed at maximal inspiration. It is best that the infant be breathing quietly rather than crying because there is less chance of getting "plethoric" lungs due to the infant's Valsalva maneuver. Films made in expiration or with the patient rotated may lead to an erroneous diagnosis of pneumonia (Table 9–1, Fig 9–1). The presence of a prominent thymus in an infant, breast buds in the pubescent teenager, or a long hair braid in a child can simulate pneumonia. (Fig 9–1,C).

TABLE 9–1.

Partial List of Diseases and Conditions That Can Radiographically Mimic "Primary" Pneumonia in Children*

Physiologic
  Thymus
  Breast bud
  Hair braid
Congenital (infection may be secondary)
  Adenomatoid malformation
  Bronchogenic cyst
  Sequestration
Aspiration (pneumonia *secondary*)
  Gastroesophageal reflux
  Tracheoesophageal fistula
  Neuromuscular disorders
  Familial dysautonomia
  Vascular ring
Traumatic, toxic, and iatrogenic
  Pulmonary contusion
  Hydrocarbon inhalation
  Smoke inhalation
  Near-drowning
  Drug reaction
  Radiation pneumonitis
  Adult respiratory distress syndrome
Pulmonary embolus and infarction
Metastatic neoplasm
Collagen-vascular disease
Sarcoid
Histiocytosis
Pulmonary hemosiderosis, pulmonary hemorrhage
Pulmonary edema
Chronic lung disease
  Bronchopulmonary dysplasia
  Cystic fibrosis
  Asthma with atelectasis (plugging off)

*Modified from Feigin RD, Cherry JD: *Textbook of Pediatric Infectious Diseases*, ed 2. Philadelphia, WB Saunders, 1987, p 294.

A review of the available earlier films is essential to make certain that one is not dealing with a residual or recurrent problem that might suggest an underlying abnormality. In most cases, all that is needed for diagnosis are good-quality frontal and lateral radiographs. However, in equivocal cases oblique or decubitus views may help in clarifying a suspected pulmonary abnormality. On the decubitus films, the "up" side is the inspiratory side while the "down" side is expiratory (Fig 9–2). In unexplained pulmonary or airway disease, evaluation of the esophagus can provide crucial information (tracheoesophageal fistula, vascular ring, esophageal foreign body, etc.) (Fig 9–3). Mediastinal shifts and diaphragmatic movement are assessed at fluoroscopy for the esophagogram. High-resolution, thin-section computed tomography (HRCT) is of value in some complicated cases or in cases of suspected bronchiectasis.

The use of thin-section (1–2 mm) HRCT with high spatial frequency reconstruction (a bone algorithm) and targeting of tissues provides the most detailed view of lung parenchyma. The chest film shows the normal main stem bronchus while the CT reveals the normal secondary lobule, i.e., the region distal to a single terminal bronchiole, the last purely conducting airway. The secondary lobule is a unit of lung parenchyma made up of less than 12 acini (the acinus is the largest unit in which the airways contribute to gas exchange and is 6–10 mm in diameter). The secondary lobule is best developed in the periphery of the lung, is irregularly polyhedral in shape (1.0–2.5 cm per side), and is marginated by the interlobular septa which contain pulmonary veins and lymphatics. In the center of each secondary lobule is an intralobular artery and bronchus. It is to be noted that the pulmonary septa are seen inconsistently and are best visualized at pleural surfaces. The intralobular artery is noted as a linear branch or a dot, but the accompanying bronchus frequently is not seen (Fig 9–4).

EPIDEMIOLOGY OF CHILDHOOD PNEUMONIA

It is not possible to determine from the radiograph whether a child is suffering from a bacterial or viral infection, or to make more than an educated guess as to what agent might be causing a specific radiographic pattern. However, knowledge of the likely organisms and their usual clinical and radiologic behavior can be useful while the clinician awaits the results of serum antibody screens and cultures (Table 9–2). Viruses are the most common cause of both upper and lower respiratory tract infection in

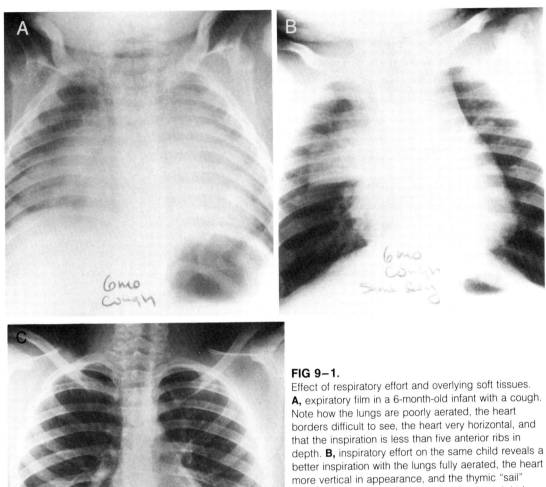

FIG 9–1.
Effect of respiratory effort and overlying soft tissues.
A, expiratory film in a 6-month-old infant with a cough.
Note how the lungs are poorly aerated, the heart
borders difficult to see, the heart very horizontal, and
that the inspiration is less than five anterior ribs in
depth. **B,** inspiratory effort on the same child reveals a
better inspiration with the lungs fully aerated, the heart
more vertical in appearance, and the thymic "sail"
sign is easily seen on the right. This region might be
considered a pneumonia on the previous film. The
inspiratory depth is almost seven anterior ribs.
C, bilateral hazy densities in the lower lung fields of a
teenage girl. A lateral film revealed these to be
breast buds.

infancy and childhood. Despite this fact, however, the most common *single* agent that produces pneumonia in childhood is neither a virus nor bacteria but *Mycoplasma pneumoniae*, the smallest free-living organism. It is distinguished from bacteria by lacking a cell wall and from viruses by growing on cell-free media. *Mycoplasma* causes about 30% of all childhood pneumonias and, in school-age children, is responsible for 40% to 60% of pneumonias. In children under the age of 3 years, however, the incidence of *Mycoplasma* pneumonia drops to about 5%.

True viruses account for 65% of pneumonias throughout childhood but over 90% in children less than 2 years old. Respiratory syncytial virus (RSV) is responsible for about one third of all cases. RSV tends to occur in epidemics in the winter and early spring and affects mostly infants and preschool children. In addition to its role as a leading cause of viral pneumonia, it is also the most common cause of bronchiolitis. Other viruses are also commonly pathogenic in the lower respiratory tract.

Bacteria account for about 5% of childhood pneumonias. They tend to occur in neonates and other hospitalized children at least as often as they do in the community. The most common bacterial infections are those due to *Streptococcus pneumoniae* (pneumococcus) and *Haemophilus influenzae*, followed by *Streptococcus pyogenes*, *Staphylococcus aureus*, *Klebsiella*, and various other gram-negative organisms.

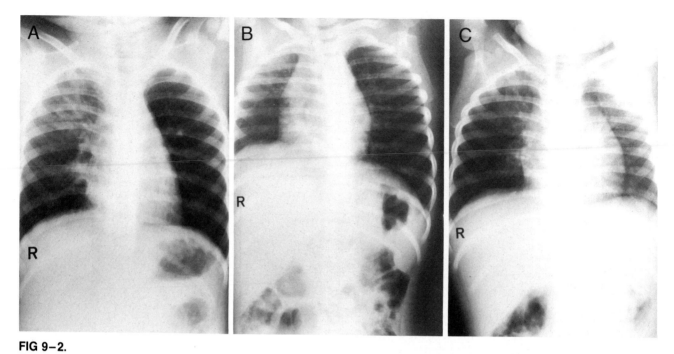

FIG 9–2.
The advantage of using decubitus films. **A,** erect radiograph showing air trapping on the left and infiltrate in the right upper lobe. **B,** with the right side down, the right lung empties entirely while the left lung remains hyperexpanded. **C,** with the left side down, the right lung expands while the left lung empties. There is no fixed obstruction and therefore there is no bronchial foreign body. This child was an asthmatic and had right upper lobe atelectasis.

TABLE 9–2.

Common Pathogens by Age*

| Age | Pathogen | |
	Virus	Bacteria and *Mycoplasma*
Neonate	Cytomegalovirus (CMV)	Group B streptococcus
	Herpes simplex virus	Gram-negative bacilli
	Respiratory syncytial	*Escherichia coli*
	virus (RSV)	*Klebsiella pneumoniae*
		Proteus
1–3 mo	RSV	*Chlamydia*
	CMV	*Streptococcus*
		pneumoniae†
		Haemophilus influenzae
		type b†
		Staphylococcus aureus
4 mo–5 yr	RSV	*S. pneumoniae*
	Parainfluenza	*H. influenzae*
	Adenovirus	*S. aureus*‡
	Influenza	
	Rhinovirus	
>5 yr		*Mycoplasma*§
		S. pneumoniae

*Modified from Christy C, Powell KR: *J Respir Dis* 1987; 8:65–73.
†Two most common bacteria throughout childhood.
‡Usually affects infants less than 1 year of age.
§More common than either bacteria or viruses over the age of 5 years.

RADIOGRAPHIC FINDINGS IN PNEUMONIA

The radiographic appearance of pneumonia varies with the age of the patient, the extent of the disease, and the etiologic agent. A variety of unique anatomical factors in the infant's chest also contribute to the final radiographic pattern. The sum of these factors is that the smaller airways of the infant are more susceptible to obstruction by secretions and inflammatory narrowing, causing three major abnormalities: generalized hyperaeration, irregular aeration, and bronchial wall thickening.

Hyperaeration is diagnosed as described earlier. "Irregular aeration" (alternating areas of atelectasis and air trapping) is very frequently seen in lower respiratory tract infections in infants and is easy to recognize when severe (Fig 9–5), but in minimal cases it is difficult to differentiate from normal. Thickening of bronchial walls (ring shadows and tramlines) is a third feature commonly seen in children with lower respiratory tract infection. These changes are secondary to edema and inflammation in the bronchial walls and interstitium of the lung. When present between bouts of acute illness, this finding suggests chronic disease such as asthma, cystic fibrosis, immunodeficiency, or aspiration pneumonia. Although less frequent, the classic consolidative changes of bacterial pneumonia also occur

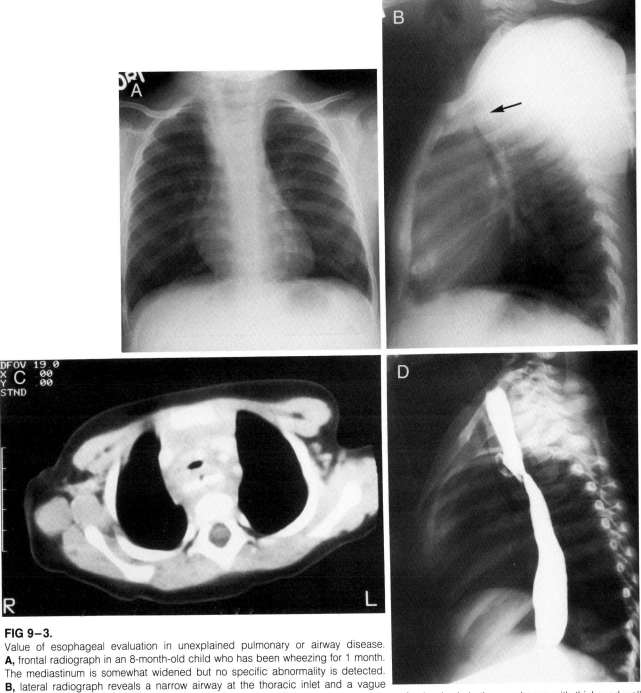

FIG 9–3.
Value of esophageal evaluation in unexplained pulmonary or airway disease.
A, frontal radiograph in an 8-month-old child who has been wheezing for 1 month.
The mediastinum is somewhat widened but no specific abnormality is detected.
B, lateral radiograph reveals a narrow airway at the thoracic inlet and a vague
opacity posterior to the narrowing *(arrow).* **C,** CT scan on this patient shows a large foreign body in the esophagus with thickened wall
between the esophagus and the airway. This foreign body proved to be a button. **D,** in this clinical situation, we usually do an esophagogram. In another child with the same history, irregularity and thickening of the anterior esophageal wall as well as the esophageal foreign
body are noted. In this instance the contrast has extended into the mediastinum and there is inflammation and edema about the airway.

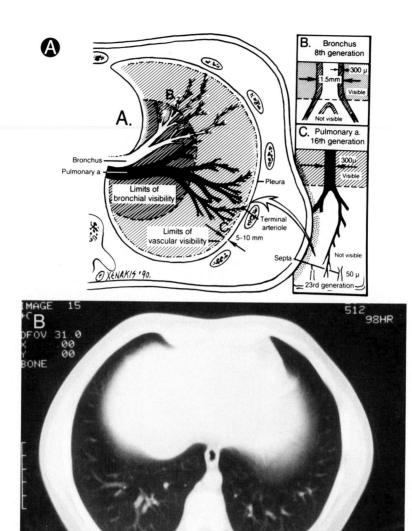

FIG 9–4.
Normal lung anatomy. **A,** limits of visibility by high-resolution CT (HRCT). It is clear the vascular and bronchial limits of visibility are different with vascular visibility noted in the periphery of the lung 5 to 10 mm from the visceral pleura. (From Naidich DP, Zerhouni EA, Siegelman SS (eds): *Computed Tomography and Magnetic Resonance of the Thorax*, ed 2. New York, Raven Press, 1991, p 340. Used by permission.) **B,** HRCT of a normal patient showing the extent of visualization of the secondary lobule.

in childhood but even here no radiographic pattern is pathognomonic of a particular organism.

Radiographic-Pathologic Correlations in Pneumonia

Radiologists generally try to classify pulmonary parenchymal patterns as interstitial or alveolar (airspace disease). Pathologists classify pneumonia as alveolar or airspace pneumonia, lobular or bronchopneumonia, and pneumonia of hematogenous origin. Unfortunately, the radiographic-pathologic correlation is imperfect. Diseases that begin in the interstitium may progress to produce airspace consolidation, in turn obscuring the radiographic signs of interstitial involvement. Conversely, diseases beginning in the airspace may develop interstitial changes later; mixed involvement is the rule late in the disease in most pulmonary disorders.

Nonetheless, analysis of the predominant roentgenographic pattern in conjunction with factors such as patient age, seasonal features, and clinical and laboratory findings will narrow the diagnostic possibilities, although the final diagnosis depends on culture of specific organisms obtained from sputum, blood, or lung aspirates.

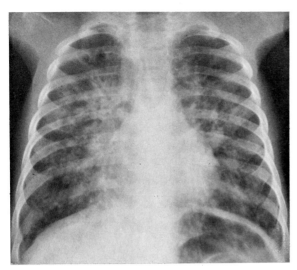

FIG 9–5.
Irregular aeration. Viral bronchopneumonia in a 10-month-old infant. Note the multiple bilateral areas of patchy consolidation (irregular aeration).

Airspace Pneumonia

Airspace pneumonia, which is classically due to *S. pneumoniae* or *K pneumoniae*, occurs after the aspiration of infected mucus into the acinus, where the bacteria injure the alveolar wall and cause edema and outpouring of fluids, or after hematogenous

transport from extrapulmonary foci of infection. Rapid centrifugal spread occurs through the pores of Kohn and the damaged alveolar wall to the terminal airspaces and to adjacent lobules. The basic morphologic change is alveolar exudation. The lumina of bronchioles in the affected areas are usually filled with inflammatory exudate, but the bronchial walls and interstitial tissues are not inflamed.

Alveolar exudate casts a shadow of increased opacity because radiolucent alveolar air is replaced by water-density inflammatory fluid. The precise nature of airspace disease is not revealed by the radiograph—blood, exudate, and edema all cast water-density shadows. The presence of airspace disease is revealed radiographically by acinar shadows and small, ill-defined nodules up to 7 mm in size. The coalescence of acinar shadows appear as a relatively homogeneous opacity with fluffy margins except where the margins abut a pleural surface or fissure; here the margin is distinct. Air bronchograms are visible within the areas of consolidation. Detection of the change of density (more opacity) is the clue to the roentgenologic diagnosis and must be sought in regions of normal opacities—behind the heart and through the liver (Fig 9–6). This change in density obliterates the normal bronchovascular markings. There is usually little if any volume loss (Fig 9–7).

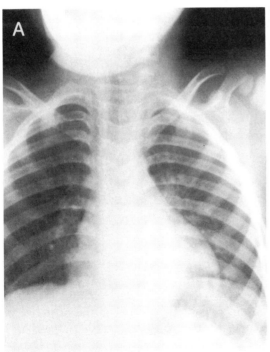

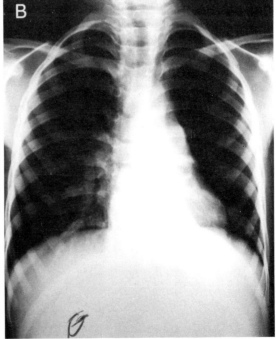

FIG 9–6.
Recognition of changes in density to detect parenchymal disease. **A,** frontal radiograph showing opacity on the left side behind the heart. This was a pneumonia which cleared within 10 days. **B,** sim-ilar opacity seen through the heart in another patient. This time the shape of the opacity suggests atelectasis of the left lower lobe.

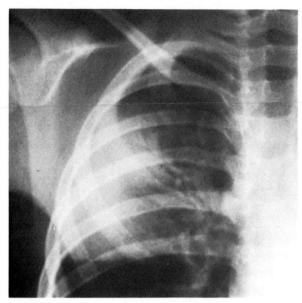

FIG 9-7.
Airspace disease without volume loss. Classic airspace pneumonia. Note the peripheral location and hazy margins (except inferiorly where the pneumonic process abuts the right minor fissure) and the air bronchogram medially.

The process may initially be segmental but usually spreads rapidly and becomes nonsegmental.

Lobar Pneumonia

Complete lobar consolidation is uncommon in infants and children; in most cases, some portion of the affected lobe remains air-containing throughout the course of the disease. When both frontal and lateral projections of the lung are viewed, it is nearly always possible to see some portion of the consolidation extending to the periphery of the lung. Massive pulmonary consolidation can usually be distinguished radiographically from pleural effusion or a thoracic mass by the presence of an air bronchogram; there is little change of volume in the consolidated lung and there is usually no significant mediastinal shift. In difficult cases, CT is beneficial in differentiating massive consolidation from other causes of pulmonary opacity.

The key to recognizing airspace disease on HRCT is the detection of poorly marginated diffuse acinar nodules. These range in size from 3 to 10 mm. The pattern is nonspecific as inflammatory as well as neoplastic disease can present in this manner. It is also true that these nodules probably originate around an airway and, in fact, represent both peribronchiolar disease and acinar disease (Fig 9-8).

Radiographic Appearance of Specific Lobar Consolidations. *Right Upper Lobe.* When consolidations in this lobe extend caudad as far as the mi-

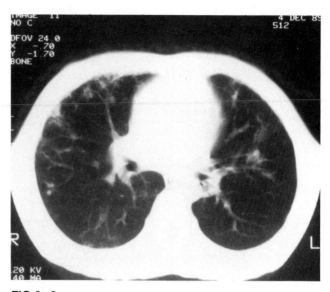

FIG 9-8.
Interstitial and airspace disease on CT. CT on this teenage boy has a mixed pattern with a few sharp interstitial nodules, but the predominant pattern is fluffy and poorly marginated nodules.

nor fissure, they are sharply defined by a horizontal (transverse) margin (Fig 9-9). The posterior portion of the right upper lobe is involved more frequently than is the anterior. Consolidations along the medial margin may resemble a large right lobe of the thymus or be obscured by the overlying thymus (see Fig 9-1).

Right Middle Lobe. There are marked normal anatomical variations in the size and shape of the middle lobe and in its relationship to the minor fissure, the anterior chest wall, and the diaphragm. For these reasons, even complete consolidation of the middle lobe produces widely different appearances in different individuals. Consolidation of the medial segment of the middle lobe in the frontal projection usually obliterates the right heart border, but occasionally fuzziness of this border is seen in consolidation in the lower lobe or even as a normal variation. The lateral view is essential for an accurate diagnosis (Figs 9-10 and 9-11).

Right Lower Lobe. The lower lobe only rarely undergoes complete consolidation; usually either the superior or the basilar segments are involved, and the rest of the lobe is normal. The middle lobe may be involved concurrently. Pneumonia in the retrocardiac area (Fig 9-12) or in the posterior portion of the lower lobe, projected through the diaphragm on the frontal view, may be overlooked if the radiograph is underpenetrated (cannot see pedicles of the spine when looking through the heart) or if a lateral view is not obtained (Fig 9-13). Basilar lobar pneumonia often presents with abdominal pain and may

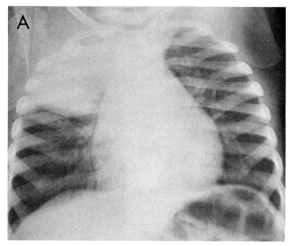
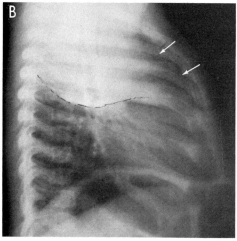

FIG 9–9.
Lobar consolidation of the right upper lobe. **A,** posteroanterior, and **B,** right lateral projections. The sharply defined lower margin parallels the minor fissure. In **A,** the entire lobe appears to be consolidated; in **B,** it is evident that a large anterior segment *(arrows)* is normally aerated. The downward bulge of the fissure could herald an incipient abscess or indicate possible *Klebsiella pneumoniae* infection.

simulate appendicitis or other abdominal pathologic conditions. The lungs must be carefully inspected on every abdominal film (Fig 9–14).

Left Upper Lobe. The left upper and lower lobes overlap in the frontal plane through the entire course of the interlobar fissure, except at the apex, so lateral projections are essential for localization. As in the right upper lobe, consolidation is usually incomplete; it is most commonly situated in the posterolateral aspect. Left upper lobe pneumonia can simulate a large thymic lobe, especially in the frontal projection. Consolidation in the lingular segment of the left upper lobe is similar radiographically to right middle lobe pneumonia and is recognized by indistinctness of the left cardiac margin and anteriorly placed densities on the lateral radiograph (Fig 9–15).

Left Lower Lobe. The pattern of consolidation resembles that of the right lower lobe (Fig 9–16). Even massive consolidations in the left lower lobe may be obscured by the cardiac shadow on an underpenetrated frontal film. To ensure adequate penetration, it is imperative to see both pedicles of the spine and the bronchovascular marking through the cardiac shadow. Consolidation will cause increased

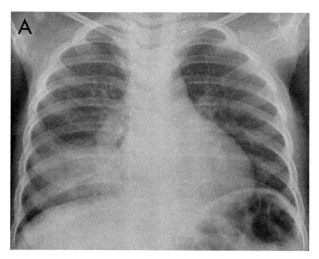
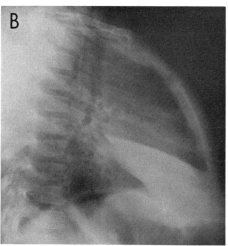

FIG 9–10.
Right middle lobe consolidation. **A,** frontal, and **B,** right lateral projections. The entire right middle lobe is opaque; its convex borders show that it is not collapsed. In **A,** one cannot be certain whether the opaque shadow above the diaphragm is in the right middle or the right lower lobe, although obliteration of the right cardiac edge does suggest that the consolidation is in the right middle lobe. In **B,** the anterior position of the shadow and its triangular shape identify it with certainty as representing the right middle lobe.

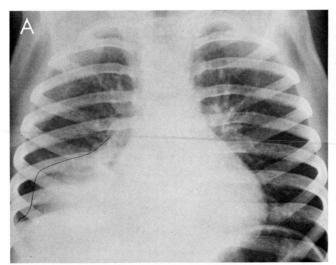
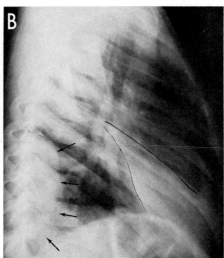

FIG 9–11.
Concurrent consolidation of the right middle and lower lobes: **A,** frontal, and **B,** right lateral projections. The two opaque shadows are superimposed and blended in **A,** but are clearly separated in **B.**

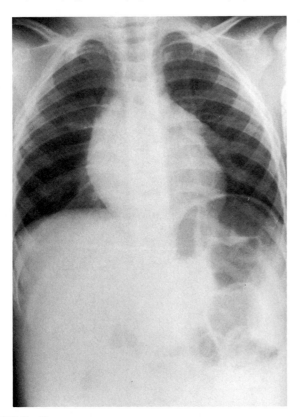

FIG 9–12.
Retrocardiac right lower lobe pneumonia. By looking through the heart, it is apparent that vessels can be seen on the left, but there is opacity behind the right heart.

opacity and silhouette the normal markings. Other common clues provided by the silhouette sign are obscuration of the descending aortic margin and the contour of the left hemidiaphragm. As in the right lower lobe, basilar consolidations are often best visualized in the lateral projections. In the normal lateral chest film, the more caudad thoracic vertebral bodies appear blacker than the cranial ones. When posterior consolidation of the lower lobe is present, the normal pattern is altered. Obscuration of the posterior portion of the diaphragmatic silhouette and increased density over the lower portion of the thoracic spine are the two most important radiographic signs (Figs 9–17 and 9–18).

In addition to the errors of diagnosis previously mentioned (including overinterpretation of expiratory and rotated films, unfamiliarity with normal variations, and a failure to observe the silhouette signs), areas of consolidation can be mistaken for tumors or vice versa (see Table 9–1). Sometimes pneumonic consolidations are so round and discrete that they are mistaken for pulmonary neoplasms (Fig 9–19). These round pneumonias may also simulate mediastinal masses (Fig 9–20). Usually, careful study reveals irregular margins and an air bronchogram. Moreover, the patient's clinical history is usually that of a child acutely ill with pneumonia rather than with symptoms suggesting neoplasm. Most round pneumonias are caused by *S. pneumoniae;* however, a follow-up examination is indicated to make certain that the round pneumonia is not, in fact, a congenital anomaly or a pulmonary neoplasm.

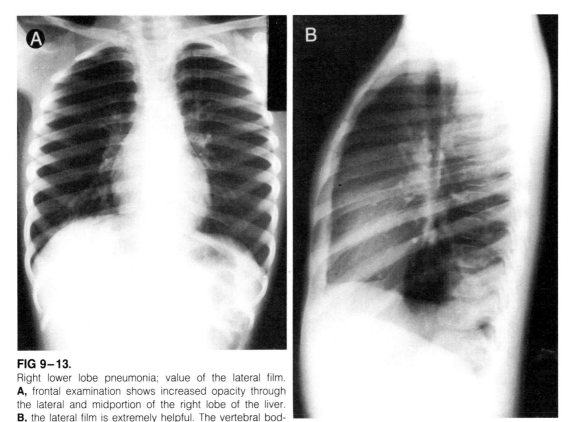

FIG 9–13.
Right lower lobe pneumonia; value of the lateral film. **A,** frontal examination shows increased opacity through the lateral and midportion of the right lobe of the liver. **B,** the lateral film is extremely helpful. The vertebral bodies normally get blacker as viewed from superior to inferior. In this instance there is clearly increased opacification in the lower thoracic vertebral bodies—the site of the right lower lobe consolidation. Note the silhouetting of the posterior aspect of the diaphragm.

Bronchopneumonia or Lobular Pneumonia

This pattern of pneumonia is commonly caused by mycoplasma and by viruses, as well as by bacteria. The initial injury occurs at the terminal and respiratory bronchioles and induces acute bronchiolitis and bronchitis. The disease then spreads to alveolar walls, with an outpouring of exudate that produces acinar filling and lobular consolidations. The radiographic pattern, often diffuse and bilateral, is one of increased peribronchial markings and small fluffy infiltrates.

Initial involvement is segmental because the disease originates in the airways rather than the airspaces (Fig 9–21). Spread to other areas and even bilateral involvement is common as the disease progresses.

Acute Interstitial Pneumonia

Acute interstitial pneumonia is usually caused by agents such as the RSV, the influenza virus, cytomegalovirus (CMV), coxsackievirus, and measles virus; mycoplasma induces this type of reaction in many patients, and occasionally, bacteria such as pneumococci can be responsible.

While there are undoubtedly other organisms that may cause pneumonia, these viruses are responsible for most of the serious lower respiratory infections in children. There is some variation in the microscopic reaction produced in the lung by the varying agents, but there is enough similarity in their gross pathologic findings that the viruses can be considered a group for the purpose of radiographic-pathologic correlation.

Viral pneumonia begins, essentially, as a surface infection with destruction of ciliated, epithelial, goblet, bronchial, and mucous gland cells throughout the respiratory tract. As these cells die, they are sloughed down to the basement membrane. The bronchiole and bronchiolar walls become edematous and infiltrated with predominantly mononuclear lymphocytic cells. Edema and cellular infiltration extend from the peribronchial tissues into the interlobular septa of the lung. Sometimes, whole lobules may be involved by the focal inflammatory reaction and associated necrosis, while at other times only the peribronchial portions of lobules may be affected. These focal changes may develop into localized or generalized hemorrhagic pulmonary edema;

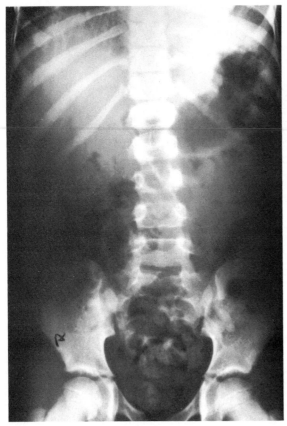

FIG 9–14.
Pneumonia detected on the abdominal film. Since lower lobe pneumonia can present as abdominal pain, it is important to always carefully examine the base of the lungs. In this instance there is increased opacity along the medial aspect of the left lung base extending from above the air shadow of the stomach to the cardiac margin.

then the alveoli become filled with edema fluid, blood, and infiltrations of polymorphonuclear leukocytes. Hyaline capillary thrombosis may supervene, and eventually necrosis and abscess may result. As the process resolves, epithelial regeneration into a "metaplastic" squamous epithelium occurs. In some cases, changes develop that are characterized by chronic well-established interstitial fibrosis.

Radiographic Appearance. If radiographic differentiation of viral and bacterial pneumonias can be made at all, it is only during the acute stages because bacterial infection is often superimposed in the later stages and because as viral infection progresses, it can cause both patchy consolidation due to atelectasis and actual airspace involvement (hemorrhage and edema). The radiographic changes in early viral pneumonia reflect the underlying pathologic changes, namely, edema and inflammatory thickening of the bronchial walls. Radiologically, therefore, one sees bronchial wall cuffing or thickening manifested as rings and tramlines. Vascular margins appear fuzzy because of edema in the bronchovascular sheaths (Fig 9–22). In mild cases, the increased bronchovascular markings are difficult to distinguish from normal, and the line separating normal, "bronchitis," and interstitial bronchopneumonia is quite nebulous. If previous films are available or if evidence of hyperaeration is present, the diagnosis is often more apparent. As pointed out by Griscom et al., air trapping and areas of irregular aeration are often the predominant radiographic features of viral lower respiratory infection, especially in infants and young children. Pleural effusion, pneumothorax, pneumatocele, and lung abscesses are rarely seen in viral pneumonia.

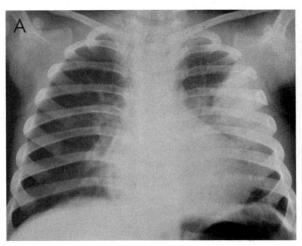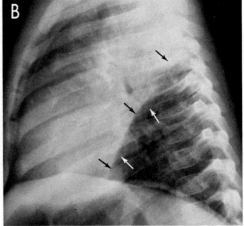

FIG 9–15.
Left upper lobe pneumonia. **A,** frontal, and **B,** left lateral projections. In **A,** the lobes overlap and it is difficult to make a lobar localization. In **B,** it is clear that all of the consolidation lies anterior to the major fissure in the left upper lobe. The small left lower lobe is emphysematous.

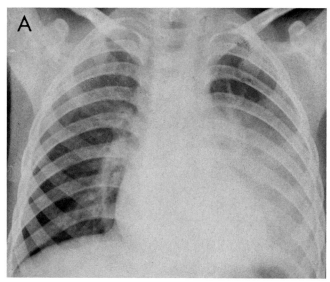
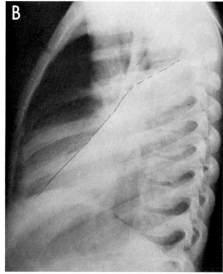

FIG 9–16.
Left lower lobe consolidation. **A,** posteroanterior, and **B,** left lateral projections. The large opaque left lower lobe is limited anteriorly by the major fissure. The left upper lobe is emphysematous. The lower cardiac edge is obliterated by this consolidation in the left lower lobe.

Interstitial pneumonia may present with nodular opacities (Fig 9–23). The figures of Conte et al. demonstrate beautifully the lobular and sublobular types of interstitial bronchopneumonia, which present rounded patches of increased density radiographically. When necrotic, these lobules may calcify, particularly in chickenpox pneumonia. The lobular phase is followed by the development of segmental and lobar edema and hemorrhage, sparse leukocytic infiltration, and some formation of hyaline membranes. During this phase, the radiographic findings simulate those of bacterial pneumonia. Later, segmental lobar edema and hemorrhage may extend to other parts of one or both lungs.

The radiographic appearance may change suddenly due to abrupt alterations in the aeration of dif-

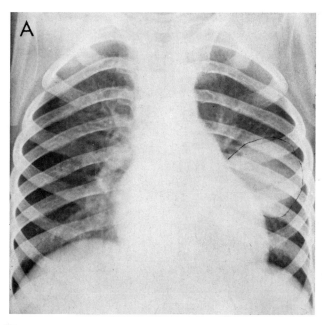
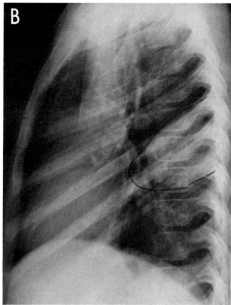

FIG 9–17.
Superior segment pneumonia of the left lower lobe. In **A,** posteroanterior projection, the rounded perihilar shadow suggests "central pneumonia"; one cannot be sure whether it is in the left upper or lower lobe except for the persisting left mediastinal border. In **B,** left lateral projection, the opaque shadow is in the superior segment of the left lower lobe and is in no sense central.

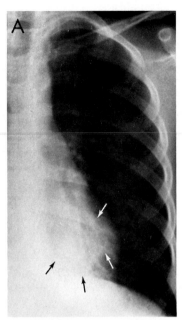

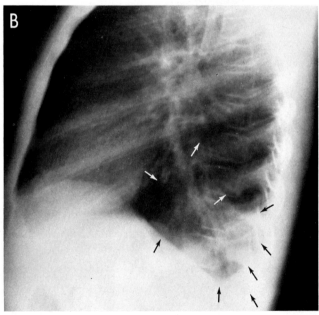

FIG 9–18.
Segmental retrocardiac pneumonia. **A,** In the frontal projection the segmental consolidation is seen through the cardiac image; it obscures the diaphragm. **B,** in the left lateral projection the consoli- dation occupies the inferior dorsal angle of the left lower lobe *(arrows)* and presents with increased opacity of the caudal vertebral bodies.

ferent portions of the lung secondary to sudden shifts of plugs of inflammatory exudate obstructing the bronchial tree. The coalescence of patches of bronchopneumonia may produce consolidations that resemble lobar pneumonia. Massive atelectasis may develop during the course of bronchopneumonia by ball-valve obstructions in the larger bronchi. In these instances, HRCT may be helpful.

The HRCT findings in interstitial lung disease are thickening of many of the septa. These include the interlobular septa and fissures. There is thickening of the interstitium surrounding vessels and bronchi and this frequently gives a nodular appearance. In addition, there may be small nodules (1–2 mm in diameter) which appear quite distinct and not hazy like those seen in airspace disease. In the severe form of interstitial lung disease there is fibrosis and lung destruction with a honeycombing pattern

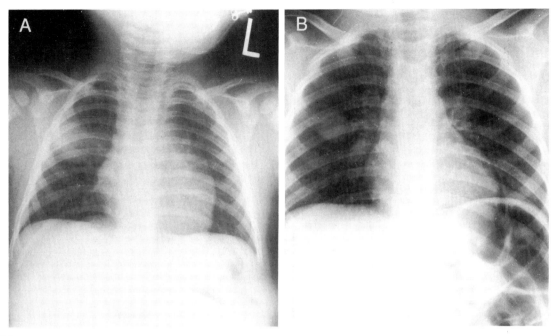

FIG 9–19.
Round pneumonia. Two children (**A** and **B**) with rounded densities in their midright lung field. It is unusual to detect pulmonary nodules or masses as the initial manifestation of metastatic disease. Repeat examination in both these children showed the infiltrate clear. The most common organism is *S.* pneumococcus.

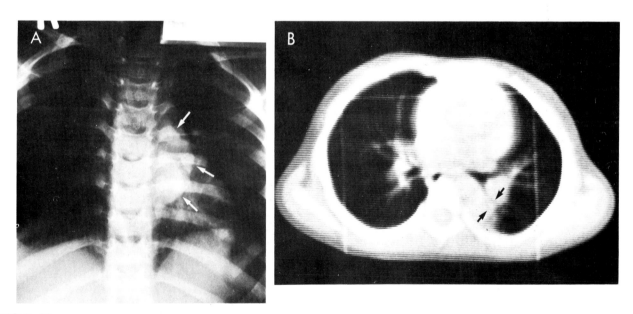

FIG 9–20.
Pneumonia suggesting a perispinal mass—the value of CT. **A,** rounded paravertebral mass density *(arrows)*. **B,** CT scan through the region of the mass density reveals that it contains an air bronchogram *(arrows)*, thus indicating that its origin is the pulmonary parenchyma. This "mass" resolved in 1 week.

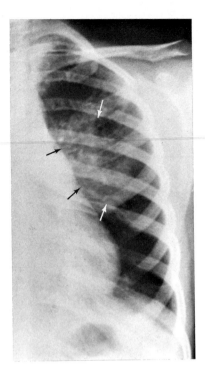

FIG 9–21.
Interstitial bronchopneumonia in the left lung of a 6-year-old girl. The pattern of the consolidation is patchy and stringy. She had cough and fever for 5 days and rales were heard posteriorly on the left side of the chest.

(Fig 9–24). An important clue both on the radiograph and the CT to interstitial lung disease is interstitial air trapping—interstitial emphysema. Table 9–3 lists the various diseases that may give an interstitial pattern.

INFECTIONS CAUSED BY SPECIFIC ORGANISMS

Bacterial Pneumonias

Gram-Positive Organisms

Streptococcus pneumoniae. This organism (one of the two most common causes of bacterial pneumonia in childhood, *H. influenzae* being the other) is a gram-positive diplococcus that infects healthy patients but also commonly attacks those with underlying illness. In the pediatric population, this includes hospitalized patients, specifically those with defective immune systems. A child with sickle cell anemia is particularly prone to pneumococcal infection, with a risk estimated at 20 to 100 times that of a normal child.

In the usual case of an infected "healthy child," the onset is acute with fever, headache, and abdominal or chest pain. The pulse and respirations are quite rapid. By the second day, respiratory symptoms of cough and expiratory grunts, as well as physical findings of rales and pleural friction rub, may appear. Rapid resolution of the clinical findings occur 24 hours after treatment with antibiotics.

The disease is usually confined to one lobe, but only rarely is the entire lobe consolidated. A pattern of homogeneous airspace consolidation is usual but is not invariable, especially in the presence of underlying lung disease. Pleural effusion and empyema occur, although their true incidence is unknown (Fig 9–25). Complications are uncommon; resolution varies but appears to be radiologically complete in about 6 weeks both in adults and children. This or-

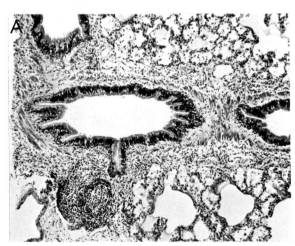

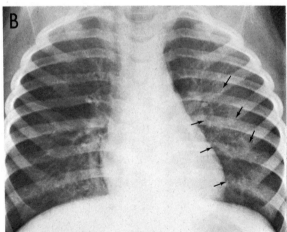

FIG 9–22.
Viral pneumonia in a child of 18 months who died within 48 hours after its onset. **A,** photomicrograph shows a bronchiole surrounded by edema fluid and mononuclear cellular infiltration. **B,** radiograph 24 hours before death shows increased bronchovascular markings in the medial segments of the bases of both lungs due to peribronchial and parabronchiolar cellular infiltrations and enlargements of the branches of the pulmonary arteries. (From Conte P, Heitzmann ER, Markarian B: *Radiology* 1970; 95:267. Used by permission.)

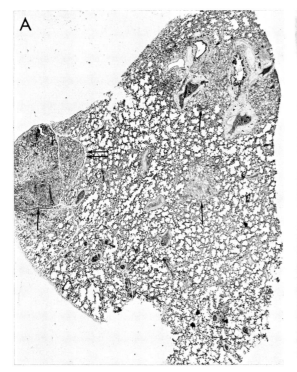

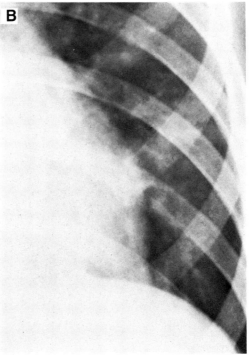

FIG 9–23.
Fatal varicella pneumonia. **A,** photomicrograph shows three peribronchiolar nodules *(single arrows).* The largest nodule represents involvement of an entire secondary pulmonary lobule; it is separated from contiguous normal nodules by a thickened interlobular septum *(double arrows).* **B,** radiograph demonstrates poorly defined nodules in the left lower lobe. (From Conte P, Heitzmann ER, Markarian B: *Radiology* 1970; 95:267. Used by permission.)

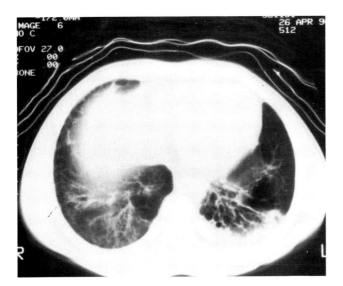

FIG 9–24.
CT of interstitial lung disease. This teenage patient with hypogammaglobulinemia reveals honeycombing at the left base. Thickening of the interlobular septum and areas of distinct sharp nodularity were seen on other sections (see Fig 9–8). Fluffy, poorly marginated airspace disease is noted at the right base.

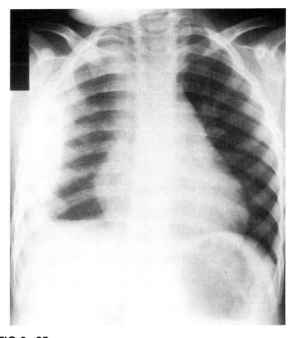

FIG 9–25.
Pneumococcal empyema in a 3-year-old child with cold and fever for 3 days. A pleural effusion is seen on the right side. The patient had a positive pleural tap and blood culture for pneumococci. The child completely recovered within 3 weeks.

TABLE 9–3.

Interstitial Lung Disease in Children*

Interstitial pneumonia
  Viral (acute)
  Chronic
  Desquamative (DIP)
  Lymphocytic (LIP)
  Giant cell
  Usual (UIP)
Interstitial pulmonary edema
  Early left-sided heart failure
  Anomalous pulmonary venous return
  Mitral stenosis
  Congenital lymphangiectasis
Asthma
Cystic fibrosis
In immunocompromised host
  Infection
    Pneumocystitis
    Tuberculosis
    Fungal
    Viral
    Bacterial
  Tumor
    Leukemic infiltrates
    Thyroid metastases
Histiocytosis
Sarcoid
Metabolic
  Gaucher disease
  Niemann-Pick disease
Collagen-vascular disease
  Rheumatoid lung
  Dermatomyositis
  Scleroderma
Neurocutaneous syndromes
  Tuberous sclerosis
  Neurofibromatosis
Idiopathic interstitial fibrosis
Idiopathic pulmonary hemosiderosis
Lymphoproliferative disorder
  Plasma cell granuloma
  Pseudolymphoma
  LIP

*Modified from Hoffer FA, Kirkpatrick JA; Radiology of interstitial lung disease in children, in Laraya-Cuasay LR, Hughes WT (eds): *Interstitial Lung Disease in Children*, vol 1. Boca Raton, Fla, CRC Press, 1988.

ganism is also responsible for most of the "round pneumonias" (see Fig 9–19).

Group A Streptococcus. This gram-positive organism was quite uncommon until the last several years as a cause of pneumonia in childhood. It can occur de novo in a healthy child or follow a viral infection. It produces bronchopneumonia of a segmental configuration with either homogeneous or patchy consolidation that frequently affects the lower lobe. It may be bilateral. Pleural effusion and empyema are common in untreated cases. Lung abscess may be a complication. Clinically and radiologically, this pneumonia is very similar to staphylococ-

cal pneumonia, although pneumatoceles are less commonly seen.

Group B Streptococcus. This infection is a leading cause of sepsis, including pneumonia and meningitis in neonates. Pneumonia may accompany or mimic hyaline membrane disease and be radiographically indistinguishable from it. These conditions are discussed in Chapter 51.

Staphylococcus aureus. This gram-positive organism is a coagulase-positive coccus that grows in clusters. It primarily affects infants under the age of 1 year (70%). In debilitated patients it occurs as a superinfection, particularly in the hospital.

As opposed to pneumococcal pneumonia, staphylococcal pneumonia is a lobular or bronchopneumonia that begins in the airways rather than in the alveoli. Consolidation of peribronchiolar acinar units occurs initially in a segmental distribution. The pneumonia can be very virulent, and severe hemorrhagic pulmonary edema may develop rapidly. Pneumatoceles are more common in this pneumonia than in any other *(S. pneumoniae, H. influenzae, E. coli)* and occur in 40% to 60% of patients. Pleural effusion and empyema are also very frequent, occurring in over 90% of children (Fig 9–26,A and B).

Pneumatoceles are defined as thin-walled air-containing cavities (Fig 9–26,C). By contrast, an abscess is a thick-walled irregular cavity. Each, however, may have an air-fluid level. There are multiple theories for the formation of pneumatoceles in children with staphylococcal pneumonia. Three leading hypotheses are: (1) a peribronchial abscess forms that subsequently communicates with the airway permitting entry of air into this abscess, and then, when the exudate clears, there is development of a large thin-walled cavity, the pneumatocele. The growth of the pneumatocele occurs because of a ball-valve obstruction at the site of the perforation of the airway to the cavity; (2) the pneumatocele is formed by distention of small bronchioles owing to a ball-valve effect secondary to the bronchial obstruction; (3) the currently most favored explanation (Boisset) for pneumatoceles is that they are subpleural collections of air formed by dissection of air from ruptured bronchi or alveoli; the dissection occurs through the interstitium of the lung. Staphylococcal pneumatoceles usually appear during the first week of the pneumonia and almost always are gone within 6 weeks. The pneumatocele occurs when the child is getting better and its presence does not denote any dire prognostic consequences. Ten percent of children with staphylococcal pneumonia will have a pneumothorax and this may result from the rupture of a pneumatocele.

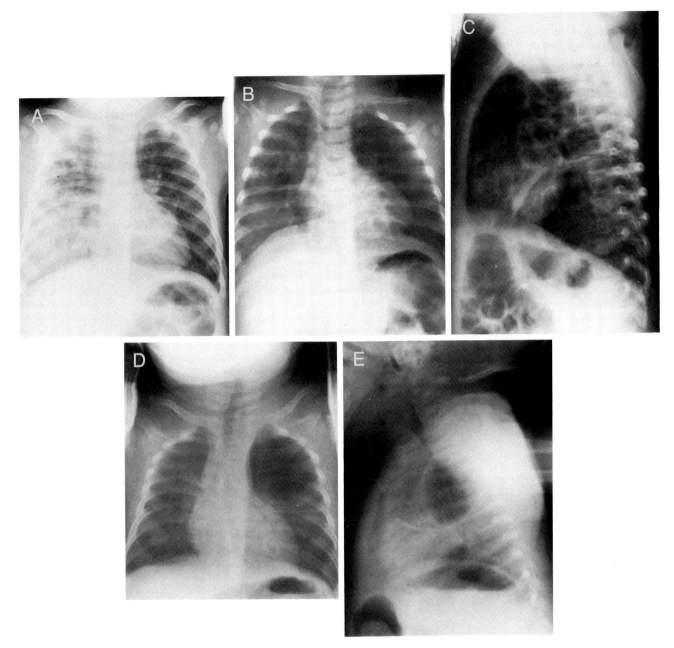

FIG 9–26.
Staphylococcal pneumonia, effusion, and pneumatocele formation. **A,** frontal radiograph of a 4-month-old child with bilateral pneumonia and a right-sided pleural effusion. Vague pneumatoceles are suggested in the right upper lobe. **B,** frontal radiograph as the child is recovering 2 weeks later reveals pneumatoceles in both right and left lungs. There is still residual density with air bronchograms in the right lower lobe. **C,** lateral view shows the pneumatoceles. **D** and **E,** frontal and lateral radiographs of a large left upper lobe thin-walled cystic structure—a pneumatocele in a child with proven *Haemophilus influenzae* type b pneumonia. Clearly, pneumatoceles are not specific for a particular organism.

The incidence of "primary" staphylococcal pneumonia has decreased since the early 1950s. However, staphylococcal pneumonia secondary to septicemia rather than inhalation of organisms is increasing and occurs in older children (67% >3 years of age). This form of "embolic" disease may present with multiple nodular masses (abscesses) (Fig 9–27). This evolving pulmonary pattern in a septic child should initiate a search for a distant source of infection, often in a bone or a joint. Despite the extensive pulmonary disease initially evident, if recovery occurs, it is usually without sequelae.

Gram-Negative Organisms

Haemophilus influenzae **Type b.** The median age of patients with *H. influenzae* pneumonia is 9.5

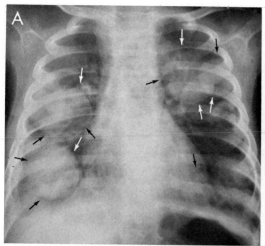
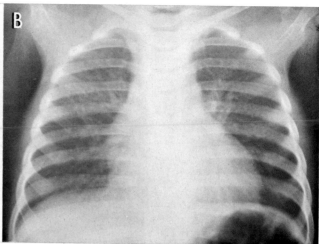

FIG 9–27.
Multiple hematogenous abscesses in an infant 4 months of age. **A,** at 4 months, several large sharply defined nodular shadows *(arrows)* are evident in both lungs. In later films, cavities were demonstrated in the sites of some of these nodular shadows. **B,** at 12 months, no pathologic changes are visible. The patient originally had pyoderma of the scalp and staphylococcal bacteremia. Staphylococci were obtained from the pleural exudate. The right pleural cavity was drained, but the pulmonary abscesses were not treated surgically; neither sulfonamides nor penicillin was available when this patient was under observation.

months and 83% of these infections occur in children less than 2 years old. *Haemophilus influenzae* pneumonia is now one of the two most common bacterial causes of pneumonia in childhood and may coexist with meningitis or epiglottitis. The radiographic pattern is nonspecific and shows infiltrates that often begin as a segmental, interstitial-appearing process, but progress to airspace consolidation (Fig 9–28). Approximately two thirds of cases have unilateral involvement, but more than one lobe is involved 25% of the time. Empyema is a common complication, occurring in about 40% of cases. The current availability of effective vaccines may reduce the frequency of *H. influenzae* type B pneumonia.

Pertussis. *Bordetella pertussis* is a gram-negative organism that causes whooping cough. The incidence of this disease has decreased significantly with immunization but is still seen in infants under 1 year of age, particularly in socioeconomic or religious groups in which immunization has been omitted. A characteristic clinical sign is paroxysmal cough (whoop). Abnormal but nonspecific roentgenographic findings are present in most patients. The classic radiographic appearance is that of the "shaggy heart" (Fig 9–29). Hyperaeration, atelectasis, segmental consolidations, and hilar lymphadenopathy are also found. Radiographic changes may persist for several weeks. Bronchiectasis can be a significant sequela.

Pseudomonas Infection. Infection due to *Pseudomonas aeruginosa* usually occurs as a superinfection in a hospitalized patient with preexisting disease; in children, this organism most often affects patients with cystic fibrosis. It is often difficult to recognize superinfection in these children because of extensive preexisting disease. In adults, different patterns of pneumonia have been reported, depending on whether the infection is acquired through sepsis or inhalation, usually from contaminated respiratory equipment. When the patient is infected by the airway contamination, the process tends to involve both lung bases with extensive bilateral paren-

FIG 9–28.
Haemophilus influenzae type B pneumonia. Lobar pneumonia (right upper lobe) in a 6-month-old infant.

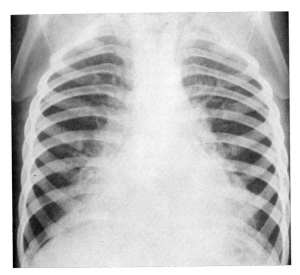

FIG 9–29.
Pertussis bronchopneumonia. Bilateral basilar bronchopneumonia during the active phase of whooping cough. The heart contours are irregular ("shaggy heart").

chymal consolidation, patchy areas of disease with small abscess formation, or small regions of lobular emphysema. In the bacteremic form, widespread patchy or nodular shadows may be found throughout both lungs.

Chlamydia Pneumonia

Chlamydia trachomatis is an intracellular bacteria commonly found in the genital tract where it causes urethritis in men and cervicitis in women. In neonates, it causes conjunctivitis which is contracted during passage through an infected birth canal. *Chlamydia* is a relatively common cause of pneumonia in infancy. The characteristic onset occurs between 2 and 14 weeks of age. The infant is affected with a staccato-like cough and may have conjunctivitis and eosinophilia, although these are not invariable findings. Usually the patient is afebrile, with a radiographic appearance suggesting an illness much more severe than the clinical findings indicate.

The radiographic findings alone are nondiagnostic, although when analyzed in conjunction with the clinical findings, the disease may be suspected (Fig 9–30). Bilateral involvement is usual and occurred in all of the 125 cases studied by Radkowski and associates. The lungs are hyperaerated with increased linear density and patchy areas of consolidation, probably representing subsegmental atelectasis. Lobar consolidation was seen in only 5 of 125 cases; pleural effusion, cardiomegaly, and signs of congestive heart failure were not seen in this series. The clinical response to appropriate therapy is usually rapid.

Spirochetal Infections

The primary spirochetal disease that may infect the respiratory system is congenital syphilis—important here because of its resurgence. Austin and Melhem recently reported persistent diffuse pulmonary infiltrates in three out of seven newborns with congenital syphilis. Visceromegaly and bone changes were also present.

Mycoplasma Pneumonia

Mycoplasma pneumoniae is the most common single cause of pneumonia in childhood (30%), although it has a low incidence in children less than 3 years old (5%). It is spread via the respiratory route but probably needs prolonged personal contact for infection. For this reason, it is prevalent in confined settings such as military recruits and families. This disease is often mild, with low-grade malaise, headache, cough, and fever being the main symptoms. Stevens-Johnson syndrome (erythema multiforme) appears to be a complication in some cases. The diagnosis is established by culturing the organisms from the sputum or by demonstration of rising specific mycoplasma titers. A rise in the titer of *cold agglutinins* is seen in about 50% of cases but is nonspecific; of greater diagnostic value are the immunofluorescent techniques and complement fixation tests for specific antibodies.

In early cases, radiologic findings are those of a fine reticular pattern suggestive of interstitial inflammation (Fig 9–31). This tends to be of segmental distribution and in some cases progresses to airspace consolidation suggestive of bacterial infection (Fig 9–32). Small pleural effusions are seen in up to 20% of patients but hilar adenopathy is common. Bilateral involvement occurs in approximately one third of cases. The radiograph, frequently more ominous than the patient's clinical condition, is slow to clear and lags behind clinical improvement.

Nonbacterial Pneumonia

Viral Pneumonia

Respiratory Syncytial Virus (RSV) Pneumonia. RSV is the major cause of lower respiratory infection in infants and young children, particularly those under 2 years of age. The disease can be virulent and is fatal in young infants in up to 6% of cases. Clinical signs range from mild coryza to severe respiratory distress with wheezing, tachypnea, cyanosis, dyspnea, and retractions. Hypoxemia, possibly due to a ventilation-perfusion imbalance, can be profound and last for several weeks. Bronchiolitis, bronchitis, and viral pneumonia all occur, and it can be difficult

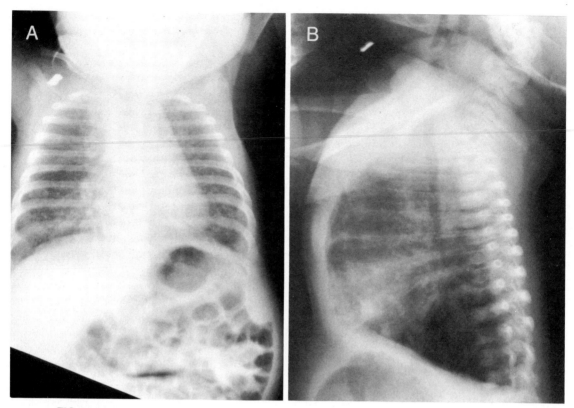

FIG 9–30.
Chlamydia pneumonia in a 1-month-old infant. **A** and **B,** frontal and lateral radiographs reveal hyper-expansion and bilateral basilar densities.

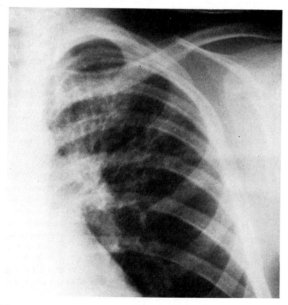

FIG 9–31.
Mycoplasmal pneumonia, interstitial presentation: a teenage boy with left upper lobe mycoplasmal pneumonia. There is bronchial wall thickening, and a linear and somewhat reticular infiltrate.

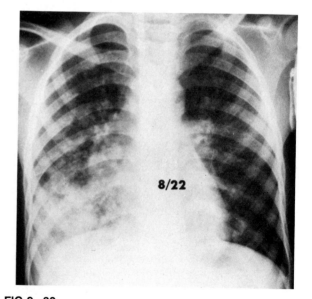

FIG 9–32.
Mycoplasmal pneumonia, airspace presentation. Airspace consol-idation in the right lower lobe, right hilar lymphadenopathy, and a patchy acinar infiltrate in the right upper lobe are visible.

in an individual case to separate one from the other. Children with bronchopulmonary dysplasia are at increased risk for RSV infection. RSV infection is rapidly diagnosed by examining nasoepithelial cells with immunofluorescent antibody techniques.

Radiologic findings are not specific and are quite similar to those in other viral infections of infancy (Fig 9–33) and also to the findings in *Chlamydia* pneumonia, although children with RSV infection tend to be much sicker. Radiologic findings, in our experience, clear slowly and lag behind clinical improvement.

Adenovirus Pneumonia. Adenovirus pneumonia is responsible for about 5% of respiratory tract disease in infants and children, with the peak age being 6 months to 5 years. It is the third most common cause of viral pneumonia behind RSV and parainfluenza virus. Adenovirus has also been associated with a pertussis-like syndrome. While often relatively benign, adenoviral infection may be severe and even fatal in young infants. It can cause necrotizing bronchopneumonia, bronchitis, or bronchiolitis. Radiographic features are nonspecific but usually include bronchial wall thickening, peribronchiolar

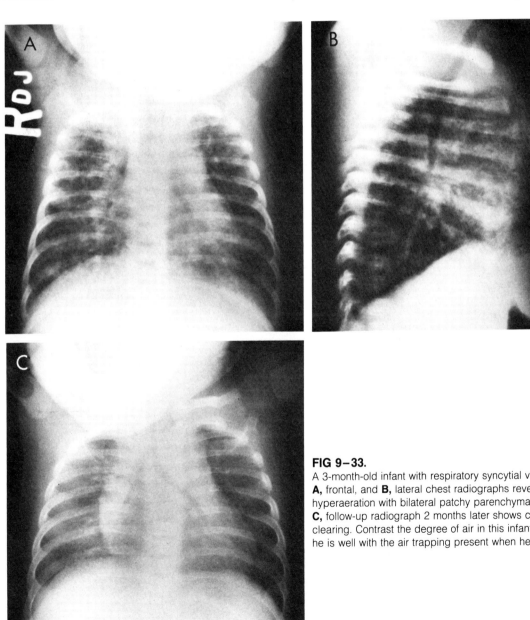

FIG 9–33.
A 3-month-old infant with respiratory syncytial virus pneumonia. **A,** frontal, and **B,** lateral chest radiographs reveal pulmonary hyperaeration with bilateral patchy parenchymal consolidation. **C,** follow-up radiograph 2 months later shows complete clearing. Contrast the degree of air in this infant's lungs when he is well with the air trapping present when he was ill.

densities, air trapping, and patchy or confluent infiltrates. Adenopathy may be more common than in other viral pneumonias. Bronchiectasis or bronchiolitis obliterans may be permanent sequelae. In a series of patients with epidemic adenovirus 21 infection, Osborne and White noted definite residual disease in 13 of 21 patients, 5 of whom had bronchiectasis. Other authors have reported similar complications. Eskimo and Indian children may be at particular risk.

Infectious Mononucleosis (Epstein-Barr Virus). Infectious mononucleosis is believed to be caused by the Epstein-Barr virus. It is a relatively common cause of disease in children and young adults but does not usually cause pneumonia. In teenagers, the disease may be suspected if the tonsils and adenoids are markedly enlarged. On the chest film, one may find hilar and mediastinal lymph node enlargement, often associated with splenomegaly (Fig 9–34). Pulmonary involvement may be seen as bilateral reticular perihilar infiltrates. Small pleural effusions are infrequently seen.

Measles Pneumonia. Pneumonia as a complication of childhood measles is diminishing in frequency because of the use of measles vaccine, but it is still occasionally seen in nonimmunized or immunosuppressed children. Measles virus is thought to

be the cause of giant cell pneumonia, which produces a radiologic picture of a diffuse reticulonodular pattern (Fig 9–35). Hilar node enlargement is common, as is superimposed bacterial infection, usually affecting the lower lobes.

Measles pneumonia in children who have been immunized with *killed* measles vaccine (1960s), and who are then exposed either to measles or who receive live vaccine, has a different course. This "atypical measles" is characterized by a prodromal period of rash and flulike illness associated with radiographic findings of extensive nonsegmental parenchymal consolidation. One or more pulmonary nodules may be present. Hilar lymph node enlargement and pleural effusion are common. Residual nodules may persist for up to 2 years following the acute illness and may be mistaken for pulmonary neoplasms (Fig 9–36).

Chickenpox Pneumonia (Varicella). In children with chickenpox, pneumonia is a relatively rare complication, but immunocompromised children are at risk for progressive varicella and more severe pulmonary involvement as well as meningoencephalitis and hepatitis. These patients tend to be severely ill with extensive rashes and high fever; chest pain and hemoptysis are frequent. Radiographic findings are similar to those of measles pneumonia. Multiple focal calcifications frequently develop following severe chickenpox pneumonia (Fig 9–37).

Cytomegalovirus (CMV) Pneumonia. CMV is the cause of congenital infection of the lungs, liver, central nervous system, and hematologic changes of petechiae, purpura, hemolytic anemia, and atypical lymphocytes. These same systems are involved in acquired disease but the disease is less severe. Children with a compromised immune status are at lifelong risk for CMV infection, and it is frequently seen in patients with the acquired immunodeficiency syndrome (AIDS) and those treated with cyclosporine. In these children, primary infection is often progressive interstitial pneumonitis. The clinical and radiographic pattern is quite similar to that seen with *Pneumocystis carinii* infection.

Protozoan Infections

Pneumocystis carinii **Pneumonia (PCP).** *Pneumocystis carinii,* a protozoan, most often affects immunodeficient children. The clinical onset is variable but often abrupt, with tachypnea, cough, and cyanosis. There is a marked decrease in the arterial oxygen saturation with a normal carbon dioxide level. Perivascular edema progressing to a granular or reticulogranular pattern, especially in the perihilar area, is typical (Fig 9–38). The disease tends to be bi-

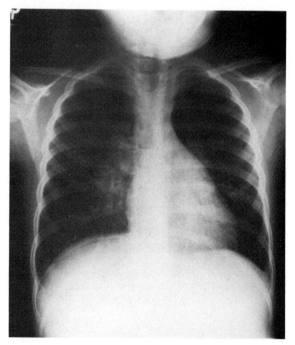

FIG 9–34.
Mononucleosis: a teenager with hepatosplenomegaly and lymphadenopathy. Chest film reveals marked bilateral hilar adenopathy. Lymphoma was considered, but infectious mononucleosis was diagnosed. (Courtesy of Dr. Jack Sty, Milwaukee.)

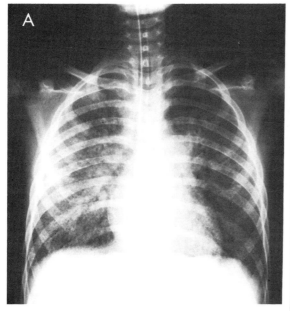

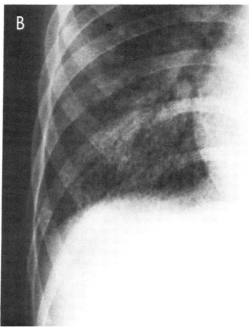

FIG 9–35.
A 12-year-old girl with leukemia and measles pneumonia. **A,** initial radiographic examination shows a diffuse bilateral reticulonodular infiltrate reflecting the interstitial distribution of the disease. **B,** a close-up of the right lower lobe shows the reticulonodular pattern to better advantage.

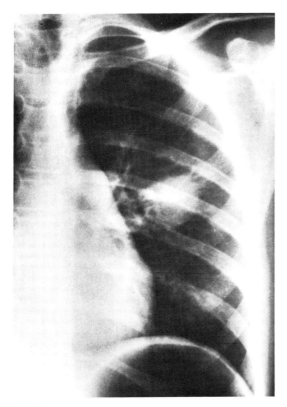

FIG 9–36.
Atypical measles pneumonia. Radiograph shows a persistent pulmonary nodule in a teenage girl recovering from atypical measles pneumonia.

lateral with increasingly confluent areas of airspace consolidation that may resemble pulmonary edema. Terminally, massive consolidation may occur, often complicated by pneumothorax and pneumomediastinum. Pleural effusions are rare. The radiographic findings are nonspecific, and tracheal washings or lung biopsy when positive will show the organisms on microscopic examination after silver methenamine stain (see below).

ACQUIRED IMMUNODEFICIENCY SYNDROME (AIDS)

"Conservative estimates project that there will be more than 3,000 children with AIDS in the United States by 1991" (Falloon et al.). Vertical transmission (mother to child across the placenta) occurs in the majority of affected children. Eighty percent have had a parent with AIDS or AIDS-related complex (ARC). Thirteen percent received AIDS from contaminated blood products. The term *human immunodeficiency virus (HIV) infection* covers the entire spectrum from healthy to critically ill children. AIDS is the most severe form of HIV disease.

The pulmonary complications of AIDS fall into three groups: (1) infectious, (2) noninfectious and non-neoplastic, and (3) neoplastic. In children, neoplasms such as Kaposi sarcoma and HIV-associated

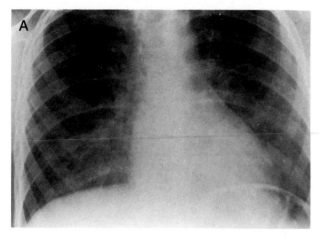

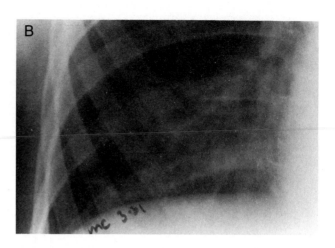

FIG 9–37.
Chickenpox pneumonia in a 6-year-old child with leukemia. **A,** frontal chest radiograph early in the disease reveals nodules at the right base. **B,** close-up of this area shows the nodules to advantage.

lymphomas are uncommon. However, "rapidly growing well defined nodules, hilar and/or mediastinal adenopathy, and pleural effusion" should suggest the possibility of HIV-associated lymphoma (Haskal et al.).

On the other hand, infectious complications in the AIDS patient are common. Bacterial infestation occurs with *S. pneumoniae, H. influenzae, Salmonella, S. aureus, Enterobacter,* and *Pseudomonas.* These infections may be primary or superimposed on a child with viral infection or with lymphocytic interstitial pneumonitis and pulmonary lymphoid hyperplasia (LIP/PLH) (see below).

Infections with RSV, adenovirus, herpes simplex, and varicella-zoster virus occur and may be devastating. Isolated CMV infection is unusual in these patients; rather, CMV occurs with PCP (see below).

Tuberculosis is increasing, especially in HIV-positive patients over 2 years of age. The pathogenesis of tuberculosis in these patients reflects the fail-ure of the normal handling of the organism *Mycobacterium tuberculosis.* In the immunocompetent host, macrophages ingest the organism and present the antigen to the T cells. "CD4 cells secrete lymphokines that enhance the capacity of macrophages to ingest and kill mycobacteria" (Barnes et al.). Since there is both progressive dysfunction of CD4 cells and defects in macrophage and monocyte function in HIV patients, it is not surprising that tuberculosis is prevalent in this population. The chest film findings of hilar adenopathy, pleural effusion, and cavitation are extremely helpful in making this diagnosis in these patients who may have anergy and not have a positive skin test (Table 9–4). Gastric washings and even bronchoalveolar lavage may be necessary to establish the correct diagnosis with certainty.

The most common opportunistic organism is PCP; it occurs in up to half of the children with AIDS. In these patients, PCP may have very atypical and rare manifestations such as enlarged calcified hilar and mediastinal lymph nodes (Groskin et al.).

TABLE 9–4.
Clinical-Radiographic Correlations in AIDS Patients*

	Clinical Onset	Clinical Toxicity	Pulmonary Nodules	Airspace Changes	Adenopathy	Effusion
Bacterial	Rapid	Moderate–severe	0	+	0	±
Viral†	Variable	Mild	±	±	0	0
Tuberculosis	Indolent	Moderate–severe	+	+	+	+
PCP‡	Rapid	Severe	±	±	0	0
LIP/PLH§	Indolent	Mild	Poorly marginated	0	+	0
Non-Hodgkin lymphoma	—	—	Well marginated	±	+	+

*PCP = *Pneumocystis carinii* pneumonia; LIP/PLH = lymphocytic interstitial pneumonitis–pulmonary lymphoid hyperplasia.
†Adenovirus; may have adenopathy.
‡Can have a negative chest film. Effusion and adenopathy can be seen on CT.
§Most children over 1 year of age are likely to have generalized lymphadenopathy and salivary or parotid gland enlargement.

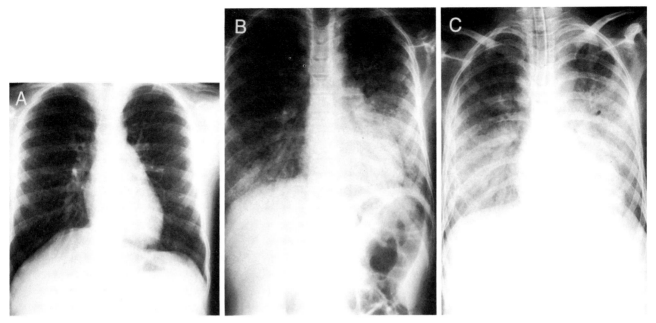

FIG 9–38.
Fatal *Pneumocystis carinii* pneumonia in a 10-year-old child with leukemia. **A,** normal chest film obtained 1 year before infection. **B,** bilateral diffuse reticulogranular pattern involving both lungs dif-

fusely, but with greater involvement of the bases. **C,** there is progression of the disease with confluent airspace involvement. A right chest tube and endotracheal tube are present.

PCP typically is seen in infants of several months of age as the first serious sign of HIV infection. Hypoxia is severe. Air-space densities are seen, and can rapidly progress; intubation and ventilatory support may lead to complications of barotrauma with pneumothorax and air leak. Survivors can show progressive clearing of the chest findings. Unlike in adults, it is the rare pediatric PCP that progresses to cysts and bleb formation, although high-resolution CT no doubt would show more examples of this. (The paucity of CT studies in pediatric AIDS reflects the clustering of cases in urban ghetto areas. Immatron high-speed CT is not available in such hospital facilities.)

The most common (over 50%) pulmonary complication in a child with AIDS is noninfectious and non-neoplastic. It is LIP/PLH. LIP is a chronic condition of "exquisitely interstitial infiltrates of the lung, predominantly lymphocytes with varying mixtures of plasma cell and other elements" (Heitzman). PLH, formerly called hyperplasia of the bronchus-associated lymphoid tissue (BALT) is so commonly associated with LIP in these patients that LIP and PLH are considered one entity.

PLH originally was described as a "perfect" correlation of pathology and radiology, with fine small nodular densities and hilar nodes typical. Such findings do exist, and can be confused with TBC or even histiocytosis-X. LIP-PLH can assume any pattern, from prominent markings to small nodules to large confluent masses. Since biopsies are done less and

less often, the diagnosis often is clinical, based on such findings as chronicity or coexistent clubbing. Cystic changes have appeared in some survivors, similar to the pattern seen in histiocytosis-X. *Bronchiectasis* also has been noted in areas of massive lobar involvement; it is impossible to exclude supervening bacterial infection as the cause of the bronchiectasis, although the history of such infections often is lacking. The HIV virus itself, with production of massive CD8 infiltration of lung parenchyma and airways, could lead to such dilated bronchi in areas of nonaerated lung.

The lymphoid nodules compress the terminal airspaces. These patients have an indolent onset of symptoms leading eventually to dyspnea, hypoxia, and because of the chronicity, digital clubbing of the extremities often develops.

Thus in this myriad of pulmonary diseases the chest film can be confusing. The best way to help clarify the pulmonary changes is to closely correlate the patient's clinical condition with the radiograph (see Table 9–4). While HRCT is not pathognomonic of PCP infection, recent reports in adults (Kuhlman et al., Bergin et al.) suggest the two most common patterns are (1) diffuse perihilar airspace disease and (2) a patchwork pattern of areas of both airspace and interstitial disease as well as spared areas (Fig 9–39). Most striking, air cysts and bullae were found in 40% and effusions or adenopathy, or both, were seen in 18% of patients. When bullae and cysts are present, the reports suggest they represent lung de-

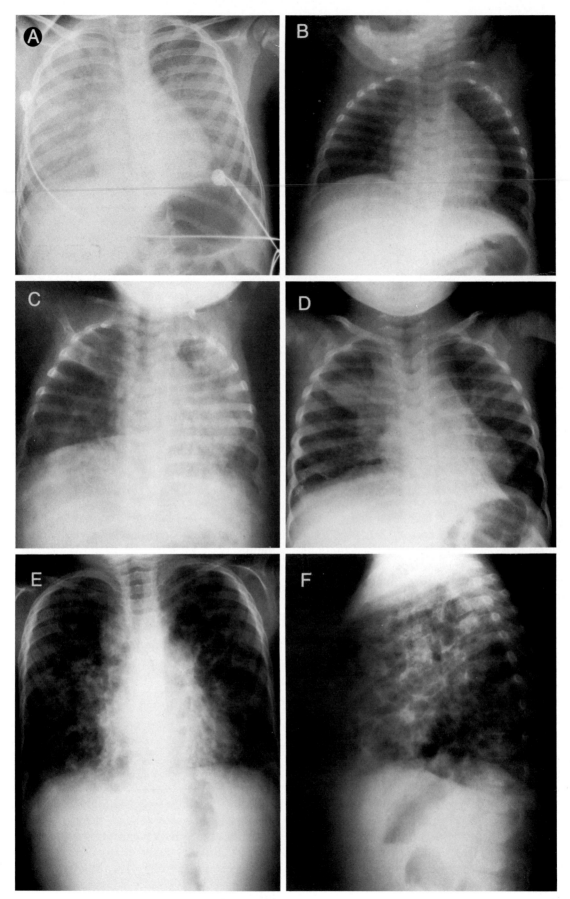

FIG 9–39.
See legend, p 539.

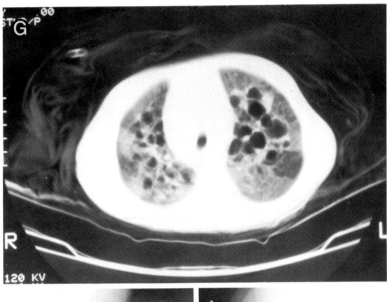

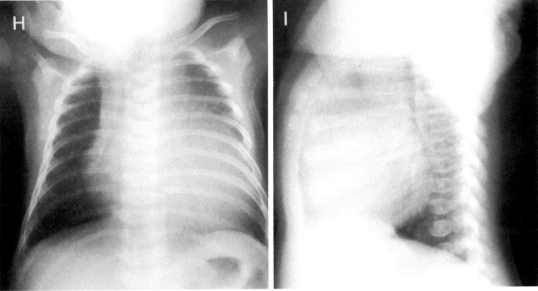

FIG 9–39.
Pulmonary and cardiac manifestations of AIDS. **A,** this 4-year-old child had diffuse airspace disease symmetrically involving both lungs. The child was quite sick with rapid clinical onset of severe disease. At autopsy *Pneumocystis carinii* was found. **B,** and **C,** young infant with *P. carinii* infection. The child was asymptomatic **(B)** but several months later **(C)** he had both airspace disease and interstitial disease. There is atelectasis of the right upper lobe. **D,** a young infant with lymphocytic interstitial pneumonitis (LIP). The child was not very sick. He had areas of atelectasis as well as poorly marginated small nodules throughout both lung fields.

There are clips from a lung biopsy in the right lower lobe. **E–G,** a 6-year-old boy had diffuse pulmonary disease, though he was not very sick. There were multiple cysts. The CT scan **(G)** demonstrates the cysts to advantage. The child at autopsy had LIP with no evidence of *P. carinii* pneumonia. **H** and **I,** frontal lateral radiographs of a child with marked cardiomegaly. There was no evidence of effusion. At autopsy, myocarditis was demonstrated. (Courtesy of Jack O. Haller, M.D., Downstate Medical Center, Brooklyn, N.Y.)

struction from multiple episodes of mixed infections.

Pericardial effusion as well as cardiac disease occurs in AIDS patients. In the study by Haller, 7 of the 26 patients had pericardial effusion without cardiac dysfunction and 18 had concomitant cardiac problems, though only 9 had an enlarged heart. The etiology for the cardiac disease is multifactorial, but at autopsy, myocytolysis, pericarditis, and myocarditis were found. HIV was cultured from the peri-

cardial fluid. All 26 patients had lung disease at some stage of their disease.

Tuberculosis and *Mycobacterium Avium-Intracellulare*

Conventional tuberculosis (TBC) is beginning to appear in HIV-infected patients, with such symptoms as marked adenopathy and atelectasis. Its radiographic appearance is no different than primary TBC, seen pre-HIV infection. Mycobacterium avium-intracellulare (MAI) has been seen with hilar adenopathy (without lung changes), sometimes with coexistent abdominal nodal enlargement. Diagnosis of MAI can be made from blood culture, so biopsy proof of the nodal disease often is lacking.

Leiomyoma/Leiomyosarcoma

Nodules in lung and airways have been seen with pathologic evidence of spindle cell tumors, thought to be of smooth muscle origin. They have been termed, therefore, leiomyoma/leiomyosarcoma. There has been some recent suggestion that they may represent a pseudo-leiomyoma reaction to MAI.

PULMONARY TUBERCULOSIS

Epidemiology

Tuberculosis is caused by *M. tuberculosis*. There are over 23,000 new cases per year (1989) and this number is rising. Young adults ranging in age from 20 to 40 years as well as children (9% of new cases) are being newly infected. Forty percent of new childhood infection occurs in children 0 to 4 years old. There are a significant number of new patients in the immunosuppressed population, particularly the AIDS group. The primary site of involvement in children and adolescents is pulmonary (76%) followed by lymphatic (peripheral adenopathy in 14%), pleural (3.3%), meningeal (2.4%), and miliary tuberculosis (1.2%).

"The portal of entry of the tubercle bacillus in children is by inhalation in 90% of the cases" (Smith). Since children produce little sputum, spread of tuberculosis is seldom from child to child; most often the child is infected by the sputum of an adult caretaker. Congenital infection is extremely rare and is most often secondary to maternal lymphohematogenous spread during pregnancy or to contamination from maternal endometriosis at birth. To document congenital infection, the organism needs to be isolated from the liver as the pathophysiology of both lymphohematogenous spread and endometrial contamination is through venous drainage into the portal vein and liver.

Primary Infection

The length of the incubation period depends on the size of the initial inhaled inoculum. In environments with proven 1-day exposure to an infected person, the incubation period varied from 19 to 56 days (Feigin and Cherry). The incubation period ends when the patient becomes "sensitized," i.e., has a positive skin test.

There is usually a single small primary focus (70%) and it is located most often in the subpleural region (Fig 9–40). From the primary foci the bacilli spread through the lymphatics and to hilar and mediastinal lymph nodes and then to regional lymph nodes. The term *primary complex* refers to combined

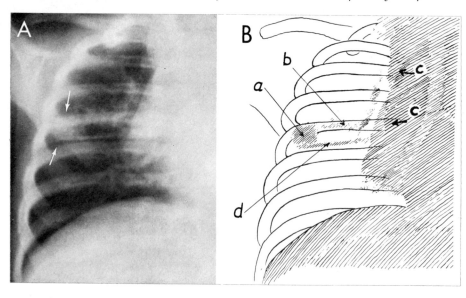

FIG 9–40.
Primary tuberculous complex in an infant 4 months of age. The pulmonary focus is the small shadow of increased density *(arrows)* in the inferolateral segment of the right upper lobe. **A,** roentgenogram. **B,** schematic drawing: *a,* primary focus; *b,* lymphangitis; *c,* enlarged hilar and mediastinal nodes; *d,* loculated pleural exudate.

findings in the pleura, lung parenchyma, lymphatics, and lymph nodes that are associated with the inhalation and implantation of the bacilli in the lung. All the components of the primary complex, including atelectasis and pleural exudate, are shown in Figure 9–40. Once the lymph nodes enlarge, the incubation period is ended. There are three striking features to the incubation period: (1) the patient is usually asymptomatic, (2) the primary foci are quite small relative to the large hilar nodes, and (3) the primary foci can look like any pneumonia and be situated anywhere— all areas of the lungs are involved.

The large lymph nodes may cause bronchial obstruction by extrinsic airway compression (Fig 9–41) with either air trapping or atelectasis, or both (Fig 9–42). Chronic obstruction can lead to bronchiectasis. Calcification occurs after caseation of the primary lesion and is seen earlier in infants (6 months after infection) than in older children (2–3 years after infection). In Payne's study of 299 children with tuberculosis, 165 had calcified lesions within 2 years (Fig 9–43). "The calcium may persist or be reabsorbed" (Smith). Lymphohematogenous spread of "tubercle bacilli from the lymphadenitis of the primary complex are probably disseminated during the incubation period in all cases" (Feigin and Cherry). The host response to the lymphohematogenous spread is varied (clearly immunosuppressed patients do the worst job of containment). The vast majority of *immunocompetent* patients are asymptomatic. A few children present with high spiking fevers, hepatomegaly, and have a positive blood culture (Smith). This presentation represents chronic tuberculous bacteremia. Least often, in very young children, miliary dissemination occurs (Fig 9–44).

Endothoracic Aspects of Primary Tuberculosis

The clinical and radiographic endothoracic response to primary tuberculosis is divided into five categories: (1) asymptomatic primary tuberculosis, (2) endobronchial tuberculosis, (3) pleurisy, (4) progressive primary pulmonary tuberculosis, and (5) miliary tuberculosis.

Asymptomatic Primary Tuberculosis. The child is well and the disease detected because of a "routine" skin test. The American Academy of Pediatrics suggests skin testing in high-risk groups *yearly*. Skin testing at 12–15 months, at 4–6 years, and in adolescence is a reasonable approach to the low-risk child. The child with a positive skin test should have a frontal and lateral chest examination. Most often (80%–90% of children older than 1 year) the results will be normal, indicating adequate host response to the organism. In some patients there will be enlarged hilar nodes or even a parenchymal lesion. Most important, since most children do not transmit the disease to one another, a search for the infected adult must be undertaken. The index child is always treated with antibiotics. There is no convincing evidence that children with positive reactions to the tuberculin test and normal chest radiographic findings have a clinical course or prognosis different from that in children with abnormal chest radiographs. Zarabi and associates analyzed the records and chest radiographs of 180 children with tuberculous meningitis. Almost half (43%) of the affected children had normal chest radiographs. Chest radiography is most useful in following the course of children with recent conversion to tuberculin sensitivity for the early detection of miliary tuberculosis. Occasionally the findings of miliary tuberculosis can be seen on a chest roentgenogram before there is overt clinical manifestations of the disease (see Fig 9–44).

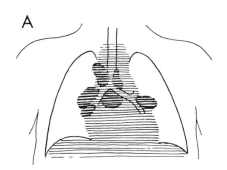
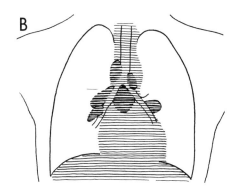

FIG 9–41.
Lymph node distribution. Relative position of enlarged lymph nodes in infants and children. **A,** during infancy, the nodes are located more laterally and are more conspicuous roentgenographically because they project farther laterad into the radiolucent lungs. **B,** in childhood, more of the enlarged nodes lie medially and are partially concealed by the opaque mediastinum, heart, vertebral column, and sternum. (Redrawn from Stoloff.)

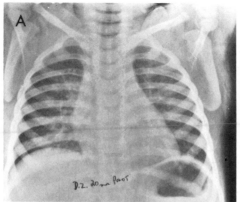

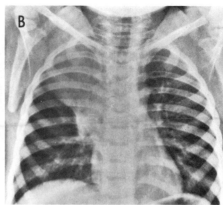

FIG 9–42.
Extrinsic airway compression causing atelectasis. **A,** posteroanterior chest film of an asymptomatic child 20 months of age with a strongly positive tuberculin skin test shows normal findings. **B,** 4 months later there are large shadows of increased density in the region of the right upper lobe. The child was asymptomatic. The findings in her right upper lobe almost certainly reflect atelectasis and resulted from swelling of a regional lymph node during a period of upper respiratory infection.

Endobronchial Tuberculosis. The bronchi are affected in several different ways: exogenous lymph node compression, intrinsic granuloma formation, or both. The presence of obstruction (air trapping or atelectasis in a segmental fan shape always in the segment of the primary complex) in a child who does not appear to be sick suggests the possibility of an inhaled foreign body (Fig 9–45). In these instances recognition of adenopathy on the chest examination or a positive skin test will most often lead to the correct diagnosis. A few patients will require bronchoscopy to diagnose the initial intrabronchial lesion (Fig 9–46). This group of patients will have steroids most often added to the antibiotic regimen. Bronchiectasis is a rare complication of this phase of disease (Fig 9–47).

Pleurisy. These children are usually over 2 years of age and present with fever, chest pains, and symptoms of pneumonia. On the chest film there is a pleural effusion (unilateral or bilateral) and a primary parenchymal lesion (Fig 9–48). The pleural fluid has few organisms, many white cells, high protein, and low glucose content. This fluid is not a good source for culturing the organism.

Progressive Primary Pulmonary Tuberculosis. This is a rare serious complication with progressive

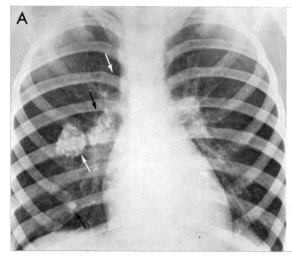

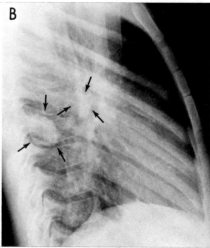

FIG 9–43.
A huge calcifying primary tuberculous focus in the right lower lobe that dwarfs the rest of the complex in an asymptomatic girl 6 years of age. The healing and calcification of this huge necrotic focus without manifest clinical disease at any time demonstrates the often benign clinical aspects of severe structural tuberculous disease. In **A,** frontal projection, the large calcifying focus appears to be perihilar, but in **B,** lateral projection, this focus lies far behind the lung roof in a dorsal subsegment of the right lower lobe near the dorsal pleura.

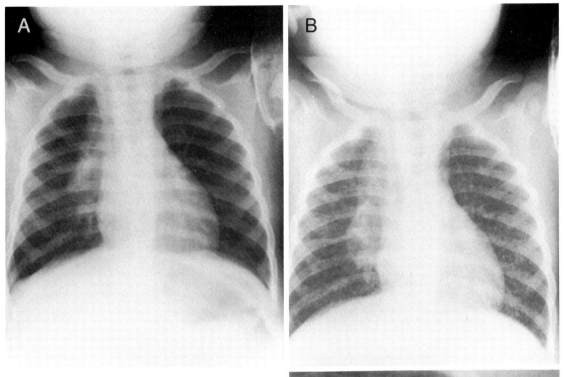

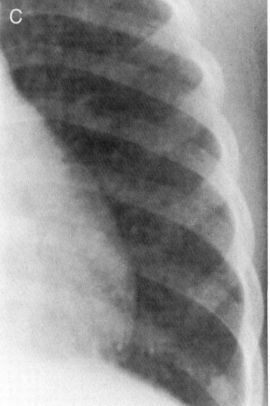

FIG 9–44.
Miliary tuberculosis in an 8-month-old infant. **A,** frontal radiograph
reveals right hilar lymphadenopathy. The airway is shifted to the
left. **B,** repeat radiograph 20 days later shows a diffuse nodular
pattern throughout lung fields as well as the adenopathy.
C, close-up of the nodularity.

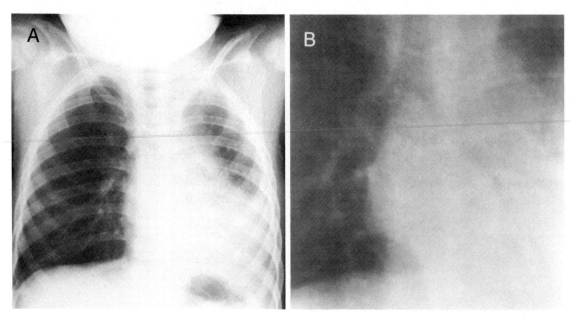

FIG 9–45.
Extrinsic lymph node compression of the airway in a 2-year-old child with tuberculosis. **A,** frontal film shows reduced volume of the left lung with atelectasis at the left base. **B,** high-kilovoltage magnification film shows compression of the approximal left main stem bronchus.

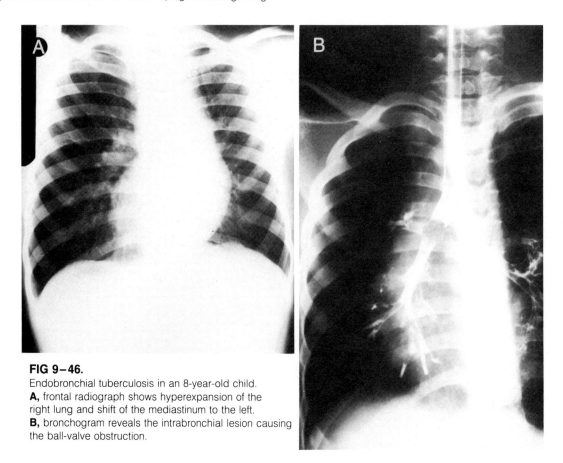

FIG 9–46.
Endobronchial tuberculosis in an 8-year-old child.
A, frontal radiograph shows hyperexpansion of the right lung and shift of the mediastinum to the left.
B, bronchogram reveals the intrabronchial lesion causing the ball-valve obstruction.

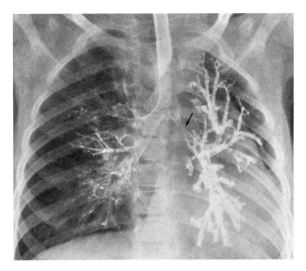

FIG 9–47.
Saccular and tubular bronchiectasis in primary tuberculosis of the left lung and bronchial tree. The left main bronchus *(arrow)* is stenosed proximal to the bronchial dilatation. Shrinkage of the left lung has displaced the heart to the left. This stenosis is probably due to compression by hypertrophied tuberculous lymph nodes. The internal edge of the bronchial wall in the segment of the stenosis is smooth. This boy was 7 years of age.

enlargement of the primary complex, caseation of the lesion, and then liquefaction. The lesion ruptures into a bronchus creating a primary cavity (Fig 9–49). These children are quite ill, have weight loss, and since this complication occurs in the immunosuppressed group it may be difficult to distinguish from bacterial infection.

Miliary Tuberculosis. Once the incubation period has ended, the multiple pulmonary lesions that were present during the lymphohematogenous spread may enlarge giving a "snowstorm" pattern in the lung, liver, and spleen. The younger patients are more prone to this complication and present with hepatosplenomegaly and varying degrees of toxicity. The diagnosis is suggested by the plain film (see Fig 9–44).

Extrathoracic Sites of Primary Infection

Extrathoracic sites account for 20% of tuberculosis in children and include superficial mycobacterial lymphadenitis (70%) (often the atypical mycobacterium and *Mycobacterium avium-intracellulare*, meningitis (10%), miliary tuberculosis (5%), bone and joint tuberculosis (5%), genitourinary tuberculosis (1.4%), and peritoneal spread (1.4%). Though extrathoracic disease is seeded during the lymphohematogenous

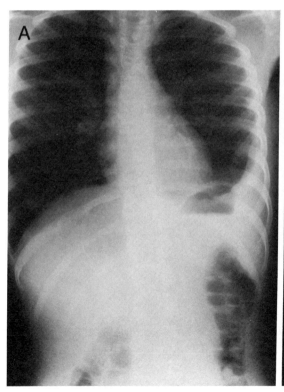

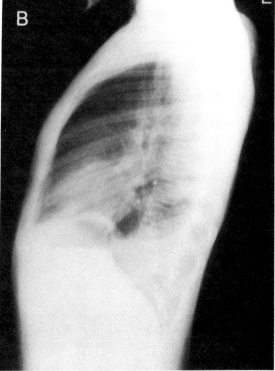

FIG 9–48.
Pleural effusion in a 10-year-old child with a positive skin test. **A,** frontal radiograph reveals a left-sided pleural effusion and a paratracheal right lymph node. **B,** lateral film again shows the effusion and fullness at the hilum.

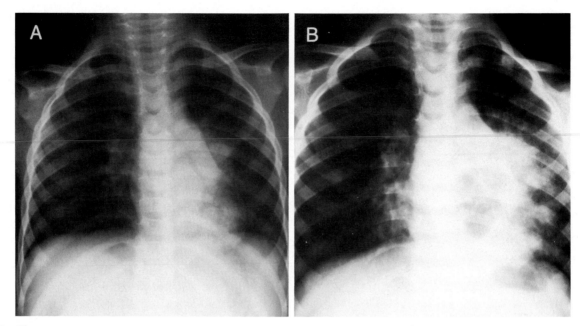

FIG 9–49.
Progressive pulmonary tuberculosis. **A,** frontal radiograph shows consolidation of the left lower lobe with left hilar as well as paratra- cheal adenopathy. **B,** follow-up film shows increased diffuse dis- ease on the left with a cavitation centrally.

spread of the incubation period, manifestation of re- mote disease does not occur for 3 months (miliary and meningeal) to 20 years (genitourinary) after seeding.

Another extrathoracic primary focus results from inoculation with bacille Calmette-Guérin (BCG). This vaccine attempts to replace "a potentially dangerous primary infection" with an innocuous infection which will "activate host cell mediated immunity" (Feigin and Cherry). There is an enlargement of the regional lymph nodes and calcification may occur (Fig 9–50).

Reactivation or Postprimary Tuberculosis

This is the classic "adult" or adolescent form. How- ever, it should be noted that primary tuberculosis is now increasing in this age group (10%–30% of pri- mary tuberculosis occurs in adults). All available in- formation indicates that postprimary pulmonary tu- berculosis is the result of growth of previously dor- mant bacilli in the apices of the lung (Fig 9–51). The reactivated lesion in the apical and posterior seg- ments of the upper lobes are composed of foci of caseous necrosis with surrounding edema, hemor- rhage, and mononuclear cells. These caseous lesions may liquefy and rupture into a bronchus, spreading the bacilli. Cavitation occurs. Reactivation tuberculo- sis is rare in children that were infected with pri- mary tuberculosis before the age of 2 years. It is much more frequent in children whose primary in-

fection occurred after 7 years of age and particularly if they were initially infected near puberty.

SARCOIDOSIS

Intrathoracic sarcoidosis and intrathoracic primary tuberculosis share many roentgenographic features. Some believe that sarcoid disease is actually a non- necrotic, noncaseating type of tuberculosis; others hold that sarcoidosis is a separate morbid entity. Tu- bercle bacilli are rarely demonstrated by staining or animal inoculations, and results of tuberculin skin tests are negative.

The roentgenographic findings are variable and never diagnostic of themselves; a definitive diagno- sis can be made only after microscopic examination of affected tissues, usually excised lymph nodes. In some cases the hilar and peritracheal nodes are greatly enlarged when the lungs are normal (Fig 9–52); in others; the pulmonary changes dominate.

In the report of Merten et al. of 26 children with sarcoidosis, 24 had abnormal chest radiographs. All 24 had lymph nodal enlargement. Decrease in pul- monary function was not necessarily correlated with the extent of pulmonary involvement. Pulmonary function was decreased in the two children with normal chest films. The changes in the lungs may simulate widespread bronchopneumonia (Fig 9–53), or consist of a fine stippling that looks like miliary tuberculosis and some types of silicosis. Tissues

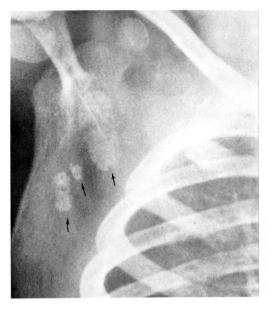

FIG 9–50.
Calcified lymph nodes in the right axilla induced by subcutaneous injection of BCG vaccine into the upper part of the right arm of a boy 4 years of age. Calcifications of this magnitude developed after several months. Similar calcifications appeared in the inguinal lymph nodes following injection of BCG into the thigh.

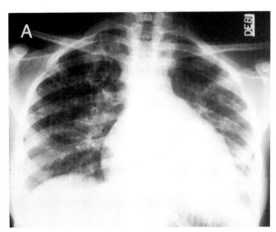

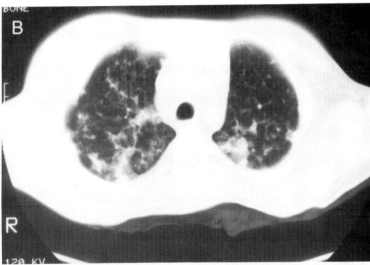

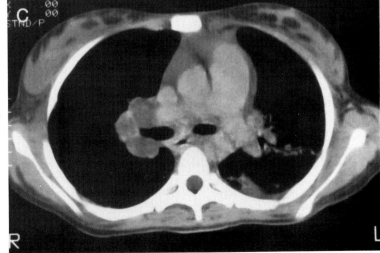

FIG 9–51.
Reactivation, or postprimary tuberculosis. **A,** frontal chest film reveals abundant apical and upper lobe disease as well as hilar adenopathy. **B,** CT scan with bone windows shows the confluent upper lobe and apical disease. **C,** contrast-enhanced CT at the hilum shows the bilateral adenopathy as well as pleural disease. There is calcification present (seen also in precontrast examination).

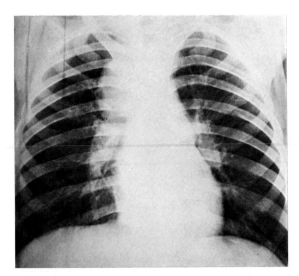

FIG 9–52.
Sarcoidosis of the mediastinum with adenopathy in an 11-year-old boy. The lymph nodes in both hila and in the right supracardiac segment of the mediastinum are greatly enlarged. The diagnosis was confirmed by microscopic findings in the affected nodes. Three years later a radiograph of the thorax was normal.

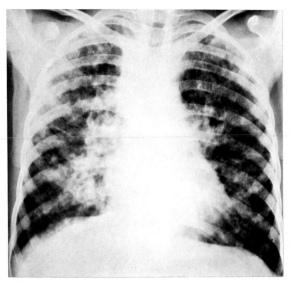

FIG 9–53.
Sarcoidosis with pulmonary and hilar disease. Widespread inflammatory changes in both lungs and enlargement of the hilar shadows are visible. Microscopic examination of a supraclavicular lymph node disclosed changes characteristic of sarcoidosis.

other than the lungs may be affected, especially the uveal body of the eye, the lacrimal and parotid glands, and the skin. Enlargement of the liver and spleen is common. Lytic lesions of tubular bones, frequently seen in adults, are rare in children with sarcoidosis.

PULMONARY MYCOSIS

In general, mycotic changes in the lung resemble tuberculous lesions and include primary complexes, perifocal shadows, necrosis with calcifications, and chronic proliferative inflammatory reactions. There is no conclusive roentgenographic differential between pulmonary tuberculosis and pulmonary mycosis or among the different mycotic diseases in the thorax.

Actinomycosis

Pulmonary actinomycosis is characterized by a chronic inflammatory reaction in the lungs and regional lymph nodes; the pleural layers are also frequently affected. The overlying thoracic wall is often invaded, and both the ribs and the soft tissues may be destroyed (see Chapter 6).

Blastomycosis

The striking feature of intrathoracic blastomycosis is a disproportionate enlargement of the mediastinal

nodes, which may reach a magnitude suggestive of lymphoma or sarcoidosis. The pulmonary lesions are usually inconspicuous save in the case of hematogenous spread, when the pulmonary stippling resembles miliary tuberculosis.

Cryptococcosis

Massive consolidation is common in pulmonary cryptococcosis; cavity formation and mediastinitis are rare. Miliary and bronchopneumonia types have also been found at necropsy. Cryptococcosis may be a rare cause of pulmonary, mediastinal, and abdominal calcifications.

Candidiasis

The diagnosis of pulmonary candidiasis is justified only when the fungus is found repeatedly in sputum that is free of other pathogenic organisms because *Candida albicans* is often a saprophyte in pulmonary tuberculosis and chronic lung abscess.

Pulmonary candidiasis was studied at autopsy in 15 patients by Kassner et al. While they found three distinctive histologic patterns (embolic, disseminated, bronchopulmonary), they were unable to correlate the pathologic findings with any distinctive radiographic appearances. The usual radiographic pattern was one of progressive airspace consolidation. Small lung nodules, which are classically the earliest histologic evidence of candidiasis, were not discernible radiologically, perhaps because of the presence of superimposed disease and the limitations imposed by the small size of the patients and the use of portable equipment. Unilateral or bilateral lobar or segmental patterns also occur. Affected patients are usually immunocompromised hosts or have leukemia or lymphoma.

Pulmonary Aspergillosis

Pulmonary aspergillosis exhibits a great variety of lesions that include consolidation, abscesses, and scattered nodulations. Aspergillus is often present in tuberculous and other lesions, and it may be difficult, even at necropsy, to determine whether aspergillus infection is primary or secondary. These infections of the lungs are uncommon in children. They may affect the immunosuppressed and those who suffer from chronic granulomatous disease. Contiguous infection may spread from the lungs and involve the chest wall. Aspergillosis may be a cause of IgE-mediated asthma. Allergic bronchopulmonary aspergillosis is discussed in Chapter 10.

Primary Pulmonary Coccidioidomycosis

The benign primary phase of pulmonary coccidioidomycosis resembles primary tuberculosis and was first recognized in 1937 by Dickson after the chronic granulomatous stages were well known. The infection is acquired by aspiration of the casual organism *Coccidioides immitis* into the lungs. Endemic areas in the United States include the semiarid regions of California, Arizona, New Mexico, and West Texas. The first infection may occur in infants, children, or adults. Roentgenographic findings and experimental observations suggest that the morbid anatomy parallels that of the tuberculous complex very closely in all phases of the infection.

Roentgenographic examination during the early stages of the clinical disease usually shows a massive airspace consolidation in the lungs with enlargement of the regional lymph nodes. The massive pulmonary shadow of primary coccidioidomycosis is similar to the large perifocal shadow of primary tuberculosis; in view of the absence of physical signs in the chest it seems likely that both alveolar exudate and atelectasis play their parts in the production of this shadow. The massive shadow of coccidioidal infection clears after a few weeks—its duration is usually much shorter than in tuberculosis—and residual calciferous opaque foci appear later in the sites of both the pulmonary and the lymph node lesions. Small localized or large free pleural effusions may be

visualized early. Small, sharply defined, thin-walled pulmonary cavities have been found in many cases (Fig 9–54); these heal by fibrosis and in some instances, ultimate calcification. A conclusive diagnosis of pulmonary coccidioidomycosis can be made only by positive reaction to the coccidioidin skin test or by positive culture of the sputum or gastric washings. There is said to be no mortality in the early benign phase of pulmonary coccidioidomycosis.

Primary Pulmonary Histoplasmosis

Infection of the lungs and tracheobronchial lymph nodes by *Histoplasma capsulatum* is a common and important disease in many parts of the United States, especially in Kentucky, Missouri, Ohio, Tennessee, and Alabama. Extensive surveys by simultaneous skin tests with tuberculin and histoplasmin along with chest films indicate that mild subclinical pulmonary infections with *H. capsulatum* are widely prevalent in these regions. It is also evident that the intrathoracic calciferous foci demonstrated roentgenographically in the tuberculin-negative residents of these areas are, for the most part, the residual healed lesions of earlier benign histoplasmosis rather than lesions of tuberculosis in anergic persons (Figs 9–55 and 9–56).

The early exudative phase is not nearly so well known as the healed stage. The studies of Christie and Peterson in Tennessee describe the initial stage

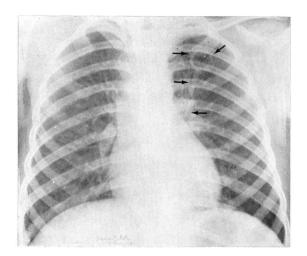

FIG 9–54.
Coccidioidomycosis of the lung: a primary complex in a girl 4 years of age whose skin reaction was positive to coccidioidin. The primary pulmonary focus is excavated into a thin-walled cavity, which is one of the most distinctive radiologic changes in this disease. The strands of increased density between the pulmonary focus and the hilar nodes represent lymphangitis. The regional hilar nodes are enlarged. (Courtesy of Dr. Hugh C. Thompson, Tucson, Ariz.)

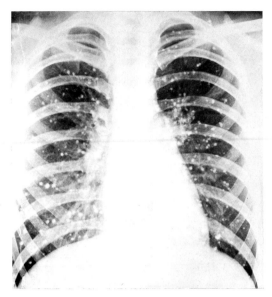

FIG 9–55.

The lesions of disseminated calcifying histoplasmosis were an incidental finding in a boy 15 years of age who was sensitive to histoplasmin but insensitive to tuberculin; the patient was asymptomatic and had never had recognized disease in the chest. The calciferous pulmonary foci may all represent multiple aspirational primary foci, secondary hematogenous foci, or a mixture of or primary and secondary foci. (Courtesy of Drs. A. Christie and J.C. Peterson, Nashville, Tenn.)

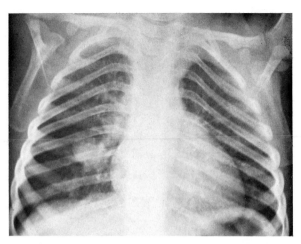

FIG 9–57.

Histoplasmosis of the peribronchial lymph nodes with a presentation similar to tuberculosis; the pulmonary focus is not visible. The shadows at the right hilum are enlarged, and the base of the right lung is emphysematous. The infant had had attacks of dyspnea and was histoplasmin-positive and tuberculin-negative. *Histoplasma capsulatum* was cultured from excised lymph nodes from the right hilum and was identified on microscopic examination of the nodes. (Courtesy of Drs. A. Christie and J.C. Peterson, Nashville, Tenn.)

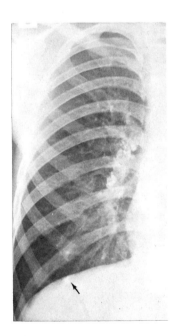

FIG 9–58.

Single calcifying primary complex of histoplasmosis just below the diaphragm *(arrow)* in a boy who was asymptomatic, histoplasmin-positive, and tuberculin-sensitive. Several large calciferous foci are visible in the regional nodes at the right hilum. The changes are identical roentgenographically with those seen in primary tuberculosis. (Courtesy of Drs. A. Christie and J.C. Peterson, Nashville, Tenn.)

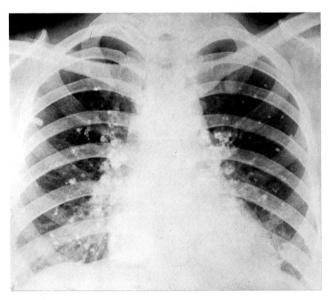

FIG 9–56.

Primary pulmonary histoplasmosis. Large and small calciferous foci in the lungs and tracheobronchial lymph nodes in a boy 14 years of age who was histoplasmin-positive and tuberculin-negative. Intrathoracic calcifications had been demonstrated when he was 5 years old. In repeated tests, he had always had negative cutaneous reactions to as much as 10 mg of tuberculin. (Courtesy of Drs. A. Christie and J. C. Peterson, Nashville, Tenn.)

of the infection in infants and children and its relation to the healed calcified lesions found in older people. The morbid anatomy appears to be similar to that of the primary tuberculous complex, with the important exception that in histoplasmosis large numbers of pulmonary foci are the rule. Occasionally a single primary complex is present in histoplasmosis, and then the roentgenographic findings are identical with those found in primary tuberculosis (Figs 9–57 and 9–58). Disseminated histoplasmosis has been observed during the exudative stage in an infant, and the roentgenographic findings are similar to those in miliary tuberculosis (Fig 9–59).

The diagnosis of pulmonary histoplasmosis rests on the positive cutaneous reaction of histoplasmin and the culture of *H. capsulatum* or its identification in a microscopic examination of excised tissue. The roentgenographic findings appear to be similar to those of tuberculosis in all phases of these diseases, and in some cases they resemble the roentgenographic changes in coccidioidomycosis. Massive hepatosplenomegaly is common in clinically disseminated cases; widespread dissemination is the rule even in clinically inapparent cases. Granulomatous

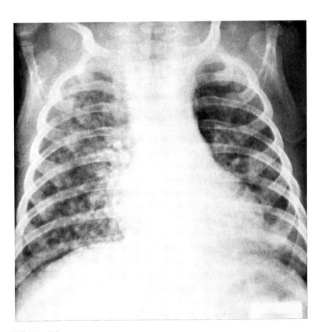

FIG 9–59.
Disseminated histoplasmosis of the lungs in an infant 5 months of age. Numerous foci of water density are visible in both lungs, with the greater concentration in the right lung. It is possible that the pulmonary lesions represent both multiple primary foci from aspiration and secondary foci from hematogenous dissemination. Antemortem culture of the blood yielded *Histoplasma capsulatum* after 3 weeks. At necropsy, disseminated histoplasmosis was demonstrated in the lungs, bone marrow, spleen, liver, and alimentary tract. (Courtesy of Drs. A. Christie and J.C. Peterson, Nashville, Tenn.)

or calcified foci are found regularly in the spleen in endemic regions. In patients that are sensitive to both tuberculin and histoplasmin, abnormal shadows found in the thorax may represent either or both of these infections; in some cases tuberculous and histoplasmal complexes are visualized side by side in the same thorax.

PARASITIC INFESTATIONS OF THE LUNGS

Pulmonary Paragonimiasis

The lung fluke *Paragonimus westermani* is endemic in parts of South America, Africa, and the Far East. Humans are infected after the ingestion of infested freshwater crabs and crayfish. The diagnosis of pulmonary paragonimiasis depends on identification of ova in the stool or from the sputum.

In the Orient, infestation of the lungs by *P. westermani* is said to be a common cause of necrosis and calcification of the lungs in children (Fig 9–60). It seems doubtful that these lesions could be satisfactorily differentiated from calcifying tuberculosis and some of the fungal diseases on radiographic grounds alone.

Pulmonary paragonimiasis has affected refugee Indochinese children in the United States. The clinical manifestations include chronic cough, chest pain, and hemoptysis. The findings in chest radiographs are nonspecific. There are localized segments of increased density in the lungs, which may include small cystic areas.

Echinococcus Disease of the Lung
Echinococcus or hydatid disease is caused by infestation with *Echinococcus granulosus* or *Tinea echinococcus* (dog tapeworm). The radiographic findings depend on whether the cysts are intact or ruptured. If intact, they present as round or oval pulmonary mass lesions of homogeneous density. They may be single or multiple, unilateral or bilateral. Pericystic emphysema may be a sign of impending rupture of the cyst. Following rupture of the cysts, cavitation or abscess formation and bronchiectasis may occur. Cyst walls may calcify.

Other Parasites
Several other types of parasitic infestation may produce clinical and radiographic signs of lung involvement in children. Practically all do so as a consequence of the human lung passage of larval forms in the course of the parasite's life cycle. These include *Ascaris lumbricoides*, *Necator americanus*, and *Ancylostoma duodenale* (hookworms), *Toxocara canis* and *Toxocara cati* (causing visceral larva migrans), and (rarely)

TABLE 9–5.

Conditions Commonly Responsible for Recurrent Infection

Anatomical and physical disorders
  Aspiration syndromes
    Swallowing disorders
      Neurogenic abnormalities, neuromuscular disorders
      Riley-Day syndrome
      Immaturity
      Cleft palate
    H-type fistula, bronchobiliary fistula
    Esophageal stricture or obstruction (e.g., foreign body, tumor, achalasia, vascular ring)
    Gastroesophageal reflux
  Congenital cardiopulmonary abnormality
    Congenital heart disease
    Bronchopulmonary foregut malformation
  Airway abnormality
    Tracheal-bronchial
      Foreign body
      Stenosis
      Anomaly
      Neoplasm
    Bronchiectasis
    Bronchopulmonary dysplasia
    Chronic atelectasis
    Immotile cilia disease
    Alpha-antitrypsin deficiency
    Asthma
    Cystic fibrosis
    Chronic upper respiratory infection (includes sinusitis)
Altered immune mechanisms
  AIDS
  T cell disorders (cellular)
    DiGeorge syndrome
    Hodgkin lymphoma
  B cell disorders (humoral)
    Congenital agammaglobulinemia
    Selective IgA
    IgM secretory component deficiency
    Leukemia
    Hodgkin lymphoma
  White blood cell disorders
    Chronic granulomatous disease
    Chédiak-Higashi disease
    Myeloperoxidase deficiency
    Wiskott-Aldrich syndrome
  Combined B cell and T cell disorders
    Severe combined deficiencies
    Swiss-type agammaglobulinemia
    Ataxia telangiectasia
    Graft-versus-host disease
  Iatrogenic disorders
    Drug therapy
    Radiation therapy

others. There are no specific diagnostic radiographic findings when the lungs are involved.

CHRONIC RECURRENT PULMONARY INFECTION

Specific causes of recurrent pneumonia shown in Table 9–5 have been discussed elsewhere in this chapter. The radiologist's role in the investigation of chronic recurrent pulmonary infection begins with a careful evaluation of the plain chest films, with particular emphasis on reviewing all earlier films and trying to discern whether there is any underlying pattern, if the disease always affects the same area of the lung, an underlying anatomical abnormality or foreign body should be suspected. Recurrent or persistent right upper lobe involvement suggests chronic aspiration. Bronchial wall thickening suggests disease affecting the airways such as asthma, cystic fibrosis, and primary ciliary dyskinesia syndromes. Careful inspection of the bony thorax is indicated to exclude rickets and other nutritional disturbances, chronic trauma, and neoplastic processes.

The airway must be thoroughly evaluated with filtered high-kilovoltage films and fluoroscopy. An esophagogram with a nasogastric tube should be carefully performed to rule out H-type fistula. An esophagogram with swallowing should be done to detect aspiration and other physiologic and anatomical abnormalities. Swallowing function, esophageal peristalsis, and the gastroesophageal sphincter region should be examined closely. The most sensitive test to detect gastroesophageal reflux is a technetium 99m GER scan. It is indicated in cases of suspected reflux-induced aspiration and bronchospasm.

Absence of adenoidal tissue in the nasopharynx after 6 months of age suggests B cell deficiency. The paranasal sinuses are nearly always opaque in cystic fibrosis and frequently in the primary ciliary dyskinesia syndromes. The absence of tooth buds suggest ectodermal dysplasia (Fig 9–61).

HRCT may be used to differentiate between interstitial and airspace patterns and also to exclude underlying bronchiectasis. CT also can determine the presence or absence of hilar and mediastinal adenopathy. CT or magnetic resonance (MR) can also resolve the question of whether a thymus is present e.g., it is absent in DiGeorge syndrome. A ^{99m}Tc-labeled white blood cell scan can be useful to determine whether an infiltrate represents fibrosis or infection.

COMPLICATIONS OF PNEUMONIA

During acute pneumonia, disturbances in pulmonary aeration are frequent. With viral pneumonia, which primarily affects the airways, the lungs are commonly hyperinflated. With airspace disease such as bacterial pneumonia, either hyperinflation or hypoaeration may be noted. Atelectasis is a common accompaniment of infection because secretions fill

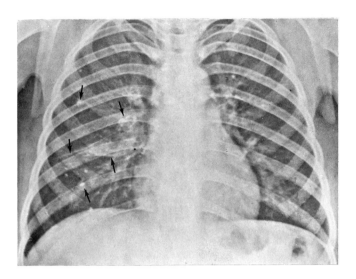

FIG 9–60.
Calcifying paragonimiasis in the lungs of a Korean boy, 12 years of age, whose sputum had contained *Paragonimus westermani* for 4 years. There are multiple calciferous foci in the right lung and hilum that are identical with the findings in some cases of primary tuberculosis. Marciniak found radiographic signs of calcifying paragonimiasis in 60 of 1,000 Korean refugee children examined by him in Poland. (Courtesy of Dr. Roman Marciniak, Wroclaw, Poland.)

the small airways and cause obstructive atelectasis. Empyema is a common complication of bacterial pneumonia, particularly those due to staphylococcus, *H. influenzae* type b, and *Diplococcus pneumoniae*. Less common complications include pneumatocele, lung abscess, bronchiectasis, and bronchiolitis obliterans.

Pneumatoceles

In addition to the general disturbances in aeration accompanying pulmonary infection, localized air collections (pneumatoceles) may develop, particularly in bacterial infections. (See under *Staphylococcus aureus*.)

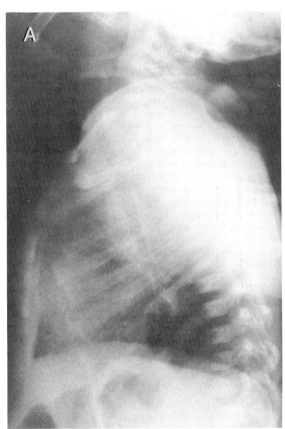

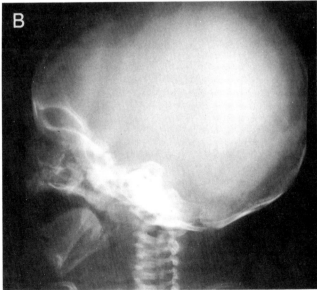

FIG 9–61.
Ectodermal dysplasia. **A,** lateral radiograph of the chest in a 6-month-old infant with recurrent pulmonary infections shows mild strandy densities of the chest but there are no tooth buds present in the jaw. **B,** lateral skull radiograph confirms these findings and leads to the diagnosis of ectodermal dysplasia.

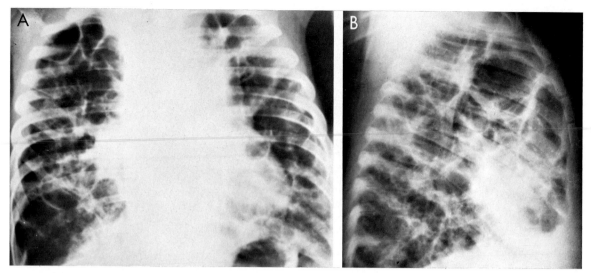

FIG 9–62.
Pneumatoceles with histiocytosis. Bilateral acquired multiple cystic emphysema (honeycomb lung) associated with histiocytosis X of the lungs (necropsy) in a child 3½ years of age. (Courtesy of Dr. R. Parker Allen, Denver.)

Although pneumatoceles are most characteristic of staphylococcal pneumonia, they also form in pneumonia caused by other bacteria such as pneumococcus, *H. influenzae,* streptococcus, *M. tuberculosis,* and *E. coli.* Pneumatoceles have also been identified after hydrocarbon ingestion (kerosene pneumonias) and occur, often multiply and extensive, in histiocytosis X of the lung (Fig 9–62). Differentiation of pneumatoceles from congenital lung cysts may be impossible, particularly if the latter have been secondarily infected.

When pneumatoceles develop in infected areas, inflammatory exudate may seep into them and produce air-fluid levels that simulate lung abscesses (Fig 9–63). Experience suggests that such cavities with air-fluid levels are more common than true lung abscesses. The majority of pneumatoceles are self-limited and disappear without surgical treatment. Even large pneumatoceles with air-fluid levels may disappear within a few days, especially when they develop in pneumonic consolidations. There is no foolproof roentgenographic method for differentiating pneumatoceles from lung abscesses. Necrosis and air trapping probably operate concurrently in the production of many pulmonary cavities. A thin, smooth wall suggests that the cavity is not due to pulmonary necrosis, and conversely, a thick irregular wall is often demonstrable in a true lung abscess.

Lung Abscess

Abscesses are areas of necrosis surrounded by zones of inflammatory consolidation. Their radiographic appearance is determined by the relative amounts of

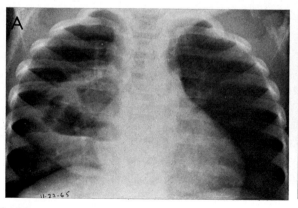
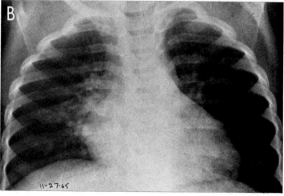

FIG 9–63.
Multiple loculated pneumatoceles. Complete disappearance over a period of 5 days of a large multiloculated pneumatocele in a segment of alveolar consolidation. In **A,** there is a large cavity with two air-fluid levels in a segment of alveolar pneumonia in the right upper lobe. In **B,** 5 days later, the cavity and most of the pneumonic consolidation have disappeared.

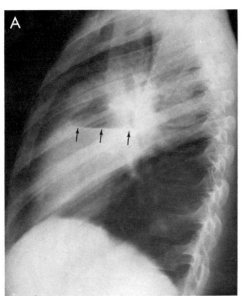
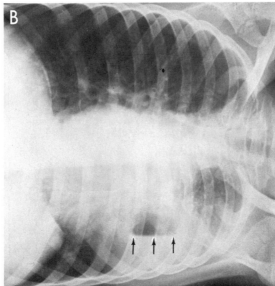

FIG 9–64.
Lung abscess. Large solitary pulmonary abscess in the left upper lobe. **A,** left lateral projection with the patient erect. **B,** posteroanterior projection with the patient horizontal and the left side down.

A large necrotic cavity filled with fluid and gas and surrounded by a large area of consolidation is located in the left lung. Shift of the gas-fluid level with change in position of the patient is evident.

necrosis and consolidation and the amount of gas in the necrotic cavity (Fig 9–64). In early stages of abscess formation, a discrete pneumonic consolidation is apparent, with no definite cavity visualized. Contrast-enhanced CT at this stage may show a low-

density center and presage the development of an abscess. When a cavity reaches sufficient size and is filled with gas, a gas-fluid level will be demonstrated that shifts with a change in the position of the patient.

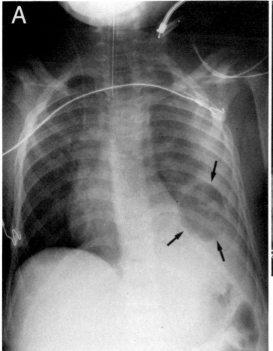
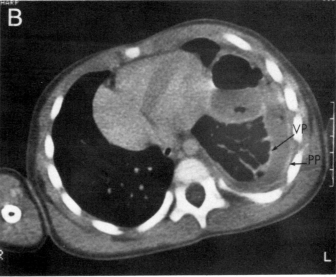

FIG 9–65.
Bronchopleural fistula and empyema simulating a lung abscess. **A,** a 4-year-old mentally retarded patient developed a cavitary lesion *(arrows)* in the left lower lobe that was associated with pleural disease. The patient was being treated for a lung abscess. **B,** contrast-enhanced CT scan reveals the air and fluid–containing cavity to be in the pleural space, thus demonstrating the lesion to be a bronchopleural fistula and empyema rather than a lung abscess. This was subsequently drained with a tube thoracotomy. *VP,* visceral pleura; *PP,* parietal pleura.

The resemblance of lung abscesses to pneumatoceles can be confusing in some cases. Pneumatoceles may also contain gas-fluid levels, but a true lung abscess has a thicker, somewhat shaggy wall. An abscess can also be confused with empyema complicated by a bronchopleural fistula. CT is a reliable method of distinguishing the two, as discussed in Chapter 6 (Fig 9–65). Multiple small lung abscesses are commonly present in children with cystic fibrosis; with this exception, lung abscesses are now quite uncommon in children.

For a discussion of empyema, see Chapter 6.

CHRONIC EFFECTS OF PNEUMONIA

Most cases of pneumonia in childhood resolve completely, even in the presence of the complications discussed above. However, a few children do develop chronic complications from the primary infections. Increased susceptibility to infection in the same region of the lung occurs in some children and may be the result of underlying damage to the airways in this region. Following a severe viral pneumonia, especially adenovirus, a postobliterative bronchiolitis may develop (Swyer-James syndrome). This is discussed more completely in Chapter 8. Bronchiectasis may also occur as a result of chronic recurrent pulmonary infection and is particularly frequent in cystic fibrosis and primary ciliary dyskinesia syndromes, as well as in chronically atelectatic and infected lobes.

REFERENCES

Alario AJ, McCarthy PL, Markowitz R, et al: Usefulness of chest radiographs in children with acute lower respiratory tract disease. *J Pediatr* 1987; 111:187.

Barrett FF: Bacterial pneumonia of infants and children in Laraya-Cuasay LR, Hugh WT (eds): *Interstitial Lung Diseases in Children*, vol. 1. Boca Raton, Fla, CRC Press, 1988.

Bessis L, Callard P, Gotheil C, et al: High-resolution CT of parenchymal lung disease: Precise correlation with histologic findings. *RadioGraphics* 1992; 12:45.

Christy C, Powell KR: Pneumonia in children: Tracking the cause. *J Respir Dis* 1987; 8:65.

Conte P, Heitzman ER, Markarian B: Viral pneumonia: Roentgen-pathological correlation. *Radiology* 1970; 95:267.

Crain EF, Bulas D, Bijur P, et al: Is a chest radiograph necessary in the evaluation of every febrile infant less than 8 weeks of age? *J Pediatr* 1991; 88:821.

Eggleston DE, Slovis TL, Watts FB: Update on pediatric chest imaging. *Pediatr Pulmonol* 1988; 5:158.

Friis B, Eiken M, Hornsleth A, et al: Chest x-ray appearances in pneumonia and bronchiolitis. *Acta Paediatr Scand* 1990; 7:219.

Galvin JR, Mori M, Stanford W: High-resolution computed tomography and diffuse lung disease. *Curr Probl Diagn Radiol* 1992; 21(2).

Griscom NT: Pneumonia in children and some of its variants. *Radiology* 1988; 167:297.

Griscom NT: Respiratory problems of early life now allowing survival into adulthood: Concepts for radiologists. *AJR* 1992; 158:1-8.

Griscom NT, Wohl MEB, Kirkpatrick JA: Lower respiratory infections: How infants differ from adults. *Radiol Clin North Am* 1978; 16:367.

Haller JO, Slovis TL: *Introduction to Radiology in Clinical Pediatrics.* St Louis, Mosby–Year Book, 1984.

Hoffer FA, Kirkpatrick JA: Radiology of interstitial lung disease in children, in Laraya-Cuasay LR, Hugh WT (eds): *Interstitial Lung Diseases in Children*, vol I. Boca Raton Fla, CRC Press, 1988.

Katz JA, Bash R, Rollins N, et al: The yield of routine chest radiography in children with cancer hospitalized for fever and neutropenia. *Cancer* 1991; 68:940.

Kuhn JP: Pediatric thorax, in Naidich DP, Zerhouni EA, Siegelman SS (eds): *Computed Tomography and Magnetic Resonance of the Thorax*, ed. 2, New York, Raven Press, 1991.

Heulitt MJ, Ablow RC, Santos CC: Febrile infants less than 3 months old: Value of chest radiography. *Radiology* 1988; 167:135.

McGuiness G, Naidich DP, Jagirdar J, et al: High resolution CT findings in miliary lung disease. *J Comput Assist Tomogr* 1992; 16:384.

Maheshwari A, Nelson DR, Sharma OP: Acute empyema: Down but not out. *J Respir Dis* 1992; 13:47.

Mayo JR: The high-resolution computed tomography technique. *Semin Roentgenol* 1991; 26:104.

Meza MP, Slovis TL: Pediatric chest CT. *J Respir Dis* 1992; 13:240–250.

Müller NL: Clinical value of high-resolution CT in chronic diffuse lung disease. *AJR* 1991; 157:1163.

Murphy TF, Henderson FW, Clyde WA Jr, et al: Pneumonia: An eleven year study in pediatric practice. *Am J Epidemiol* 1981; 113:12.

Naidich DP, Zerhouni EA, Siegelman SS: *Computed Tomography and Magnetic Resonance of the Thorax*, ed 2, New York, Raven Press, 1991.

Nishimura K, Kitaichi M, Izumi T, et al: Unusual interstitial pneumonia: Histologic correlation with high-resolution CT. *Radiology* 1992; 182:337.

Pare JAP, Fraser RG: *Diseases of the Chest.* Philadelphia, WB Saunders, 1983.

Patterson RJ, Bissett GS III, Kirks DR, et al: Chest radiographs in the evaluation of the febrile infant. *AJR* 1990; 155:833.

Poznanski A: *Practical Techniques in Pediatric Radiology.* St Louis, Mosby–Year Book, 1976.

Rose RW, Ward BH: Spherical pneumonias in children simulating pulmonary and mediastinal masses. *Radiology* 1973; 106:179.

Stern EJ, Webb WR, Golden JA, et al: Cystic lung disease associated with eosinophilic granuloma and tuberous sclerosis: Air trapping at dynamic ultrafast high-resolution CT. *Radiology* 1992; 182:325.

Suchet IB, Horwitz TA: CT in tuberculous constrictive pericarditis. *J Comput Assist Tomogr* 1992; 16:391.

Swensen SJ, Aughenbaugh GL, Douglas WW, et al: High-resolution CT of the lungs: Findings in various pulmonary diseases. *AJR* 1992; 158:971.

Theros EG: Value of radiologic-pathologic correlation in the education of the radiologist. Hickey lecture. *Am J Roentgenol* 1969; 107:235.

Webb WR: High-resolution computed tomography of the lung: Normal and abnormal anatomy. *Semin Roentgenol* 1991; 26:110.

Wood BP, Anderson VM, Mauk JE, et al: Pulmonary lymphatic air: Locating "pulmonary interstitial emphysema" of the premature infant. *Am J Roentgenol* 1982; 138:809.

Zwirewich CV, Mayo JR, Müller NL: Low-dose high-resolution CT of lung parenchyma. *Radiology* 1991; 180:413–417.

Infections Caused by Specific Agents

Asmar BI, Slovis TL, Reed JO, et al: *Haemophilus influenzae* type B pneumonia in 43 children. *J Pediatr* 1978; 93:389.

Austin R, Melhem RE: Pulmonary changes in congenital syphilis. *Pediatr Radiol* 1991; 21:404.

Boisset GF: Subpleural emphysema complicating staphylococcal and other pneumonias. *J Pediatr* 1972; 81:259.

Buff SJ, McClelland R, Gallis HA: *Candida albicans* pneumonia: Radiographic appearance. *AJR* 1982; 138:645.

Eriksson J, Nordshus T, Carlson KH, et al: Radiological findings in children with respiratory syncytial virus infection: Relationship to clinical and bacterial findings. *Pediatr Radiol* 1986; 16:120.

Felman AH, Shulman ST: Staphylococcal osteomyelitis, sepsis and pulmonary disease: Observation of 10 patients with combined osseous and pulmonary infections. *Radiology* 1975; 117:649.

Gold R, Wilt JC, Adhikari PK, et al: Adenoviral pneumonia and its complications in infancy and childhood. *J Can Assoc Radiol* 1969; 20:218.

Gouliamos AD, Kalovidouris A, Papailion J, et al: CT appearance of pulmonary hydatid disease. *Chest* 1991; 100:1578.

Gruenbaum M: Radiological manifestation of lung *Echinococcus* in children. *Pediatr Radiol* 1975; 3:65.

Hall CB, Hall WJ, Speers DM: Clinical and physiological manifestations of bronchiolitis and pneumonia: Outcome of respiratory syncytial virus. *Am J Dis Child* 1979; 133:798.

Hanparin UV, Cramblett HG: Viral etiology of respiratory illness, in Kendig EL, Chernig V (eds): *Disorders of the Respiratory Tract in Childhood.* Philadelphia, WB Saunders. 1983.

Kassner EG, Kaufman SL, Yoon JJ, et al: Pulmonary candidiasis in infants: Clinical, radiologic, and pathologic features. *Am J Roentgenol* 1981; 137:707.

Lunicao GG, Heggie AD: Chlamydial infection. *Pediatr Clin North Am* 1979; 26:269.

McCarthy PL, Spiesel SZ, Stachwick CA, et al: Radiographic findings and etiologic diagnosis in ambulatory childhood pneumonias. *Clin Pediatr (Phila)* 1981; 20:686.

Osborne D: Radiologic appearance of viral disease of the lower respiratory tract in infants and children. *Am J Roentgenol* 1978; 130:29.

Osborne E, White P: Radiology of epidemic adenovirus 21 infection of the lower respiratory tract in infants and young children. *Am J Roentgenol* 1979; 133:397.

Radkowski M, Pranzler JK, Beem MO: Chlamydia pneumonia in infants: Radiography in 125 cases. *Am J Roentgenol* 1981; 137:703.

Schultz G: Unusual roentgen manifestations of primary staphylococcal pneumonia in infants and young children. *Am J Roentgenol* 1959; 81:290.

Swischuk LE, Hayden CK: Viral vs bacterial pulmonary infections in children (is roentgenographic differentiation possible?). *Pediatr Radiol* 1986; 16:278.

Wildin SR, Chonmaitree T, Swischuk LE: Roentgenographic features of common pediatric viral respiratory tract infections. *Am J Dis Child* 1988; 142:43.

Acquired Immunodeficiency Syndrome (AIDS)

Ambrosino MM, Genieser NB, Krasinski K, et al: Opportunistic infections and tumors in immunocompromised children. *Radiol Clin North Am* 1992; 30:639–658.

Amorosa JK, Miller R, Cuasay L, et al: Bronchiectasis in children with LIP and AIDS. *Pediatr Radiol,* in press.

Ball F: X-ray diagnosis of immunologically induced lung diseases in children and adolescents. *RADIOLOGE* 1990; 30:303–309.

Balsam D, Segal S: Multiple smooth muscle tumors in an HIV infected child. *Pediatr Radiol,* in press.

Barnes PF, Bloch AB, Davidson PT, et al: Tuberculosis in patients with human immunodeficiency virus infection. *N Engl J Med* 1991; 324:1642.

Bergin CJ, Wirth RL, Berry GJ, et al: *Pneumocystis carinii* pneumonia: CT and HRCT observations. *J Comput Assist Tomogr* 1990; 14:756.

Bradford BF, Abdenour GE Jr, Frank JL, et al: Usual and unusual radiologic manifestations of acquired immunodeficiency syndrome (AIDS) and human immunodeficiency virus (HIV) infection in children. *Radiol Clin North Am* 1988; 26:341.

Bye MR, Bernstein LJ: Identifying pulmonary sequelae in children with AIDS. *J Respir Dis* 1989; 10:27.

Connor E, Bagarazzi M, McSherry G, et al: Clinical and laboratory correlates of *Pneumocystis carinii* pneumonia in children infected with HIV. *JAMA* 1991; 265:1693.

Falloon J, Eddy J, Wiener L, et al: Human immunodeficiency virus infection in children. *J Pediatr* 1989; 114:1.

Goldman HS, Ziprokowski MN, Charyton M, et al: Lymphocytic interstitial pneumonitis in children with AIDS: A perfect radiologic-pathologic correlation. Presented at 28th Annual Meeting of the Society for Pediatric Radiology, April 18–21, 1985.

Goodman PC: Pulmonary disease in children with AIDS. *J Thorac Imaging* 1991; 6:60–64.

Groskin SA, Massi AF, Randall PA: Calcified hilar and mediastinal lymph nodes in an AIDS patient with *Pneumocystis carinii* infection. *Radiology* 1990; 175:345.

Grattan-Smith D, Harrison LF, Singleton ED: Radiology of AIDS in the pediatric patient. *Curr Probl Diagn Radiol* 1991; 21:(3).

Haller JO: Pericardial effusion and its relationship to cardiac disease in children with AIDS. Presented at the American Roentgen Ray Society Annual Meeting, Boston, May 1991.

Haney PJ, Yal-Loehr AJ, Nussbaum AR, et al: Imaging of infants and children with AIDS: Review. *Am J Roentgenol* 1989; 152:1033.

Haskal ZJ, Lindan CE, Goodman PC: Lymphoma in the immunocompromised patient. *Radiol Clin North Am* 1990; 28:885.

Heitzman ER: Pulmonary neoplastic and lymphoproliferative disease in AIDS: A review. *Radiology* 1990; 177:347.

Joshi VV: Pathology of childhood AIDS. *Pediatr Clin North Am* 1991; 38:97–120.

Kuhlman JE, Kavuru M, Fishman EK, et al: *Pneumocystis carinii* pneumonia: Spectrum of parenchymal CT findings. *Radiol* 1990; 175:711.

Marolda J, Pace B, Bonforte RJ, et al: Pulmonary manifestations of HIV infection in children. *Pediatr Pulmonol* 1991; 19:231–235.

Marquis J: Further observations of interstitial patterns in chest x-rays of HIV infected children. Presented at the 35th Annual Meeting, Society for Pediatric Radiology Orlando, Fla, May 14–17, 1992.

Naidich DP, McGuinness G: Pulmonary manifestations of AIDS CT and radiographic correlations. *Radiol Clin North Am* 1991; 29:999–1017.

Nicholas SW: Management of the HIV-positive child with fever. *J Pediatr* 1991; 119:S21.

Panicek DM: Cystic pulmonary lesions in patients with AIDS. *Radiology* 1989; 173:12.

Saldana MJ, Mones JM: Lymphoid interstitial pneumonia in HIV infected individuals. *Prog Surg Pathol* 1992; 12:181–215.

Sandhu JS, Goodman PC: Pulmonary cysts associated with *Pneumocystis carinii* pneumonia in patients with AIDS. *Radiology* 1989; 173:33–35.

Tovo PA, DeMartino M, Gabiano C, et al: Prognostic factors and survival in children with perinatal HIV-1 infection. *Lancet* 1992; 2:1249–1253.

Zimmerman BL, Haller JO, Price AP, et al: Children with AIDS—is pathologic diagnosis possible based on chest radiographs? *Pediatr Radiol* 1987; 17:303.

Pulmonary Tuberculosis and Sarcoidosis

American Academy of Pediatrics Committee on Infectious Diseases: Chemotherapy for tuberculosis in infants and children. *Pediatrics* 1992; 89:161.

Abdulla F, Dietrich KA: Endobronchial tuberculosis manifested as obstructive airway disease in a 4 month old infant. *South Med J* 1990; 83:715.

Buckner CB, Leithiser RE, Walker CW, et al: The changing epidemiology of tuberculosis and other mycobacterial infections in the United States: Implications for the radiologist. *Am J Roentgenol* 1991; 156:255.

Caglayan S, Coteli I, Ascar U, et al: Endobronchial tuberculosis simulating foreign body aspiration. *Chest* 1989; 95:1164.

Cameron C: The point of entry of tuberculous infection. *Lancet* 1943; 2:1275.

Choe KO, Jeong HJ, Sohn HY: Tuberculous bronchial stenosis: CT findings in 28 cases. *AJR* 1990; 155:971.

Daly FJ, Brown DS, Lincoln EM, et al: Endobronchial tuberculosis in children. *Dis Chest* 1952; 22:380.

Feigin RD, Cherry JD: *Textbook of Pediatric Infectious Diseases,* ed 2. Philadelphia, WB Saunders, 1987.

Ghon A: *The Primary Lung Focus of Tuberculosis in Children.* London, J & A Churchill, 1916.

Harris VJ, Schauf V, Duda F, et al: Fatal tuberculosis in young children. *Pediatrics* 1979; 63:912.

Joffe N: Cavitating primary tuberculosis in infancy. *Br J Radiol* 1960; 33:430.

Kendig L: The clinical picture of sarcoidosis in children. *Pediatrics* 1974; 54:289.

Kennedy DH, Fallon RJ: Tuberculous meningitis. *JAMA* 1979; 241:264.

Kuess G: De l'hérédité parasitaire de la tuberculose humaine (thesis). Paris, Asselin & Houzeau, 1898.

Lamont AC, Cremin BJ, Pelteret RM: Radiological patterns of pulmonary tuberculosis in the paediatric age group. *Pediatr Radiol* 1986; 16:2.

Leung AN, Muller NL, Pineda PR, et al: Primary tuberculosis in childhood: Radiographic manifestations. *Radiology* 1992; 182:87.

Lincoln EM, Sewell EM: *Tuberculosis in Children.* New York, McGraw-Hill, 1963.

Matsaniotis H, Kattamis C, Economou-Mavrou E, et al: Bullous emphysema in childhood tuberculosis. *J Pediatr* 1967; 71:703.

Merten DF, Kirks DR, Grossman H: Pulmonary sarcoidosis in childhood. *Am J Roentgenol* 1980; 135:673.

Payne M, cited in Miller FJW, Scale RME , Taylor MD: *Tuberculosis in Children.* Boston, Little, Brown, 1963.

Smith MHD: Tuberculosis in children and adolescents. *Clin Chest Med* 1989; 10:381.

Smith MHD, Marquis JR: Tuberculosis and other mycobacterial infections in Feigin RD, Cherry JD (eds): *Textbook of Pediatric Infectious Diseases.* ed 2. Philadelphia, WB Saunders, 1987.

Terplan K: Anatomical studies in human tuberculosis. *Am Rev Tuberc* 1940; 42(suppl):1.

Veneeklas GMH: Cause and sequela of intrapulomonary shadows in primary tuberculosis. *Am J Dis Child* 1952; 83:271.

Wallgren A: Primary tuberculosis in childhood. *Am J Dis Child* 1935; 49:1105.

Wallgren A: Pulmonary tuberculosis: Relation of childhood infection to disease in adults. *Lancet* 1938; 1:1417.

Zarabi M, Sane S, Girdany BR: The chest roentgenogram in the early diagnosis of tuberculous meningitis in children. *Am J Dis Child* 1971; 121:389.

Pulmonary Mycosis

Boroff CP: Acute pulmonary blastomycosis. *Radiology* 1950; 54:157.

Conant NF, Martin DS, Smith DT, et al: *Manual of Clinical Mycology, Military Manuals, National Research Council.* Philadelphia, WB Saunders, 1944.

Grief A, Moscuna M, Suprun H, et al: Fatal childhood pulmonary aspergillosis from contact with pigeons. *Clin Pediatr (Phila)* 1981; 20:357.

Kassner EG, Kauffman SL, Yoon JL, et al: Pulmonary candidiasis in infants: Clinical, radiologic, and pathologic features. *AJR* 1981; 137:707.

Middleton E Jr, Reed CE, Ellis EF: *Allergy Principles and Practice,* vol 2. St Louis, Mosby–Year Book, 1978.

Mintzer RA, Rogers LF, Kruglik GD, et al: The spectrum of radiologic findings in allergic bronchopulmonary aspergillosis. *Radiology* 1978; 127:301.

Siewers CMF, Cramblett HG: Cryptococcosis (torulosis) in children: Report of four cases. *Pediatrics* 1964; 34:393.

Primary Pulmonary Coccidioidomycosis

Dickson EC: Coccidioides infection. *Arch Intern Med* 1937; 59:1920.

Greendyke WH, Resnick DL, Harvey WC: The varied roentgen manifestations of primary coccidioidomycosis. *AJR* 1970; 109:491.

Pinckney L, Parker BR: Primary coccidioidomycosis in children presenting with massive pleural effusion. *Am J Roentgenol* 1978; 130:247.

Richardson HB Jr, Anderson JA, McKay BM: Acute pulmonary coccidioidomycosis in children. *J Pediatr* 1967; 79:376.

Primary Pulmonary Histoplasmosis

Christie A: Histoplasmin sensitivity. *J Pediatr* 1946; 29:417.

Christie A: The relationship of sensitivity to histoplasmin tuberculin and haplosporangin to pulmonary calcification. *JAMA* 1946; 131:658.

Christie A, Peterson JC: Pulmonary calcification and sensitivity to histoplasmin. *Am J Public Health* 1945; 35:1131.

Schwarz J: *Histoplasmosis.* New York, Praeger, 1981.

Parasitic Infestations of the Lungs

Burton K, Yogev R, London N, et al: Pulmonary paragonimiasis in Laotian refugee children. *Pediatrics* 1982; 70:246.

Wall MA, McGhee G: Paragonimiasis. *Am J Dis Child* 1982; 136:828.

10

Immune Disorders and the Lung

Normal immune system
Immunodeficiency disorders
  Disorders of cellular immunity
    DiGeorge syndrome
  Defective humoral immunity (antibody deficiency
    disorders)
      Congenital agammaglobulinemia (Bruton disease)
      Selective IgA deficiency
      "Acquired" or common variable agammaglobulinemia
      X-linked lymphoproliferative syndrome (Duncan
      syndrome)
      Hyperimmune globulinemia E syndrome
  Severe combined immunodeficiency disorders (SCID)
  Partial combined immunodeficiency disorders

Wiskott-Aldrich syndrome
Ataxia telangiectasia
Cartilage-hair hypoplasia
Disorders of phagocytosis
  Chronic granulomatous disease
  Chédiak-Higashi syndrome
  Shwachman syndrome
Malignancy and immunodeficiency
Immunosuppressive therapy
  Bone marrow transplants
Acquired immunodeficiency syndrome (AIDS)
Immunologic diseases of the lung
  Complex immunoreactions

NORMAL IMMUNE SYSTEM

Disorders of the immune response often result in chronic recurrent pulmonary infections which may be caused by common or uncommon bacterial, viral, or fungal agents. Radiologists may be the first to suspect an immune disorder, or they may be called upon to detect infection in a patient known to have altered immunity.

Primary immunodeficiency syndromes are all quite rare; it has been estimated, for instance, that agammaglobulinemia occurs with a frequency of 1 in 50,000 live births. IgA deficiency is probably the most frequent disorder; its reported incidence ranges between 0.03% and 0.97%. Secondary or acquired immunodeficiency syndromes are much more common, particularly AIDS, but immune disorders also occur frequently after therapy for malignancies and organ transplants.

The immune system comprises the lymphocytes and the antibodies they secrete, phagocytes, and the complement system. There are two populations of lymphocytes: T cells, which are derived from the thymus, and B cells, which are derived from bone marrow stem cells. T lymphocytes are responsible for cell-mediated immunity (CMI), control of delayed hypersensitivity reactions, immunologic memory, killer cells in graft rejection, immune surveil-

lance for malignancy, and the release of cytotoxic, chemotactic, and macrophage-reactive factors. B lymphocytes are responsible for the body's humoral immune protection by producing antibodies or immunoglobulins. They are found in the germinal centers of the lymph nodes and in the spleen. Upon antigenic stimulation, they become plasma cells and produce one of the five classes of immunoglobulins: IgG, IgA, IgM, IgE, or IgD. The primary role of humoral immunity is to aid in repelling bacterial invaders.

Complement acts to neutralize viruses and to opsonize and lyse bacteria. Phagocytic cells engulf and destroy invading bacteria and aid in antigen preparation. Disorders occur in which either the phagocytic or bactericidal function of the white blood cell is impaired.

The radiologist should suspect an immune disturbance in patients with unusual or recurrent pulmonary infections, persistent or progressive sinus infections, monilial esophagitis, or pronounced lymphoid hyperplasia of the gastrointestinal tract. In children over 6 months of age the soft-tissue mass of the adenoids is normally visible posteriorly in the lateral view of the posterior nasopharynx. If no tissue is seen and adenoidectomy has not been performed, defective B cell (humoral) immunity may be suspected (Fig 10–1). Absence of the thymic shadow

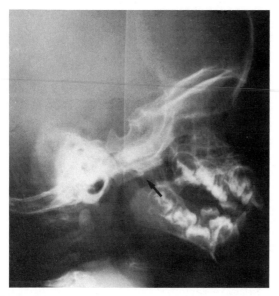

FIG 10–1.
Absent adenoid tissue in a patient with congenital agammaglobulinemia. Lateral film of the nasopharynx in this 6-month-old baby shows that there is a lack of soft tissue in the region of the adenoid *(arrow)*. Normally by this age a measurable amount of soft tissue should be present in the nasopharynx.

suggests T cell (cellular) immune defects, but this sign is severely compromised by the fact that the thymus involutes with stress so that, unless films are available in the first few days of life, the diagnosis of thymic absence is unreliable.

IMMUNODEFICIENCY DISORDERS

The immune disorders are discussed as though they were pure in form, but the immune mechanism is extremely complex and impairments of immune responses are usually mixed, although certain features predominate.

Disorders of Cellular Immunity

DiGeorge Syndrome
In the DiGeorge syndrome there is congenital absence of the thymus and parathyroid glands. Both glands arise from the third and fourth pharyngeal pouches during the sixth gestational week. Other congenital malformations frequently present include a hypoplastic mandible, ear deformities, esophageal atresia, and complex congenital heart disease, especially anomalies of the great vessels. If these infants do not succumb to neonatal tetany or congenital heart disease, they are prone to develop infection from acid-fast bacteria, viruses, fungi, and *Pneumocystis carinii*. Immunoglobulin levels are normal, but cellular immunity is defective. One should suspect this syndrome in all infants with severe congen-

ital heart disease, especially those with great-vessel anomalies (Fig 10–2) and bizarre upper mediastinal contours.

Nezelof Syndrome
Nezelof syndrome is characterized by decreased lymphoid tissue, abnormal thymic architecture, and normal or increased serum levels of most of the immunoglobulins. Patients present in infancy with pulmonary infections, diarrhea, failure to thrive, candidiasis, and a host of infections. The thymus is small but present. This disorder could be confused clinically with AIDS because of the presence of normal or increased immunoglobulins; however, AIDS patients have lymphadenopathy rather than the lymphopenia and lymphocyte depletion that are characteristic of the Nezelof syndrome.

Defective Humoral Immunity (Antibody Deficiency Disorders)

Congenital Agammaglobulinemia (Bruton Disease)
This is an X-linked recessive condition in which there is a marked decrease in the amount of serum immunoglobulins and therefore virtual absence of humoral immunity, although cellular immunity remains intact. Patients generally are well until they are 6 to 9 months of age, presumably being protected by transplacental antibodies. Chronic recurrent pneumonias caused by common pyogenic organisms are likely to ensue. The pneumonias may be complicated by slow resolution, atelectasis, bronchiectasis, and empyema. Characteristically, hilar lymphadenopathy is not present, and nasopharyngeal lymphoid tissue is absent, but the thymus is present. In later stages, the chest film may resemble that seen in cystic fibrosis, although hilar enlargement is usually not present. Chronic sinus infection is common. There is an increased risk of lymphoma and leukemia, the most common immunodeficiency.

Selective IgA Deficiency
This disorder is the most common immunodeficiency; it is characterized by isolated absence or near-absence of serum and secretory IgA. In one series, IgA deficiency was present in 1 in 333 blood donors. Patients may be healthy or susceptible to recurrent infections in the respiratory, gastrointestinal, and urogenital tracts, which are usually bacterial in nature. There is a frequent association with atopic diseases, collagen-vascular and autoimmune diseases, and nodular lymphoid hyperplasia of the gastrointestinal tract. Pulmonary hemorrhage has been reported as a complication.

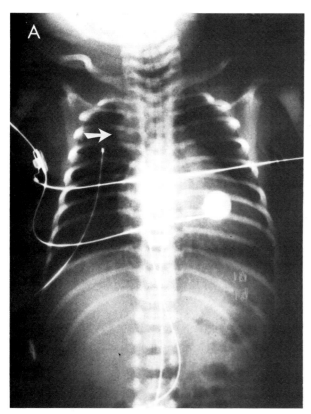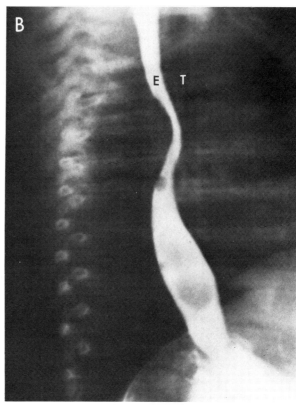

FIG 10–2.
DiGeorge syndrome in a 1-day-old infant with cyanotic congenital heart disease. **A,** frontal chest radiograph shows cardiomegaly and a large right paratracheal density *(arrow)* that could represent the thymus but, in fact, was due to a large right-sided aortic arch as seen on the lateral radiograph. **B,** because of the large right arch, recognition of the absent thymus is not easy. Some retrosternal radiolucency was visible on the lateral chest radiograph, but the cardiomegaly partially obscured this finding as well. *E,* esophagus; *T,* trachea.

"Acquired" or Common Variable Agammaglobulinemia

This disorder affects a heterogeneous group of patients of both sexes and all ages but usually occurs in late childhood or early adult life. The B cells may be normal in number but defective in function. Tonsils, adenoids, and lymph nodes may be enlarged. Patients are predisposed to pulmonary and sinus infections and may develop noncaseating granulomas in the lungs, skin, liver, and spleen. Findings on chest films are diverse and nonspecific but include pneumonia, atelectasis, and bronchopneumonia. There is an increased incidence of malignancy estimated at 8%; about one third of patients develop nonlymphoid malignancies, half of which are gastric carcinomas.

X-Linked Lymphoproliferative Syndrome (Duncan Syndrome)

X-linked lymphoproliferative syndrome (Duncan syndrome) is a recessive trait characterized by an inadequate immunoreaction to infection by the Epstein-Barr virus. The male patients characteristically are well until after a bout of infectious mononucleosis which appears to induce a B cell proliferation which is followed by hypogammaglobulinemia or B cell lymphoma.

Hyperimmune Globulinemia E Syndrome

Merten et al. reported on a group of patients with *hyperimmune globulinemia E syndrome* in whom large, persistent pneumatoceles developed following pneumonia. Wood and Young reported similar radiographic findings in patients with systemic leukocyte abnormalities and postulated that altered leukocyte response to infection leads to fibroblastic sequestration of the pneumatoceles (Fig 10–3). Both males and females are affected with recurrent severe staphylococcal infections.

Severe Combined Immunodeficiency Disorders (SCID)

These disorders are thought to be due to a defect in the maturation of the stem cell itself, leading to defi-

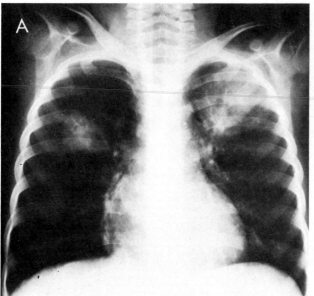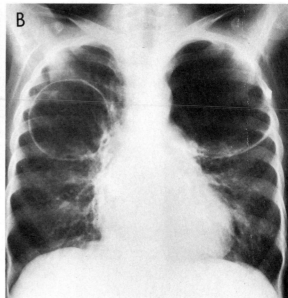

FIG 10–3.
Persistent pneumatoceles in a patient with hyperimmune globuline-mia syndrome. **A,** bilateral upper lobe pneumonias. **B,** 18 months later, large pneumatoceles remain in both upper lobes. (From Wood BP, Young LW: *Pediatr Res* 1976; 5:10. Used by permission.)

ciencies in both humoral and cellular immunity. Swiss-type agammaglobulinemia is an autosomal recessive disorder occurring in both sexes. The condition is severe, and most patients die in the first year (Fig 10–4). Monilial infection of the skin, lungs, and gastrointestinal tract may be the presenting complaint (Fig 10–5). *Pneumocystis carinii* and viral pneumonias are frequent fatal sequelae. The thymus is small or absent and lymphoid tissue is absent. There is also an X-linked autosomal recessive form which is probably more common than the Swiss type. Approximately 40% of the patients with the autosomal recessive form of SCID have been shown to have adenosine deaminase (ADA) deficiency. Some of these patients, in infancy, have skeletal abnormalities consisting of flared ribs, costovertebral separation, squared scapulae, and metaphyseal cupping, but in contrast to rickets, there is no excess osteoid. A response to enzyme replacement therapy has been documented with regression of the bony changes (Chakravaiti et al.). A third type, associated with leukopenia, is less frequent. Clinically and immunologically, the types are very similar. Bone marrow transplant may be curative.

Partial Combined Immunodeficiency Disorders

Wiskott-Aldrich Syndrome

This is an X-linked recessive condition in which a triad of thrombocytopenia, severe eczema, and marked susceptibility to pyogenic infection is present. Infections usually begin in the first year of life. The basic defect is in cellular immunity, but humoral immunity is also compromised. Serum IgM levels are low. This condition is usually fatal in the first few years of life. If patients survive, there is an 8% to 12% risk for lymphoreticular malignancies.

Ataxia Telangiectasia

The patients affected with this autosomal recessive syndrome have scleral and cutaneous telangiectasia and progressive cerebellar ataxia. Most develop acute pneumonia and severe recurrent sinusitis secondary to severe defects in cellular and humoral immunity. In most patients IgA is either absent or very low. Patients that survive the first decade are at high risk for malignancies, most of which are lymphoid. The thymus is hypoplastic.

Cartilage-Hair Hypoplasia

Cartilage-hair hypoplasia is a severe short-limbed dwarfism, the skeletal aspects of which are described in Chapter 43. These children can have a variety of immune disorders, the most common of which is defective cellular immunity, but defective antibody-mediated and severe combined immunodeficiency have also been reported. Varicella, progressive vaccinia, and vaccine-associated poliomyelitis have been observed.

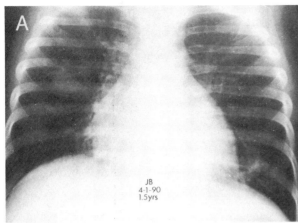

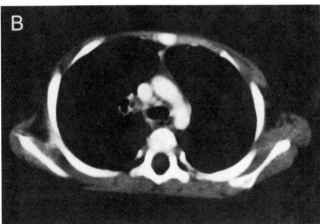

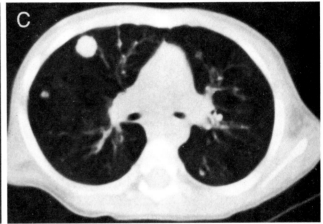

FIG 10–4.
Severe combined immunodeficiency with absent thymus and lymphoid interstitial pneumonia. **A,** frontal chest film in an 18-month-old infant shows ill-defined nodular opacities bilaterally. **B,** contrast-enhanced CT at the level of the aortic arch reveals the thymus to be absent. **C,** unenhanced CT image at a lower section reveals discrete nodular opacities bilaterally which were proved on biopsy to be localized nodules of lymphoid interstitial pneumonia (pseudolymphoma). The patient subsequently died of vaccine-induced poliomyelitis.

Disorders of Phagocytosis

Chronic Granulomatous Disease

The most common phagocytic disorder is chronic granulomatous disease (CGD). The white cells are able to phagocytize normally, but the engulfed organisms are not killed. There appear to be two forms—the more common is X-linked, but there is also an autosomal recessive form that can occur in either sex.

The pathologic organisms in this condition all produce catalase. They include *Staphylococcus aureus*, *Staphylococcus epidermidis*, and some gram-negative bacteria. The reaction to infection is granulomatous. Chest film findings are typically those of recurrent pneumonia that is slow to resolve and may progress to abscess formation. Hilar lymphadenopathy is often present. Fungal infections occur in about 20% of children. Pulmonary aspergillosis may appear as a chronic reticulonodular pneumonia or as a more aggressive infection with chest wall invasion. Osteomyelitis, liver abscess, and gastric antral involvement are other features of the disease. The granulomas may calcify (Fig 10–6). Diagnosis is established by the nitroblue tetrazolium (NBT) test.

Chédiak-Higashi Syndrome

Chédiak-Higashi syndrome is a rare, autosomal recessive condition characterized by partial albinism, frequent recurrent bacterial infections, and abnormal granulocytes which have characteristic, deeply staining granules. There is neutrophil dysfunction and abnormal chemotaxis. The patients are prone to Epstein-Barr viral infections, which often appear to accelerate the disease, as well as bacterial infections. Death usually occurs by age 10 years although bone marrow transplantation has been curative in a few cases.

Shwachman Syndrome

Shwachman syndrome is characterized by pancreatic dysfunction and malabsorption, but also manifests leukopenia and defective neutrophil mobility which are associated with recurrent, often bacterial sinopulmonary infections. Skeletal abnormalities are frequent and include metaphyseal rarefactions and

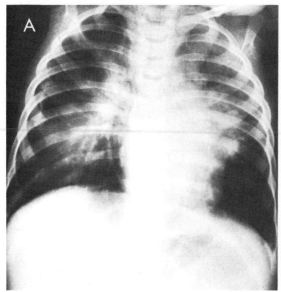
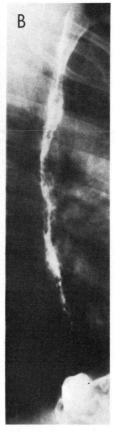

FIG 10–5.
Severe combined immunodeficiency complicated with monilial esophagitis in a 10-month-old boy presenting with cough and dyspnea. **A,** chest film shows a central bilateral airspace consolidation that, on lung biopsy, was shown to be due to *Pneumocystis carinii* pneumonia. **B,** an esophagogram, same patient, shows marked mucosal irregularity secondary to monilial esophagitis.

V-shaped deformities of the growth plates, especially at the knees.

MALIGNANCY AND IMMUNODEFICIENCY

The immune system is not only responsible for defense against infection, but also plays an important role in the prevention of malignancy. Both primary and acquired immunodeficiency disorders are associated with an increased risk of malignancy ranging from 100 to 10,000 times that of a control population. The six primary immunodeficiency disorders for which there is the highest risk of malignancy are X-linked agammaglobulinemia, combined immunodeficiency, common variable immunodeficiency, Wiskott-Aldrich syndrome, selective IgA deficiency, and ataxia telangiectasia. The greatest risk is present in patients with the last condition, but because IgA deficiency is so much more common, this group is actually responsible for the greatest number of malignancies. Lymphoma and leukemia are the commonest malignancies, but gastrointestinal carcinomas and sarcomas also are frequent. Lymphoproliferative malignant disorders are common complications of cyclosporine therapy given to suppress the immune response following organ transplantation. Non-Hodgkin lymphoma and Kaposi sarcoma are common complications of AIDS in children.

IMMUNOSUPPRESSIVE THERAPY

Children in whom organ transplants have been performed and in whom immunosuppressive therapy is used extensively are at risk for infection and also for malignancies. In patients with malignancies, it may be difficult to determine whether decreased resistance to infection results from primary disease or the therapy. Prompt detection of an infectious complication and identification of the responsible organism are critical so that appropriate therapy can be started. Bacterial infections in these patients are commonly due to gram-negative organisms or staphylococci. The presence of lobar or segmental consolidation on the radiographs suggests bacterial infection. Rapidly enlarging multiple nodules may result from septic emboli. Fungal infections include aspergillosis, candidiasis, cryptococcosis, histoplasmosis, mucormycosis, and nocardiosis. Retrieval of organisms is essential, since the radiographic findings are nonspecific. Viral infections, including varicella and measles, are relatively common complica-

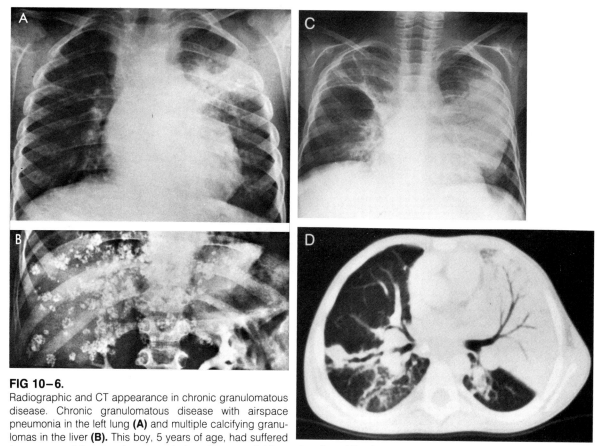

FIG 10–6.
Radiographic and CT appearance in chronic granulomatous disease. Chronic granulomatous disease with airspace pneumonia in the left lung **(A)** and multiple calcifying granulomas in the liver **(B)**. This boy, 5 years of age, had suffered from recurrent fever and pneumonia from the age of 10 months. **C** and **D**, airspace consolidation in chronic granulomatous disease in an 8-year-old boy. **C**, frontal radiograph reveals massive consolidation in the left midlung involving primarily the upper lobe. Loss of volume is noted in the right upper lobe. **D**, CT scan reveals, in addition to the massive airspace consolidation in the left lobe, extensive subcarinal adenopathy, perihilar nodes on the right side, and cylindric bronchiectasis involving the lateral segmental bronchus of the right lower lobe. A more superior CT image (not shown) showed extensive bronchiectasis of the right upper lobe. (**A** and **B** courtesy of Dr. Melvin Becker, Bellevue Hospital, New York.)

tions in children with leukemia and lymphoma. The radiographic pattern is nonspecific; often initially it is reticulonodular, but confluence may occur (Fig 10–7). Computed tomography (CT) is useful for early detection of infection and to direct lung biopsy.

Bone Marrow Transplants

Transplantation of allogeneic bone marrow is used increasingly for treatment of aplastic anemia, leukemia, neuroblastoma, and certain immunodeficiencies. Four major complications occur following bone marrow transplantation: (1) toxicity from the preparatory regimen of irradiation and chemotherapy; (2) graft-versus-host disease; (3) posttransplant infections; and (4) recurrence of the primary disease. Pulmonary complications are common following this procedure; 2 to 4 weeks after transplantation, a pattern consistent with interstitial pulmonary edema

frequently seen. At about this same time, diffuse alveolar hemorrhage may occur; it commonly presents radiographically as abrupt onset of either interstitial or extensive bilateral alveolar consolidation. These abnormalities may be related to damage to the capillary bed resulting from the aggressive preoperative chemotherapeutic regimen. Obliterative bronchiolitis has also been noted; the radiographs in these patients may only show air trapping. This complication usually occurs 90 to 180 days after transplantation. It may represent a postviral complication or be due to graft-versus-host disease. Pneumonia is the most common complication, and cytomegalovirus is the most common pathogen. Mixed infections are frequent. Radiographic appearances are nonspecific, but the presence of nodular or masslike infiltrates, with or without cavitation in a neutropenic patient or in one being treated for graft-versus-host disease, should suggest pulmonary fungal infection. *Aspergillus* and *Candida* are the most frequent organisms.

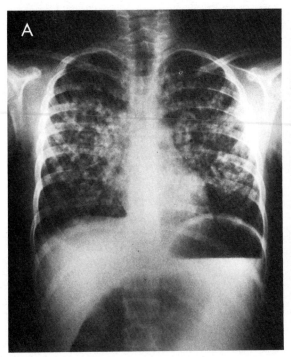
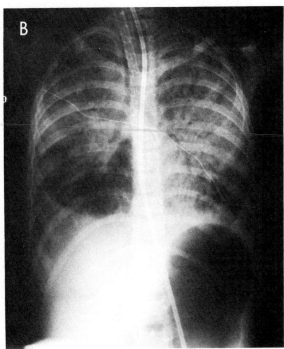

FIG 10–7.
Varicella pneumonia developing in a 13-year-old patient with leukemia. **A,** patchy acinar nodules are visible throughout both lungs. **B,** 12 hours later, massive pulmonary consolidation has developed. There is a large area of interstitial emphysema at the right lung base. The patient died shortly after this examination.

ACQUIRED IMMUNODEFICIENCY SYNDROME (AIDS)

This topic is discussed in Chapter 9. AIDS is increasingly common in the larger cities of the United States and is affecting ever-greater numbers of children, especially infants. Two factors put children at risk: blood transfusions and mothers who are intravenous drug users. Clinical features of pediatric AIDS are nonspecific and include failure to thrive, lymphadenopathy, hepatosplenomegaly, chronic diarrhea, oral thrush, parotitis, and pneumonia. Pyogenic bacterial infections are also frequently present. Morbidity and mortality from AIDS in children most commonly are related to pulmonary involvement, as discussed in Chapter 9.

IMMUNOLOGIC DISEASES OF THE LUNG

Normally, the antigen-antibody response is beneficial to the host, warding off infection and malignancy, but in certain cases, especially when there is an immunologic response to the body's own antigens (autoimmune response), the immune response can be harmful and cause disease. There are four recognized types of immune response (antigen-antibody reaction). Three involve humoral immunity, and the fourth is cell-mediated. The responses are summarized in Table 10–1.

Type 1 is an IgE-mediated immediate hypersensitivity response that is typified by *extrinsic asthma.* The mast cell is stimulated by an antigen such as ragweed pollen to release histamine and other vasoactive substances, thereby producing an increase in capillary permeability, edema, and smooth muscle contraction. The primary effect is on the tracheobronchial tree and small airways where obstruction typical of bronchial asthma occurs. This disease is described in detail in Chapter 8.

Type 2, or cytotoxic responses in the lung, are typified by *Goodpasture syndrome,* in which it is theorized that the alveolar basement membrane is damaged, perhaps by a virus, becomes antigenic, and is attacked by the body's own IgG and IgM antibodies, with pulmonary hemorrhage as a result. In contrast to asthma, Goodpasture syndrome is a disease of the pulmonary parenchyma but not the airways. Damage to the renal glomerular basement membrane leads to glomerulonephritis, which usually follows the onset of pulmonary disease. Diagnosis can be made by a renal biopsy and the finding of linear staining of the glomerular basement membranes for IgG and complement by immunofluorescent techniques. Goodpasture syndrome is relatively un-

TABLE 10–1.

The Immune Responses*

Type	Antibody	Skin Test	Transferable	Cytotoxic	Clinical Examples
IgE-dependent	E	Immediate	Yes (Prausnitz-Küstner reaction)	No	Extrinsic asthma, anaphylaxis
Tissue-specific antibody	G,M		Yes		Goodpasture syndrome
Immune complexes	G,M	Arthus (6-hr delay)	Yes	Yes	Extrinsic alveolitis: organic dust, inorganic dust. Intrinsic alveolitis: collagen-vascular disease, fibrosing alveolitis
Cell-mediated (delayed) hypersensitivity	None	Delayed (24–48 hr)	Transfer factor	Yes	Intracellular infection, graft rejection, cancer suppression

*Modified from Roberts SR Jr: *Semin Roentgenol* 1975; 10:7.

common in children and tends to involve young adult males. Symptoms include hemoptysis, iron deficiency anemia, and hematuria. Radiographic findings in the acute stage are those of airspace disease which may resemble pulmonary edema. Acinar nodules appear, and a reticular pattern is often seen after the alveolar pattern clears and before the chest film shows a return to normal. Following multiple episodes of hemorrhage, interstitial fibrosis may occur.

Idiopathic pulmonary hemosiderosis is probably better called idiopathic pulmonary hemorrhage (IPH) because it is the hemorrhage and not the hemosiderosis which is the major clinical feature. IPH is more common than Goodpasture syndrome in children. It affects both sexes equally and occurs mainly in children under the age of 10 years. While its exact cause is unknown, its clinical and radiologic similarities to Goodpasture syndrome warrant its discussion here. It may well be an autoimmune disorder, with some cases related to sensitivity to the proteins in cow's milk. Hemosiderin-laden macrophages are present in both the interstitium and the alveolar spaces of the lung. The diagnosis of idiopathic pulmonary hemosiderosis is based on the presence of hemoptysis and iron deficiency anemia, the absence of renal disease, and the absence of anti–glomerular basement membrane (anti-GBM) antibodies on immunofluorescent staining techniques. Hemorrhage may be confined to the peripheral airspaces without the presence of hemoptysis, or severe hemoptysis and hematemesis may occur. Symptoms depend on the severity of the pulmonary hemorrhage but include cough, dyspnea, fever, pallor, and fatigue (Fig 10–8). The radiologic findings are identical to those described above in Goodpasture syndrome.

Albelda and associates have reviewed the topic of *diffuse pulmonary hemorrhage (DPH)* and devised a useful classification. Six groups of pulmonary hemorrhage are described in Table 10–2. Not all DPH is related to disturbance of the immune system, but several are, and thus the topic is discussed in this chapter.

DPH is characterized by widespread hemorrhage from the microvasculature of the lung into the alveolar spaces. It occurs in association with a wide variety of diseases, many of which have overlapping features of glomerulonephritis, immune complex, and anti-GBM disease. Hemoptysis, anemia, and diffuse alveolar consolidation are the typical triad of findings. Not all features, however, are present in all patients, but the radiographic findings classically are those of rapid onset of a diffuse alveolar filling pattern that is often perihilar or basilar. If the patient survives, resolution of the radiographic findings is rapid and may revert to normal in less than 2 weeks. In more chronic cases the radiograph may show primarily interstitial changes. It may be necessary to resort to fiberoptic bronchoscopy or open lung biopsy to establish a diagnosis.

Type 3 immune responses (immune complex disease) are thought to occur when an airborne or blood-borne antigen reacts with an antibody, to produce immune complexes that activate complement and injure tissue. The reaction site may be either alveolar wall or vascular wall, where alveolitis, vasculitis, or granuloma formation may occur. An example thought to typify this reaction is *extrinsic fibrosing alveolitis*, which includes the diseases listed in Table 10–3.

Most of these occupationally related conditions are uncommon in children. Farmer's lung is most frequently seen and is typical of the other disorders. After exposure to the antigen, onset may be either

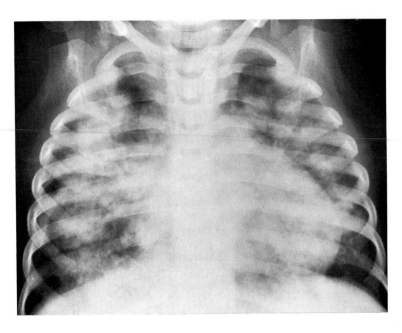

FIG 10–8.
Diffuse pulmonary hemorrhage which was thought to be due to id-iopathic pulmonary hemosiderosis in a boy 3 years of age. Frontal radiograph reveals bilateral airspace consolidation which is some-what patchy in nature. Tracheal washing contained large numbers

of macrophages filled with hemosiderin. Ten days later, most of the consolidative changes in the lungs had cleared. The patient's ane-mia was successfully treated with blood transfusion. (Courtesy of Dr. Bertram Girdany, Pittsburgh.)

acute or insidious with dyspnea, cough, and malaise among the common symptoms. Radiographic mani-festations vary with the stage of the disease. Small

TABLE 10–2.
Diffuse Pulmonary Hemorrhage (DPH)*

1. DPH plus glomerulonephritis and anti–glomerular basement membrane (anti-GBM) antibody (e.g., Goodpasture syndrome)
2. DPH with nonimmunologic renal disease (e.g., end-stage uremia with hemorrhage; adult respiratory distress syndrome [ARDS] with renal failure)
3. DPH with glomerulonephritis and immune complex disease (e.g., systemic lupus erythematosus [SLE]; Wegener granulomatosis)
4. DPH and immune complex disease without nephritis (e.g., unusual but can occur in SLE or Wegener granulomatosis)
5. DPH and anti-GBM antibodies without renal disease (e.g., early Goodpasture syndrome and ? idiopathic pulmonary hemosiderosis [IPH])
6. IPH or DPH alone or IPH and DPH associated with disseminated intravascular coagulopathy (DIC) or ARDS

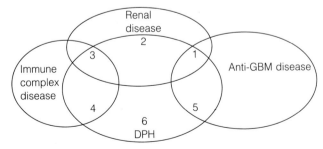

*Modified from Albelda SM, Gefter WB, Epstein DM, et al: *Radiology* 1985; 154:289.

nodular opacities (Fig 10–9) are the most common abnormalities. Hilar lymph node enlargement is variable but usually is not present. If the patient is removed from the adverse environment, the radio-graph tends to become normal in days to weeks, but with continued exposure, a reticular pattern charac-teristic of diffuse interstitial fibrosis may develop.

Intrinsic fibrosing alveolitis includes diseases in which the antigen is unknown or is a tissue compo-nent of the body (autoimmune disease). These con-ditions, also uncommon in children, include col-lagen-vascular diseases and a large group of idio-pathic interstitial pulmonary fibroses. The role of the altered immune response in this group of diseases is poorly understood.

Rheumatoid arthritis is the most common col-lagen-vascular disease in childhood. It may have an acute systemic or polyarticular presentation. Recur-rent pleural effusion may be the first manifestation of the disease. Pleuritic pain may be present, with or without visible pleural fluid on radiographic exami-nation. Yousefzadeh and Fishman have stressed the occurrence of pleural effusion, pericarditis, and pul-monary infiltrates as characteristic of juvenile rheu-matoid arthritis (JRA). Rheumatoid nodules, which may cavitate, are seen more frequently in adults than in children. Rarely DPH related to dissemi-nated intravascular coagulopathy *(DIC)* and hepatic failure is seen in JRA (Fig 10–10).

Systemic lupus erythematosus (SLE) is a collagen-vascular disease that is most common in young

TABLE 10–3.

Hypersensitivity Pneumonitis*

Disease	Antigen	Environmental Source of Antigen
Allergic aspergillosis	*Aspergillus fumigatus*	Malting operations, etc.
Bagassosis	*Micropolyspora faeni* or *Thermoactinomyces vulgaris*	Moldy sugar cane
Farmer's lung	*M. faeni* or *T. vulgaris*	Moldy hay
Pandora's pneumonitis	*T. vulgaris* (?)	Heating or air-conditioning systems
Mushroom picker's lung	*M. faeni* or *T. vulgaris*	Mushroom compost
Maple bark disease	*Cryptostroma corticale*	Moldy maple bark
Sequoiosis	*Graphium* sp.	Redwood dust
Suberosis	*Graphium* sp.	Moldy cork dust
Cheese washer's lung	*Penicillium*	Cheese
Paprika splitter's lung	*Mucor stolonifer*	Paprika beans
Malt worker's lung	*Aspergillus clavatus*	Malt dust
Bird breeder's lung	Avian proteins	Pigeons or other birds
Pituitary snuff user's lung	Pituitary powder	
Woodworker's lung	Wood dust (oak, mahogany, boxwood, other?)	Wood-processing plant

*Modified from Feigin D: Handout from Refresher Course, "Allergic Diseases of the Lungs." Presented at the Radiological Society of North America Annual Meeting, Chicago, November 1982.

women, but 20% of cases begin in girls 16 years of age or younger. It affects blacks more often than whites and women about eight times more often than men. SLE has protean manifestations including a photosensitive facial rash, arthritis, renal disease, pleural and pericardial effusions, vasculitis, and stroke. Pulmonary involvement is common, most frequently presenting as nonspecific infiltrates or small pleural effusions, but on occasion has been noted to present with massive, DPH, sometimes as the initial manifestation of the disease.

The cause of *idiopathic interstitial pulmonary fibrosis*

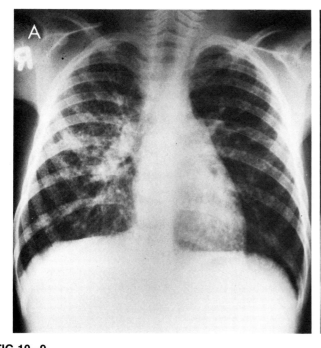
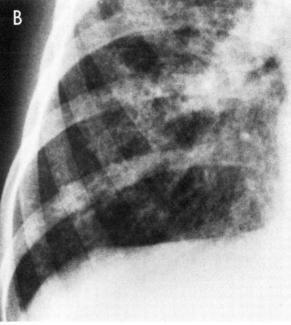

FIG 10–9.

Extrinsic allergic alveolitis in a 10-year-old boy with cough and dyspnea. Blood eosinophilia was also present. **A,** radiographic examination shows the bilateral reticulonodular infiltrate to be more pronounced on the right side. Some hilar adenopathy is also noted. **B,** a close-up of the right lower lobe shows the reticulonodular infiltrate to better advantage. The radiographic findings cleared in 1 week.

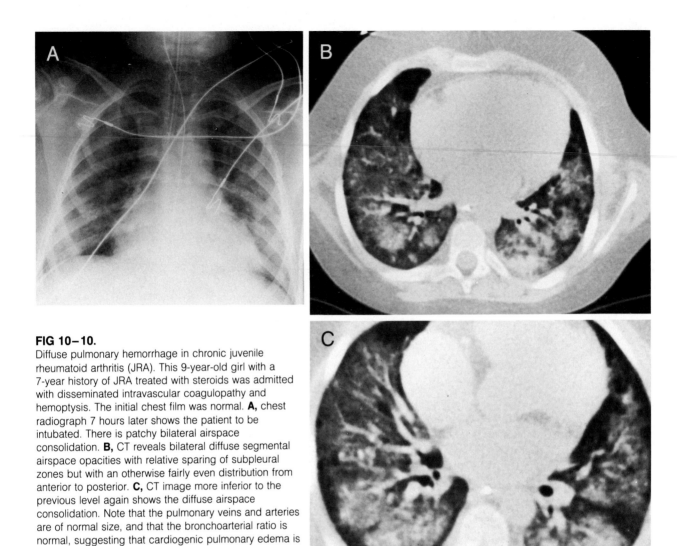

FIG 10–10.
Diffuse pulmonary hemorrhage in chronic juvenile rheumatoid arthritis (JRA). This 9-year-old girl with a 7-year history of JRA treated with steroids was admitted with disseminated intravascular coagulopathy and hemoptysis. The initial chest film was normal. **A,** chest radiograph 7 hours later shows the patient to be intubated. There is patchy bilateral airspace consolidation. **B,** CT reveals bilateral diffuse segmental airspace opacities with relative sparing of subpleural zones but with an otherwise fairly even distribution from anterior to posterior. **C,** CT image more inferior to the previous level again shows the diffuse airspace consolidation. Note that the pulmonary veins and arteries are of normal size, and that the bronchoarterial ratio is normal, suggesting that cardiogenic pulmonary edema is unlikely. Autopsy subsequently revealed evidence of bilateral pulmonary hemorrhage.

is unknown, although there appears to be a relationship to collagen-vascular diseases. A number of patients with these conditions have antinuclear antibodies or positive rheumatoid factor, and some authors think that there may be an autoimmune component to some or all of these disorders. Chronic interstitial lung disease of unknown cause is uncommon in adults and rare in children. Hogg has recently proposed a classification based on pathogenesis which is a convenient way to discuss this group of diseases about which little is known in childhood. He suggests that these be divided into those conditions due to an inflammatory and those to a neoplastic cause (Fig 10–11). In the inflammatory group, after the initial alveolar wall injury, there can be either a granulomatous or a nongranulomatous response. The nongranulomatous response can be further subdivided into a "usual" and a

"variant" response. Either response may lead to healing or go on to end-stage lung. The typical response is that called by Liebow et al. "usual interstitial pneumonia" (UIP) or "cryptogenic fibrosing alveolitis" by British authors. This condition is regarded by American authors as being separate from desquamative interstitial pneumonitis (DIP) although the British authors feel that DIP is an earlier stage of UIP. The conditions cannot be distinguished radiologically or clinically. Both are rare in children. There appears to be a familial form and onset is often in infancy. Symptoms are nonspecific, with cough and hyperpnea frequent. The disease is thought to start with an alveolitis and progress to interstitial fibrosis (Fig 10–12). The radiograph may be normal or may show a diffuse, reticulonodular infiltrate. CT findings in adults have been reported to show septal thickening, ground-glass

Inflammatory Process   Neoplastic Process

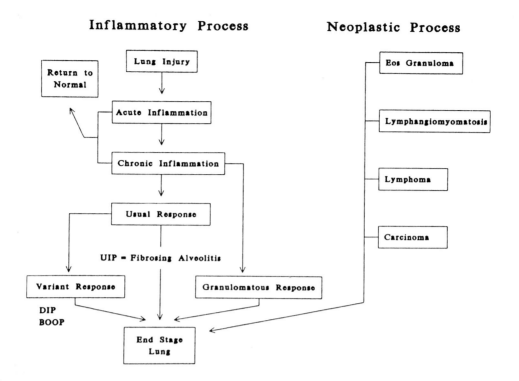

FIG 10–11.
Schema with three main pathogenetic pathways for development of end-stage lung disease. Pathways of chronic nongranulomatous inflammation (usual form of interstital pneumonia *[UIP]*/fibrosing alveolitis) and chronic granulomatous inflammation can be subdivided, and account for most cases of interstital lung disease. Third pathway is produced by expansion of lung interstitial space by desmoplastic reaction to benign, borderline, or frankly malignant cells. *Eos* = eosinophilic, *DIP* = desquamative interstitial pneumonia, *BOOP* = bronchiolitis obliterans with organizing pneumonia. (From Hogg JL: *AJR* 1991; 156:225–233. Used by permission.)

opacities, and subpleural cysts. Diagnosis requires open lung biopsy. Steroid therapy is helpful in early cases.

The second or variant type of response is diagnosed when inflammatory exudate is seen filling the alveolar space and alveolar ducts. This group is called cryptogenic organizing pneumonia by the British authors and bronchiolitis obliterans with organizing pneumonia (BOOP) by American authors. Pathologically, in BOOP, granulation tissue fills the alveolar sacs, ducts, and terminal bronchioles. It differs from UIP by having a more rapid onset, better response to steroids, and a differing radiographic appearance, the hallmark of which is bilateral, nodular, or subsegmental opacities, which are often quite peripheral. BOOP is known to occur as a response to infections, silo-filler's disease, drugs, collagen-vascular disease, bronchial obstruction, chronic aspiration, and idiopathic conditions (Katzenstein et al.). It also occurs in patients being treated for malignancy (Fig 10–13). The granulomatous response to inflammation occurs in sarcoidosis (see Chapter 9) and extrinsic allergic alveolitis (see above and Table 10–3). Neoplastic etiologies for interstitial lung disease that terminate in end-stage lung include histiocytosis X, lym-

phoma, and carcinoma. Lymphangiomyomatosis is also included in this group of diseases although it is extremely rare in children. Any of these conditions, whether the initial inciting factor be inflammatory or neoplastic, can lead to diffuse, chronic interstitial fibrosis (end-stage lung), which is marked by cysts and a reticular pattern, both on chest film and on high-resolution CT (HRCT).

Type 4 immune responses are cell-mediated, i.e., the cell itself and not the antibody reacts with the antigen. Delayed hypersensitivity is typical. Type 4 reactions are thought to be involved in the formation of pulmonary granulomas; pulmonary tuberculosis is typical of this reaction and is discussed in detail in Chapter 9.

COMPLEX IMMUNOREACTIONS

Certain diseases have more than one immune component involved. Among these diseases are allergic bronchopulmonary aspergillosis, Wegener granulomatosis, and some of the eosinophilic pneumonias.

Allergic bronchopulmonary aspergillosis (ABPA) combines type 1 and type 3 reactions. There is a strong history of asthma in most patients; in chil-

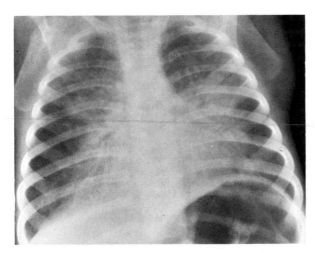

FIG 10–12.
Desquamative interstitial pneumonia (DIP) in a 14-month-old male
infant. Patchy airspace consolidation with some streaky opacities
occupy the medial portions of the lower two thirds of both lungs.
The lateral and apical segments of both lungs are spared. Pulmonary biopsy revealed DIP which responded favorably to steroid
therapy.

dren, cystic fibrosis is also a commonly associated
disease. This condition is discussed in Chapter 8.

Vasculitis, inflammation, and necrosis of small
blood vessels may affect the lung and produce a
granulomatous response. These diseases are uncommon in children but do occur, especially in teenagers. Diseases in this group include Wegener granulomatosis, probably the most common; allergic angiitis and granulomatosis (AAG) of Churg and
Strauss; necrotizing sarcoid granulomatosis (NSG);
and bronchocentric granulomatosis.

Wegener granulomatosis is a granulomatous
vasculitis that is thought to represent a combination
of type 3 and type 4 responses. The classic Wegener
granulomatosis includes a triad of necrotizing lesions in both the upper and lower respiratory tract
as well as glomerulonephritis. Additional involvement may occur in the skin, spleen, and joints. The
diagnosis appears to be established by the finding of
antineutrophil cytoplasmic autoantibodies (ANCA).
A much less common form of Wegener granulomatosis (the limited form) occurs in which lesions are
present only in the lung. Diffuse pulmonary hemorrhage may occur in either form. The radiographic
appearance of the lung is identical in both forms and
includes nodules and small masses, often with cavitation (Fig 10–14). Segmental and lobar consolidation may also be present. On CT, lesions may be
connected to vessels, although a bronchocentric
form also has been reported. The disease may have
an acute and fulminating course, but steroid and cy-
clophosphamide therapy has been successful in
some cases.

AAG is distinguished by a history of allergy,
usually asthma, pulmonary involvement, and blood
and tissue eosinophilia. Pulmonary infiltrates are
nonspecific; nodules are common, but cavitation is
rare. Katzenstein et al. believe that cases of polyarteritis nodosa with lung lesions probably are AAG.
NSG may be a variant of sarcoidosis except that extrapulmonary involvement is rare and hilar adenopathy is uncommon. Radiographs show multiple or
solitary nodules or infiltrates. The disease is rare in
childhood. Bronchocentric granulomatosis can occur

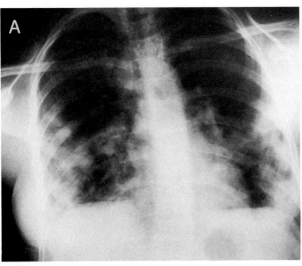

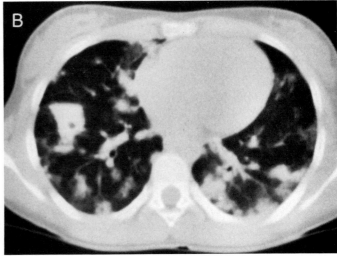

FIG 10–13.
Bronchiolitis obliterans with organizing pneumonia. An 11-year-old
girl 5 years post therapy for leukemia developed cough and dyspnea. **A,** chest radiograph reveals diffuse, poorly defined, bilateral
airspace consolidation. **B,** unenhanced CT scan reveals bilateral
airspace opacities which are patchy, peripheral, posterior, and
lobular in distribution. Biopsy revealed bronchiolitis obliterans with
organizing pneumonia (BOOP).

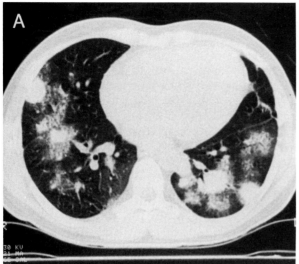
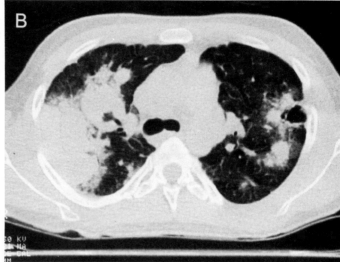

FIG 10–14.
Wegener granulomatosis: a 17-year-old boy with renal failure. A chest radiograph, not shown, shows ill-defined bilateral airspace consolidation. High-resolution CT (**A** and **B**) reveals airspace consolidation with a halo sign similar to that described in invasive as-pergillosis. There is also septal thickening and a single cavitary lesion. Biopsy revealed vasculitis consistent with Wegener granulomatosis. Antineutrophil cytoplasmic autoantibodies test was positive.

rarely in older teenagers, usually associated with asthma, eosinophilia, and upper lobe infiltrates. There are radiographic and clinical similarities to APBA. Diagnosis is made by lung biopsy and requires exclusion of fungal and mycobacterial infection.

Eosinophilic pneumonias, or pulmonary infiltrates with eosinophilic pneumonias, are now considered not a single disease but several different diseases, all with a combination of pulmonary infiltrates and blood eosinophilia. These include *Aspergillus* sensitivity, asthma, extrinsic allergic alveolitis, Hodgkin disease, Löffler syndrome, and parasitic disease. Most of these conditions have been discussed above. Löffler syndrome is a condition in which transient nonsegmental areas of pulmonary consolidation appear in patients who have eosinophilia. Patients usually have a history of atopy. They may be asymptomatic or may present with considerable dyspnea. Radiographic features include multiple, peripheral, subsegmental areas of consolidation that are transient and shifting.

REFERENCES

Immune disorders
Buckley RH: Immunodeficiency diseases. *JAMA* 1987; 258:2841.

Capitanio MA, Kirkpatrick JA: Nasopharyngeal lymphoid tissue: Roentgen observations in 247 children two years of age or less. *Radiology* 1970; 94:323.

Chakravarti VS, Borns P, Lobelle J, et al: Chondroosseous dysplasia in severe combined immunodeficiency due to adenosine deaminase deficiency (chondroosseous dysplasia in ADA deficiency SCID). *Pediatr Radiol* 1991; 21:447.

Chusid MJ, Sty JR, Wells RG: Pulmonary aspergillosis appearing as chronic nodular disease in chronic granulomatous disease. *Pediatr Radiol* 1988; 18:232–234.

Fitch SJ, Magill HL, Herrod HG, et al: Hyperimmunoglobulinemia E syndrome: Pulmonary imaging considerations. *Pediatr Radiol* 1986; 16:285.

Hong R: The immunologic system: Diseases due to immunologic deficiency, in Behrman RE, Vaughan VC II (eds): *Nelson Textbook of Pediatrics*, ed 13. Philadelphia, WB Saunders, 1987, pp 455–467.

Hughes WT: *Pneumocystis carinii* pneumonitis, in Kendig EL, Chernik V (eds): *Disorders of the Respiratory Tract in Children*, ed 4. Philadelphia, WB Saunders, 1983, pp 314–322.

Merten DF, Buckley RH, Pratt PC, et al: Hyperimmunoglobulinemia E syndrome: Radiographic observations. *Radiology* 1979; 132:71.

Provisor AJ, Iacuone JJ, Chilcote RR, et al: Acquired agammaglobulinemia after a life-threatening illness with clinical and laboratory features of infectious mononucleosis in three related male children. *N Engl J Med* 1975; 293:62.

Purtilo DT: Epstein-Barr virus–induced diseases in the X-linked lymphoproliferative syndrome and related disorders. *Biomed Pharmacother* 1985; 39:52.

Purtilo DT, et al: Epstein-Barr virus–induced diseases in males with the X-linked lymphoproliferative syndrome (XLP). *Am J Med* 1982; 73:49.

Sullivan JL: Epstein-Barr virus and the X-linked lymphoproliferative syndrome. *Adv Pediatr* 1983; 30:365–399.

Wood BP, Young LW: Persistent pneumatoceles associated with systemic leukocyte abnormalities. *Pediatr Radiol* 1976; 5:10.

Malignancy and immunodeficiency

Shackelford GD, McAlister WH: Primary immunodeficiency diseases and malignancy. *Am J Roentgenol* 1975; 123:144.

Immunosuppresive therapy

Allan BT, Patton D, Ramsey NKC, et al: Pulmonary fungal infections after bone marrow transplantation. *Pediatr Radiol* 1988; 18:118–122.

Blank N, Castellino RA: The diagnosis of pulmonary infection in patients with altered immunity. *Semin Roentgenol* 1975; 10:63.

Buff SJ, McClelland R, Gallis HA: *Candida albicans* pneumonia: Radiographic appearance. *Am J Roentgenol* 1982; 138:645.

Graham NJ, Müller NL, Miller RR, et al: Intrathoracic complications following allogeneic bone marrow transplantation: CT findings. *Radiology* 1991; 181:153–156.

Green R: Opportunistic pneumonias. *Semin Roentgenol* 1980; 15:50.

Kassner EG, Kaufman SL, Yoon JJ, et al: Pulmonary candidiasis in infants: Clinical, radiologic, and pathologic features. *Am J Roentgenol* 1981; 137:707.

Moore EH, Webb WR, Amend WFC: Pulmonary infections in renal transplantation patients treated by cyclosporine. *Radiology* 1988; 167:97–103.

Witte RJ, Gurney JW, Robbins RA, et al: Diffuse pulmonary alveolar hemorrhage after bone marrow transplantation: Radiographic findings in 39 patients. *Am J Roentgenol* 1991; 157:461.

Acquired immune deficiency syndrome

Amodio JB, Abramson S, Berdon WE, et al: Pediatric AIDS. *Semin Roentgenol.* 1987; 32:66.

Zimmerman BI, Haller JO, Price AP, et al: Children with AIDS: Is pathological diagnosis possible based on chest radiography? *Pediatr Radiol* 1987; 17:303.

Immunologic diseases of the lungs

Ahmad M, Dar MA, Weinstein AJ, et al: Thoracic aspergillosis (part II): Primary pulmonary aspergillosis, allergic bronchopulmonary aspergillosis, and related conditions. *Cleve Clin Q* 1984; 51:631.

Albelda SM, Gefter WB, Epstein DM, et al: Diffuse pulmonary hemorrhage: A review and classification. *Radiology* 1985; 154:289.

Alberle DR, Gamsu G, Lynch DA: Thoracic manifestations of Wegener granulomatosis: Diagnosis and course. *Radiology* 1990 174:703.

Baldree LA, Gaber LW, McKay CP: Anti-neutrophil cytoplasmic autoantibodies in a child with pauci-immune necrotizing and crescentic glomerulonephritis. *Pediatr Nephrol* 1991; 5:296.

Boat TF, Polmar SH, Whitman SV, et al: Hyperreactivity to cow's milk in young children with pulmonary hemosiderosis and cor pulmonale secondary to nasopharyngeal obstruction. *J Pediatr* 1975; 87:23.

Chandler PW, Shin MS, Friedman SE, et al: Radiographic manifestations of bronchiolitis obliterans with organizing pneumonia vs usual interstitial pneumonia. *Am J Roentgenol* 1986; 147:899.

Chetty A, Bhuyan UN, Mitra KK, et al: Cryptogenic fibrosing alveolitis in children. *Ann Allergy* 1987; 58:336.

Epstein DM, Bennett MR: Bronchiolitis obliterans organizing pneumonia with migratory pulmonary infiltrates. *AJR* 1992; 158:515–517.

Foo SS, Weisbrod GL, Herman SJ, et al: Wegener granulomatosis presenting on CT with atypical bronchovasocentric distribution. *J Comput Assist Tomogr* 1990; 14:1004.

Friedman PJ: Idiopathic and autoimmune type 3–like reactions. Interstitial fibrosis, vasculitis, and granulomatosis. *Semin Roentgenol* 1975; 10:43.

Hadchouel M, Prieur AM, Griscelli C: Acute hemorrhagic, hepatic, and neurologic manifestations in juvenile rheumatoid arthritis: Possible relationship to drugs or infection. *J Pediatr* 1985; 106:561.

Hakala M, Paakko P, Huhti E, et al: Open lung biopsy of patients with rheumatoid arthritis. *Clin Rheumatol* 1990; 9:452.

Helton KJ, Kuhn JP, Fletcher BD, et al: Bronchiolitis obliterans–organizing pneumonia (BOOP) in children with malignant disease. *Pediatr Radiol*, accepted for publication.

Hogg JC: Chronic interstitial lung disease of unkown cause: A new classification based on pathogenesis. *AM J Roentgenol* 1991; 156:225.

Katzenstein AL, Liebow AA, Friedman PJ: Bronchocentric granulomatosis, mucoid impaction and hypersensitivity reaction to fungi. *Am Rev Respir Dir* 1975; 111:497.

Kuhlman JE, Fishman EK, Burch PA, et al: CT of invasive pulmonary aspergillosis. *Am J Roentgenol* 1988; 150:1015.

McHugh K, Manson D, Eberhard BA, et al: Wegener's granulomatosis in childhood. *Pediatr Radiol* 1991; 21:552–555.

Levy J, Wilmott RW: Pulmonary hemosiderosis. *Pediatr Pulmonol* 1986; 2:384–391.

Liebow AA, Carrington CB, Friedman PJ: Lymphomatoid granulomatosis. *Hum Pathol* 1972; 3:457.

Muller NL, Miller RR, Webb WR, et al: Fibrosing alveolitis: CT-pathologic correlation. *Radiology* 1986; 160:585.

Muller NL, Staples CA, Miller RR, et al: Disease activity in idiopathic pulmonary fibrosis: CT and pathologic correlation. *Radiology* 1987; 165:731.

O'Brodovich HM, Way CR, Andrew M, et al. Noninvasive

diagnosis of pulmonary hemorrhage in rheumatoid arthritis. *Pediatrics* 1983; 72:720.

Onomura K, Nakata H, Tanaka Y, et al: Pulmonary hemorrhage in patients with system lupus erythematosus. *J Thorac Imaging* 1991; 6:57.

Orsvath P, Paldy L, Bencze G, et al: Autoimmune pneumonitis and Hamman-Rich syndrome. *Helv Paediatr Acta* 1973; 28:28.

Ramirez RE, Glasier C, Kirks D, et al: Pulmonary hemorrhage associated with systemic lupus erythematosus in children. *Radiology* 1984; 152:409.

Singer J, Suchet I, Horwitz T: Paediatric Wegener's granulomatosis: Two case histories and a review of the literature. *Clin Radiol* 1990; 42:50.

Specks U, Wheatley CL, McDonald TJ, et al: Anticytoplas-mic autoantibodies in the diagnosis and follow-up of Wegener's granulomatosis. *Mayo Clin Proc* 1989; 64:28.

Stillwell PC, Norris DG, O'Connell EJ, et al: Desquamative interstitial pneumonitis in children. *Chest* 1980; 77:165.

Travis WD, Colby TV, Lombard C, et al: A clinopathologic study of 34 cases of diffuse pulmonary hemorrhage with lung biopsy confirmation. *Am J Surg Pathol* 1990; 14:1112.

Weisbrod GL: Pulmonary angiitis and granulomatosis: A review. *J Can Assoc Radiol* 1989; 40:127.

Young LW, Smith DI, Glasgow LA: Pneumonia of atypical measles pneumonia. *Am J Roentgenol* 1970; 134:257.

Yousefzadeh DK, Fishman PA: The triad of pneumonitis, pleuritis, and pericarditis in juvenile rheumatoid arthritis. *Pediatr Radiol* 1979; 8:147.

11

Disorders of Pulmonary Circulation

NORMAL ANATOMY AND PHYSIOLOGY

The normal anatomy and the physiology of the major pulmonary vessels are discussed in Chapter 7.

CONGENITAL ABNORMALITIES

Pulmonary Arteries

Congenital abnormalities affecting the pulmonary arteries are listed in Chapter 16. Most of these conditions are discussed in that chapter. Absence of a pulmonary artery usually occurs on the side opposite the aortic arch and is associated with a defect in pulmonary development; the ipsilateral lung may be either absent or hypoplastic. If the lung is present, absence of the pulmonary artery is more accurately called proximal interruption of the pulmonary artery, because there are pulmonary arterial branches present in the lung. The blood supply of the lung is either from a patent ductus arteriosus which inserts distal to the atretic segment, or more commonly, from bronchial or transpleural collateral vessels. The chest film shows a small, hyperlucent lung with an absent or diminutive hilar shadow (Fig 11–1). This appearance can be confused with the Swyer-James syndrome; it is differentiated by lack of expiratory air trapping which is present in the Swyer-James syndrome.

The pulmonary artery is hypoplastic in the hypogenetic lung syndrome which is discussed in Chapter 7; pulmonary artery hypoplasia can also occur as an isolated finding, although the lung is nearly always hypoplastic.

Pulmonary artery aneurysms are rare in children; aneurysmal dilatation is seen with congenital absence or dysplasia of the pulmonary valve; the vessel can become so large that it causes airway obstruction, especially in the neonate. The pulmonary arteries can become markedly enlarged in longstanding pulmonary hypertension.

Pulmonary Arteriovenous Malformations

Pulmonary arteriovenous malformations are abnormal connections between a pulmonary artery and a pulmonary vein. The malformation may be single or multiple and discrete and may present as a nodule or a mass lesion, or may be tiny and diffuse (telangiectatic). The fistula occurs in the lower lobes in approximately 60%, is single in 65%, and is unilateral in approximately 75% of patients. The diagnosis is made in childhood in only 4% to 6% of patients.

579

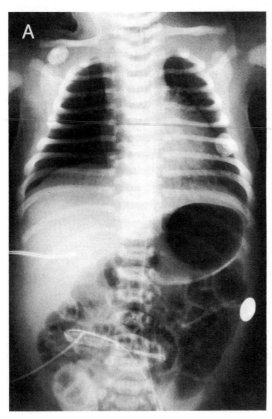

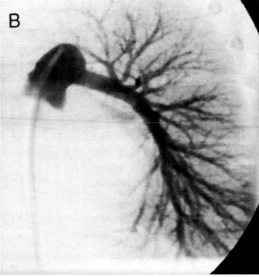

FIG 11–1.
Absence of the right pulmonary artery in a neonate with mild respiratory distress. **A,** frontal radiograph reveals a hyperlucent right lung of normal size. There is a visible left pulmonary artery seen through the cardiac shadow but no right pulmonary artery can be recognized. **B,** pulmonary angiogram confirms the absence of the right pulmonary artery. This finding can also be documented by contrast-enhanced CT scanning or MRI.

About 30% to 40% of patients with pulmonary telangiectasia have Rendu-Osler-Weber disease; arteriovenous malformations (AVM) are found in the skin, mucous membranes, and the lungs. This condition, also known as hereditary hemorrhagic telangiectasia, is transmitted as an autosomal dominant trait. Patients may be asymptomatic or have hemoptysis, clubbing, and cyanosis as a result of the right-to-left shunt. Radiographic findings range from completely normal to the presence of one or more various-sized nodules which are seen on computed tomography (CT) to be related to blood vessels. Magnetic resonance imaging (MRI) may be useful in differentiating between a solid mass and an AVM, especially using flow-sensitive gradient-echo techniques. Contrast echocardiography is sensitive for detection of the associated right-to-left shunt, but pulmonary angiography is required if surgery or embolization procedures are contemplated because many small fistulas may otherwise go unrecognized.

Patients with hepatic cirrhosis may develop cyanosis, clubbing, and hypoxemia associated with pulmonary arteriovenous communications through which right-to-left shunting occurs. The chest film and pulmonary angiographic appearances are similar to those seen in pulmonary telangiectasia, as described above. Chronic active hepatitis can also be associated with primary pulmonary hypertension.

Pulmonary Veins

The most common abnormality of the pulmonary veins is anomalous venous return, which may be either partial or complete. This topic is discussed in Chapter 16, although anomalies of venous return are also common in bronchopulmonary foregut malformations. If anomalous venous return is complete, the common pulmonary vein may drain in a supracardiac location, usually into a persistent left superior vena cava, a cardiac location, usually emptying into the coronary sinus, or be infradiaphragmatic and drain usually into the portal vein. Partial anomalies of venous return are often associated with an atrial septal defect; on the right side, drainage is usually into the superior vena cava. Radiographs may show signs of pulmonary venous congestion; the anomalous veins may be demonstrated occasionally on the chest radiograph, but are more reliably seen on CT or magnetic resonance (MR) scanning (Fig 11–2). Pulmonary angiography remains the definitive diagnostic procedure.

Pulmonary Vein Atresia

Unilateral absence of the pulmonary veins has been reported. The condition is thought to be congenital although in some cases it is difficult to exclude an acquired etiology. The pulmonary veins draining the

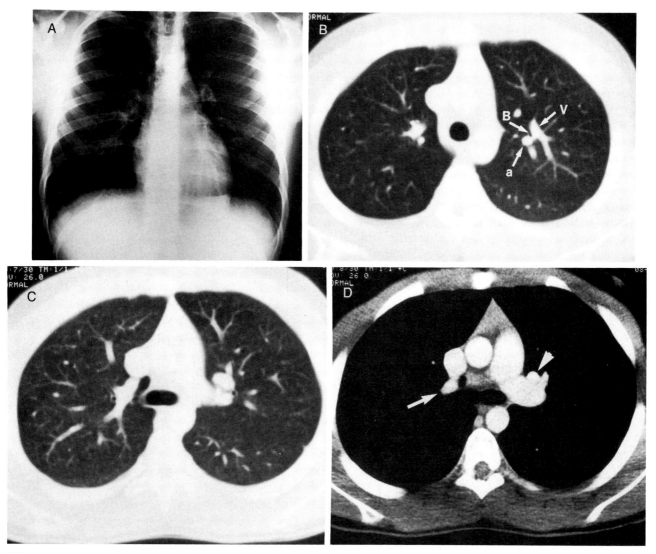

FIG 11–2.
Partial anomalous venous return demonstrated by computed tomography. Thirteen-year-old boy with cardiac murmur. **A,** normal chest radiograph. **B,** 6-mm thick CT scan through the upper lobes demonstrates prominent vessels in both upper lung zones, with arteries *(a)* larger than their accompanying bronchi *(B)*. *V* = vein. **C,** 6-mm contrast-enhanced CT scan at the level of the carina shows that the large upper lobe vessel demonstrated in **B** is a pulmonary vein that enters the posterior wall of the superior vena cava. **D,** 6-mm contrast-enhanced CT scan, 8 mm inferior to **B,** reveals that the anomalous vein *(arrow)* has entered the posterior wall of the superior vena cava. A relatively large superior pulmonary vein also is noted in the left lung *(arrowhead)*. Lower images confirmed the presence of a sinus venosus defect and a secundum atrial septal defect, which were confirmed at cardiac catheterization and surgery. A 3-to-1 left-right shunt was present, which accounted for the increased size of the pulmonary artery in comparison with its accompanying bronchus.

involved lobe are atretic and show intimal thickening and fibrosis. The lung shows chronic pulmonary edema, superimposed infection, and pulmonary venous infarction. Patients present with either hemoptysis or infection. Cyanosis and right-to-left shunting is usually absent. Radiographs show findings ranging from total opacity of a lung to a relatively normal but hypoplastic-appearing lung. Kerley B lines and an interstitial pattern are frequent findings. Definitive diagnosis requires pulmonary angiography, CT, or MRI.

PULMONARY EDEMA

Pulmonary edema is the excessive extravascular accumulation of water and solute in the lung tissues. It may be due to (1) increased hydrostatic pressure in the pulmonary veins; (2) decreased osmotic pressure gradient across the capillary wall; (3) increased capillary permeability; or (4) diminished lymphatic drainage.

For purposes of discussion, the causes of pulmonary edema can be divided into those cases associated with elevated microvascular pressure (cardiogenic), those associated with increased capillary permeability with normal microvascular pressure (noncardiogenic), and those due to overhydration, either because of renal disease or iatrogenic causes.

CARDIOGENIC EDEMA

Cardiogenic pulmonary edema in childhood has a number of causes, which are discussed in detail in Chapter 16. Most of the lesions are related to impaired left ventricular function or obstruction to the pulmonary venous return.

The radiographic diagnosis of early pulmonary edema requires a high-quality chest radiograph made with a short exposure time to minimize blurring. Pulmonary edema is divided into three stages of increasing severity: (1) pulmonary vascular redistribution, (2) interstitial edema, and (3) alveolar edema.

Pulmonary Vascular Redistribution

Pulmonary vascular redistribution or pulmonary vascular congestion are terms often used interchangeably. In this condition, which may be considered as a pre-edema phase, the pulmonary capillary wedge pressure (PCWP) is 15 to 20 mm Hg (normal <10 mm Hg). In the upright position, the upper lobe vessels become distended, and the relative caliber of the pulmonary vessels are larger, since gravity directs blood flow through the more dependent vessels. This sign, however, is difficult to interpret in infants and children in whom many radiographs are made in the supine position. The use of arterial-bronchus ratios may prove useful in detection of increased pulmonary flow and pulmonary congestion in adults and older children. In the normal erect patient, the upper lobe vessels are equal to or smaller than their companion bronchus and they are smaller than the lower lobe arterial branches, which in turn are larger than their companion bronchus. In the normal supine patient both the upper and lower lobe vessels are nearly the same size as their respective bronchi. When blood flow is redistributed, the upper lobe vessels become relatively larger and the lower lobe ones smaller.

Interstitial Edema

Interstitial pulmonary edema is often the first recognizable sign of cardiac decompensation. It develops as PCWP reaches 20 to 25 mm Hg. Interstitial edema can be divided into perivascular and septal components.

Perivascular Edema. Intrapulmonary vessels should be sharply marginated against adjacent aerated lungs. Since the vessels lie in the same interstitial planes as the lymphatics and the bronchioles, their margins can be expected to lose their usual sharp definition if excess fluid occurs in the surrounding tissues. Bronchial wall thickening also occurs; this may be due not only to edema in the loose interstitial tissue surrounding the bronchi but also to edema of the bronchial walls themselves.

Septal Edema. Interstitial edema is also manifested by septal thickening (Fig 11–3). Kerley A lines are due to thickening of the interlobular septa, which are thin, nonbranching lines extending from the hila. They are 2 to 6 cm long and are generally best seen in the upper lungs midway between the hilum and the lung periphery. They represent the central pulmonary septa. Kerley B lines are straight lines, no longer than 2 cm, that are peripheral and perpendicular to the pleural surface and are usually best seen in the lower lungs anteriorly and laterally. They are produced by thickened interlobular septa and first develop when the pulmonary venous pressure is 17 to 20 mm Hg or higher. The cause of Kerley C lines is uncertain. They are shorter and tend to form a reticulum in the central basilar portion of the lung. They may represent superimposition of many Kerley B lines.

Our experience is that in children Kerley lines are often best seen in the retrosternal space on the lateral view of the chest. Frequently seen in association with Kerley lines is slight thickening of the interlobar fissures of the lungs owing to subpleural edema. Fissural thickening is much more easily recognized in children than are Kerley lines.

Alveolar Edema

Alveolar edema becomes recognizable when air in the alveoli is replaced by edema fluid and is thought to occur as the PCWP reaches 25 to 30 mm Hg. Although the temporal sequence is not always obvious radiologically, alveolar edema usually occurs after development of interstitial edema. Its onset may be quite sudden; fluid in the distended alveolar walls may pour into the alveoli as the pulmonary venous pressure rises to critical levels. The radiographic findings vary with the extent of the involvement. Initially, one may see multiple small acinar shadows becoming confluent and creating multiple areas of patchy opacity throughout both lungs. An air bronchogram pattern occurs as the shadows consolidate. The classic appearance of acute alveolar edema is a central or "butterfly" distribution in which edema is marked centrally while the lung peripheries remain

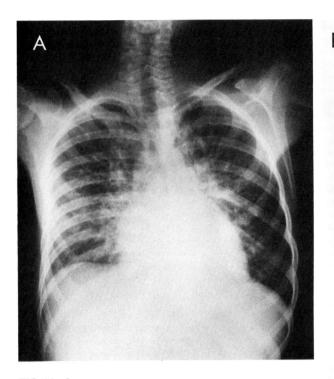
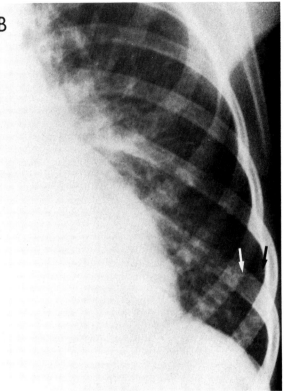

FIG 11–3.
Acute myocarditis with predominantly interstitial pulmonary edema with some airspace component in an 8-year-old patient.
A, frontal chest radiograph reveals mild cardiomegaly and prominent but ill-defined pulmonary vascular markings. **B,** close-up of the left costophrenic angle reveals multiple small Kerley B lines *(arrows).*

relatively clear (Fig 11–4). On rare occasions, pulmonary edema is asymmetric or unilateral. The factors causing this atypical distribution are thought to be either the position of the patient or the presence of preexisting pulmonary disease.

Milne has been able, in adults, to differentiate cardiogenic, noncardiogenic, and overhydration types of pulmonary edema based on their radiographic appearances. He analyzed distribution of blood flow, distribution of the pulmonary edema, and the width of the vascular pedicle. Helpful ancillary signs were septal lines, peribronchial cuffing, air bronchograms, heart size, and pleural effusions. It remains to be proved that these findings can be applied to children. The structures are smaller, the vascular pedicle width is difficult to assess because of the thymus, and most films are made in the supine position.

Noncardiogenic Edema

In most cases, the radiographic appearance of noncardiogenic pulmonary edema, or normal microvascular pressure edema, is similar to cardiogenic pulmonary edema, except that cardiomegaly is usually not present. Classically, there is no redistribution of blood flow, no pleural effusion, and no peribron-

chial cuffing. The clinical hallmark is increased protein concentration in the edema fluid relative to plasma protein levels. Important causes of noncardiogenic pulmonary edema to be discussed here include neurogenic pulmonary edema, acute glomerulonephritis, upper airway obstruction, pulmonary edema after the intravenous administration of contrast media, and adult respiratory distress syndrome (ARDS). Other causes of pulmonary edema include Mendelson syndrome (aspiration pneumonia), neardrowning, hydrocarbon pneumonia, smoke inhalation, and drug reactions.

Adult Respiratory Distress Syndrome

ARDS is a syndrome of acute alveolar damage incited by a diverse group of either pulmonary or systemic conditions including sepsis, shock, neardrowning, burns, trauma, pneumonia, and neurologic disasters. Despite its name, ARDS occurs frequently in children, even in infants. It is characterized by a clinical, functional, and radiographic tetrad: (1) acute, severe, and progressive respiratory distress; (2) refractory hypoxemia; (3) increasing stiffness of the lungs leading to respiratory failure; and (4) diffuse radiographic lung opacification.

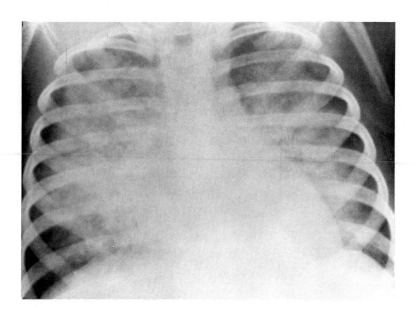

FIG 11–4.
Massive pulmonary edema with predominant airspace pattern in a 7-year-old boy with renal failure and azotemia. The heart is at the upper limits of normal in size. There is a "butterfly" pattern of cen- tral pulmonary edema with peripheral sparing. No pleural effusion is present.

The pathophysiology is complex and multifactorial, but a common denominator is acute alveolar capillary membrane damage causing pulmonary edema. Leukocyte accumulation in the pulmonary microvessels may result in release of oxygen radicals and other toxic products. However, leukocytes are not the only mediating factor; even severely neutropenic children can develop ARDS. Surfactant deple-

tion causing alveolar atelectasis also appears to be an important factor. The clinical, pathologic, and radiographic stages are summarized in Table 11–1.

The initial chest film findings are often normal unless there is an underlying pulmonary abnormality; within 24 to 48 hours diffuse, bilateral airspace opacities develop (Fig 11–5). They may increase in severity and then, often, partially clear. It has been

TABLE 11–1.

Typical Characteristics of Adult Respiratory Distress Syndrome (ARDS)*

Characteristic	Stage		
	I	II	III
Duration of pathologic findings	First 12–24 hr: capillary congestion, endothelial cell swelling	Days 2–5: fluid leakage, fibrin deposition, vascular obstruction	After day 5: alveolar cell hyperplasia, collagen deposition, microvascular destruction
Clinical findings	Acute respiratory failure, shunt due to microatelectasis, hypoxemia relieved by positive end-expiratory pressure (PEEP)	Respiratory failure, shunt due to consolidation, hypoxemia not relieved by PEEP	Respiratory failure, hypoxemia due to ventilation-perfusion imbalance
Prototypical radiographic appearance	Low lung volumes, clear lungs	Diffuse consolidation, pulmonary artery filling defects on angiography	Less dense, ground-glass, opacification; cortical lucencies if ischemic infarcts are present
Radiographic modifiers	Opacities if pulmonary inciting process	Local lucencies or densities if complicated by infection or hemorrhage	Same as stage II
Differential diagnosis	Neuromuscular hypoventilation, airway obstruction, pulmonary embolism	Cardiogenic pulmonary edema, fluid overload, massive aspiration, nosocomial infection, lung hemorrhage	Same as stage II

*Adapted from Greene R: *Radiology* 1987; 163:57–66.

shown by CT that a change in position produces a change in the position of the opacities which appear in the new dependent position, suggesting that the weight of the lung may be causing compressive atelectasis. The opacities shift too rapidly to be due solely to focal edema. CT shows the opacities to be much more unevenly distributed than would be suspected from the chest film. Pleural effusion is not commonly seen and should suggest an associated complication. In children, air leak complications develop in over half the cases at a mean of 6 days post injury. These usually persist until the patient is weaned from the respirator. The mortality rate in children varies from 40% to 93%.

The long-term effects of ARDS on the pediatric lung are not known, but recurrent respiratory symptoms and abnormal pulmonary function tests are common in survivors. Oxygen toxicity is thought to

be the cause of the changes of alveolar duct fibrosis noted on biopsy (Fig 11–6).

Neurogenic Edema

Neurogenic pulmonary edema may occur in children after cranial trauma, seizures, or neoplasms that produce increased intracranial pressure. A sudden increase in intracranial pressure seems to be the most likely precipitating factor, but insidious onset of intracranial hypertension has also been implicated.

It has been theorized that there is a marked but transient increase in both systemic and pulmonary vascular pressures, resulting in a shift of blood from the systemic to the low-resistance, pulmonary circulation. The sharply increased pulmonary capillary pressure leads to capillary wall damage and in-

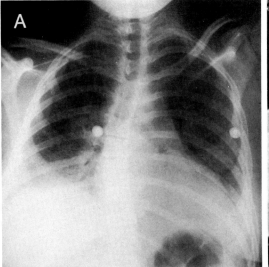
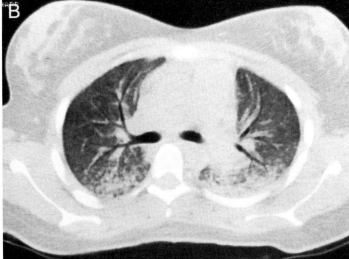
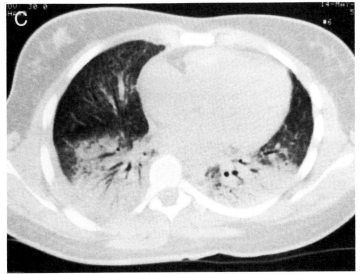

FIG 11–5.
ARDS, probably due to acute viral pneumonia, in a 13-year-old patient with sudden onset of severe respiratory distress. **A,** chest radiograph reveals hazy, ill-defined basilar opacities with faint air bronchograms seen through the cardiac silhouette. A radiograph taken 24 hours earlier (not shown) had been normal. **B,** 6-mm, 0.1-second, unenhanced CT scan reveals ground-glass opacities and diffuse air bronchograms in the anterior three fourths of each lung. Ill-defined, coalescent, nodular airspace lesions are seen posteriorly. The intrapulmonary vessels are of normal size. **C,** 0.1-second, unenhanced CT scan through the lung base reveals extensive bilateral lower lobe consolidation. A small pleural effusion is present on the right side and ill-defined airspace opacities and faint ground-glass opacification are noted anterior in the right lung. Lung biopsy revealed diffuse alveolar damage consistent with ARDS. The patient deteriorated rapidly and died before lung transplantation could be performed. Autopsy revealed no specific etiologic agent.

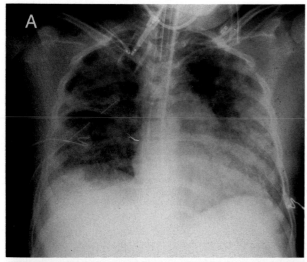

FIG 11–6.
Pulmonary fibrosis following ARDS. A 10-year-old patient with a complicated history of overwhelming sepsis developed severe ARDS but survived. **A,** chest radiograph reveals a right-sided pneumothorax, consolidation of the right upper lobe, which is partly atelectatic, and patchy airspace consolidation throughout the remainder of both lungs with the changes somewhat peripheral in the left lung. This radiograph was made 2 weeks after the onset of ARDS and after the subsequent development of air block phenomenon. **B,** CT scan through the lung base on the same day of the chest radiograph **(A)** showed marked cystic areas present in both lungs, probably due to areas of interstitial pulmonary emphysema. The interspersed lung is markedly abnormal with ground-glass opacification. **C,** 1 month later, 3-mm CT scan through the level of the bronchus intermedius shows the development of extensive pulmonary fibrosis with accentuation of interlobular septa and destruction of lung parenchyma.

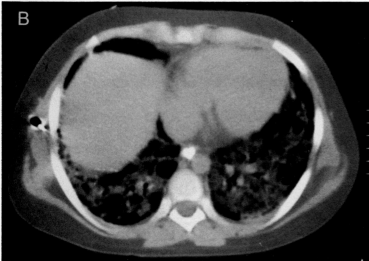

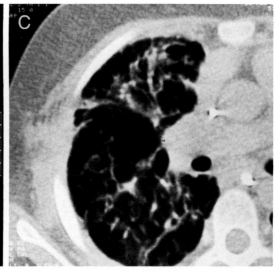

creased permeability, which persists and causes ongoing pulmonary edema. As the vascular pressures subsequently return to normal, heart failure is averted.

The radiographic features of neurogenic pulmonary edema are indistinguishable from other types of pulmonary edema. The distribution is unpredictable; it is sometimes asymmetric and may be unilateral. Pleural effusions are uncommon; the edema may disappear within hours after intracranial pressure is lowered, or it may persist for several days. Aspiration or severe hypoxia may complicate the radiographic presentation.

Acute Glomerulonephritis

Acute glomerulonephritis is characterized by systemic hypertension, periorbital and peripheral edema, renal failure, and blood, protein, and red blood cell casts in the urine. Pulmonary edema occurs commonly in children with acute glomerulonephritis. The edema is multifactorial in origin, includ-

ing fluid retention due to renal failure, increased capillary permeability, hypoproteinemia, and, in some cases, left ventricular failure.

Radiographic features of acute glomerulonephritis are often sufficiently characteristic for the radiologist to suggest the correct diagnosis (Fig 11–7). Commonly seen are cardiomegaly, pulmonary vascular congestion, small pleural effusions, septal edema, and subcutaneous edema. Frank airspace edema occurs in about 25% of patients.

The nephrotic syndrome may often be differentiated radiologically from acute glomerulonephritis when one sees a heart that is normal to small in size, relatively clear lungs, and, usually, a much greater accumulation of pleural fluid than is present in glomerulonephritis.

Pulmonary Edema Secondary to Upper Airway Obstruction

Croup and epiglottitis can cause acute onset of pulmonary edema in childhood. The mechanism is un-

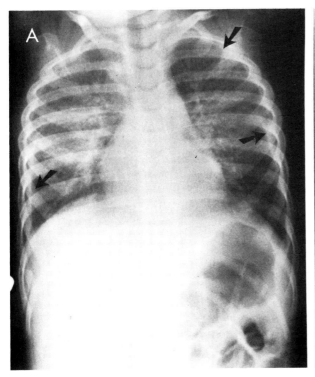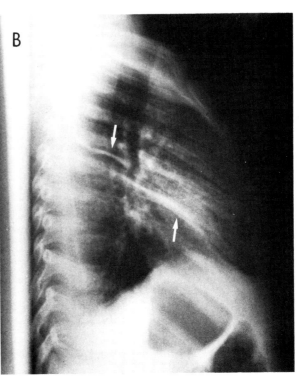

FIG 11–7.
Pulmonary edema in acute glomerulonephritis. This 3-year-old child was thought by the examining physicians to have bilateral pneumonia. **A,** frontal radiograph reveals small bilateral pleural effusions and patchy airspace consolidation in both lungs, especially the central portion of the right lung, findings which are consistent with pulmonary edema. **B,** lateral radiograph reveals subpleural edema or interlobar fluid collections or both, with fissural widening *(arrows).* Pleural effusion is also noted posteriorly on this cross-table lateral film. The radiographic findings suggested the correct diagnosis of acute glomerulonephritis.

known, although it has been suggested that there may be a common mechanism of a sudden increase in the negative intrathoracic pressure that is caused by violent inspiration against a closed glottis. This may interfere with the clearance of pulmonary fluid by the lymphatics and result in pulmonary edema. Capillary permeability may also be increased by the sudden drop in intrathoracic pressure. An upper lobe distribution of the edema is often seen. A similar cause is implied for the occasional case of pulmonary edema that is seen after rapid expansion of a pneumothorax or removal of a large collection of pleural effusion.

Chronic upper airway obstruction, usually due to enlarged tonsils and adenoids, has been found to cause cor pulmonale and cardiac failure in some children.

Pulmonary Edema After Intravenous Administration of Contrast Media

Acute pulmonary edema has been reported both in infants and young adults following the administration of standard amounts of intravenous contrast media. The edema could not be explained by anaphylactic reaction to contrast media, overdose, or other obvious cause. Hypertonicity of the contrast material, causing an increase in intravascular volume and possible damage to the alveolar capillary bed, has been suggested.

Other Causes of Pulmonary Edema

Other causes of pulmonary edema are rare in childhood, but edema may follow inhalation of a variety of noxious fumes or soluble aerosols including nitrogen dioxide (silo-filler's disease), carbon monoxide, sulfur dioxide, oxygen, ozone, ammonia, chlorine, phosgene, and organophosphates. Aspiration of hypertonic water-soluble contrast agents or the newer nonionic contrast media can also produce pulmonary edema. Pulmonary edema has also occurred following blood transfusion in the absence of fluid overload.

PULMONARY HYPERTENSION

Pulmonary hypertension is defined as a prolonged increase above the normally accepted values for pressure of 30 mm Hg systolic and 18 mm Hg mean arterial pressure in the main pulmonary artery. Pathologically, the changes in the pulmonary vessels are most striking in the small arterioles. In children, pulmonary hypertension most often results from pulmonary vasoconstriction secondary to hypoxia. There are multiple known etiologies but in some cases (primary pulmonary hypertension) no apparent cause can be documented. A common classification is to divide pulmonary hypertension into precapillary (arterial) and postcapillary (venous) causes. Among precapillary causes are left-to-right shunts, thromboembolic disease, lung disease (cystic fibrosis, bronchopulmonary dysplasia), and causes of alveolar hypoventilation such as obesity and neuromuscular diseases. Postcapillary causes are essentially those diseases associated with venous obstruction. There are some combined cases in which abnormalities of vessels on both sides of the capillary bed contribute to pulmonary hypertension. Depending on the etiology, pulmonary hypertension may be reversible or irreversible; if irreversible, it ultimately leads to right ventricular hypertrophy, cor pulmonale, and death. Radiographic findings are complicated by the presence of the underlying causative pulmonary or cardiac disease and thus are variable and relatively insensitive. In pulmonary arterial hypertension, enlargement of the main, right, and left pulmonary arteries is usually present. In the frontal view, the normal right pulmonary artery should be about the same size as the trachea; on the lateral view, the left pulmonary artery should also be of similar size to the trachea. Classically, in pulmonary hypertension, the vessels taper rapidly in size toward the periphery of the lung, providing a "pruned tree" appearance. In postcapillary hypertension, signs of venous congestion predominate, including Kerley lines, interstitial edema, and blood flow redistribution.

Pulmonary veno-occlusive disease is a rare idiopathic disorder which can occasionally be seen in children. There is a gradual downhill course over a period of a year or longer, marked by the development of pulmonary hypertension and cor pulmonale. The radiograph may show cardiomegaly and signs of interstitial edema with prominent Kerley B lines. It is not known whether the condition is due to a thromboembolic phenomenon or endothelial injury and subsequent subintimal fibrosis. There is often a history of preceding respiratory infection. Left atrial enlargement and blood flow redistribution are usually absent.

PULMONARY VASCULITIS

Pulmonary vasculitis (angiitis) is quite rare in children. Often there is an associated granulomatous reaction. After fungal and mycobacterial infections

have been excluded, there is a rare group of diseases, presumably immunologic in origin, which can be responsible. They include Wegener granulomatosis, allergic angiitic granulomatosis of Churg and Strauss, bronchocentric granulomatosis, necrotizing sarcoid granulomatosis, and lymphomatoid granulomatosis. This last-named condition is now believed by many authors to be a form of malignant lymphoma. Wegener granulomatosis is the most common in this group. Orlowski et al. reported on 17 patients, all adolescents. The disease is described as limited, involving only the lung, or classic, in which case there is multiorgan disease with glomerulonephritis, paranasal sinusitis and pulmonary involvement. The lungs show diffuse, bilateral, nodular, or masslike opacities; some may cavitate, and segmental and lobar consolidation may also occur (see Fig 10–13).

Other conditions that rarely may be associated with vasculitis in children include polyarteritis nodosa, systemic lupus erythematosus, Henoch-Schönlein purpura, and Takayasu and Kawasaki syndromes. Radiographic findings are nonspecific but include ill-defined perihilar and perivascular haze. Diffuse pulmonary hemorrhage may also rarely occur in this group of diseases. These diseases are discussed elsewhere in this text.

PULMONARY THROMBOEMBOLIC DISEASE

Pulmonary thromboembolic disease is much less common in children than in adults. Its incidence is unknown, but pulmonary embolism or infarction is diagnosed only a few times a year in most pediatric radiology practices. Pulmonary thromboemboli in children, as in adults, most often originate from intravascular thrombi in veins in the leg or pelvis (Fig 11–8,A). Other common sites include indwelling catheters, especially ventriculoatrial shunt catheters. Slowing of the circulation secondary to immobilization is a frequent predisposing factor. Children with hypercoagulable states such as sickle cell anemia and nephrotic syndrome are at increased risk of thromboembolic disease.

Radiographic Manifestations

Even in adults, most episodes of pulmonary embolism are asymptomatic and produce no detectable changes on the plain chest film; this is probably even more often the case in children. Radiographic findings can be separated into those occurring with thromboembolism alone and thromboembolism associated with pulmonary infarction. If the embolic

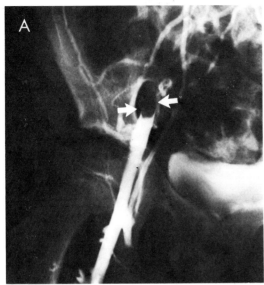

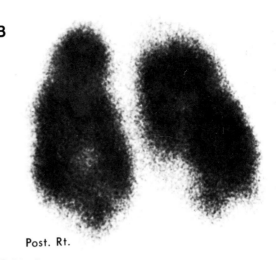

FIG 11–8.
Pelvic thrombophlebitis and pulmonary thromboembolism. **A,** a venogram in a patient with a suspected pulmonary embolism shows complete occlusion of the right iliac vein (arrows). **B,** a posterior perfusion lung scan shows bilateral perfusion defects consistent with multiple pulmonary thromboemboli. The patient died shortly after this study, and bilateral emboli were found at autopsy.

episode occurs without infarction, the chest film, most often, is normal. If abnormal, it may show localized or generalized oligemia, an enlarged pulmonary artery, changes of acute cor pulmonale, or loss of lung volume. Pulmonary infarction may be accompanied by any or all of the above signs in addition to changes of pulmonary consolidation. Classically, consolidation is in the shape of a truncated cone of homogeneous opacity located at the lung periphery, abutting the pleural surface, although in fact this pattern is uncommon. A small pleural effusion and mild elevation of the hemidiaphragm are often present. Contrast-enhanced CT reveals an irregularly hypo- or avascular region of peripheral pulmonary consolidation and ultrafast CT and fast-spiral CT have demonstrated emboli in central, and occasionally in smaller, peripheral vessels. Definitive diagnosis can be established by pulmonary angiography, although radionuclide scanning reveals a fairly characteristic pattern of single or multiple focal segmental or lobar perfusion defects (Fig 11–8,B). Ventilation scans are classically normal.

Septic Embolism

Septic emboli are the most frequently recognized form of pulmonary embolic disease in children. Common sites of origin include an infected venous catheter, grafts, artificial heart valves, and so forth. Staphylococcal osteomyelitis may be the primary

site of septic embolic disease. Radiologic manifestations are those of multiple, ill-defined, round, or wedge-shaped densities in the periphery of both lungs (Fig 11–9). They may be of uniform or variable size, and cavitation is not unusual. CT may show the lesions to be connected to a vessel. Hilar lymph node enlargement is frequent and can be striking.

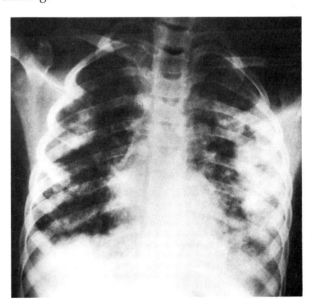

FIG 11–9.
Staphylococcal pneumonia with septic emboli in a teenage boy with acute fulminating staphylococcal septicemia. Extensive bilateral peripheral pulmonary infiltrates are seen. The patient died 12 hours after this study. Multiple staphylococcal emboli were found throughout both lungs.

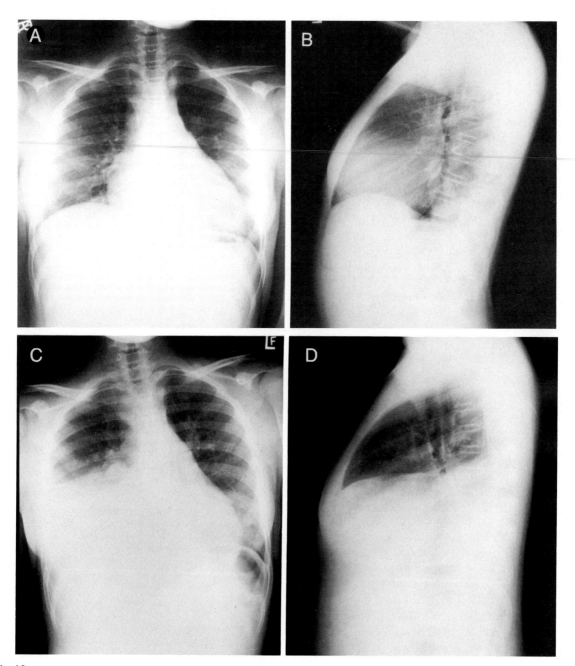

FIG 11–10.
Probable pulmonary infarction in a 15-year-old patient with sickle cell anemia. **A,** frontal and **B,** lateral radiographs show consolidation and a small pleural effusion posteriorly in the right lower lobe which is best appreciated on the lateral radiograph. **C,** frontal and **D,** lateral radiographs made less than 24 hours later show massive right middle and lower lobe consolidation and effusion. No organisms could be cultured. Diagnosis of probable pulmonary infarction was established clinically. (Courtesy of Dr. Thomas Slovis, Children's Hospital of Michigan.)

Pulmonary Infarction in Sickle Cell Disease

Patients with sickle cell disease are at increased risk of pulmonary infarction. Infarcts were present in 12% of the patients in one clinical series. Haupt et al. reported an incidence of alveolar wall necrosis in 12 (17%) of an autopsy series of 72 patients. These areas of infarcted lung parenchyma were in regions where the alveoli were filled with fluid or exudate, which suggested that intravascular sickling had occurred in regions of the lung where gas exchange was impaired. In addition to infarction, thrombotic vascular occlusion may lead to pulmonary hypertension and cor pulmonale.

Pulmonary thromboembolism occurs in children

with sickle cell anemia chiefly as a result of embolism of necrotic bone marrow. Haupt et al. recorded a 13% incidence of this complication in their series. While differentiation of infarction from infection in these patients is always difficult, these authors suggest that the clinical syndrome of bone marrow infarction associated with symptoms suggestive of pulmonary embolization should raise the possibility of bone marrow embolization.

Pneumonia is a frequent complication in these children, particularly pneumococcal pneumonia. Fever, upper or middle lobe disease, and lack of symptoms of sickle crisis are findings favoring infection over infarction (Fig 11–10). Perfusion lung scanning can be helpful; if diminished perfusion is seen in areas that appear normal on the radiograph, ischemia is more likely than infection. Chest pain and symptoms suggestive of pulmonary infarction can also be produced by infarction of a rib.

Pulmonary Fat Embolism

Pulmonary fat embolism is characterized by a triad of progressive pulmonary insufficiency, cerebral dysfunction, and petechiae. Nearly all pulmonary fat emboli occur following trauma, especially in patients with fractures of the femora and tibias. Fat droplets, probably from the marrow cavity, appear in the blood and lodge in the capillaries of the lungs, brain, and other organs. Autopsy studies have shown an incidence of 60% to 97%, but in one series of 670 patients with leg fractures only 1.2% had clinical evidence of fat embolism. If symptoms develop, usually they do not appear until 24 to 48 hours after injury. Dyspnea, cyanosis, and tachycardia with cough and fever are common. Fat globules in the urine and extra large fat globules in the blood can usually be demonstrated. A reduction in alveolar oxygen pressure (P_{AO_2}) to 50 mm Hg or less within 72 hours of injury is an early indication of pulmonary fat embolism.

Radiographic Findings. Most often the chest film is normal. Abnormalities, when present, include widespread airspace consolidation due to alveolar hemorrhage and edema. The distribution may be peripheral rather than central, usually involving the basilar regions to a greater degree than does pulmonary edema of cardiac origin. The time lapse between trauma and the development of radiographic signs is usually 1 to 2 days. This delay differentiates fat embolism from traumatic lung contusion; in the latter, the radiograph is abnormal initially. Changes due to fat embolism usually disappear gradually within a week to 10 days. Pleural effusion is uncommon.

REFERENCES

Anomalies and Disorders of Pulmonary Vessels

Currarino G, Willis KW, Johnson AF Jr, et al: Pulmonary telangiectasia. *Am J Roentgenol* 1976; 127:775.

Dinsmore BJ, Gefter WB, Hatabu H, et al: Pulmonary arteriovenous malformations: Diagnosis by gradient-refocused MR imaging. *J Comput Assist Tomogr* 1990; 14:918.

Dubois RS, Slovis TL, Tolia V, et al: Chronic active hepatitis and pregnancy: A report of two cases in adolescence. *Am J Gastroenterol* 1982; 77:649.

Ellis K: Developmental abnormalities in the systemic blood supply to the lungs. *Am J Roentgenol* 1991; 156:669.

Greene R, Miller SW: Cross-sectional imaging of silent pulmonary venous anomalies. *Radiology* 1986; 159:279.

Higgins CB, Wexler L: Clinical and angiographic features of pulmonary arteriovenous fistulas in children. *Radiology* 1976; 119:171.

Murakami T, Nakanishi M, Konishi T, et al: Diffuse pulmonary arteriovenous fistula shown by contrast echocardiography and pulmonary angiography. *Pediatr Radiol* 1991; 21:128.

Oh KS, Bender TM, Bowen A, et al: Plain radiographic, nuclear medicine and angiographic observations of hepatogenic pulmonary angiodysplasia. *Pediatr Radiol* 1983; 13:111.

Simon M: The pulmonary vessels: Their hemodynamic evaluation using routine radiographs. *Radiol Clin North Am* 1963; 2:363.

Swischuk LE, L'Heureux PL: Unilateral pulmonary vein atresia. *Am J Roentgenol* 1980; 135:667.

Swischuk LE, Stansberry SD: Pulmonary vascularity in pediatric heart disease. *J Thorac Imaging* 1989; 4:1.

Thorsen MK, Erickson SJ, Mewissen MW, et al: CT and MR imaging of partial anomalous pulmonary venous return to the azygos vein. *J Comput Assist Tomogr* 1990; 14:1007.

Weibel ER, Taylor CR: Design and structure of the human lung, in Fishman AP (ed): *Pulmonary Diseases and Disorders*, Vol 1. New York, McGraw-Hill, 1988.

White CW, Sondheimer HM, Crouch EC, et al: Treatment of pulmonary hemangiomatosis with recombinant interferon alpha$_{2a}$. *N Engl J Med* 1989; 320:1197.

Pulmonary Edema

Alford BA, Dee P, Feldman P: Effects of metrizamide on the lung. *Pediatr Radiol* 1983; 13:5.

Effman EL, Merten DF, Kirks DR, et al: Adult respiratory distress syndrome in children. *Radiology* 1985; 157:69.

Felman A: Neurogenic pulmonary edema: Observations in six patients. *Am J Roentgenol* 1971; 112:393.

Gattinoni L, Pesenti A, Baglioni S, et al: Inflammatory pulmonary edema and positive end-expiratory pressure: Correlations between imaging and physiologic studies. *J Thorac Imaging* 1988; 3:59.

Greene R: Adult respiratory distress syndrome: Acute alveolar damage. *Radiology* 1987; 163:57.

Katz R: Adult respiratory distress syndrome in children. *Clin Chest Med* 1987; 8:635.

Luke MJ, McKrinzi A, Folger GM, et al: Chronic nasopharyngeal obstruction as a cause of cardiomegaly, cor pulmonale, and pulmonary edema. Part I. *Pediatrics* 1966; 37:762.

Maltby JD, Gouverne ML: CT findings in pulmonary venoocclusive disease. *J Comput Assist Tomogr* 1984; 8:758.

Milne ENC: Correlation of physiologic findings with chest roentgenology. *Radiol Clin North Am* 1973; 11:17.

Milne ENC, Pistolesi M, Miniati M, et al: The radiologic distinction of cardiogenic and noncardiogenic edema. *Am J Roentgenol* 1985; 144:879–894.

Murata K, Herman PG, Khan A, et al: Intralobar distribution of oleic acid–induced pulmonary edema in the pig: Evaluation by high-resolution CT. *Invest Radiol* 1989; 24:647.

Newman B, Park SC, Oh KS: Coexistent transient pulmonary edema and pericardial effusion. *Pediatr Radiol* 1988; 18:455.

Pfenninger J, Tschaeppeler H, Wagner BP, et al: The paradox of adult respiratory distress syndrome in neonates. *Pediatr Pulmonol* 1991; 10:18.

Pistolesi M, Giuntini C: Assessment of extravascular lung water. *Radiol Clin North Am* 1978; 16:551.

Rigler LG, Supernant EL: Pulmonary edema. *Semin Roentgenol* 1967; 2:33.

Royal JA, Levin DL: Adult respiratory distress syndrome in pediatric patients. I. Clinical aspects, pathophysiology, pathology, and mechanisms of lung injury. *J Pediatr* 1988; 112:169.

Sivan Y, Mor C, Al-Jundi S, et al: Adult respiratory distress syndrome in severely neutropenic children. *Pediatr Pulmonol* 1990; 8:104.

Stark P, Greene R, Kott MM, et al: CT-findings in ARDS. *Radiologe* 1987; 27:367.

Stark P, Jasmine J: CT of pulmonary edema. *Crit Rev Diagn Imaging* 1989; 29:245.

Wood BP, Smith WL: Pulmonary edema in infants following injection of contrast media for urography. *Radiology* 1981; 139:377.

Woodring JH: Pulmonary artery–bronchus ratios in patients with normal lungs, pulmonary vascular plethora, and congestive heart failure. *Radiology* 1991; 179:115.

Other Pulmonary Vascular Disease

Balakrishnan J, Moulay AM, Siegelman SS, et al: Pulmonary infarction: CT appearance with pathologic correlation. *J Comput Assist Tomogr* 1991; 15:941–945.

Barrett-Conner E: Pneumonia and pulmonary infarction in sickle cell anemia. *JAMA* 1973; 224:977.

Batra P: The fat embolism syndrome. *J Thorac Imaging* 1987; 2(3):12–17.

Geraghty JJ, Stanford W, Landas SK, et al: Ultrafast computed tomography in experimental pulmonary embolism. *Invest Radiol* 1992; 27:60–63.

Gumbs RV, McCauley DI: Hilar and mediastinal lymphadenopathy in septic pulmonary embolic disease. *Radiology* 1982; 142:313.

Hampton AO, Castleman B: Correlation of post mortem chest teleroentgenograms with autopsy findings with special reference to pulmonary embolism and infarction. *Am J Roentgenol* 1940; 43:305.

Haupt MM, Moore GW, Bauer TW, et al: The lung in sickle cell disease. *Chest* 1982; 81:3.

Karayalcin G, Rosner F, Kim KY, et al: Sickle cell anemia: Clinical manifestations in 100 patients and review of the literature. *Am J Med Sci* 1974; 269:51.

Orlowski JP, Clough JD, Gyment PG: Wegener's granulomatosis in the pediatric age group. *Pediatrics* 1978; 61:83.

Saltzman HA, Alavi A, Greenspan RH, et al (PIOPED investigators): Value of the ventilation/perfusion scan in acute pulmonary embolism: Results of the prospective investigation of pulmonary embolism diagnosis (PIOPED). *JAMA* 1990; 263:33.

Sherrier RH, Chiles C, Newman GE: Chronic multiple pulmonary emboli: Regional response of the bronchial circulation. *Invest Radiol* 1989; 24:437.

Woodruff WW III, Merten DF, Wagner ML, et al: Chronic pulmonary embolism in children. *Radiology* 1986; 159:511.

12

Disorders Due to Effects of Physical Agents on the Lungs

Blunt and penetrating injuries
  Rib fractures
  Hemothorax
  Pneumothorax
  Pneumomediastinum
  Airway injury
  Pulmonary parenchymal injury
  Lung torsion
  Mediastinal widening
  Trauma to the diaphragm
Postoperative abnormalities
  Gas collection
  Pleural effusion
  Mediastinal widening
  Atelectasis
  Parenchymal opacities
  Postpneumonectomy syndrome
Complications of tubes and catheters
  Endotracheal tubes
  Chest tubes
  Nasogastric tubes
  Central venous lines
Bronchopulmonary dysplasia

Drug reactions and the lungs
  General effects
  Effects of antineoplastic agents
    Methotrexate toxicity
    Cyclophosphamide (Cytoxan)
    Busulfan and bleomycin
  Other drugs having pulmonary toxicity
    Cyclosporine
    Amiodarone
    Nitrofurantoin
Pulmonary radiation damage
Inhalation injuries
  Nitrogen dioxide
  Beryllium
  Talcum powder
  Smoke inhalation
Aspiration pneumonia
  Acute aspiration pneumonia
  Chronic aspiration pneumonia
  Hydrocarbon pneumonia
  Near-drowning

BLUNT AND PENETRATING INJURIES

Blunt trauma, caused primarily in children by vehicular accidents, is also discussed in Chapter 6. *Penetrating trauma*, due mainly to gunshot and knife wounds, is fortunately less common in children than in adults and is not discussed separately here.

Supine, anteroposterior (AP), portable chest radiographs are often the first and sometimes the only radiographic investigation of the child with thoracic trauma. Recognition of abnormal fluid and air collections can be difficult under these conditions and therefore, whenever possible, a horizontal-beam radiograph should be obtained. Sivit and associates have shown that 38% of all abnormalities detected on computed tomography (CT) scanning were missed by chest radiography. They suggest that when a child with blunt abdominal trauma is imaged by CT, a few images should be made through the lower thorax with specific lung windows. The entire thorax should be imaged if abnormalities are seen on the initial images. In their series of patients imaged primarily for blunt abdominal trauma, they found that chest injuries were most frequent in children under 7 years of age. Mortality was greater in children with combined thoracoabdominal injury than in those with only abdominal injury.

Rib Fractures

Rib fractures occur in thoracic trauma, but because of the pliability of the child's rib cage, it is possible to have severe intrathoracic injury without actual disruption of the bony thorax. Fractures of the first, second, or third ribs (uncommon in children) should suggest the likelihood of severe injury to cardiovascular structures, the tracheobronchial tree, or even the spinal cord. Fractures of the three lower ribs should prompt a careful search for injury to the liver, spleen, and diaphragm. Detection of rib fractures without a history of trauma raises the possibility of child abuse.

Hemothorax

After thoracic injury, blood extravasates from tears in the pulmonary parenchyma and visceral pleura. When lacerations are small, bleeding often stops spontaneously. Evidence of continued accumulation of large amounts of fluid should raise the possibility of a serious vascular tear. Large pleural fluid collections can be distinguished from underlying pulmonary contusion by the use of real-time ultrasound or CT. It should be remembered that in the supine position fluid will layer posteriorly and produces a diffuse pulmonary haze rather than being seen as a meniscus laterally. Pneumothorax often accompanies pleural injury, and air-fluid levels are quite common if a horizontal-beam radiograph is obtained.

Pneumothorax

A small pneumothorax may be difficult to recognize in a limited AP supine examination, although a unilateral lucent lung or a medial radiolucency may be useful clues. No matter how sick the patient, it usually is possible to get a lateral decubitus film to diagnose even a relatively small pneumothorax. In the series of Sivit et al., 50% of pneumothoraces and pleural fluid collections were missed on the initial radiographic examination.

The diagnosis of tension pneumothorax is a clinical one, but the radiographic findings of a large amount of gas in the pleural space, shift of the mediastinal structures away from the affected side, and a depressed ipsilateral hemidiaphragm usually require that a chest tube be placed. Should a pneumothorax not respond to the usual management measures, an underlying tracheobronchial or esophageal laceration should be considered.

Pneumomediastinum

Pneumomediastinum is seen frequently after chest injury, as is subcutaneous emphysema. It is a less ominous finding than pneumothorax and often re-

quires no therapy. Posterior paramediastinal gas cysts, which may be accumulations of gas in the pulmonary ligaments or posttraumatic pneumatoceles, have been described.

Airway Injury

Major airway trauma, including laceration or rupture of the tracheobronchial tree, is life-threatening. Two thirds of patients have an associated pneumothorax. Bronchial fracture in children can occur without rib fracture or torn lung parenchyma (Fig 12–1). Fractures most commonly occur near the carina. A fracture of the tracheobronchial tree should be considered in any patient who has a pneumothorax (with or without a pneumomediastinum) following blunt chest trauma. The diagnosis often is strongly suggested if the air leak continues despite a satisfactorily functioning thoracostomy tube. Chest CT is indicated in such cases. The lung may be collapsed initially, or atelectasis may not develop until days or weeks after the original trauma. If no infection occurs, bronchial reconstruction may be possible even months to years after initial injury.

Pulmonary Parenchymal Injury

Pulmonary contusion is seen radiologically because of accumulation of blood or fluid in the alveoli and

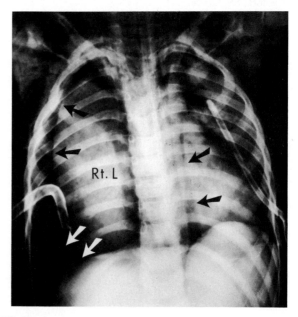

FIG 12–1.
Right mainstem bronchial fracture. Note the large bilateral pneumothorax *(arrows)* despite the presence of chest tubes. Pneumomediastinum and subcutaneous emphysema are also present. There is consolidation and incomplete atelectasis of the stiff right lung *(Rt. L).*

the perivascular and peribronchial spaces. Contusion usually presents with patchy airspace consolidation detected at the initial radiographic examination; the findings clear rapidly, often by the third day. This injury is not commonly followed by pneumonia or other complications (Fig 12–2).

A *pulmonary laceration* is diagnosed when a spherical or linear accumulation of air is seen in the pulmonary parenchyma. CT is much more sensitive than plain radiography. In the series of Sivit et al., one third of parenchymal lesions detected by CT were missed on radiography. It has been suggested that pulmonary laceration is the basic component in the mechanism of injury in pulmonary contusion, hematoma, cyst, or pneumatocele. A traumatic pneumatocele is an air-filled lung space which may be single or multiple (Fig 12–3) and range in size from tiny to quite large. A traumatic pulmonary hematoma is a blood-filled posttraumatic lung space; it can initially simulate a pulmonary contusion except that it resolves much more slowly and may persist for months (Fig 12–4).

Chest CT can also be used to quantitate the amount of parenchymal injury. The approximate percentage of opacified parenchyma is estimated and compared to the lobar volume calculations of Horsfield et al. and the total percentage of opacified lung is derived (Fig 12–5). If, for instance, half of the left lower lobe and half of the right lower lobe are consolidated, a total of 24.5% of lung volume is compromised. Using this method for determining pulmonary injury in adults, Wagner et al. determined that if there was greater than 28% total lung consolidation, then mechanical ventilation was required. Conversely, if the amount of consolidation was less than 18%, ventilator support was not required.

Other *pulmonary opacities* can appear after trauma. These may be due to aspiration, atelectasis, or pulmonary edema, either cardiogenic or noncardiogenic (the adult respiratory distress syndrome, ARDS). Usually, abnormal radiographic findings do not appear until 24 hours after injury. They may progress rapidly over the next 24 hours and then stabilize. In posttraumatic ARDS, approximately 50% eventually resolve, but 50% of patients die. This disorder is discussed in Chapter 11.

Lung Torsion

Torsion of the lung following sudden compressing injuries of the thorax, especially crushing of the chest by an automobile wheel, has been reported in children; this lesion is probably overlooked frequently. The upper lobe is most frequently involved; it twists 180 degrees, which results in the apex being pointed inferiorly. As a result, the normal bronchovascular markings are inverted. Decrease in lobar volume, consolidation, and hilar displacement are the most frequent findings. Twisting and obstruction of the bronchus may be demonstrated by CT

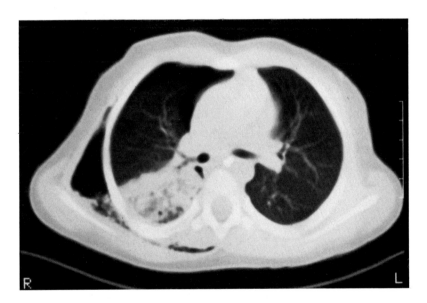

FIG 12–2.
CT scan of pulmonary contusion. Six-year-old child struck by an automobile. Nonenhanced CT scan section, 6 mm thick, shows a pneumothorax anteriorly. This was not appreciated on the AP supine portable chest radiograph. There is a large amount of subcutaneous emphysema present, which was noted radiologically. The posterior segment of the right upper lobe shows patchy diffuse air space consolidation, consistent with pulmonary contusion. A small intrapulmonary air collection, probably due to pulmonary laceration, also is noted.

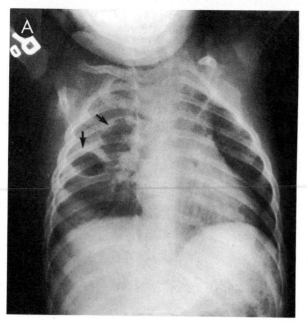

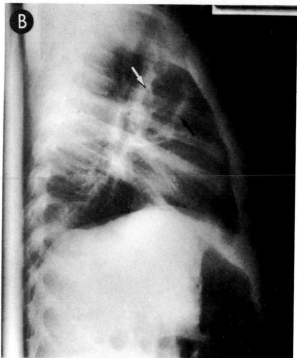

FIG 12–3.

Posttraumatic pneumatoceles. Two traumatic pneumatoceles *(arrows)* are present in the anterior segment of the right upper lobe. Pulmonary contusion is visible throughout the right lung as an area of increased opacity. **A,** frontal, and **B,** lateral projections.

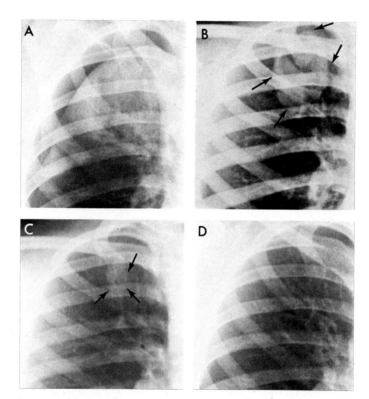

FIG 12–4.

Pulmonary contusion and hemorrhage. **A,** intrapulmonary hemorrhage and pneumothorax are noted in the right upper lobe on a film made immediately after an automobile accident. **B,** 18 days later, the patch of increased density that represents the intrapulmonary hematoma has shrunk and is now quite sharply defined *(arrows).* The pneumothorax has resolved. Without the history or other preceding radiographs, one might suspect a neoplasm or cyst. **C,** 3 months later, the patch of increased opacity has now shrunk to a small fraction of its former size and probably represents contracting fibrous scar *(arrows).* **D,** 12 months later, the right upper lobe appears completely normal.

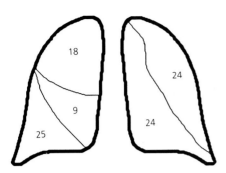

FIG 12–5.
Schematic drawing of segmental lung volume (%). (Drawn by C. Jonas.)

scanning. Lung torsion can also occur as a complication of pneumothorax or following lobectomy.

Mediastinal Widening

This may be due to single or multiple injuries and suggests aortic or other major vessel laceration. Findings suggestive of aortic laceration include tracheal deviation to the right, deviation of the esophagus or nasogastric tube to the right, obscuration of the sharpness of the aortic knob, a left extrapleural apical cap, depression of the left mainstem bronchus, a left hemothorax, left rib fractures, and widening of the right paratracheal stripe. Plain film findings are sensitive but not specific. Mediastinal hemorrhage detected by CT is an indication for aortography. Approximately 95% of all aortic ruptures occur at the ligamentum arteriosum; the remainder occur in the supravalvular area.

Trauma to the Diaphragm

Diaphragmatic injury may initially be masked by pulmonary or mediastinal damage. Pleural effusion, left lower lobe atelectasis, loss of the diaphragmatic contour, contralateral mediastinal shift, or diaphragmatic hernia may all be indicators of trauma to the hemidiaphragm. Ninety percent of the time, the left side is affected; usually the central tendon is torn anteriorly and transversely. Plain chest films can establish or suggest the correct diagnosis in approximately two thirds of patients. Elevation of the diaphragm is the most sensitive finding but it is quite nonspecific. The CT diagnosis of diaphragmatic rupture is also difficult. Intrathoracic herniation of intra-abdominal fat or organs is the most frequent finding (Fig 12–6). An "absent" or disrupted diaphragm is a specific finding when present. Magnetic resonance imaging (MRI) may prove very useful because of the direct coronal and sagittal views and the fact that the

diaphragm can be directly imaged as a low-signal band.

POSTOPERATIVE ABNORMALITIES

The appearance of the thorax following surgery is quite variable, depending on what type of procedure was performed and for what condition. We concern ourselves here with common postoperative pulmonary complications secondary to cardiovascular or thoracic surgery. The thoracic roentgen abnormalities appearing in the immediate postoperative period have been reviewed in detail by Goodman and Putnam, and the problems in interpreting radiographs made in the intensive care unit (ICU) were reviewed by Swensen et al.

Gas Collection

Subcutaneous emphysema is commonly present for 2 to 3 days after surgery. If the gas increases in amount, it may be dissecting from a large pneumomediastinum or leaking around a chest tube. A large pneumothorax may indicate a bronchopleural fistula or an improperly positioned or otherwise malfunctioning chest tube. A large, posterior pneumomediastinum can be seen after tracheal rupture. A later appearance of gas may herald a lung abscess.

Pleural Effusion

Effusion is commonly seen in small amounts but is usually adequately drained by a chest tube. Fluid may reaccumulate after the tube is removed. Rapid accumulation of pleural effusion may indicate bleeding and, of course, effusion can be associated with pulmonary infection. In children that have had cardiac surgery, a large fluid accumulation postoperatively is often due to chylothorax secondary to thoracic duct trauma.

Mediastinal Widening

Some widening of the mediastinum is commonly seen postoperatively. If not due to rotation or to AP portable radiographic technique, it is most often caused by hemorrhage. Mediastinal abscesses, which occur later in the postoperative period, also present with widening of the mediastinum. CT is required for satisfactory evaluation of postoperative mediastinal abnormalities, but even with CT distinction between postoperative edema and diffuse infection or hemorrhage can be difficult.

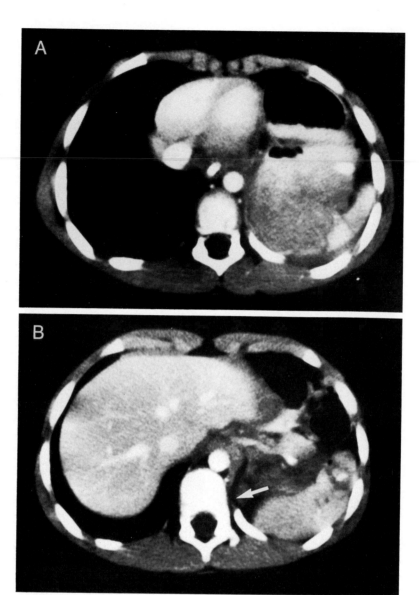

FIG 12–6.
Diaphragmatic rupture and gastric herniation. This 6-year-old patient was struck by a motor vehicle. Chest film (not shown) revealed the gastric bubble in the left hemithorax. **A,** contrast-enhanced CT scan reveals the stomach, which is filled with air, contrast media, and food, to be in the left hemithorax. The superior portion of the spleen is visible posterolaterally. **B,** CT scan 4 cm inferior to **A** reveals the inferior portion of the spleen which is fractured anterolaterally; the diaphragmatic crus *(arrow)* is noted to be disrupted.

Atelectasis

Atelectasis is the most common postoperative complication and is seen in most patients. It is especially likely to involve the left lower lobe after cardiac surgery. In patients who have undergone cardiopulmonary bypass procedures, its cause is thought to be a combination of mucous plugging and surfactant deficiency. The reason for the predominance in the left lower lobe is uncertain. If an air bronchogram is present, bronchoscopy is unlikely to improve the atelectasis; absence of an air bronchogram suggests bronchial obstruction due to mucous plug or thrombus.

Parenchymal Opacities

Parenchymal opacities are most commonly due to atelectasis; but pneumonia, localized edema, hemorrhage, or infarction must be differentiated. Inadvertent ligature of the pulmonary veins may result in severe congestion or hemorrhagic infarction following surgery. A lobar or segmental distribution of parenchymal opacity and pleural effusion are commonly seen, but differentiation from bacterial lobar pneumonia is difficult from the appearance of the radiograph alone. Postoperative bleeding, either into the lung or the pleural space, can produce large areas of consolidation. This complication may be indicated clinically by falling hemoglobin levels, shock, or hemoptysis. Cardiogenic and noncardiogenic (adult respiratory distress syndrome, ARDS) edema are common findings; their appearances are discussed in Chapter 11.

Postpneumonectomy Syndrome

Following right pneumonectomy, especially in infants and children, there is marked displacement and rotation of the heart into the right hemithorax. This can cause recurrent infection and airway obstruction, particularly involving the distal trachea and left main bronchus which are compressed by the left pulmonary artery and aorta (Fig 12–7). Similar findings can occur following left pneumonectomy, especially if there is a right-sided aorta.

COMPLICATIONS OF TUBES AND CATHETERS

Endotracheal Tubes

Rarely, an endotracheal tube is misplaced in the esophagus; this complication is best seen on lateral x-ray films. Marked abdominal gaseous distention may be present. An endotracheal tube placed too low may cause atelectasis or obstructive emphysema. Most commonly, the tube is in the right main bronchus and the left main bronchus is partially or completely obstructed. The tip of the endotracheal tube should be one to two vertebral bodies above the carina with the patient's head in neutral position. Donn and Kuhns have shown that the position of the head is important when assessing endotracheal tube position in infants. With the head extended, the tube moves cephalad (toward the glottis). This apparently paradoxical motion occurs because the skull, from the maxilla to C1, acts as a lever arm moving about a fulcrum centered at the upper cervical spine. When the neck is flexed, the lever arm is rotated inferiorly and forces the endotracheal tube to a more caudal position. Rotating the head laterally draws the tip cephalad.

Tracheal stenosis following intubation is discussed in Chapter 8 and is a chronic rather than an acute complication. Erosion of the trachea from a long-standing tracheostomy or endotracheal tube can have disastrous consequences, but this complication cannot be predicted on the basis of the chest radiograph.

Chest Tubes

Chest tubes may occasionally be placed subcutaneously or may have one or more holes outside the thorax. A tube may also be inadvertently wedged in

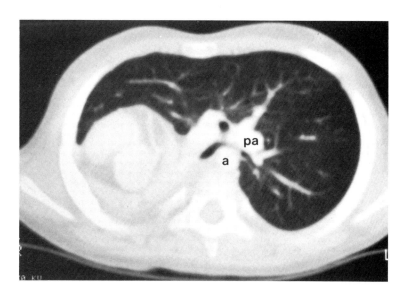

FIG 12–7.
Postpneumonectomy syndrome in an 18-month-old whose right lung was resected at birth because of pulmonary infarction secondary to agenesis of the pulmonary artery. This 6-mm thick contrast-enhanced CT scan reveals the heart to occupy the posterior half of the right hemithorax. The left lung is herniated anteriorly. With this marked distortion of the cardiopulmonary anatomy the left mainstem bronchus is compressed between the aorta (a) and the pulmonary artery (pa).

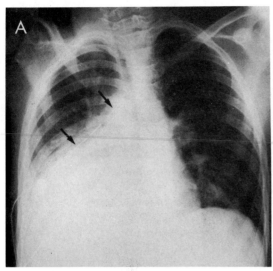

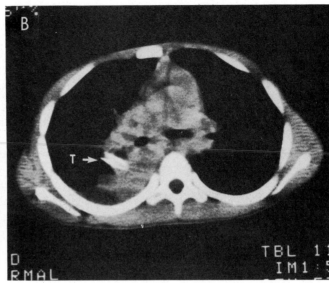

FIG 12–8.
Malpositioned chest tube demonstrated on radiography and CT in a 12-year-old boy with pneumonia and empyema. **A,** chest tube is not draining satisfactorily. Its upward oblique course is consistent with a position in the major fissure. **B,** CT scan demonstrates that the chest tube *(T)* has traversed obliquely across the major fissure. Its tip is lodged in the lung parenchyma posteriorly.

a fissure (Fig 12–8). This diagnosis is suggested if the tube is seen to follow the course of the fissure; a lateral view is especially helpful. The AP position of the tube is important. A posteriorly positioned tube will drain an effusion satisfactorily in the supine position, but not a pneumothorax, which tends to accumulate anteriorly. Therefore, a lateral film is needed for complete assessment of satisfactory chest tube position. In fact, CT may be necessary in some cases when loculated collections do not respond adequately to chest tube drainage. On occasion, the tube may perforate the lung. Machin reported, in an autopsy study, that 9 of 70 infants who had chest tubes inserted had suffered pulmonary laceration. This complication can be suspected when a pneumothorax persists despite chest tube drainage and also if there appears to be atelectasis or infiltrate around the tip of the tube. In neonates, a thoracic tube inserted too far medially can obstruct the thoracic aorta.

Nasogastric Tubes

The most common problem with a nasogastric tube is that it may be coiled in the nasopharynx or the esophagus, or, on occasion, be inadvertently placed in the tracheobronchial tree rather than in the esophagus. Tubes in place for a long period of time can perforate the gastrointestinal tract. Perforation of the esophagus by a feeding tube may also occur (Fig 12–9), and be suspected by unusual tube placement.

Central Venous Lines

Central venous lines are usually placed in the superior vena cava (SVC). If they are inserted into a smaller vein, perforation or thrombosis is more likely, and hydrothorax can occur (Fig 12–10).

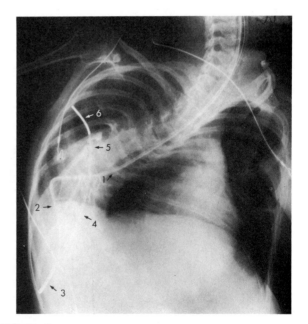

FIG 12–9.
Esophageal perforation by a feeding tube. The bizarre course of the tube is readily apparent by following the numbers. The tip of the tube *(6)* was apparently in the right pleural space because pleural fluid developed when the patient was given liquids through the tube.

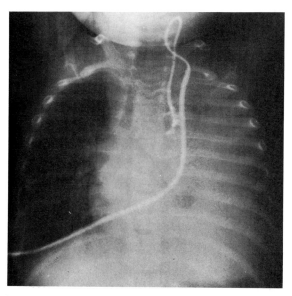

FIG 12–10.
Hydrothorax as a complication of vascular perforation in a 1-year-old child with cystic fibrosis who had been sustained with long-term hyperalimentation therapy. The catheter had previously been positioned in the vena cava at the time of the last radiograph, 2 months earlier. Respiratory distress occurred after fluid administration. This film taken subsequent to the feeding reveals the tube in an aberrant location, probably in a superior intercostal vein which has perforated. Two hundred milliliters of hyperalimentation fluid was removed from the pleural space.

Thrombophlebitis, either bland or septic, can occur, and an SVC syndrome may develop. Kramer et al. reported three cases of lethal chylothorax in newborns who had SVC thrombosis due to long-standing central lines. Placement in the right atrium is sometimes used but is associated with a greater risk of cardiac arrhythmias.

BRONCHOPULMONARY DYSPLASIA

Bronchopulmonary dysplasia (BPD) is a term introduced in 1967 by Northway et al. to describe the chronic lung disease which developed in infants treated with high oxygen concentrations and mechanical ventilation for respiratory distress syndrome (RDS). The disorder was initially described as occurring in four distinct radiographic and pathologic stages. Perhaps because of advances in neonatal care, BPD as seen today seldom progresses through stereotyped stages, and is usually more insidious in onset and milder in its clinical and radiographic manifestations than initially described. Still, despite considerable research and the passage of 25 years, the exact pathophysiology of BPD remains unclear and the disease still cannot be prevented.

BPD, which is now the most common chronic lung disease of infants, is characterized by the triad of oxygen dependence, clinical respiratory compromise, and radiographic abnormalities that persist beyond 28 days of life in infants with respiratory failure treated with positive pressure ventilation at birth. Although originally described in infants of average 34 weeks' gestation, today BPD is uncommon in infants above 32 weeks' gestation. Incidence is increased with decreased birth weight, exceeding 50% in infants weighing under 1,000 g; thus the incidence rises as neonatologists increasingly are able to save infants of very low birth weight.

At least three factors appear to be important in the development of BPD. The first is immaturity of the lungs, which is greatest in smaller infants, although there is considerable variability; some infants with less than 1,000-g birth weight do not develop BPD, while some larger infants do. The second major factor is oxygen. This is usually understood to be high concentrations of inspired oxygen, but it is speculated that some very immature infants suffer lung damage from oxygen levels at or only slightly greater than that of room air. The third major factor is mechanical ventilation (*barotrauma*). The mechanism by which this occurs is uncertain, but may involve *lung stretch*, which is the term used to describe the finding that there is relatively greater dilatation of the bronchioles than of the alveoli during positive pressure ventilation. This cyclic bronchiolar stretching may result in terminal airway ischemia and necrosis, which in turn may lead to pulmonary interstitial emphysema and possibly pneumothorax, leading to further lung injury.

Several other factors have also been implicated in the pathogenesis of BPD, including shunting through a patent ductus arteriosus (PDA), the presence of pulmonary air leaks, familial tendency, nutritional deficiencies, excessive influx of inflammatory cells, superimposed pneumonia, and colonization with the organism *Ureaplasma urealyticum*. It is also known that the preexisting condition of RDS is not necessary for the development of BPD, although the vast majority of BPD cases arise in this setting.

Pathologic findings in BPD have been reviewed extensively, and are only summarized here. In the acute phases of the disease, the findings are those of the underlying RDS. In days to weeks, there is extensive necrosis of distal airway lining cells and global edema. The picture that then ensues is a mixture of continued lung injury and ongoing reparative changes, the latter including airway squamous metaplasia, interstitial fibroplasia, and increasing irregularity of aeration with focal areas of bronchiolitis obliterans. At the end of the primarily reparative phase, at about 1 to 2 months, the lungs often show uneven aeration to the extent that the surface of the lung may have a cobblestone appearance. Some alveoli appear normal, whereas others are dysplastic and compressed by regions of fibrosis.

The focal nature of the changes has led Stocker to speculate that complete bronchiolar obstruction may actually protect some alveolar units from the effects of hyperoxia and stretch injury, and that the repair process will be more complete in these units because the initial damage is less.

Less is known about the pathologic findings in older patients who have survived their initial course of RDS and BPD, because autopsy material is limited. A morphometric analysis of a few such BPD patients (Margraf et al.) revealed a decrease in the total number of alveoli present, with a relatively increased size of the remaining functioning alveolar units and increased central bronchial smooth muscle and glands. It is likely that repair continues for months to years. In the relatively severely affected patients, Stocker has noted marked septal fibrosis, thick pseudofissures, and a cobblestone appearance of the lung surface. Tracheomegaly, tracheomalacia, and ciliary dysfunction may occur either diffusely or focally, and cardiac and pulmonary changes of pulmonary hypertension are also frequent. Clinically, the older survivors by school age commonly have no pulmonary symptoms or handicap, although abnor-

malities of pulmonary function testing remain at least into young adulthood.

Radiographic manifestations of BPD vary widely among individual patients and within the same patient. Within a single patient, this variation is greatest in the early phases of the disease. The initial presentation is generally RDS of greater or lesser severity and that appearance is in turn modified by the use of exogenous surfactant therapy, ventilator pressure, and the appearance of complications such as air leaks and left-to-right shunting through the PDA. Overall, the radiograph is a poor tool for monitoring the early stages of BPD; however, by about 2 to 3 weeks, consideration should be given to the diagnosis of BPD if the radiograph has not cleared and the abnormalities present are relatively stable from film to film rather than evanescent.

The radiographic changes of chronic BPD vary substantially from patient to patient. At their mildest, there is a fine increase in interstitial markings and perivascular fuzziness. Sometimes infection, shunting through the PDA, fluid overload, or persistent pulmonary interstitial emphysema may cause such findings, and may be impossible to distinguish from BPD radiographically. In more severe cases, the diffuse findings may be more coarse, often with localized or generalized hyperinflation (Figs 12–11 and 12–12). In the most severe cases, there are gross, irregular cystic changes and substantial hy-

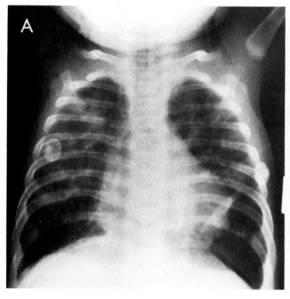
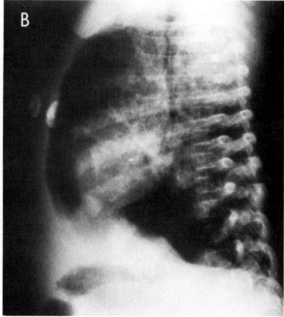

FIG 12–11.
Bronchopulmonary dysplasia in an 8-month-old infant who had severe hyaline membrane disease and persistent need for oxygen. **A,** frontal, and **B,** lateral radiographs show that the lungs are hy- perinflated, especially at the bases. Streaky upper lobe parenchymal opacities are seen bilaterally. This appearance was baseline normal for this patient.

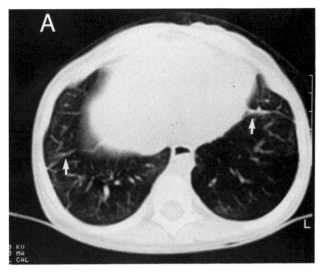

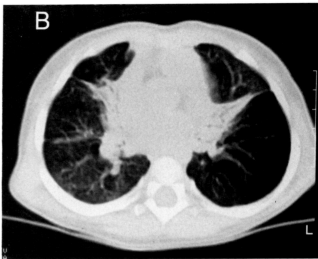

FIG 12–12.
HRCT findings in bronchopulmonary dysplasia. Two-year-old boy. **A,** 3-mm thick section through the lung base reveals parenchymal bands *(arrows)*, numerous areas of interlobular septal thickening, and areas of air trapping, especially in the left lower lobe, associated with disruption of the normal branching vascular pattern. No bronchial wall thickening is observed. **B,** CT scan through the mid-lung zones reveals a similar pattern posteriorly in the left lung. There is atelectasis and presumably fibrosis of the lingula and the right middle lobe. The right lower lobe also is diffusely abnormal, with subsegmental areas of air trapping and interstitial thickening.

perinflation; pulmonary architecture is markedly disarrayed; fortunately this pattern, as initially described by Northway et al. (1967), is presently relatively uncommon. Air trapping is variable, and is more apparent in the lower lobes. Tracheomalacia and tracheomegaly may be present as well. In severe cases, changes reflecting pulmonary hypertension may be seen, with prominence of the main pulmonary artery segment, right ventricular hypertrophy, and episodes of pulmonary edema. Superimposed areas of atelectasis and infectious consolidation are common in the subacute and chronic phases of disease.

As the child matures, the radiographic abnormalities tend to become less apparent, although this tendency toward clearing may be interrupted during the first years of life by viral pneumonias to which these children are susceptible. Ultimately, in some patients, the radiographs may become normal, although Griscom et al. have shown abnormalities of varying degree persisting into middle childhood in about two thirds of patients; a frequent abnormality was the presence of line shadows, which may represent fibrosis or pleural pseudofissures. Peribronchial cuffing is also common. Affected infants and children also tend to have rather narrow AP diameters of the chest, unlike the usually increased AP diameter associated with most other causes of air trapping; the cause and significance of this finding are unknown. Radionuclide scans show marked ventilation-perfusion imbalances and loss of the normal gravity-dependent flow distribution. Pulmonary function abnormalities persist into young adulthood, with hyperaeration, airflow obstruction, and hyperreactive airways.

At present, the only cure for BPD would seem to be its prevention, primarily by avoiding preterm delivery and secondarily by minimizing elevated inspired oxygen concentration and ventilator pressures as much as possible. The use of steroids during the early recovery phases has not been tested in a controlled, blinded manner, and thus its validity is unknown. Despite this, the use of steroids has rapidly become ingrained in clinical neonatology. It is difficult to speculate about the overall effects of this therapeutic maneuver, if any. As it presently stands, BPD is the most common chronic lung disease of infancy, and all efforts to date have succeeded at best in ameliorating its effects.

DRUG REACTIONS AND THE LUNGS

The adverse effects of multiple drugs on the lungs have been extensively reviewed and are only briefly summarized here.

General Effects

Asthma or *bronchospasm* has been associated with ingestion of aspirin, penicillin, tetracycline, and several other antibiotics. Changes of air trapping or pulmonary infiltrates (with eosinophils) can be seen.

Aspirin-sensitive asthmatics also frequently have severe nasal polyposis.

Hypersensitivity pneumonias may be produced by reactions to sulfonamides, nitrofurantoin, *p*-amino-salicylic acid, and penicillin. The pattern can be similar to that of extrinsic allergic alveolitis with a diffuse nodular infiltrate; occasionally, infiltrates may be more patchy. They may affect the lower lobes primarily, and pleural effusion can be seen.

Noncardiogenic pulmonary edema can occur secondary to overdoses of heroin and morphine and methadone. Idiosyncratic reactions to aspirin and contrast agents have also been associated with radiographic findings of pulmonary edema.

Effects of Antineoplastic Agents

Interstitial pneumonia and *pulmonary fibrosis* are the most frequent manifestations of drug reactions in the lungs. Offending agents include the cytotoxic drugs, especially bleomycin and methotrexate. This topic has been reviewed by Batist and Andrews. These agents can produce interstitial or alveolar disease, but the pulmonary reaction can be difficult to separate from the primary malignant disease or superimposed pulmonary infection. High-resolution CT (HRCT) can be useful in the early diagnosis of pulmonary drug toxicity.

Methotrexate Toxicity

Methotrexate appears to cause an acute allergic granulomatous reaction that may progress to chronic interstitial fibrosis. Wall and colleagues studied 38 patients receiving high-dose methotrexate therapy and concluded that there was no dose-related effect of methotrexate on the lungs of children. They suggest the true incidence of methotrexate-induced lung disease is infrequent, probably less than 10%. Methotrexate pulmonary consolidation must be differentiated from opportunistic infections and complications of the underlying neoplastic disease. The radiographic appearance is a nodular or reticulonodular pattern.

Cyclophosphamide (Cytoxan)

This alkylating agent, used in a variety of pediatric malignancies, can cause pulmonary alveolitis and fibrosis, although these effects appear to be rare.

Busulfan and Bleomycin

Other drugs implicated in pulmonary fibrosis include busulfan and bleomycin, which produce a radiologic pattern of reticulonodular findings that progress to alveolar consolidation and pulmonary fibrosis. Nodules and masses can be seen. Frequency and severity of toxicity increases with increasing dose.

Other Drugs Having Pulmonary Toxicity

Cyclosporine

Cyclosporine is a fungal metabolite which has become widely used for immunosuppression in transplant patients. A number of patients treated with this drug have developed a lymphoproliferative disorder with pulmonary manifestations including a mass or multiple pulmonary nodules and hilar adenopathy. This B cell disorder appears to develop after infection with the Epstein-Barr virus. The disorder may be reversible if the drug therapy is stopped, but a malignant clone may develop.

Amiodarone

Amiodarone is used for therapy of severe cardiac dysrhythmias. About 5% of patients treated develop pulmonary toxicity which can manifest patchy, peripheral airspace opacities which on CT are noted to be of high attenuation. Other patients have a diffuse, poorly defined interstitial pattern.

Nitrofurantoin

Nitrofurantoin is an antimicrobial agent used for urinary tract infections. Pulmonary reactions are relatively frequent and can be one of two patterns. There can be an acute flulike syndrome associated with a dry cough and either a normal x-ray film or one that shows bilateral interstitial or alveolar infiltrates. The less common, more chronic presentation includes a gradual onset of dyspnea and cough with a radiographic pattern of diffuse interstitial infiltrate.

PULMONARY RADIATION DAMAGE

Lung damage may follow radiation therapy given primarily to the lungs, any part of the mediastinum, or the chest wall. While changes in pulmonary function may be present in many patients, symptoms are present in only a minority. The important factors in determining whether or not the lungs are damaged are the amount of tissue radiated, the dose given, the length of time of therapy, and the relative biologic effectiveness of the therapy employed. Doses under 2,000 rad (20 Gy) do not usually produce radiation pneumonia, whereas doses of 5,000 to 6,000 rad (50–60 Gy) given over a 5- to 6-week period almost universally produce severe radiation pneumonia. Preexisting lung diseases and associated pulmonary toxicity of chemotherapeutic agents such as actinomycin D also contribute to the likelihood of pulmonary damage. Radiation given to the lung of a young child can cause pulmonary hypoplasia.

Radiographic changes, if present, usually appear 1 to 2 months after the cessation of x-ray therapy. CT is more sensitive than chest radiography is in their detection. If the mediastinum has been irradiated, a central, sharply delineated area of linear, increased opacity corresponding to the radiation portal may be seen. Parenchymal disease, produced by radiation, occurs in three stages: (1) an early exudative phase, characterized by edema fluid in both the airspaces and the interstitium; (2) an intermediate, or organizing phase, in which hyaline membranes form and are incorporated into the interstitium, and there is gradual infiltration of the interstitium by collagen fibers; and (3) a fibrotic stage with well-organized bands of collagen, honeycombing, and obliteration of the terminal portion of the respiratory tree and vasculature. Radiographic stages correspond with an initial picture of an ill-defined alveolar process. As the process extends, it becomes more interstitial in appearance until changes recognized as radiation fibrosis appear (Fig 12–13). Occasionally, a discrete mass suggesting recurrent tumor may be seen as a form of local radiation pneumonitis.

INHALATION INJURIES

These generally occupationally related diseases are uncommon in childhood. Some, including farmer's lung and other causes of extrinsic allergic alveolitis, are considered in Chapter 10.

Nitrogen Dioxide

NO_2 inhalation causes a condition known as "silo-filler's disease." Three to 10 days after a silo has been filled, the fresh silage begins to produce nitric oxide, which on contact with air forms NO_2. Anyone entering the silo during this period is at risk of developing serious pulmonary disease, its severity being in direct proportion to the duration of exposure. Acute pulmonary edema may develop and prove fatal. In moderate-to-severe disease, which is not fatal, the initial pulmonary edema may clear and the chest film remains normal for 2 to 5 weeks, but the acute bronchiolitis of the first stage may then progress to bronchiolitis obliterans and cause progressive pulmonary insufficiency.

In rural districts during the silo-filling season, silo-filler's disease should be considered in the radiographic diagnosis of pneumonia in both children and adults.

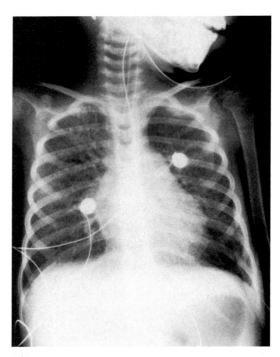

FIG 12–13.
Radiation fibrosis developing after therapy for Wilms tumor. Chest radiograph reveals diffuse bilateral linear interstitial pattern.

Beryllium

Beryllium dust and fumes have been identified as toxic agents both to workers in beryllium plants and to others, including children, living nearby. The roentgen changes in the lungs resemble those in silicosis and asbestosis. Pneumothorax may be a complicating feature.

Talcum Powder

Since talcum powder (magnesium hydrous silicate 95%, magnesium carbonate 5%) largely replaced zinc stearate years ago as a dusting powder for babies in the United States, deaths from aspiration of dusting powder are all but unknown. However, death from the aspiration of talcum powder still occurs on rare occasions. The cause of death is usually acute obliterative bronchiolitis that produces mixed atelectasis and emphysema.

Smoke Inhalation

Children are often trapped in their burning homes. If rescued, they may still suffer severe pulmonary abnormalities. In the first 24 hours, complications result primarily from upper airway edema caused by direct heat injury or toxic products.

Teixidor et al. reported abnormal radiographs in 35 of 56 patients with significant smoke inhalation. Radiographic abnormalities consisted of a combination of interstitial and alveolar edema, most commonly in the upper lobes and perihilar areas. In only 2 of 35 patients were infiltrates confined to the lower lobes. Interstitial edema was seen as perivascular fuzziness or peribronchial cuffing. Septal lines were not seen.

New infiltrates may develop in the 24 hours after the insult, but are almost always accompanied by abnormal physical findings. Infiltrates appearing after 48 hours are usually related to a complication of the injury or its treatment. Pneumonia and ARDS are present in a vast majority of the patients who die.

Passive smoking is associated with an increased rate of respiratory illness in infancy and childhood; the frequency of reactive airway disease also appears to be increased.

ASPIRATION PNEUMONIA

Aspiration pneumonia results from the inhalation of materials that have been swallowed or regurgitated from the upper gastrointestinal tract. The disease may be acute and massive, or smaller repeated bouts of aspiration may result in chronic, recurrent pneumonia (Fig 12–14). Gravity is the major determinant affecting the anatomical distribution of the pneumonic changes. Most commonly, the posterior segments of the upper and lower lobes are involved.

Acute Aspiration Pneumonia

Acute aspiration pneumonia, or Mendelson syndrome, refers to aspiration of liquid gastric contents. Classically, the aspiration occurs in a comatose or somnolent patient. The liquid aspirate passes to the peripheral air spaces and is widely distributed through the lungs, often as a result of coughing. The

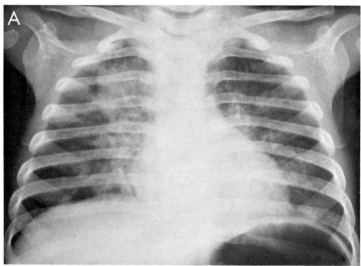

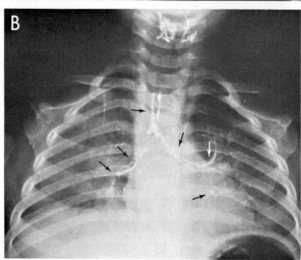

FIG 12–14.
Chronic aspiration pneumonia in a marasmic, retarded 1-year-old infant. **A,** conventional frontal film shows an extensive patchy increase in opacity in the right lung with increase in perivascular and peribronchial markings in the left lung as well. **B,** film made 30 minutes after an esophagogram shows aspiration with contrast material outlining the proximal tracheobronchial tree.

gastric acids damage the capillary walls and produce increased capillary permeability and the radiographic findings of acute pulmonary edema. The chest film shows rapid onset of airspace consolidation and some areas of confluence (Fig 12–15). While the findings may otherwise resemble acute pulmonary edema, heart size is normal and clearing of the radiographic changes is relatively slow, taking from 7 to 10 days. Secondary infection or ARDS may complicate the picture.

Chronic Aspiration Pneumonia

In chronic, recurrent, aspiration pneumonia, there may be no history of vomiting. The whole subject of gastroesophageal reflux and its relationship to apnea, asthma, and other chronic lung diseases of childhood is currently the subject of considerable controversy concerning how large a role aspiration may play in these conditions. The clinical manifestations of recurrent pulmonary disease associated with gastroesophageal reflux may include wheezing, nocturnal wheezing or cough, anemia, failure to thrive, and bouts of recurrent pneumonia.

The nature of the pathologic findings depends on the aspirated material, but usually a mixture of gastric acid and milk, or a formula containing lipid materials is the culprit. The radiologic manifestations include hyperaeration of the lungs; subsegmental or segmental areas of consolidation, due ei-

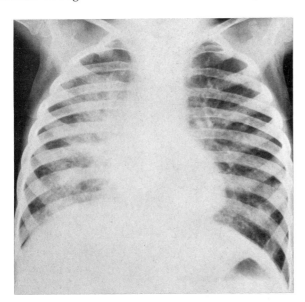

FIG 12–15.
Extensive aspiration pneumonia. A bilateral patchy increase in density is present; a combination of airspace and interstitial disease appears to be present. These findings could be due to infectious bronchopneumonia or even pulmonary edema. However, lipoid pneumonia was found at autopsy.

ther to pneumonia or to atelectasis; and a changing pattern of "bronchopneumonia" with slow clearing and recurrent involvement. Secondary signs of growth failure may be noted. Lung abscesses are uncommon in this condition in children.

Lipid aspiration pneumonia has been associated previously with aspiration of oily nose drops. Recently, Wolfson et al. reported a case of lipid aspiration pneumonia due to gastroesophageal reflux and aspiration of a medium-chain triglyceride solution which is commonly used in infant nasogastric feeding. The radiographic abnormalities varied from diffuse bilateral interstitial infiltrates to a diffuse bilateral alveolar pattern at the time of lung biopsy.

The diagnosis of gastroesophageal reflux is discussed in detail in Chapter 25. There are two major radiologic tests used to diagnose reflux. The first is the barium esophagogram, which allows one to study swallowing function, exclude H-type fistula, evaluate esophageal motility, and confirm the presence or absence of hiatal hernia and major or minor gastroesophageal reflux. The second test, the radionuclide "milk scan," is performed by adding ^{99m}Tc-labeled sulfur colloid to routine formula feedings. Reflux into the esophagus can be documented and quantified. Gastric emptying time can be measured. An additional advantage of this test is the possibility of detecting aspiration into the lungs, though the accuracy of this portion of the test is controversial. The radionuclide test is probably more physiologic than the esophagogram since it uses milk rather than barium. However, no information is gained about the physiology of swallowing and the anatomical detail is considerably less than that seen on an esophagogram.

Aspiration may occur not only as a result of gastroesophageal reflux but also because of swallowing dysfunction. There are multiple causes of swallowing disorders; these are discussed in Chapter 25.

Hydrocarbon Pneumonia

Hydrocarbon pneumonia results from the aspiration of halogenated aromatic hydrocarbons. Kerosene and gasoline are the most common causes of hydrocarbon pneumonia, although furniture polish, lighter fluid, cleaning fluid, floor waxes, and other household materials also are causative agents.

Most authors now agree that in the majority of cases, hydrocarbon pneumonia in children is the result of aspiration of the ingested material and gastric contents rather than absorption of the material from the gastrointestinal tract and secretion through the capillary bed.

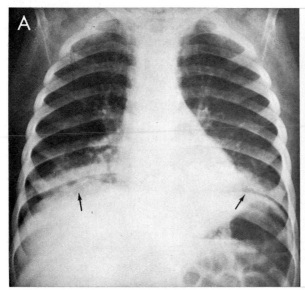
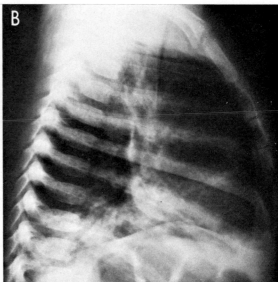

FIG 12–16.
Hydrocarbon pneumonia. Patchy, nodular airspace disease with some air bronchograms is noted in the bases of both lungs in an infant 18 months of age who had ingested gasoline 18 hours earlier. **A,** frontal, and **B,** lateral projections.

Abnormal physical findings are elicited in about one fourth of cases, while in three fourths there are radiographic changes. The radiographic opacities usually occur shortly after ingestion. It is unusual to find pulmonary abnormalities if a film 6 hours after ingestion is normal. The typical radiographic pattern is one of patchy airspace consolidation, characteristic of alveolar edema involving predominantly the medial, basilar portions of the lungs; usually bilateral symmetric involvement is noted (Fig 12–16).

Resolution of the radiographic changes tends to be slow and usually lags behind clinical improvement. Pneumatoceles, pleural effusion, pneumothorax, pneumomediastinum, pneumopericardium, and subcutaneous emphysema have developed in some cases.

Near-Drowning

Drowning is the second most frequent cause of accidental death in children over age of 5 years in the United States. Sixty-five percent of those who die in swimming pools in this country are children under 10 years of age. Whether the drowning occurs in seawater, freshwater, or the bathtub, the basic pathophysiologic abnormalities leading to death are hypoxemia and metabolic acidosis.

Abnormal chest radiographs are found in up to 60% of patients. The chest radiograph is usually abnormal when first obtained and may worsen over the next several days (Fig 12–17). Putman et al., however, have reported delays of up to 48 hours be-

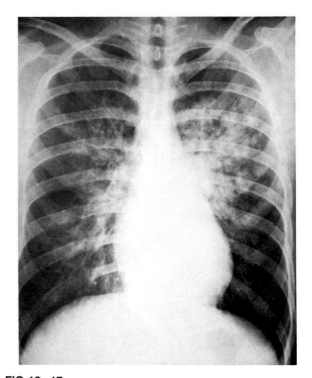

FIG 12–17.
Near-drowning. A bilateral perihilar patchy increase in density is seen in this 16-year-old boy who had been removed unconscious 2 hours before from a swimming pool where he had suffered from submersion. (Courtesy of Dr. R. Parker Allen, Denver.)

fore radiographic abnormalities develop. The basic radiographic finding is one of pulmonary edema, the severity of which presumably depends on the amount of water inhaled. Delayed radiographic abnormalities may be caused by the development of ARDS. Clearing of the lungs may occur within 3 to 5 days and complete resolution by 7 to 10 days.

REFERENCES

Blunt and Penetrating Injuries

Bender TM, Oh KS, Medina JL, et al: Pediatric chest trauma. *J Thorac Imaging* 1987; 2:60.

Fagan CJ, Swischuk LE: Traumatic lung and paramediastinal pneumatoceles. *Radiology* 1976; 120:11.

Gelman R, Mirvis SE, Gens D: Diaphragmatic rupture due to blunt trauma: Sensitivity of plain chest radiographs. *Am J Roentgenol* 1991; 156:51.

Greene R: Lung alterations in thoracic trauma. *J Thorac Imaging* 1987; 2:1.

Horsfield K: Morphology of the human bronchial tree (thesis), quoted in Pierce RJ, Brown DJ, Denison DM: Radiographic, scintigraphic, and gas-dilution estimates of individual lung and lobar volumes in man. *Thorax* 1980; 35:773–780.

Mahboubi S, O'Hara AE: Bronchial rupture in children following blunt chest trauma: Report of five cases with emphasis on radiologic findings. *Pediatr Radiol* 1980; 10:1.

Munk PL, Vellet AD, Zwirewich C: Torsion of the upper lobe of the lung after surgery: Findings on pulmonary angiography. *Am J Roentgenol* 1991; 157:471.

Schild HH, Strunk H, Weber W, et al: Pulmonary contusion: CT vs plain radiograms. *J Comput Assist Tomogr* 1989; 13:417.

Sidhu GS, Radcliffe WB, Wagner RB: Lung laceration in blunt chest trauma. *Appl Radiol* 1990; 19:45.

Sivit CJ, Taylor GA, Eichelberger MR: Chest injury in children with blunt abdominal trauma: Evaluation with CT. *Radiology* 1989; 171:815.

Spouge AR, Burrows PE, Armstrong D, et al: Traumatic aortic rupture in the pediatric population: Role of plain film, CT and angiography in the diagnosis. *Pediatr Radiol* 1991; 21:324.

Wagner RB, Crawford WO Jr, Schimpf PP: Classification of parenchymal injuries of the lung. *Radiology* 1988; 167:77.

Wagner RB, Crawford WO Jr, Schimpf PP: Quatitation and pattern of parenchymal lung injury in blunt chest trauma: Diagnostic and therapeutic implications. *J Comput Tomogr* 1988; 12:270–281.

Postoperative Abnormalities

Garniek A, Morag B, Schmahmann S, et al: Aortobronchial fistula as a complication of surgery for correction of congenital aortic anomalies. *Radiology* 1990; 175:347.

Goodman LR, Putman CE: *Critical Care Radiology,* ed 3. Philadelphia, WB Saunders, 1991.

Henry DA, Jolles H, Berberich JJ, et al: The post-cardiac surgery chest radiograph: A clinically integrated approach. *J Thorac Imaging* 1989; 4:20.

Quillin SP, Shackelford GD: Postpneumonectomy syndrome after left lung resection. *Radiology* 1991; 179:100.

Shepard JAO, Grillo HC, McLoud TC, et al: Right-pneumonectomy syndrome: Radiologic findings and CT correlation. *Radiology* 1986; 161:661.

Swensen SJ, Peters SG, LeRoy AJ, et al: Radiology in the intensive care unit. *Mayo Clin Proc* 1991; 66:296.

Complications of Tubes and Catheters

Balogh GJ, Adler SJ, VanderWoude J, et al: Pneumothorax as a complication of feeding tube placement. *Am J Roentgenol* 1983; 141:1275.

Donn SM, Kuhns LR: Mechanism of endotracheal tube movement with change of head position in the neonate. *Pediatr Radiol* 1980; 9:37.

Kramer SS, Taylor GA, Garfinkel DJ, et al: Lethal chylothoraces due to superior vena caval thrombosis in infants. *Am J Roentgenol* 1983; 133:559.

Kuhlman JE, Teigen C, Ren H, et al: Amiodarone pulmonary toxicity: CT findings in symptomatic patients. *Radiology* 1990; 177:121.

Machin GA: Lung perforation by chest tubes in the neonate. *Pediatr Pathol* 1984; 2:103.

Maurer JR, Freidman PJ, Wing VW: Thoracostomy tube in an interlobar fissure: Radiologic recognition of a potential problem. *Am J Roentgenol* 1982; 139:1155.

Ren H, Kuhlman JE, Hruban RH, et al: CT-pathology correlation of amiodarone lung. *J Comput Assist Tomogr* 1990; 14:760.

Stark DD, Federle MP, Goodman PC: CT and radiographic assessment of tube thoracostomy. *Am J Roentgenol* 1983; 141:253.

Strife JL, Smith P, Dunbar JS, et al: Tube perforation of the lung in premature infants: Radiographic recognition. *Am J Roentgenol* 1983; 141:73.

Bronchopulmonary Dysplasia

Bhutani VK, Ritchie WG, Shaffer TH: Acquired tracheomegaly in very preterm neonates. *Am J Dis Child* 1986; 140:449.

Bush A, Busst CM, Knight WB, et al: Changes in pulmonary circulation in severe bronchopulmonary dysplasia. *Arch Dis Child* 1990; 65:739.

Edwards DK, Colby TV, Northway WH Jr: Radiographic-pathologic correlation in bronchopulmonary dysplasia. *J Pediatr* 1979; 95:834.

Edwards DK, Hilton SvW: Flat chest in chronic bronchopulmonary dysplasia. *Am J Roentgenol* 1987; 14P:1213.

Edwards DK, Jacob J, Gluck L: The immature lung: Radiographic appearance, course, and complications. *Am J Roentgenol* 1980; 135:659.

Fitzgerald P, Donoghue V, Gorman W: Bronchopulmonary dysplasia: A radiographic and clinical review of 20 patients. *Br J Radiol* 1990; 63:444s.

Frey EE, Smith WL, Wagener J, et al: Chronic airway obstruction in children; Evaluation with cine-CT. *Am J Roentgenol* 1987; 148:347.

Griscom NT, Wheeler WB, Sweezey NB, et al: Bronchopulmonary dysplasia: Radiographic appearance in middle childhood. *Radiology* 1989; 171:811.

Heneghan MA, Sosulski R, Baquero JM: Persistent pulmonary abnormalities in newborns: The changing picture of bronchopulmonary dysplasia. *Pediatr Radiol* 1986; 16:180.

Margraf LR, Tomashefski JF Jr, Bruce MC, et al: Morphometric analysis of the lung in bronchopulmonary dysplasia. *Am Rev Respir Dis* 1991; 143:391.

McCubbin M, Frey EE, Wagener JS, et al: Large airway collapse in bronchopulmonary dysplasia. *J Pediatr* 1989; 114:304.

Myers MG, McGuinness GA, Lachenbruch PA, et al: Respiratory illnesses in survivors of infant respiratory distress syndrome. *Am Rev Respir Dis* 1986; 133:1011.

Northway WH Jr: Bronchopulmonary dysplasia; then and now. *Arch Dis Child* 1990; 65:1076.

Northway WH Jr, Moss RB, Carlisle KB, et al: Late pulmonary sequelae of bronchopulmonary dysplasia. *N Engl J Med* 1990; 323:1793.

Northway WH Jr, Rosan RC: Radiographic features of pulmonary oxygen toxicity in the newborn: Bronchopulmonary dysplasia. *Radiology* 1968; 91:49.

Northway WH Jr, Rosan RC, Porter DY: Pulmonary disease following respiratory therapy of hyaline membrane disease. *N Engl J Med* 1967; 267:357.

Parker BR, Northway WH Jr, Carlisle RPT, et al: Radiographic sequelae of stage IV bronchopulmonary dysplasia in teenagers and young adults (abstract). Presented at Annual Meeting, Radiological Society of North America, Chicago, December 1991.

Sanchez PJ, Regan JA: *Ureaplasma urealyticum* colonization and chronic lung disease in low birth weight infants. *Pediatr Infect Dis* 1988; 7:542.

Shankaran S, Szego E, Eizert D, et al: Severe bronchopulmonary dysplasia: Predictors of survival and outcome. *Chest* 1984; 86:607.

Stocker JT: Pathologic features of long standing healed bronchopulmonary dysplasia. *Hum Pathol* 1986; 17:943–961.

Williams JO, Cummings WA: Bronchopulmonary dysplasia. *J Thorac Imaging* 1986; 1:16.

Drug Reactions and the Lungs

Aronchick JM, Gefter WB: Drug-induced pulmonary disease: An update. *J Thorac Imaging* 1991; 6:19.

Batist G, Andrews JL Jr: Pulmonary toxicity of antineoplastic drugs. *JAMA* 1981; 246:1449.

Demeter SL, Ahmad M, Tomashefski JF: Drug induced pulmonary disease: I. Patterns of response. II. Categories of drugs. III. Agents used to treat neoplasms or alter the immune system including a brief review of radiation therapy. *Cleve Clin Q* 1979; 46:89.

Everts CS, Westcott JL, Bragg DG: Methotrexate therapy and pulmonary disease. *Radiology* 1973; 107:539.

Gefter WB: Drug-induced disorders of the chest, in Taveras JM, Ferrucci JT (eds): *Radiology: Diagnosis, Imaging, Intervention,* vol 1. Philadelphia, JB Lippincott, 1991, pp 1–17.

Gregory SA, Grippi MA: The clinical diagnosis of drug-induced pulmonary disorders. *J Thorac Imaging* 1991; 6:8.

Im JG, Lee KS, Han MC, et al: Paraquat poisoning: Findings on chest radiography and CT in 42 patients. *Am J Roentgenol* 1991; 157:697.

McCarroll KA, Roszler MH: Lung disorders due to drug abuse. *J Thorac Imaging* 1991; 6:30.

O'Driscoll BR, Hasleton PS, Taylor PM, et al: Active lung fibrosis up to 17 years after chemotherapy with carmustine (BCNU) in childhood. *N Engl J Med* 1990; 323:378.

Wall MA, Wohn MEB, Jaffe N, et al: Lung function in adolescents receiving high dose methotrexate. *Pediatrics* 1979; 63:741.

Pulmonary Radiation Damage

Fennessy JJ: Irradiation damage to the lung. *J Thorac Imaging* 1987; 2:68.

Inhalation Injuries

Dutra FR: The pneumonitis and granulomatosis peculiar to beryllium workers. *Am J Pathol* 1948; 24:1137.

Olson ET: Occurrence of silo-filler's disease in children. *J Pediatr* 1964; 64:724.

Teixidor HS, Rubin E, Novick GS, et al: Smoke inhalation: Radiologic manifestations. *Radiology* 1983; 149:383.

Wright AL, Holberg C, Martinez FD, et al: Relationship of parental smoking to wheezing and nonwheezing lower respiratory tract illnesses in infancy. *J Pediatr* 1991; 118:207.

Aspiration Pneumonia

Arasu TS, Franken EA, Wyllie R: Gastroesophageal scintiscan in detection of gastroesophageal reflux and pulmonary aspiration in children. *Ann Radiol (Paris)* 1980; 23:187.

Berquist WE, Rachelefsky GS, Cadden M: Gastroesophageal reflux associated recurrent pneumonia and chronic asthma in children. *Pediatrics* 1981; 68:29.

Darling DB, McCauley RG, Leonidas J: Gastroesophageal reflux in infants and children: Correlation of radiologic severity and pulmonary pathology. *Radiology* 1978; 127:735.

Griffin JW, Daeschner CW, Collins VP, et al: Hydrocarbon

pneumonitis following furniture polish ingestion. *J Pediatr* 1954; 45:13.

Harris VJ, Brown R: Pneumatoceles as a complication of chemical pneumonia after hydrocarbon ingestion. *Am J Roentgenol* 1975; 125:531.

Heyman S, Kirkpatrick JA, Winter HS: An improved radio-nuclide method for the diagnosis of gastroesophageal reflux and aspiration in children. *Radiology* 1979; 131:479.

Jimenez JP, Lester RG: Pulmonary complications following furniture polish ingestion: Report of 21 cases. *Am J Roentgenol* 1966; 98:323.

Laughlin JJ, Eigen H: Pulmonary function abnormalities in survivors of near drowning. *J Pediatr* 1982; 100:26.

Martin ME, Groomstein MM, Larsen GL: A relationship of gastroesophageal reflux to nocturnal wheezing in children with asthma. *Ann Allergy* 1982; 49:318.

Molnar JJ, Nathanson G, Edberg S: Fatal aspiration of talcum powder by a child. *N Engl J Med* 1962; 266:36.

Putman CE, Tummillo AM, Meyerson DA, et al: Drowning: Another plunge. *Am J Roentgenol* 1975; 125:543.

Williams HE, Freeman M: Milk inhalation pneumonia: The significance of fat-filled macrophages in tracheal secretions. *Aust Paediatr J* 1973; 9:286.

Wolfe BM, Brodeur AE, Shields JB: The role of gastrointestinal absorption of kerosene in producing pneumonitis in dogs. *J Pediatr* 1970; 76:876.

Wolfson BJ, Allen JL, Panitch HB, et al: Lipid aspiration pneumonia due to gastroesophageal reflux: A complication of nasogastric lipid feedings. *Pediatr Radiol* 1989; 19:545.

13

Pulmonary Neoplasms and Miscellaneous Conditions

Primary malignant tumors
    Bronchial adenomas
    Primary mesenchymal tumors and cystic neoplasms
    Bronchogenic carcinoma
    Epithelioid hemangioendothelioma
  Metastatic malignancy
    Specific metastatic disease
      Leukemia
      Lymphomas
      Malignant histiocytosis
  Nonlymphomatous lymphoid disorders
  Benign pulmonary neoplasms
    Laryngeal papillomatosis
    Hamartomas

    Hemangiomas
    Pseudotumors
  Miscellaneous conditions
    Histiocytosis X (Langerhans cell histiocytosis)
    Sinus histiocytosis
    Gaucher disease
    Juvenile xanthogranulomatosis
    Pulmonary alveolar microlithiasis
      Radiographic findings
    Pulmonary alveolar proteinosis
      Radiologic findings
    Pulmonary calcifications

Primary pulmonary neoplasms are uncommon in children, but may present with respiratory or systemic symptoms or be detected as incidental findings on a chest radiograph. Approximately 20% of children are totally asymptomatic (Hartman and Sochat). A neoplasm may present radiologically as a tiny nodule, a parenchymal mass, or as a totally opaque thorax; however, most nodules and masses seen on chest radiography are not neoplasms at all, but have congenital or inflammatory causes. The history, prior radiographic studies, and laboratory tests will clarify the cause of many pulmonary mass lesions. Computed tomography (CT) is probably the most helpful imaging technique, but in many cases the exact diagnosis may not be clear until biopsy is performed. In a review published in 1983, malignant tumors outnumbered benign ones by about 2 to 1, although benign lesions are probably less likely to be reported (Hartman and Sochat).

PRIMARY MALIGNANT TUMORS

Primary malignant lung tumors are rare in children. Their classification is confusing since they are so infrequent and often different names are used for

what may be the same tumor or variants of the same tumor.

Bronchial Adenomas

Bronchial adenomas are probably the most frequent primary malignant respiratory tumor in childhood. They can be separated into two groups: the carcinoid and salivary gland types. The lesion most often occurs in the tracheobronchial tree and is therefore discussed in Chapter 8. Rarely, peripheral lesions can be seen in the lung parenchyma where they present as solitary pulmonary nodules round or oval in shape, ranging in size from 1 to 10 cm, and located most often in the right upper lobe, the right middle lobe, and the lingula (Good and Harrington).

Primary Mesenchymal Tumors and Cystic Neoplasms

This is a fascinating group of rare neoplasms about which much is yet to be learned. As is true in the kidney with Wilms tumor, there may well prove to be a relationship between teratogenesis and onco-

613

genesis in pulmonary tumors (Bolande; Manivel et al.).

Mesenchymal tumors (sarcomas) of childhood contain primitive mesenchyme and varying degrees of more mature cartilage, skeletal and smooth muscle, and fibrous tissue. Depending on the predominant tissues, these tumors may be called malignant mesenchymoma, rhabdomyosarcoma, leiomyosarcoma, fibrosarcoma, mesenchymal sarcoma, and pleural-pulmonary (pulmonary) blastoma. The histogenesis of these tumors is speculative and how they relate to one another is not known; however, since there clearly is some overlap and since the radiographic features are similar, they are discussed together here.

The subject is further complicated by the increasing awareness that these tumors can be associated with developmental cystic lesions such as bronchogenic cyst, cystic adenomatoid malformation, congenital pulmonary cyst, and cystic mesenchymal hamartoma. Cystic mesenchymal hamartoma has recently been described by Mark, who believed that this lesion was distinguished by the presence of a subepithelial layer of poorly differentiated mesenchyme, the cambium layer. Mesenchymal sarcomas may arise from this layer. Hedlund and associates recently described two cases of mesenchymal sarcoma arising in congenital cystic mesenchymal hamartoma and reviewed 14 other reported cases of concurrent cysts and neoplasms.

The largest group of malignant mesenchymal tumors in childhood is described under the name *pleural pulmonary blastoma*, a rare malignant tumor which usually presents in adults, although approximately 25% of the reported cases have occurred in children. The tumor was first described by Barnard in 1952, who named it "embryoma" because of its similarity to fetal lung tissue. In 1961, Spencer suggested that "blastoma" was a more accurate term because he postulated that the tumor arose from pulmonary blastema (primitive pluripotent mesoderm) and that its development was analogous to the renal nephroblastoma (Wilms tumor) which arises from renal nephroblastema. Recently, two groups (Manivel et al. and Cohen et al., 1991) have described features of the childhood blastoma which suggest that it is a distinctly different tumor from that seen in adults. The childhood pulmonary blastoma usually presents in patients under 5 years of age and its histologic features differ from those seen in the adult tumor. In the pediatric tumor, the malignant elements are mesenchymal and blastematous but the epithelial elements appear benign and entrapped by the mesenchymal tumor growth rather than being malignant, as is true in the adult tumor, which some authors have suggested represents a carcinosarcoma. The pediatric blastoma (pulmonary blastoma) appears to be an embryonal tumor which recapitulates the morphogenesis of the fetal lung at about 3 months of gestation.

Mesenchymal sarcomas and pleural pulmonary blastomas, regardless of their histologic differences, may present as solid, cystic, or multicystic lesions. There may be a huge mass which is sometimes locally invasive occupying the hemithorax (Fig 13–1). Rarely, the tumor may appear as a nodule or small

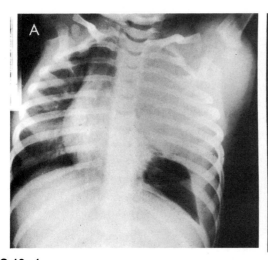 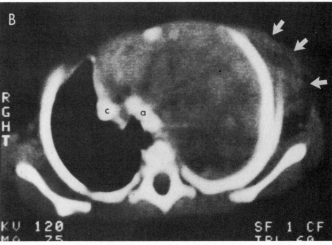

FIG 13–1.
Pulmonary rhabdomyosarcoma. **A,** a chest radiograph of a 2-year-old girl with a swollen left shoulder shows opacity of the left hemithorax with displacement of the left lower lobe bronchus inferiorly and the heart and mediastinal structures to the right. Increased soft-tissue density is seen in the region of the left shoulder. **B,** a contrast-enhanced CT scan shows displacement of the aorta (a) and the vena cava (c) by a huge, irregularly enhancing mass (arrows) filling the left hemithorax and extending into the soft tissues of the anterior portion of the chest wall.

mass and rapidly progresses in size with appearance suggestive of an empyema. Contrast-enhanced CT (CECT) is useful in the differential diagnosis as the blastoma has a characteristic CT appearance which, interestingly, resembles a Wilms tumor with a solid rim and an area of central necrosis (Fig 13–2). These lesions may also present as a cyst which may appear quite benign and be suggestive of a congenital pulmonary cyst or a pneumatocele. Some of these children may present with a pneumothorax (Fig 13–3). Some tumors have presented as a combination of solid and cystic mass lesions and solid elements may be present in the cyst wall or may protrude into the cyst lumen (Fig 13–4).

When this last presentation occurs, surgery is usually performed promptly, but when the lesion appears as a benign cyst, delay in diagnosis has resulted. It is probably prudent, therefore, when a child presents with a pulmonary cyst that is not clearly shown to be post inflammatory, that this le-

sion be followed closely or else surgically removed. It is of interest that Sumner reported a case in which a tumor arose 4 years later at the site of a previously resected cyst so that even surgery may not always totally eliminate the risk of neoplasia developing in these cystic malformations.

The prognosis for survival in pulmonary blastoma is relatively poor, with approximately 50% of children dying of metastatic disease which involves most commonly the liver and the central nervous system. The metastases commonly show only mesenchymal and not epithelial elements, further strengthening the case that this is a distinctly different tumor from the adult variant.

Bronchogenic Carcinoma

Bronchogenic carcinoma is very rare in childhood. In a review of 4,307 cases of bronchogenic carcinoma in the literature, Auxner et al. found that 0.16% oc-

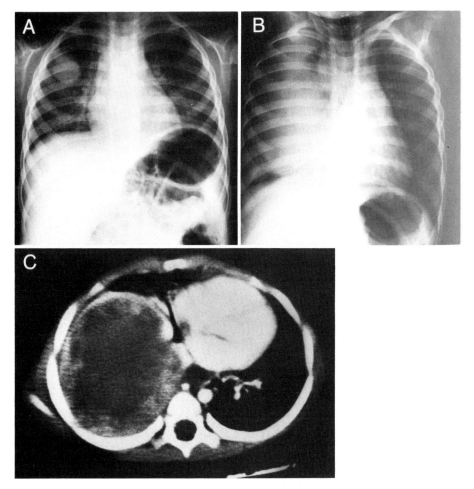

FIG 13–2.
Pulmonary blastoma. **A,** this chest radiograph of a 1-year-old infant with fever was interpreted as round right upper lobe pneumonia. **B,** a follow-up radiograph 1 month later reveals a large mass occupying most of the right hemithorax and displacing the heart and mediastinal structures from right to left. **C,** a contrast-enhanced CT scan reveals a necrotic mass with an enhancing rim occupying most of the right thorax. At surgery, a pulmonary blastoma was removed. The child subsequently developed cerebral metastases.

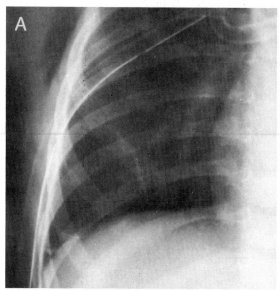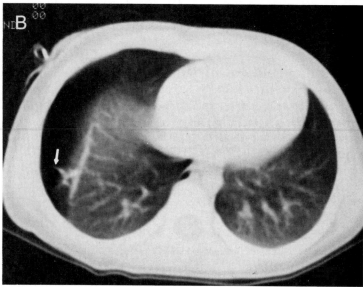

FIG 13–3.
Cystic mesenchymal sarcoma presenting as a pneumothorax. **A,** frontal radiograph made 2 days following treatment of the pneumothorax with a chest tube shows a multilocular cystic lesion in the right lower lobe. **B,** unenhanced CT scan reveals the presence of a multilocular cyst *(arrow)* without evidence of mural nodules. At sur-gery, a mesenchymal sarcoma arising in a cystic mesenchymal hamaratoma was removed. The child is being treated with chemotherapy and is doing well 1 year following resection. (Courtesy of Dr. Gary Hedlund, Cincinnati.)

curred in the first decade and 0.7% in the second decade. In adults, primary bronchogenic carinoma is ten times as common as primary sarcoma of the lung. In children, this relationship is reversed (Dargeon et al.). A review of the world literature in 1974 showed 29 cases of bronchogenic carcinoma in children under age 16 years; 5 of these were of the squamous cell type (Yasutka et al.). Shelley and Lorenzo reported an additional case recently. Bronchogenic carcinoma of childhood has an unusually rapid course with early metastases, and there is only a short span between the onset of symptoms and death.

Epithelioid Hemangioendothelioma

Epithelioid hemangioendothelioma of the lung was described by Dail and colleagues in 1983 under the name of intravascular bronchioalveolar tumor (IVBAT), but subsequent investigation by Weiss and

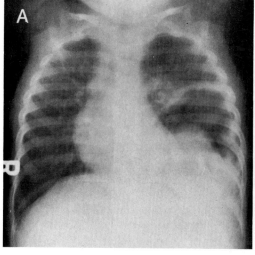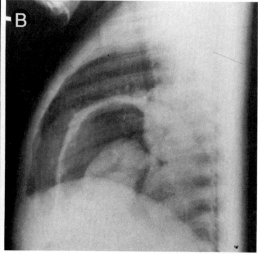

FIG 13–4.
Cystic pulmonary blastoma. An 18-month-old child presented with mild tachypnea. **A,** frontal, and **B,** lateral radiographs reveal a multiloculated cystic and solid mass at the left lung base. At surgery, a pulmonary blastoma was resected. The child is doing well 5 years later with no evidence of metastatic disease.

Enzinger resulted in the name being changed to more accurately reflect the origin of the tumor. It is now apparent that the tumor occurs in soft tissue, bone, and the liver as well as in the lungs. Affected patients are most often asymptomatic young women, but the tumor does occur in childhood. The tumor most often is seen radiologically as small nodular opacities in both lungs. Loss of lung volume may occur unilaterally and be associated with pleural and bony involvement (Fig 13–5). Liver lesions are often seen at diagnosis and it is not known if the tumor is multifocal, or, if not, which site represents the primary tumor and which the metastatic site. The tumor is relatively slow-growing, with a mean survival of 4.6 years in the series of Dail et al. Its clinical course is intermediate between a hemangioma and an angiosarcoma. Death occurs by slow respiratory failure secondary to extensive pulmonary involvement.

METASTATIC MALIGNANCY

Metastatic disease is by far the most common cause of a pulmonary malignancy in childhood. Metastatic spread most commonly occurs hematogenously via the pulmonary arterial system, but can also occur via the lymphatics, the airway, or by direct invasion. Pediatric tumors that have a propensity to metastasize to the lung are listed in their approximate order

TABLE 13–1.

Pediatric Tumors That Metastasize to the Lung

Wilms tumor	Neuroblastoma
Osteosarcoma	Germ cell tumors
Ewing sarcoma	Ovarian tumors
Rhabdomyosarcoma	Thyroid carcinoma
Lymphoma, leukemia	Pheochromocytoma
Hepatocarcinoma	

of frequency in Table 13–1. The metastatic focus may be solitary or multiple (Fig 13–6); usually spherical in shape, they range in size from a tiny nodule barely visible on a CT scan to a huge mass filling the entire thorax. Less commonly, a lymphangitic pattern of spread may be present.

It is relatively uncommon for an abnormal chest film to be the first manifestation of malignancy; therefore, if a nodule or a mass is detected incidentally, one should consider other causes for the finding before embarking on a search to detect an occult primary malignancy. If a patient is known to have a malignancy that may spread to the lungs, frontal and lateral or both oblique films of the chest should be made. Further imaging investigation may not be needed if the chest film shows multiple, bilateral lesions. If the chest film is normal and if the detection of pulmonary metastases would alter either the staging or the therapy of the primary disease, then CT examination of the chest is indi-

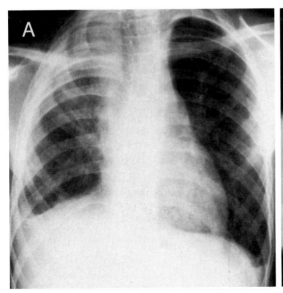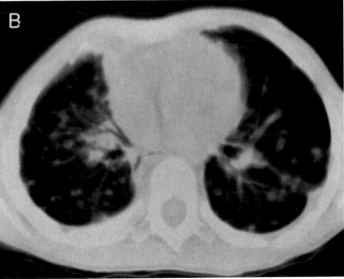

FIG 13–5.
Epithelial hemangioendothelioma in an 8-year-old black girl. **A,** chest radiograph shows mild scoliosis, a smaller right hemithorax, and extensive pleural thickening. Nodular parenchymal opacities are present in both lungs. **B,** computed tomography section through the mid-lung shows multiple noncalcified, parenchymal nodules, greater in number on the right; associated hilar adenopathy; and right-sided volume loss. Other sections revealed bilateral pleural thickening, greater on the right than on the left; and extensive periosteal reaction involving several of the right ribs. (Courtesy of Dr. Robert Kaufmann, Memphis.)

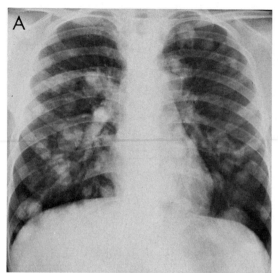
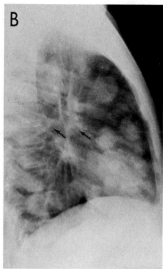

FIG 13–6.
Metastatic disease presenting as multiple bilateral pulmonary nodules. Ewing sarcoma in a boy 9½ years of age. **A,** frontal and **B,** lateral projections. The primary lesion was in the ileum.

cated. The CT scan is performed with sedation if necessary, but general anesthesia should be avoided, not only because it is usually unnecessary but also because when a child is given a general anesthetic, extensive atelectatic changes develop in the lungs that make the identification of small nodules impossible (Fig 13–7).

There is no uniform way to perform chest CT when searching for metastatic disease. Most authors agree that contiguous slices should be used. In small children the slice thickness should be less than 1 cm but will vary with the equipment available and the size of the patient. Using 1.5-mm slices is generally disadvantageous because it becomes difficult to discriminate between tiny nodules and vessels sectioned transaxially which appear nodular on a very thin slice. A reconstruction algorithm maximizing spatial resolution is optimal. Contrast enhancement is usually not necessary, but since some tumors may spread to the hilum or the mediastinum, this choice also must be individualized. On CT examination a metastatic lesion is most often round, sharply defined, and usually of homogeneous, soft-tissue attenuation. Metastases of osteosarcoma may ossify and cases of cavitary metastatic Wilms tumor, Hodgkin disease, and osteosarcoma have been reported. Other nodular lesions that may cavitate and simulate a cavitary metastasis are listed in Table 13–2.

CT will demonstrate the majority of metastases to be subpleural or in the outer two thirds of the lung. They are often seen to be directly continuous with a pulmonary artery branch which reflects their hematogenous origin (Fig 13–8). More are seen at the lung bases than in the upper lobes. Occasionally, it may be difficult to determine whether one is visualizing a nodule or a vessel sectioned transversely; it may be helpful to make a thinner slice through the suspicious area and, in some cases, placing the child in either a prone or lateral decubitus position may help to distinguish a vessel from a nodule. HRCT can demonstrate the hematogenous origin of a metastatic nodule by demonstrating continuity of a nodule with a vessel, oligemia peripheral to the nodule, and beading of the interlobular septa. Lymphangitic spread is manifest radiologically by a reticular or reticulonodular pattern on the chest x-ray film, but it is better visualized on CT where nodules, thickening of interlobular and interlobar septa, and uneven thickening along bronchovascular bundles are typically seen (Fig 13–9). Tumors likely to show lymphangitic spread include the lymphoma group, rhabdomyosarcomas, and neuroblastoma.

Unfortunately, although CT is quite sensitive in detecting pulmonary nodules, it is not specific, and not all nodules discovered are metastatic. In a retrospective study of nodules developing in the lungs of children with known malignancy, Cohen et al. (1981) discovered that one third of the nodules were

TABLE 13–2.

Nodular Lesions That May Cavitate or Simulate Cavitary Metastasis

Septic emboli	Vasculitis
Laryngeal papillomatosis	Histoplasmosis
Histiocytosis X	Aspergillosis
Tuberculosis	

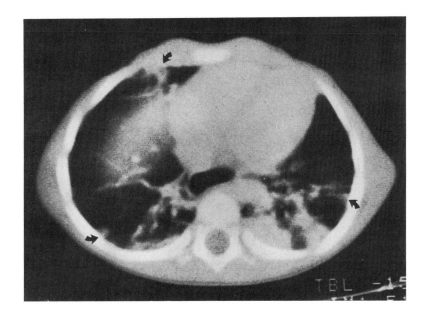

FIG 13–7.
Atelectasis simulating metastatic disease. CT scan of the chest done under general anesthesia following a metrizamide myelogram reveals multiple areas of atelectasis scattered throughout both lungs, including the three peripheral areas *(arrows)*. These could not be distinguished from metastatic lesions, but a follow-up scan 2 days later was completely normal, indicating that all the changes were anesthesia-induced atelectasis.

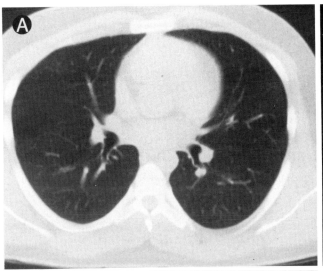

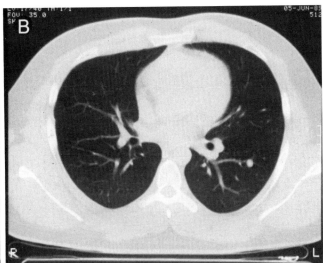

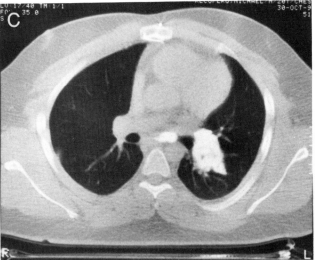

FIG 13–8.
Hematogenous and nodal metastases in osteogenic sarcoma.
A, CT scan of the chest initially was normal. **B,** 6 months later, a repeat CT scan image at nearly the same level shows a 5-mm nodule in the left lower lobe posteriorly that is at the end of a small pulmonary arterial branch, indicating its hematogenous origin. Not appreciated on the unenhanced CT scan at that time were small nodal metastases surrounding the left lower lobe bronchus. Compare with **A. C,** follow-up unenhanced CT scan of the chest 16 months after resection of the apparent solitary metastasis in the left lower lobe shows a huge, ossified, recurrent hilar mass. Subcarinal nodes are also involved and ossified.

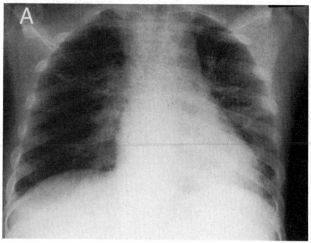

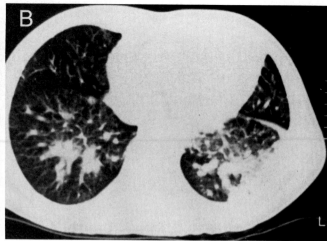

FIG 13–9.
Metastatic rhabdomyosarcoma presenting with a lymphangitic (interstitial) pattern. **A,** chest x-ray shows bilateral interstitial linear opacities, more on the left than on the right. **B,** 6-mm thick CT image shows marked thickening of the bronchovascular bundles and accentuation of the interlobular septa on the right lung. On the left side marked thickening is seen along the major fissure. Thickened bronchovascular opacities are noted in the lower lobe, where there also is peripheral pleural involvement.

not metastatic. This study did not use CT, which probably would have been of differential value in some of these cases, but most granulomas cannot be differentiated from metastases by CT. Our experience in a geographic area with a low incidence of granulomatous disease suggests that over 95% of nodules found by CT in children with primary malignancies do, in fact, prove to be caused by metastatic disease. Also, granulomas even in endemic regions are relatively uncommon in very young children. However, even after therapy, some metastases do not disappear completely and can be seen as persistent abnormalities on CT scans. Surgery, however, has shown only residual fibrous tissue. Magnetic resonance (MR) is theoretically superior to CT in separating vessels from metastases because of the high contrast between lung and tumor. However, motion unsharpness has thus far precluded widespread use of MR in this role.

Specific Metastatic Disease

The metastases of *osteosarcoma* may ossify, calcify, or cavitate and are more likely than most pediatric metastases to cause pneumothorax. Hilar nodal metastases also commonly occur in osteosarcoma. The metastases of *thyroid carcinoma* most commonly present as multiple small bilateral nodular densities. The disease is not common in children. The nodules may function and take up iodine 131. *Pheochromocytoma metastases* may also function and cause a recurrence of symptoms of the primary disease.

Neuroblastoma is not commonly considered to involve the lung, but Towbin and Gruppo found pulmonary metastases at autopsy in 7 of 30 patients with neuroblastoma. Pulmonary metastatic disease was present in 3 of their patients at initial presentation. The lesions spread by direct extension, via hematogenous and lymphatic pathways. Radiographs may show multiple nodules, Kerley B lines, and a fine nodular and linear density throughout the lungs. Mediastinal, hilar, and pleural involvement is commonly present.

Leukemia

Leukemia may present with diffuse, bilateral, nodular, or interstitial infiltrates even before clinical evidence of the disease is present (Fig 13–10). The highest incidence of leukemic infiltrates is in acute monocytic leukemia. Rapid development of infiltrates has been reported, with extensive disease appearing within 36 hours. Most of the time, however, when infiltrates are seen in the lungs of children with leukemia, they are due to opportunistic infection. Transfusion reaction, pulmonary edema, hemorrhage, and drug reactions may also produce diffuse pulmonary abnormalities and lung biopsy is required for an accurate diagnosis.

Another manifestation of leukemia in the chest is pleural thickening; hilar and mediastinal lymphadenopathy are frequently seen but cannot be distinguished from lymphoma on radiographic examination.

Lymphomas

Pulmonary involvement in *Hodgkin lymphoma* may be present at initial diagnosis or may result from a relapse. A combined series from St. Jude Children's

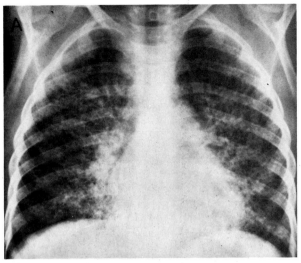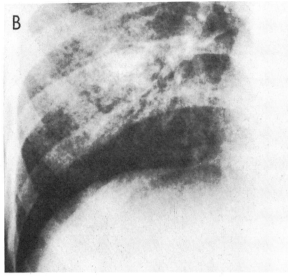

FIG 13–10.
Pulmonary leukemia. **A,** leukemia of the lungs in a boy 7 years of age (microscopic diagnosis). Both lungs show a reticulonodular pattern with central confluence. There is relative sparing of the apices and the lateral segments of both lungs. No obvious adenopathy is noted. **B,** close-up of the right hemithorax in another patient shows a reticulonodular infiltrate. Lung biopsy revealed acute monocytic leukemia.

Research Hospital and Stanford University Medical Center had 60 intrathoracic relapses in 497 patients. Pulmonary parenchymal disease usually is not seen without hilar lymph node involvement (Fig 13–11). Disease may be contiguous or noncontiguous with the affected mediastinal nodes. It extends in a peribronchovascular fashion into the lung. Parenchymal disease is usually bilateral and may be nodular or infiltrative in appearance. Pulmonary masses larger than 1 cm are the most frequent finding. Large nodules may cavitate. Pleural effusion is found in less than 5% of children. A diffuse interstitial pattern suggestive of pulmonary involvement may actually be due to large mediastinal nodes obstructing the lymphatic and venous drainage of the lung. Non-Hodgkin lymphoma may involve the lung with or without associated mediastinal adenopathy. Nodules and a lymphangitic pattern may occur. The radiographic and CT appearances cannot be distinguished from Hodgkin disease. Rapid spread of large cell (histiocytic) lymphoma is frequent (Fig 13–12).

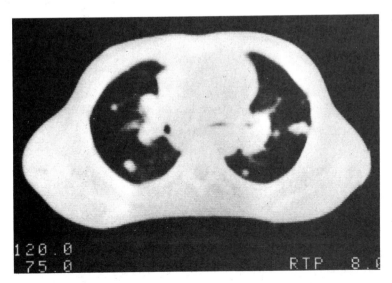

FIG 13–11.
Hodgkin disease with hilar and parenchymal involvement in a 13-year-old boy. CT scan shows pulmonary parenchymal nodular disease associated with obvious bilateral hilar lymph node enlargement.

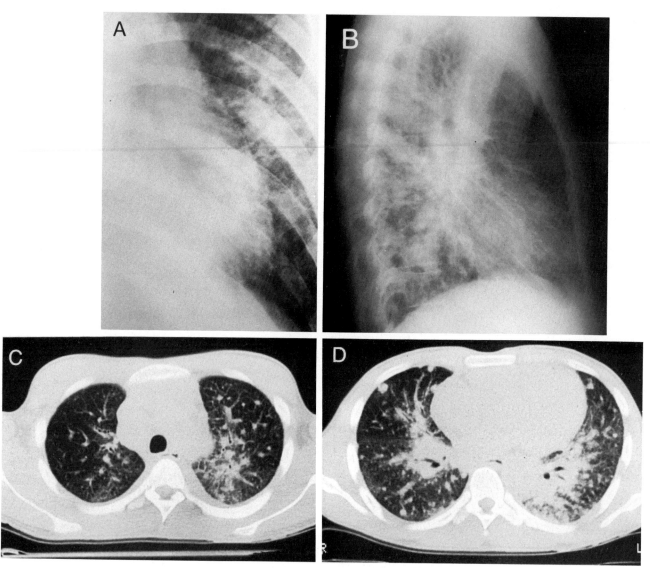

FIG 13–12.
Large cell (histiocytic) lymphoma presenting with a pattern of rapid onset of lymphangitic spread. A chest film 6 days earlier (not shown) had been completely normal although a CT scan of the abdomen at that time showed retroperitoneal lymphadenopathy. **A,** close-up view of the left lower lobe in frontal projection shows bilateral reticular nodular infiltrates. **B,** lateral radiograph reveals hilar adenopathy, thickening of the fissures, and an interstitial pattern. **C,** 6-mm, 0.1-second ultrafast CT scan through the upper mediastinum reveals marked mediastinal widening and bilateral effusions. In the left lung, multiple small interstitial nodules are seen, many of which appear to be at the end of vessels. Marked thickening is noted along bronchovascular bundles and there is an accentuation of the interlobular pattern, especially posteriorly and medially. Similar though less marked changes are seen in the right upper lobe. **D,** 6-mm CT scan through the lower lobes reveals more extensive changes bilaterally, with a pattern of multiple small nodules; marked thickening along the bronchovascular bundles, especially apparent anteriorly where the lung involvement is less severe; and a generalized accentuation of the interstitial pattern of the lung. Lung biopsy revealed extensive lymphangitic spread of histiocytic lymphoma.

Malignant Histiocytosis

Malignant histiocytosis is a lymphoreticular malignancy, probably of the large cell lymphoma variety, that presents with fever, malaise, lymphadenopathy, and hepatosplenomegaly. It is important to diagnose this disorder because of its reported responsiveness to combined chemotherapy. Primary pulmonary symptoms are not common, but lung involvement is frequent as the disease progresses.

Stempel and colleagues reported three children who had pulmonary symptoms and radiographic findings of reticulonodular infiltrates and Kerley lines.

NONLYMPHOMATOUS LYMPHOID DISORDERS

Nonlymphomatous lymphoid disorders of the lung consist of several entities, none of which is common in childhood. Their clinical and histologic behavior makes them difficult to classify, but they are discussed briefly in this section because some of them have neoplastic behavior. Six conditions are considered in this group; they have recently been discussed and classified by Glickstein et al.

Plasma cell granuloma is the most frequently occurring lesion of this group in childhood. It is discussed below and is not believed to have any malignant behavior, although it can be locally invasive. *Castleman disease,* benign lymph node hyperplasia, is divided into a hyaline form, which accounts for about 90% of cases, and a plasma cell type. It presents most often as an incidental hilar or mediastinal mass which shows marked enhancement on CT (see Fig 14–43). It probably is a postinflammatory lesion, perhaps with an immunologic basis in its pathogenesis (Chen). *Pseudolymphoma* is rare in children. Patients generally are not ill but may have nonspecific respiratory symptoms. Radiographs show discrete lesions, often with air bronchograms ranging from 2 to 5 cm in size. Lymphoma has been reported to develop in some cases of pseudolymphoma. There can be considerable difficulty in separating pseudolymphoma from a true lymphoproliferative condition, even using modern immunofluorescence techniques, and authors differ over whether pseudolymphoma should be considered a premalignant or a postinflammatory condition (Holland et al.); however, there is agreement that the lesion should be treated aggressively with complete surgical excision, radiotherapy, or immunosuppressive chemotherapy.

In the pediatric age group, *lymphoid interstitial pneumonia* is seen commonly in children with acquired immunodeficiency syndrome (AIDS) or in children who are immunosuppressed or immunocompromised. This topic is discussed in Chapter 9. Diffuse, interstitial, and reticulonodular infiltrates are noted on chest film.

Lymphomatoid granulomatosis is a poorly understood entity that was formerly grouped with the angiodestructive lesions such as Wegeners granulomatosis, but now is considered to be more closely related to the lymphoproliferative diseases. It is rare in children but has been reported in a 10-year-old child. Multiple organs, including the lungs, are involved with the typical radiographic findings including multiple nodules and masses which frequently cavitate. The disease has a fulminant course, a poor prognosis, and may progress to a frankly malignant pulmonary lymphoma.

Angioimmunoblastic lymphadenopathy presents with parenchymal infiltrates, adenopathy, and pleural effusion. It has a high likelihood of malignant transformation, but is rare in childhood.

BENIGN PULMONARY NEOPLASMS

Laryngeal Papillomatosis

Papillomas are the most common laryngeal tumors in children. When multiple, they may seed along the tracheobronchial tree into the lungs. The papillomas may be cauliflower-like, pedunculated, or sessile; microscopically a papilloma is seen to be composed of irregular folds of well-differentiated, stratified squamous epithelium with a core of vascular connective tissue stroma and a well-defined basement membrane. Malignant transformation is rare, but the prognosis is poor if pulmonary involvement occurs.

Laryngeal tracheopapillomatosis spreads to involve the lungs in less than 1% of cases. Kramer et al. described radiographic findings of both cystic and solid pulmonary lesions. Pathologic examination proved them to be papillomas with central cavities containing debris or air. The lesions appeared to grow peripherally, using the alveolar walls as scaffolding, producing coalescence and, ultimately, lung destruction. Some patients developed symptoms of restrictive lung disease in addition to the more common problem of recurrent upper airway obstruction. The lung lesions of papillomatosis may be widely scattered and can be subpleural. It has been postulated that fragments detached from the airway during endoscopic resection are carried farther down the airways (Kramer et al.). Those that lodge proximal to the respiratory bronchioles are removed by mucociliary action; those that travel farther are poorly cleared and are likely to grow into cystic papillomas (Fig 13–13).

Hamartomas

A pulmonary hamartoma is a congenital tumor composed of the lung's normal elements in an abnormal mixture. All pulmonary hemangiomas and chondromas could also be properly classified as pulmonary hamartomas because they usually contain bronchial anlagen along with vascular, muscular, epithelial, lymphoid, neural, and fibrotic elements. Hamartomas occasionally are calcified radiologically; they vary in size from pinpoint to large masses occupying all or most of a lobe (Fig 13–14), but most often they are 0.5 to 2.0 cm in diameter. Their usual radiographic appearance is that of a smooth, oval, and sharply defined mass. Bronchial obstruction is not

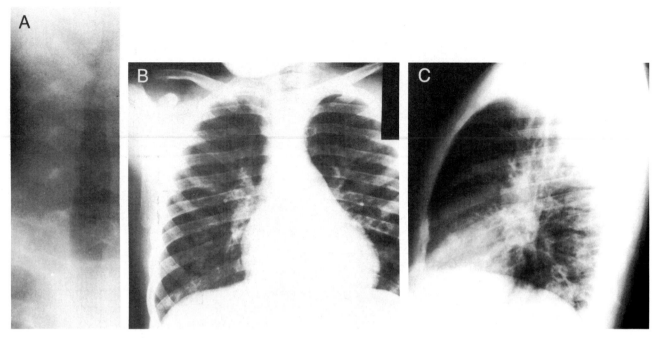

FIG 13–13.
Laryngeal papillomatosis with intrapulmonary spread. **A,** high-kilo voltage film of the airway reveals multiple small nodules along the right lateral aspect and in the subglottic region of the cervical tra- chea. **B,** frontal and **C,** lateral radiographs reveal cavitary pulmo- nary nodules involving both lungs. (Courtesy of Dr. Thomas Slovis, Detroit.)

usually associated with these tumors as less than 10% are endobronchial. Pulmonary chondroma has been reported in young females with gastric smooth muscle tumors and extra-adrenal paragangliomas (Carney triad). It has been suggested that well-dif- ferentiated pulmonary blastoma may mature into a hamartoma much as a neuroblastoma matures into a ganglioneuroma (Fisher et al.).

Hemangiomas

Hemangiomas rarely occur in the lung. When they do, they are usually solitary nodular lesions that may be quite large (Fig 13–15). Diffuse involvement of the lungs by benign hemangiomas is quite rare but occurs most commonly in the newborn. Rowen et al. presented three cases in children with charac- teristic clinical and radiographic findings. Unre- solved recurrent pneumonia was the initial diagno- sis. Hemoptysis occurred in some patients. Each pa- tient later developed thrombocytopenia because of platelet trapping by hemangiomas. Chest radio- graphs showed hyperaerated lungs and widespread "interstitial" infiltration followed by increasing pleu- ral effusion. At thoracotomy, the pleural effusions were found to be bloody. Lesions in the lung were primarily in the pleural and interlobular septa, dis-

tributed along bronchi and arteries and within the septa along the course of veins.

Pseudotumors

Not all discrete mass lesions in the lung parenchyma are neoplastic—in fact, most are not. The common- est of these pseudotumors, the *round pneumonia* of childhood, is discussed and illustrated in Chapter 9.

Plasma cell granuloma, also known as fibrous his- tiocytoma, fibrous xanthoma, xanthogranuloma, xanthofibroma, and postinflammatory pseudotumor is the most common benign neoplasm of the lung in children. Its cause is unknown, although it is be- lieved to be of inflammatory origin, representing a reactive response to various, but mostly infectious, insults. Most children in whom the lesion occurs are older than 5 years, although it has been reported in a 12-month-old infant. Approximately 25% of pa- tients are asymptomatic; the rest have a variety of nonspecific respiratory symptoms. Fever and a his- tory of prior respiratory infection are present in only about 25% of patients. Laboratory findings are most often normal, although several children have been noted to have elevated sedimentation rates, hyper- gammaglobulinemia, and thrombocytosis. The tu- mor arises in the lung parenchyma but may invade the mediastinum or pleura, although it does not ap-

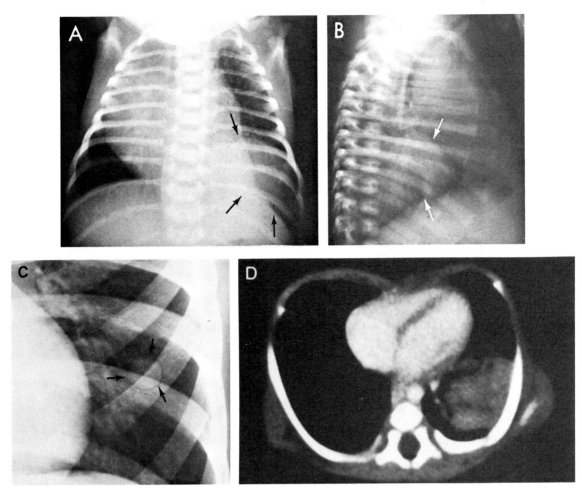

FIG 13–14.

Range of findings in pulmonary hamartoma. A large hamartoma *(arrows)* is in the left lower lobe of an infant 2 months of age. In **A,** frontal projection, there is a large mass lesion in the left lower lobe. The heart and mediastinum were displaced to the right. In **B,** lateral projection, the mass is noted to lie posterior. At surgery the mass was found to be within the visceral pleura of the left lower lobe. Microscopically, it was a hamartoma. The patient did well after excision of the mass and the mediastinum returned to normal position. **C,** a small, rounded hamartoma of the lung *(arrows)* in an asymptomatic girl 6 years of age. This lesion had been followed for 4 years with the only change being slight enlargement. **D,** CT appearance of neonatal pulmonary hamartoma in a 2-week-old infant with a left-sided thoracic mass. Contrast-enhanced CT revealed a solid mass displacing the bronchi. The mass showed mild but uniform increase in attenuation following contrast enhancement. At surgery a benign pulmonary hamartoma was removed.

pear to metastasize. It is solid, well demarcated, and ranges in size from a nodule of 1 cm to a huge tumor occupying most of the thorax. Calcification is present in 15% to 25% of cases. The pathologic appearance of the tumor is varied. Lymphocytes, histiocytes, spindle cells, and plasma cells are commonly present in a fibrous or vascular stroma. The variety of names the lesion is known by reflects the predominant cell type and stroma. Plasma cell granuloma is now the most widely accepted term.

The radiographic appearance reflects the gross pathologic features of the tumor. Usually the lesion shows no evidence of growth but, on occasion, the nodule may increase in size (Fig 13–16). When the mass is large, it may be difficult to know if its origin

was the lung parenchyma or the mediastinum (Fig 13–17). If the mediastinum is involved and the mass contains calcifications, it may simulate a germ cell tumor, neuroblastoma, or metastatic osteosarcoma. On CT, the calcifications may be dense and quite striking or mottled and subtle; the mass usually does not show much enhancement but some cases have been noted to have a thick, enhancing rim. Therapy consists of total surgical removal; if this can be accomplished, the prognosis is excellent.

Pulmonary granulomas, following histoplasmosis or tuberculosis infection, can simulate primary or metastatic lesions in the lung. These conditions are discussed in Chapter 9. History, skin tests, and the presence of calcification in either primary focus or

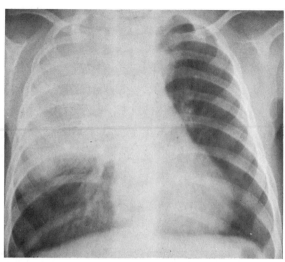

FIG 13–15.
Massive hemangioma of the right upper lobe in an infant 4 months of age. The trachea is displaced to the left. Hemangiomas were present in several other structures (necropsy).

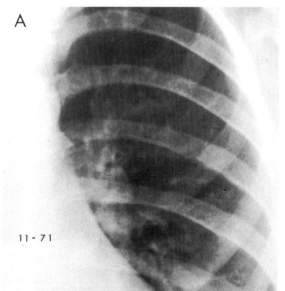

FIG 13–16.
Plasma cell granuloma showing signs of interval growth. **A,** an initial chest radiograph in an 8-year-old boy shows no abnormality. **B,** 2 years later, a small pulmonary nodule is projected near the end of the fourth anterior rib. This nodule was only seen in retrospect. **C,** a radiograph 2½ years after **B** shows that the nodule (arrows) has approximately doubled in size. Thoracotomy at this time revealed a plasma cell granuloma.

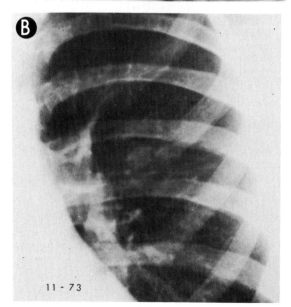

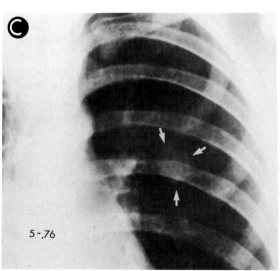

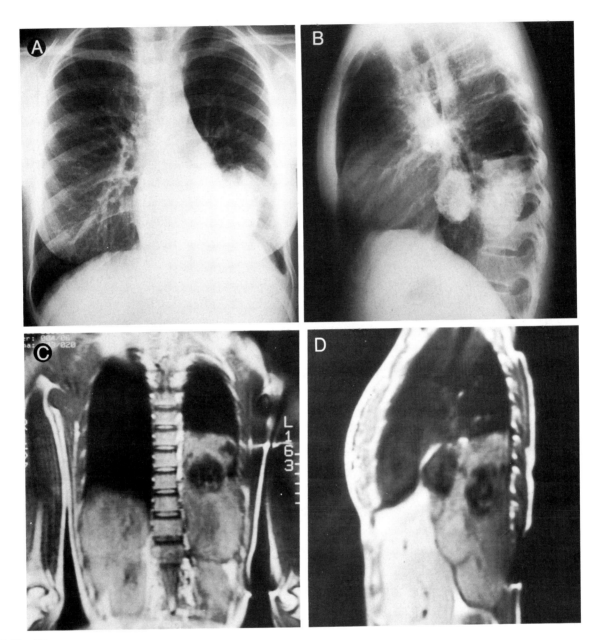

FIG 13–17.
Massive plasma cell granuloma with calcification simulating a mediastinal mass. The patient was an 18-year-old woman who presented with a fever and sore throat. **A,** frontal and **B,** lateral radiographs revealed a huge calcified, lobulated left lower lobe or mediastinal mass. **C,** coronal and **D,** sagittal T1-weighted MR imaging studies revealed a huge lobulated mass containing two areas of signal void corresponding to the calcification seen on the plain film and CT (not shown). The mass is inverting the hemidiaphragm and extending inferiorly as far as the upper pole of the left kidney. At surgery the mass was adherent to the pericardium and left hilum. A left pneumonectomy was performed and the mass was completely removed without complication. An eventual diagnosis of plasma cell granuloma was made at the Duke University Medical Center and at the Armed Forces Institute of Pathology. (Courtesy of Dr. Eric Effman, Seattle.)

hilar nodes may aid in differentiation. Sarcoidosis can have hilar and paratracheal adenopathy with pulmonary infiltrates simulating malignancy. This condition is also discussed in Chapter 9.

In adults, CT is of value to differentiate benign from malignant pulmonary nodules. Detection of small foci of calcification, by a print-out of Hounsfield numbers or use of a reference phantom, suggests the nodule is granulomatous. No work has been published in children to confirm or refute this experience, although our personal observations suggest some difficulty with this method unless the nodule measures at least 1 cm.

Vascular lesions, such as an arteriovenous malformation, either solitary or multiple, can produce a masslike lesion in the lung parenchyma (Fig 13–18).

CECT will show the lesion to be vascular and MR will reveal a flow void. *Mucoid impaction of a bronchus,* especially in a "bronchocele" associated with bronchial atresia, may produce a pulmonary nodule, most commonly the apical superior branch of the left upper lobe. *Round atelectasis* occurs most commonly in the left lower lobe. When the basilar segment collapses and separates from the diaphragm, the margin of the collapsed lung becomes rounded, simulating a mass.

Pulmonary hematoma following trauma can produce a rounded, masslike lesion that may remain solid or may cavitate. Usually, the history or the radiologic detection of rib fractures aids in the diagnosis. *Sequestration of the lung* can produce a basilar opacity simulating a mass lesion. Its radiographic

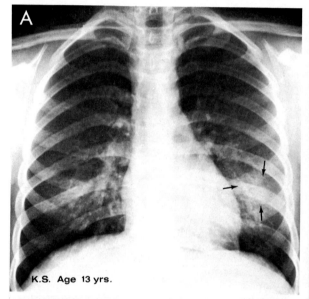

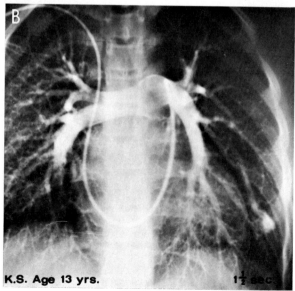

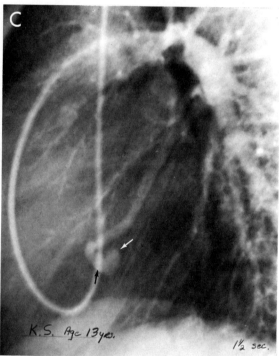

FIG 13–18.
Arteriovenous malformation simlating a mass lesion in a girl 13 years of age. **A,** frontal radiograph of the chest reveals a sharply circumscribed mass *(arrows)* in the left lower lung zone. **B,** frontal and **C,** lateral radiographs of a pulmonary angiogram depict the malformation and the afferent and efferent vessels. A segmental resection of the lingual was performed and the patient has done well since. (Courtesy of Drs. Frederic N. Silverman and Avery D. Pratt, Children's Hospital, Cincinnati.)

features are discussed in Chapter 7. *Intrathoracic ectopy* of abdominal organs, especially the kidney, may simulate a mass lesion. The cranial aspect of the mass is sharply outlined, and often a small amount of bowel gas can be detected above the diaphragm on close observation (see Chapter 14). The diagnosis can be established by intravenous urography, ultrasound, CT, MR, or nuclear medicine. *Chest wall lesions* such as Ewing sarcoma may simulate an intrapulmonary mass, pneumonia, or a mediastinal mass lesion. CT can usually correctly identify the origin of the mass, but biopsy is necessary for histologic diagnosis.

Multiple pulmonary nodules can occur from septic emboli; fungal infections, especially histoplasmosis and *Candida;* vasculitis; and lipid emboli in patients receiving total parenteral alimentation.

MISCELLANEOUS CONDITIONS

Langerhans Cell Histiocytosis (Histiocytosis X)

Histiocytosis X is the name given by Lichtenstein in 1953 to three diseases with similar morphologic characteristics, previously called Letterer-Siwe disease, Hand-Schüller-Christian disease, and eosinophilic granuloma. The sometimes tenuous separation of these three disease varieties is based on differences in involvement; all are characterized by an abnormal proliferation of histiocytes or Langerhans cells in which Bierbeck granules can be demonstrated by electron microscopy. *Letterer-Siwe disease* occurs in infants and young children. It is an aggressive, widespread disease with a fulminating, often fatal course. Hepatosplenomegaly, lymphadenopathy, cutaneous lesions, otitis media, anemia, leukopenia, and thrombocytopenia occur in addition to pulmonary involvement. *Hand-Schüller-Christian disease* tends to occur in older children and is more indolent. It presents with a classic triad of diabetes insipidus, exophthalmos, and osteolytic lesions of the skull. Other skeletal lesions are present in more than 80% of cases. *Eosinophilic granuloma* is usually confined to bone or lung but can occur in both simultaneously. It occurs more frequently in older children and young adults, especially males.

Pulmonary involvement occurs in Langerhans cell histiocytosis, with an incidence approaching 50%. Pulmonary involvement does not appear to have an adverse prognostic effect (Ha et al.; Lahey; Melhem et al.). Granulomatous lesions occur in the peribronchial and perivascular interstitial tissues and in the septa beneath the pleura. Alveolar wall invasion occurs later in the disease, and pulmonary fibrosis may replace the granulomatous process, with development of multiple small cysts giving the lung a honeycomb appearance.

Radiologic findings vary widely with the extent of the disease. The initial chest film may be normal. Nodules ranging in size from 1 to 10 mm in diameter may be seen (Basset et al.). As in other granulomatous diseases, upper lobe involvement may be equal to or more extensive than lower lobe involvement (Fig 13–19). Pneumatoceles may develop secondary to bronchiolar wall involvement, and may resolve either spontaneously or following therapy (Fig 13–20). Extensive bilateral cystic lung changes may develop; indeed, histiocytosis X is the most common cause of extensive cystic lung disease in children (MacDonald and Shanks). Mediastinal and hilar lymph node involvement can be seen, but only rarely as the presenting finding. Cavitation may develop as healing occurs, but it may be difficult to determine if these cysts are subpleural and intrapulmonary or mediastinal (see Fig 14–32). HRCT studies in adults have shown that histiocytosis X of recent onset is characterized by nodules and cavitated nodules. More advanced disease is characterized by an increasing number of cysts and eventual formation of complexes of cysts. The reticular appearance noted on chest film is often due to multiple small cysts. The cysts are distributed throughout the lung parenchyma with a tendency to be more numerous in the upper lobes.

The pleura is thickened and sometimes replaced by a thick layer of granulomatous tissue. Many of the cells in the pleura and the granulomatous nodules in the interstitial tissue of the lung contain fat droplets that retain scarlet red. Despite the frequent pleural lesions, pleural effusions are rare. Matlin and associates reported effusions in two children

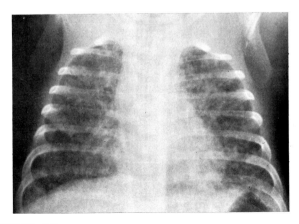

FIG 13–19.
Histiocytosis X of the lungs in a boy 3½ months old (microscopic diagnosis). Both lungs show a coarse reticulonodular pattern. Later, pneumatoceles developed in both lungs.

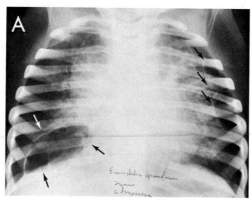

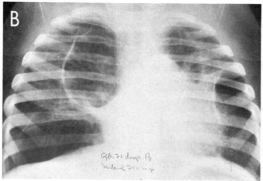

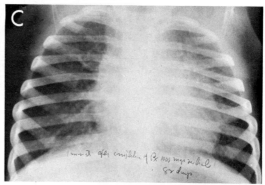

FIG 13–20.
Histiocytosis X of the thymus, mediastinal lymph nodes, and both lungs of a boy 2 years of age. **A,** before treatment, the mediastinum is widened and the medial zones of both lungs are filled with patches of increased density. In both lungs are large radiolucent patches that probably represent pulmonary blebs secondary to bronchial obstructions caused by multiple granulomas in the bronchial walls. **B,** after 21 days of prednisone (total of 250 mg), the mediastinal mass has shrunk and most of the pulmonary granulomas have disappeared; at the same time the pulmonary blebs have increased in volume. **C,** 1 month after completion of a total course of 82 days of prednisone (1,000 mg), the blebs have disappeared but the mediastinum is beginning to rewiden. Small nodules are also visible in the lungs.

but found only three cases in the literature. However, spontaneous pneumothorax occurs in about 10% of patients with pulmonary involvement, and may be the first indicator of pulmonary disease.

Sinus Histiocytosis

Sinus histiocytosis with massive lymphadenopathy (SHML) was described by Rosai and Dorfman as a histiocytic syndrome distinct from histiocytosis X; the disease was comprehensively reviewed by McAlister et al. recently. It is of unknown etiology but is thought to be a disorder of immune response to an unknown, probably viral, infectious agent manifested primarily by massive cervical lymphadenopathy due to proliferation of the sinusoidal histiocytes. It is believed to be a benign, reactive process rather than a neoplastic one. Some of the patients have an associated immunodeficiency syndrome. In addition to massive cervical lymphadenopathy, which is present in over 90% of patients, mediastinal and hilar adenopathy occurs in 30% to 40% of patients; extrinsic airway compression is also known to occur. When the lung parenchyma is involved, there is extension from the hila into the interstitium of the lung, although reticulonodular infiltrates are unusual. The disease has a protracted, indolent clinical course. The nodes may involute spontaneously; chemotherapy, steroids, and radiation therapy have all been used. There is a reported mortality rate of 7%.

Gaucher Disease

Gaucher disease is caused by an abnormality of the enzyme β-glucosidase, the deficiency of which results in an accumulation of glucosylceramide in reticuloendothelial cells. Hepatosplenomegaly, lymphadenopathy, and bony deformities occur. Pulmonary involvement is not frequent but has been documented. Wolson reported two children and found ten others previously described in the literature. A recent large autopsy series (Lee and Yousem) found pulmonary involvement in one third of cases. Three patterns were observed: (1) interstitial infiltrates of Gaucher cells with fibrosis; (2) alveolar consolidation with Gaucher cells; and (3) capillary plugging with secondary pulmonary hypertension. The radiographs show a diffuse reticulonodular appearance with irregular opacities that may be in a miliary pattern.

Lung disease results from the deposit of Gaucher cells in alveolar walls, sacs, and capillaries as well as in the hilar and mediastinal lymph nodes. Recurrent pulmonary infections are common. Pulmonary hypertension has been reported and thought to be due to the pulmonary cellular infiltration; however, a recent case had pulmonary hypertension without pulmonary infiltration, raising the possibility that a vasoactive factor from the liver might be responsible for the pulmonary hypertension.

Niemann-Pick disease produces similar radiographic findings (Fig 13–21).

Juvenile Xanthogranulomatosis

Juvenile xanthogranulomatosis is a diffuse xanthoma belonging to the broad category of diseases of histiocytes. It is normally a benign condition occurring in newborns and young infants and is characterized by cutaneous and ophthalmologic manifestations. Visceral involvement is uncommon.

Diard et al. reported an infant with pulmonary, extrapleural, and hepatic involvement. The chest film showed multiple bilateral round pulmonary

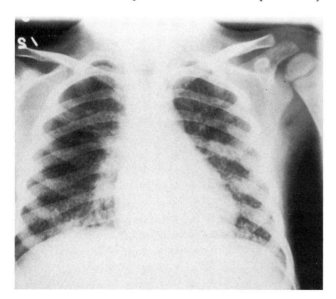

FIG 13–21.
Niemann-Pick disease. Frontal radiograph reveals bilateral nodular pattern in both lungs in one of male siblings known to have Niemann-Pick disease. (Courtesy of Dr. Ronald Holzman, New York, N.Y.)

nodules varying in size from 10 to 25 mm. A pleural mass was also present. The radiographic abnormalities gradually resolved over the first 8 months of life. In a review of the literature, the authors found a 7% incidence of pulmonary involvement. Typical pulmonary manifestations resembled those of pulmonary metastatic disease. The diagnosis is established by biopsy of the skin lesion, and the prognosis is excellent.

Pulmonary Alveolar Microlithiasis

This rare disease of unknown etiology is characterized by the presence of innumerable calcium phosphate microliths in the alveoli. These tiny stones measure from 0.01 to 3.0 mm in size and are similar to bone. In fact, bone tracer has reportedly been picked up in the lung by these lesions (Brown et al.). Many cases are familial. The disease has been reported in premature twins, suggesting that it may start in utero (Caffre and Altman). A review in 1987 found a total of 168 reported cases, 40 of which were in children.

The disease is chronic with the radiographs much more striking late, when pulmonary fibrosis may become severe and induce right heart failure. Microscopically, the alveoli are filled with microcalculi which are made up of irregularly concentric calcium rings, some of which surround a central nidus. Occasionally, the microcalculi contain metaplastic new bone. The number and size of the calculi and the amount of interstitial reaction increase with the age of the patient and the duration of the disease.

Many patients are asymptomatic despite startling radiographic abnormalities. A very characteristic finding is a fine, dense, nodular infiltration involving both lungs. The lesions are very sharply defined and usually are under 1 mm in diameter. The opacity may be so great as to render the lungs white in a normally exposed radiograph. Marked opacity of the lungs can produce an illusion of a black pleural line peripherally. As the microliths enlarge, they become confluent. In the bases of the lungs, Kerley lines appear, the cardiac borders may become obliterated, and blebs form. Sharp radiopaque lines become evident at the pleural surface, at the interlobar fissures, and at the bases (Sosman et al.).

Pulmonary Alveolar Proteinosis

Pulmonary alveolar proteinosis is a rare disease of unknown etiology first described by Rosen et al. in 1958. It is characterized by intra-alveolar deposition

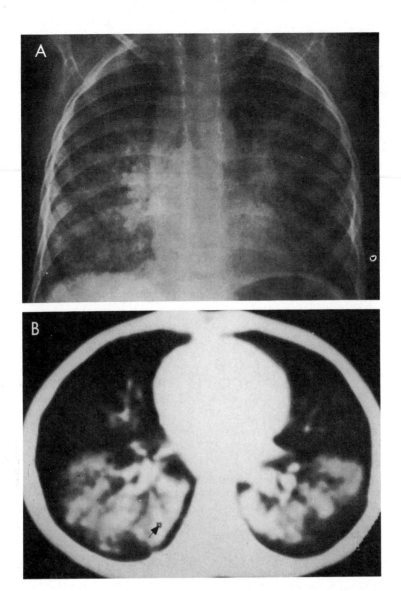

FIG 13–22.
Pulmonary alveolar proteinosis in an 8-month-old girl with a history of failure to thrive and recurrent upper respiratory infections. Open lung biopsy revealed changes diagnostic of pulmonary alveolar proteinosis. **A,** chest radiograph shows bilateral, widespread reticulonodular densities with some confluence in the right midlung. **B,** chest CT examination showing bilateral confluent alveolar densities sparing the cortex of the lung. Densities *(arrow)* measure 0 Hounsfield units (HU) compared with normal lung, which measured −550 HU (Courtesy of Dr. Donald Kirks. Duke Medical Center, Durham, NC.)

of material high in protein and lipids. It occurs both in infants and children and has been noted in siblings, although a mode of inheritance has not been documented (McCook et al., Wilkinson et al.).

Colon et al. noted thymic alymphoplasia in 30% of 23 children and speculated that a defective immune system may contribute to the etiology of the disease. The histologic changes resemble those of *Pneumocystis* infection; silver staining is necessary to eliminate the presence of this opportunistic organism.

Clinically, respiratory symptoms are present in only about half of affected children, and symptoms usually are less striking than the radiographic findings. Failure to thrive, dyspnea, and cyanosis are among the typical clinical findings. Bronchopulmonary lavage and extracorporeal membrane oxygenation have been successful in some cases, and spontaneous remission has also occurred (McCook et al.). Survival is uncommon (14%) if the disease presents in the first year of life.

McCook et al. reported three differing radiographic patterns: (1) reticulonodular, (2) small acinar nodules mimicking miliary disease, and (3) coalescence of acinar nodules leading to focal consolidation. Absence of cardiomegaly, pleural effusions, or

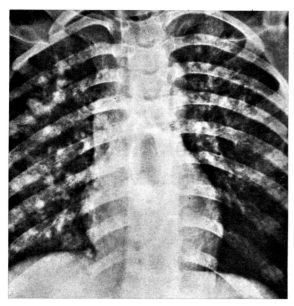

FIG 13–23.
Pulmonary calcifications in leukemia. Multiple patchy calcifications in the lungs of a girl 10 years of age who died of leukemia. At necropsy, almost all of this calcification was in the walls of the alveoli. (Courtesy of Dr. Frank Sherman, Children's Hospital, Pittsburgh.)

lymphadenopathy was a consistent observation helping to differentiate the radiographic findings from cardiogenic pulmonary edema. Varying combinations of airspace and interstitial disease have been seen on CT. Airspace disease ranged from ill-defined nodules to patchy consolidation to large areas of confluence. Air bronchograms were not a prominent feature (Fig 13–22). McCook et al. theorized that progressive growth of the acinus during childhood might account for the variable pattern of pulmonary alveolar proteinosis in children as compared with adults.

Pulmonary Calcifications

Pulmonary calcifications may be either focal or diffuse and dystrophic or metastatic. Focal pulmonary calcifications in childhood are usually due to granu-lomatous infection, most commonly tuberculosis or histoplasmosis. Diffuse calcifications, which are probably dystrophic, occur in patients with leukemia (Fig 13–23) as well as following varicella infection. Metastatic calcification is due to abnormal calcium and phosphorous metabolism, usually in one of the following clinical situations: chronic renal failure and secondary hyperparathyroidism, acute renal failure or following renal transplantation, and following cardiac surgery (Fig 13–24). Calcifications tend to occur in the anterior portions of the lung in supine patients, probably because these portions are relatively more alkalotic. Initially the radiograph shows airspace consolidation which may be mistaken for pneumonia, but which may show a progressive increase in opacity. Definite diagnosis can be made by CT or ^{99m}TC diphosphonate scanning.

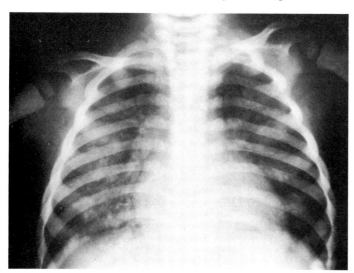

FIG 13–24.
Metastatic calcification in renal failure. Frontal radiograph reveals mildly sclerotic bone. Diffuse bilateral pulmonary calcifications are noted, somewhat more severe in the right than in the left lung. (Courtesy of Dr. Thomas Slovis, Detroit.)

REFERENCES

Primary Malignant Tumors

Auxner A, Dixon JL, Debakey M: Primary bronchogenic carcinoma: An analysis of 190 cases, 58 of which were successfully treated by pneumonectomy with a review of the literature. *Clinics* 1945; 3:1187.

Barnard WG: Embryoma of the lung. *Thorax* 1952; 7:299.

Bolande RP: Teratogenesis and oncogenesis, in Wilson JG, Fraser FC (eds): *Handbook of Teratology,* vol 2. New York, Plenum Press, 1974, pp 293–325.

Cohen M, Emms M, Kaschula ROC: Childhood pulmonary blastoma: A pleuropulmonary variant of the adult-type pulmonary blastoma. *Pediatr Pathol* 1991; 11:737.

Dail DH, Liebow AA, Gmelich JT, et al: Intravascular, bronchiolar, and alveolar tumor of the lung (IVBAT). *Cancer* 1983; 51:452.

Dargeon H: American Academy of Pediatrics roundtable discussion on tumors, benign and malignant. *J Pediatr* 1947; 30:716.

Dehner LP: *Pediatric Surgical Pathology,* ed 2. Baltimore, Williams & Wilkins, 1987, pp 284–293.

Fisher JE, Khan AR, Jewett TC, et al: Childhood pneumoblastoma (pulmonary blastoma) and adult chondroid hamartoma of the lung—a unifying concept (abstract). *Pediatr Pathol* 1986; 5:94.

Good CA, Harrington SW: Asymptomatic bronchial adenoma. *Proc Mayo Clin* 1953; 28:577.

Hartman GE, Sochat SJ: Primary pulmonary neoplasms of childhood: A review. *Ann Thorac Surg* 1983; 36:108.

Hedlund GL, Bissett GS III, Bove KE: Malignant neoplasms arising in cystic hamartomas of the lung in childhood. *Radiology* 1989; 173:77.

Kassner EG, Goldman HS, Elguezabal A: Cavitating lung nodules and pneumothorax in children receiving cytotoxic chemotherapy. *Am J Roentgenol* 1978; 126:728.

Maennle DL, Grierson HL, Gnarra DG, et al: Sinus histiocytosis with massive lymphadeonpathy: A spectrum of disease associated with immune dysfunction. *Pediatr Pathol* 1991; 11:399.

Manivel JC, Priest JR, Watterson J, et al: Pleuropulmonary blastoma: The so-called pulmonary blastoma of childhood. *Cancer* 1988; 62:1516.

Mark EJ: Mesenchymal cystic hamartoma of the lung. *N Engl J Med* 1986; 15:1255.

Nessi R, Ricci PB, Ricci SB, et al: Bronchial carcinoid tumors: Radiologic observations in 49 cases. *J Thorac Imaging* 1991; 6:47.

Ohtomo K, Araki T, Yashiro N, et al: Pulmonary blastoma in children. *Radiology* 1983; 143:101.

Rock MJ, Kaufman RA, Lobe TE, et al: Epitheloid hemangioendothelioma of the lung (intravascular bronchioalveolar tumor) in a young girl. *Pediatr Pulmonol* 1991; 11:181.

Ross GJ, Violi L, Friedman AC, et al: Intravascular bronchioalveolar tumor: CT and pathologic correlation. *J Comput Assist Tomogr* 1989; 13:240.

Senac MO, Wood BP, Isaacs H, et al: Pulmonary blastoma: A rare childhood malignancy. *Radiology* 1991; 179:743.

Shelley BE, Lorenzo RL: Primary squamous cell carcinoma of the lung in childhood. *Pediatr Radiol* 1983; 13:92.

Solomon A, Rubenstein ZJ, Rogoff M, et al: Pulmonary blastoma. *Pediatr Radiol* 1982; 12:148.

Spencer H: Pulmonary blastoma. *J Pathol* 1961; 82:161.

Spencer H: The pulmonary plasma cell/histiocytoma complex. *Histopathology* 1984; 8:903.

Stark P, Smith DC, Watkins GE, et al: Primary intrathoracic extraosseous osteogenic sarcoma: Report of three cases. *Radiology* 1990; 174:725.

Stempel DA, Volberg FM, Parker BR: Malignant histiocytosis presenting as interstitial pulmonary disease. *Am Rev Respir Dis* 1982; 126:726.

Sumner TE, Phelps CR II, Crowe JF, et al: Pulmonary blastoma in a child. *AJR* 1979; 133:147.

Weinberg AG, Currarino GA, Moore GC: Mesenchymal neoplasia and congenital pulmonary cysts. *Pediatr Radiol* 1980; 9:179.

Weiss SW, Enzinger FM: Epithelioid hemangioendothelioma: A vascular tumor often mistaken for a carcinoma. *Cancer* 1982; 50:970.

Yasutka N, Hideo K, et al: Lung cancer (squamous cell carcinoma in adolescents). *Am J Dis Child* 1974; 127:108.

Metastatic Disease

Armstrong P, Dyer R, Alford BA, et al: Leukemic pulmonary infiltrates: Rapid development mimicking pulmonary edema. *Am J Roentgenol* 1980; 135:373.

Castellino RA: The non-Hodgkin lymphomas: Practical concepts for the diagnostic radiologist. *Radiology* 1991; 178:315.

Castellino RA, Bellani FF, Gasparini M, et al: Radiographic findings in previously untreated children with non-Hodgkin's lymphoma. *Radiology* 1975; 117:657.

Chang PJ, Parker BR, Donaldson SS, et al: Dynamic probabilistic model for determination of optimal timing of surveillance chest radiography in pediatric Hodgkin disease. *Pediatr Radiol* 1989; 173:71.

Cobby M, Whipp E, Bullimore J, et al: CT appearances of relapse of lymphoma in the lung. *Clin Radiol* 1990; 41:232.

Cohen M, Smith WL, Wheetman R: Pulmonary pseudometastases in children with malignant tumors. *Radiology* 1981; 141:371.

Davis SD: CT evaluation for pulmonary metastases in patients with extrathoracic malignancy. *Radiology* 1991; 180:1.

Hait WN, Farber L, Cadman E: Non-Hodgkin's lymphoma for the nononcologist. *JAMA* 1985; 253:1431.

Heitzman ER: Pulmonary neoplastic and lymphoproliferative disease in AIDS: A review. *Radiology* 1990; 177:347.

Hidalgo H, Korobkin M, Kinney TR: Problem of benign pulmonary nodules in children receiving cytotoxic chemotherapy. *Am J Roentgenol* 1983; 140:21.

Kuhlman JE, Fishman EK, Teigen C: Pulmonary septic emboli: Diagnosis with CT. *Radiology* 1990; 174:211.

Landry BA, Melhem RE: Pulmonary nodules secondary to total parenteral alimentation. *Pediatr Radiol* 1989; 19:456.

Lewis ER, Caskey CI. Fishman EK: Lymphoma of the lung: CT findings in 31 patients. *Am J Roentgenol* 1991; 156:711.

Magill HL, Sackler JP, Parvey LS: Wilms' tumor metastatic to the mediastinum. *Pediatr Radiol* 1982; 12:62.

Muhm JR, Brown LR, Crowe JK: Detection of pulmonary nodules by computed tomography. *Am J Roentgenol* 1977; 128:267.

Munk PL, Muller NL, Miller RR, et al: Pulmonary lymphangitic carcinomatosis: CT and pathologic findings. *Radiology* 1988; 166:705.

Ren H, Hruban RH, Kuhlman JE, et al: Computed tomography of inflation-fixed lungs: The beaded septum sign of pulmonary metastases. *J Comput Assist Tomogr* 1989; 13:411.

Siegel MJ, Shackelford GD, McAlister WN: Pleural thickening: An unusual feature of childhood leukemia. *Radiology* 1981; 128:367.

Siegelman SS, Zerhouny EA, Leo FP: CT of solitary pulmonary nodule. *Am J Roentgenol* 1980; 135:1.

Smith SD, Rubin CM, Horvath A, et al: Non-Hodgkin's lymphoma in children. *Semin Oncol* 1990; 17:113.

Towbin R, Gruppo RA: Pulmonary metastases in neuroblastoma. *Am J Roentgenol* 1982; 138:75.

Nonlymphomatous Lymphoid Disorders

Chen KT: Multicentric Castlemen's disease and Kaposi's sarcoma. *Am J Surg Pathol* 1984; 8:287.

Colby TV: Lymphomatoid granulomatosis, in Dail DH, Hammar SP (eds): *Pulmonary Pathology.* New York, Springer-Verlag, 1987.

de Terlizzi M, Toma MG, Santostasi T, et al: Angioimmunoblastic lymphadenopathy with dysproteinemia: Report of a case of infancy with review of literature. *Pediatr Hematol Oncol* 1989; 6:37–44.

Glickstein M, Kornstein MJ, Pietra GG, et al: Nonlymphomatous lymphoid disorders of the lung. *Am J Roentgenol* 1986; 147:227.

Holland EA, Ghahremani GG, Fry WA: Evolution of pulmonary pseudolymphomas: Clinical and radiologic manifestations. *J Thorac Imaging* 1991; 6:74.

Libson E, Fields S, Strauss S, et al: Widespread Castleman disease: CT and US findings. *Radiology* 1988; 166:753.

Myers JL: Lymphomatoid granulomatosis: Past, present, ... future? *Mayo Clin Proc* 1990; 65:274.

Pearson ADJ, Kirpalani H, Ashcroft T, et al: Lymphomatoid granulomatosis in a 10 year old boy. *Br Med J* 1983; 286:1313.

Pisani RJ, DeRemee RA: Clinical implications of the histopathologic diagnosis of pulmonary lymphomatoid granulomatosis. *Mayo Clin Proc* 1990; 65:151.

Benign Neoplasms

Bahadori M, Liebow A: Plasma cell granuloma of the lung. *Cancer* 1973; 31:191.

Hammer J, Gradel E, Signer E, et al: Plasma cell granuloma of the lung: Associated laboratory findings and ultrastructural evidence of inflammatory origin. *Pediatr Pulmonol* 1991; 10:299.

Imperato JP Folkman J, Sagerman RH, et al: Treatment of plasma cell granuloma with radiation therapy. *Cancer* 1986; 57:2127.

Kaufman RA: Calcified postinflammatory pseudotumor of the lung: CT features. *J Comput Assist Tomogr* 1988; 12:653.

Knake JE, Gross MD: Extra-adrenal paraganglioma, pulmonary chondroma and gastric leiomyoblastoma: Triad in young females. *Am J Roentgenol* 1979; 132:448.

Kramer SS, Wehunt WD, Stocker TJ: Pulmonary manifestations of juvenile laryngotracheal papillomatosis. *AJR* 1985; 144:687.

Kubicz ST, Poradowska W, Czarnowski-Nastula B: Pseudotumor of the lungs in children. *Ann Radiol* 1975; 18:447.

Laufer L, Cohen Z, Mares AJ, et al: Pulmonary plasma-cell granuloma. *Pediatr Radiol* 1990; 20:289.

Matsubara O, Tan-Liu NS, Keney RM, et al: Inflamatory pseudotumors of the lung: Progression from organizing pneumonia to fibrous histiocytoma or to plasma cell granuloma in 32 cases. *Hum Pathol* 1988; 19:807.

Monzon CM, Gilchrist GS, Burgert EO, et al: Plasma cell granuloma of the lung in children. *Pediatrics* 1982; 70:268.

Pearl M, Woolley MM: Pulmonary xanthomatous postinflammatory pseudotumors in children. *J Pediatr Surg* 1973; 8:255.

Perle M: Post-inflammatory pseudotumor of the lung in children. *Radiology* 1972; 105:391.

Rowen M, Thompson JR, Williamson RA, et al: Diffuse pulmonary hemangiomatosis. *Radiology* 1978; 127:445.

Schwartz MD, Katz SM, Mandell GA: Postinflamatory pseudotumours of the lung: Fibrous histiocytoma and related lesions. *Radiology* 1980; 136:609.

Shapiro MP, Gale ME, Carter BL: Variable CT appearance of plasma cell granuloma of the lung. *J Comput Assist Tomogr* 1987; 11:49.

Taybi H: Pseudoneoplastic masses (pseudotumors) in children. *Med Radiogr Photogr* 1978; 54:2.

Miscellaneous Conditions

Abramson SJ, Berdon WE, Reilly BJ, et al: Cavitation of anterior mediastinal masses in children with histiocytosis-X: Report of four cases with radiographic-pathologic findings and clinical follow up. *Pediatr Radiol* 1987; 17:10.

Bassett F, Corrin B, Spencer H, et al: Pulmonary histiocytosis X. *Am Rev Respir Dis* 1978; 118:811.

Brauner MW, Grenier P, Mouelhi MM, et al: Pulmonary histiocytosis X: Evaluation with high-resolution CT. *Radiology* 1989; 172:255.

Brown ML, Swee RG, Olson RJ, et al: Pulmonary uptake of 99m technetium diphosphonate in alveolar microlithiasis. *Am J Roentgenol* 1978; 131:703

Caffre PR, Altman RS: Pulmonary alveolar microlithiasis occurring in premature twins. *J Pediatr* 1965; 66:758.

Chalmers AG, Wyatt J, Robinson PJ: Computed tomographic and pathological findings in pulmonalveolar microlithiasis. *Br J Radiol* 1986; 59:408.

Colon AR Jr, Lawrence RD, Mills SD, et al: Childhood pulmonary alveolar proteinosis. *Am J Dis Child* 1971; 121:481.

Diard F, Cadier L, Billaud C, et al: Neonatal juvenile xanthogranulomatosis with pulmonary, extrapleural, and hepatic involvement: One case report. *Ann Radiol (Paris)* 1982; 25:113.

Garty I, Giladi N, Flatau E: Bone scintigraphy in two siblings with pulmonary alveolar microlithiasis. *Br J Radiol* 1985; 58:763.

Godwin J, Muller NL, Takasugi JE: Pulmonary alveolar proteinosis: CT findings. *Radiology* 1988; 169:609.

Ha SY, Helms P, Fletcher M, et al: Lung involvement in Langerhans' cell histiocytosis: Prevalence, clinical features, and outcome. *Pediatrics* 1992; 89:466.

Kuhlman JE, Ren H, Hutchins GM, et al: Fulminant pulmonary calcification complicating renal transplantation: CT demonstration. *Radiology* 1989; 173:459.

Lahey ME: Prognosis in reticuloendotheliosis in children. *J Pediatr* 1962; 60:664.

Lallemand D, Lacombe P, Garel P: Metastatic pulmonary calcifications in children. *Ann Radiol (Paris)* 1982; 25:106.

Lee RE, Yousem SA: Frequency and type of lung involvement in patients with Gaucher disease. *Lab Invest* 1988; 58:54A.

Lenoir S, Grenier P, Brauner MW, et al: Pulmonary lymphangiomyomatosis and tuberous sclerosis: Comparison of radiographic and thin-section CT findings. *Thorac Radiol* 1990; 175:329.

Lichtenstein L: Histiocytosis-X: Integration of eosinophilic granuloma of bone, "Letter-Siwe disease" and "Schüller-Christian disease" as related manifestations of a single nosologic entity. *Arch Pathol* 1953; 56:84.

MacDonald AM, Shanks RA: Honeycomb lung and xanthomatosis. *Arch Dis Child* 1954; 29:127.

Mani TM, Lallemand D, Corone S, et al: Metastatic pulmonary calcifications after cardiac surgery in children. *Radiology* 1990; 174:463.

Matlin AH, Young LW, Klemperer MR: Pleural effusion in two children with histiocytosis-X. *Chest* 1972; 61:33.

McAlister WH, Herman T, Dehner LP: Sinus histiocytosis with massive lymphadenopathy (Rosai-Dorfman disease). *Pediatr Radiol* 1990; 20:425.

McCook TA, Kirks DR, Merten DF, et al: Pulmonary alveolar proteinosis in children. *Am J Roentgenol* 1981; 137:1023.

Melhem RE, Hajjar JJ, Balassanian N: Histiocytosis-X: A report of 15 cases in the pediatric age group. *Br J Radiol* 1964; 37:898.

Merten DF, Kirks DR, Grossman H: Pulmonary sarcoidosis in childhood. *Am J Roentgenol* 1980; 135:673.

Miro JM, Moreno A, Coca A, et al: Pulmonary alveolar microlithiasis with unusual radiologic pattern. *Br J Dis Chest* 1982; 76:91–96.

Moore ADA, Godwin JD, Muller NL, et al: Pulmonary histiocytosis X: Comparison of radiographic and CT findings. *Radiology* 1989; 172:249.

Newell JD, Underwood GH Jr, Russo DB, et al: Computed tomographic appearance of pulmonary alveolar proteinosis in adults. *CT: J Comput Assist Tomogr* 1984; 8:21.

Nussbaum E, Groncy P, Finklestein J, et al: Early onset of childhood pulmonary lymphangiomyomatosis. *Clin Pediatr* 1988; 27:279.

Paul K, Muller KM, Oppermann HC, et al: Pulmonary alveolar lipoproteinosis in a seven-year-old girl. *Acta Paediatr Scand* 1991; 80:477.

Prakash UBS, Barham SS, Rosenow EC III, et al: Pulmonary alveolar microlithiasis: A review including ultrastructural and pulmonary function studies. *Mayo Clin Proc* 1983; 58:290.

Rosai J, Dorfman RF: Sinus histiocytosis with massive lymphadenopathy. A newly recognized benign clinicopathologic entity. *Arch Pathol* 1969; 87:63–70.

Rosen SH, Castleman B, Liebow AA: Pulmonary alveolar proteinosis. *N Engl J Med* 1958; 258:1123.

Schumacher RE, Marrogi AJ, Heidelberger KP: Pulmonary alveolar proteinosis in a newborn. *Pediatr Pulmonol* 1989; 7:178.

Sindel LJ, Blackburn WR, Grogdon BG, et al: Progressive pulmonary lymphangiectasia. *Pediatr Pulmonol* 1991; 10:57.

Slovis TL, Chand N, Shavanos TO, et al: Pulmonary calcification in a child with renal failure. *Pediatr Radiol* 1977; 6:112.

Sosman MC, Dodd GD, Jones WD, et al: The familial occurrence of pulmonary alveolar microlithiasis. *Am J Roentgenol* 1957; 77:947.

Teja K, Cooper PH, Squires JE, et al: Pulmonary alveolar proteinosis in four siblings. *N Engl J Med* 1981; 305:1390.

Theise ND, Ursell PC: Pulmonary hypertension and Gaucher's disease: Logical association or mere coincidence? *Am J Pediatr Hematol Oncol* 1990; 12:74.

Volle E, Kaufmann HJ: Pulmonary alveolar microlithiasis in pediatric patients—review of the world literature and two new observations. *Pediatr Radiol* 1987; 17:439.

Wilkinson RH, et al: Pulmonary alveolar proteinosis in three infants. *Pediatrics* 1059; 41:510.

Wolson AH: Pulmonary findings in Gaucher's disease. *Am J Roentgenol* 1975; 123:712.

Mediastinum

NORMAL MEDIASTINUM

The mediastinum occupies the thoracic cavity between the medial aspects of the pleurae, posterior to the sternum and anterior to the vertebral column. It is bounded above by the thoracic inlet and below by the diaphragm. For purposes of description, it is arbitrarily divided into four major parts (Fig 14–1,A).

The *superior mediastinum* is the space above the line drawn between the T4–5 intervertebral disk and the manubrial-sternal junction. The space below the superior mediastinum is divided into three compartments by the heart and pericardium.

The *anterior mediastinum* is a shallow space between the sternum and the pericardium; it contains the thymus, the transverse thoracic muscle, the internal mammary vessels, and loose areolar tissue in which a few lymph nodes are embedded.

The *middle mediastinum* is limited by the pericardial reflections and contains the heart, aortic arch, superior and inferior vena cava, brachiocephalic vessels, pulmonary arteries and veins, phrenic and vagus nerves, trachea, main bronchi, and lymph nodes.

The *posterior mediastinum* lies behind the pericardium and classically extends only to the prevertebral area, but for purposes of discussion, it is practical to consider that it extends to the chest wall posteriorly so as to include the paravertebral space. It contains the descending aorta, esophagus, thoracic duct, azygos and hemiazygos veins, sympathetic nerve trunks, and lymph nodes.

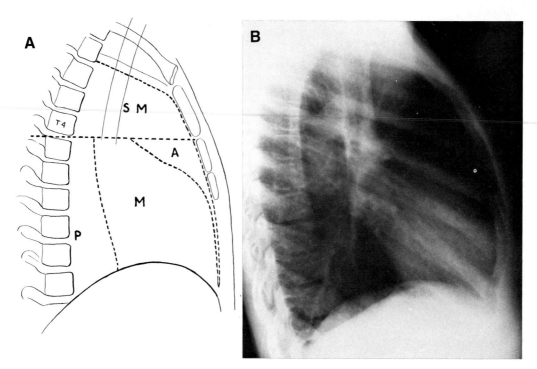

FIG 14–1.
A, schematic representation of the subdivisions of the mediastinum as viewed in a lateral projection. *SM,* superior mediastinum; *A,* anterior mediastinum; *M,* middle mediastinum; *P,* posterior mediastinum. **B,** thorax and mediastinum in lateral projection. Compare with **A** for the relative positions of the mediastinal segments.

Radiographic Appearance

The relationship of the four subdivisions is best visualized in lateral projection (Fig 14–1,B). The superior mediastinum is divided into anterior and posterior portions by the trachea. The anterior mediastinum is the triangular space between the sternum and the anterior surface of the pericardium. In older children, this space is clear; in infants, it is opaque because of the thymus. The middle mediastinum is opaque except for the tracheobronchial tree because it is filled with the water-density shadows of the heart and great vessels. The posterior mediastinum appears as a deep, clear space behind the heart. Normally, the only structures visible in this area, in addition to the vertebral bodies, are the larger superimposed bronchovascular trunks of both lower lobes.

Mediastinal Lines and Margins

Adult radiologists have placed great importance on the recognition and understanding of the multiple lines and contours of the normal mediastinum. These have been described in beautiful detail in Heitzman's book and elsewhere, and will only be summarized here. They have less importance in children than they do in adults, not only because neoplastic masses are so much less common in children

but also because the presence of the thymus and the lack of mediastinal fat in children makes many of the lines and contours less consistently visible in the young child.

Mediastinal contours are best recognized on high-kilovoltage or slightly overpenetrated films and can be best understood by correlating their appearance on chest film with the cross-sectional anatomy as seen on the computed tomography (CT) scan (Fig 14–2,A–H).

The anterior junction line is a hairline shadow representing visceral and parietal pleura of the contiguous upper lobes. It measures only 1 to 2 mm in diameter, can be seen projected over the air column of the trachea for several centimeters, and can often be followed from the level of the manubrium to the carina. It is often not visible in radiographs of children because the thymus prevents apposition of the right and left lungs. In infants it can be visualized in the presence of a bilateral pneumothorax, and in older children it becomes visible when the lungs are hyperinflated.

Also present in the upper mediastinum is the supra-aortic posterior junction line, or superior esophageal pleural stripe. It is formed where the visceral and parietal pleural layers of the lungs come into contact above the aortic arch, behind the trachea and esophagus, and in front of the thoracic spine. This line extends higher than the anterior junction line and usually bows slightly to the left. This line is rarely seen in infants but may be visible in x-ray films of teen-agers, especially if the lungs are hyperaerated.

As the azygos vein extends up the vertebral column, it is intimately related to the pleura of the right lung and to the esophagus just anterior to it. Between the esophagus and the vein is a space termed the "azygoesophageal recess" by Heitzman et al. The interface seen radiologically represents the medial extent of the azygoesophageal recess outlined by air-containing lung. Patriquin et al. called this the pleuroesophageal line and found it visible in 83% of children. CT clearly delineates the azygoesophageal recess, which is almost always concave in adults but may be slightly convex in children.

Two additional interfaces—the descending aortic and the paraspinal—are visible in the posterior mediastinum. The descending aortic interface is formed by the contact of the air-containing left lower lobe with the lateral aspect of the descending thoracic aorta. In children, this vertical line is usually barely visible just to the left of the spine. The paraspinal interface on the left side appears in some children as a line projected about midway between the outer border of the descending thoracic aorta and the vertebral column, extending from the aortic arch down to the diaphragm. It represents an interface between the lung and the paraspinal soft tissues. A corresponding small, short right paraspinal line is occasionally seen in older children.

Right Mediastinal Margins. The lateral margin of the right upper mediastinum varies greatly in appearance, depending on the size of the thymus and the age of the patient. In older children, when the thymus is no longer visible, the right upper mediastinal margin is due to the interface of lung with the superior vena cava. The right tracheal wall stripe is seen in older children if the lung contacts the tracheal wall. Pathologic conditions that can obliterate the tracheal wall stripe include mediastinal fluid or hematoma, paratracheal lymphadenopathy, pleural effusion in the supine patient, or consolidation of the apical segment of the right upper lobe.

The arch of the normal azygos vein is often visible in children. The arch is the terminal segment of the vein that bends forward and laterad on the ventral surface of either T4 or T5 and then curves over the right main bronchus and right main pulmonary artery to descend slightly before it opens into the posterior wall of the superior vena cava. It is visualized en face next to the right tracheobronchial junc-

tion and often blends with the tracheal wall stripe. It enlarges in congestive heart failure and conditions associated with increased azygos blood flow such as interruption of the inferior vena cava.

The thymus may overlie the right hilum and partially obscure but not silhouette it. As the child grows, the hilar shadow becomes more visible because the inferior extension of the thymus decreases with age. The right upper lobe bronchus is the first branch of the bronchial tree. Directly above it, in the tracheobronchial angle, the arch of the azygos vein may be seen. The bronchus intermedius, or interlobar bronchus, is visible immediately inferior to the right upper lobe bronchus. Parallel and lateral to it is the main source of the right hilar shadow, the lower division of the right pulmonary artery. In many older children, this vessel may be followed inferiorly and be seen as a straight structure with parallel walls outlined by the lung laterally, and by air in the interlobar bronchus medially.

Adenopathy may give the usually smooth lateral vascular margins a nodular appearance. The right upper lobe pulmonary vein is normally small but may enlarge in patients with congestive heart failure and cause a conspicuous convexity as it crosses the pulmonary artery on its way to the left atrium. The hilar notch is seen as a concavity between the lower division of the right pulmonary artery and the combination shadow of the right superior pulmonary vein and the right upper lobe branches of the pulmonary artery. Lymphadenopathy or pulmonary venous hypertension can cause the notch to fill in or become convex. A clearly defined notch, however, is often not visible in infants and young children. Inferior to the hilar shadow the right lateral mediastinal margin is usually due to the right atrium which intersects variably with the medial aspect of the right hemidiaphragm. In the subcarinal region, a rounded shadow is sometimes seen medial and inferior to the hilum projected through the cardiac shadow. In some patients this may be the left atrium; in others, the normal confluence of the pulmonary veins.

Left Mediastinal Margins. In infancy, the appearance of the left upper mediastinum is also dominated by the overlying thymus. The thymus causes the "hilum overlay" sign of Felson, which is produced by an anterior mediastinal structure extending farther laterad than the hilar shadow does, but not silhouetting the hilar shadow because it does not touch it. The thymus, since it is located anteriorly, usually is not visible on a frontal radiograph above the level of the sternoclavicular joint.

The aortic arch may or may not be visible in in-

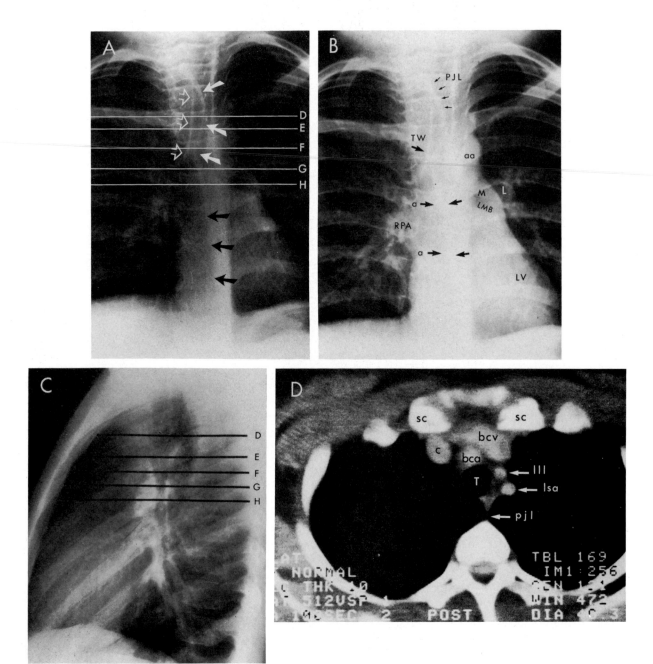

FIG 14–2.

A, frontal radiograph showing normal mediastinal lines. *Black arrows* indicate the esophageal pleural line (azygoesophageal recess). *Solid white arrows* indicate the posterior junction line. *Open arrows* indicate the right tracheal wall stripe. Lines *D* through *H* indicate corresponding CT planes seen in **D** through **H. B,** normal mediastinal lines and contours in a teen-age boy. *PJL,* posterior junction line; *TW,* tracheal wall; *a,* azygoesophageal recess; *aa,* aortic arch; *M,* main pulmonary artery; *L,* left pulmonary artery; *LMB,* left main bronchus; *LV,* left ventricle; *RPA,* right pulmonary artery, lower division. **C,** normal lateral chest radiograph. Lines *D,* through *H,* indicate the mediastinal planes seen in **D,** through **H.** Plane *D,* is above the aortic arch through the origin of the great vessels. Plane *E,* extends through the level of the aortic arch. Plane *F* is through the region of the aortic pulmonary window. The left pulmonary artery is just below this plane; the inferior portion of the arch of the aorta is just superior to it. Plane *G* is through the

origin of the right upper-lobe bronchus, which can be seen as a small additional radiolucency in the tracheobronchial air column. Note the decrease in caliber of the trachea at this level. Also note the visible wall of the bronchus intermedius posteriorly. The shadow anterior to the trachea at this level is cast primarily by the right pulmonary artery. A portion of the left pulmonary artery is visible posteriorly both at this section and the next lowest section. Plane *H* passes through the bronchus intermedius, the azygoesophageal recess, the left main-stem bronchus, and the left pulmonary artery. **D,** contrast-enhanced CT scan at the level of the sternoclavicular joints *(sc);* vascular structures visible include the vena cava *(c),* brachiocephalic vein *(bcs),* brachiocephalic artery *(bca),* left innominate artery *(III),* and left subclavian artery *(lsa).* The posterior junction line *(pjl)* is visible in this teen-age patient. A study of this image shows how the vena cava and left subclavian artery are the border-forming structures of the upper mediastinum.

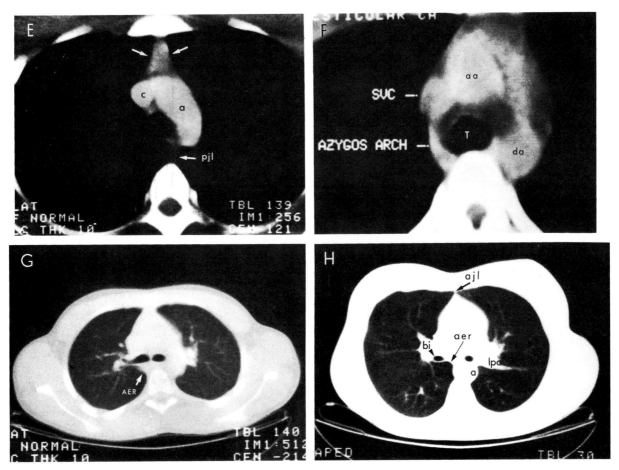

FIG 14–2   (cont.).

E, CT scan image through the arch of the aorta *(a)* and superior vena cava *(c)* reveals a small amount of thymus seen anterior to the innominate vein, which is entering the superior vena cava from the left. When the lungs are hyperinflated, a posterior junction line can be visible at this level. The esophagus is seen to lie between the trachea and the posterior portion of the aortic arch. **F,** CT scan section through the aortic pulmonary window, which is the clear space between the ascending aorta *(aa)* and the descending aorta *(da).* Also at this level, the azygos vein arches anteriorly to enter the posterior aspect of the superior vena cava *(svc).* At this level, the tracheal wall *(T)* is silhouetted by the azygos arch. **G,** CT scan level through the carina. The left main stem bronchus and right upper lobe bronchus are visible. The azygos vein is seen as a small opacity in the azygoesophageal recess *(arrow).* The left pul-

monary artery is just beginning to cross over the left upper lobe bronchus; the right pulmonary artery lies anterior to the right upper lobe bronchus. The thymus is still visible in this 6-year-old child both in the right and the left anterior mediastinum. **H,** CT scan image at a slightly inferior level reveals that the left pulmonary artery has crossed over the left main-stem bronchus and is now descending posterior to the left upper lobe bronchus. The azygos vein is still visible in the azygoesophageal recess *(arrow)* as a slight convexity, a normal variant in childhood. The right pulmonary artery is seen to lie anterior to the bronchus intermedius. Lung contacts the posterior wall of the bronchus intermedius at this level. *bi,* bronchus intermedius; *t,* thymus; *ra,* right pulmonary artery; *la,* left pulmonary artery; *svc,* superior vena cava; *az,* azygos vein; *aa,* ascending aorta; *da,* descending aorta.

fants owing to its more ventral-dorsal course in this age group. In older children, the arch becomes visible (Fig 14–2,B). Above it, the medial border of the upper mediastinum is formed by the left subclavian artery. Just below the aortic arch is a generally quite shallow, but usually visible concavity, the aortico-pulmonary window (Fig 14–2,F). An aortic "nipple" due to the left superior intercostal vein is occasionally seen in children.

The main pulmonary artery produces a smooth convexity continuous with the heart border at the level of the left pulmonary artery above the left main

bronchus (Fig 14–2,G). Laterally, at this level, the left pulmonary artery is seen as it arches posteriorly over the left main bronchus. The diameter of the left pulmonary artery is not usually greater than that of the aortic arch unless pulmonary arterial hypertension is present. The left lower lobe division of the artery is lateral to the corresponding bronchus. The convexity of an enlarged left atrial appendage is nearly always visible below the level of the left main bronchus. The left heart border often appears straight in children owing to inferior extension of the thymus rather than being a sign of left atrial enlargement. The most inferior portion of the left mediastinal margin is usually the left ventricle, which characteristically extends below the plane of the left hemidiaphragm.

Mediastinal Anatomy in the Lateral Projection

The anatomy of the chest as seen on the lateral radiograph has been elegantly detailed by Proto and Speckman and only a few common findings are summarized here.

In many healthy children, right lateral projections of the thorax show a retrosternal strip of water density (Fig 14–3) that parallels the dorsal edge of the sternum and is partially superimposed on the ventral edge of the heart. This retrosternal image is characteristically widest at its base near the diaphragm and tapers to a point cephalad, which may suggest pleural exudate to the inexperienced ob-

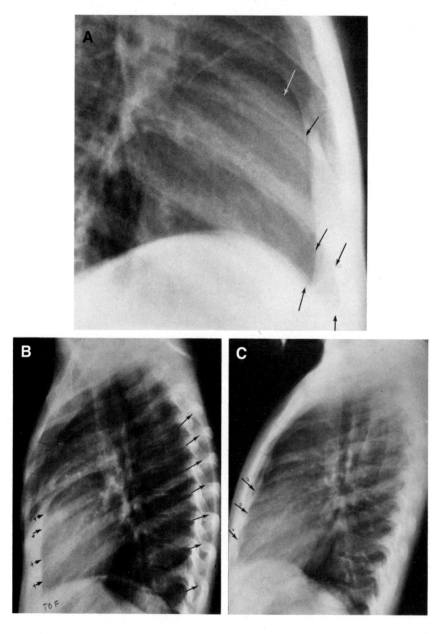

FIG 14–3.
A, normal retrosternal strip *(arrows)* in right lateral projection of the thorax of a healthy girl 7 years of age. The strip is thickest at its base and tapers cephalad to a sharp apex, which fades out at the level of the upper edge of the heart. The dorsal edge of the strip represents the ventral edge of the left lung, which is prevented from reaching the ventral thoracic wall, as the right lung does, by the normal cardiac mass on the left side of the thorax. **B,** thickening of the retrosternal strip *(arrows)* by slight rotation of the thorax **(B)** in comparison with the narrower strip in more direct lateral projection **(C).** This healthy girl was 6 years of age.

server. Whalen and associates, in careful anatomical radiographic studies, demonstrated conclusively that this retrosternal strip represented the difference in the complete forward extension of the normal right lung and the incomplete forward extension of the left lung, due to presence of the heart in the left hemithorax (Fig 14–4).

The key to identifying adenopathy or other hilar masses on the lateral radiograph is to be able to recognize the normal vessels. To do this, one must first be able to satisfactorily identify the airways, which can be difficult in children, especially if the child has not been filmed in full inspiration. The tracheal air column appears to narrow at the level of the lower border of the aortic arch (Fig 14–5; see also Fig 14–40,A and B). This change in caliber marks the level of the bifurcation. The mainstem bronchi are, of course, smaller in diameter than the trachea itself. The right upper lobe bronchus is often seen end-on as a circular radiolucency, usually projected through the arch of the left pulmonary artery as it swings posteriorly over the left main bronchus. It is made more conspicuous by bronchial wall thickening, a finding commonly seen in cystic fibrosis. Just distal to the tracheal bifurcation, the interlobar bronchus (bronchus intermedius) on the right has a linear posterior wall where lung touches the bronchial wall.

Changes in appearance of the normal posterior wall of the bronchus intermedius provide clues to the presence of lymphadenopathy, peribronchial edema or infection, or consolidation of the superior segment of the right lower lobe. A short segment of the right middle lobe bronchus can often be seen extending anteriorly and inferiorly at the level of the lower portion of the bronchus intermedius. The right pulmonary artery is seen as a soft-tissue opacity just above the right middle lobe bronchus.

The contribution of the left-sided vascular structures to the appearance of the lateral film can also be studied by reference to the airways. The arch of the left pulmonary artery may be outlined by lung above, and below by the left mainstem bronchus as the artery curves over this structure. When visible, the horizontal portion of the left upper lobe bronchus is seen as a dark circular shadow because of its end-on projection. It is inferior to the similar shadow of the right upper lobe bronchus. A subcarinal mass or left upper lobe atelectasis can elevate the left main bronchus and cause this to become the horizontal structure rather than the left upper lobe bronchus. A short segment of the posterior wall of the left upper lobe bronchus can be seen in about 40% of adult lateral chest films but is less commonly seen in children; its wall is usually obscured by the

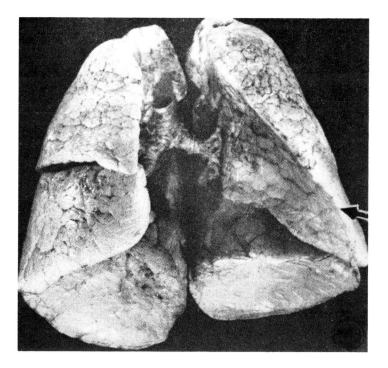

FIG 14–4.
Frontal photograph of two inflated, companion, normal lungs. The right lung extends forward to the ventral wall of the thorax and then curls mediad and is flush with the ventral wall for several centimeters. The ventral edge of the left lung, in contrast, does not reach the ventral thoracic wall and is prevented from curling forward by the cardiac mass. (From Whalen JP, *Am J Roentgenol* 1973; 117:861. Used by permission.)

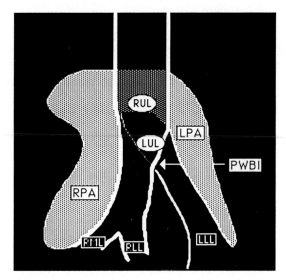

FIG 14–5.
Schematic representation of normal hilar anatomy as seen on a lateral radiograph. *RPA,* right pulmonary artery and veins; *LPA,* left pulmonary artery; *RUL,* right upper lobe bronchus; *PWBI,* posterior wall of bronchus intermedius; *RML,* right middle lobe bronchus; *RLL,* right lower lobe bronchus; *LUL,* left upper lobe bronchus; *LLL,* left lower lobe bronchus. (Drawn by C. Jonas.)

left pulmonary artery. The left lower lobe bronchus continues posteriorly beyond the level at which the end-on bronchus is seen. The anterior wall may be visible where outlined by lung, but the posterior wall is usually silhouetted by the descending left pulmonary artery. The artery parallels the left lower lobe bronchus and points toward the posterior costophrenic sulcus. Therefore, a convex shadow anterior or inferior to the airways below the level of the arc of the left pulmonary artery is usually an abnormal mass lesion. The major vascular shadows form a horseshoe-like density around the airway in the lateral view; the left pulmonary artery forms the top and posterior portion, and the right pulmonary artery and upper lobe veins form its anterior portion. There should be, therefore, a relatively lucent region inferiorly in line with the airways. Adenopathy or venous engorgement can fill in this space, transforming the horseshoe into a circle.

The diaphragms are normally clearly visible on the lateral radiograph. The anterior one third of the left diaphragm is usually silhouetted by the heart. The posterior border of the heart is usually formed by the left ventricle; it and a short portion of the inferior vena cava normally outline the anterior edge of the posterior mediastinum. The anterior cardiac margin, the right ventricular outflow tract, and ascending aorta are normally silhouetted by the thymus and are inseparable from it. The vertebral bodies and disk spaces are the major structures visible

in the posterior mediastinum; they should normally be increasingly radiolucent from superior to inferior. The anterior margin of the scapulae are seen as long, slightly concave (anteriorly) opacities in the upper one third of the posterior medastinum. In older children, portions of the ascending aorta and occasionally the descending aorta may be visible.

Mediastinal Displacement

The midline position of the mediastinal structures in the thorax depends on the equilibrium of intrathoracic pressures maintained by the lungs. Abnormal intrapulmonary or intrapleural pressures may cause deformation and displacement of the normal mediastinum. It may be widened in cases of unilateral pulmonary atelectasis and narrowed in cases of unilateral emphysema; the shift of the mediastinum is toward a collapsed, atelectatic lung and away from an expanded, emphysematous lung. Large pleural effusions may compress the mediastinum on the affected side and displace it toward the opposite normal side. In bilateral, severe pulmonary hyperaeration, as seen in asthmatics and children with cystic fibrosis, the mediastinal and cardiac shadows remain in the midline but are compressed by the hyperexpanded lungs.

When the diaphragm is paralyzed on one side, the mediastinum is drawn toward the normal side during inspiration as a result of the negative pressure produced by the descent of the functioning half of the diaphragm.

DISEASES OF THE MEDIASTINUM

Pneumomediastinum

Pneumomediastinum, gas in the mediastinal space, is seen commonly in infants but much less frequently in older children. Its appearance and significance in neonates is discussed in Chapter 51. Pneumomediastinum in a child usually develops following a sudden increase in intra-alveolar pressure. It has been suggested that, when alveolar rupture occurs, gas may pass into the interstitium of the lung and travel along the perivascular space to the hilum and into the mediastinum. At least in some cases, it travels in the lymphatics and may extend to the visceral pleura and rupture into the pleural space to cause a pneumothorax. A pneumothorax can also result from rupture of the mediastinal pleura if sufficient tension occurs. A pneumothorax is a common complication of a pneumomediastinum but not a cause of it. Usually, however, except in infancy, the mediastinum is decompressed as the gas extends into the subcutaneous tissues of the neck, upper part of the trunk, and the retropharyngeal area. Occasionally, severe pneumomediastinum may dissect into the abdomen and cause intra-abdominal extraperitoneal gas or even a pneumoperitoneum.

Pneumomediastinum may be spontaneous in origin, although frequently it follows a bout of increased intra-alveolar pressure, as may occur with coughing or vomiting. After infancy, it is most commonly seen in asthmatic children but it also occurs in patients in the intensive care unit, following tracheostomy, or in patients on ventilator therapy, especially those with interstitial pulmonary emphysema and diffuse bilateral lung disease such as *Pneumocystis carinii* pneumonia or adult respiratory distress syndrome. A patient with an aspirated foreign body may present with a pneumomediastinum; therefore, in a child less than 2 years of age with no history of trauma, the findings of a pneumomediastinum should prompt investigation for an aspirated foreign body (Burton et al.). Regardless of the etiology, the patient may present with a feeling of retrosternal fullness, dysphagia, or sore throat; occasionally, chest pain and dyspnea are present. Rarely, a pneumomediastinum is detected in a relatively asymptomatic person as an incidental radiographic finding. The condition is nearly always self-limited.

Radiologic diagnosis of pneumomediastinum is usually not difficult (Fig 14–6,A and B). Air in the mediastinum displaces the mediastinal pleura later-ally. The thymus is separated from the cardiac silhouette. Subtle signs include a "sliver of air" adjacent to the cardiac border, usually on the left side or outlining the arch and descending aorta, on the lateral view. Sometimes, even when the chest findings are not striking, a lateral radiograph of the nasopharynx reveals a large amount of retropharyngeal gas (Fig 14–6,C). In infants, large collections of gas elevate the thymus both on the frontal and lateral radiographs to produce a "spinnaker" sign. When the mediastinal gas collection is large, confusion with a medial pneumothorax can occur. A decubitus film can resolve the issue. The mediastinal gas does not move, whereas a pneumothorax will move superiorly in the elevated thorax.

The CT scan in Figure 14–7 shows that mediastinal gas is not limited to the anterior mediastinum but commonly is widely diffuse.

When gas is interposed between the heart and the diaphragm, the usually obscured central portion of the diaphragm can be seen, resulting in the "continuous diaphragm" sign (Fig 14–8). In some cases, gas may dissect into the extrapleural space and appear as a loculated, lucent strip between the parietal layer of the pleura and the diaphragm.

Usually, mediastinal air presents in the anterosuperior mediastinum, but on occasion, collections of air can be seen in the lower half of the thorax; their exact location is not always clear. Large, loculated midline collections, posterior to the heart, are seen in association with tracheal lacerations as well as occurring in some children being treated with

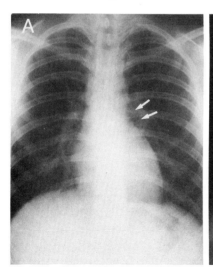 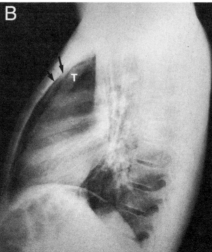 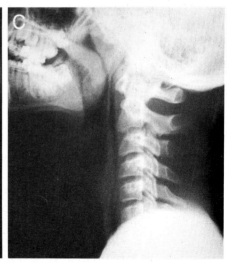

FIG 14–6.

Pneumomediastinum in a teen-age male with asthma. **A,** frontal radiograph shows subtle findings of pneumomediastinum with mediastinal pleura and thymus faintly outlined by air *(arrows)* **B,** lateral radiograph reveals the findings to be more apparent as the thymus *(T)* is more clearly outlined as is the mediastinal pleura *(arrows).* **C,** lateral radiograph of the neck in the same patient reveals extensive dissection of air into the retropharyngeal soft tissues. Often this is the most convincing film that can be obtained to document a pneumomediastinum.

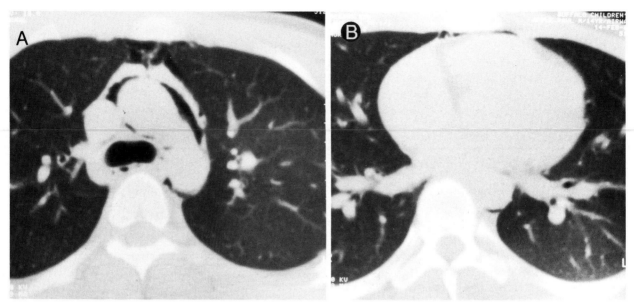

FIG 14–7.
CT appearance of pneumomediastinum in the same patient as Figure 14–6, demonstrating that air in the pneumomediastinum dissects freely throughout the mediastinum. CT examination was obtained because the patient had given a history of trauma and there was concern over a possible tracheal laceration. **A,** CT scan at the level of the aortic arch reveals that air is seen in the anterior mediastinum surrounding the thymus but also has dissected into the middle mediastinum medial to the aortic arch and is seen in the posterior mediastinum posterior to the trachea and around the descending aorta. **B,** more inferior CT scan section at the level of the pulmonary veins reveals that there is still air in the anterior mediastinum in a retrosternal location as well as air seen around the descending aorta. No airway laceration was found and the patient recovered uneventfully.

positive pressure respiration. These collections have been called infrazygos pneumomediastinum. Inferior paravertebral collections of air can also develop in similar clinical situations but are also are seen following trauma. It was at one time thought that these were collections of air loculated in or by the pulmonary ligaments, but in most cases the collections are probably too posterior for that to be the explanation. They may represent posttraumatic pneumatoceles or, alternatively, either loculated pneumothorax or loculated pneumomediastinum. CT clearly visualizes the collections, but even with CT there can be difficulty in deciding exactly where the collections are located (Fig 14–9). The collections are usually self-limited, although posttraumatic pneumatoceles can persist for weeks or months, gradually decreasing in size. Other gas collections can be confused with pneumomediastinum, particularly a medial pneumothorax. A decubitus film readily differentiates these two conditions. Without the use of a decubitus film, it can be difficult or impossible to distinguish between a small subpulmonary pneumothorax and extrapleural dissection of air along the diaphragm. A pneumopericardium can also superficially resemble a pneumomediastinum, but the pericardial air should outline the pericardium, have a dome-shaped superior margin, and be limited to the peri-cardial sac. The thymus and the arch of the aorta will therefore not be outlined by intrapericardial air collections. In most patients, pneumopericardium and pneumomediastinum coexist.

Mediastinal Fluid Collections

Mediastinal hemorrhage most commonly occurs after blunt trauma that has caused venous bleeding and, sometimes, radiographically visible fractures of the ribs or sternum. Aortic and other great-vessel lacerations may rarely occur after severe trauma. Aortic rupture may be suspected on plain film and sometimes diagnosed by contrast-enhanced CT (CECT) but definitive exclusion of the diagnosis still requires angiography. Medical procedures are the common cause of perforating trauma—the placement of venous catheters, sternal marrow aspirations, pericardiocentesis, intracardiac injections, arteriography, cardiac catheterizations, and cervical and thoracic surgery. Especially in hemophilic children, hemorrhage can occur in the retropharyngeal space, and as with infection, may dissect into the mediastinum. Mediastinal widening commonly occurs following cardiac surgery, but without the use of CT its exact nature cannot be determined.

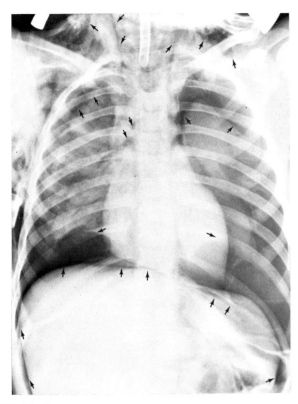

FIG 14–8.
Continuous diaphragm sign of pneumomediastinum. This patient developed a pneumomediastinum, bilateral pneumothorax, pneumoperitoneum, and subcutaneous emphysema following an attempted lumbar subarachnoid puncture for a pneumoencephalogram. Note that the diaphragm is not silhouetted medially by the heart as is normally seen. This continuous diaphragm sign results from mediastinal air interposing itself between the inferior border of the heart and the diaphragm.

Mediastinal Infection

Acute Mediastinitis

Mediastinal pus may be localized (abscess) or diffuse (cellulitis), and most commonly results from perforation of the esophagus or trachea. Perforations may be spontaneous or be secondary to the passage of instruments, impacted foreign bodies, child abuse, or leakage at the sites of surgical anastomoses. After esophageal rupture, small amounts of mediastinal gas are usually evident, followed by rapid extension of suppurative mediastinitis after spillage of esophageal and, sometimes, gastric content. Pyothorax and pyopneumothorax may then develop. Abscesses may develop almost anywhere in the mediastinum; they vary greatly in size and shape (Fig 14–10). Abscesses in the posterior mediastinum are usually due to extension of infections of the spine, and abscesses in the superior mediastinum, secondary to cervical infection or sternoclavicular osteomyelitis. Retropharyngeal abscesses can extend inferiorly into the me-

diastinum (Fig 14–11). Abscesses may be revealed by a positive gallium 67 a citrate scan and localized by CT.

Plain film findings are nonspecific. Mediastinal widening and obliteration of normal mediastinal contours may be recognized. The trachea may be displaced or narrowed. The diagnosis is much clearer if gas can be recognized in the mediastinum in the appropriate clinical setting. Carrol et al. reviewed the CT evaluation of mediastinal infection. Focal mediastinal abscesses and abscesses associated with empyema or subphrenic abscess were readily diagnosed by CT. Diffuse mediastinitis, however, could not be reliably separated from postoperative changes in the absence of mediastinal gas.

Chronic Fibrosing Mediastinitis

Fibrosing mediastinitis usually follows tuberculous or *Histoplasma* infection but is rare in childhood. Radiographic examination shows widening of the upper half of the mediastinum with a lobulated paratracheal mass that may be calcified. Extrinsic obstruction of the tracheobronchial tree and occlusion of the vascular structures may result. CT or magnetic resonance (MR) imaging may demonstrate subcarinal adenopathy, and obstruction of the pulmonary veins and arteries have been seen, but obstruction of the superior vena cava is more common.

MEDIASTINAL MASSES

Evaluation

Most authors analyze mediastinal masses by their location and classify them into those arising from the anterior, middle, and posterior compartments. Since these compartments are not anatomical spaces, masses may often involve more than one compartment. The center of the mass may be considered the likely region of origin. The masses most commonly arising in these compartments are tabulated in the appropriate subdivisions of this section.

Radiology

Radiologic evaluation has consisted of frontal and lateral chest radiographs, fluoroscopy, esophagrams, high-kilovoltage films, tomography, and, occasionally, myelography and angiography. Most of the studies previously performed after the initial chest film now can be replaced by CT or MRI which provide much more specific diagnostic information, although fluoroscopy with an esophagogram is still a simple and useful initial procedure.

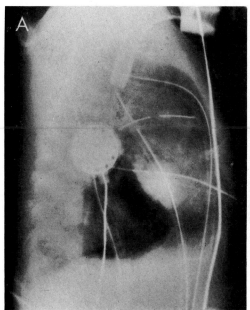

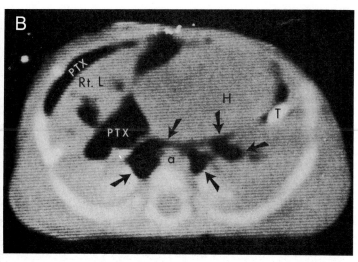

FIG 14–9.
Infraazygos pneumomediastinum. **A,** lateral radiograph in an infant shows a large triangular accumulation of gas posterior to the heart. **B,** postmortem CT scan made in an attempt to localize the abnormal gas collections. A central, somewhat lobulated gas collection *(arrows)* extends freely across the midline anterior to the aorta *(a)* and posterior to the heart *(H)* Pneumothorax *(PTX)* surrounds the atelectatic right lung *(Rt. L)* A left chest tube is still in place anteriorly *(T).* At necropsy a tracheal laceration was discovered. The gas collection was in the mediastinum but not loculated in the pulmonary ligaments.

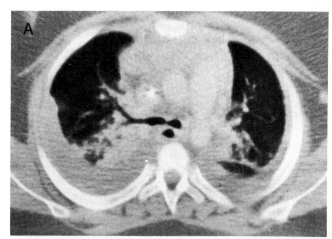

FIG 14–10.
Mediastinitis. Contrast-enhanced CT (CECT) image in a 10-year-old female suffering from mediastinitis and septic shock. The patient had group A beta-hemolytic streptococcal infection as well as varicella. **A,** CECT scan image through the right upper lobes shows bilateral pleural effusions; marked mediastinal widening and edema are present. **B,** CT scan image slightly superior to **A** reveals ill-defined areas of increased attenuation in the anterior mediastinum but particularly in the right paratracheal region, which is massively enlarged. **C,** follow-up CT scan 3 weeks later shows the mediastinum has returned to nearly normal appearance. Some residual thymic tissue is noted anteriorly.

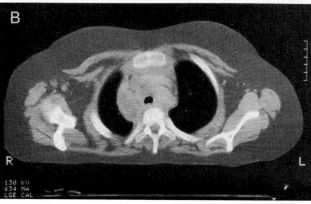

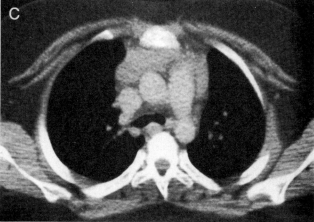

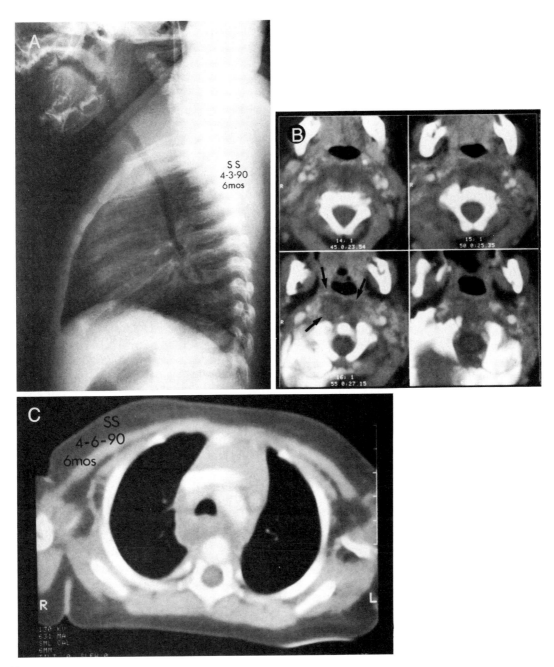

FIG 14–11.
Retropharyngeal abscess with mediastinal extension of infection. **A,** a 6-month-old infant with retropharyngeal abscess. Note the widening of the retropharyngeal space and the slight but definite anterior displacement of the tracheal air column. **B,** series of contrast-enhanced CT (CECT) images of the neck from inferior to superior. A poorly defined, low-attenuation collection is seen in the retropharyngeal area extending slightly toward the right side in the parapharyngeal space *(arrows).* Diffuse, poorly marginated, low attenuation is seen in the remainder of the retropharyngeal area. **C,** CECT image of the thorax in the same patient reveals poorly marginated, low attenuation in the posterior mediastinum displacing the trachea anteriorly. The infection was successfully treated with antibiotics without surgical drainage.

Computed Tomography

CT of the mediastinum is critical in the evaluation of a mass lesion detected on a chest film. One can differentiate a mass from normal structures, measure its attenuation values, and determine its exact location and whether it is vascular or avascular.

An adequate CT examination of the mediastinum requires equipment capable of scan times of 2 seconds or less. Ideal imaging of the pediatric mediastinum is provided by the use of ultrafast CT (UFCT) scanning (Imatron, San Francisco). This scanner uses electron-beam technology to allow scan times as short as 0.1 second in the high-resolution mode. The short scan time makes it practical to get high-quality images of the mediastinum even in infancy. Cardiac pulsation artifact is virtually eliminated. Regardless of the equipment available, contiguous 0.3- to 1.0-cm slices are made, depending on the age of the patient and the suspected abnormality. Contrast enhancement is mandatory for evaluation of most mediastinal pathologic conditions. An intravenous (IV) bolus of contrast medium given during scanning provides optimal visualization of vessels and vascular structures.

While not specific, attenuation coefficients measured in Hounsfield units (HU) are accurate enough to determine whether a lesion is fatty, water density, soft tissue, vascular, or calcified. *Fatty masses* are of the lowest attenuation, measuring from −20 to −100 HU. Benign mediastinal lipomatosis in children usually is related to steroid therapy or Cushing disease. Fat can be present in focal quantities in teratomas. Intrathoracic lipomas and lipoblastomas, although rare, can be suspected because of their CT appearances. *Water-density masses* with attenuation values near water are usually cysts of benign or developmental origin. Characteristically, they measure between 0 and +20 HU. A clearly defined wall is usually not seen. Some cysts, notably bronchogenic cysts, may be thought to be solid because of high Hounsfield numbers ranging between +50 and +100 due to calcium and proteinaceous material in the cyst fluid. However, the avascular and presumably cystic nature of the mass should be diagnosed if the Hounsfield values do not increase following contrast enhancement. *Soft-tissue* masses range in attenuation from +10 to +60 HU. Many of these masses are somewhat vascular and therefore show an increase in attenuation values after contrast enhancement that may be either homogeneous or inhomogeneous. If necrosis is present, areas of low attenuation simulating a cystic lesion may be noted. *Calcification* can occur in both benign and malignant masses, but calcification in lymph nodes strongly suggests granulomatous disease. CT is able to show calcifications not visible on plain films. Vascular masses are near soft-tissue attenuation prior to contrast enhancement but show as much enhancement or nearly so as the vessels.

Ultrasound

Ultrasound is the simplest and least invasive modality for evaluation of mediastinal abnormalities but is often limited by intervening bone or lung, depending on the location of the suspected abnormality. As elsewhere in the body, ready distinction between cystic and complex masses can be made. Doppler flow characteristics and color flow Doppler aid in the evaluation of suspected vascular masses and in the evaluation of aberrant vessels. Associated pulmonary changes, however, are not consistently well imaged.

Scintigraphy

Scintigraphy, though useful, has a limited role in the evaluation of mediastinal abnormalities. The thyroid gland can be definitively localized. Abscesses and some neoplasms can be detected with ^{67}Ga citrate scanning. Some neuroblastomas and lesions containing ectopic gastric mucosa will be localized by ^{99m}Tc pertechnetate scanning.

Magnetic Resonance Imaging

MRI has become an important modality for the evaluation of mediastinal lesions. The availability of sagittal and coronal views in addition to the transaxial view offered by CT is a significant advantage, as is the fact that no contrast injection is necessary to define vascular structures. The fact that no ionizing radiation is used is another significant benefit, although the time-consuming nature of the examination, at present, with its attendant requirement for sedation is a major disadvantage. MRI has largely eliminated the need for CT metrizamide myelography in evaluation of posterior mediastinal lesions. Vascular structures are seen as areas of no signal owing to the flow void phenomenon. Thymus and lymph nodes on T1-weighted images are slightly less bright than fat is but considerably more intense than muscle. Hilar and subcarinal nodes are clearly demonstrated in contrast to the adjacent vascular structures. Inflammatory and neoplastic processes tend to have a prolonged T1 and T2, which means that they are near muscle density on T1-weighted images but brighter on T2-weighted images. Hemorrhagic lesions older than 48 hours are bright on T1-weighted images and somewhat variable in appearance on T2-weighted images. Other than the technical difficulties in getting a good examination in a sick child, the major drawbacks of MRI are that the lungs are not as well imaged as they are by CT and that calcifications cast no signals on MRI. This latter limitation could be important in evaluation of adenopathy where calcification would strongly suggest granulomatous involvement rather than a more ominous condition.

Anterior Mediastinal Masses

Masses occurring most commonly in the anterior mediastinum are classified in Table 14–1 according to their CT characteristics.

Thymus

The thymus is a soft organ occupying the midline of the superior mediastinum. It is formed of two asymmetric lobes. Its embryology is discussed in Chapter 5. In infancy its cephalad margin extends nearly to the thyroid gland, while its lower margins commonly overlap the upper half of the heart. It normally lies entirely anterior to the great vessels of the upper mediastinum. In relation to body size, the thymus is largest at birth but attains its greatest actual size just before puberty. It normally weighs about 15 g at birth and 35 g at puberty. It may weigh as much as 60 g in children dying suddenly, but is much smaller in those who die following a prolonged illness. Any type of stress can cause a rapid decrease in the size of the gland, presumably because of the lympholytic effects of steroids. According to Caffey and Silbey, the thymus is larger in males than in females during the first 2 years of life. The function of the thymus appears to be to stock the spleen and lymph nodes by liberating its lymphocytes (T cells) into the bloodstream and thence to their eventual homes where they mature into populations of lymphocytes responsible for developing cellular immunity. This critical thymic function appears to be completed during the first days of life.

Radiographic Appearance. The thymus is extremely variable in its radiographic appearance. It widens on expiration and elongates and narrows during inspiration (Fig 14–12). It changes in relative size and shape with the age and, sometimes, with the health of the patient. Characteristically, it is a prominent soft-tissue density in the anterosuperior mediastinum until the age of 3 years or so, and is often visible after that time. It fills the anterior mediastinum, on the lateral radiograph, with a soft-tissue opacity inseparable from the superior cardiac margin. On frontal films, the left lobe produces widening of the mediastinum and usually overlaps the left pulmonary artery, which can be seen through the thymus. The anterolateral margins of the gland often show smooth indentations from the overlying ribs and costal cartilages (the "wave" or "ripple" sign) (Fig 14–13). A small notch may mark the inferior border between the thymus and the heart (Fig 14–14). A normal gland may obscure anywhere from a third to all of the left upper lobe. The right lobe exhibits similar features except that its inferior

TABLE 14–1.
Computed Tomography Characteristics of Anterior Mediastinal Masses

I. Solid
  A. Thymus
    1. Normal
    2. Thymic enlargement
      a. Physiologic
      b. Pathologic
        (1) Thymic cyst
        (2) Lymph hemangioma
        (3) Thymolipomas
        (4) Massive thymic hyperplasia
        (5) Thymic neoplasm
  B. Lymphadenopathy
    1. Lymphoma
    2. Histiocytosis
    3. Sarcoidosis
    4. Infectious mononucleosis
    5. Mediastinitis/abscess
  C. Germ cell tumor/teratoma (may contain fat/fluid)
  D. Thyroid (may enhance)
  E. Chest wall tumor
  F. Morgagni hernia (liver)
II. Cystic/avascular
  A. Cystic hygroma
  B. Thymic cyst
  C. Abscess
III. Vascular
  A. Aneurysm of sinus of Valsalva
IV. Fatty
  A. Lipoma, thymolipoma, lipoblastoma
  B. Teratoma
V. Calcified
  A. Granulomatous infection
  B. Teratoma
  C. Seminoma

margin is more likely to be flattened and produce the "sail sign." In the younger patient, the prominence of one or both thymic lobes can simulate cardiomegaly, but the lateral radiograph is usually reassuring as it can be seen that the posterior margin of the left ventricle is not displaced posteriorly as would be the case with true cardiomegaly. In the infant, a prominent or large thymus is not only nearly always normal, but, indeed, a reflection of good health and nutrition; however, a prominent thymic lobe can either simulate or obscure an upper lobe pneumonia (see Chapter 9). A lateral or oblique film will usually clarify any confusion. Some of the most bizarre variations of normal thymic size and shape are seen as a result of a rebound growth phenomenon following stress-induced atrophy such as cardiac surgery, a prolonged stay in the intensive care nursery, or chemotherapy (Fig 14–15).

Appearance on Other Imaging Modalities. *Ultrasound* performed through the sternum of the

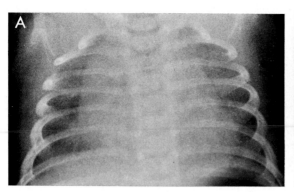

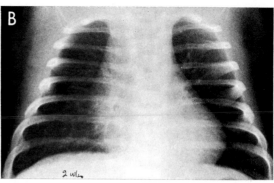

FIG 14-12.
Changes in size and shape of the thymus during the respiratory cycle. **A,** wide flat thymus and mediastinum near the end of expi-

ration. **B,** narrow elongated thymus and mediastinum near the end of inspiration. This was an asymptomatic boy 2 weeks of age.

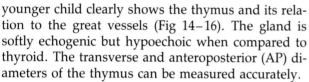

younger child clearly shows the thymus and its relation to the great vessels (Fig 14–16). The gland is softly echogenic but hypoechoic when compared to thyroid. The transverse and anteroposterior (AP) diameters of the thymus can be measured accurately.

On *CT and MR studies,* the normal thymus is seen as a soft-tissue structure in the anterosuperior mediastinum. The thymus is relatively soft and insinuates itself behind the sternum and along the cardiac margins. It normally lies anterior to the great vessels, although its left lobe often extends posteriorly and laterally along the arch of the aorta to the plane of the descending aorta. On MRI studies, in approximately 10% of children we have seen a small nubbin of what appears to be normal thymus poste-

rior to the superior vena cava; although this could be a retrocaval lymph node, the appearance on the sagittal MR scan suggests that this is a tongue of thymic tissue (Fig 14–17,A and B). Superiorly, the thymus may extend as high as the thyroid gland. It extends an average of 1.7 cm superior to the innominate vein (Fig 14–18) where it may simulate adenopathy when seen on axial imaging. Its inferior extension is variable. In infancy, it is commonly seen to the level of the pulmonary arteries or below, but since the thorax elongates faster than the thymus, its relative inferior extension decreases with age.

In the axial plane, the gland is of quadrilateral shape in infants and younger children, becoming more triangular as the child grows. Its margins are sharp and smooth, slightly convex in infants, and become straight or concave in older children.

The size of the gland is variable and has been measured with both CT and MRI. Cranial-caudal measurements (length) increase with age; the width, and AP and transverse diameters show little change. On CT, the average thickness of the thymus appears to decrease with advancing age, diminishing from an average of 1.4 cm in children aged 0 to 5 years to

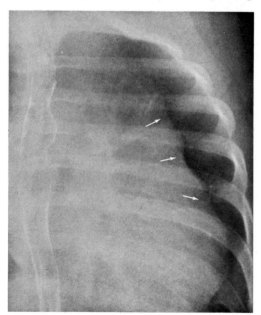

FIG 14-13.
Thymic wave sign, right anterior oblique projection. Indentations of the anterolateral edge of a large left lobe of the thymus opposite the contiguous costal cartilage produce scalloping of the thymic edge—the thymic wave sign.

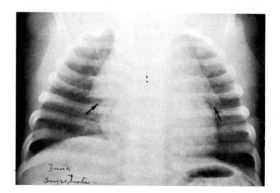

FIG 14-14.
Normal thymus with wide right and left lobes *(arrows)* that produce notches at their junctions with the cardiac image.

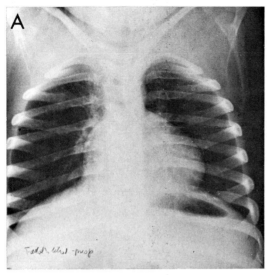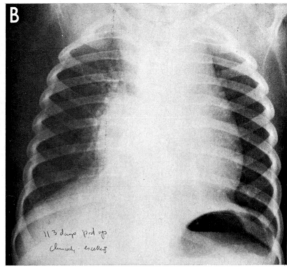

FIG 14–15.
Rebound hypertrophy of the thymus after surgical correction of tetrology of Fallot. **A,** deformed heart with a small thymus before surgery when this girl was 33 months of age. **B,** widening of the cardiac and supracardiac images 113 days later and after surgical treatment. Cyanosis had disappeared, and she was thriving despite the factitious radiographic enlargement of the heart (enlarged cardiothymic image).

1.0 cm in children aged 10 to 19 years. In 59 children studied with MR, slightly different findings were noted (Table 14–2, Fig 14–19). There was a slight but definite increase in the transverse dimension of the thymus but a marked decrease in the ratio of the size of the thymus relative to both the transverse and cranial-caudal measurements of the thorax, accounting for the thymus appearing relatively less prominent with advancing age. The width of the left lobe increased, but MR failed to reveal any age-related change in the thickness of the thymus. On MR, the thymus had slightly greater thickness than was noted by CT, with an average of 1.8 cm for the right lobe and 2.1 cm for the left lobe. The cranial-caudal length of the thymus was found to increase from an average of 5.6 cm to 8.5 cm for children aged 0 to 1 year compared with the age group 15 to 19 years. It is likely that the differing measurements reflect the fact that the MR scans were made during quiet breathing, whereas CT, especially in older children, was commonly performed at inspiration, possibly producing some flattening of the thymus. Using UFCT, we have demonstrated this change in thymic shape with respiration (Fig 14–20).

On CT, the thymus is of slightly higher attenuation than the vessels, but approximately the same as muscle tissue. The mean Hounsfield units of the thymus have been found to be 36. Using UFCT, it is possible to distinguish between thymus and vessels even without contrast enhancement, but contrast enhancement is required to optimally delineate the gland, which shows homogeneous enhancement of 20 to 30 HU after bolus injection (Fig 14–21). MR clearly distinguishes the thymus from the vascular structures in the mediastinum. On T1-weighted images, the signal intensity of the thymus appears slightly brighter than muscle; on intermediate, gated sequences, it appears slightly less intense than fatty tissue; and on T2-

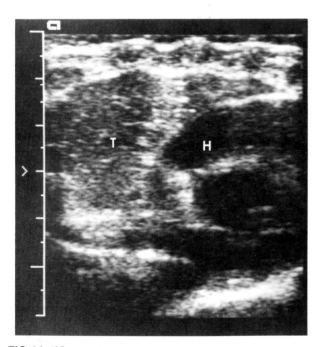

FIG 14–16.
Normal thymus seen by ultrasound. A sagittal real-time ultrasound shows the thymus *(T)* to be smoothly tapered inferiorly. It lies anterior to the heart *(H)* and is homogeneously hypoechoic with a pattern somewhat resembling that of normal spleen.

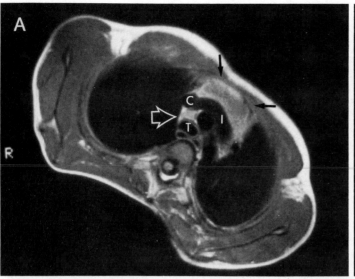

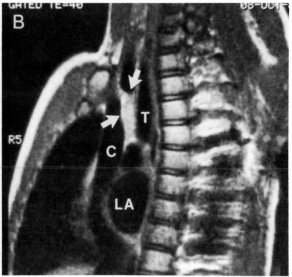

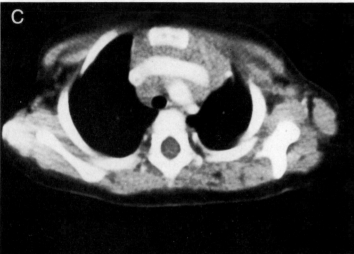

FIG 14–17.
Probable retrocaval thymic tissue. **A,** transaxial gated, T1-weighted MR image reveals thymic tissue both anterior to the innominate vein (I) in its normal position as well as a small nubbin of tissue of similar signal intensity noted between the superior vena cava (C) and the trachea (T) (arrow). **B,** oblique sagittal image in the same patient reveals this tissue to have continuous cephalad extension, suggesting that it is a tongue of thymic tissue rather than a lymph node. *LA,* left atrium. **C,** presumed retrocaval thymic tissue in a different patient, demonstrated by CECT. Note the nubbin of tissue posterior to the innominate vein on the left and vena cava on the right.

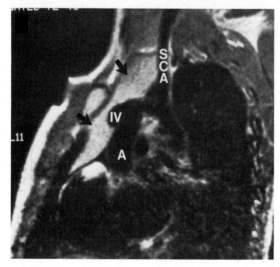

FIG 14–18.
Normal extension of thymic tissue into the neck. Gated oblique MR image. Note that on this mildly T1-weighted image the thymus is clearly distinguished from vessels; it is of intermediate signal intensity, less than fat but greater than muscle. Note how far cephalad to the innominate vein the thymic tissue extends. *SCA,* subclavian artery; *IV,* innominate vein; *A,* aorta.

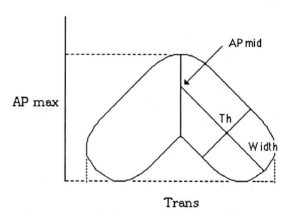

FIG 14–19.
Diagramatic representation of points at which MRI thymus (Th) measurements were taken. (From Naidich DP, Zerhouni EA, Siegelman SS (eds): *Computed Tomography and Magnetic Resonance of the Thorax,* ed 2. New York, Raven Press, 1991. Used by permission.)

TABLE 14-2.
Magnetic Resonance Measurements of Thymic Dimensions in 59 Children*

	Age (yr)						SD
	0-1 (n = 18)	2-4 (n = 12)	5-9 (n = 10)	10-14 (n = 10)	15-19 (n = 9)	0-19 (n = 59)	
Maximum transverse width	4.9	5.0	5.4	6.3	5.8	5.4	1.1
Thymic thoracic ratio	.51	.41	.34	.35	.28	.41	.11
AP diameter in midline	1.7	1.7	1.6	1.7	2.0	1.7	.5
AP diameter, maximum left	3.5	4.1	4.2	4.5	5.0	4.1	1.0
AP diameter, maximum right	2.8	2.7	2.6	2.8	3.1	2.7	.9
Right lobe width	2.5	2.4	2.8	3.0	3.0	2.7	.6
Left lobe width	2.9	3.3	3.6	4.2	4.4	3.5	1.0
Right lobe thickness	1.9	1.7	1.8	1.8	1.6	1.8	.06
Left lobe thickness	2.2	2.1	1.8	2.2	1.9	2.1	.5
Length	5.6	6.6	7.6	8.0	8.5	7.2	1.9

*From Naidich D, Zerhouni EA, Siegelman SS (eds): *Computed Tomography and Magnetic Resonance of the Thorax,* ed 2. New York, Raven Press, 1991, p 506. Used by permission.)

weighted images, it becomes brighter than both the surrounding fat and muscle (Fig 14–22). In children the normal thymus, regardless of size, should be homogeneous on MRI, CT, or ultrasound. Fatty infiltrate, common in adults, is unusual in children and inhomogeneity in the thymus in childhood should be regarded as probably pathologic.

Congenital Abnormalities and Normal Variants. The thymus is absent in the DiGeorge syndrome in which absence of the parathyroid glands and congenital heart disease are other important features. These infants suffer from hypocalcemia and immunodeficiency due to T cell abnormalities.

Absence or hypoplasia of the thymus may be suggested from plain film findings, but CT or MR will often reveal that the thymus is present. There are no known reliable criteria for diagnosis of thymic hypoplasia because the gland is known to decrease in size as a normal response to stress.

A variant of normal thymic position and size is the retrocaval or ectopic thymus. As illustrated in Figure 14–17, a small amount of what appears to be thymic tissue is seen posterior to the superior vena cava in some normal infants, but we believe that on occasion this portion of thymus may enlarge disporportionately and be perceived on the plain film as a possible mediastinal mass, leading to further investigation. CT or MR reveal tissue with characteristics identical to normal thymus that extends contiguously into the middle and even the posterior mediastinum, extending posteriorly to the superior vena cava when the enlargement is on the right side (Fig

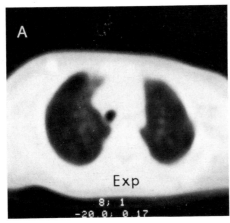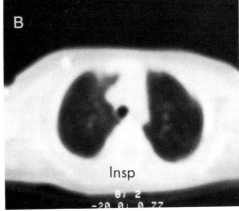

FIG 14-20.
Change in thymic shape with respiration demonstrated in an infant by ultrafast CT (UFCT). Images taken from a 0.05-second cine sequence reveal the thymus to appear thicker and wider on expiration *(Exp).* (From Naidich DP, Zerhouni EA, Siegelman SS (eds): *Computed Tomography and Magnetic Resonance of the Thorax,* ed 2. New York, Raven Press, 1991. Used by permission.)

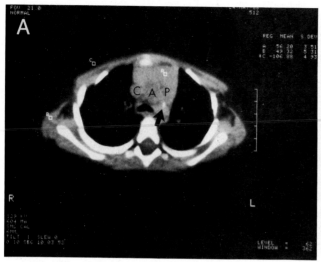

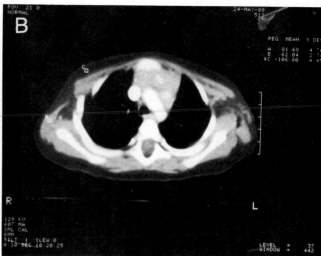

FIG 14–21.
Normal CT appearance of the thymus in a 10-month-old child. **A,** thymus (*A* cursor) measures 56 Hounsfield units (HU) and is seen to be denser than the superior vena cava (*C*), aorta (*A*) and pulmonary artery (*P*). A small linear calcification is incidentally noted in the ductus (*arrow*). Muscle (*B* cursor) measures 49 HU; fat (*C* cursor) measures −106 HU. **B,** after contrast enhancement, the thymus (*A* cursor) is more easily distinguished from the great vessels; its attenuation has increased from 56 to 81 HU. Following IV contrast administration, muscle (*B* cursor) measures 62 HU; fat (*C* cursor) still measures −106 HU. (From Naidich DP, Zerhouni EA, Siegelman SS (eds): *Computed Tomography and Magnetic Resonance of the Thorax,* ed 2. New York, Raven Press, 1991. Used by permission.)

14–23). On the left side, direct extension posteriorly, parallel to the aortic arch, may occur with the gland extending all the way into the posterior mediastinum (Fig 14–24). While no imaging procedure can provide a histologic diagnosis, this appearance is so characteristic that in the absence of any atypical clinical or imaging features, it appears to be justified to observe patients with these findings rather than to resort to biopsy. Most cases in our experience, and most of the published cases, have been in children 2 years of age or younger. If there is evidence of airway or vascular compression, or if the child has other significant clinical abnormalities, biopsy may be warranted.

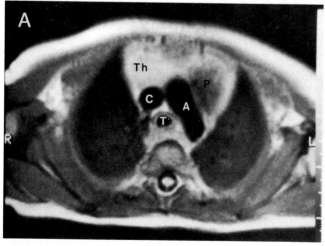

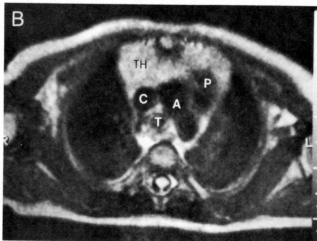

FIG 14–22.
MR appearance of normal thymus in a 10-month-old child. **A,** intermediate weighted, gated transaxial image reveals the thymus (*Th*) to be slightly brighter than the muscle tissue but less bright than the subcutaneous fat. (From Naidich DP, Zerhouni EA, Siegelman SS (eds): *Computed Tomography and Magnetic Resonance of the Thorax,* ed 2. New York, Raven Press, 1991. Used by permission.) **B,** nongated T2-weighted image (TR/TE = 2,000/80) is less sharp than the gated image. The thymus (*TH*) is now slightly brighter than the subcutaneous fat and has considerably greater signal intensity than the skeletal muscle. *A,* aorta; *C,* superior vena cava; *P,* pulmonary artery; *T,* trachea.

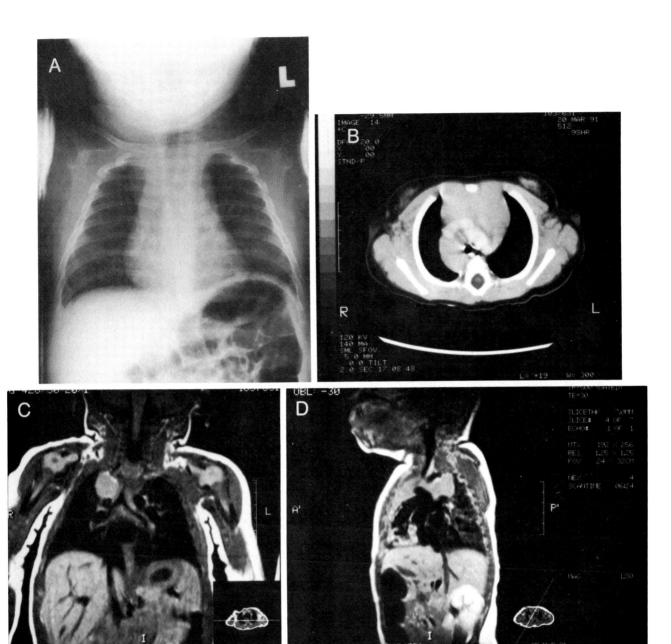

FIG 14–23.

Right ectopic (retrocaval) posterior mediastinal thymic tissue. **A,** frontal radiograph reveals a double density in the right upper lobe with extension to the level of the first rib which is higher than the normal thymus usually extends. The findings are suggestive of a mediastinal mass. **B,** CECT reveals a soft-tissue attenuation mass extending from the retrocaval region into the posterior mediasti-num. It is of the same attenuation as normal thymic tissue. **C,** coronal T1-weighted, gated MR image at the level of the trachea reveals thymic tissue more posterior in location than normal. **D,** oblique sagittal MR image reveals continuity of the posterior mediastinal thymus with normal anterior mediastinal thymus.

Ectopic thymic tissue may either be contiguous with or separate from normal thymus. Ectopic thymic tissue has been reported in the neck, usually on the left side, and also in the trachea. Ectopic thymic tissue, in contradistinction to normal thymus, has been reported to cause airway obstruction.

Bizarre forms of thymic enlargement occur as a rebound phenomenon after severe stress. This most commonly occurs in infants who have had severe respiratory distress syndrome or its complications; surgery for congenital heart disease is another common clinical history. Usually, despite the bizarre size and shape of the thymus, there is little, if any, difficulty in establishing the correct diagnosis of rebound thymic enlargement. These children only need CT or MR examination in unusual circumstances (Fig

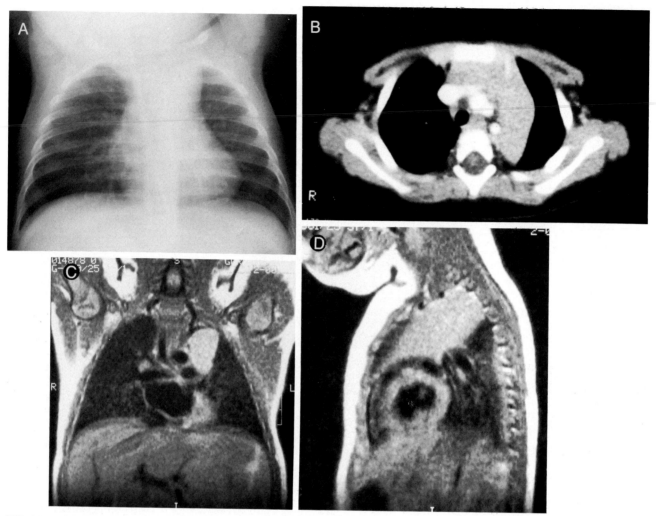

FIG 14–24.
Left-sided ectopic (posterior mediastinal) thymus. It appears less frequently than right-sided posterior mediastinal thymus. **A,** frontal radiograph reveals an unusually opaque appearance to the thymus on the left with apparent extension to the posterior aspect of the first rib, higher than would be expected for a normal thymus. **B,** CECT reveals tissue of identical attenuation as the thymus with di-rect continuity with it. **C,** T1-weighted, gated MR scan at the level of the trachea reveals a large amount of thymic tissue present at this slice. **D,** sagittal oblique T1-weighted gated image reveals extension of the thymus all the way from the anterior to the superior posterior mediastinum.

14–25). Greater diagnostic difficulty occurs when thymic enlargement occurs as a rebound phenomenon following therapy for malignancy. If imaging characteristics are all consistent with normal thymus, it may be possible to observe the patient, but biopsy is the only certain way of establishing the correct diagnosis (Fig 14–26).

Thymic hyperplasia may occur in association with hyperthyroidism or therapy for hypothyroidism. It may also be seen in association with myasthenia gravis and red cell aplasia, and may rarely occur as an isolated finding. Biopsy is required for definitive diagnosis (Fig 14–27).

Pathologic Causes of Thymic Enlargement. In the newborn, acute thymic enlargement, particularly when associated with pleural effusion, should suggest acute thymic hemorrhage. Thymic cysts are relatively unusual causes of thymic enlargement; they probably are of developmental origin, representing persistent tubular remnants of the third pharyngeal pouch. The cysts may vary in size from microscopic to several centimeters, and they may be unilocular or multicular. Ultrasound and CECT have been used in diagnosis. The cyst may present in the neck, mediastinum, or in both regions (Fig 14–28). Thymic cysts are more frequent in children with various forms of bone marrow aplasia; acute hemorrhage into a thymic cyst has been reported in children with

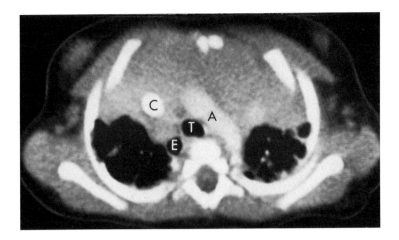

FIG 14–25.
Rebound thymic enlargement. Six-month-old prematurely born infant with bronchopulmonary dysplasia presented with a bizarre cardiomediastinal silhouette. Contrast-enhanced UFCT (0.1 sec), reveals marked enlargement of the thymus filling the anterosuperior mediastinum. *A,* aorta; *C,* superior vena cava; *E,* esophagus; *T,* trachea. (From Naidich DP, Zerhouni EA, Siegelman SS (eds): *Computed Tomography and Magnetic Resonance of the Thorax,* ed 2. New York, Raven Press, 1991. Used by permission.)

aplastic anemia. Thymic cysts have also been reported to occur following thoractomy and treatment for Hodgkin disease.

Thymic enlargement may also occur as a result of a thymic hemangioma or lymphangioma, the nature of which can be strongly suggested from the CT and MR studies which show abnormal vessels in the thymus (Fig 14–29). Thymolipoma can cause marked thymic enlargement and is diagnosed by seeing streaky, low attenuation in a whorled pattern throughout the thymus (Fig 14–30).

Thymomas are rare in infancy and childhood. There appears to be little association between thymomas and myasthenia gravis in children. Radiographic features resemble those of lymphoma. Calci-

fication is seen somewhat more commonly in thymoma than in untreated lymphoma, but this alone is not a reliable differential point; biopsy is required. Carcinoids may occur in the thymus and present as cases of Cushing syndrome due to adrenocorticotropic hormone (ACTH) production by the tumor (Fig 14–31).

Lymphomas, especially Hodgkin disease, often involve both the anterior and middle mediastinum and are discussed below under Middle Mediastinal Masses. Anterior and mediastinal lymph node enlargement may occur not only in lymphoma but with histiocytosis X, sarcoidosis, infectious mononucleosis, and as a result of direct spread of infection. These subjects are further discussed below under

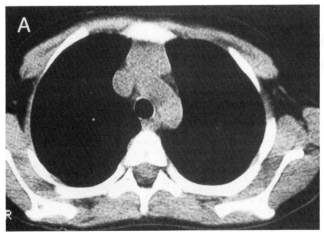
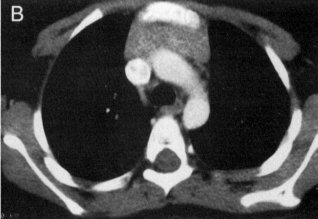

FIG 14–26.
Rebound thymic hypertrophy in a patient treated for rhabdomyosarcoma. **A,** unenhanced CT scan at the level of the aortic arch reveals a normal-sized thymus. **B,** CECT scan, same patient. Three months later, after cessation of chemotherapy, the thymus is approximately twice the volume seen on the earlier study, but imaging characteristics are all consistent with a normal thymus. This is a 6-year-old boy.

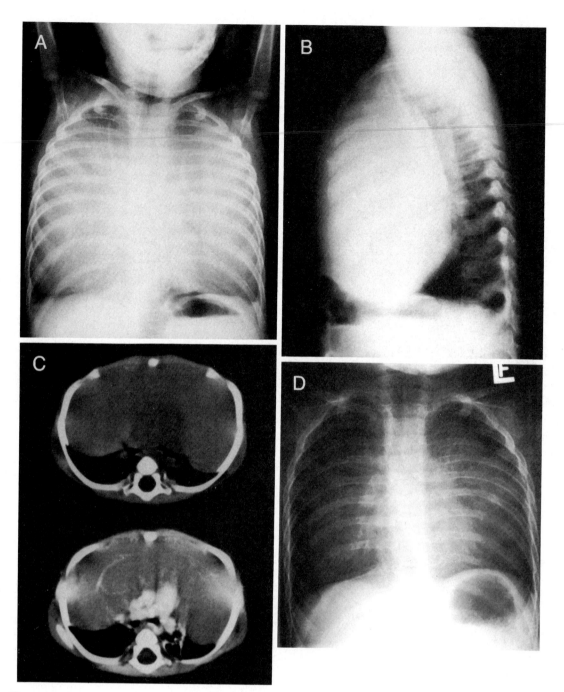

FIG 14–27.
Massive thymic hyperplasia of unknown cause. **A,** frontal, and **B,** lateral radiographs reveal a huge mediastinal mass occupying the anterior and middle mediastinum. **C,** unenhanced *(above)* and enhanced *(below)* CT images at the same level reveal the thymus to be of higher attenuation than the cardiac structure. Following contrast enhancement, a few vessels are noted in the thymus but it appears otherwise of homogeneous attenuation. **D,** biopsy revealed thymic hyperplasia. The patient was treated with steroids. This frontal radiograph shows some interval decrease in the size of the mass of the thymic hyperplasia.

Lymph Node Enlargement. Histiocytosis X is of particular interest because the lymph node enlargement has been noted to cavitate (Fig 14–32).

Cystic hygromas (lymphangioma) may be classified as simple, cavernous, or cystic. Most lesions arise in the neck and are located in the posterior cervical space behind the sternocleiodomastoid muscle. About 10% may extend into the mediastinum. Sumner et al. found 24 cases in the literature in which the malformation arose in the mediastinum without any associated disease in the neck. Most are in the anterior or middle mediastinum but posterior ones

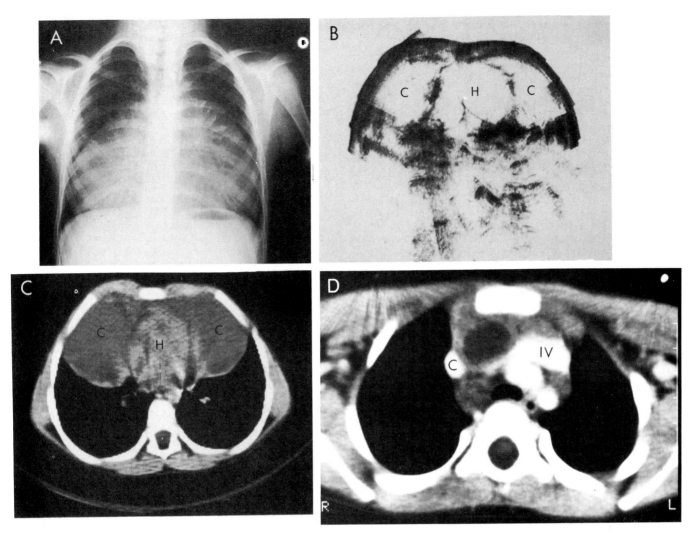

FIG 14–28.

Thymic cyst. **A,** a frontal radiograph shows a large cardiothymic silhouette. **B,** an ultrasound study shows a bilobed cystic mass *(C)* located on either side of the heart *(H)*. **C,** unenhanced CT scan shows identical findings in this surgically proven thymic cyst *(C)*. (Courtesy of Dr. Beverly Wood, Los Angeles.) **D,** cervical thymic cyst in a different patient. A contrast-enhanced CT scan in a 4-year-old child reveals a cystic lesion in the thymus anterior to the vena cava *(C)* that is displacing the innominate vein *(IV)* posteriorly. More cranial sections revealed that this cystic mass originated in the neck. At surgery, a thymic cyst extending from the neck inferiorly into the thymus was removed.

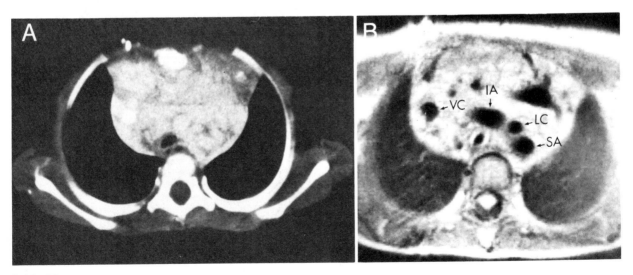

FIG 14–29.

Thymic hemangioma. This 1-year-old child had respiratory distress and a large mediastinal mass. **A,** CT scan, and **B,** gated MR image reveal diffuse thymic enlargement with multiple vascular channels. At surgery a thymic hemangioma was partially resected. *VC,* superior vena cava; *IA,* innominate artery; *LC,* left carotid artery; *SA,* subclavian artery.

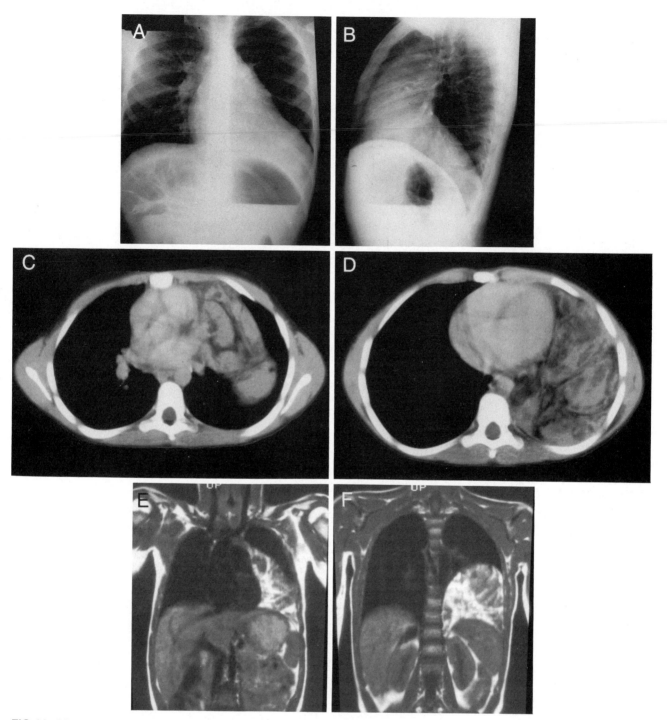

FIG 14–30.
Thymolipoma. **A,** frontal, and **B,** lateral radiographs reveal an anterior left-sided mediastinal mass. **C** and **D,** CECT images show a large mass of mixed attenuation with multiple low- attenuation streaks and whorls within it. **E** and **F,** coronal T1-weighted MR images show multiple fatty streaks in this surgically proven thymolipoma. (Courtesy of Dr. Shashikant Sane, Minneapolis.)

do occur. The lesions may present with symptoms of airway compression, especially in infancy, but 50% of children over the age of 2 years are asymptomatic.

Radiographic findings range from normal, in the case of a small lesion in the neck, to a large mediastinal mass. Chest radiography shows the lesion to be sharply demarcated; its borders have little, if any, lobulation, and the mass is of homogeneous appearance. CT, MR, or ultrasound can aid in distinguish-

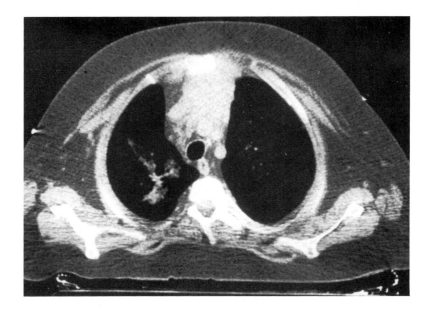

FIG 14–31.
Malignant thymic carcinoid tumor with ectopic ACTH production. This teenage boy presented with Cushing syndrome. Nonenhanced CT image reveals extensive deposition of subcutaneous fat as well as excess fatty tissue in the mediastinum. An irregularly shaped nodular mass is seen in the anterior mediastinum. Metastatic disease is visible in the right upper lobe posteriorly. A thymic carcinoid tumor was partially removed and extensive metastatic disease subsequently developed.

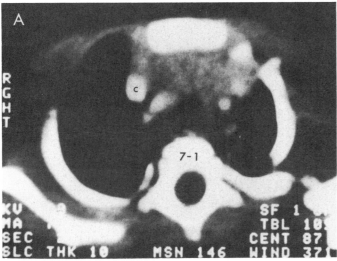

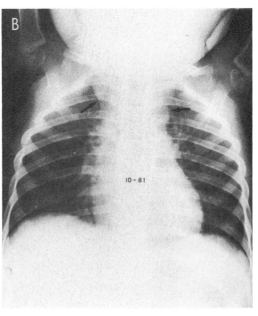

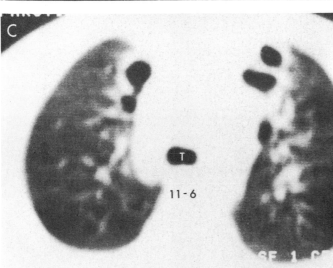

FIG 14–32.
Eighteen-month-old girl with a history of draining ears and cervical lymphadenopathy. **A,** CT scan performed because of questionable mediastinal widening on the plain film shows what could be normal thymus, but the pattern of enhancement is somewhat unusual, with multiple small nodular densities suggested. c = vena cava. **B,** follow-up chest radiograph 3 months later shows persistent mediastinal widening *(arrows).* **C,** follow-up CT scan 1 month later shows multiple cystic lesions located bilaterally and medially. It was difficult on both the CT scan and the chest radiograph to be certain whether these were in the mediastinum or subpleural in the lungs. Follow-up 1 year later showed that the cystic lesions had regressed completely, and the child now is well. A diagnosis of histiocytosis X was established on the basis of skin lymph node biopsy findings. *T* = trachea.

ing mediastinal extension from cervical lesions and in establishing the multicystic nature of the mediastinal lesion. Ultrasound examination shows a multicystic mass, sometimes containing internal echoes, and CT reveals a well-circumscribed lesion of low attenuation that molds to the mediastinal contours and envelops the great vessels. Contrast enhancement is usually minimal and, if present, suggests a hemangiomatous component. In some patients,

marked venous dilatation is noted—either the superior vena cava or the jugular vein may be involved. It has been suggested that the venous dilatation is part of the malformation (Joseph et al.) (Fig 14–33).

A *mediastinal thyroid* is an uncommon cause of an anterosuperior mediastinal mass in children. A mediastinal thyroid gland may displace the trachea but usually does not cause any significant symptoms (Fig 14–34). It may be diagnosed by thyroid scintig-

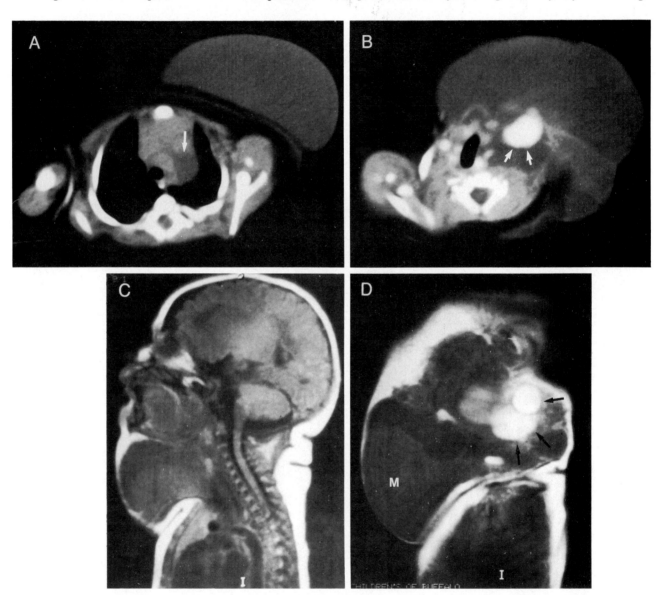

FIG 14–33.

Cystic hygroma of the neck, anterior chest wall, and mediastinum associated with venous aneurysm. This 2-day-old infant had a huge cervical mass. **A,** unenhanced CT scan reveals a water attenuation mass extending down over the left anterior chest wall from the cervical region. Also noted is extension of the mass into the upper middle mediastinum posterior to the thymus and lateral to the aortic arch *(arrows)*. **B,** CECT reveals aneurysmal enlargement of the left jugular vein *(arrows)*. The rest of the mass remains primarily avascular except for a few enhancing septa. **C,** sagittal

T1-weighted, MR scan shows the cervical mass extending posterior to the thymus into the upper mediastinum. **D,** parasagittal T1-weighted MR image reveals the large mass *(M)* anteriorly. The aneurysm of the jugular vein is bright (arrows) on this image, resulting from flowing blood. (From Naidich DP, Zerhouni EA, Siegelman SS (eds): *Computed Tomography and Magnetic Resonance of the Thorax*, ed 2. New York, Raven Press, 1991, p. . Used by permission.)

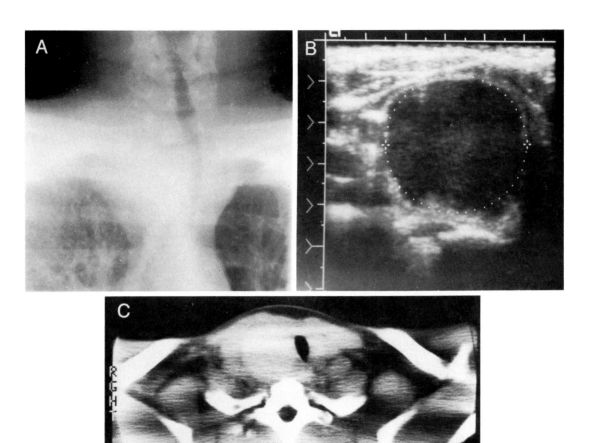

FIG 14–34.
Substernal thyroid. Sixteen-year-old female presented with dysphasia. **A,** frontal radiograph shows a superior mediastinal mass displacing the trachea to the left. **B,** CECT reveals an enhancing mass consistent with thyroid tissue displacing and flattening the trachea. **C,** ultrasound image reveals a well-demarcated, hypoechoic mass consistent with a colloid mass.

raphy, but can also be recognized on CT; marked prolonged enhancement is seen following injection of iodine-containing IV contrast media.

Germ Cell Neoplasms

Primary germ cell tumors arise from primitive germ cell rests whose journey along the urogenital ridge to the gonadal ridge was interrupted in the mediastinum. Included in this group of lesions are teratoma and teratocarcinoma, seminoma, embryonal carcinoma, choriocarcinoma, and endodermal sinus or yolk sac tumor (Fig 14–35).

Teratomas are embryonal neoplasms that contain tissue of ectodermal, endodermal, and mesodermal origins. They are most commonly found in the sacrococcygeal area, but about 10% arise in the mediastinum. They may be benign or malignant, cystic or solid; 21% were found to be malignant in a review by Thompson and Moore. In infants, the mediastinal masses tend to be symptomatic, but often very large asymptomatic masses are discovered in older children. Symptoms seen in a minority of children include sudden onset of pain, dyspnea, or cough. The teratoma may rupture into the tracheobronchial tree and cause expectoration of hair. Radiographic recognition from plain film examination is not possible unless teeth or skeletal elements are seen. A teratoma can be difficult to separate from a normal thymus or even the normal cardiac silhouette. In fact, lesions can be intrapericardiac and present as apparent cardiomegaly (Fig 14–36). CT can be diagnostic of teratomas by revealing pathognomonic findings of fat and calcific densities (Fig 14–37). While usually anterior in location, mediastinal teratomas can occur in virtually any area. The term *dermoid cyst* is usually reserved for those lesions of only ectodermal origin, but this separation from teratoma has been abandoned by several authors.

Primary seminomas of the mediastinum are rare. There is an apparent predominance in males. The

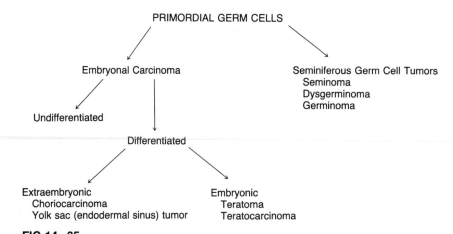

PRIMORDIAL GERM CELLS

Embryonal Carcinoma

Seminiferous Germ Cell Tumors
Seminoma
Dysgerminoma
Germinoma

Undifferentiated

Differentiated

Extraembryonic
Choriocarcinoma
Yolk sac (endodermal sinus) tumor

Embryonic
Teratoma
Teratocarcinoma

FIG 14–35.
Classification of germinal cell neoplasms. (From O'Sullivan P, Daneman A, Chan HSL, et al: *Pediatr Radiol* 1983; 13:249. Used by permission.)

tumor radiologically is indistinguishable from a lymphoma unless extensive calcification is present (Fig 14–38). Mediastinal metastatic disease from an occult gonadal lesion must always be excluded; therefore, careful ultrasound examination of the testicles is indicated.

Yolk sac tumors or *endodermal sinus cell tumors* may arise from poorly differentiated embryonal carcinoma. These lesions occur most often in males, present with systemic symptoms, and are associated with an elevated level of serum alpha-fetoprotein. No distinguishing radiologic features are present in

these patients with large anterior mediastinal masses. The prognosis is poor, with survival rates of below 20%.

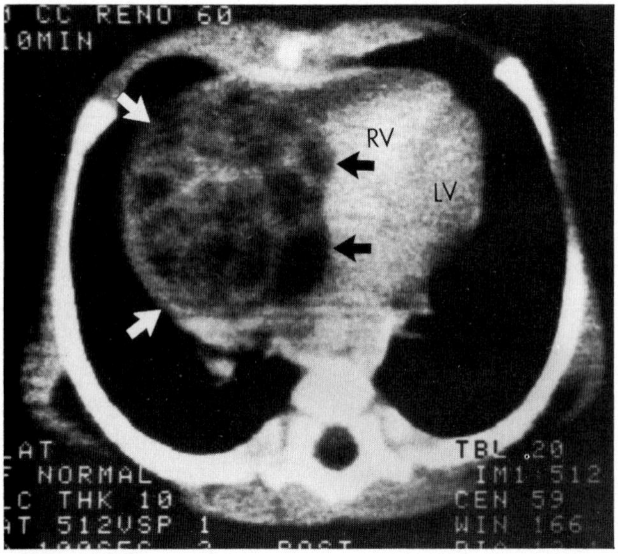

Mediastinal lymph node enlargement is discussed under Middle Mediastinal Masses although there are lymph nodes present in the anterior and posterior mediastinum as well.

Middle Mediastinal Masses

Lesions of the middle mediastinum are classified by their CT characteristics in Table 14–3.

Lymph Node Enlargement

Hilar and mediastinal lymph node enlargement are considered together for purposes of this discussion. Adenopathy may be caused by any pulmonary infection but is most marked in tuberculosis and histoplasmosis. Sarcoidosis, a common cause of adenopathy in adults, is infrequent in children. Children with cystic fibrosis, in our experience, frequently have extensive adenopathy. The most common causes of marked lymphadenopathy are lymphoma and leukemia. Lymph node enlargement also occurs in infectious mononucleosis and histiocytosis X. Castleman disease is a rare cause of massive mediastinal adenopathy. Neoplasms such as neuroblastoma in the young child and testicular carcinoma in the teen-ager metastasize to mediastinal nodes.

Radiographic Diagnosis of Adenopathy. Seven groups of lymph nodes may be visible on chest radiography when they become enlarged. They are (1) anterior mediastinal, (2) paratracheal, (3) tracheobronchial, (4) bronchopulmonary (hilar), (5) subcarinal, (6) posterior mediastinal, and (7) paracardiac.

A plain film diagnosis of enlarged nodal groups

FIG 14–36.
Intrapericardiac teratoma in a newborn. Patient presented with what was thought to be pericardial effusion. Echocardiography, however, revealed a possible intracardiac mass. CECT reveals a hypoattenuating mass with enhancement of the septa. At surgery an intrapericardiac teratoma was successfully removed. *RV*, right ventricle; *LV*, left ventricle.

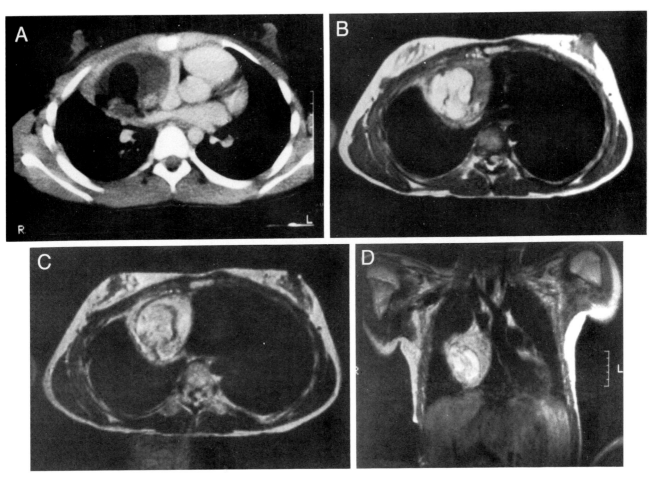

FIG 14–37.
Mediastinal teratoma. A twelve-year-old girl presented with what was initially thought to be right middle lobe pneumonia. **A,** contrast-enhanced UFCT scan reveals a right-sided anterior and middle mediastinal mass composed of fat, fluid, and solid elements. **B,** axial T1-weighted MR image reveals the fatty components of the mass to have high signal intensity. **C,** T2-weighted MR image shows chemical shift, artifact, and decreased signal intensity of the fatty portion of the mass. **D,** coronal T1-weighted MR image clearly reveals the relationship of the mass to the cardiac structures.

is difficult unless the nodes are calcified after a granulomatous infection or unless enlargement is striking. The findings depend on the degree of enlargement and on which groups are involved. High-kilovoltage films aid in delineating these mediastinal nodes, although they are best seen on CT or MRI.

Because there is so little mediastinal fat in most children, if one wishes to visualize nodes on CT it is nearly always necessary to use bolus contrast enhancement to separate mediastinal nodes from the other soft-tissue structures. Unenhanced CT is indicated prior to CECT to detect calcified nodes that would suggest granulomatous disease. Nodes are seen as discrete or confluent rounded masses of soft-tissue density. As in adults, discrimination between normal and abnormal nodes is made by criteria of visibility (present where none are usually seen), size (<1 cm), and abnormalities of enhancement. MR

more readily separates nodes from vessels than does CT. On T1-weighted images, nodes are similar in intensity to muscle; on T2-weighted images, they are brighter than muscle and become similar in signal intensity to surrounding fat. Their MR signal characteristics are quite similar to those of normal thymus. Regardless of the pulse sequence used, they are clearly distinguished from vessels that show no signal.

Paratracheal nodes can be identified on the right side as soft-tissue masses obliterating the right paratracheal stripe. Adenopathy is easier to detect in the older child when the thymus is smaller and the normal structures of the mediastinum and hilum are more easily identified. In the younger child, separation from normal thymus is possible on cross-sectional imaging techniques but not on conventional chest radiography. Large nodes in this area are eas-

I. Solid
  A. Lymph node enlargement
    1. Malignant
      a. Lymphoma
        (1) Hodgkin
        (2) Non-Hodgkin
      b. Leukemic
      c. Metastatic
    2. Benign inflammatory
      a. Bacterial infection
      b. Viral infection
        (1) Infectious mononucleosis
        (2) Pertussis
        (3) Viral pneumonia
      c. *Mycoplasma* infection
      d. Granulomatous infection
        (1) Tuberculosis
        (2) Histoplasmosis
        (3) Other granulomatous infections
    3. Miscellany
      a. Histiocytosis X
      b. Sarcoid
    4. Reactive
      a. Castleman disease
      b. Sinus histiocytosis
II. Cystic
  A. Bronchogenic or other foregut cyst
  B. Pericardial cyst
  C. Pancreatic pseudocyst
  D. Intrapericardial teratoma (multicystic)
III. Vascular
  A. Venous
    1. Azygos
    2. Superior vena cava
    3. Total anomalous pulmonary venous return
    4. Arteriovenous malformations
  B. Arterial
    1. Aortic aneurysm
      a. Mycotic
      b. Connective tissue
    2. Coronary artery aneurysm
    3. Pulmonary artery aneurysm
IV. Miscellaneous
  A. Esophagus
    1. Hiatal hernia
    2. Achalasia
  B. Neurofibromatosis

ily seen by chest radiography or CT. Smaller paratracheal nodes, posterior to the superior vena cava, can be identified on contrast-enhanced CT scans but not on plain chest films.

Anterior mediastinal nodes usually cannot be differentiated from the normal thymus on the chest film until they have become very large; then their size and lobulated borders may reveal their presence. On CT, confusion with the normal thymus can occur, but an uneven pattern of enhancement is often seen in patients with lymph node enlargement. Moreover, in the older child, the nodes are much larger than the normal thymus would be and, on occasion, they are discrete, separate masses without the triangular configuration of the normal thymus. The margins may be rounded or lobular instead of angular. Anterior mediastinal nodes often are in continuity with enlarged nodes in either the neck or the lower mediastinum, thus aiding differentiation from normal thymus. Anterior mediastinal adenopathy is most frequent and massive in lymphoma, but has been noted in histiocytosis X, infectious mononucleosis, granulomatous infections, and metastatic malignancies.

Enlarged ductus nodes can alter the aorticopulmonary window, which normally appears as a concavity between the aorta and the left pulmonary artery on the plain film. In children, minimal concavity is normal, but the "window" should not be convex. This area is well seen on CT just inferior to the aortic arch and superior to the left pulmonary artery. However, because of the small size of this region in children, partial volume averaging is a problem. Coronal MRI and the use of UFCT have made evaluation of this region more reliable.

On chest radiography, *hilar nodes* can be difficult to distinguish from prominent hilar vessels, but filling in of the hilar notch between the right superior pulmonary vein and the descending right pulmonary artery and a lobulated contour to the descending pulmonary artery on each side can be seen (Fig 14–39). Increased opacity of the hilum may also be a clue to the presence of a hilar mass. Lateral radiographs should normally show the posterior wall of the bronchus intermedius as a sharp line; obliteration or thickening of this line suggests the presence of a mass or enlarged nodes. The vessels on the lateral film normally form a horseshoe-shaped opacity; there should usually be a clear space inferior to the trachea and between the vessels. Conversion of this horseshoe to a circle by a soft-tissue opacity suggests subcarinal adenopathy (Fig 14–40). On CT, hilar nodes are readily distinguished from vessels following contrast enhancement as well as by familiarity with normal hilar contours (Fig 14–41). A notch between the descending branch of the left pulmonary artery and the aorta, and the posterior wall of the bronchus intermedius are normal landmarks that can be obliterated by enlarged nodes. MRI easily distinguishes nodes from vessels because of the different signal characteristics (Fig 14–42). Striking hilar adenopathy can occur in lymphoma, granulomatous infection, infectious mononucleosis,

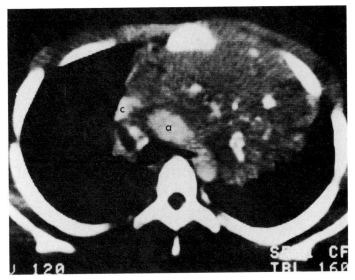

FIG 14–38.
Mediastinal seminoma in a 17-year-old boy. A large, irregularly enhancing mass with calcification is present. *a*, aorta; *c*, vena cava.

and Castleman disease (Fig 14–43). Lesser degrees of adenopathy are frequent in acute and chronic pulmonary infections, both of viral and bacterial origin.

Subcarinal nodes can be suspected on the lateral chest film in the infratracheal areas, as described above, and by seeing a soft-tissue mass in the azygoesophageal recess on a well-penetrated frontal film. On CT, the azygoesophageal recess is concave in adults but slightly convex in many children.

Nonetheless, nodes are clearly visible as a relatively unenhancing soft-tissue mass on contrast-enhanced CT. In addition to being a common site for adenopathy associated with lymphoma, we have seen several children with pulmonary infections that have had a moderate amount of subcarinal adenopathy (Fig 14–44).

Granulomatous infections, particularly tuberculosis and histoplasmosis, can produce significant adenopathy. CECT reveals nodes of low attenuation,

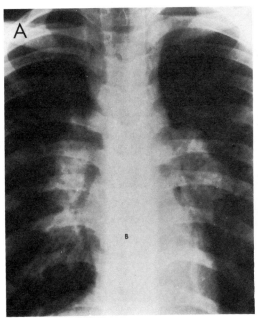

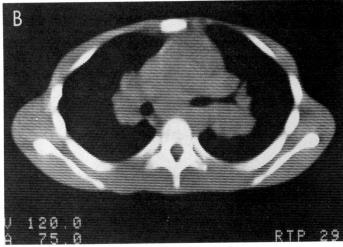

FIG 14–39.
Bilateral hilar lymphadenopathy in a 15-year-old boy with Hodgkin lymphoma. **A,** a chest radiograph shows bilateral hilar and paratracheal adenopathy. **B,** an unenhanced CT scan through the level of the bronchus intermedius and left upper lobe bronchus. Anterior mediastinal, bilateral hilar, and subcarinal adenopathy are obvious. Compare with normal CT anatomy (see Fig 14–2,G and H).

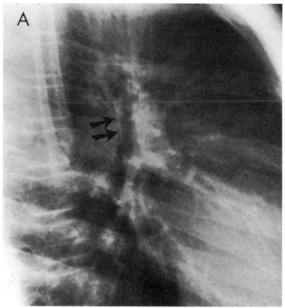

FIG 14–40.
Diagnosis of hilar lymphadenopathy on a lateral radiograph. **A,** normal lateral radiograph of a teenage girl. Posterior wall of bronchus intermedius is indicated by *arrows*. **B,** same patient during acute atypical measles pneumonia with hilar adenopathy. Note the rounded configuration of the perihilar soft tissues as well as the obliteration of the posterior wall of the bronchus intermedius.

peripheral rim enhancement, and septation (Rollins and Currarino) (Fig 14–45).

Posterior mediastinal nodes can be enlarged in chronic infection, particularly reflux esophagitis (Siegel), but they are much more frequently enlarged by metastatic retroperitoneal malignancy, most commonly neuroblastoma. They are retrocrural in location and displace the crura laterally and anteriorly, and produce widening of the paraspinal line on the chest roentgenogram (Fig 14–46). On CT, they ap-

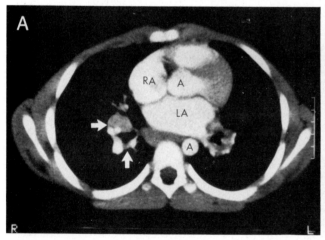

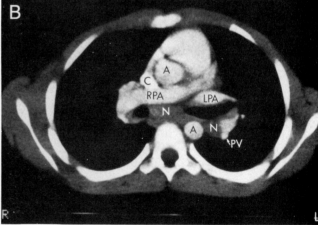

FIG 14–41.
Bilateral hilar and subcarinal adenopathy in a 10-year-old patient with asthma and chronic recurrent infection. **A,** contrast-enhanced UFCT (0.1 sec), reveals bilateral hilar adenopathy, more prominent in the right *(arrows)*. *A,* aorta; *LA,* left atrium; *RA,* right atrium. **B,** UFCT section, 16 mm superior to **A,** reveals subcarinal adenopathy as well as bilateral hilar adenopathy, more prominent in the left side in this patient with recurrent infections. *N,* peribronchial nodes; *C,* superior vena cava; *LPA,* left pulmonary artery; *PV,* pulmonary vein; *RPA,* right pulmonary artery. (From Naidich DP, Zerhouni EA, Siegelman SS (eds): *Computed Tomography and Magnetic Resonance of the Thorax,* ed 2. New York, Raven Press 1991. Used by permission.)

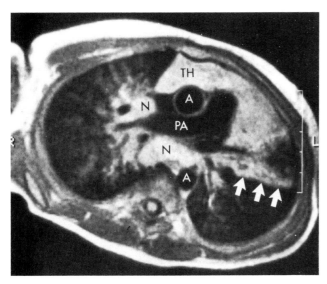

FIG 14–42.
Hilar and subcarinal adenopathy in a 9-month-old patient examined with MR for a vascular ring and recurrent pulmonary infections. Gated axial T1-weighted MR image reveals extensive subcarinal and right hilar adenopathy. Lingular atelectasis *(arrows)* is present but is difficult to separate from the thymus *(TH)* because of similar signal intensity. *A,* aorta; *N,* nodes; *PA,* pulmonary artery. (From Naidich DP, Zerhouni EA, Siegelman SS (eds): *Computed Tomography and Magnetic Resonance of the Thorax,* ed 2. New York, Raven Press, 1991. Used by permission.)

pear as retrocrural masses and their presence usually signifies involvement in both the abdominal and thoracic cavities.

Paracardiac nodes may present as lobulated masses at the cardiophrenic angle on either side. Non-Hodgkin lymphoma is the most common cause. They may simulate a pericardial cyst or fat pad.

Lymphomas

Lymphomas are the third most common group of malignant diseases in childhood after leukemia and central nervous system (CNS) tumors. The Hodgkin group of lymphomas are divided into four groups: (1) nodular sclerosing, (2) mixed cellularity, (3) lymphocyte depletion, and (4) lymphocyte predominance. The classification depends on the relative amounts of lymphocytes, Reed-Sternberg cells, and the type of connective tissue proliferation present. For example, in the lymphocyte predominance type, the number of lymphocytes is high and the number of Reed-Sternberg cells is low; the reverse is true in the lymphocyte depletion type. The nodular sclerosing and mixed cellularity types account for more than 90% of the cases seen in childhood.

Non-Hodgkin lymphoma is a more heterogeneous group of diseases but includes T cell, histiocytic, mixed cell, and B cell types (including the Burkitt type).

Hodgkin lymphomas were once thought to be in-

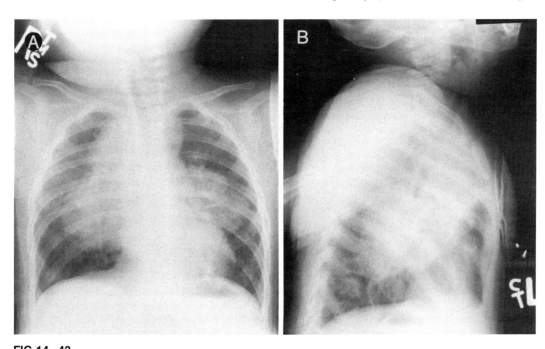

FIG 14–43.
Castleman disease. **A,** frontal, and **B,** lateral chest radiographs reveal massive hilar adenopathy proved by biopsy to be Castleman disease. This infant's mother had suffered from the same disorder.

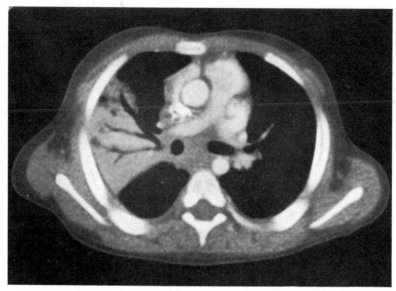

FIG 14–44.
Subcarinal adenopathy. CECT in a patient with acute bacterial right upper lobe
pneumonia. Marked subcarinal adenopathy is noted.

curable but now are apparently cured in a large
number of cases. The patients most commonly
present with asymptomatic cervical lymph node enlargement. Systemic symptoms of fever, fatigue,
weight loss, and night sweats may develop. Knowledge that the disease tends to spread in a contiguous fashion has aided staging and therapy.

Approximately one third of children with lymphoma have mediastinal adenopathy at the time of
diagnosis. Involvement tends to be bilateral but
asymmetric. Mediastinal involvement at the time of
presentation had an adverse prognostic significance

in one series. The 5-year survival rate was 88% for
patients in stage I or stage II with mediastinal involvement, compared with a 98% 5-year survival in
the same groups of patients without mediastinal adenopathy. Anterior mediastinal nodes are frequently
involved, in contrast to sarcoidosis, which usually
has bilateral hilar and paratracheal adenopathy.

Nodal involvement can occur anywhere in the
thorax and may range from a solitary node to huge,
bulky masses of tumor. All of the mediastinal
groups of nodes with the exception of the paracardiac and posterior mediastinal groups are more com-

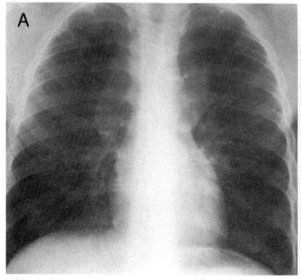

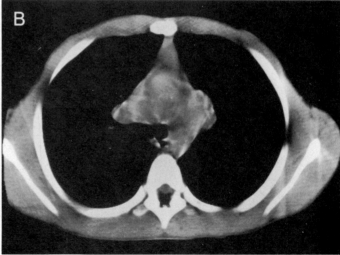

FIG 14–45.
Mediastinal adenopathy due to histoplasmosis. **A,** chest radiograph reveals bilateral hilar and paratracheal as well as subcarinal
adenopathy. **B,** CECT reveals inhomogeneous mixed attenuation
subcarinal adenopathy. (Courtesy of Dr. Nancy Rollins, Dallas.)

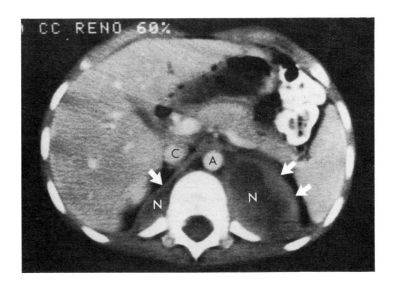

FIG 14–46.
Posterior mediastinal and retrocrural adenopathy secondary to rhabdomyosarcoma in a 10-year-old boy. CECT reveals bilateral retrocrural nodal masses *(N)* displacing the crura *(arrows)* laterally. *A,* aorta; *C,* superior vena cava.

monly affected by Hodgkin than they are by non-Hodgkin disease. In Hodgkin lymphoma, involvement tends to spread in a contiguous fashion so that if there is disease present in the cervical region, unless the paratracheal and anterior mediastinal nodes are involved, it is unusual for hilar nodes to be diseased.

The chest film may be normal or show a huge mediastinal mass. CT is indicated for detection and staging of disease. It is not unusual for the chest film to appear normal and for the CT scan to reveal adenopathy (Fig 14–47). Anterior mediastinal adenopa-

thy can simulate the normal thymus, particularly in younger children, but it is nearly always possible using CT to differentiate normal thymus from anterior mediastinal adenopathy as was discussed above in the section on the thymus.

CT findings of lymphoma are those of lymph node enlargement, usually in the anterior mediastinum, but involvement of hilar and subcarinal nodes is common. Nodes may range in size from 1 cm to huge masses filling the mediastinum. Nodes may be seen as discrete nodular masses or as confluent masses of tumor. Calcification is rare in untreated

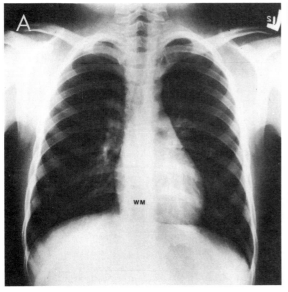

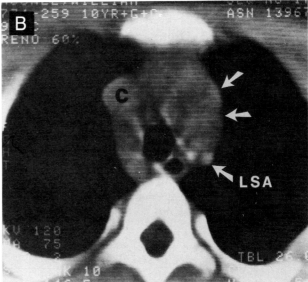

FIG 14–47.
Value of CT in diagnosing mediastinal disease in Hodgkin lymphoma. **A,** chest radiograph interpreted as normal. **B,** CECT reveals marked widening of the mediastinum by an irregular enhancing mass *(arrows)* which is displacing the great vessels posteriorly. Right-sided paratracheal adenopathy is also present posterior to the superior vena cava *(C)*. *LSA,* left subclavian artery.

cases (Panicek); areas of necrosis are commonly seen, particularly following contrast enhancement (Fig 14–48). In our experience, about 1 patient in 4 shows a homogeneous mass of tumor which could be mistaken for normal thymus except for its abnormal size; usually, other areas of disease are noted, commonly adenopathy in the neck or elsewhere in the mediastinum, simplifying the differential diagnosis (Heron et al.). Morphology of the nodal masses on MR (Fig 14–49) is similar to that seen with CT, although the coronal view gives a clearer idea of the cephalocaudad extent of disease. Signal characteristics on MR are somewhat variable but the mass tends to be intermediate on T1-weighted images and somewhat brighter on T2-weighted images. As on CT, some are homogeneous and some are very heterogeneous. Research is ongoing to try to correlate signal patterns with the degree of cellularity and aggressiveness of the tumor. There is also some evidence that as the tumor responds to therapy, changes in the signal intensity are more helpful than changes in size in determining whether the residual masses often seen following therapy represent fibrosis or active tumor.

Complications. Tracheobronchial compression of some degree occurred in 55% of the children with Hodgkin disease reported by Mandel et al. This complication is seen better by CT than by airway films. Superior vena cava obstruction is readily diagnosed by CT or MR; findings include extensive collateral flow and failure to visualize the superior vena cava (Fig 14–50).

Pulmonary involvement is rarely seen as the sole manifestation of Hodgkin disease. Typically, it tends to occur as the disease spreads contiguously from the mediastinal nodes to the hilar nodes, to the lung parenchyma. A nodular or infiltrative pattern may be seen, and pleural masses may also be present. These findings are better demonstrated by CT than by conventional x-ray studies.

Residual masses are often seen in the mediastinum following therapy, and it is difficult to know if they represent fibrotic areas or residual tumor. Calcifications seen on CT suggest fibrosis as do areas of shortened T2 on MR. Gallium 67 citrate scanning can be helpful in some of these patients, particularly if the tumor has previously shown gallium avidity.

Non-Hodgkin Lymphoma. *Non-Hodgkin lymphoma* does not refer to a single disease entity, but rather to a more heterogeneous group of diseases generally having a more aggressive course and a worse prognosis than Hodgkin lymphoma.

The Burkitt type of non-Hodgkin lymphoma is characterized by abdominal involvement with relatively infrequent involvement of the mediastinum.

The poorly differentiated lymphocytic variety of non-Hodgkin lymphoma has a high association of leukemic transformation and may, in fact, be part of the same disease process.

Findings on CT and MR are nonspecific and cannot be differentiated from Hodgkin disease. The masses may be larger, and airway and vascular compression tends to be more frequent and more severe; pulmonary parenchymal involvement is reported in only 2% of cases, but pleural effusion is seen in approximately 1 in 7 children (Parker and Castellino). The posterior mediastinal and paracardiac nodes are more frequently involved by non-Hodgkin lymphoma than by Hodgkin lymphoma.

Cystic Mediastinal Masses

Bronchogenic Cysts. Bronchogenic cysts, thought to result from an abnormal budding of the ventral diverticulum of the foregut, may present in the pulmonary parenchyma or the mediastinum (Ramenofsky). They are thin-walled cysts lined with respiratory epithelium and filled with mucoid material. Usually, there is no direct communication of mediastinal cysts with the tracheobronchial tree.

Most mediastinal bronchogenic cysts are situated near the carina, and are often attached by a stalk or common wall to one of the major airways. Radiographic examination shows a round or oval mass of homogeneous density with clearly defined margins. The mass varies in size and often extends slightly to the right side. In infants, the masses are usually discovered because associated airway compression causes symptoms such as wheezing, stridor, and cough. Usually, the cyst is obvious on a radiographic examination, although subcarinal cysts may be hidden and difficult to diagnose (see Fig 8–8 in Chapter 8). An esophagram may be helpful as the esophagus may be deviated by the subcarinal mass.

CT is helpful to determine the nature and extent of a suspected bronchogenic cyst (Fig 14–51) (Hernandez). Although usually not frankly calcified on plain radiographic examination, some cysts have CT numbers much higher than water. Although the high numbers suggest the possibility of a solid mass, contrast enhancement reveals the true avascular, cystic nature of the mass. Mild airway obstruction, not apparent on plain radiography, may be obvious on CT examination (Fig 14–52). MR demonstrates the anatomy well in additional planes. Fluid-filled masses tend to have prolonged T1 and T2 relaxation times; on T1-weighted images the mass may blend with the pulmonary parenchyma, but T2-weighted images reveal increased signal from the cyst fluid. Sagittal and coronal sections are helpful in establishing the geography of the mass; airway obstruction

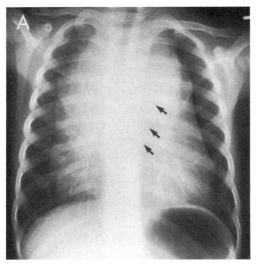

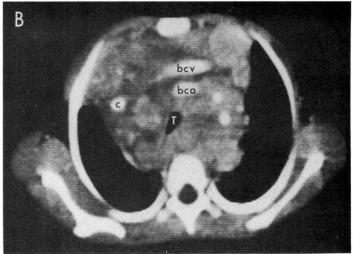

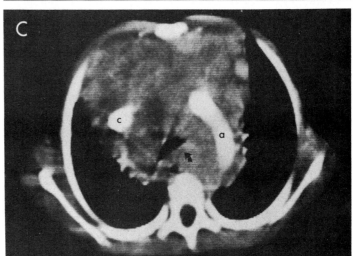

FIG 14–48.
An 8-year-old boy with non-Hodgkin lymphoma. **A,** huge anterior mediastinal mass is present. Suggestion of posterior mass *(arrows)* is also seen. The trachea appeared normal on this and his lateral radiograph. **B,** CECT scan, same patient at the level of the upper mediastinum. The trachea *(T)* is narrowed from side to side and its area diminished. Note the huge irregularly enhancing mass surrounding the great vessels. *(c),* vena cava; *bca,* brachiocephalic artery; *bca,* brachiocephalic vein. **C,** same patient, CT scan, lower section. The trachea is again severely compressed and narrowed *(arrow). c,* vena cava; *a,* aorta.

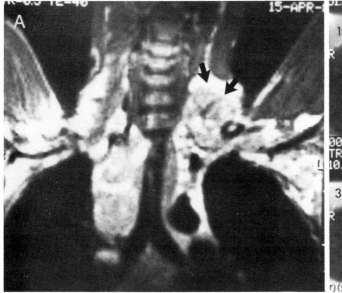

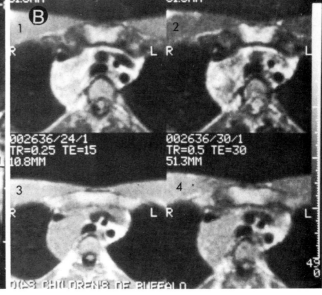

FIG 14–49.
MR appearance of Hodgkin lymphoma in a 15-year-old boy. **A,** coronal T1-weighted MR image reveals right paratracheal adenopathy with extension into the left supraclavicular region *(arrows).* **B,** axial images acquired with progressively greater T1-weighting. Level *1,* TR/TE-2,000/80; level *2,* TR/TE-2,000/40; Level *3,* TR/TE-5,000/30; level *4,* TR/TE-250/15. Note that the right paratracheal mass becomes progressively brighter in relation to the muscle tissue with increased T2 weighting and also becomes less homogeneous. (From Naidich DP, Zerhouni EA, Siegelman SS (eds): *Computed Tomography and Magnetic Resonance of the Thorax,* ed 2. New York, Raven Press, 1991. Used by permission.)

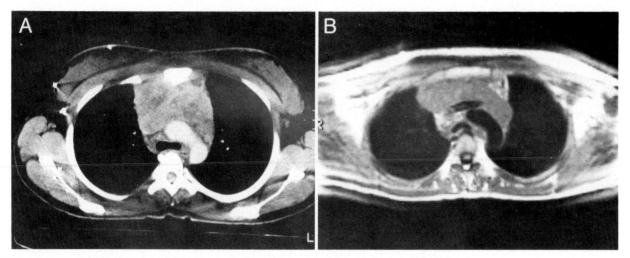

FIG 14–50.
Superior vena caval obstruction due to Hodgkin lymphoma in a 15-year-old girl. **A,** CECT scan reveals gross enlargement of the thymus for age. The mediastinal mass is irregularly nodular and shows uneven contrast enhancement. Superior vena caval ob- struction is also present. **B,** T1-weighted MR scan, same patient. The lymphomatous mass is of a relatively homogeneous nature with a long T1. Note the absence of flow void from the superior vena cava.

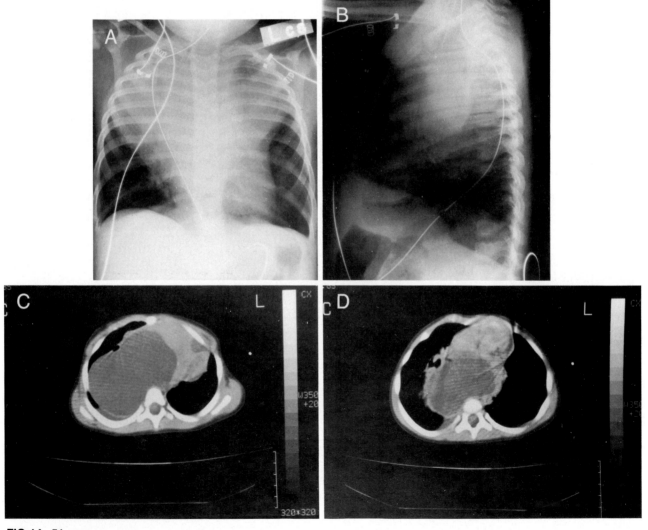

FIG 14–51.
Infected bronchogenic cyst in a 14-month-old infant. This patient retrospectively had a mediastinal mass since birth. At several months of age she had some wheezing as her only symptom. **A,** frontal, and **B,** lateral radiographs reveal a large diffuse mass crossing the midline in the upper chest. The patient is intubated and the airway is stretched anteriorly. **C** and **D,** CT scan reveals the enormous nature of the cystic structure. Note the anterior posi- tion of the airway. The presence of a thin, enhancing visible wall suggests that this may be infected, a finding documented at sur- gery.

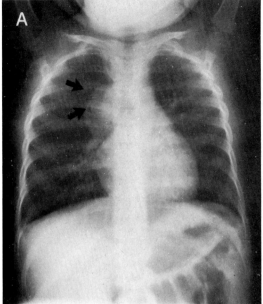

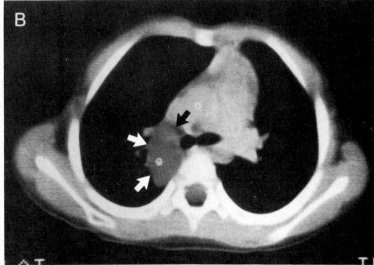

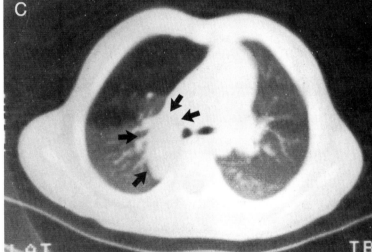

FIG 14–52.
Paratracheal mediastinal bronchogenic cyst. **A,** chest radiograph reveals a paratracheal mass *(arrows).* **B,** CECT scan shows the middle and posterior mediastinal location of the avascular mass *(arrows).* No enhancing rim is noted. **C,** same level viewed at lung windows reveals obstructive emphysema of the anterior segment of the right upper lobe *(arrows).*

and air trapping are less well visualized than on CT. Some foregut cysts have been reported to involute spontaneously.

Vascular Lesions

On plain radiography, vascular malformations of the mediastinum may simulate other mediastinal masses of solid or cystic origin. Vascular malformations are discussed more fully in Part III, but those which may present as masses are summarized here. Accurate diagnosis of these lesions requires the use of CECT or MR. In some cases, confirmation by angiography may be required.

Venous abnormalities. The *azygos vein* is seen end-on as a small oval opacity in the right tracheobronchial angle. It may increase in size in congestive heart failure and intrahepatic interruption or thrombosis of the inferior vena cava. A change in size and position with breathing differentiates it from an en-

larged azygos node or other solid mass. A right-sided paravertebral mass produced by the dilated azygos vein is often visible (Fig 14–53). Consolidation of an azygos lobe can simulate a mediastinal mass (Fig 14–54).

The *superior vena cava* may dilate and produce a right superior mediastinal mass. The dilatation is usually of unknown cause. Aneurysmal dilatation of the superior vena cava has been noted with cystic hygroma. Right upper lobe atelectasis may simulate an enlarged vena cava (see Chapter 8). There may be absence of the right superior vena cava with a persistent left superior vena cava, or both veins may be present. The persistent left superior vena cava usually drains into the coronary sinus. *Total anomalous pulmonary venous return* of the supradiaphragmatic type produces a figure-8 or snowman appearance of the upper mediastinum and cardiac structures that could be mistaken for a mediastinal mass on plain film. In the scimitar syndrome (pulmonary

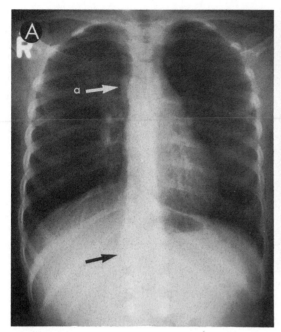

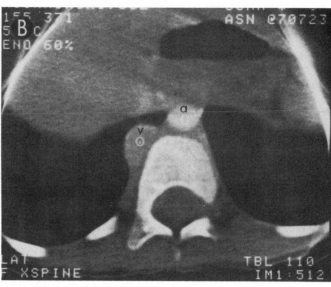

FIG 14–53.

Infrahepatic interruption of the inferior vena cava with azygos continuation resulting in a right paravertebral mass. **A,** chest radiograph in an 11-year-old girl with a heart murmur shows a right paravertebral mass *(black arrow)* and a second mass in the region of the azygos vein *(white arrow).* **B,** CECT confirms the suspected diagnosis of infrahepatic interruption of the inferior vena cava with azygos continuation. The dilated azygos vein *(v)* is causing the right paraspinal mass. *a,* aorta.

venolobar syndrome), an anomalous right pulmonary vein may drain into the right atrium or may extend below the diaphragm and insert into the inferior vena cava, or the hepatic or portal veins. The superior vena cava may be obstructed by masses, most commonly lymphoma. Thrombosis as a complication of central venous lines are not uncommon. The diagnosis can be established by venography, CECT, or MRI.

Arterial Abnormalities. Pulmonary Arteries. The pulmonary arteries are well seen by MR in three views and can also be well demonstrated by CT in the transaxial plane with the use of bolus contrast enhancement. The left and right pulmonary

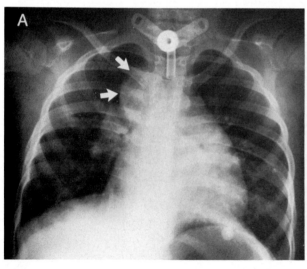

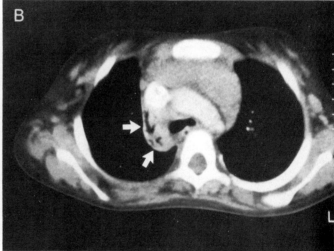

FIG 14–54.

Consolidation of an azygos lobe simulating a mediastinal mass. Note the similarity between this patient's chest radiograph and the patient with a bronchogenic cyst illustrated in Figure 14–52. This 6-year-old child had chronic lung disease. **A,** chest radiograph reveals a right paratracheal mass *(arrows).* **B,** CECT reveals consolidation with an air bronchogram of an azygos lobe *(arrows).*

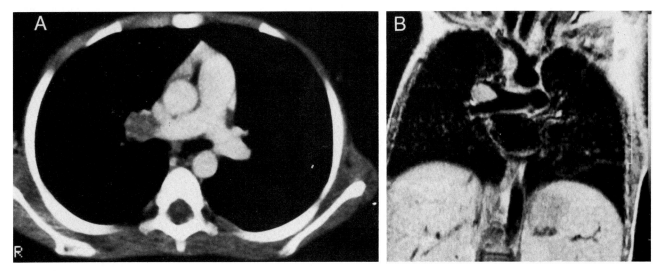

FIG 14–55.
A, CECT reveals a right hilar mass in or near the pulmonary artery. **B,** coronal MR image reveals CT findings to be due to hilar adenopathy from metastatic rhabdomyosarcoma.

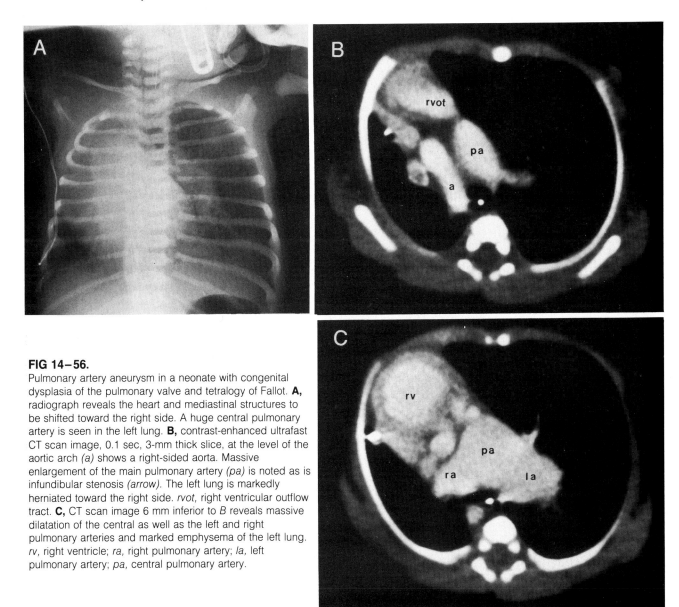

FIG 14–56.
Pulmonary artery aneurysm in a neonate with congenital dysplasia of the pulmonary valve and tetralogy of Fallot. **A,** radiograph reveals the heart and mediastinal structures to be shifted toward the right side. A huge central pulmonary artery is seen in the left lung. **B,** contrast-enhanced ultrafast CT scan image, 0.1 sec, 3-mm thick slice, at the level of the aortic arch *(a)* shows a right-sided aorta. Massive enlargement of the main pulmonary artery *(pa)* is noted as is infundibular stenosis *(arrow)*. The left lung is markedly herniated toward the right side. *rvot,* right ventricular outflow tract. **C,** CT scan image 6 mm inferior to *B* reveals massive dilatation of the central as well as the left and right pulmonary arteries and marked emphysema of the left lung. *rv,* right ventricle; *ra,* right pulmonary artery; *la,* left pulmonary artery; *pa,* central pulmonary artery.

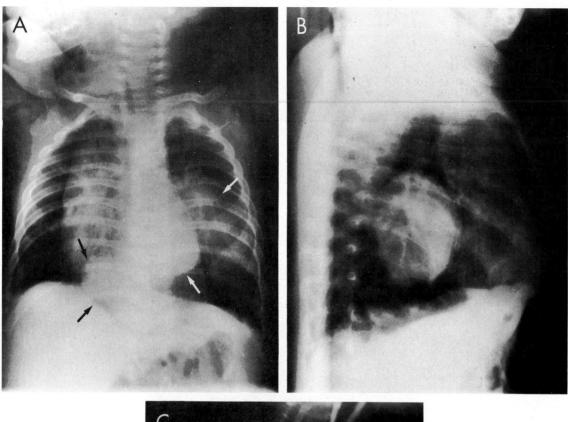

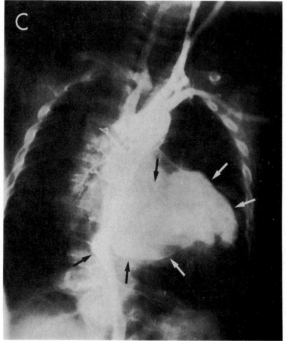

FIG 14–57.
Mycotic aneurysm. This 8-month-old boy had had an umbilical artery catheterization as a neonate. He developed staphylococcal sepsis but did well until 3 months of age when chest films were obtained because of a failure to thrive and a heart murmur. **A,** frontal and **B,** lateral films disclosed a large, rounded mass lesion in the left midlung (*white arrows*) and a smaller one in the right cardiophrenic angle (*black arrows*). **C,** a thoracic aortogram confirms the presence of several large aortic aneurysms (*arrows*). These were treated successfully surgically, and the patient has done well to date.

arteries are approximately equal in size but there is a lack of normal CT standards for size in the pediatric patient. Anomalies of the pulmonary arteries are listed in Chapter 17 and discussed also in Chapter 11.

Enlargement of the pulmonary arteries occurs with pulmonary hypertension and with large left-to-right shunts. Ready recognition of pulmonary artery enlargement and separation from questionable hilar adenopathy is easily performed with either CT or MR (Fig 14–55).

Rarely, the pulmonary arteries may be aneurysmally dilated in the neonate. This usually occurs with congenital absence of the pulmonary valve, as with a variant of the tetralogy of Fallot. The enlarged pulmonary artery may cause bronchial compression resulting in either delayed clearance of neonatal lung liquid or, in older life, segmental or lobar air

trapping (Fig 14–56). A tumor thrombus or pulmonary thromboembolism of any cause is rare in children but can be detected by CECT, MRI, or angiography. The pulmonary artery may, on occasion, be compressed by a mediastinal mass, most commonly lymphoma.

Aorta. Vascular rings are significant because they cause airway compression and frequently require surgical correction. They are described in more detail in Chapter 17. A prominent right-sided aortic arch can simulate plain film findings of a mediastinal mass (see Chapter 8).

An *aneurysm of the ductus arteriosus* may produce a mass in the region of the aorticopulmonary window. This lesion may be due to delayed closure of the aortic end of the ductus, which produces a diverticulum that undergoes myxoid degeneration and aneurysmal dilatation as a result of continued expo-

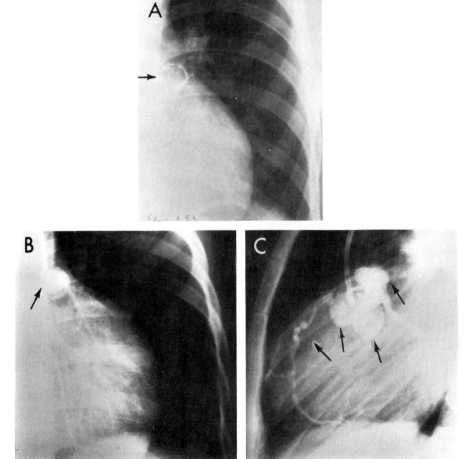

FIG 14–58.
Kawasaki disease (mucocutaneous lymph node syndrome) in a Japanese boy of 9 years. In **A,** frontal projection, an aneurysm of the left coronary artery is completely calcified *(arrow)*. In **B** and **C,** arteriograms of the coronary arteries disclose the dilated lumen of the left coronary artery and tortuosities of the anterior descending interventricular branch of the left coronary artery *(anterior arrow),* **C,** the two *middle arrows* point to two normal cusps of the aortic valve. The superior and inferior *arrows* indicate coronary artery aneurysms.

sure to arterial pressures. Calcification is occasionally seen in the wall of the aneurysm.

Aneurysms of the aorta are uncommon in childhood but may occur following trauma, infection, or in some connective tissue disorders such as Marfan or Ehlers-Danlos syndromes. With increasing use of arterial catheters in the newborn, mycotic lesions are seen more often. The radiologic appearance depends on the size and location, but lesions can become huge (Fig 14–57). Coronary artery aneurysms, which can calcify, are a complication of Kawasaki disease (Fig 14–58).

An *arteriovenous malformation* may be centrally located and present as a mediastinal mass. A murmur, cyanosis, and right-to-left shunting may be noted clinically. The typical mass is 2 to 4 cm in size, oval, and sharply defined.

Neurofibromatosis

Neurofibromatosis is usually associated with posterior mediastinal masses but can occur in the middle mediastinum and simulate lymphoma. On CT, lesions are of lower attenuation than muscle and characteristically show little contrast enhancement (Fig 14–59).

Mediastinal Calcification

Calcifications in the mediastinum are infrequent and usually are detected only by CT examination with

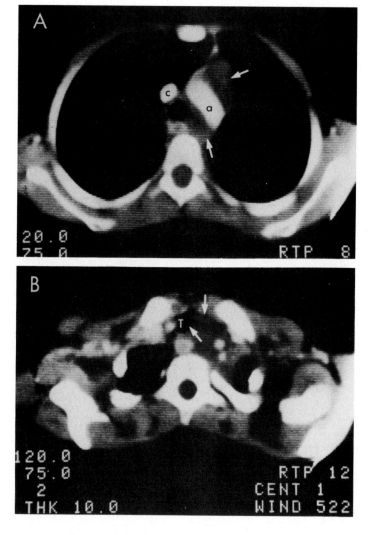

FIG 14–59.
Mediastinal neurofibromatosis simulating lymphoma. **A,** CECT scan performed because of plain radiographic findings of a lobulated middle mediastinal mass thought to represent lymphoma. CT examination reveals the presence of a homogeneous, relatively low-density mass surrounding the aorta *(a) (arrows).* (c, vena cava.) **B,** higher CT section, same patient, shows the mass extending into the neck on the left side *(arrows)* and slightly compressing the trachea *(T).* A family history and the presence of café au lait spots suggested the correct diagnosis of neurofibromatosis.

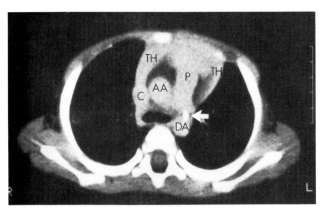

FIG 14–60.
Calcification of the ligamenum arteriosum. Unenhanced UFCT (0.1 sec) in a 2-year-old infant reveals curvilinear calcification *(arrow)* at the level of the aortic pulmonary window. *AA,* ascending aorta; *C,* superior vena cava; *DA,* descending aorta; *P,* pulmonary artery; *TH,* thymus. (From Naidich DP, Zerouni EA, Siegalman SS (eds): *Computed Tomography and Magnetic Resonance of the Thorax,* ed 2. New York, Raven Press, 1991. Used by permission.)

which small linear or curvilinear calcification is seen in the ductus arteriosus (ligamentum arteriosum) in approximately 30% of children (Fig 14–60). Calcification, usually specklike or rounded, occurs in mediastinal nodes in granulomatous infections. Mediastinal neoplasms that may contain calcifications in-

clude germ cell tumors, teratomas, neuroblastomas, ganglioneuroblastomas, and ganglioneuromas (Fig 14–61). Calcifications are very rare in untreated lymphoma, but may develop following radiation therapy. One case of calcification recently was reported in an otherwise normal but hyperplastic thymus.

Posterior Mediastinal Masses

Posterior mediastinal masses that occur in children are classified according to their CT characteristics in Table 14–4. By far, the most common lesions are neurogenic, which account for 30% to 40% of the total mediastinal masses in most pediatric series.

Neoplasms of neural origin can be divided into three groups: (1) those arising from sympathetic ganglia, including neuroblastoma, ganglioneuroblastoma, and ganglioneuroma (the first two are malignant lesions that tend to occur in children under 4 years of age); (2) those arising from peripheral nerves, such as neurofibromas and neurilemmomas (these lesions are benign; neurofibromas, when found in the mediastinum, are often associated with neurofibromatosis); (3) lesions arising from the paraganglion cells (these neoplasms are rarely seen in children).

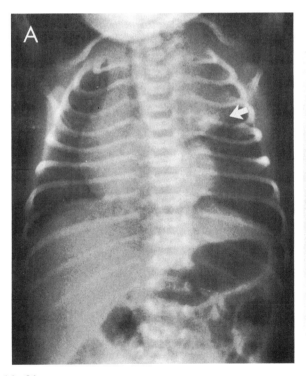

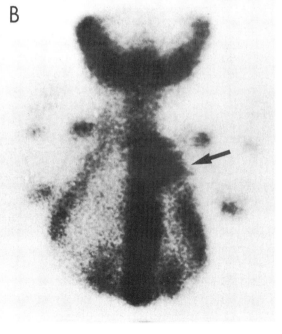

FIG 14–61.
Mediastinal neuroblastoma in a neonate with Horner syndrome. **A,** initial chest radiograph was interpreted as prominent left lobe of the thymus until a small area of calcification *(arrow)* was recog-

nized. **B,** technetium 99m pyrophosphate bone scan shows marked uptake in the mediastinal neuroblastoma *(arrow).*

TABLE 14–4.

TABLE 14–4.

Computed Tomography Characteristics of Posterior Mediastinal Masses

I. Solid
  A. Neurofibroma
  B. Ganglioneuroma
  C. Neuroblastoma (primary or metastatic)
  D. Lymphoma
  E. Ectopic thymus
  F. Chest wall tumor
  G. Paraspinal abscess/diskitis
  H. Hamartoma, mesenchymoma
  I. Extramedullary hematopoiesis
  J. Germ cell tumor
  K. Castleman disease
II. Cystic
  A. Neuroenteric cyst
  B. Gastroenteric cyst
  C. Meningocele
III. Vascular
  A. Descending aorta aneurysm
  B. Dilated azygos vein
IV. Fatty
  A. Lipoblastoma
  B. Teratoma
V. Calcified
  A. Neuroblastoma (primary)
  B. Ganglioneuroma
VI. Miscellaneous
  A. Bochdalek hernia

Neurogenic Tumors of Sympathetic Nervous System Origin

Included in this group are neuroblastoma, ganglioneuroblastoma, and ganglioneuroma. Approximately 16% of all neuroblastomas are of mediastinal origin, and these are nearly always in the posterior mediastinum. *Neuroblastoma* is found 40% of the time before the age of 2 years, and most of the rest of the tumors are discovered in preschool children. A posterior mediastinal mass found in these age groups should be considered neuroblastoma until proved otherwise. *Ganglioneuroblastoma* and *ganglioneuroma* are more commonly found in somewhat older children. Those tumors with undifferentiated histologic features are more malignant than better-differentiated types. The ganglioneuroma is regarded as an essentially benign tumor which may represent a matured neuroblastoma.

While many neurogenic lesions are incidentally discovered on chest radiography, the neuroblastoma may present with a wide variety of signs and symptoms, including fever, malaise, back pain, anemia, and other nonspecific findings. Horner syndrome may be present in apical lesions (see Fig 14–61). Lower limb weakness can be seen in lesions involving the spinal canal. Patients may have respiratory symptoms, and a few may present with a relatively distinct neurologic syndrome, the opsoclonus cerebellar ataxia syndrome.

Radiologic Findings. Bar-Ziv and Nogrady reviewed 23 cases of mediastinal neuroblastoma: 6 were primary; 12 were metastatic; 1 was a ganglioneuroblastoma; 4 were ganglioneuromas. The borders of the primary neuroblastomas were often indistinct ("ghost tumor"), and rib spreading and erosion were more marked. This lesion may be mistaken for pneumonia or, if superiorly located, for a normal thymus or upper lobe atelectasis (Fig 14–62). Borders of the more mature ganglioneuromas and ganglioneuroblastomas were sharper, and rib erosion and costal separations were more subtle. Calcification was present in both benign and malignant tumors. Metastatic tumors were bilateral, paravertebral, triangular masses found in the lower posterior mediastinum. Rib erosion and calcifications were not seen in the metastatic group. CT and MRI are essential to localize the mass, determine its solid nature, and evaluate its extent.

On CT neuroblastomas are soft-tissue masses, approximately 40% of which may contain speckled or curvilinear calcification (Armstrong et al.). The masses show variable, usually inhomogeneous enhancement following contrast injection. They are located in the paravertebral region where they may extend superiorly and inferiorly for several centimeters. Extradural extension is frequent, even in the absence of neurologic signs and symptoms; one of the important aims of the imaging procedure is to diagnose or exclude such spread (Kirks et al., Armstrong et al.). In the past this has been achieved by the use of CT metrizamide myelography. Our experience has been that high-quality, bolus IV. CECT provides equivalent information, as the extradural spread of tumor nearly always enhances (Fig 14–63). Even though MR fails to demonstrate the calcification often associated with neuroblastoma, it is likely that MR will become the modality of choice for staging because of the accuracy with which this modality demonstrates intraspinal spread of tumor. In sagittal and coronal views, tumor spread along nerves can be seen extending into neural foramina. On T2-weighted images, the signal intensity of the tumor is increased. MR has the additional benefits of separating tumor from other surrounding soft tissues more readily than CT, as well as being more accurate in the recognition of bone marrow involvement which is seen as areas of prolonged T1.

Though extradural spread and marrow involvement are more frequent, neuroblastoma can also ex-

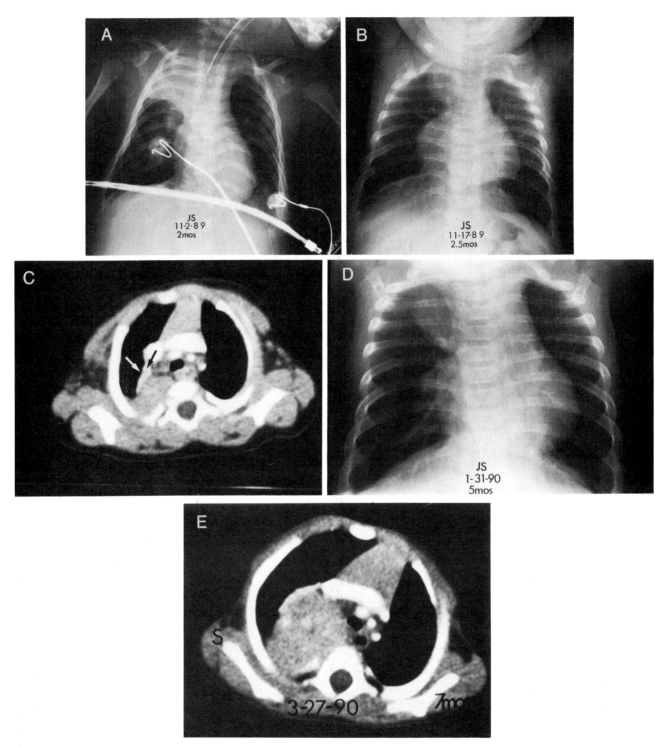

FIG 14–62.
Posterior mediastinal neuroblastoma mistaken for chronic right upper lobe atelectasis. **A,** portable radiograph at 2 months of age reveals right upper lobe atelectasis in this neonate with mild bronchopulmonary dysplasia. **B,** repeat radiograph, 2 weeks later reveals residual right upper lobe opacity thought to be continued atelectasis. **C,** CECT scan reveals a posterior mediastinal mass which is of approximately the same attenuation as muscle tissue. A small wedge of atelectatic enhancing lung is noted just anterior to the mass *(arrows)*. **D,** repeat radiograph approximately 2 months later shows enlargement of the right upper mediastinal opacity with questionable calcification in its inferior portion. **E,** repeat CT scan shows marked increase in the size of the mass, which was finally biopsied and found to be neuroblastoma.

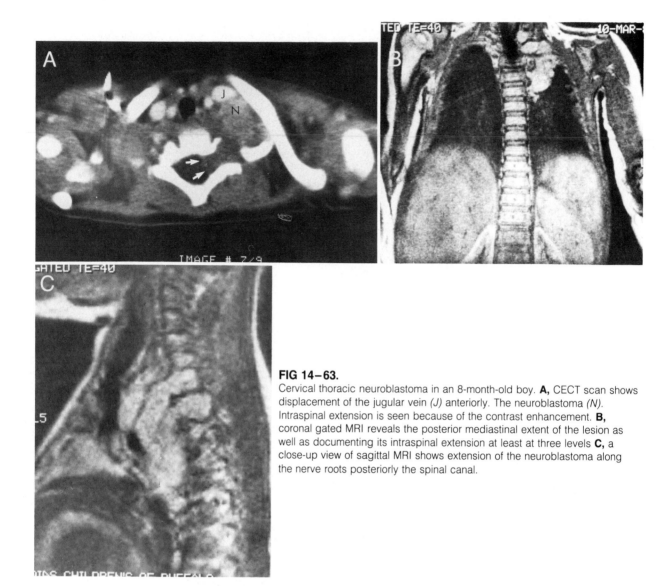

FIG 14–63.
Cervical thoracic neuroblastoma in an 8-month-old boy. **A,** CECT scan shows displacement of the jugular vein (*J*) anteriorly. The neuroblastoma (*N*). Intraspinal extension is seen because of the contrast enhancement. **B,** coronal gated MRI reveals the posterior mediastinal extent of the lesion as well as documenting its intraspinal extension at least at three levels **C,** a close-up view of sagittal MRI shows extension of the neuroblastoma along the nerve roots posteriorly the spinal canal.

tend directly into the mediastinal lymph nodes, and even into the hilar vessels. Either CT or MR can document this extension. Neuroblastoma may extend from a primary site in the abdomen into the thorax. Most commonly, this occurs by direct invasion through the retrocrural space and into the lower paravertebral regions, often bilaterally. Metastatic spread to lung parenchyma or pleura tends to be a late complication; the metastases can, on occasion, be large enough to be recognized on CT but frequently are microscopic.

Ganglioneuroblastomas are regarded as malignant neuroblastomas which have partially matured. Their imaging characteristics are similar to neuroblastoma, and approximately 20% have calcification (Armstrong et al.). Ganglioneuromas are benign tumors which may be the end result of the maturation process. They present either as a large, smooth spherical mass or as a small, elongated sausage-shaped mass. Some of the large ones are of low, homogeneous attenuation and show little, if any, contrast enhancement; neuroblastoma tends to appear more inhomogeneous following contrast enhancement, but these masses cannot be reliably distinguished from one another by CT. Experience with MR is limited, but it seems unlikely that there will be enough difference in signal characteristics to allow confident differentiation of a benign from a malignant mass (Fig 14–64).

Malignant sarcomas arising from the chest wall may simulate neurogenic tumors. We have seen intraspinal extension not only in neurogenic tumors but also in rhabdosarcoma and Ewing sarcoma (Fig 14–65). Inflammatory lesions such as actinomycosis must also be considered in the differential diagnosis.

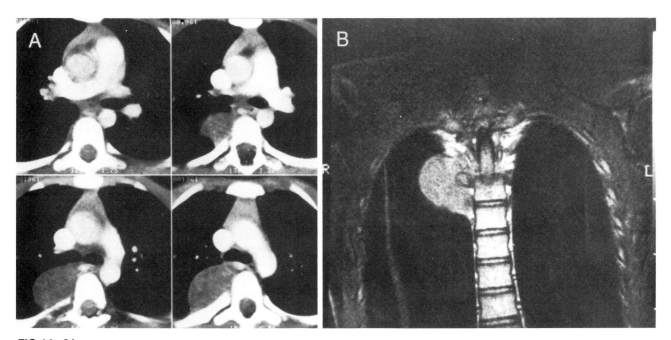

FIG 14–64.
Ganglioneuroma in a teen-age boy. **A,** contiguous 3-mm CECT images reveal a low-attenuation mass in the posterior mediastinum.

B, coronal T2-weighted MR image shows the mass to be brighter than muscle tissue and of fairly homogeneous character.

Neurogenic Tumors of Peripheral Nervous System Origin: Neurofibromas

Neurofibromas occur predominantly in patients with systemic neurofibromatosis rather than as isolated lesions. These tumors arise most often in the superior and posterior mediastinum; they are more often bilateral than other neurogenic lesions. In addition

to revealing the mass, a chest radiograph is often diagnostic because of the presence of other stigmata of neurofibromatosis such as scoliosis or typical "ribbon-like" rib deformities. On CT, the masses are smooth and typically homogeneous, of slightly lower attenuation than muscle (Fig 14–66). Little contrast enhancement is usually present. In addition

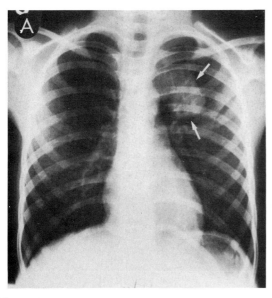
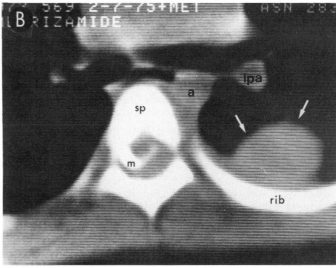

FIG 14–65.
Rhabdomyosarcoma. This 8-year-old girl presented with back pain. **A,** a chest radiograph reveals a soft-tissue density in the left upper part of the thorax *(arrows).* There is slight spreading of the left fourth and fifth ribs posteriorly. A neurogenic tumor was suspected. **B,** metrizamide-enhanced CT scan, same patient. The

mass is seen to lie slightly lateral to the paravertebral region *(arrows).* However, intraspinal extension is apparent from the displacement of the metrizamide *(m)*-enhanced spinal subarachnoid space. The operative diagnosis was rhabdomyosarcoma. *sp,* spine; *a,* aorta; *ipa,* left pulmonary artery.

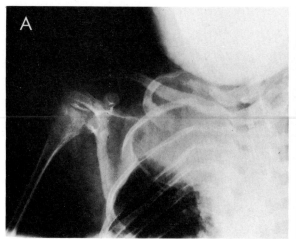

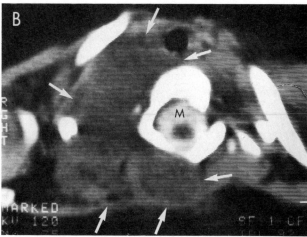

FIG 14–66.
Neurofibromatosis. **A,** radiograph of the upper part of the thorax reveals a large posterior mediastinal mass with extensive rib abnormalities characteristic of neurofibromatosis. **B,** metrizamide-enhanced CT scan through the neck of the same patient. A huge mass extends into the soft tissues *(arrows)* No intraspinal component is visualized at this level. *M,* metrizamide in the spinal subarachnoid space.

to dumbbell extension, extension into the neck has been present in several of our cases and airway compression has occurred. Involvement of the middle mediastinum suggesting lymphoma has been seen. It has been suggested that detection of an area of low attenuation in the mass may indicate fibrosarcomatous degeneration, but fat in the tumor may cause an identical appearance on CT, although it should be possible to make the distinction on MR examination.

Other Posterior Mediastinal Lesions

Cystic duplications, either of enteric or foregut origin, are the second most common type of posterior mediastinal mass. Neurenteric cysts contain both neural and gastrointestinal elements. The cyst is connected by a stalk to the meninges and is associated with a vertebral anomaly as part of the so-called split notochord syndrome. Vertebral anomalies include hemivertebrae, fusion anomalies, and spina bifida (Geremia et al.).

Esophageal Duplication Cysts. *Esophageal duplication cysts* may result from failure of the solid esophageal tube to vacuolate completely to form a hollow tube or from abnormal budding of the dorsal foregut. Approximately 10% to 15% of all gastroenteric duplications are located in the thorax adjacent to the esophagus. The lesions rarely communicate with the esophageal lumen. Many are asymptomatic, but they may present with symptoms relating to respiratory distress or difficulty in swallowing. The mass tends to have smooth outlines and usually impinges on the barium-filled esophagus. Although

usually small, the cysts may be quite large, often attaining a size of 10 cm or more. Technetium 99m pertechnetate scanning can demonstrate gastric mucosa in the cyst, aiding in preoperative diagnosis. The lesions are cystic and avascular on CT (Fig 14–67); MR shows a prolonged T2 relaxation time and clearly separates the mass from the aorta (Fig 14–68). These modalities may contribute valuable

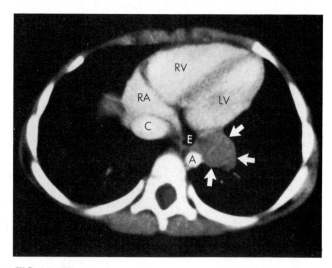

FIG 14–67.
Esophageal duplication cyst. UFCT in a 2-year-old girl with a past history of repair of a tracheoesophageal fistula. A mediastinal mass was noted on a routine radiographic follow-up examination. On this CT scan image an avascular mass *(arrows)* is seen anterolateral to the aorta and lateral to the esophagus. The mass shows no contrast enhancement and does not have a definable wall. At surgery an esophageal duplication cyst was removed. *C,* superior vena cava; *E,* esophagus; *A,* aorta; *RA,* right atrium; *RV,* right ventricle; *LV,* left ventricle.

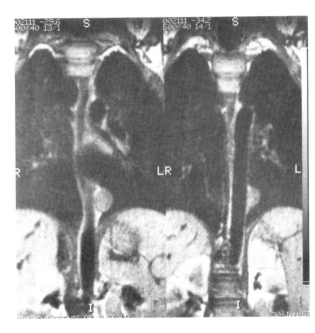

FIG 14–68.
Esophageal duplication cyst. Coronal MRI, 5 mm apart, shows a 1.5-cm oval mass adjacent to but separate from the descending aorta. An esophageal duplication cyst was removed at surgery.

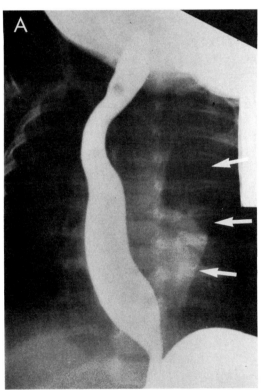

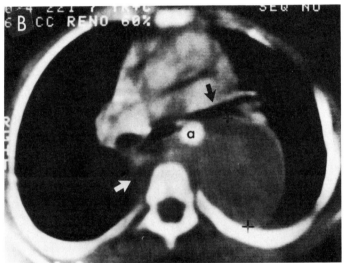

FIG 14–69.
Cystic hygroma (lymphangioma). **A,** infant with a posterior mediastinal mass *(arrows)*. Note the displacement of the esophagus. **B,** CT scan, same patient, at 1 year of age after attempted surgical removal of the mass, which was found to be a lymphangioma. A large mass displacing the left mainstem bronchus *(black arrow)* anteriorly is noted. The mass (+) surrounds the aorta *(a)* and extends across the midline *(white arrow)*.

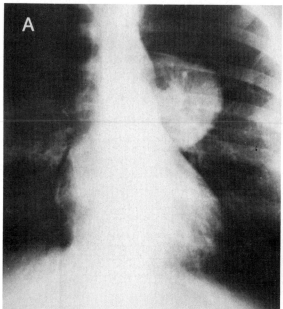 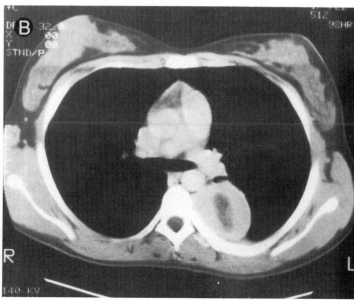

FIG 14–70.
Hyaline vascular type of Castleman disease. This 15-year-old girl presented with a respiratory history and a posterior mediastinal mass. **A,** frontal chest radiograph reveals a sharply marginated central mediastinal mass which on the lateral radiograph (not shown) was posterior in location. **B,** CECT scan reveals the poste-rior mediastinal location of the mass which shows marked periph-eral enhancement with central low attenuation. Marked enhance-ment is typical of Castleman disease. The diagnosis was surgically proved. (Courtesy of Dr. Eric Effman, Seattle, and Duke University Medical Center, Durham, NC.)

preoperative information by demonstrating the pre-cise size and location of the lesion, its anatomical re-lationship to other organs, and, perhaps most im-portant, its transdiaphragmatic extent into the abdo-men.

Lymphangiomas can occur in the posterior me-diastinum, although they are more commonly found anteriorly. Their avascular nature and extent can be nicely demonstrated on CECT. These lesions may extend across the midline (Fig 14–69).

Non-Hodgkin lymphoma, metastatic neuroblas-toma, and, rarely, other types of metastatic malig-nancy can involve the posterior mediastinal and ret-rocrural nodes. These lesions present with paraspi-nal widening, suggesting disease both above and be-low the diaphragm. The adenopathy of Castleman disease can rarely present in the posterior mediasti-num (Fig 14–70).

Siegel et al. (1981) described two cases of poste-rior mediastinal mass due to inflammatory lymphad-enopathy secondary to severe esophagitis and gas-troesophageal reflux. Probably more common is an inflammatory mass due to diskitis or spondylitis. The mass is often relatively small and may be associ-ated with disk space narrowing and vertebral body destruction, which is well demonstrated by either CT or MR. Spondylitis with a paravertebral mass from tuberculosis has been rarely seen in children in the United States, but with a recurrence of tubercu-losis, this may change.

Vascular lesions can present as posterior medias-tinal masses. These occur less commonly in children than in adults, but aortic aneurysms of either my-cotic or connective tissue origin can be seen. Dilata-tion of the azygos and hemiazygos veins serving as collateral channels can be seen if the inferior vena cava is congenitally absent or obstructed.

Posteriorly situated pneumonias can simulate mediastinal masses. The clinical picture or follow-up radiographs usually establish the diagnosis. A se-questration of the lung may appear on chest radiog-raphy to arise in the mediastinum. CT is helpful in these cases.

Chest wall masses due to benign, malignant, or inflammatory lesions may simulate mediastinal le-sions if they arise either anteriorly or posteriorly; when they are more lateral, an intrapulmonary pro-cess may be mimicked. Lipomas, lipoblastomas, and benign or malignant mesenchymal tumors occur. Ewing sarcoma and rhabdosarcoma are the malig-nant lesions that occur most frequently. Actinomy-cosis may extend to the chest wall from a pulmonary lesion, and primary osteomyelitis of the rib can also be seen. Plain film findings are usually limited to vi-sualization of the mass itself; bone destruction may be noted in either the malignant or inflammatory le-

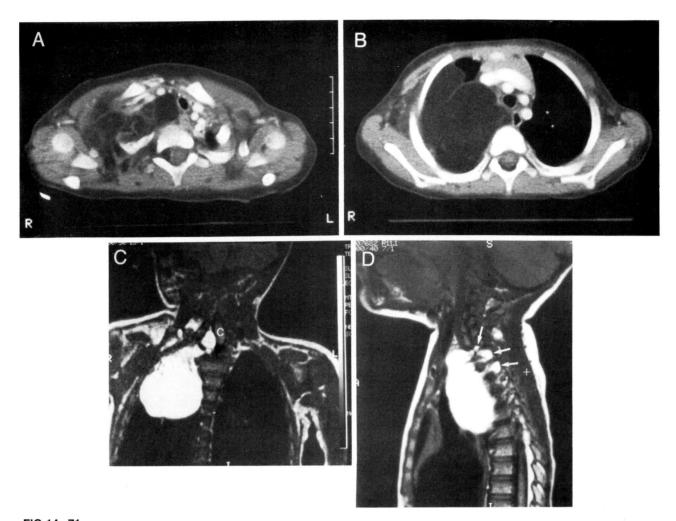

FIG 14–71.

Lipoblastoma in an 18-month-old boy who presented with a right cervical mass and mediastinal mass on the chest roentgenogram. **A,** UFCT at the level of the thoracic inlet reveals a low-density multiseptated mass that is infiltrating the soft tissues of the neck and displacing the trachea *(T)*. Intraspinal extension *(arrows)* is also noted. **B,** lower section through the upper thorax reveals a huge multiseptated mass of fat density infiltrating the mediastinum. No intraspinal extension is present at this level. **C,** coronal T1-weighted, 2.5 mm MR image reveals intraspinal extension with slight displacement of the cord *(C)* **D,** sagittal T1-weighted image to the right of the midline reveals intraspinal extension at three levels *(arrows)*. Note the pattern of extension along the nerve roots similar to that seen in the patient with neuroblastoma (see Fig 14–63,C).

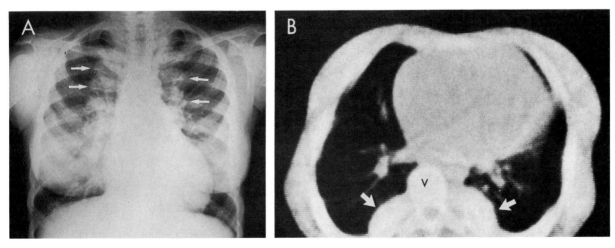

FIG 14–72.

Extramedullary hematopoiesis presenting as paravertebral masses. **A,** 17-year-old girl with known thalassemia. Note large paravertebral masses *(arrows)*. **B,** CT scan in same patient. *(Arrows)* indicate areas of extramedullary hematopoiesis. *V* = vertebral body.

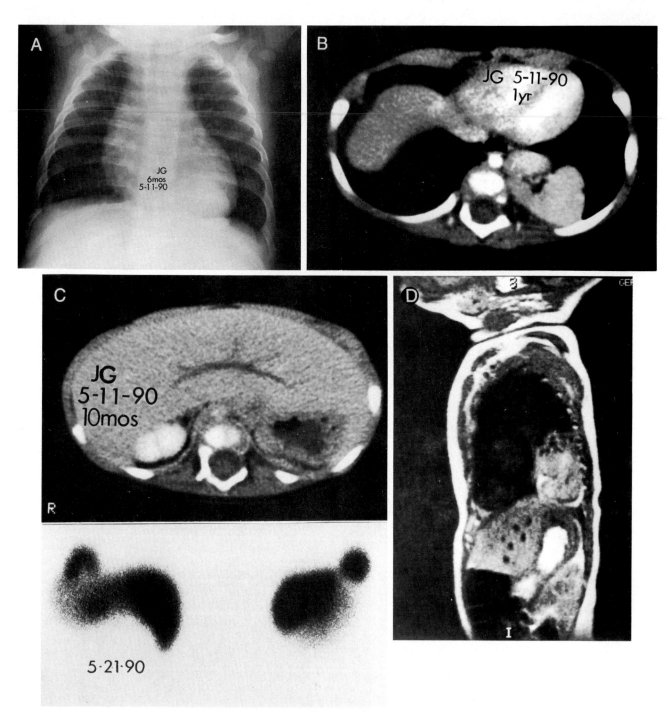

FIG 14–73.
Mediastinal mass caused by intrathoracic spleen. **A,** frontal radiograph at 6 months of age shows an apparent posterior mediastinal mass. **B,** contrast-enhanced CT scan reveals a posterior mass with a lobulated appearance that resembles a kidney, but the mass does not opacify as much as the kidney normally does. **C,** CT scan image at a level inferior to **B** through the liver fails to document the presence of an intra-abdominal spleen. Interestingly, the liver has a transverse position, similar to that identified in patients with asplenia. **D,** sagittal, T1-weighted MRI reveals the mass to imaging characteristics consistent with splenic tissue. **E,** technetium sulfur colloid scan reveals the mass to accumulate radionuclide, consistent with splenic tissue.

sions. Fatty tumors may be recognized on CT by their low density, and on MR by their short T1, but the other lesions cannot be distinguished from one another, although cross-sectional imaging is of value in determining location and extent of disease (Fig 14–71).

Extramedullary hematopoiesis should be considered a possible cause for a mediastinal mass in any patient with severe anemia. The characteristic radiographic findings are multiple smooth or lobulated paravertebral masses (Fig 14–72).

Anterior or lateral meningoceles are rare mediastinal masses due to spinal canal anomalies in which the leptomeninges herniate through the neural foramina. These lesions occur mostly in patients with neurofibromatosis, usually in conjunction with kyphoscoliosis, with the meningocele at the convex apex of the curve. MRI is the diagnostic method of choice.

Organs extending through the diaphragm through a posterior Bochdalek hernia or under an eventration such as ectopic kidney, liver, or spleen may simulate mediastinal masses or pulmonary lesions (Fig 14–73). A large hiatal hernia may project either as a middle or posterior mediastinal mass.

REFERENCES

General References

Felman AH: *Radiology of the Pediatric Chest.* New York, McGraw-Hill, 1987.

Felson B: *Principles of Chest Roentgenology.* Philadelphia, WB Saunders, 1973, p 251.

Fraser RG, Pare JAP: *Diagnosis of Diseases of the Chest.* ed 2. Philadelphia, WB Saunders, 1977, p 149.

Glasier CM, Leithiser RE Jr, Williamson SL, et al: Extracardiac chest ultrasonography in infants and children: Radiographic and clinical implications. *J Pediatr* 1989; 114:540.

Heitzman ER: The mediastinum: *Radiologic correlations with Anatomy and Pathology,* ed 2. New York, 1988, Springer Verlag.

Heitzman ER, Scrivani JV, Martino J, et al: The azygos vein and its pleural reflections: Normal roentgen anatomy. *Radiology* 1971; 101:249.

King MR, Telander RL, Smithson W, et al: Primary mediastinal tumors in children. *J Pediatr* 1982; 17:512.

Kirks DR, Effmann EL, Osborn D: Chest masses in infants and children: A selective overview. In Putman CD (ed): *Pulmonary Diagnosis.* New York, Appleton-Century-Crofts, 1981.

Liu P, Daneman A, Stringer DA: Real-time sonography of mediastinal and juxtamediastinal masses in infants and children. *J Can Assoc Radiol* 1988; 39:198.

Merten DF: Diagnostic imaging of mediastinal masses in children. *AJR* 1992; 158:825–832.

Parker B, Castellino R: *Pediatric Oncologic Radiology.* St Louis, Mosby–Year Book, 1977.

Patriquin H, Beauregard G, Dunbar JS: The right pleuromediastinal reflection in children. *J Can Assoc Radiol* 1976; 27:9.

Proto AV, Speckman JM: The left lateral radiograph of the chest. *Med Radiogr Photogr* 1979; 55:30.

Siegel MJ: Chest applications of magnetic resonance imaging in children. *Top Magn Reson Imaging* 1990; 3:1.

Wernecke K, Vassallo P, Potter R, et al: Mediastinal tumors: Sensitivity of detection with sonography compared with CT and radiography. *Radiology* 1990; 175:137.

Whalen JP, et al: The retrosternal line: A new sign of an anterior mediastinal mass. *Am J Roentgenol* 1973; 117:861.

Diseases of the Mediastinum

Ablin DS, Reinhart MA: Esophageal perforation with mediastinal abscess in child abuse. *Pediatr Radiol* 1990; 20:524.

Bowen A, Quattromani FL: Infraazygous pneumomediastinum in the newborn. *Am J Roentgenol* 1980; 135:1017.

Burton EM, Riggs W Jr, Kaufman RA, et al: Pneumomediastinum caused by foreign body aspiration in children. *Pediatr Radiol* 1989; 20:45.

Carrol CL, Jeffrey RB Jr, Federle MP, et al: CT evaluation of mediastinal infections. *J Comput Assist Tomogr* 1987; 11:449.

Cohen MD, Weber TR, Sequeira FW, et al: The diagnostic dilemma of the posterior mediastinal thymus: CT manifestations. *Radiology* 1983; 146:691.

Macklin MT, Macklin CC: Malignant interstitial emphysema of the lungs and mediastinum as an important occult complication in many respiratory diseases and other conditions: An interpretation of the clinical literature in the light of laboratory experience. *Medicine (Baltimore)* 1944; 23:281.

Pollack MS: Staphylococcal mediastinitis due to sternoclavicular pyarthrosis: CT appearance. *J Comput Assist Tomogr* 1990; 14:924.

Quattromani FL, Foley LC, Bowen A, et al: Fascial relationship of the thymus: Radiologic-pathologic correlation in neonatal pneumomediastinum. *Am J Roentgenol* 1981; 137:1209.

Anterior Mediastinal Masses

Abramson SJ, Berdon WE, Reilly BJ, et al: Cavitation of anterior mediastinal masses in children with histiocytosis-X: Report of four cases with radiographic-pathologic findings and clinical follow-up. *Pediatr Radiol* 1987; 17:10.

Bar-Ziv J, Barki Y, Itzchak Y, et al: Posterior mediastinal accessory thymus. *Pediatr Radiol* 1984; 14:165.

Bode U, Scheidt W: Change of thymic size during and following cytotoxic therapy in young patients. *Pediatr Radiol* 1988; 18:20.

Caffey J, Silbey R: Regrowth of the thymus after atrophy induced by the oral administration of adrenocorticosteroids to human infants. *Pediatrics* 1960; 26:761.

Castellino RA, Blank N, Hoppe RT, et al: Hodgkin disease: Contributions of chest CT in the initial staging evaluation. *Radiology* 1986; 160:603.

Cory DA, Cohen MD, Smith JA: Thymus in the superior mediastinum simulating adenopathy: Appearance on CT. *Radiology* 1987; 162:457.

Day DL, Gedgaudas E: The thymus. *Radiol Clin North Am* 1984; 22:519–538.

deGeer G, Webb WR, Gamsu G: Normal thymus: Assessment with MR and CT. *Radiology* 1986; 158:313.

Faerber EN, Balsara RK, Schidlow DV, et al: Thymolipoma: Computed tomographic appearances. *Pediatr Radiol* 1990; 20:196.

Fagin CJ, Swischuk LE: Traumatic lung and paramediastinal pneumatoceles. *Radiology* 1976; 120:11.

Fox MA, Vix VA: Endodermal sinus (yolk sac) tumor of the anterior mediastinum. *Am J Roentgenol* 1980; 135:291.

Glenn LD, Kumar PP: The residual mediastinal mass following radiation therapy for Hodgkin's disease. *Am J Clin Oncol* 1991; 14:16.

Han BK, Babcock DS, Oestreich AE: Normal thymus in infancy: Sonographic characteristics. *Radiology* 1989; 170:471–474.

Heiberg E, Wolverson MK, Sundaram M, et al: Normal thymus: CT characteristics in subjects under age 20. *Am J Roentgenol* 1982; 138:491.

Heron CW, Husband JE, Williams MP: Hodgkin disease: CT of the thymus. *Radiology* 1988; 167:647.

Ishii K, Maeda K, Hashihira M, et al: MRI of mediastinal cavernous hemangioma. *Pediatr Radiol* 1990; 20:556.

Jaramillo D, Perez-Atayde A, Griscom NT: Apparent association between thymic cysts and prior thoracotomy. *Radiology* 1989; 172:207.

Johnson PM, Berdon WE, Baker D, et al: Thymic uptake of gallium 67 citrate in a healthy four-year-old boy. *Pediatr Radiol* 1978; 7:243.

Joseph AE, Donaldson JS, Reynolds M: Neck and thorax venous aneurysm: Association with cystic hygroma. *Radiology* 1989; 170:109.

Kuhn JP, Neeson H: Magnetic resonance imaging of the normal thymus, in Naidich DP, Zerhouni EA, Siegelman SS (eds): *Computed Tomography and Magnetic Resonance of the Thorax,* ed 2. New York, Raven Press, 1991.

Lanning P, Heikkinen E: Thymus simulating left upper lobe atelectasis. *Pediatr Radiol* 1980; 9:177.

Lemaitre L, Leclerc F, Dubos JP, et al: Thymic hemorrhage: A cause of acute symptomatic mediastinal widening in an infant with late haemorrhagic disease. Sonographic findings. *Pediatr Radiol* 1989; 19:128.

Levine C: Cervical presentation of a large thymic cyst: CT appearance. *J Comput Assist Tomogr* 1988; 12:656.

Levitt RG, Husband JE, Glazer HS: CT of primary germ-cell tumors of the mediastinum. *Am J Roentgenol* 1984; 142:73.

Molina PL, Siegel MJ, Glazer HS: Thymic masses on MR imaging. *Am J Roentgenol* 1990; 155:495.

Odagiri K, Nishihira K, Hatekeyama S, et al: Anterior mediastinal masses with calcifications on CT in children with histiocytosis-X (Langerhans cell histiocytosis). *Pediatr Radiol* 1991; 21:550–551.

O'Sullivan P, Daneman A, Chan HS, et al: Extragonadal endodermal sinus tumors in children: Review of 24 cases. *Pediatr Radiol* 1983; 13:249.

Palmer WE, Rivitz SM, Chew FS: Bilateral bronchogenic cysts. *Am J Roentgenol* 1991; 157:950.

Polanski SM, Brawick DW, Ravin CE: Primary mediastinal seminoma. *Am J Roentgenol* 1979; 132:21.

Rollins NK, Currarino G: MR imaging of posterior mediastinal thymus. *J Comput Assist Tomogr* 1988; 12:518.

Salonen OLM, Kivisaari ML, Somer JK: Computed tomography of the thymus of children under 10 years. *Pediatr Radiol* 1984; 14:373.

Seline TH, Gross BH, Francis IR: CT and MR imaging of mediastinal hemangiomas. *J Comput Assist Tomogr* 1990; 14:766.

Siegel MJ, Glazer HS, Wiener JL. et al: Normal and abnormal thymus in childhood: MR imaging. *Radiology* 1989; 172:367.

Sumner TE, Volbert FM, Kiser PE, et al: Mediastinal cystic hygroma in children. *Pediatr Radiol* 1981; 11:160.

Thompson DP, Moore TC: Acute thoracic distress in childhood due to spontaneous rupture of a large mediastinal teratoma. *J Pediatr Surg* 1969; 4:416.

Tobias JD, Bozeman PM: Pneumococcal abscess presenting as an anterior mediastinal mass in an eight-year-old child. *Pediatr Infect Dis J* 1990; 9:916.

Toye R, Armstrong P, Dacie JE: Lymphangiohaemangioma of the mediastinum. *Br J Radiol* 1991; 64:62.

Wernecke K, Vassallo P, Rutsch F, et al: Thymic involvement in Hodgkin disease: CT and sonographic findings. *Radiology* 1991; 181:375.

Yeh H, Gordon A, Kirschner PA, et al: Computed tomography and sonography of thymolipoma. *Am J Roentgenol* 1983; 14:1131.

Middle Mediastinal Masses

Bourgouin PM, Shepard JO, Moore EH, et al: Plexiform neurofibromatosis of the mediastinum: CT appearance. *Am J Roentgenol* 1988; 151:461.

Crombleholme TM, deLorimier AA, Adzick NS, et al: Mediastinal pancreatic pseudocysts in children. *J Pediatr Surg* 1990; 25:843.

Filly R, Blank N, Castellino RA: Radiographic distribution of intrathoracic disease in previously untreated patients with

Hodgkin's and non-Hodgkin's lymphoma. *Radiology* 1976; 120:277.

Im J, Song KS, Kang HS, et al: Mediastinal tuberculous lymphadenitis: CT manifestations. *Radiology* 1987; 164:115.

Khoury MB, Godwin JD, Halvorsen R, et al: Role of chest CT in non-Hodgkin lymphoma. *Radiology* 1986; 158:659.

Landay MJ, Rollins NK: Mediastinal histoplasmosis granuloma: Evaluation with CT. *Radiology* 1989; 172:657.

Mandel GA, Lantieri R, Goodman LR: Tracheobronchial compression in Hodgkin lymphoma in children. *Am J Roentgenol* 1982; 139:1167.

Martin KW, Siegel MJ, Chesna E: Spontaneous resolution of mediastinal cysts. *Am J Roentgenol* 1988; 150:1131.

Panicek DM, Harty MP, Scicutella CJ, et al: Calcification in untreated mediastinal lymphoma. *Radiology* 1988; 166:735.

Park C, Webb WR, Klein JS: Inferior hilar window. *Radiology* 1991; 178:163.

Ramenofsky ML, Leape LL, McCauley RGK: Bronchogenic cyst. *J Pediatr Surg* 1979; 14:219.

Sharma S, Puri S, Chaturvedi P, et al: Mediastinal pancreatic pseudocyst and rupture of diaphragm. *Pediatr Radiol* 1988; 18:337.

Weiner M, Leventhal B, Cantor A, et al: Gallium-67 scans as an adjunct to computed tomography scans for the assessment of a residual mediastinal mass in pediatric patients with Hodgkin's disease. *Cancer* 1991; 68:2478–2480.

Posterior Mediastinal Masses

Armstrong EA, Harwood-Nash DCF, Fitz CR, et al: CT of neuroblastomas and ganglioneuromas in children. *Am J Roentgenol* 1982; 139:571.

Bar-Ziv J, Nogrady MB: Mediastinal neuroblastoma and ganglioneuroma: Differentiation between primary and secondary involvement of the chest radiograph. *Am J Roentgenol* 1975; 125:380.

Geremia GK, Russell EJ, Clasen RA: MR imaging characteristics of a neurenteric cyst. *AJNR* 1988; 9:978.

Grosfeld JL, O'Neal J, Clatworthy HW: Enteric duplication in infancy and childhood: 18-year review. *Ann Surg* 1970; 172:83.

Kawashima A, Fishman EK, Kuhlman JE, et al: CT of posterior mediastinal masses. *Radiographics* 1991; 11:1045.

Malmgren N, Laurin S, Ivancev K, et al: Mediastinal pseudomass: Pneumonia and atelectasis behind the left pulmonary ligament. *Pediatr Radiol* 1987; 17:451.

Siegel MJ, Shackelford GD, McAlister WH: Posterior mediastinal masses secondary to lymphadenitis from esophagitis. *Radiology* 1981; 140:277.

So CB, Li DKB: Anterolateral cervical meningocele in association with neurofibromatosis: MR and CT studies. *J Comput Assist Tomogr* 1989; 13:692.

Solomon GE, Chutorian AM: Opsoclonus: An occult neuroblastoma. *N Engl J Med* 1968; 279:475.

Weiss LM, Fagelman D, Warhit JM: CT demonstration of esophageal duplication cyst. *J Comput Assist Tomogr* 1983; 7:716.

Whyte AM, Powell N: Case report: Mediastinal lipoblastoma of infancy. *Clin Radiol* 1990; 42:205.

PART III

The Heart and Great Vessels

VIRGIL R. CONDON

RICHARD B. JAFFE

15

Introduction: Overview of Heart Disease

SECTION 1

Overview of Heart Disease

Heart disease is the fifth most common cause of death in infants and children. Congenital cardiac lesions account for approximately 90% of these fatalities. Congenital heart disease (CHD) occurs in approximately 1% of all live births. Ventricular septal defect (VSD) is the most common CHD (28%), followed by atrial septal defect (ASD) (10%), pulmonary valvular stenosis (PVS) (10%), patent ductus arteriosus (PDA) (10%), tetralogy of Fallot (10%), aortic stenosis (AS) (7%), coarctation (5%), transposition (5%), and miscellaneous lesions (15%) (Keith) (Table 15–1).

Other factors that play an important role in the incidence of CHD relate to genetic and environmental factors, parental age, chromosomal aberrations, and syndrome-related lesions.

Two thirds of infants who die of CHD do so within the first year of life, one third within the first month. The most common cause of death in the first year relates to hypoplastic left heart syndrome. Severe coarctation, critical AS, and transposition of the great arteries are other important causes of death in this age group.

CLINICAL PRESENTATIONS

The primary clinical presentation of congenital and acquired heart disease is (1) congestive heart failure (CHF) or (2) cyanosis, or both. CHF, particularly in infants, is frequently diagnosed late and often mistaken for infection or other pulmonary processes. Other manifestations in the neonate include (1) failure to thrive, (2) tachypnea, and (3) poor feeding. CHF usually relates to (1) pressure overload from

TABLE 15–1.

Incidence of Congenital Heart Disease (%)

Diagnosis	Keith et al.*	Bound and Logan†	Mitchell et al.‡	Kenna et al.§	Rose et al.¶	Hoffman‖	Average
Ventricular septal defect—all types	28	27	29	30	33	31	29
Atrial septal defect—all types	10	15	11	8	12	10	11
Secundum	(7)	(8)	(7)	(6)		(6)	7
Primum/atrioventricular canal	(3)	(7)	(4)	(2)		(4)	4
Pulmonary stenosis—all types	10	2	10	8	11	13	9
Patent ductus arteriosus	10	6	7	10	7	6	8
Tetralogy of Fallot	10	8	5	4	8	4	6
Aortic stenosis—all types	7	4	3	5	9	4	5
Coarctation of aorta	5	5	3	5	3	6	5
Transposition of great vessels	5	4	3	6	3	4	4
Dextrocardia	2	—	—	—	1	—	2
Common ventricle	2	1	1	—	—	1	1
Hypoplastic left-heart syndrome	2	3	3	—	—	1	2
Total anomalous pulmonary venous return	1	2	—	—	2	1	2
Partial anomalous pulmonary venous return	1	—	—	—	—	—	1
Vascular rings	1	—	1	—	—	—	1
Tricuspid atresia	1	1	1	1	1	—	1
Endocardial fibroelastosis	1	—	2	—	1	—	1
Hypoplastic right heart syndrome	1	—	1	—	—	1	1
Truncus arteriosus	1	1	2	1	—	2	1
Double-outlet right ventricle	1	—	—	—	—	1	1
Miscellaneous (aortic insufficiency; Ebstein anomaly, coronary artery anomaly; mitral stenosis; mitral insufficiency; aorticopulmonary window; interrupted aortic arch; pulmonary hypoplasia; etc.)	3	13	6	22	6	18	11

*Keith JD, Rowe RD, Vlad P: *Heart Disease in Infancy and Childhood,* ed 3. New York, Macmillan, 1978.
†Bound JP, Logan WFWE: Incidence of congenital heart disease in Blackpool, 1957–1971. *Br Heart J* 1977; 39:445–450.
‡Mitchell SC, Korones SB, Berendes HW: Congenital heart disease in 56,109 births: Incidence and natural history. *Circulation* 1971; 43:323.
§Kenna AP, Smithells RW, Fielding DW: Congenital heart disease in Liverpool, 1960–1969. *Q J Med* 1975; 44:17–44.
¶Rose V, Boyd ARJ, Ashton TE: Incidence of heart disease in children in the city of Toronto. *Can Med Assoc J* 1964; 91:95.
‖Hoffman JIE: Congenital heart disease in 19,502 births. *Am J Cardiol* 1978; 42:641.

obstructive lesions; (2) volume overload, i.e., high output states, left-to-right shunt, or valvular insufficiency; and (3) myocardial damage, i.e., hypoxia and infection. The patient's age at the time of presentation with CHF is of considerable value in predicting the cause of failure (Table 15–2). In the first few hours, CHF usually relates to (1) volume overload or (2) arrhythmia. Hypoplastic left heart syndrome (aortic valve atresia) with pressure overload is the most common etiology in the first week of life. Coarctation is the usual cause in the second and third weeks. After 1 month, as the pulmonary resistance decreases, left-to-right shunts are the primary cause for failure.

Cyanosis may relate to either CHF or CHD with right-to-left or admixture shunting (Table 15–3). Severe cyanosis in the first week of life is usually associated with (1) transposition of the great arteries, (2) hypoplastic right heart syndrome with pulmonary atresia, or (3) total anomalous pulmonary venous re-

turn with obstruction. In the first few weeks of life, less severe cyanosis is more likely associated with (1) tetralogy of Fallot, (2) truncus arteriosus, or (3) total anomalous pulmonary venous return without obstruction.

Roentgenographic manifestations of CHD with CHF include (1) cardiomegaly, (2) diffuse haziness of vascular structures, (3) hyperinflation, (4) thymic atrophy, and (5) interstitial and minor pleural fluid (Fig 15–1).

DEVELOPMENT AND GROWTH

An in-depth discussion of the development and embryology of the heart is beyond the scope of this text. Those interested in a more complete discussion are referred to Moore's *The Developing Human* and Patten's *Human Embryology.*

The heart tube develops in the primitive embryo from fusion of a pair of vessels arising from the me-

TABLE 15–2.

Congestive Heart Failure Etiologies, by Patient Age

0–24 hours
   Intrauterine arrhythmia
   Placental transfusion
   Hypoplastic left heart syndrome (rare)
1–7 days
   Hypoplastic left heart syndrome—most common (usually
      appears within 24–48 hr)
   Total anomalous pulmonary venous return with obstruction
   Persistent fetal circulation
   Diabetic mother
   Myocardial dysfunction—hypoxia, acidosis, sepsis
   Arteriovenous malformation (and other volume overload)
2–4 weeks
   Coarctation syndrome (with ventricular septal defect/patent
      ductus arteriosus)—most common (usually appears within
      7–14 days)
   Critical aortic stenosis
   Tachyarrhythmia
   Transposition of the great arteries
   Cardiomyopathies—endocardial fibroelastosis
   Anomalous left coronary artery
   Large left-to-right shunts
   Complex malformation, common ventricle, etc.
1–4 months
   Left-to-right shunts
      Ventricular septal defect
      Atrial septal defect
      Patent ductus arteriosus
      Atrioventricular canal
   Truncus arteriosus
   Transposition of the great arteries (other forms, e.g., double-
      outlet right ventricle)
   Cardiomyopathies (endocardial fibroelastosis)
   Total anomalous pulmonary venous return without obstruction

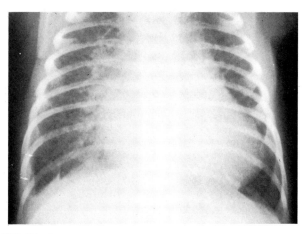

FIG 15–1.
Congestive heart failure at 10 days, secondary to coarctation. Pulmonary venous congestion with interstitial fluid lines in the costophrenic angle and minor pleural fluid *(arrows)* can be seen. Note cardiomegaly and hyperinflation.

cephalic wall of the primitive atrium and grows ventrocaudad toward a septum originating from the atrioventricular canal. The initial passage between these two developing septa will form the foramen primum of the interatrial septum. During the sixth week of embryonic life, the cephalic portion of the septum primum divides to form the ostium secundum. A second septum (septum secundum) appears in the sixth embryonic week as a fold from the ventrocephalic wall of the atrium and grows dorsocephalad to overlap the ostium secundum and eventually form the foramen ovale. Failure of this septum to form properly produces the ostium secundum ASD. The common ventricle is divided into left and right ventricles by a crescentic ridge that appears near the apex of the common ventricle, with ridges extending on the dorsal and ventral aspect to the atrioventricu-

TABLE 15–3.

Etiologies of Cyanotic Congenital Heart Disease, by Patient Age

0–7 days—severe cyanosis
   Transposition of the great arteries
   Hypoplastic right heart syndrome
   Hypoplastic left heart syndrome
   Ebstein malformation and tricuspid insufficiency
   Tricuspid atresia
   Total anomalous pulmonary venous return with obstruction
1–4 weeks
   Tetralogy of Fallot—most common
   Truncus arteriosus
   Total anomalous pulmonary venous return without obstruction
   Left-to-right shunts (large) with congestive heart failure (usually
      subclinical cyanosis)
1 month and older
   Pulmonary hypertension with reversing shunt
   Pulmonary arteriovenous malformations

soderm that covers the ventral aspect of the foregut. Rapid growth of this tube leads to a marked ventral flexure, proceeding to a series of dilatations. The most cephalic of these, the bulbus cordis and the ventricle, lie on the ventrocephalic side of this redundant loop; the more dorsocaudal dilatation is the developing atrium. These dilatations are connected by a constricted portion to become the atrioventricular canal. The truncus arteriosus arises from the cephalic end of the bulbus cordis, while the systemic venous drainage of the embryo empties into the dorsal portion of the atrium. In the fourth embryonic week, the bulboventricular loop twists sharply to the right; the bulbus cordis now joins the ventricle at a right angle before passing up on the ventral aspect of the heart.

Before this common tubular heart can become a four-chambered structure, septation must occur at the atrial and ventricular level. Two primary septa form to develop the interatrial septum. The first, or septum primum, develops as a fold from the dorso-

lar cushion. The atrioventricular cushion similarly has developed in the fifth week of intrauterine life from two cushions that have appeared and begun to grow from the dorsal and ventral aspects of the atrioventricular constriction. The fusions of these atrioventricular septa give rise to the primitive tricuspid and mitral valves. Defects in the normal growth pattern of the dorsal and ventral atrial ventricular canal septa lead to the variety of atrioventricular canal defects noted clinically. Eventual closure of the common ventricle results from the fusion of the right and left ridges of the apical ridge; this continued growth proceeds into the cavity of the bulbus cordis, dividing it into an infundibular portion and the aortic vestibule. Simultaneous with the development of the interventricular septum occurs a torsion of the bulbus cordis and ventricles. Final fusion of the interventricular septum occurs as an extension of tissue arising from the inferior atrioventricular cushion and forms the fibrous or membranous portions of the interventricular septum.

In addition to the division of the ventricular chambers, two additional developing ridges continue the division of the bulbus cordis into the aortic vestibule and infundibulum. During the fifth week of embryonic life, the outlines of the pulmonary and aortic valve become evident at the apex of the infundibulum and aortic vestibule, respectively. By the eighth week, the pulmonary and aortic valves have fairly well demarcated cusps and leaflets. Developmental failures in these areas result in the various forms of valvular and subvalvular aortic and pulmonary stenosis. Anomalous development in the bulboventricular area with abnormal torsion causes the various forms of transposition. The final stages in cardiac development are the division of the truncus arteriosus into the ascending aorta and pulmo-

nary arteries, along with the development of aortic arches, which are discussed with the various anomalies of these arches in Chapter 17. Separation of the truncus arteriosus into the ascending aorta and pulmonary artery results from an outgrowth of mesenchymous tissue from both sides of the truncus toward the bulbus cordis. This division takes a spiral course so that the final aortic pulmonary septum represents a relative spiral with the base of the pulmonary artery originating to the left of the aortic root. Failure in the spiral development of this truncus arteriosus septum leads to various forms of truncus arteriosus, aortic pulmonary windows, and transposition of the great arteries.

The mean weight of the heart in a full-term newborn is approximately 17 g, with a disproportionate prominence of the right ventricle. During the first month of life there is a 25% increase in cardiac weight, primarily due to an increase in left ventricular mass. Subsequently, the rate of growth is less than that of the body as a whole and of most other organs. The heart doubles in weight during the first year, and is four times its birth weight after 5 years.

REFERENCES

Development and Growth

Dawes GS: *Fetal and Neonatal Physiology.* St Louis, Mosby–Year Book, 1968.

Duckworth JWA: Embryology of congenital heart disease, in Keth JD, Rowe RD, Vlad P (eds): *Heart Disease in Infancy and Childhood.* New York, Macmillan, 1978, pp 129–152.

Moore KL: *The Developing Human.* Philadelphia, WB Saunders, 1974.

Patten BN: *Human Embryology,* ed 3. New York, Blakiston, 1968.

SECTION 2

Cardiac Evaluation

ROUTINE CHEST ROENTGENOGRAPHY

Posteroanterior (PA) or anteroposterior (AP) and lateral chest roentgenograms should be the initial imaging modality for suspected cardiac disease. Critical attention to good inspiration, motion, exposure factors,

and position and rotation are mandatory. Oblique views and barium swallow have little place in the evaluation of the cardiac patient except for anomalies of the aortic arch and pulmonary arteries. Chest fluoroscopy is useful for the evaluation of cardiac calcifications and prosthetic valve motion.

Roentgenographic manifestations of CHF and CHD vary considerably, particularly in the neonate, and recognition is often complicated by pulmonary disease, atelectasis, and increased pulmonary blood flow. Cardiomegaly is usually present, although the configuration of the heart is frequently nonspecific. In rare situations (e.g., obstructed total anomalous pulmonary venous return), the heart size may be normal or even small. In the neonate, plain films usually show loss of sharp definition of the broncho-vascular structures (see Fig 15–1). Rarely is there evidence of interstitial or interlobular fluid or significant pleural effusion unless severe pulmonary venous obstruction is present, as in obstructed total anomalous pulmonary venous return. The thymus is usually atrophic, and exaggerated inspiratory effort (air hunger) produces flattening of the diaphragm. In the older child, findings may be similar to those in the adult with pulmonary vascular redistribution into the upper lungs, interstitial septal (Kerley B) lines, fluid retention, and pleural effusion.

The differential diagnosis of the patient with CHD and congestive failure from an infant or child with pneumonia or other diffuse pulmonary process may be very difficult. Group B streptococcal sepsis in the neonate may be particularly confusing, with most of the clinical and roentgenographic findings quite similar. Differentiation will necessitate the use of other diagnostic methods, including blood culture (and other laboratory tests) and echocardiography. Another primary differential consideration is transient tachypnea of the newborn where interstitial fluid, minor pleural fluid, and mild cardiomegaly may also present a very similar roentgenographic pattern. In the older infant, diffuse interstitial pulmonary disease, as frequently seen with viral infection, may produce some of the roentgenographic findings similar to CHF, including poor definition of vascular markings, hyperinflation, and thymic atrophy. Heart size and shape, however, remain normal and Kerley B lines or pleural effusion is rarely seen. It must be recognized that pulmonary disease frequently is present in patients with left-to-right shunts, especially those with Down syndrome.

Pulmonary Vasculature

Evaluating the pulmonary vasculature is the most important and difficult step in the systematic review of the chest roentgenogram in CHD. Difficulty is

TABLE 15–4.

Congenital Heart Disease Related to Pulmonary Blood Flow and Cyanosis

Cyanosis	Increased Flow	Normal Flow	Decreased Flow

Acyanotic	Ventricular septal defect (VSD)
	Patent ductus arteriosus
	Atrial septal defect (ASD)
	  Secundum
	  Primum
	Atrioventricular canal
	Partial anomalous pulmonary venous
	  return
	Levotransposition of the great arteries
	  with VSD
		Pulmonary stenosis
		Aortic stenosis
		Coarctation (interrupted aortic arch)
		Levotransposition of the great arteries
		  without associated defects
		Ebstein anomaly (without large ASD)
		Neonatal high pulmonary resistance
		  with left-to-right shunt lesions
			Cerebral arteriovenous malformation
			  (occasionally)

Cyanotic	Admixture lesions
	  Transposition of the great arteries,
	    with or without a single ventricle
	    with tricuspid atresia
	  Double-outlet right ventricle
	  Truncus arteriosus
	  Total anomalous pulmonary venous
	    return
		Pulmonary arteriovenous malformation
		Neonatal high pulmonary resistance
		  with admixture shunt lesions
			Severe pulmonary stenosis
			  VSD, tetralogy of Fallot
			  ASD or patent foramen ovale
			Pulmonary atresia
			  With VSD (pseudotruncus)
			  Without VSD (hypoplastic right
			    heart syndrome)
			Tricuspid atresia with small
			  VSD/pulmonary atresia
			Transposition of the great arteries
			  with pulmonary stenosis or
			  pulmonary atresia
			Common ventricle or double-outlet
			  right ventricle with pulmonary
			  stenosis
			Right-to-left atrial shunt, Ebstein
			  anomaly, congenital tricuspid
			  insufficiency

caused, in part, by the factors noted previously—overexposed, underexposed, or expiratory films—all of which may produce faulty interpretation.

Pulmonary flow may appear normal in the presence of clinical heart disease (Table 15–4). It should be emphasized that pulmonary flow in the presence of CHD is an age-related factor. The normally elevated pulmonary vascular resistance in the neonate may prevent the diagnosis of increased flow even in the presence of a typical left-to-right anatomical shunt lesion. It is also difficult to differentiate pulmonary arteries from veins in the neonate and young infant, whereas they become more discrete in the older child and the adult. The pulmonary vessels should be evaluated both centrally and peripherally. Centrally, the right pulmonary artery should be compared with the size of the trachea in the PA (AP) projection and normally should be of approximately equal size (Coussement and Gooding). In the lateral view, the left pulmonary artery should be compared with the trachea; they should be of similar size. In the end-on projection, the peripheral pulmonary vessels should be related to an accompanying bronchus (Fig 15–2). The transverse diameter of the vessels should not exceed the internal diameter of the bronchus in a patient with normal pulmonary flow. An increase in vessel size indicates a left-to-right shunt (volume overload), although occasionally the vessel appears enlarged secondary to pulmonary

venous hypertension and failure (pressure overload). Increased pulmonary flow is rarely seen with lesions where the ratio of pulmonary to systemic flow is less than 2:1. In patients with a left-to-right shunt, the main pulmonary artery is characteristically enlarged. A large central pulmonary artery is common in all children, particularly in teen-age females. Therefore, the size of the main pulmonary artery is probably of less diagnostic value than the size of the right and left segment or peripheral pulmonary vessels. It is important to learn to evaluate the hilar vasculature on a lateral chest film, especially in the neonate. Recognizing increased flow may be difficult on the AP film because of the overlying thymus or a large cardiac silhouette (Fig 15–3).

Decreased, like increased, pulmonary vascularity is difficult to recognize with a small right-to-left shunt. In lesions with major right-to-left shunt, there is a decrease in size of the central pulmonary arteries in relation to the trachea and, in general, a decrease in the prominence of the hilar vessels on both the frontal (Fig 15–4) and the lateral views. The peripheral lung appears unusually clear and hyperlucent, and one is rarely able to evaluate an end-on artery with accompanying bronchus. The diaphragm is frequently depressed as a secondary manifestation of hypoxemia. In severe disease, or in older patients with right-to-left shunting, increased bronchial artery flow may appear as a disorganized vascular pattern. Asymmetry in pulmonary vascularity may relate to unilateral peripheral pulmonary stenosis, pulmonary aplasia-hypoplasia, surgically created systemic-pulmonary shunts, patent ductus inserting peripherally into the left, or occasionally right pulmonary artery, and directional flow created by anatomical relationships of the right ventricular outflow tract, as in tetralogy of Fallot and transposition of the great vessels.

CHD is frequently complicated by the presence of CHF or pulmonary disease and may obscure the shunt vascularity until failure has been treated and the vessels become more discrete. Similarly, the pulmonary flow pattern may be obscured in the premature infant with respiratory distress syndrome.

Cardiomediastinal Silhouette

Evaluation of the cardiomediastinal silhouette in the infant is difficult for a variety of reasons. A large normal thymus is frequently present (see Fig 15–3). Its size is exaggerated on the supine AP projection and on a less-than-optimal inspiratory film. It is usually possible to distinguish the thymus by its slightly different and more radiolucent density. The caudal

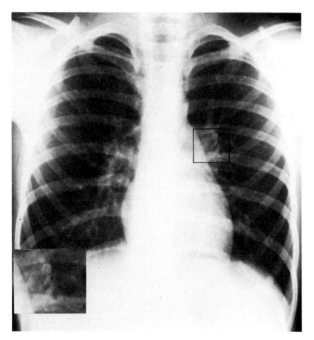

FIG 15–2.
Ventricular septal defect with left-to-right shunt. Mild enlargement of the central pulmonary arteries demonstrates reversed pulmonary artery bronchial size relationship *(inset).*

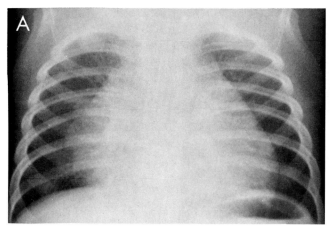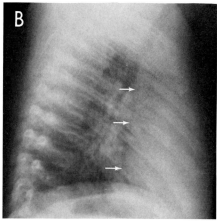

FIG 15–3.

Normal thymus: frontal **(A)** and lateral **(B)** chest films demonstrate a large cardiomediastinal silhouette caused predominantly by the large thymus, which obliterates the cardiac silhouette in the frontal view and fills in the anterior mediastinal space *(arrows)* in the lateral projection. The posterior cardiac contour is not enlarged.

margin can usually be identified as a minor indentation where it blends with the cardiac silhouette. The lateral film is also of considerable value in the differentiation of the thymus from an enlarged heart. The thymus may totally obscure the retrosternal space, and yet the posterior cardiac silhouette will be normal. Left ventricular–inferior vena caval relationships and left mainstem bronchial–cardiac relations will remain normal. Failure to visualize a normal thymic silhouette in children with CHD may indicate significant stress, related to CHF or hypoxemia, or both, with right-to-left shunts. Absence of the thymus is also a sign in a number of syndromes (e.g., DiGeorge syndrome).

Cardiac position, of course, should be critically

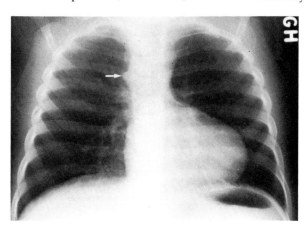

FIG 15–4.

Tetralogy of Fallot with decreased pulmonary blood flow. Central pulmonary arteries are small, and the peripheral lungs are hyperlucent; the diaphragm is depressed and the thymus atrophic, which is consistent with hypoxia. The right aortic arch pushes the trachea to the left and displaces the azygos vein lateral to the aortic arch *(arrow).*

evaluated; a major increase in CHD is frequent in patients having dextrocardia with situs solitus or levocardia with situs inversus (see Chapter 18). Mesocardia is a frequent finding that may or may not be related to CHD. Evaluation of systemic venous return from both the inferior and superior vena cava is helpful in diagnosing congenital heart problems (asplenia, polysplenia).

The size of the heart varies considerably with the age of the patient. In the neonate, a cardiac silhouette greater than 57% of the thoracic diameter on an AP 40-in. supine film with good inspiration indicates cardiomegaly and, therefore, heart disease (Edwards et al.). The cardiothoracic ratio gradually decreases during the first year of life and in the second year should not exceed 50% in an upright 6-ft. PA or AP chest film. A film obtained during good inspiration is vital when the cardiothoracic ratio is used as an index. The evaluation of specific heart chambers is particularly difficult in the infant, whereas prominence of any portion of the cardiac silhouette in the older child has the same implication for cardiac enlargement that one expects in the adult.

While the shape or silhouette of the heart is frequently nonspecific, certain classic configurations may well be indicative of a specific lesion. Classically, the coeur en sabot or boot-shaped heart is typical of tetralogy of Fallot (see Fig 15–4). The configuration results from the underlying pathologic condition, with the transversely orientated heart related to the right heart enlargement, and the concavity in the upper left heart border secondary to the small pulmonary artery resulting from the right-to-left shunt. In supracardiac total anomalous pulmonary venous return, the typical "snowman" configuration

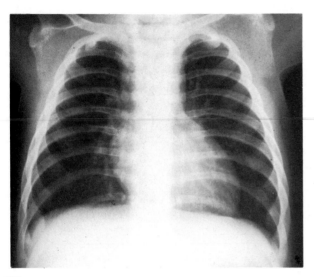

FIG 15–5.
Transposition of the great vessels. An egg-shaped cardiac silhouette secondary to transposition of the great vessels can be seen. The main pulmonary artery is inconspicuous because its medial position produces a narrow base for the heart. Thymic atrophy and hyperinflation secondary to hypoxia is evident. Pulmonary flow is only mildly increased in this patient without a VSD.

(see Fig 16–71) is due to a large left vertical vein and a dilated right superior vena cava. A prominent convex left upper heart border may be a fairly good indicator of levotransposition of the great arteries (see Fig 16–68) or a juxtaposed atrial appendage (see Fig 16–92), as frequently seen with tricuspid atresia and transposition. The egg-shaped or egg-on-side configuration, while certainly nonspecific, is suggestive of transposition of the great arteries (Fig 15–5) and is occasionally seen with truncus arteriosus. The triangular cardiac silhouette, indicative of a prominent right ventricle and right atrium with a small superior vena cava, may be quite suggestive of an ostium secundum ASD. Poststenotic dilatation of the ascending aorta is characteristic of valvular AS (Fig 15–6). The configuration seen in scimitar syndrome, showing the typical changes related to partial anomalous pulmonary venous return to the inferior vena cava (with associated pulmonary hypoplasia), is another classic cardiopulmonary silhouette (Fig 15–7).

It is particularly important to define the position of the aortic arch in vascular rings and congenital cardiac lesions associated with a right aortic arch (Table 15–5). In the infant, the aortic arch location can usually be determined by evaluating minor deviation of the trachea at the level of the aortic arch. An overpenetrated or filtered chest film may be necessary to see the trachea optimally (Fig 15–8). With these techniques, it can usually be identified ade-

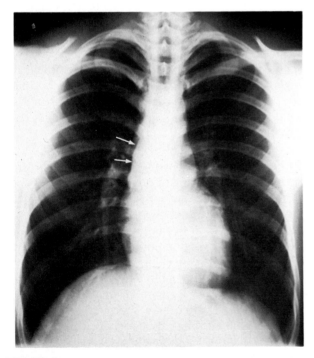

FIG 15–6.
Valvular aortic stenosis. Poststenotic dilatation of the ascending aorta *(arrows)* secondary to valvular aortic stenosis (AS). Dilatation of the aorta produces a slight prominence of the aortic arch, but not the more striking enlargement seen in patients with combined AS and aortic insufficiency.

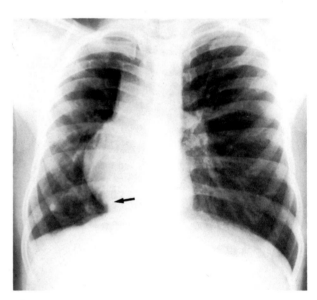

FIG 15–7.
Scimitar syndrome. Hypoplasia of the right lung and pulmonary artery with partial anomalous pulmonary venous return of the right lung to the inferior vena cava *(arrow)* and compensatory increased pulmonary blood flow to the left lung are evident.

TABLE 15–5.

Congenital Lesions Associated With a Right Aortic Arch

Tetralogy of Fallot
Tricuspid atresia
Truncus arteriosus
Dextrotransposition of great arteries with pulmonary stenosis
Ventricular septal defect
Aortic arch anomalies

TABLE 15–6.

Congenital Lesions Associated With a Prominent Main Pulmonary Artery

Valvular pulmonary stenosis
Left-to-right shunts
Truncus arteriosus—type I
Total anomalous pulmonary venous return

quately down to the level of the carina. While the trachea often deviates considerably in the extrathoracic segment, the deviation in the intrathoracic segment is almost always to the side opposite that of the aortic arch. If there is no tracheal deviation in the presence of CHD, interruption of the aortic arch is an important consideration (Jaffe). The presence of a right-sided aortic arch is suggestive of tetralogy of Fallot (30%), truncus arteriosus (25%), tricuspid atresia, (20%), VSD (5%), and transposition of the great vessels with pulmonary stenosis. The visual-

ization of a right aortic arch in the absence of intrinsic CHD usually indicates some form of double aortic arch or arch anomaly.

The configuration of the aorta also merits special attention in relation to coarctation of the aorta. The figure-3 sign is usually evident on plain films, showing indentation due to the coarctation and the poststenotic segment of the aorta immediately below it (Fig 15–9,*A*). The proximal segment may or may not appear dilated, depending upon whether it represents an isolated discrete coarctation or is associated with a hypoplastic aortic isthmus. The converse manifestation can be seen on an esophagram, where an E sign can be observed, with the lower portion of the E secondary to the dilatation of the poststenotic segment of the aorta (Fig 15–9,*B*). The proximal ascending aorta also should be closely examined. It has more significance in children than in adults because minor dilatation may be highly suggestive of valvular AS with poststenotic dilatation, aortic insufficiency, or systemic hypertension (see Fig 15–6).

The main pulmonary artery likewise plays an important role in the cardiac silhouette and may be highly indicative of CHD (Tables 15–6 and 15–7). A large pulmonary artery secondary to poststenotic dilatation is the classic finding of PVS (Fig 15–10); the dilatation usually extends into the left pulmonary artery, as seen on the lateral chest roentgenogram. With tetralogy of Fallot and corrected transposition of the great arteries the main pulmonary artery is inconspicuous but directional flow may enlarge the right pulmonary artery. The pulmonary artery is enlarged in all left-to-right shunts, as well as in admixture shunts (e.g., truncus arteriosus type I and double-outlet right ventricle) (see Table 15–6). Massive

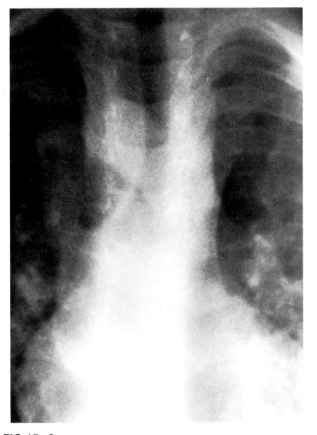

FIG 15–8.
High-kilovoltage peak and added-filtration film of the mediastinal area. Note the deviation of the trachea to the left with a right aortic arch traversing behind the trachea and esophagus in a patient with a circumflex aortic arch (right ascending aorta with posterior left descending aorta).

TABLE 15–7.

Congenital Lesions Associated With a Concave (Small) Main Pulmonary Artery

Tetralogy of Fallot
Pulmonary atresia
Tricuspid atresia with pulmonary stenosis
Pulmonary artery malpositions (i.e., transposition)

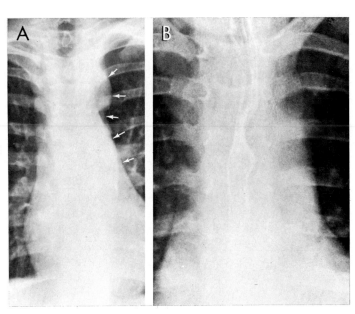

FIG 15–9.
Coarctation of the aorta. A figure-3 sign **(A)** indicates coarctation between the large proximal segment of the aorta and/or a prominent left subclavian artery above the narrowing and the poststenotic dilatation of the descending aorta below it *(arrows)*. Barium esophagogram **(B)** demonstrates the reversed 3 (E sign) impression on the barium-filled esophagus adjacent to the coarcted aorta that is produced by the medial aspect of the same structures described in **A.**

enlargement of the main or left and right pulmonary arteries is also present with congenital absence of the pulmonary valve, a variant of tetralogy of Fallot (Fig 15–11). Idiopathic dilatation may be a normal variant, particularly in the teen-age female. A concave left upper heart border may indicate a hypoplastic pulmonary artery, as in all patients with right-to-left shunts, or a malposition of the pulmonary artery in admixture lesions, as in transposition and truncus type II or III (see Table 15–7).

Skeletal Manifestations of Congenital Heart Disease

Other changes on chest roentgenograms that may indicate CHD include the following:

1. Eleven pairs of ribs, frequently seen in Down syndrome.
2. Variations in sternal ossification centers.

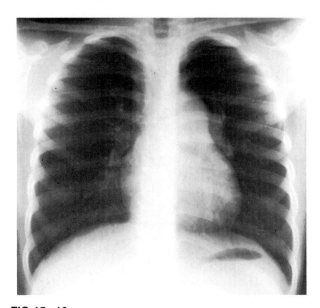

FIG 15–10.
Pulmonary valvular stenosis. Poststenotic dilatation of the main and left pulmonary artery, normal pulmonary flow, and a prominent slightly elevated apex secondary to right ventricular hypertrophy can be seen.

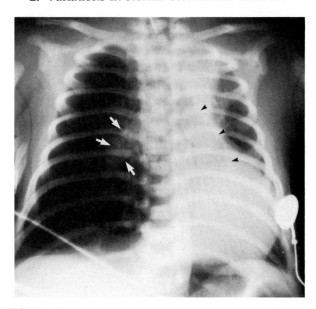

FIG 15–11.
Congenital absence of the pulmonary valve. Aneurysmal dilatation of the right main pulmonary artery *(white arrows)* secondary to congenital absence of the pulmonary valve (tetralogy of Fallot variant). Air trapping the right lung is caused by compression of the right mainstem bronchus by the pulmonary artery and herniation of the lung across the mediastinum to the left *(black arrowheads)*.

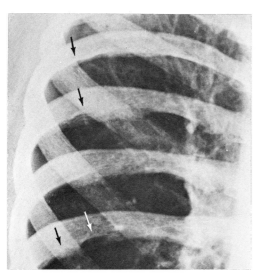

FIG 15–12.
Coarctation of the aorta. Notching on the inferior aspects of the posterolateral ribs is related to collateral flow through intercostal arteries secondary to coarctation of the aorta *(arrows)*. Note the characteristic, somewhat sclerotic margin, which differentiates this lesion from the normal subcostal groove.

3. Metaphyseal osseous irregularities related to rubella.

4. Pectus carinatum, particularly common in Marfan syndrome.

5. Rib notching. Rib notching is evaluated best in the posterolateral inferior margin of the ribs. The posteromedial rib has a very thin cortical surface with undulation, and rib notching is difficult to dif-

TABLE 15–8.

Causes of Rib Notching

Bilateral
  Coarctation
  Aortic arch interruption, type I
  Neurogenic tumors*
  Intercostal collateral flow to the lungs with chronic pulmonary
    oligemia*
  Superior vena cava obstruction*
Right-sided
  Right Blalock-Taussig anastomosis
  Coarctation with stenotic left subclavian artery
  Aortic arch interruption, types II, III
  Right thoracotomy
  Vascular malformations
Left-sided
  Left Blalock-Taussig anastomosis
  Coarctation with aberrant right subclavian artery
  Aortic arch interruption, type I with aberrant right subclavian
    artery
  Left thoracotomy
  Vascular malformations
*May also be unilateral.

ferentiate from the normal subcostal groove. In children and adolescents, rib notching is often well defined (Fig 15–12), but in young children may be manifest only as cortical sclerosis. Rib notching typically involves the third through ninth ribs, and may be unilateral, right- or left-sided, or bilateral (Table 15–8). Rib notching is only present when there is antegrade flow in the subclavian and internal mammary artery.

6. Thin ribs, particularly in trisomies 13, 18, and 21.

7. Shoulder or arm anomalies in Holt-Oram syndrome.

Spine abnormalities may be seen in tetralogy of Fallot, truncus arteriosus, VATER syndrome (*v*ertebral defects, imperforate *a*nus, *t*racheo*e*sophageal fistula, *r*adial and *r*enal dysplasia), and storage diseases, with straight back syndrome in which a functional venous hum or murmur of mitral prolapse may be present, and increased vertebral body height (Marfan syndrome and homocystinuria).

ANGIOCARDIOGRAPHY

Although the noninvasive evaluation of the heart with echocardiography, cine–computed tomography (cine-CT) and magnetic resonance imaging (MRI) defines the cardiac anatomy in many cases, cardiac catherization and angiocardiography are usually necessary at some point in the evaluation of most patients. Catheterization is important in (1) determining shunts, (2) evaluating gradients, (3) measuring systemic and pulmonary artery flow, (4) evaluating cardiac output, and (5) determining pulmonary vascular resistance. Angiocardiography still provides optimal anatomical detail and is particularly important prior to attempted surgical correction of CHD. Biplane-image–intensified fluoroscopy and biplane angiocardiography are essential if cardiac catheterization is performed. Biplane videotape or direct digital recording is mandatory for immediate review of injections in order to evaluate which further studies may be necessary. Digital subtraction angiography (DSA) or cineangiography at 30 to 60 frames per second better visualizes shunt lesions, while obstructive malformations may be better visualized with filming at 12 frames per second. Angiocardiography is performed in differing projections, including (1) AP and lateral projections in critically ill infants assisted by respirators; (2) long-axis (Fig 15–13,A) or four-chambered projections (Fig 15–13,B) for septal anatomy and great-vessel relations; and (3) 45-degree "sitting-up"

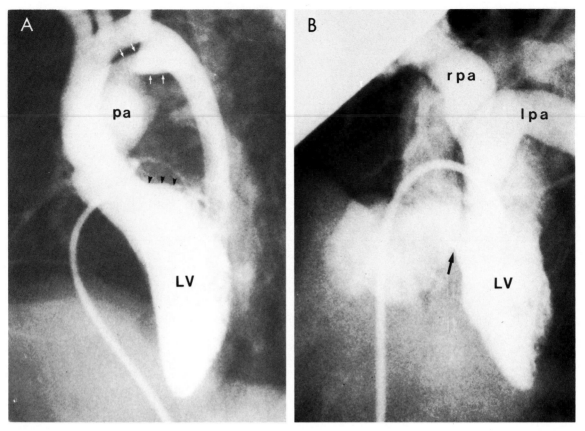

FIG 15–13.
A, long-axis left ventriculogram elongates the left ventricular *(LV)* outflow tract and optimally shows the interventricular septum as well as the subaortic and aortic areas. The left atrium projects well posterior to the outflow tract, and the mitral-aortic relationship is easily identified *(arrowheads); pa,* pulmonary artery. Patent ductus arteriosus with a moderate left-to-right shunt *(arrows).* **B,** four-chamber left ventriculogram in a patient with transposition and a VSD *(arrow)* identifies the left ventricular *(LV)* pulmonary artery relationship and ideally shows the right and left pulmonary arteries *(RPA, LPA).*

AP (Fig 15–14) or a steep left anterior oblique (LAO) projection with maximum cranial-caudal angulation (Garcia-Medina et al.) and lateral projections, or a steep left anterior oblique (LAO) projection with maximum cranial-caudal angulation (Garcia-Medina et al.) for pulmonary valve, pulmonary artery, and right ventricular outflow tract disorders.

Most venous cardiac catheterizations are performed from the percutaneous femoral approach utilizing a Berman-type, double-lumen balloon catheter. When the atrial septum is intact or when other indications warrant left heart evaluation, percutaneous retrograde arterial catheterization with a thin-walled pigtail catheter is usually performed. In infants, low osmolar or nonionic contrast is usually used in a dose of 1 to 2 mL/kg injected in less than 1 second per injection with a total volume limited to 4 mL/kg. The use of low osmolar or nonionic contrast may permit the use of larger volumes up to 6 mL/kg. If DSA is utilized, concentrations of contrast may be decreased to 180 to 240 mg/mL. In older children,

ionic hyperosmolar contrast is usually used if no allergic problems exist. In patients with small cardiac chambers or obstructive lesions, a dose of 1 mL/kg per injection is usually sufficient. Mortality related to heart catheterization and angiocardiography is low (less than 1%) and usually relates to (1) cardiac perforations, (2) severe arrhythmia, and (3) contrast reaction. Morbidity relates to (1) hypertonic solutions and electrolyte imbalance, (2) renal or hepatic damage, and (3) direct myocardial injury.

ECHOCARDIOGRAPHY

The development of real-time (two-dimensional) and Doppler echocardiography probably represents the most important advance in the noninvasive evaluation of CHD over the past two decades. Ultan et al. first described the use of echocardiography in CHD in 1967, and Meyer and Kaplan in 1973 pointed out the specificity of echocardiographic findings in certain conditions (e.g., hypoplastic left heart syn-

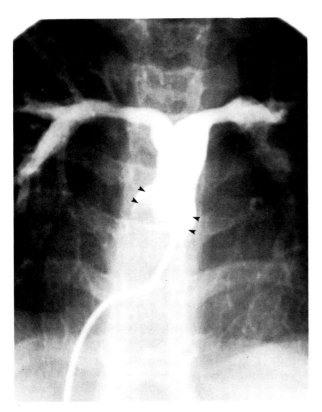

FIG 15–14.
Sitting-up AP pulmonary arteriogram in a patient with peripheral pulmonary hypoplasia produces a central beam tangential to the pulmonary valve leaflets *(arrows)*. The main pulmonary artery is relatively elongated. The right and left pulmonary arteries are easily distinguished, and the left pulmonary artery is not obscured by the main pulmonary artery, as in the conventional AP projection.

drome), making a definitive diagnosis possible without further invasive procedures, except in unusual clinical situations. Specific diagnostic criteria for various CHDs have been developed with real-time echocardiography by Lange, Bierman, Silverman, and Henry and their colleagues. The utilization of Doppler, and more recently two-dimensional Doppler color-flow mapping, allows the examiner to obtain both anatomical and physiologic information in real time.

Technical Factors

Echocardiography is performed with a pulsed ultrasound beam of less than 1-μs duration repeated 2,000 to 3,000 times per second; the intervals between pulsations are used for recording the returning echo. At present, no significant reproducible harmful effects have been demonstrated with the energies and frequencies used. The earlier techniques utilizing M-mode evaluation enabled some determination of chamber size and function, along with anatomical relations and ventricular and septal thicknesses. With the development of two-dimensional equipment utilizing either sector scanners, linear phased array scan, or multicrystal rays, a much more vivid, dynamic image of intracardiac anatomy can be obtained. The two-dimensional study is commonly recorded on videotape for delayed slow-motion, or stop-action evaluation. Relations of the great vessels to cardiac chambers, as well as to the intracardiac anatomy, are easily recorded.

Currently, a combined M-mode, real-time, and Doppler examination is performed in nearly all patients with serious CHD. M-mode evaluation uses the window of the left fourth parasternal intercostal space perpendicular to the chest and heart for optimal visualization of the aorta, septum, mitral valve, left ventricle, and posterior left ventricular wall (Fig 15–15). Slight angulation allows visualization of the tricuspid valve and the pulmonary valve, although the latter may require changing to a more cephalad interspace. A sweep from the aortic root through the aortic valve and into the left ventricle gives optimal points of measurement of the left atrium and defines the relations of the aortic root to the septum and the anterior leaflet of the mitral valve.

In real-time echocardiography, a more complex series of maneuvers is carried out with the trans-

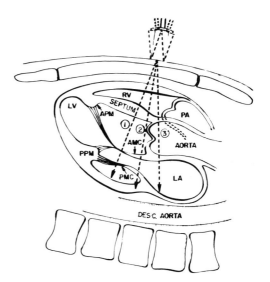

FIG 15–15.
Diagram of M-mode echocardiogram performed in the left parasagittal (long-axis) projection. The transducer sweeps from the mid–left ventricular area *(1)* cephalad toward the level of the aortic root *(3)*. *AMC,* anterior mitral leaflet. *APC,* anterior papillary muscle. *LA,* left atrium. *LV,* left ventricle. *PA,* pulmonary artery. *PMC,* posterior mitral valve leaflet. *PPM,* posterior papillary muscle. *RV,* right ventricle. **(Courtesy of Dr. Richard A. Meyer and F.A. Davis Co, Philadelphia.)**

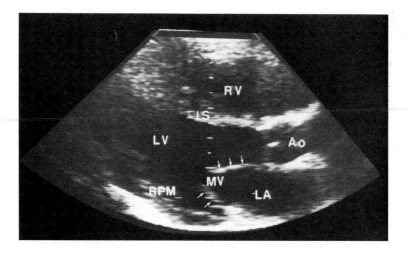

FIG 15–16.
Normal two-dimensional long-axis parasternal echocardiogram identifying the left atrium *(LA)*, left ventricle *(LV)*, and ascending aorta *(Ao)* with appropriate valve structures. There is normal continuity of the interventricular septum *(IS)* with the anterior annulus of the aortic valve and the anterior leaflet of the mitral valve *(MV) (ar-* rows) with the posterior aortic annulus *(RPM,* right papillary muscle). Anatomical relationships are very similar to the levoangiocardiogram as seen in the long-axis LAO projection (see Fig 15–13,A).

ducer. Initially, the heart is evaluated in a long-axis view, with the transducer scan orientated from the right shoulder toward the left hip to the left of the sternum (Fig 15–16). Clockwise or counterclockwise rotations identify the tricuspid valve, aorta, and pulmonary valve. Utilizing a transverse position of the transducer, and sweeping from the apex of the heart cephalad through the level of the mitral valve into the root of the great vessels, gives a short-axis view of the heart. The great vessels can also be evaluated in this position, with both the aortic and pulmonary valve identifiable. The transducer is then placed at the apex of the heart, with the central beam parallel to the plane of the ventricular and atrial septa, producing a four-chamber configuration that shows both atrioventricular valves as well as the cardiac chambers. Next, a subxiphoid projection produces a modified four-chamber configuration demonstrating the interventricular and intra-atrial septa and, with angulation, the aortic and pulmonary root and left and right ventricular outflow tracts (Fig 15–17). Pulmonary venous return is also best seen in this projection, while systemic venous return can be seen in a modified long-axis view. Finally, the aortic arch is evaluated from the suprasternal notch, where the origin of the great vessels can be seen, along with the aortic isthmus beyond the level of the left subclavian artery. The aortic arch also may be evaluated from the subxiphoid view, although, in our experience, this has been somewhat more difficult than with the suprasternal notch view.

Doppler Echocardiography

According to the Doppler principle, the frequency of a sound wave that is reflected off a moving object will differ with the frequency of the incident wave. Frequency will increase or decrease depending on the object's direction and velocity relative to the incident wave. This change in frequency is called the *Doppler shift.* When an ultrasonic beam is parallel to the expected direction of flow, Doppler shift is proportional to blood flow velocity. This principle is the basis of Doppler echocardiography.

With this technique, a burst of ultrasonic signals is transmitted into the heart at very high frequency. The signals are reflected back by the moving erythrocytes, producing the Doppler shift signals. By convention, flow toward the transducer shifts the velocity upward above the baseline, whereas motion away from the transducer shifts the frequency downward.

While there are several types of ultrasonic transmission and processing techniques, current Doppler echocardiography utilizes one of three techniques, each with its own advantages and disadvantages. These include pulsed, continuous-wave, and high pulse repetition frequency Doppler.

Pulsed Doppler is similar to M-mode echocardiography in which a burst of ultrasonic waves is transmitted to the tissues and reflected back to the same transducer. However, unlike M-mode, the pulsed repetition frequency is varied, depending on the depth of sampling. The pulse mode system offers a great advantage in that it permits range reso-

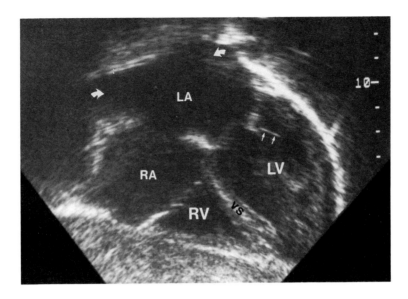

FIG 15–17.
Two-dimensional subxiphoid echocardiogram produces a four-chamber cardiac silhouette visualizing both atria *(RA, LA)*, both ventricles *(RV, LV)*, atrioventricular valves, and interventricular *(VS)* and interatrial septa. Minor rotation from this view makes it possible to sweep into the aortic and pulmonary outflow tract and visu-alize these great vessels. Pulmonary veins enter the left atrium *(curved arrows)* and posterior papillary muscle and chordae and proceed to the mitral valve *(arrows)*. Angiography in the hepato-clavicular (four-chamber) view closely simulates this echocardio-graphic projection (see Fig 15–13,*B*).

lution so that flow can be characterized in any se-lected location in a given cardiac chamber or great vessel. Utilizing a simultaneous two-dimensional echocardiogram, the examiner can place the sample volume within a chamber or great vessel of interest, and determine its velocity and direction of flow (Fig 15–18; see also Fig 16–18). Its major disadvantage is that there are significant velocity measurement limi-tations. High velocities, particularly those encoun-tered across stenotic valves, result in an aliasing er-ror, which makes the determination of the true Dop-pler shift ambiguous.

Continuous-wave Doppler utilizes two crystals, one that continuously sends, and the other that con-tinuously receives ultrasound. Since ultrasound is transmitted continuously, range gating is not possi-ble. The continuous-wave Doppler receives informa-tion all along the beam and does not allow determi-nation of the depth at which the frequency shift oc-curred (range ambiguity). Unlike pulsed mode there is no limit on the maximum velocity that can be measured by this technique. Therefore, continuous-wave Doppler is excellent for the analysis of high ve-locities, particularly across stenotic orifices.

High pulse rate frequency Doppler represents an intermediate between continuous-wave and pulsed Doppler that has been developed to allow measure-ments of higher velocities than is possible for stan-dard pulsed Doppler. Multiple sample volumes can be placed simultaneously at different depths within the heart. Summation of velocities at each sample volume permit measurement of higher velocities than can be measured from a single, more distant sample volume.

In the evaluation of patients with CHD, Doppler

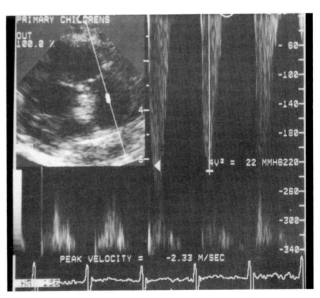

FIG 15–18.
Pulmonary valvular stenosis with Doppler estimation of pulmonary valve gradient. In the short-axis projection the Doppler sample is placed in the pulmonary artery in the jet of laminar flow distal to the stenotic pulmonary valve *(upper left corner)*. The recorded peak velocity is 2.33 m/sec. The calculated pulmonary valve gradient utilizing the modified Bernoulli equation ($4V^2$) is 22 mm Hg.

echocardiography is most utilized in the recognition of flow disturbances, flow computation, and Doppler measurement of pressure gradients. Doppler echocardiography can distinguish laminar or normal flow from disturbed or turbulent flow. Laminar flow is characterized by a well-defined flow profile while turbulent flow is incoherent with wide spectral dispersion, both positively and negatively. Flow computation is possible by Doppler echocardiography. The average velocity of blood flow multiplied by the area through which the blood passes enables determination of flow volume. Determination of aortic, pulmonary artery, tricuspid valve, and mitral valve flow permits determination of cardiac output, calculation of left-to-right shunts, and determination of regurgitant fractions. The greatest utilization of Doppler echocardiography is in the estimation of pressure gradients across areas of obstruction. The pressure gradient across an obstruction to blood flow can be estimated noninvasively by measuring the maximum velocity (V) beyond the obstruction with Doppler echocardiography, then utilizing the simplified Bernoulli equation (pressure gradient = $4V^2$). The maximal gradient obtained by utilizing the modified Bernoulli equation has an excellent correlation with the maximal instantaneous pressure gradient measured at catheterization. Recall that most catheterization laboratories report a peak-to-peak gradient, whereas Doppler echocardiography measures instantaneous velocities and instantaneous gradients. Because of the high-velocity flows typically encountered across stenotic valves, continuous-wave Doppler is the optimal method for use in quantitation of valve gradients. With use of Doppler echocardiography, gradients can be estimated across areas of pulmonary obstruction such as PVS, infundibular pulmonic stenosis, and pulmonary artery band (Fig 15–18). The gradient can be estimated across the left ventricular outflow tract permitting estimation of the severity of subaortic, valvular, or supravalvular AS. The severity of coarctation can be estimated by placing the sample volume distal to the site of coarctation.

The recent utilization of real-time two-dimensional Doppler color-flow mapping permits the rapid determination of anatomical and physiologic information. The Doppler velocities present within any particular spatial location are determined separately and rapidly by digital electronic processing using an autocollator which estimates velocities and passes them to a digital scan convertor where they are read out into a color convertor for display. In several systems, flow toward the transducer has been coded in increasing brightness of red to yellow and flow away from the transducer in increasing brightness of blue.

Turbulent, or abnormal flow, with spectral broadening has been shown in green. This method provides excellent spatial orientation of flow. One can rapidly define the location and distribution of the area where normal or abnormal flows occur, such as regurgitant or stenotic jets. One can rapidly localize the maximal velocity area of a jet through stenotic orifices, and can quantitate valvular insufficiency (Figs 15–19, 15–20, and 15–21) rather than continually sampling with single-pulse Doppler around the cavity receiving the regurgitant flow. Recognition of left-to-right shunts, especially ASDs (Fig 15–22), membranous (Fig 15–23) and muscular VSDs (Fig 15–24), and PDA (Fig 15–25) is also facilitated.

FETAL ULTRASONOGRAPHY

High resolution ultrasound equipment can readily examine the fetal heart. The transabdominal approach may be used as early as 14 weeks' gestation. The transvaginal approach may be used during the first trimester. Those groups in whom a careful fetal cardiac ultrasound examination should be performed are: a mother, a sibling, or first-degree relative with a history of CHD; predisposing maternal conditions, such as insulin-dependent diabetes, connective tissue disease, advanced maternal age; exposure to teratogens such as phenytoin, lithium, alcohol, the rubella virus, and antihypertensive drugs. Others that should be examined include those who have an abnormal pregnancy as defined by multiple gestations, persistent malpresentations, fetal cardiac arrhythmias, and known or suspected fetal anomalies based on ultrasound, amniotic fluid volume, fetal growth, or chromosomal aberrations.

Both abnormalities in fetal cardiac structure and fetal cardiac function may be detected. An evaluation of the fetal heart requires an understanding of the difference between the fetal heart and the adult heart. The fetal heart should have a patent foramen ovale with blood flow from right atrium to left atrium. The ductus arteriosus should be patent with blood flowing from pulmonary artery to aorta. The right and left ventricles are of equal size or the right ventricle is slightly larger. The ventricular walls and intraventricular septum are of equal thickness.

In the evaluation of fetal cardiac anatomy, the right atrium is identified by the entry of the inferior and superior venae cavae. Enlargement of the right atrium is often seen with tricuspid valve regurgitation, Ebstein anomaly, CHF, and tricuspid atresia. The tricuspid valve and mitral valves are usually well visualized. Endocardial cushion defects may be recognized. The atrial septum, the patent foramen

FIG 15–19.

Color Doppler documentation of severe rheumatic mitral regurgitation. Utilizing the apical four-chamber projection the color field is positioned in the region of the mitral valve and left atrium. A systolic image *(ECG, arrow)* demonstrates severe mitral regurgitation with turbulent flow producing a mosaic pattern throughout the left atrium. In this illustration the flow toward the transducer is colored red with the highest velocities in yellow; flow away from the transducer is blue with the highest velocities in light blue. Turbulent flow produces a mosaic pattern. *RA,* right atrium; *LA,* left atrium; *RV,* right ventricle; *LV,* left ventricle.

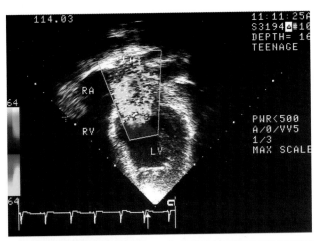

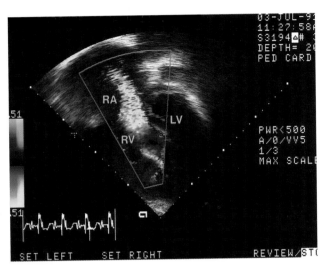

FIG 15–20.

Color Doppler documentation of moderate tricuspid regurgitation. In the subcostal four-chamber projection the color field is positioned in the right ventricle and right atrium. A systolic image *(ECG, arrow)* documents turbulent blood flow through the tricuspid valve producing a mosaic pattern of blue and yellow in the medial right atrium. In this illustration flow toward the transducer is in shades of red with the highest velocities in yellow; flow away from the transducer is in shades of blue with the highest velocities in light blue. Turbulent flow produces a mosaic pattern. *RA,* right atrium; *RV,* right ventricle; *LV,* left ventricle.

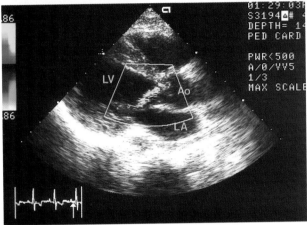

FIG 15–21.

Color Doppler documentation of mild aortic regurgitation. In the long-axis projection the color field is positioned in the region of the aortic valve and left ventricular outflow tract. This diastolic image *(ECG, arrow)* demonstrates a mosaic pattern of turbulent blood flow through the aortic valve directed against the anterior mitral valve leaflet. In this illustration flow toward the transducer is in shades of red with the highest velocities in yellow; flow away from the transducer is in shades of blue with the highest velocities in light blue. Turbulent flow produces a mosaic pattern. *LV,* left ventricle; *Ao,* aorta; *LA,* left atrium.

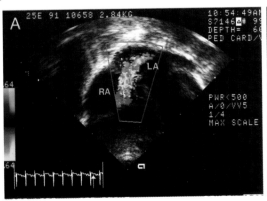

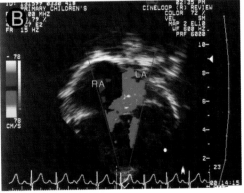

FIG 15–22.

A, color Doppler documentation of ostium secundum atrial septal defect (ASD). In the subcostal four-chamber projection, the color field is positioned in the region of the atrial septum. This image recorded during ventricular systole (atrial diastole) *(ECG, arrow)* documents a moderate-sized ostium secundum ASD with left-to-right shunt flow. In this illustration flow toward the transducer is in shades of red with the highest velocities in yellow; flow away from the transducer is in shades of blue with the highest velocities in light blue. Turbulent flow produces a mosaic pattern. *RA,* right atrium; *LA,* left atrium. **B,** color Doppler documentation of ostium primum ASD. In the apical four-chamber projection, the color field is positioned in the region of the atrial septum. This image recorded during atrial systole *(ECG, arrow)* documents a moderate-sized ostium primum ASD with left-to-right shunt flow. Early diastolic filling of the right and left ventricles is also noted. The color legend is similar to **A.** *RA,* right atrium; *LA,* left atrium.)

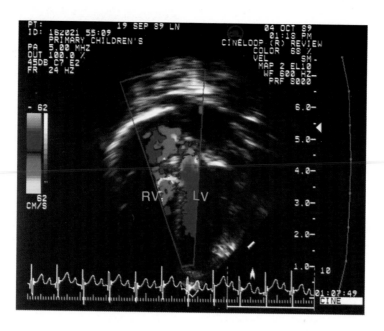

FIG 15–23.

Color Doppler documentation of small membranous VSD. In the apical four-chamber projection the color field is positioned in the region of the membranous and anterior muscular septum. This image at end-ventricular systole *(ECG, arrow)* demonstrates high-velocity flow through a small membranous VSD into the upper medial right ventricle. In this illustration, flow toward the transducer is in shades of red with highest velocities in yellow; flow away from the transducer is in shades of blue with the highest velocities in light blue. Turbulent flow produces a mosaic pattern. *RV,* right ventricle; *LV,* left ventricle. **(From Jaffe RB: Ventricular septal defect—echocardiography, in Elliott LP (ed):** *Cardiac Imaging in Infants, Children, and Adults.* **Philadelphia, JB Lippincott, 1991, p 575. Used by permission.)**

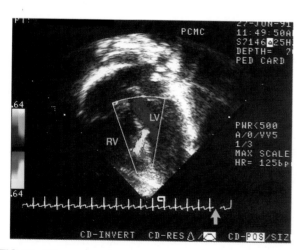

FIG 15–24.

Color Doppler documentation of small mid-muscular VSD. In the apical four-chamber projection the color field is positioned in the region of the muscular septum. This systolic image *(ECG, arrow)* demonstrates high-velocity, left-to-right shunt flow through an oblique mid-muscular VSD. In this illustration flow toward the transducer is in shades of red with highest velocities in yellow; flow away from the transducer is in shades of blue with highest velocities in light blue. Turbulent flow produces a mosaic pattern. *RV,* right ventricle; *LV,* left ventricle.

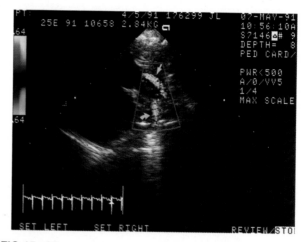

FIG 15–25.

Color Doppler documentation of patent ductus arteriosus (PDA). In the short-axis projection, the color field is positioned in the region of the main pulmonary artery. This image at end diastole *(ECG, arrow)* demonstrates a jet of turbulent flow into the main pulmonary artery at end diastole *(arrow)* confirming the presence of a PDA with left-to-right shunt flow. Turbulent blood flow also is seen in the left pulmonary artery *(curved arrow).* Although a PDA may not be visualized directly on two-dimensional examination in some patients, the color documentation of retrograde turbulent blood flow in the main pulmonary artery during diastole confirms the presence of a PDA with left-to-right shunt flow. In this illustration, flow toward the transducer is in shades of red with highest velocities in yellow; flow away from the transducer is in shades of blue with highest velocities in light blue. Turbulent flow produces a mosaic pattern.

ovale, and the ventricular septum may be visualized. Defects of the muscular and inlet ventricular septum may be recognized. Defects of the membranous aspect of the septum are difficult to visualize, but may be detected by Doppler techniques, including color-flow Doppler. The origins of the aorta and pulmonary artery with their respective semilunar valves may be identified. The aortic arch and the origin of the brachiocephalic vessels may be visualized, as well as the pulmonary artery.

The four-chamber view is the easiest to obtain. This view allows assessment of the size of the right and left ventricles and the size of the right and left atria (Fig 15–26). One may determine if the heart is in the left thorax and if the stomach is on the same side as the fetal heart. This allows for exclusion of situs abnormalities. Functional cardiac abnormalities may be present, such as those that present with fetal arrhythmias. Supraventricular tachycardia or ventricular tachycardia may cause fetal hydrops secondary to fetal congestive failure. Two-dimensional imaging may assess for the association of fetal structural cardiac defects. Specific delineation of the cardiac arrhythmia and selection of appropriate therapy depends on detailed M-mode echocardiographic and Doppler studies of the relationship of atrial and ventricular contraction.

In addition to the four-chamber view, one may obtain a five-chamber view, a left parasternal view, a short-axis view, and a view of the aorta and of the aortic arch. M-mode echocardiography may be recorded and ventricular chamber dimensions, thickness of the ventricular walls and intraventricular septum, and aortic and pulmonary root and valve dimensions may be determined. The shortening fraction may be calculated from the M-mode. M-mode also may be useful in detecting pericardial effusions and documenting cardiac activity in the fetus.

Doppler echocardiography may be used as an adjunctive technique in the establishment of fetal structural or functional defects. Continuous-wave, pulsed, and color Doppler ultrasound techniques have been utilized. The umbilical artery blood flow measurements often involve comparisons of systolic and diastolic flow. The umbilical vein has been examined, and the intracerebral arteries, and tricuspid, mitral, pulmonary, and aortic valves may be examined.

There are some lesions in the neonate that are difficult or impossible to exclude with fetal echocardiography. These include a patent foramen ovale, PDA, small VSDs, small ASDs, mild valvular abnormalities, and pulmonary venous abnormalities. If a structural cardiac abnormality is present, a karyotypic abnormality may be present in 12% to 35% of the fetuses. Karyotypic analysis is indicated if a fetal cardiac abnormality has been detected. If karyotypic abnormality has been detected, there is a significant likelihood that a cardiac abnormality may be present. If another fetal abnormality has been detected, there is also a significant likelihood that the heart is also abnormal. Detection of fetal cardiac abnormalities can result in better care for the fetus. It also allows for better preparation of the parents, obstetricians, neonatologists, and pediatric cardiologists caring for the child. Detection of fetal cardiac abnormalities can allow for proper selection of time, location, and personnel for the delivery.

COMPUTED TOMOGRAPHY

Computed tomography, particularly ultrafast (cine) CT with contrast enhancement, provides opportunities for cross-sectional evaluation of cardiac malformations. When this is used with a cine-loop technique, cardiac function and shunts can be evaluated. Arch anomalies with associated abnormalities of the tracheobronchial tree may be one of the primary uses of ultrafast CT. These arch and tracheal anomalies are also well demonstrated with MRI.

MAGNETIC RESONANCE IMAGING

During the past several years, electrocardiographic (ECG)-gated MRI of the heart has been used to evaluate selected patients with CHD. Whereas two-dimensional, Doppler, and color-flow Doppler echocardiography provide excellent anatomical and he-

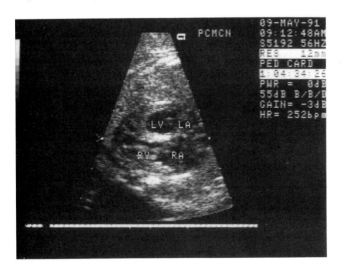

FIG 15–26.
Fetal ultrasound examination at 24 weeks' gestation demonstrates a variant of hypoplastic left heart syndrome. The left ventricle *(LV)* is abnormally small in size. *LA,* left atrium; *RV,* right ventricle; *RA,* right atrium. **(Courtesy of Dr. Victoria E. Judd.)**

TABLE 15–9.

Sedation Protocol for MRI

Patient	Drug	Initial Dose and Administration	Supplemental Dose
Infants and small children	Chloral hydrate	75 mg/kg po Maximum dose 2,000 mg including supplemental dose	25 mg/kg
Small and large children	Sodium pentobarbital (Nembutal)	6 mg/kg IV Administer ½ total dose, observe 30 sec, administer ½ of the remaining dose, observe 30 sec, administer remainder of dose	1–2 mg/kg
Older children and adolescents	Nalbuphine (Nubain) plus midazolam (Versed)	0.1 mg/kg mixed with 0.1 mg/kg Infuse IV in 1–2 min Maximum dose midazolam—5 mg	Repeat initial dose if necessary

modynamic information about almost all intracardiac lesions, MRI is largely limited to imaging of extracardiac anatomy and a few intracardiac lesions.

High-quality ECG-gated MRI depends on the contrast between rapidly flowing blood, which produces little or no signal, and stationary cardiac structures and vessel walls. The major advantages of MRI are the ease with which large fields of view can be obtained, and an ability to image orthogonal planes at any angle.

Contraindications

Patients with ferromagnetic foreign bodies in or around the orbit, intracranial metallic aneurysm clips, and epicardial or intracardial pacemakers must be excluded from MRI studies. Patients with prosthetic valves, sternal wires, or small metallic hemostatic clips in the thorax or abdomen can be imaged safely.

Obtaining high-quality images of the heart and great vessels requires sedation in infants and children to avoid motion artifact. Sleep deprivation is a helpful adjunct when used before sedation, and in older children who are not sedated. We sleep-deprive all patients under 12 years of age and those older patients who are hyperactive, mentally retarded, or emotionally unstable. Our sedation protocol is listed in Table 15–9. Infants and children under the age of 6 years are routinely sedated before examination. We administer chloral hydrate to infants and small children, sodium pentobarbital (Nembutal) to small and large children, and a mixture of nalbuphine (Nubain) and midazolam (Versed) to older children and adolescents.

TABLE 15–10.

Imaging Parameters for Spin-Echo Imaging (1.5 T)*

	Infants	Small Children	Large Children
TE (ms)	20–25	20–25	20–25
TR (ms)	Dependent on the R-R interval (R-R − 150 = TR)		
Signal average	4	3–4	3–4
Coil			
Siemens	CP-head	CP-head or LP-linear head	Body
GE	Quadrature head coil	Quadrature head coil or body	
Field of view	180–240 mm	240–320 mm	320–480 mm
Slice thickness	2–3 mm	3 mm	3–6 mm
Interslice gap	2–3 mm	3 mm	3–6 mm
Matrix	192 × 256	192 × 256	192 × 256

*TE = echo time; TR = repetition time.

Imaging Protocol

ECG-gated images are dependent on a high-quality ECG tracing for accurate gating. Lead placement varies with each patient and with different machines. Some vendors have an optional retrospective ECG-gating program. Our standard imaging technique uses multisection spin-echo imaging. Imaging parameters for 1.5-tesla (1.5-T) scanning are listed in Table 15–10. When performed as two separate sequences of interleaved images, tomographic sections at 3- or 5-mm intervals with no gap are obtained throughout the heart and great vessels at varying times during the cardiac cycle. To evaluate blood flow, turbulence, and valvular regurgitation, gated cine-MRI is utilized. Imaging parameters are listed in Table 15–11.

Indications for Scanning

Aortic Anomalies

The entire thoracic aorta, brachiocephalic vessels, and their relationship to the airway are well visualized in patients of any age. The large fields of view obtainable in any plane make MRI the imaging modality of choice for the aorta and brachiocephalic vessels. Vascular rings and their relationship to the tracheobronchial tree, are exceptionally well depicted in the coronal and axial planes (see Figs 17–8, 17–10, 17–16, and 17–17). Patients with coarctation are imaged best in the sagittal, LAO, and axial planes to visualize the dilated ascending aorta (secondary to an associated bicuspid valve), transverse arch, coarctation, and poststenotic descending aorta (see Fig 16–52). MRI is the modality of choice to serially follow the results and recognize associated complications and development of recoarctation following operation or balloon dilatation (see Fig 16–53). In these patients the coronal plane is also imaged after sagittal and axial images have been obtained. In patients with cystic medial necrosis, MRI in the sagittal, axial, and coronal oblique planes clearly depicts the thoracic aorta in its entirety (see Fig 18–6). It is the preferred modality for following these patients for serial changes in aortic size and for complications, such as dissection. Patients with supravalvular aortic stenosis and associated peripheral pulmonary artery stenosis can be imaged accurately in the sagittal and coronal planes (see Fig 16–44). After surgery, imaging in the sagittal, coronal, and axial planes should be obtained. In patients with dissection, spin-echo imaging (Fig 15–27) should be followed by cine-MRI to best evaluate abnormalities in flow in the true and false lumina. Abnormalities involving the descending thoracic aorta, such as mycotic aneurysms, are well visualized in the sagittal, coronal, and axial planes (see Fig 19–11).

Pulmonary Arteries

Although the central pulmonary arteries and veins can be visualized well by echocardiography, they cannot be seen to the level of the pulmonary hila with a high degree of confidence. These vessels can be imaged in multiple planes with MRI and their relation to the tracheobronchial tree well depicted. The pulmonary artery origin and central confluence are evaluated best in the axial projection with 3- to 5-mm interleaved scans. Aberrant origin of the left pulmonary artery from the right pulmonary artery (pulmonary sling) is well visualized in the axial and sagittal projections (see Fig 17–25). Cine-MRI can be helpful in identifying pulmonary flow in small

TABLE 15–11.

Imaging Parameters for Gated Cine-MRI

	Infants	Small Children	Large Children
TE (ms)	12–16	12–16	12–16
TR (ms)			
GE	20–30	20–30	20–30
Siemens	50	50	50
Signal average	3	3	3
Coil			
Siemens	CP-head coil	CP-head coil	CP-head coil
GE	Quadrature head coil	Quadrature head or body coil	
Field of view	200–240 mm	240–320 mm	320–480 mm
Interslice gap	0%–100%	0%–100%	0%–100%
Matrix	128 × 256	128 × 256	128 × 256
Flip angle	30 degrees	30 degrees	30 degrees
Phases		No. of phases = R-R − 100/25	
Locations	2	2	2

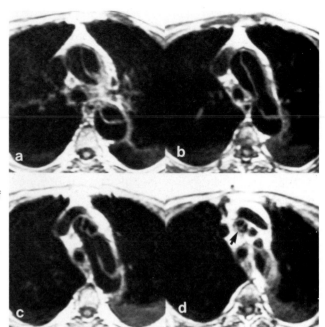

FIG 15–27.
MRI aortic arch. Type I aortic dissection. *(a)* Axial spin-echo image demonstrates the intimal flap in the ascending and descending aorta. *(b* and *c)* The intimal flap is seen at the level of the aortic arch. *(d)* The dissection with intimal flap extends into the right innominate artery *(arrow)*. Left pleural fluid is also noted. **(Courtesy of George S. Bisset III, M.D.)**

vessels, distinguishing them from bronchi. Evaluation of pulmonary size, before and after systemic–pulmonary artery shunts, is best performed in the axial and axial-oblique planes with interleaved 3- to 5-mm images (Fig 15–28). The main right pulmonary artery also is well visualized in the coronal plane, and the left pulmonary artery in the sagittal plane. In patients with pulmonary artery stenosis, axial and coronal oblique planes permit identification of peripheral pulmonary artery stenosis in the

supravalvular region, at the pulmonary bifurcation (see Figs 21–13 and 21–29), and in the right and left pulmonary arteries to the level of the hila. Aneurysmal enlargement of the central pulmonary arteries, typically seen in patients with tetralogy of Fallot and absent pulmonary valve, and their relation to the tracheobronchial tree can be evaluated in all planes with 3- to 5-mm interleaved images. In other patients, aneurysmally dilated pulmonary arteries (see Fig 21–11) can be distinguished from hilar masses

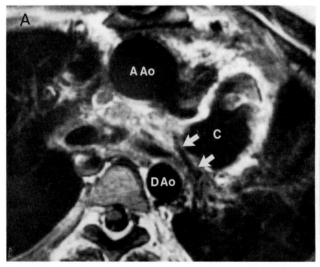

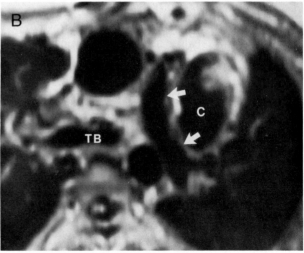

FIG 15–28.
MRI heart. A 16-year-old child with tetralogy of Fallot, post right ventricular–right pulmonary artery conduit *(C)*. The left pulmonary artery could not be identified at angiography. **A,** axial 5-mm spin-echo image demonstrates a 3-mm left pulmonary artery *(arrows)* passing between the conduit (C) and left bronchus; *(AAo,* ascending aorta; *DAo,* descending aorta. **B,** follow-up axial 3-mm scan 6 months after Blalock-Taussig anastomosis demonstrates interval growth of the central left pulmonary artery now measuring 10 to 11 mm *(arrows); C,* right ventricular–right pulmonary artery conduit; *TB,* tracheal bifurcation.

such as bronchogenic cysts, tumors, or adenopathy (see Fig 16–31). While most patients with anomalies in pulmonary venous return can be accurately evaluated on two-dimensional echocardiography, certain patients with partial or total anomalous pulmonary venous drainage may benefit from MRI (see Fig 16–31). Since patients with complex cyanotic CHD related to asplenia invariably have anomalies in pulmonary venous return, MRI may permit evaluation of systemic and pulmonary venous return, and complex intracardiac anomalies in a single study (see Fig 18–2). Patients with suspected focal pulmonary venous stenosis should be studied in both axial and coronal planes with thin 3-mm interleaved images.

Complex Heart Disease

MRI is an excellent modality for visualizing both extracardiac and intracardiac anomalies in patients with complex heart disease related to abnormality in situs and those with asplenia or polysplenia syndrome (see Fig 18–2). Scans in the coronal plane allow analysis of the tracheobronchial tree for symmetry (see Fig 18–2, A), and determination of abdominal situs. Coronal and sagittal images may be utilized to locate the inferior vena cava and aorta within the abdomen, and to document azygos and hemiazygos continuation of the inferior vena cava (see Fig 18–2, B). Atria, unilateral, or bilateral superior venae cavae, and their relation to the coronary sinus are easily identified on coronal and axial images (see Fig 18–2, C). Segmental analysis of complex intracardiac anomalies can then be performed in multiple planes.

Pericardiac and Intracardiac Masses

MRI can identify primary and secondary myocardial and pericardiac masses in the axial and coronal planes. Differentiating mediastinal masses from the aorta, central pulmonary arteries, atria, and ventricles is facilitated by the contrast between flowing blood in these structures (see Fig 16–31). The fibrous pericardium is of low signal intensity and provides a cleavage plane between mediastinal tissue and cardiac structures. Pericardial tumor involvement may be visualized as focal thickening of the pericardium or disruption of the low-intensity pericardial line. Pericardial effusions and vascular extension of tumor in either the inferior vena cava or superior vena cava can be recognized in any imaging plane. While most intracardiac masses can be recognized on echocardiography (see Fig 20–2), those lesions involving myocardial walls are best evaluated

by MRI with its large field of view. Multiple imaging planes, including true long- and short-axis images of the ventricles are suggested (see Fig 20–3). Cine-MRI is helpful in showing tumor motion between atria and ventricles and associated valvular regurgitation.

Postoperative Evaluation

Surgical correction of complex CHD is often accomplished by creating geometrically complex structures or by creating pathways within the mediastinum that are difficult to interrogate by ultrasound. MRI is a particularly useful modality to evaluate patients with many systemic–pulmonary artery shunts (Fig 15–29), conduits between the right atrium and right ventricular outflow tract or pulmonary artery (see Fig 21–17), and atrial baffles (Mustard or Senning procedure) (see Fig 21–20). MRI is also useful in evaluation of the central pulmonary arteries following pulmonary artery band (see Fig 21–13), or systemic–pulmonary artery shunt (see Figs 15–29, 21–11), and for all operations involving the aorta.

NUCLEAR CARDIOLOGY

The use of radionuclides in pediatric cardiovascular studies is varied and includes detection of shunts, functional cardiac evaluation, myocardial perfusion,

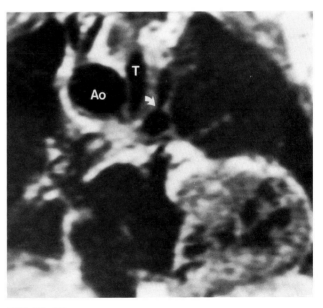

FIG 15–29.
MRI heart. Stenotic left Blalock-Taussig shunt in a 10-year-old girl with single ventricle, transposition, and pulmonic and mitral atresia. Coronal 3-mm MRI spin-echo image demonstrates stenosis of the left Blalock-Taussig shunt *(arrow)* at the anastomosis with the left pulmonary artery. *Ao,* right aortic arch; *T,* trachea.

regional metabolism, identification of myocardial necrosis, and the presence of inflammation.

Shunt Detection

First-pass radionuclide scintigraphy has been used in pediatric cardiology primarily for detection and quantitation of cardiac shunts. This examination requires meticulous technique involving placement of a 21- or 19-gauge catheter in the superior vena cava to obtain an adequate bolus. Cardiac output and ejection fractions can be calculated with first-pass radionuclide scintigraphy. The radiation dose to the patient is negligible. However, this examination is seldom performed today, having been replaced by Doppler echocardiography and color-flow imaging.

Cardiac Function Imaging

Gated blood pool angiography or multiple gated acquisition (MUGA) blood pool scans permits evaluation of both global and regional ventricular function. Most commonly, autologous red cells are labeled with^{99m}Tc in vitro and reinjected into the patient. The scintillation data acquisition is synchronized with the R-R interval from the ECG which is divided into a number (usually 16 or 32) of chronological segments. The scintillation data acquired during hundreds of cardiac angles are partitioned by the computer into these segments which results in a single sequence spanning the entire cardiac cycle. The images produced may be played back sequentially at any speed to produce a cine display for evaluating wall motion. Imaging should be performed in anterior, LAO, and left lateral projections. Cardiac output, right and left ventricular ejection fractions, stroke volume, and end-diastolic and end-systolic volumes can be obtained from this study. Unlike the first-pass scintigraphy, injection technique is unimportant and the counting statistics and spatial resolution are much better. Sedation may be necessary for the uncooperative child but, because time is not a limiting factor as far as the radioactive tracer is concerned, sleep deprivation, feeding, and patience may help to achieve a diagnostic study. The gated radionuclide study has been used to evaluate wall motion and ejection fractions in cardiac trauma and, since the right ventricle can be evaluated, it is better than myocardial perfusion. It is also used in cardiac transplants.

Myocardial Perfusion

Myocardial perfusion scintigraphy (Fig 15–30) is used to detect myocardial ischemia and infarction as

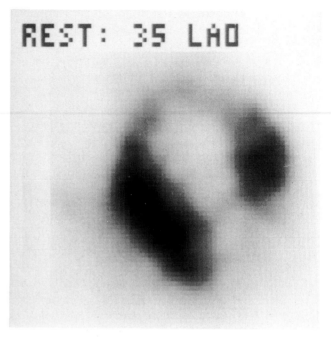

FIG 15–30.
A 3-week-old infant 2 weeks after arterial switch for transposition. Planar myocardial perfusion image performed at rest in the 35-degree LAO projection demonstrates a significant perfusion defect in the anterolateral and apical musculature. Biplane cineangiocardiogram performed the same day showed good visualization of all the major branches of the right and left coronary arteries.

may be seen with anomalous left coronary artery, cardiomyopathy produced by glycogen storage disease, and thalassemia. It can be used to evaluate perfusion in septal hypertrophy and postoperative arterial switch for transposition. Thallium 201 as thallous chloride is the most widely used imaging agent. Thallium acts as a potassium analog and is extracted by the myocardial cells proportionate to coronary flow. In adults a single injection is made when the patient is stressed while using the treadmill or other form of exercise such as a bicycle. In children it is difficult to obtain adequate stress. For this reason pharmacologic stress may be used such as dipyridamole which produces vasodilation. The flow in normal coronary arteries will increase three to five times; abnormal coronary arteries will not dilate, resulting in detectable regional differences in perfusion. Intravenous dipyridamole is currently approved as a pharmacologic stress agent. Adenosine may soon be approved as another pharmacologic stress agent.

The patient should be fasting for 3 to 4 hours to decrease flow to the splanchnic bed since sedation will be necessary in some children. Planar ^{201}Tl images are obtained in anterior, LAO, and left lateral projections and repeated 3 to 4 hours or even later to evaluate redistribution of ^{201}Tl. In noninfarcted myo-

cardium, satisfactory perfusion should be obtained. Cine playback of resting myocardial perfusion images will demonstrate specific areas of decreased ventricular contraction.

Single photon emission computed tomography (SPECT) acquisition increases the contrast resolution of the images and increases the sensitivity of the study. Reconstruction of the images in the short axis, vertical long axis, and horizontal long axis are performed and the coronary artery territories are well defined.

Recently new ^{99m}Tc-labeled compounds have been approved, such as ^{99m}Tc sestamibi and ^{99m}Tc teboroxime, which are distributed to the myocardium, proportionate to blood flow, like ^{201}Tl. The difference is that ^{99m}Tc sestamibi does not redistribute and if images are obtained at rest, a repeat injection must be given at a later interval for stress imaging. Technetium 99m teboroxime redistributes quickly and is less well suited for SPECT imaging and use in pediatrics. The lack of redistribution allows for long acquisition times with sestamibi. The physical half-life is less for ^{99m}Tc sestamibi than ^{201}Tl and the radiation dose for the same activity is less. Because the photon energy of technetium (140 keV) is ideal for current scintillation cameras and the injected dose can contain more activity, there is improved count density with improved image quality and spatial resolution.

Metabolic Function Evaluation

Positron emission tomography (PET) imaging can evaluate and quantify regional metabolic rates and regional blood flow in the myocardium. The development of new metabolic tracers such as N-13 ammonia for perfusion, C-11 hydroxyephedrine for heart neuronal studies, and fluorine 18-fluorodeoxyglucose (F-18 FDG) for metabolic assessment of the myocardium assesses functions for which there are no other means of evaluation available. The value of PET is the ability to identify viable myocardium on the basis of intact metabolic activity in regions of otherwise underperfused and dysfunctional myocardium. Currently there are centers investigating cardiomyopathies with PET. Although it may be clinically useful, PET is available only at centers with a cyclotron.

Myocardial Necrosis Evaluation

Technetium 99m pyrophosphate is the current standard for myocardial necrosis imaging. Peak activity in an area of myocardial necrosis is seen at approximately 48 hours following chest trauma and changes

may be present for up to a week. However, this study is relatively insensitive and not often performed in pediatric situations. Indium 111 antimyosin monoclonal antibody Fab will be a more sensitive and specific alternative test when approved in the United States, especially with the addition of SPECT imaging. The antimyosin antibody adheres to myosin which is exposed to extracellular fluid only with cell death. The extent and intensity of antimyosin uptake may be used as an indicator of necrotic myocardial tissue.

Inflammation

Indium 111–labeled autologous white blood cells as well as ^{67}Ga is useful in identifying those patients with myocarditis and Kawasaki disease in the acute phase. SPECT imaging identifies the tracer in the myocardium or pericardium. Technetium 99m–labeled white blood cells with hexamethylpropyleneamine oxime (HMPAO) are approved and will be useful for detecting infection in the heart. Antimyosin imaging is effective for the detection of myocyte necrosis associated with active myocarditis. Antimyosin uptake in the heart has been seen in a large number of cases of dilated cardiomyopathy. It has a negative predictive value which may obviate the need for endomyocardial biopsy in suspected myocarditis and in patients post transplant.

ELECTROCARDIOGRAPHY

Electrocardiography has been useful in the diagnosis and management of arrhythmias. Twenty-four-hour continuous ambulatory ECG (cardioscan) allows for adequate evaluation of a child that complains of palpitations, dizziness, or syncope. It also allows for evaluation of premature ventricular contractions to determine the frequency, timing, and morphology. Knowledge of the baseline heart rate in all activities is essential for management of patients with congenital complete heart block. The presence of ventricular arrhythmias is a poor prognostic sign in patients with cardiomyopathy and the 24-hour cardioscan monitor allows detection. Antiarrhythmic drug therapy can be followed with serial cardioscans. Many corrective operations for congenital heart malformations have cardiac arrhythmias as a subsequent complication. The cardioscan allows for detection and proper management of these. Transtelephonic ECG monitoring is also useful in the management of patients with CHD. It allows for evaluation of permanently implanted pacemakers. It has become an important tool for arrhythmia detection. It also allows for the evaluation of the efficacy of antiarrhythmic therapy. Exercise stress ECG (treadmill) is also used for evaluation of cardiac arrhythmias in children and to assess for functional abnormalities. Exercise treadmill testing in combination with nuclear medicine imaging may allow for detection of functional abnormalities.

REFERENCES

Routine Chest Roentgenography

Burbank F, Parish D, Wexler L: Echocardiographic-like angled views of the heart by MR imaging. *J Comput Assist Tomogr* 1988; 12:181.

Coussement AM, Gooding CA: Objective radiographic assessment of pulmonary vascularity in children. *Radiology* 1973; 109:649.

Edwards DK, Higgins CB: Radiology of neonatal heart disease. *Radiol Clin North Am* 1980; 18:369.

Edwards DK, Higgins CB, Gilpin EA: The cardiothoracic ratio in newborn infants. *Am J Roentgenol* 1981; 136:907.

Elliott LP: An angiocardiographic and plain film approach to complex congenital heart disease: Classification and simplified nomenclature. *Curr Probl Cardiol* 1978; 3:1–64.

Farmer DW, Lipton JJ, Webb WR, et al: Computed tomography in congenital heart disease. *Radiology* 1985; 155:284.

Gyppes MT, Bensant WR: Severe congenital heart disease in the neonatal period. *Am J Roentgenol* 1972; 116:490.

Jaffe RB: Complete interruption of the aortic arch. I: Characteristic radiographic findings in 21 patients. *Circulation* 1975; 52:714.

Keith JD, Rowe RD, Vlad P: *Heart Disease in Infancy and Childhood,* ed 3. New York, Macmillan, 1978, p 5.

Nitz L: Roentgenographic evaluation of pulmonary arteries in normal babies and roentgen appearance of pulmonary vascularity in young infants with congenital heart disease. *Ann Radiol* 1975; 18:465.

Rosario-Medina W, Strife JL, Dunbar JS: Normal left atrium: Appearance in children on frontal chest radiographs. *Radiology* 1986; 161:345.

Angiocardiography

Arciniegas JG, Soto B, Coghlan HC, et al: Congenital heart malformations: Sequential angiographic analysis. *Am J Roentgenol* 1981; 137:673.

Bargeron LM Jr, Elliott LP: Axial cineangiocardiography in congenital heart disease. I. Concept, technical and anatomic considerations. *Circulation* 1977; 56:1075.

Ceballos R, Roto B, Bargeron LM Jr: Angiographic anatomy of the normal heart through axial angiography. *Circulation* 1981; 64:351.

Elliott LP, Bargeron LM Jr, Soto B, et al: Axial cineangiog-

raphy in congenital heart disease. *Radiol Clin North Am* 1980; 15:515.

Fellows KE, Keane JF, Freed MD: Angled views in cineangiography of congenital heart disease. *Radiology* 1977; 56:485.

Garcia-Medina V, Bass J, Braunlin E, et al: A useful projection for demonstrating the bifurcation of the pulmonary artery. *Pediatr Cardiol* 1990; 11:147–149.

Mitchell SW, Kan J, White RI: Interventional techniques in congenital heart disease. *Semin Roentgenol* 1985; 20:290.

Tonkin ILD: Digital subtraction angiography in congenital heart disease. *Semin Roentgenol* 1985; 20:283.

Echocardiography

Allen HD, Goldberg SJ, Sahn DJ, et al: Suprasternal notch echocardiography: Assessment of its clinical utility in pediatric cardiology. *Circulation* 1977; 55:605.

Bierman FZ, Williams RG: Subxiphoid two-dimensional imaging of the interatrial septum in infants and neonates with congenital heart disease. *Circulation* 1979; 60:80.

Gramiak R, Nanda NC: New techniques in cardiac imaging with ultrasound: State of the art. *Radiology* 1979; 133:609.

Henry WL, Maron BJ, Griffiths JM: Cross-sectional echocardiography in the diagnosis of congenital heart disease: Identification of the relation of the ventricles and great arteries. *Circulation* 1977; 56:267.

Kelley MJ, Jaffe CC, Shoum SM, et al: Radiographic and echocardiographic approach to cyanotic congenital heart disease. *Radiol Clin North Am* 1980; 18:411.

Kotler MN, Mintz GS, Segal BL, et al: Clinical uses of two-dimensional echocardiography. *Am J Cardiol* 1980; 45:1061.

Lange LW, Sahn DJ, Allen HD, et al: Subxiphoid cross-sectional echocardiography in infants and children with congenital heart disease. *Circulation* 1979; 59:513.

Lee RT, Bhatia SJS, St John Sutton MG: Assessment of valvular heart disease with Doppler echocardiography. *JAMA* 1989; 262:2131.

Ludomirsky A, Huhta JC (eds): *Color Doppler of Congenital Heart Disease in the Child and Adult.* Mount Kisco, NY, Futura Publishing, 1987.

Maron BJ, Henry WL, Griffiths JM, et al: Identification of congenital malformations of the great arteries in infants by real-time two dimensional echocardiography. *Circulation* 1975; 52:671.

Meyer RA, Kaplan S: Non-invasive techniques in pediatric cardiovascular disease. *Prog Cardiovasc Dis* 1973; 15:341.

Miyatake K, Okamoto M, Kinoshita N, et al: Clinical applications of a new type of real-time two-dimensional Doppler flow imaging system. *Am J Cardiol* 1984; 54:857–868.

Popp RL, Fowles RE, Collart DJ, et al: Cardiac anatomy

viewed systematically with two-dimensional echocardiography. *Chest* 1979; 75:579.

Sahn DJ: Real-time two-dimensional Doppler echocardiographic flow mapping. *Circulation* 1985; 71:849.

Silverman NH, Schiller NB: Apex echocardiography: Two-dimensional technique for evaluating congenital heart disease. *Circulation* 1978; 57:503.

Snider AR, Silverman NH: Suprasternal notch echocardiography: A two-dimensional technique for evaluating congenital heart disease. *Circulation* 1981; 63:165.

Tajik AJ, Seward JB, Hagler DJ, et al: Two-dimensional real-time ultrasonic imaging of the heart and great vessels: Technique, image orientation, structure identification and validation. *Mayo Clin Proc* 1978; 53:271.

Ultan LB, Segal BL, Likoff W: Echocardiography in congenital heart disease—preliminary observations. *Am J Cardiol* 1967; 19:74.

Computed Tomography

Lackener K, Thurn P: Computed tomography of the heart: ECG gated and continuous scans. *Radiology* 1981; 140:413.

Morehouse CC, Brody WR, Guthaner DF, et al: Gated cardiac computed tomography with a motion phantom. *Radiology* 1980; 134:213.

Ritman EL, Harris LD, Kinsey JH, et al: Computed tomographic imaging of the heart: The dynamic spatial reconstructor. *Radiol Clin North Am* 1980; 18:547.

Magnetic Resonance Imaging

Amparo EG, Higgins CB, Farmer D, et al: Gated MRI of cardiac and paracardiac masses: Initial experience. *Am J Roentgenol* 1984; 143:1151–1156.

Burbank F, Parish D, Wexler L: Echocardiographic-like angled views of the heart by MR imaging. *J Comput Assist Tomogr* 1988; 12:181–195.

Burrows PE: Magnetic resonance imaging of the aorta in children. *Semin Ultrasound CT MR* 1990; 11:221–233.

Didier D, Higgins CB, Fisher MR, et al: Congenital heart disease: Gated MR imaging in 72 patients. *Radiology* 1986; 158:227–235.

Formanek AG, Witcofski RL, D'Souza VJ, et al: MR imaging of the central pulmonary arterial tree in conotruncal malformation. *Am J Roentgenol* 1986; 147:1127–1131.

Gomes AS, Lois JF, Williams RG: Pulmonary arteries: MR imaging in patients with congenital obstruction of the right ventricular outflow tract. *Radiology* 1990; 174:51–57.

Gutierrez F, Mirowitz S, Canter C: Magnetic resonance imaging in the evaluation of postoperative congenital heart defects. *Semin Ultrasound CT MR* 1990; 11:234–245.

Higgins CB: MR of the heart: Anatomy, physiology and metabolism. *Am J Roentgenol* 1988; 151:239–248.

Jaffe RB: Magnetic resonance imaging of vascular rings. *Semin Ultrasound CT MR* 1990; 11:206–220.

Julsrud PR: Magnetic resonance imaging of the pulmonary arteries and veins. *Semin Ultrasound CT MR* 1990; 11:184–205.

Rienmuller R, Tiling R: Evaluation of paracardiac and intracardiac masses in children. *Semin Ultrasound CT MR* 1990; 11:246–250.

Sechtem U, Pflugfelder PW, White RD, et al: Cine MR imaging: Potential for the evaluation of cardiovascular function. *Am J Roentgenol* 1987; 148:239–246.

Utz JA, Herfkens RJ, Heinsimer JA, et al: Valvular regurgitation: Dynamic MR imaging. *Radiology* 1988; 168:91–94.

Nuclear Cardiology

Bonow RO, Dilsizian V: Thallium 201 for assessment of myocardial viability. *Semin Nucl Med* 1991; 21:230–241.

Carrio I, Berna I, Ballester M, et al: Indium-111 antimyosin scintigraphy to assess myocardial damage in patients with suspected myocarditis and cardiac rejection. *J Nucl Med* 1988; 29:1893–1900.

Harrison KA, Dalrymple GV, Frick MP, et al: Nuclear cardiology: Current practice and future trends. *Appl Radiol* 1991; 20:17–20.

Homma S, Gilliland Y, Gurney TE, et al: Safety of intravenous dipyridamole for stress testing with thallium imaging. *Am J Cardiol* 1987; 59:152–155.

Hossack KF, Mofen CA, Vanway CW, et al: Frequency of cardiac contusion in nonpenetrating chest injury. *Am J Cardiol* 1988; 61:391–394.

Khaw BA, Yasuda T, Gold HK, et al: Acute myocardial infarct imaging with indium-111 labeled monoclonal antimyosin Fab fragments. *J Nucl Med* 1987; 28:1671–1676.

Matsura H, Ishikita T, Yamamoto S, et al: Gallium-67 myocardial imaging for the detection of myocarditis in the acute phase of Kawasaki disease (mucocutaneous lymph node syndrome): The usefulness of single photon emission computed tomography. *Br Heart J* 1987; 58:385–392.

Nakata T, Sakakibara T, Noto T, et al: Myocardial distribution of indium-111–antimyosin Fab in acute inferior and right ventricular infarction: Comparison with technetium-99m–pyrophosphate imaging and histologic examination. *J Nucl Med* 1991; 32:865–867.

Nishimura T, Nagata S, Uehara T, et al: Assessment of myocardial damage in dilated-phase hypertrophic cardiomyopathy by using indium-111–antimyosin Fab myocardial scintigraphy. *J Nucl Med* 1991; 32:1333–1337.

Roddie ME, Peters AM, Danpure HJ, et al: Inflammation: Imaging with Tc-99m HMPAO-labeled leukocytes. *Radiology* 1988; 166:767–772.

Schwaiger M, Hicks R: The clinical role of metabolic imaging of the heart by positron emission tomography. *J Nucl Med* 1991; 32:565–578.

Siffring PA, Gupta NC, Mohiuddin SM, et al: Myocardial uptake and clearance of Tl-201 in healthy subjects.

Comparison of adenosine-induced hyperemia and exercise stress. *Radiology* 1989; 173:769–774.

Strauss HW, Boucher CA: Myocardial perfusion studies: Lessons from a decade of use. *Radiology* 1986; 16:577–584.

Treves ST: Heart, in Treves ST, Hurwitz R, Kuruc A, et al (eds): *Pediatric Nuclear Medicine.* New York, Springer-Verlag, 1985.

Vogel M, Smallhorn JR, Gilday D, et al: Assessment of myocardial perfusion in patients after the arterial switch operation. *J Nucl Med* 1991; 32:237–241.

Wakasugi S, Shibata N, Kobayashi T, et al: Thallium-201 imaging in a patient with mid-ventricular hypertrophic obstructive cardiomyopathy. *J Nucl Med* 1988; 29:1738–1741.

Williams HT, Miller JH: Scintigraphy of major closed chest cardiac trauma in childhood. *Pediatr Radiol* 1988; 18:74–76.

Williamson SL, Williamson MR, Seibert JJ: Indium-111 leukocyte localization for detecting early myocarditis in patients with Kawasaki disease. *Am J Roentgenol* 1986; 146:255.

16

Congenital Heart Disease

The heart develops initially as a tube formed from the fusion of a pair of vessels in the ventral aspect of the foregut of the primitive embryo. Through a series of flexures, torsions, and focal dilatations, the several chambers are formed and become separated from one another by fusions of septa protruding into the cavities. The great vessels are similarly separated. Disturbances of the complicated simultaneous and sequential processes result in malformations involving abnormal communications, obstructions, hypoplasias, etc., that are discussed in the following sections. A detailed description of the embryology and development of the heart can be found in Moore's *The Developing Human* and Patten's *Human Embryology*.

SECTION 1

Acyanotic Congenital Heart Disease With Increased Pulmonary Flow

VENTRICULAR SEPTAL DEFECT

Ventricular septal defect (VSD) accounts for 25% of all congenital heart disease (CHD), with an incidence of between 1.3 and 2.5 per 1,000 live births. Many small VSDs close spontaneously (33%), so the incidence varies depending upon age at evaluation (see Table 15–1).

Classification

A VSD may be isolated or part of a complex congenital heart malformation, i.e. tetralogy of Fallot, truncus arteriosus, atrioventricular (AV) canal, coarctation syndrome, tricuspid atresia, transposition of the great arteries, and double-outlet right ventricle. Although many classifications of VSDs have been proposed, a common working classification divides the septum into four components: (1) *inlet* septum separating the mitral and tricuspid valves; (2) *trabecular* septum extending from the attachment of the tricuspid valve leaflets to the apex and upward to the crista supraventricularis; (3) *outlet* septum extending from the crista supraventricularis to the pulmonary valve; and (4) the *thin membranous* septum (Fig 16–1). Approximately 80% of VSDs occur in the membranous septum and may extend and involve the inlet, trabecular, or outlet septum and then are called perimembranous defects. Less commonly, VSDs occur in the inlet, trabecular, or muscular septum. These defects, their frequency, and associated malformations and complications are listed in Table 16–1. A VSD is the most common lesion in the chromosomal syndromes of trisomy 13, 18, and 21.

Pathophysiology

The pathophysiologic effect of a VSD is a high-pressure left-to-right shunt at the ventricular level. This subjects the pulmonary vasculature to high flow and high pressure, which frequently results in obstruc-

tive pulmonary vascular disease that may be irreversible in advanced stages.

Clinical Manifestations

Symptoms relate to the size of the VSD and the degree of left-to-right shunt. Failure to thrive and congestive heart failure (CHF) usually do not appear until after the first month as pulmonary vascular resistance falls. A characteristic systolic murmur is evident over the low precordium with a restricted VSD. This murmur is always holosystolic and extends to the second sound. A soft, low-pitched early diastolic murmur is also frequently heard in the apical area. With a large VSD, no murmur may be present, or there may be a midsystolic crescendo-

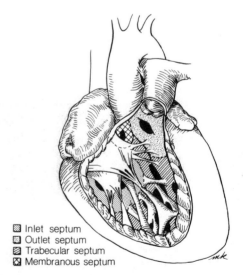

Inlet septum
Outlet septum
Trabecular septum
Membranous septum

FIG 16–1.
Schematic representation of ventricular septal defect (VSD) position as seen from the right ventricle. VSDs are illustrated in black in the four components of the ventricular septum: inlet, outlet, trabecular, and membranous septa. Multiple VSDs are illustrated in the trabecular septum. A defect in the membranous septum may extend into the inlet, outlet, or trabecular septum and is then known as a perimembranous VSD.

TABLE 16–1.

Classification of Ventricular Septal Defect

Type	Synonym	Frequency	Associated With or Complicated by	Optimal Angiographic Projection(s)*
Membranous	Perimembranous Infracristal	80%	Aneurysm of the membranous septum, and spontaneous closure Adherence of tricuspid valve tissue to defect with left ventricle–right atrial shunt Extension to trabecular, outlet septum Malalignment with subaortic stenosis	Long-axis (steep LAO)
Inlet	AV canal type	8%	Straddling tricuspid valve	Long-axis (shallow LAO)
Outlet	Conal Subpulmonary Subarterial Supracristal Infundibular	5%–7%	Aortic valve prolapse through defect with right ventricular outflow tract obstruction Aortic regurgitation Dilatation of the sinus of Valsalva Aortic–right ventricular fistula	AP, RAO, lateral
Trabecular	Muscular Central muscular Apical muscular Marginal "Swiss cheese" muscular	5%–20%		Long-axis and four-chamber (shallow and steep LAO)

*LAO = left anterior oblique; AP = anteroposterior; RAO = right anterior oblique.

decrescendo murmur. A widely split and accentuated second sound is frequently noted. With pulmonary hypertension the second sound becomes louder and fixed.

Chest Roentgenography

Roentgenographic findings vary depending upon the size of the VSD. A normal chest roentgenogram will be seen with a small VSD. Common findings with a larger defect include (1) cardiomegaly (75% under age of 2 years), (2) increased pulmonary blood flow (Figs 15–2 and 16–2) with a large main pulmonary artery segment, (3) enlargement of the left atrium and displacement of the left mainstem bronchus (Fig 16–2, *B*), and (4) right aortic arch (5%). CHF is frequent in the infant (Fig 16–2, *A*), while pulmonary hypertension becomes evident in the older child with enlarged central pulmonary arteries.

Spontaneous closure of the VSD or development of acquired infundibular pulmonary stenosis (acquired tetralogy of Fallot) results in a decrease in heart size and pulmonary blood flow. The differential diagnosis includes: (1) patent ductus arteriosus (PDA), (2) AV canal, (3) aorticopulmonary window, and (4) atrial septal defect (ASD).

Echocardiography

Real-time echocardiography allows direct imaging of larger membranous and muscular septal defects, particularly from the subxiphoid (subcostal) and parasternal projection (Fig 16–3, *A–C*). Enlargement of the left atrium, membranous septum aneurysms, and other associated lesions may also be seen. Doppler interrogation along the right ventricular margin of the ventricular septum will show a positive flow pattern (see Figs 15–23 and 15–24). Color Doppler examination also will document directional shunting and turbulence and permit more rapid indentification of muscular VSDs (see Fig 15–24).

Angiocardiography

A selective left ventriculogram performed in the long-axis or four-chamber projection, or in both projections, is preferred (Figs 16–4 and 16–5; see also Fig 15–13,B). With large defects, 2 mL/kg contrast should be injected in as short as time as possible. Catheterization can usually be performed from the venous approach although with a closed atrial septum retrograde aortic catheterization will be necessary. Because of the combined presence of membranous and muscular septal defects (see Fig 16–5), the entire septum must be adequately visualized. Su-

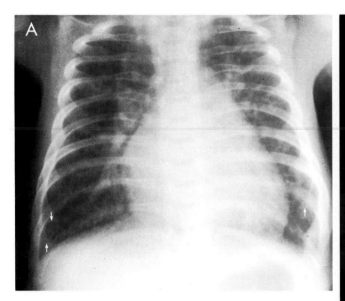

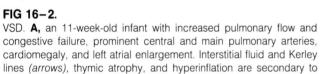

FIG 16–2.
VSD. **A,** an 11-week-old infant with increased pulmonary flow and congestive failure, prominent central and main pulmonary arteries, cardiomegaly, and left atrial enlargement. Interstitial fluid and Kerley lines *(arrows)*, thymic atrophy, and hyperinflation are secondary to failure in this acyanotic heart lesion. **B,** a lateral view shows left atrial enlargement displacing the left mainstem bronchus posteriorly *(arrows)* and prominent central pulmonary vasculature with large vessels extending into the peripheral lungs (see Fig 15–2).

pracristal VSDs may be visualized best in true AP and lateral projections or RAO projection of the long-axis view (Fig 16–6). Appropriate injections to rule out associated lesions such as coarctation, PDA, and ASD must be made. If significant pulmonary hypertension exists, contrast angiography should be performed with caution, preferably by using non-ionic media. VSD imaging with magnetic resonance imaging (MRI) has been successful.

Prognosis

The prognosis is good with an early diagnosis and operative treatment. Muscular septal defects are more difficult to close than are membranous ones. Operative correction is preferable before the age of 2 or 3 years to decrease the chance of irreversible pulmonary hypertension (Eisenmenger syndrome). In high-risk patients or patients with complex associated lesion, pulmonary artery banding may be performed as a palliative procedure. Early closure of all outlet defects is recommended to prevent development of aortic sinus prolapse and subsequent development of aortic regurgitation. Without surgery endocarditis develops in 1% to 5% of patients. Catheter closure techniques are in the experimental stages (Fig 16–7).

ATRIAL SEPTAL DEFECT

Incidence

Atrial septal defect (ASD) accounts for 10% of all CHD. The incidence in females is more than twice that in males. Most cases occur sporadically, but secundum defects have been reported in families as a genetic abnormality. Anomalies of the upper extremities and a secundum ASD (Holt-Oram syndrome) also have been reported in families (see Table 15–1).

Secundum defects account for greater than 90% of all ASDs and are usually isolated anomalies. Important associated lesions include abnormalities of the mitral valve, particularly mitral valve prolapse with or without mitral regurgitation. A sinus venosus defect accounts for 5% to 10% of ASDs, and is located posterior to the secundum defect. This defect is commonly associated with anomalous connection of the right pulmonary veins, particularly the upper lobe veins to either the right atrium or superior vena cava (SVC). The coronary sinus ASD is a rare lesion occurring at the expected site of the coronary sinus ostium. It is usually part of a developmental complex that includes absence of the coronary sinus and persistent left SVC emptying into the left atrium.

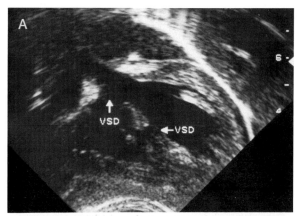

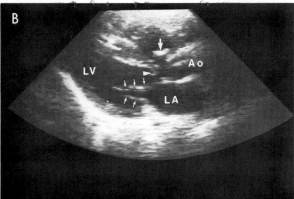

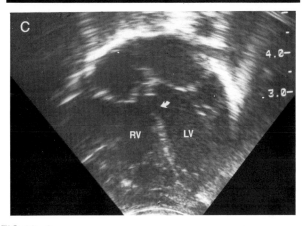

FIG 16–3.
A, subcostal four-chamber projection demonstrates a moderate-sized membranous VSD (*vertical arrow*) and a small midmuscular VSD (*horizontal arrow*). (From Jaffe RB: Ventricular septal defect—echocardiography, in Elliott LP (ed): *Cardiac Imaging in Infants, Children, and Adults.* Philadelphia, JB Lippincott, 1991, p 575. Used by permission.) **B,** a two-dimensional long-axis echocardiogram demonstrates a VSD and aneurysm of the membranous septum *(large arrow)* projecting into the right ventricular outflow tract. Membranous subaortic stenosis is present caudad to the VSD arising from the membranous septum *(arrowhead)*. *Small arrows* indicate the mitral valve. **C,** in the apical four-chamber projection, a moderate-sized inlet VSD *(curved arrow)* is present in the posterior muscular septum in the plane of the tricuspid and mitral valves. *RV,* right ventricle; *LV,* left ventricle.

Pathophysiology

Low-pressure left-to-right shunting occurs with increased right ventricular compliance and produces right atrial and right ventricular dilatation. Shunt volume relates to the size of the defect, right heart compliance, and pulmonary resistance. Pulmonary hypertension in childhood is uncommon.

Clinical Manifestations

Systolic ejection murmurs in the pulmonary region and parasternal diastolic murmurs are present. The second sound is split and does not vary with respiration. Children with a large ASD have a mild diastolic flow murmur through the tricuspid valve.

Chest Roentgenography

In the neonate the heart and pulmonary flow are usually within normal limits. Findings in later infancy and childhood include (1) mild cardiomegaly with right atrial and right ventricular enlargement, (2) mild increased pulmonary blood flow (particularly centrally), (3) a "triangular" cardiac silhouette related to right heart and main pulmonary artery enlargement, and (4) a relatively inconspicuous SVC (Fig 16–8). Primary differential diagnoses include AV canal, VSD, PDA, and other left-to-right shunts.

Echocardiography

Two-dimensional imaging reveals (1) ASD, (2) a large right atrium, and (3) a large right ventricle (Fig 16–9). M-mode and real-time evaluation demonstrate paradoxical or flat septal motion. Doppler interrogation in the right atrium demonstrates a positive flow pattern in the right atrium. Color Doppler examination permits rapid identification of left-to-right shunting at the atrial level (see Fig 15–22).

Angiocardiography

Optimal visualization is achieved with a right upper lobe pulmonary vein injection in the four-chamber projection with a biplane cineangiocardiogram. The secundum ASD and associated left-to-right shunting will be well demonstrated and differentiated from sinus venosus and ostium primum defects (Fig

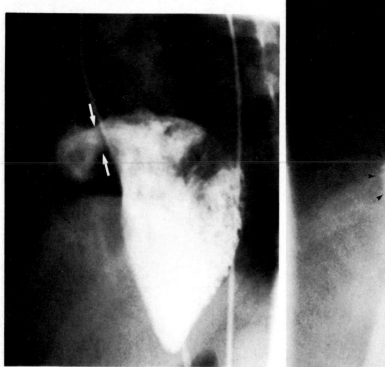

FIG 16–4.
A, membranous infracristal VSD *(arrows)* in a left ventriculogram in the long-axis projection. Note the proximity of the defect to the right aortic sinus. **B,** left ventricular long-axis angiocardiogram showing a membranous infracristal VSD with associated aneurysm of the interventricular septum *(arrowheads).* This cloverlike aneurysm bulges in systole into the right ventricle beneath the tricuspid valve.

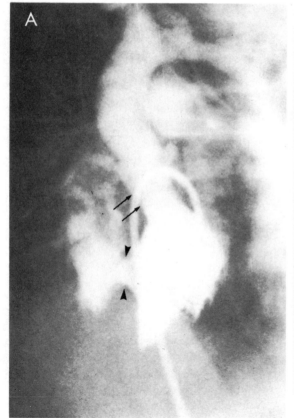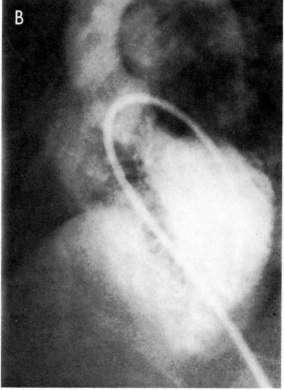

FIG 16–5.
Muscular VSD. **A,** long-axis left ventriculogram demonstrates muscular VSD in the midportion of the septum with an associated left-to-right shunt *(arrowheads).* The membranous portion of the septum is intact *(arrows).* **B,** left ventriculogram demonstrates multiple muscular VSDs with associated left-to-right shunting (Swiss cheese septum).

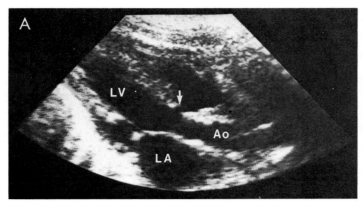

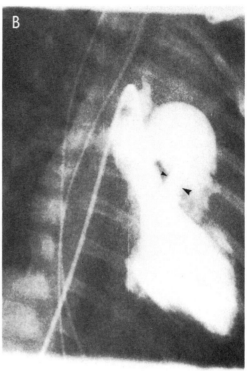

FIG 16–6.
Supracristal VSD. **A,** long-axis echocardiogram demonstrates an oblique defect *(arrow)* extending from just beneath the aortic valve into the right ventricular outflow tract below the pulmonary valve. **B,** angiocardiogram in the frontal long-axis view demonstrates the supracristal defect extending superolaterally from the left ventricle into the right ventricular outflow tract *(arrowheads).*

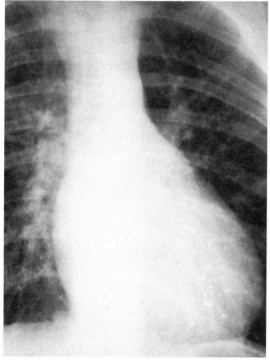

FIG 16–7.
Catheter closure of muscular VSD. Chest radiograph demonstrates experimental clamshell occlusion device across a muscular VSD prior to complete repair of double-outlet right ventricle.

16–10). Long-axis left ventriculography is important to exclude associated VSD or PDA.

Magnetic Resonance Imaging

MRI in the four-chamber projection through the atrial septum may clearly show an ASD (Fig 16–11).

Prognosis

The prognosis after surgical correction is excellent. Large left-to-right shunts should be closed in childhood. Closure of ASD by interventional catheter techniques is in the experimental stage (Fig 16–12). Closure of small defects is controversial. Complications of untreated patients mainly relate to arrhythmia and late pulmonary hypertension.

OSTIUM PRIMUM ATRIAL SEPTAL DEFECT AND ENDOCARDIAL CUSHION DEFECT (ATRIOVENTRICULAR CANAL)

These lesions result from abnormal development of the embryologic endocardial cushion that produces, in its milder form, a defect limited to the lower portion of the atrial septum and an associated cleft mitral valve (ostium primum ASD); the complete form produces an associated VSD and common AV valve (AV canal). Associated lesions include PDA, coarctation, pulmonary valvular stenosis (PVS), pulmonary

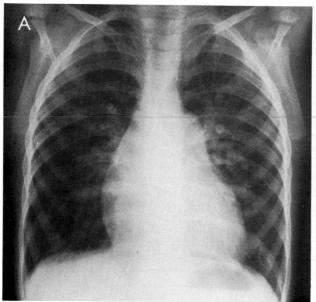

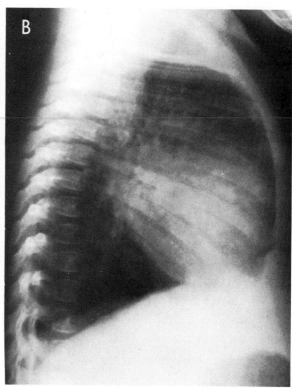

FIG 16–8.
Atrial septal defect (ASD), secundum type. AP **(A)** and lateral **(B)** chest roentgenograms show increased pulmonary vascularity and moderate cardiomegaly. Fullness of the right heart border (right atrium) and relatively inconspicuous superior vena cava and aortic arch are common findings with this lesion. Right ventricular dilatation fills in the retrosternal space in the lateral view.

atresia, tricuspid atresia, transposition of the great arteries, tetralogy of Fallot, and total anomalous pulmonary venous return.

Pathophysiology

Mild to moderate left-to-right shunting occurs predominantly at the atrial level. Pulmonary hyperten-sion develops more commonly in patients with Down syndrome than in others.

Clinical Manifestations

Clinical findings are similar to those of ostium secundum lesions, although more dramatic in the complete endocardial cushion defect and in those

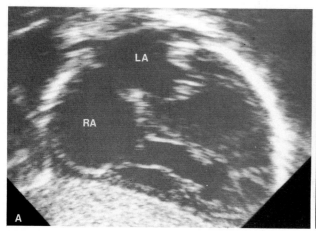

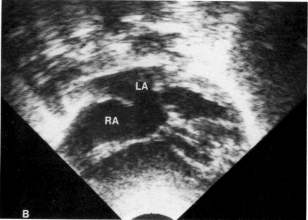

FIG 16–9.
A, ostium secundum ASD. Subxiphoid four-chamber echocardio-gram demonstrates a large defect in the midportion of the atrial septum, typical of an ostium secundum defect. Enlargement of the right atrium *(RA)* is also noted. *LA,* left atrium. **B,** ostium primum ASD. Subxiphoid four-chamber echocardiogram demonstrates a large defect in the lower portion of the atrial septum extending to the level of the mitral and tricuspid valves. Note that the mitral and tricuspid valves are at the same level, typical of an endocardial cushion defect. *RA,* right atrium; *LA,* left atrium.

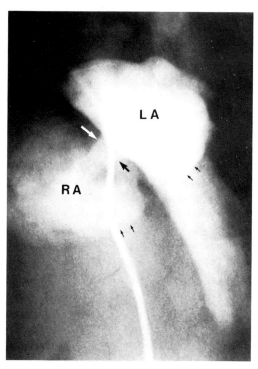

FIG 16–10.
ASD, secundum type. Four-chamber hepatoclavicular angiocardiogram with contrast injected into a right upper lobe pulmonary vein. Contrast streams along the interatrial septum and through an ostium secundum ASD *(large arrows)*. Mitral and tricuspid valves *(small arrows)* are apparent. *RA,* right atrium; *LA,* left atrium.

patients with Down syndrome (30%–40% of patients with AV canal). Failure to thrive, dyspnea, fatigue, and occasionally congestive failure and cyanosis may be seen.

Chest Roentgenography

Roentgenographic findings include (1) mild to moderate cardiomegaly with right atrial and right ventricular enlargement; (2) occasional left atrial enlargement related to mitral insufficiency; (3) moderate increased pulmonary vascularity; (4) moderate pulmonary disease; and (5) 11 pairs of ribs and accessory sternal ossification centers, frequently added findings in Down syndrome patients (Fig 16–13). The differential diagnosis includes ASD, PDA, and VSD.

Echocardiography

Real-time evaluation demonstrates echo dropout in the lower atrial septum (see Fig 16–9,A). Displacement of the anterior mitral valve leaflet into the left ventricular outflow tract may be observed along with abnormal anterior excursion of the anterior mitral valve leaflet. In complete AV canal, abnormal

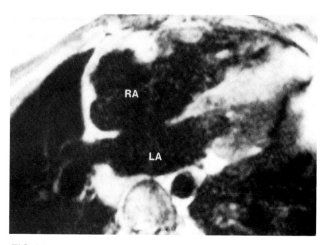

FIG 16–11.
Axial oblique MR scan in the four-chamber projection demonstrates a large secundum ASD. The defect could not be visualized well by echocardiography in this 12-year-old obese patient. *RA,* right atrium; *LA,* left atrium.

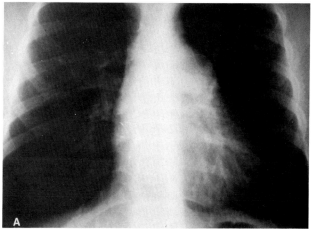

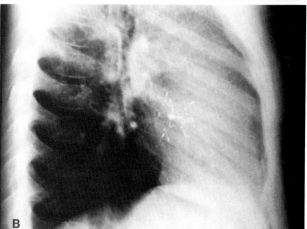

FIG 16–12.
Frontal **(A)** and lateral **(B)** chest radiographs demonstrate an experimental clamshell occlusion device utilized for catheter closure of an ostium secundum ASD.

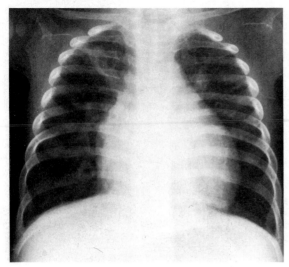

FIG 16–13.
Atrioventricular (AV) canal. A chest roentgenogram demonstrates moderate cardiomegaly with a round (globular) cardiac silhouette having a prominent right atrium and right ventricle. There is increased pulmonary flow with a relatively narrow cardiac base. Patchy right upper lobe and left lower lobe pulmonary disease is commonly seen in patients with Down syndrome.

orientation and an oval or figure-8 configuration of the AV valve are frequently seen. The adjacent membranous VSD will also be evident, with anomalous chordal attachment and prominent papillary muscles frequently noted. A common leaflet bridging the VSD may be seen (Fig 16–14, *A*). M-mode evaluation shows exaggerated anterior mitral valve leaflet motion and paradoxical septal motion (Fig 16–14, *B*). In partial AV canal (ostium primum ASD) Doppler interrogation in the right atrium demonstrates a positive flow pattern in diastole, while in those patients with complete AV canals, a similar systolic positive flow pattern will be evident in the right ventricle (see Fig 15–22,B).

Angiocardiography

In patients with an ostium primum ASD, a biplane four-chamber angiocardiogram performed with injection into the right upper lobe pulmonary vein identifies the ostium primum ASD and left-to-right shunt. A long-axial left ventriculogram will identify the left ventricular outflow tract abnormality ("gooseneck" deformity) related to the abnormal position of the mitral valve, and also demonstrate the mitral valve cleft, and severity of mitral regurgitation. No ventricular shunting should be seen. Patients with a complete AV canal will demonstrate on long-axis and four-chamber left ventriculograms a left-to-right shunt through a VSD. The common AV valve, the severity of mitral regurgitation, abnormal

chordal attachments, and left ventricular size and function will be identified on these injections (Fig 16–15). If pulmonary hypertension is present, a right ventriculogram in the axial projections to evaluate the VSD may be necessary. An aortogram will be necessary to exclude a PDA and, occasionally, coarctation. Other injections may be needed to exclude other associated lesions.

Prognosis

Simple ostium primum ASDs have an excellent prognosis with early surgery before the age of 5 years. The prognosis in complete AV canal defects is good. Early surgery is necessary prior to the development of significant pulmonary vascular disease. This may necessitate pulmonary artery banding in infancy. Residual AV valvular dysfunction is a common problem with complete AV canal defects.

PATENT DUCTUS ARTERIOSUS

PDA represents the persistence of a vital normal embryologic structure, the sixth aortic arch, that connects the pulmonary artery and the upper descending aorta. This structure may persist on either side, but normally the right involutes while the left persists. The ductus normally closes after birth and becomes a residual fibrous cord (ligamentum arteriosum) that may calcify. PDA occurs once in 2,500 to 5,000 live births, constitutes 10% to 12% of CHD, and is more common in females (see Table 15–1). PDA in premature infants may be as common as 21% to 35%.

Pathophysiology

Closure of the ductus arteriosus begins immediately after birth with the onset of normal respiration and the fall of pulmonary vascular resistance. Ninety percent of the ductus arteriosus has closed by 2 months of age. Closure is delayed in premature infants with respiratory distress and hypoxia. Persistence of the ductus is probably multifactorial, with genetic factors and rubella being contributing factors. Blood flow is predominantly left to right from the aorta into the pulmonary artery, although right-to-left shunting (persistent fetal circulation) will occur in the presence of severe lung disease and pulmonary hypertension.

Clinical Manifestations

An infant with a small patent ductus normally has no clinical manifestations except for a murmur. With

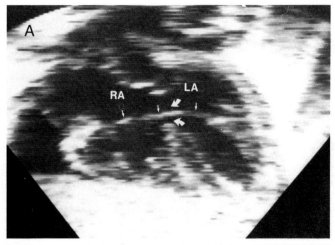

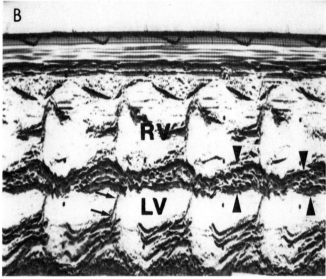

FIG 16–14.

A, complete AV canal. Subcostal four-chamber projection demonstrates the ASD and VSD *(upper* and *lower curved arrows)* and the large common anterior leaflet *(small arrows)* traversing the AV orifice. *RA,* right atrium; *LA,* left atrium. **(From Jaffe RB: Complete atrioventricular canal—echocardiography, in Elliott LP (ed):** *Cardiac Imaging in Infants, Children, and Adults.* **Philadelphia, JB Lippincott, 1991. Used by permission.) B,** M-mode echocardiogram shows the mitral valve leaflet *(arrows)* continuing into and through the plane of the interventricular septum *(arrowheads),* which is characteristic of an endocardial cushion defect. A large right ventricle and tricuspid valve are noted anteriorly. Paradoxical ventricular septal motion shows anterior (superior) septal motion with ventricular contractility characteristic of right heart volume overload.

a larger ductus, failure to thrive and CHF is seen in 40% of children under 2 years of age. Classically, a machinery-like murmur is heard in the pulmonic area, and the second sound is accentuated. PDA is often associated with such conditions as VSD, coarctation, aortic stenosis (AS), PVS, and mitral regurgitation.

Chest Roentgenography

Chest roentgenograms in patients with significant shunting will show (1) increased pulmonary blood flow (Fig 16–16, *A*), (2) cardiomegaly, (3) a prominent ascending aorta and aortic arch, (4) focal aortic dilatation (ductus bump) (Fig 16–16, *B*), and (5) left atrial enlargement. Primary differential diagnoses are VSD, aorticopulmonary window, and truncus arteriosus.

Echocardiography

Real-time echocardiography will frequently demonstrate the patent ductus from the suprasternal notch projection or modified short-axis view (Fig 16–17). Doppler interrogation of the pulmonary artery, however, has proved to be a much more sensitive diagnostic modality (Fig 16–18). Color Doppler rapidly identifies the left-to-right shunting through a PDA

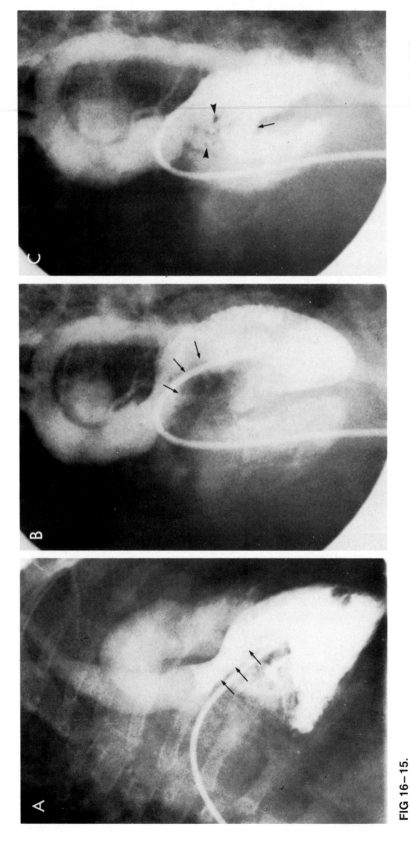

FIG 16—15.

AV canal. **A,** long-axis left ventriculogram (frontal tube view) demonstrates malposition of the mitral valve, with the anterior leaflet projecting into the left ventricular outflow tract (gooseneck deformity) (arrows). An absence or altered alignment of the normal straight segment of the proximal interventricular septum is apparent. **B,** long-axis lateral view in diastole again shows the medial malposition of the mitral valve opening into the left ventricular outflow tract (arrows). Note the VSD and common AV valve. **C,** long-axis left ventriculogram in systole shows the posterior VSD component (arrow) and chordae (arrowheads) as they attach to the interventricular septum.

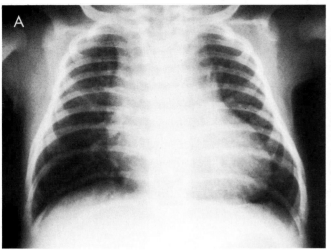
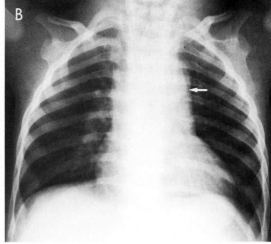

FIG 16–16.
Patent ductus arteriosus in **A,** 3-week-old infant with increased pulmonary vascularity, cardiomegaly, and a prominent right ventricle. The base of the heart is obscured by the thymus. The aortic arch pushes the trachea to the right. Enlargement of the aorta secondary to the patent ductus is not seen. **B,** enlarged left aortic arch shows a second lateral "ductus bump" *(arrow)* and a slight prominence of the descending thoracic aorta. The mildly increased prominence of the central hilar vessels is related to the left-to-right shunt, and cardiomegaly is present.

(see Fig 15–25). An increased arotic–left atrial ratio is frequent.

Angiocardiography

Biplane left ventriculography or aortography, or both, are performed, preferably in the long-axis projection (Fig 16–19; see also Fig 15–13,A). The ductus can be quantitated with respect to size and shunt in this view. Other lesions, i.e., VSD, coarctation, etc., must be ruled out. The differential angiographic diagnosis includes (1) aorticopulmonary window and (2) truncus arteriosus.

Prognosis

The prognosis is excellent with surgery before 24 months of age. Operative mortality is extremely low. Indomethacin is often a successful method of ductus closure in the neonate. Experimental nonsurgical

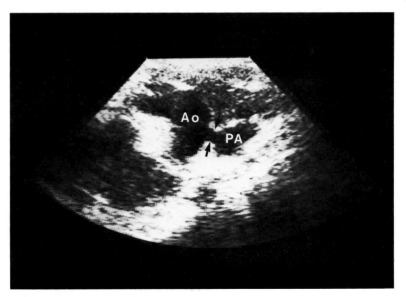

FIG 16–17.
PDA. Short-axis echocardiogram shows a defect in the aortic *(Ao)* wall and continuity between the aortic arch and pulmonary artery *(PA) (arrows).*

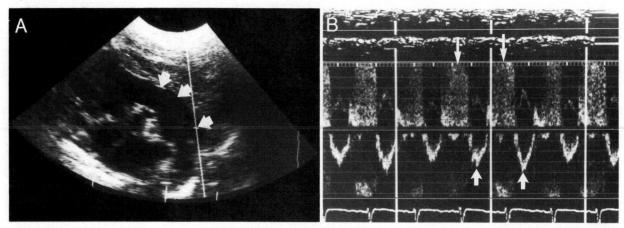

FIG 16–18.
PDA. **A,** Doppler real-time parasagittal longitudinal image demonstrates a large main pulmonary artery *(top two arrows)* with a Doppler sample marker *(bottom arrow)* at the pulmonary artery junction of the PDA. **B,** Doppler image demonstrates pandiastolic retro-grade pulmonary artery flow *(arrows)*, which represents a positive Doppler signal directed toward the transducer head. *Arrowheads* represent systolic forward pulmonary artery flow.

catheter closure has been successful in over 90% of patients (over 8 kg) and awaits Food and Drug Administration (FDA) approval (Fig 16–20). Complications of delayed surgical closure include (1) pulmonary vascular occlusive disease, (2) bacterial endocarditis and mycotic aneurysm of the left pulmonary artery, (3) aneurysm of the ductus arteriosus. Inadvertent ligation of the left pulmonary artery during attempted PDA closure is not an uncommon operative complication (Fig 16–21) in neonates and infants.

OTHER ACYANOTIC CONGENITAL HEART DISEASE WITH LEFT-TO-RIGHT SHUNTS

Aorticopulmonary Window

An aorticopulmonary window represents the failure of the septa dividing the truncus arteriosus to fuse. This leaves a communication between the ascending aorta and pulmonary artery immediately above the aortic valve. The presence of this oval defect creates a major high-pressure left-to-right shunt. An aorticopulmonary window is usually an isolated lesion but may be associated with VSD and PDA. Occasionally ASD, an interrupted aortic arch, coarctation, subaortic stenosis, and an anomalous coronary artery have been noted.

Clinical Manifestations

Tachypnea, tachycardia, and cardiomegaly are common. A systolic murmur may be heard along the left sternal border; a diastolic murmur may occur when an aorticopulmonary window is associated with pulmonary insufficiency. The pulses are frequently bounding.

Chest Roentgenography

Abnormal roentgenographic findings include (1) cardiomegaly with a nonspecific silhouette, (2) an enlarged left atrium, (3) increased pulmonary blood flow related to the left-to-right shunt, and (4) prominence of the ascending aorta and pulmonary artery. Primary differential diagnostic considerations are (1) truncus arteriosus and (2) PDA.

Echocardiography

Findings are similar to those in other left-to-right shunts with left atrial enlargement. The actual defect between the great vessels may be seen with real-time and color-flow Doppler studies.

Angiography

Aortic root injection with biplane AP and lateral cineangiography will demonstrate the left-to-right shunt near the aortic root (Fig 16–22). Differentiation from truncus arteriosus is critical and may be accomplished by identification of two separate semilunar valves. With a large shunt, at least 2 mL/kg of contrast must be injected into the aortic root or left ventricle through a relatively large catheter in minimal time.

Prognosis

The prognosis is good with early surgery prior to the development of pulmonary vascular occlusive disease.

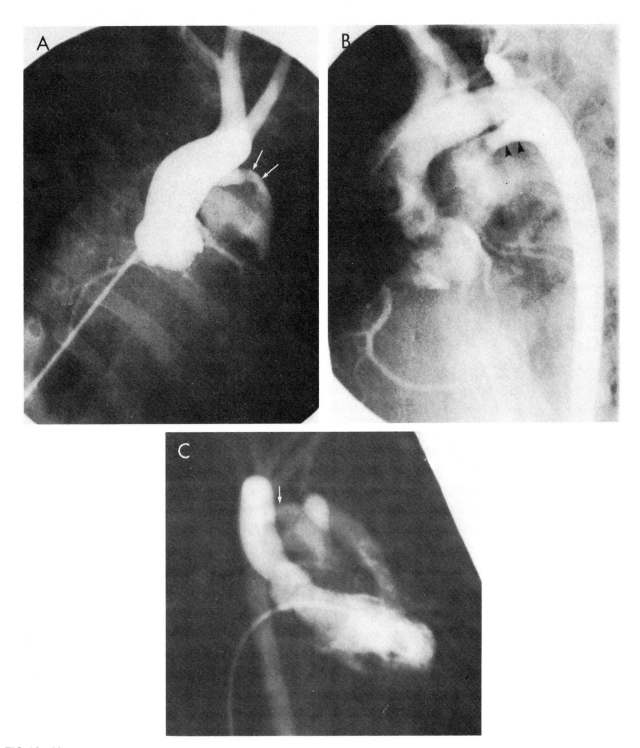

FIG 16–19.
PDA. Long-axis frontal **(A)** and lateral **(B)** films following retrograde aortography demonstrate a moderately large left-to-right shunt through a PDA with a left aortic arch *(arrows)* (see also Fig 15–13, A). Minor pulmonary insufficiency can often be seen with this examina-

tion. **C,** PDA *(arrow)* originates from the right aortic arch and extends to the left to a normal main pulmonary artery with a moderate left-to-right shunt (see Fig 15–29).

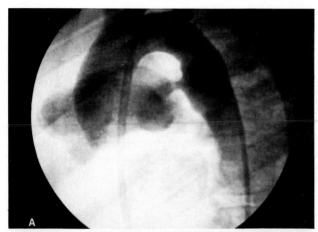

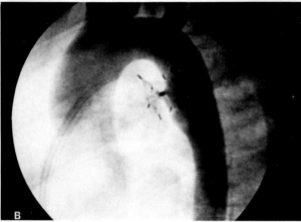

FIG 16–20.
Catheter closure of PDA in an 8-year-old girl with pulmonary hypertension. **A,** lateral digital aortogram demonstrates the PDA with filling of the pulmonary arteries. **B,** repeat lateral digital aortogram after catheter closure with an experimental clamshell occlusion device demonstrates effective closure of the PDA. One side of the occlusion device is in the pulmonary artery, the other in the aorta. A monitoring catheter is now present in the pulmonary artery.

Anomalous Origin of a Pulmonary Artery From the Aorta (Hemitruncus Arteriosus)

This rare anomaly is characterized by anomalous origin of a pulmonary artery, usually the right, from the ascending aorta. The other pulmonary artery, usually the left, is a continuation of the main pulmonary artery arising from the right ventricle. In a series of 50 patients with hemitruncus arteriosus, the right pulmonary artery arose from the ascending aorta in 44 (88%) (Table 17–1). A PDA is present in up to 80% of patients. The aortic arch is usually left-sided.

Clinical Manifestations
Clinical manifestations include, in almost all patients, the rapid development in infancy of CHF from the large left-to-right shunt. If the malforma-

tion is not recognized and corrected at an early age, pulmonary vascular obstructive disease rapidly develops in both lungs.

Chest Roentgenography
Patients with aberrant origin of the pulmonary artery from the ascending aorta show: (1) increased pulmonary blood flow to the lung supplied by the aberrant artery, unless complicated by pulmonary hypertension (Fig 16–23), (2) CHF, and (3) cardiomegaly with right heart and main pulmonary artery enlargement.

Echocardiography
The diagnosis can readily be made on two-dimensional examination. In the most common form, the main pulmonary artery continues as the left pulmonary artery, best appreciated in the short-axis high parasternal projection, while the right pulmonary artery is seen to originate from the ascending aorta.

Angiocardiography
Selective right ventricular injection will demonstrate absence of the normal pulmonary artery bifurcation (Fig 16–24,A). Typically the left pulmonary artery is a continuation of the main pulmonary artery. An aortogram or left ventricular angiogram will demonstrate origin of the aberrant pulmonary artery from the proximal ascending aorta, and confirm the presence of an associated PDA (Fig 16–24, B).

Prognosis
The prognosis is good with early recognition and operative anastomosis of the aberrant pulmonary artery to the main pulmonary artery. If diagnosis is delayed, pulmonary vascular obstructive disease rapidly develops with an extremely poor prognosis.

Anomalous Origin of the Left Coronary Artery

This rare congenital malformation creates a small left-to-right shunt as blood flows from a normal right coronary artery into the low-pressure system of the left coronary artery arising from the base of the pulmonary artery. As pulmonary resistance drops, the left coronary artery blood flow into the myocardium diminishes resulting in left ventricular hypoxemia, ventricular dilatation, and dysfunction.

Clinical Manifestations
CHF, failure to thrive, irritability, and respiratory infections usually commence in the second month of life. Pallor, sweating, and dyspnea may also be present. The electrocardiogram is probably more

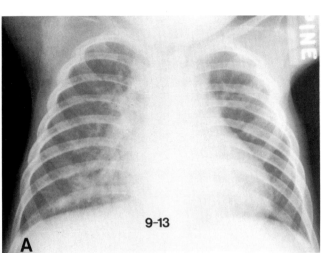

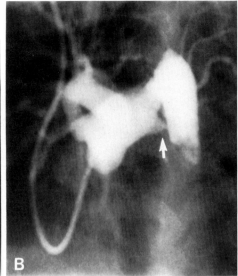

FIG 16–21.
Inadvertent ligation of the left pulmonary artery during attempted PDA closure. **A,** chest radiograph 5 months 10 days after attempted PDA closure demonstrates asymmetric pulmonary blood flow, decreased to the left lung, and increased to the right lung in this patient with Down syndrome. **B,** LAO pulmonary cineangiocardiogram demonstrates inadvertent ligation of the left pulmonary artery at its origin *(arrow)*, PDA, and filling of the proximal descending thoracic aorta. There was delayed collateral filling of the distal left pulmonary artery from the left intercostal collaterals (not illustrated). (From Jaffe RB, Orsmond GS, Veasy LG: *Radiology* 1986; 161:355–357. Used by permission.)

helpful in this condition than with most other congenital heart lesions showing a pattern of anterior myocardial infarction. Thallium radionuclide cardiac scanning can show decreased coronary perfusion and confirm the presence of myocardial ischemia.

Chest Roentgenography

Marked cardiac enlargement secondary to left ventricular dilatation and left atrial enlargement is present (Fig 16–25). Congestive failure is common

FIG 16–22.
Aorticopulmonary window. A right ventriculogram demonstrates minor right-to-left shunting through an aorticopulmonary defect and opacification of the ascending aorta *(arrows)*. The left ventriculogram (not shown) showed a much larger left-to-right shunt through the defect, but the lesion itself was less well appreciated.

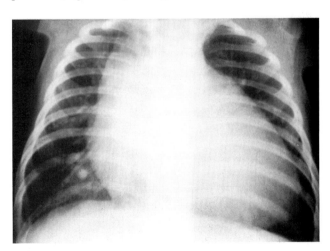

FIG 16–23.
A 1-year-old infant with anomalous origin of the right pulmonary artery from the aorta. Increased pulmonary blood flow to the right lower lung is seen with moderate cardiomegaly.

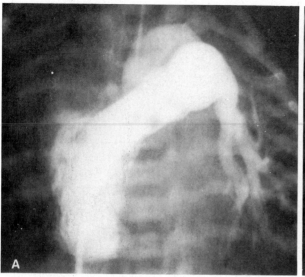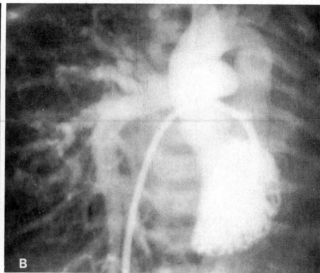

FIG 16–24.
A 2-week-old infant with anomalous origin of the right pulmonary artery from the aorta and small PDA. **A,** right ventricular injection in the frontal projection demonstrates a dextroposed right ventricle with filling of the main and left pulmonary artery. Right-to-left shunt flow through a small patent ductus opacifies the aortic arch. **B,** left ventricular injection in the frontal projection demonstrates origin of the right pulmonary artery from the ascending aorta.

and frequently associated with pneumonia. Primary differential diagnoses include (1) endocardial fibroelastosis and (2) other cardiomyopathies.

Echocardiography
Two-dimensional echocardiography demonstrates (1) left ventricular and left atrial enlargement, (2) de-creased left ventricular contractility, (3) enlargement of the right coronary artery, (4) mitral regurgitation, and (5) occasional identification of the anomalous left coronary artery arising from the base of the pulmonary artery.

Angiocardiography
Left ventriculography demonstrates (1) left ventricular dilatation, (2) diminished function, and (3) mitral regurgitation. A supravalvular aortogram demonstrates (1) enlargement of the right coronary artery, (2) an absence of a left coronary artery on early films, and (3) late visualization of the retrograde filling of the left coronary artery emptying into the pulmonary artery (Fig 16–26).

Prognosis
The prognosis is guarded depending on the severity of left ventricular dysfunction. Early surgical correction is recommended with a bypass graft or relocation of the left coronary artery to the aorta.

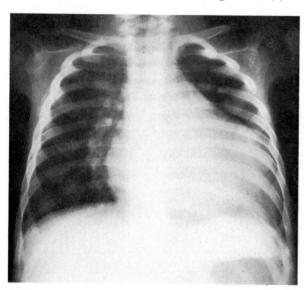

FIG 16–25.
Anomalous origin of the left coronary artery. A 6-month-old infant presented with CHF, cardiomegaly, and the left coronary artery arising from the pulmonary artery. The primary differential consideration is that of cardiomyopathy. Confirmation of the diagnosis with ultrasound or aortography is usually necessary. Compression of the left mainstem bronchus by the large left atrium and left ventricle produces left lower lobe atelectasis.

Coronary Artery Arteriovenous Fistula

This rare malformation relates to the anomalous development of a major branch coronary artery connecting directly to a large venous channel that drains directly into the right heart (90%) or occasionally into the left heart. When the anomaly drains into the right heart, a left-to-right shunt occurs.

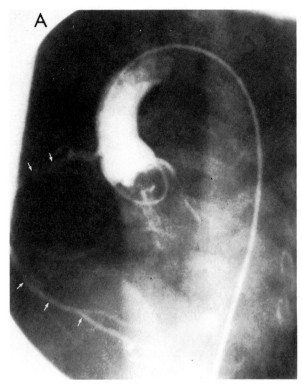

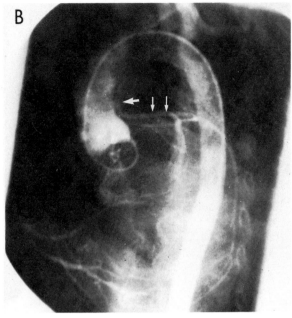

FIG 16–26.
Anomalous origin of the left coronary artery. **A,** long-axis lateral retrograde aortogram shows enlargement of the right coronary artery *(arrows)* and a failure to visualize the left coronary artery. A later film **(B)** shows retrograde filling of the left coronary artery and flow into the main pulmonary artery *(arrows).*

Clinical Manifestation

Signs are rare except when failure results from the large left-to-right shunt. A continuous murmur may be heard over the precardium and clinically PDA, AP window, VSD with aortic insufficiency, systemic arteriovenous fistulas, and ruptured sinus of Valsalva aneurysm are differential considerations.

Chest Roentgenography

Roentgenographic findings are frequently normal. Cardiomegaly may be present because of a left-to-right shunt with associated increased pulmonary blood flow. Abnormal bulges on the cardiac silhouette may relate to the aneurysmally dilated anomalous vessels. Differential diagnoses primarily involve (1) PDA, (2) aorticopulmonary window, and (3) truncus arteriosus.

Echocardiography

An echocardiogram with real-time and Doppler study easily identifies the enlarged coronary artery and left-to-right shunt. Frequently it may be followed to its point of insertion into the draining cardiac chamber. Paradoxical septal motion may occur with a large right atrial shunt.

Angiocardiography

Aortic root or selected coronary artery injections will readily demonstrate the large, dilated, and fre-quently tortuous coronary artery (Fig 16–27). The drainage point can usually be identified with biplane angiography. The normal coronary branches may be small and difficult to visualize because of differential flow through the low-resistance fistula.

Prognosis

The prognosis is good with surgical correction.

Isolated Partial Anomalous Pulmonary Venous Return (PAPVR)

Common sites of involvement are (1) right lung (two thirds) and (2) left lung (one third). Drainage occurs to the (1) SVC (50%), (2) right atrium, (3) IVC, (4) azygos vein, and (5) coronary sinus. The fairly common anomalous pulmonary venous drainage of the right lung to the IVC produces the so-called scimitar syndrome with associated (1) hypoplasia of the right lung and (2) systemic arterial supply to the right lower lung.

Clinical Manifestations

Unless more than 50% of the pulmonary flow drains to the right heart, clinical manifestations are rare. In this instance, failure related to the left-to-right shunt may be present. Most patients with scimitar syn-

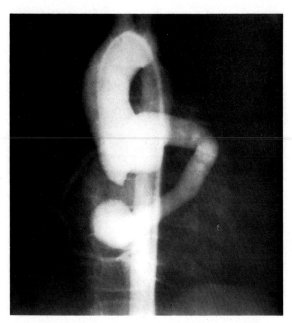

FIG 16–27.
Coronary artery—right atrial fistula. A retrograde aortogram in the AP projection shows a large aneurysmally dilated left posterior circumflex coronary artery emptying into the right atrium. Other branches of the right and left coronary arteries appear uninvolved. (From Jaffe RB, Glancy DL, Epstein SE, et al: *Circulation* 1973; 47:133. Used by permission.)

drome have a small right hemithorax and an increased incidence of pulmonary infection.

Chest Roentgenography

Patients with scimitar syndrome typically demonstrate (see Fig 15–7) (1) a crescent-shaped vessel paralleling the lower right heart border and enlarging in size as it approaches the cardiophrenic angle, (2) hypoplasia of the right lung, (3) varying degrees of cardiac dextroposition, (4) a small right pulmonary artery, and (5) systemic artery supply to the right lower lung from the aorta, or celiac artery.

Other forms of isolated PAPVR rarely show specific abnormalities on chest roentgenography. A large shunt may create cardiomegaly and right heart enlargement with increased pulmonary flow. Occasionally the horizontal anomalous course of a pulmonary vein may be specifically identified (Fig 16–28) or the vertical course of a dilated left vertical vein.

Echocardiography

With scimitar syndrome, real-time echocardiography may demonstrate (1) the anomalous vein entering the IVC, (2) a small right pulmonary artery, and (3) an anomalous artery supplying a sequestration.

Angiography

Selective biplane AP and lateral pulmonary arteriograms will demonstrate the anomalous venous drainage of the multiple types described (Figs 16–29 and 16–30). Thoracic and abdominal aortography should be performed to evaluate anomalous systemic pulmonary vasculature and sequestration.

MRI

MRI may be used to evaluate uncommon or atypical forms of PAPVR (Fig 16–31).

Prognosis

Operative correction is not indicated with small isolated PAPVR. With sequestration and infection, lobectomy may be necessary. The aberrant systemic artery to the lung, typically the right lung, may be occluded by coil embolization (Fig 16–32). Surgical correction of other large shunt lesions is also successful.

Complicated PAPVR

PAPVR probably occurs more frequently than is suspected (see Table 15–1). It usually represents a limited left-to-right shunt and is of little clinical significance unless associated with a sinus venosus ASD. Complicated PAPVR usually occurs with ASD but may be encountered with tetralogy of Fallot, tricuspid atresia, common ventricle, VSD, and PDA. Approximately 50% of complicated PAPVR is associated with an ASD. The anomalous vein usually drains into the right atrium or SVC.

Clinical Manifestations

Signs and symptoms usually relate to the underlying lesion in this complicated variant rather than to the anomalous vein per se.

Chest Roentgenography

Plain film findings result from the underlying associated cardiac malformation. In the instance of sinus venosus ASD or other ASDs they are predominantly those of (1) a left-to-right shunt, (2) right atrial dilatation, and (3) right ventricular enlargement. Differential considerations relate to the associated lesions, but most often to the ASDs.

Angiocardiography

Angiographic diagnosis is best accomplished after retrograde venous catheterization of the anomalous vein and injection into this vein with subsequent visualization of the SVC or, occasionally, direct filling of the right atrium. The latter may be difficult to differentiate from a sinus venosus defect. Four-

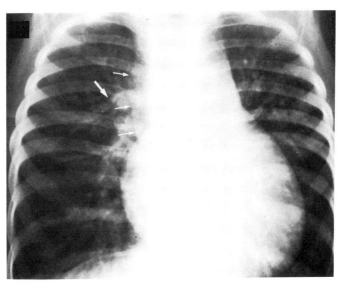

FIG 16–28.
PA chest film demonstrates anomalous pulmonary venous drainage of the right upper lobe *(large arrow)* into the dilated superior vena cava *(small arrows).*

chamber long-axis projections may be helpful in this instance. Angiography to otherwise define the other associated lesions must be appropriate for the lesions present. Selective AP and lateral pulmonary artery views may be helpful on occasion.

Prognosis

The prognosis with the associated ASD lesions is generally good. The prognosis for other variants relates primarily to the primary congenital malformation.

Sinus of Valsalva Aneurysm

Sinus of Valsalva aneurysm is a rare malformation defined as localized dilatation of one of the aortic si-

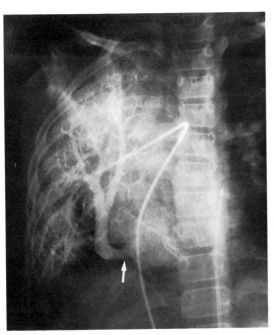

FIG 16–29.
Scimitar syndrome (see Fig 15–7). A late pulmonary venous-phase film after right pulmonary artery injection shows anomalous venous drainage below the diaphragm to the point of junction with the hepatic veins and inferior vena cava *(arrow).* Hypoplasia of the right lung is present with an associated mediastinal shift to the right.

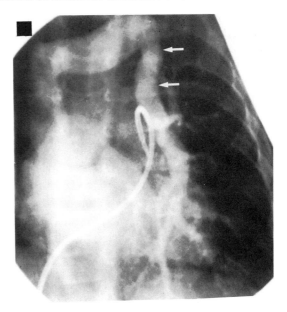

FIG 16–30.
Partial anomalous venous return (PAPVR). Left lung drains anomalously through a persistent left vertical vein *(arrows)* to the innominate vein and SVC.

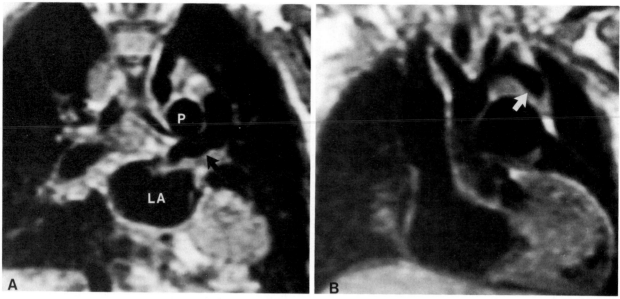

FIG 16–31.
An 8-year-old boy with mitral stenosis, coarctation, and an unusual form of partial anomalous pulmonary venous return from the left lung. **A,** coronal 3-mm MRI image demonstrates a levoatriocardinal vein *(arrow)* lateral to the pulmonary artery *(P)*. The vein communicates with the left atrium *(LA)*, and then ascends vertically in the left mediastinum receiving venous return from the left lung. Also note the paratracheal, carinal, and hilar adenopathy. **B,** the vein ascends in the left mediastinum *(arrow)* to empty into the left innominate vein.

nuses of Valsalva. The lesion may be either congenital or acquired. The incidence of this malformation has been reported from 0.1% to 3.5% of congenital heart disease.

Pathophysiology

Congenital sinus of Valsalva aneurysms are commonly associated with other congenital cardiac defects, most commonly a VSD. This is usually an outlet (supracristal) VSD (60%) with perimembranous defect significantly less frequent. Aortic insufficiency may develop in 30% to 40% of patients related to alteration in the valvular cusps secondary to prolapse of the sinus and aneurysmal expansion. Other occasionally associated congenital lesions include subaortic stenosis, ASD, infundibular pulmonary steno-

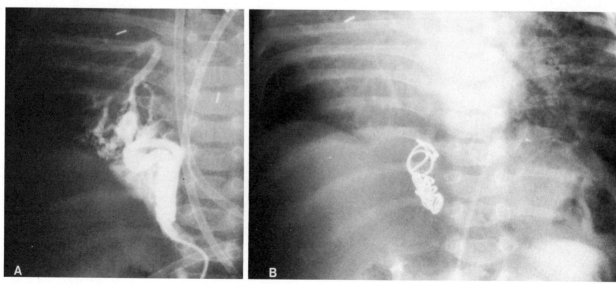

FIG 16–32.
Coil occlusion of aberrant systemic artery to the right lung in a patient with the scimitar syndrome. **A,** frontal angiogram during injection into the aberrant systemic artery after catheter passage from the abdominal aorta demonstrates opacification of the medial right lower lung and retrograde opacification of the right lower lobe pulmonary artery. **B,** frontal radiograph of the upper abdomen and lower chest demonstrates multiple coils in the aberrant systemic artery following coil occlusion.

sis, coarctation, and Marfan syndrome. Acquired sinus of Valsalva aneurysms most often relate to inflammatory disease such as endocarditis.

The aneurysm usually involves the right coronary sinus (80%–90%), and less commonly the noncoronary sinus. The aneurysm may prolapse into and occlude the VSD, particularly an outlet VSD, and occasionally extend into the intraventricular septum. Rupture of the coronary sinus is usually into the right ventricle (70%–80%) with almost all of the remainder extending into the right atrium.

Clinical Manifestations

Clinical manifestations of a nonruptured sinus of Valsalva aneurysm are rare. Occasionally a prolapsed aneurysm into the VSD or right ventricular outflow tracts may become symptomatic. Otherwise, symptoms primarily develop after rupture, which usually occurs beyond 10 years of age. Primary symptoms relate to left-to-right shunt when the rupture is into the right ventricle or right atrium. Volume overload of the left heart may also occur in the rare instances in which rupture extends into the left ventricle and, of course, is complicated by aortic in-

sufficiency. Clinical symptoms of shortness of breath, fatigue, tachycardia, and chest pain may develop and auscultation usually reveals a continuous murmur.

Roentgenographic Manifestations

Plain films in a nonruptured sinus of Valsalva aneurysm are usually normal. Following rupture one identifies increasing heart size, increased pulmonary blood flow, or CHF, or any combination of these.

Echocardiography

Two-dimensional and Doppler echocardiography are sensitive in detecting sinus of Valsalva aneurysm, especially when rupture is present. Doppler manifestations are those of left-to-right shunt and aortic valvular insufficiency.

Angiocardiography

Angiocardiograms readily demonstrate not only the sinus of Valsalva aneurysm (Fig 16–33) but also the effect of rupture and the direction of flow (Fig 16–34). Injections are usually performed in the

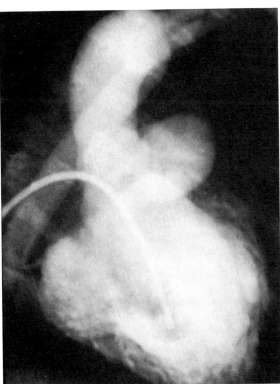

FIG 16–33.
Sinus of Valsalva aneurysm. Left ventricular injection in the axial RAO projection demonstrates an enlarged left ventricle and right sinus of Valsalva aneurysm in a 6-year-old girl. An aortogram (not shown) demonstrated marked aortic regurgitation without fistulous communication to the right heart.

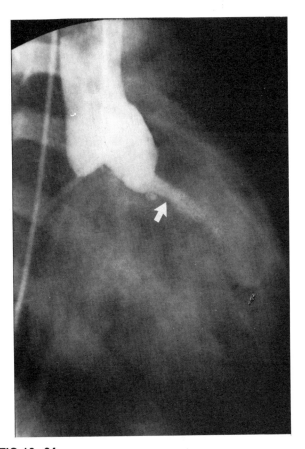

FIG 16–34.
Sinus of Valsalva to right ventricle fistula. Aortogram in the axial RAO projection demonstrates a right sinus of Valsalva aneurysm with fistulous communication (arrow) into the right ventricle.

supravalvular region with long-axis biplane angiography, possibly supplemented with AP and lateral biplane angiography. The aneurysm itself is identified as a focal dilatation of the sinus of Valsalva with the direction of protrusion variable depending upon the sinus involved. Differential diagnostic considerations include AP window, coronary arteriovenous fistula, and aorticoatrial or aorticoventricular tunnel.

Prognosis

Treatment is operative repair, usually resecting portions of the aneurysm, then utilizing patch repair of the sinus, and the VSD, if present. On occasion, depending on the valvular anatomy, aortic valve replacement is necessary. Mortality is generally listed at 3% to 4% although late death is a complication reported in some literature at 10% to 15%. Heart block is a significant complication.

REFERENCES

Ventricular Septal Defect

Azia KU, Cole RG, Paul NH: Echocardiographic features of supracristal ventricular septal defect with prolapsed aortic valve leaflet. *Am J Cardiol* 1979; 43:854.

Bierman FC, Fellows KE, Williams RG: Prospective identification of ventricular septal defects in infancy using subxiphoid two-dimensional echocardiogram. *Circulation* 1980; 62:807.

Canale JM, Sahn DJ, Allen HD, et al: Factors affecting real-time, cross-sectional echocardiographic imaging of perimembranous ventricular septal defects. *Circulation* 1981; 63:689.

Cheatham JP, Latson LP, Gutgesell HP: Ventricular septal defect in infancy: Detection with two-dimensional echocardiography. *Am J Cardiol* 1981; 47:85.

Didier D, Higgins CB: Identification and localization of ventricular septal defect by gated magnetic resonance imaging. *Am J Cardiol* 1986; 57:1363.

Didier D, Higgins CB, Fisher MR, et al: Congenital heart disease: Gated MR imaging in 72 patients. *Radiology* 1986; 158:227.

Elliott LP, Bargeron LN Jr, Soto B, et al: Axial cineangiography in congenital heart disease. *Radiol Clin North Am* 1980; 18:515.

Freedom RM, Culham JAG, Moes CAF: *Angiocardiography of Congenital Heart Disease.* New York, Macmillan, 1984, p 128.

Green CE, Elliott LP, Bargeron LN Jr: Axial cineangiographic evaluation of the posterior ventricular septal defect. *Am J Cardiol* 1981; 48:331.

Helmcke F, de Souza A, Nanda NC, et al: Two-dimensional and color doppler assessment of ventricular

septal defect of congenital origin. *Am J Cardiol* 1989; 63:1112–1116.

Jaffe RB, Scherer JL: Supracristal ventricular septal defects: Spectrum of associated lesions and complications. *Am J Roentgenol* 1977; 128:629.

Moore KL: *The Developing Human.* Philadelphia, WB Saunders, 1974.

Patten BN: *Human Embryology,* ed 3. New York, Blakiston, 1968.

Riggs T, Mehta S, Hirshfeld S, et al: Ventricular septal defect in infancy: A combined ductographic and echocardiographic study. *Circulation* 1979; 59:385.

Santamaria H, Soto B, Ceballos R, et al: Differentiation of types of ventricular septal defects. *Am J Roentgenol* 1983; 141:273.

Snider AR, Silverman HN, Schiller NB, et al: Echocardiographic evaluation of ventricular septal aneurysms. *Circulation* 1979; 59:920.

Soto B, Bargeron LM Jr, Diethelm E: Ventricular septal defect. *Semin Roentgenol* 1985; 20:200.

Soto B, Becker AE, Moulaert AJ, et al: Classification of ventricular septal defects. *Br Heart J* 1980; 43:332.

Van Praagh R, Geva T, Kreutzer J: Ventricular septal defects: How shall we describe, name and classify them? *J Am Coll Cardiol* 1989; 14:1298–1299.

Yoo S-J, Lim T-H, Park I-S, et al: Defects of the interventricular septum of the heart: En face imaging in the oblique coronal plane. *AJR* 1991; 157:943–946.

Atrial Septal Defect, Ostium Primum Atrial Septal Defect, and Endocardial Cushion Defect

Beppu S, Saito Y, Ohta M, et al: Mitral cleft in ostium primum atrial septal defect assessed by cross-sectional echocardiography. *Circulation* 1980; 62:1099.

Bleiden LC, Randall PA, Castaneda AR, et al: The "gooseneck" of the endocardial cushion defect: Anatomic basis. *Chest* 1974; 65:13.

Didier D, Higgins CB, Fisher MR, et al: Congenital heart disease: Gated MR imaging in 72 patients. *Radiology* 1986; 158:227.

Diethelm L, Dery R, Lipton MJ, Higgins CB: Atrial-level shunts: Sensitivity and specificity of MR in diagnosis. *Radiology* 1987; 162:181–186.

Elliott LP, Bargeron LM Jr, Bream PR, et al: Axial cineangiography in congenital heart disease. II. Specific lesions. *Circulation* 1977; 56:1084.

Freedom RM, Culham JAG, Moes CAF: *Angiocardiography of Congenital Heart Disease.* New York, Macmillan, 1984.

Green CE, Gottdiener JS, Goldstein HA: Atrial septal defect. *Semin Roentgenol* 1985; 20:214.

Keith JD: Atrial septal defect: Ostium secundum, ostium primum, and atrioventricularis communis, in Keith JD, Rowe RE, Vlad P (eds): *Heart Disease in Infancy and Childhood.* New York, Macmillan, 1978, p 350.

gurgitant systolic murmur secondary to tricuspid insufficiency.

Chest Roentgenography

Classic plain film findings include (1) dilatation of the main and left pulmonary artery (see Figs 15–10 and 16–35), (2) right ventricular hypertrophy with elevation and uplifting of the cardiac apex and associated filling in of the upper retrosternal space, and (3) right atrial enlargement when associated with tricuspid insufficiency. Patients with mild PVS may have a normal cardiac silhouette. The pulmonary flow is normal, and the aortic arch is on the left. Differential considerations include idiopathic dilatation of the pulmonary artery (particularly in older female children), left-to-right shunts (i.e., ASD), or pulmonary hypertension, singly or in combination.

Echocardiography

Real-time echocardiography will demonstrate (1) a thickened domed pulmonary valve, (2) a small pulmonary annulus when associated with a dysplastic valve, (3) right ventricular hypertrophy, and (4) early opening or exaggerated "a" dip of the posterior leaflet of the pulmonary valve. Doppler evaluation can accurately calculate the gradient across the valve from the modified Bernoulli equation, valve gradient = $4V^2$, where V = peak Doppler velocity beyond the obstruction (see Fig 15–18).

Angiocardiography

Biplane AP and lateral right ventriculography is preferred in the 45-degree sitting-up projection. The catheter (usually a balloon catheter) is positioned in the right ventricular outflow tract, and approximately 1 mL/kg of contrast is injected. When the left pulmonary artery cannot be adequately visualized, angled views may be a necessary supplement. Findings include (1) a thickened domed pulmonary valve (Fig 16–36), (2) poststenotic dilatation of the main and left pulmonary arteries, (3) right ventricular hypertrophy, and (4) in patients with moderate to marked PVS, dynamic infundibular narrowing in systole may be present.

Prognosis

The prognosis is good without treatment in mild cases or with pulmonary valve balloon angioplasty (Fig 16–37) or surgical intervention in the more severe cases. Correction of PVS may result in right ventricular outflow obstruction from severe infundibular hypertrophy.

VALVULAR AORTIC STENOSIS (AS)

AS, combining valvular, subvalvular, and supravalvular types, represents the second most common form of obstructive CHD and accounts for 7% of all CHD (see Table 15–1). Congenital valvular AS accounts for 70% of all forms of AS. AS is classified according to valve types as (1) unicuspid (most severe disease), (2) bicuspid, (3) quadricuspid, and (4) tricuspid valve. The unicuspid valve usually has a central orifice and no lateral commissure. The bicuspid aortic valve with stenosis is by far the most common. A bicuspid valve is present in up to 85% of patients with coarctation, but may not be stenotic.

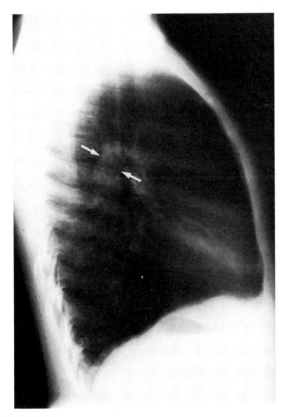

FIG 16–35.
Pulmonary valvular stenosis (see Fig 15–10). A lateral chest roentgenogram demonstrates enlargement of the left pulmonary artery as an extension of the poststenotic dilatation from the main pulmonary artery *(arrows)*.

Pathophysiology

Unicuspid valve AS presents in infancy with critical left heart obstruction and CHF. Other forms of AS develop, progress gradually with age, and lead to (1)

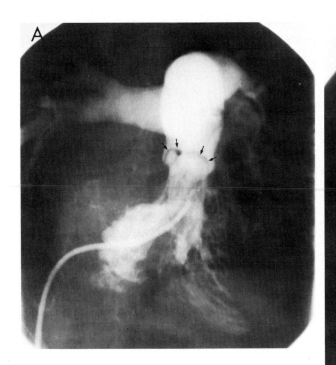

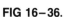

FIG 16–36.
Pulmonary valvular stenosis. AP **(A)** and lateral **(B)** sitting-up right ventriculograms show elongation of the right ventricular outflow tract with the stenotic domed pulmonary valve tangential to the central beam *(arrows)*. Characteristic thickening of the valve leaflets along with poststenotic dilatation of the main and left pulmonary arteries is apparent. A jet effect into the main pulmonary artery is evident in the lateral view *(arrows)*.

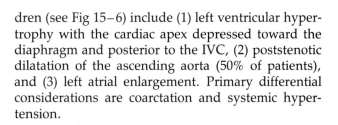

concentric left ventricular hypertrophy, (2) elevated end-diastolic pressures, (3) elevated left atrial pressures, (4) pulmonary venous congestion, and (5) CHF. Critical AS in infancy may have associated left heart hypoplasia or endocardial fibroelastosis, or both.

Clinical Manifestations

Critical AS in infancy leads to (1) failure to thrive, (2) poor feeding, (3) pneumonia, (4) dyspnea, and (5) congestive failure. From 1 year to 5 years of age, 70% of patients are asymptomatic. Physical finding is a characteristic systolic ejection murmur transmitted into the right side of the neck. Alarming findings in older patients requiring immediate evaluation and treatment include (1) dyspnea, (2) decreased exercise tolerance, (3) angina, and (4) syncope.

Chest Roentgenography

Infants with clinical AS present with (1) cardiomegaly, (2) pulmonary venous congestion, and (3) minor pleural effusion (Fig 16–38). Findings in older chil-

dren (see Fig 15–6) include (1) left ventricular hypertrophy with the cardiac apex depressed toward the diaphragm and posterior to the IVC, (2) poststenotic dilatation of the ascending aorta (50% of patients), and (3) left atrial enlargement. Primary differential considerations are coarctation and systemic hypertension.

Echocardiography

Two-dimensional real-time echocardiography demonstrates (1) thickening and doming of the aortic valve (Fig 16–39), (2) eccentric closure of the bicuspid valve, (3) concentric left ventricular hypertrophy, and (4) left atrial enlargement. Doppler evaluations can accurately determine the gradient across the aortic valve. (Modified Bernoulli equation; see Echocardiography under Pulmonary Valvular Stenosis, above.)

Angiocardiography

Left ventriculography is performed in the long-axis projection after retrograde aortic catheterization. In

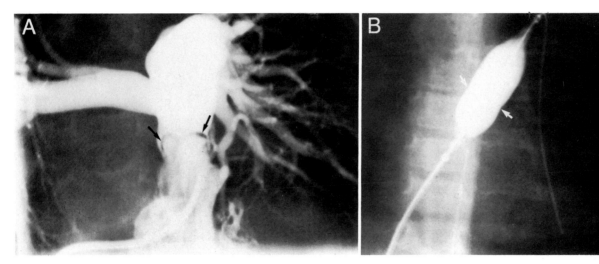

FIG 16–37.
Pulmonary valvular stenosis (PVS). **A,** an AP right ventricular angiocardiogram demonstrates doming and thickening of the pulmonary valve *(arrows)* and poststenotic dilatation of the main pulmonary artery. **B,** balloon angioplasty with the dilated balloon travers-ing the pulmonary valve with only a minimal waist *(arrows)* at the valve level and an excellent postangioplasty decrease in the PVS gradient.

infants, the left ventricle may be entered through the foramen ovale from venous catheterization. Approximately 1 mL/kg of contrast is utilized. Angiographic findings include (1) thickened and domed aortic valve leaflets (Fig 16–40), (2) poststenotic dilatation of the ascending aorta, and (3) left ventricular hypertrophy. Aortic root injection may be desirable to evaluate aortic insufficiency and rule out other frequently associated lesions such as coarctation and

PDA. The differential diagnosis includes subvalvular and supravalvular AS.

Prognosis

The prognosis is guarded in infants with severe or critical AS. In the older child with a significant (75 mm Hg) gradient, operative valvulotomy or balloon angioplasty (Fig 16–41) produces good results, al-

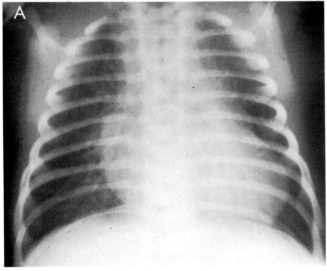

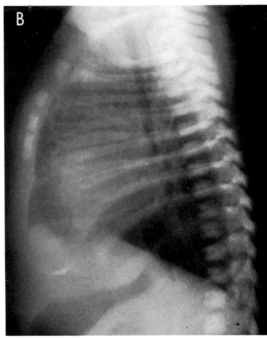

FIG 16–38.
Critical aortic stenosis (AS). AP **(A)** and lateral **(B)** chest roentgenograms in a 3-day-old infant show pulmonary venous congestion, moderate cardiomegaly, and hyperinflation. No abnormality of the ascending aorta is identified with AS at this age.

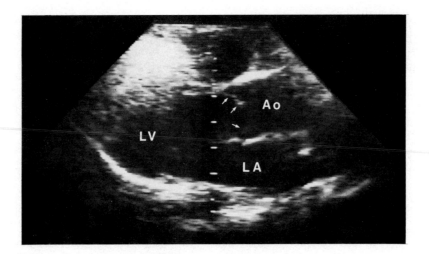

FIG 16–39.
Aortic stenosis. A long-axis two-dimensional echocardiogram centered at the aortic root shows doming of the aortic valve leaflet (arrowheads) and mild dilatation of the ascending aorta. (Ao). LV, left ventricle; LA, left atrium.

though aortic insufficiency and late recurrence are common. Valve replacement may be necessary. Sudden death occurs in 4% to 18% of older patients without surgery.

SUPRAVALVULAR AORTIC STENOSIS (SAS)

SAS may occur as an isolated lesion or be seen in SAS syndrome (Williams syndrome) (33%). Williams syndrome includes (1) SAS, (2) peripheral pulmonary stenosis, (3) elfin facies, (4) mental and physical retardation, (5) neonatal hypercalcemia, and (6) abnormal dentition.

Pathophysiology

Types of SAS include (1) hourglass narrowing immediately above the sinuses of Valsalva (66%), (2) diffuse narrowing of the entire ascending aorta (20%–30%), and (3) a diaphragm in the supravalvular area (10%). Additional pathologic findings include (1) thickening of the aortic valve cusps, (2) dilated tortuous coronary arteries, (3) left ventricular hypertrophy, and (4) occasionally associated coarctation.

Clinical Manifestations

Findings in patients with Williams syndrome include (1) feeding problems, (2) failure to thrive, (3) hypercalcemia, (4) elfin facies, (5) hoarse voice, (6) strabismus, and (7) inguinal hernia. All patients with SAS may have (1) left heart failure, (2) dyspnea, (3) angina, and (4) syncope. Physical findings include (1) an ejection systolic murmur in the aortic area, (2) increased pulses in the right arm, and (3) elevated right arm blood pressure.

Chest Roentgenography

Chest roentgenographic findings are usually normal, although left ventricular hypertrophy and dilatation may be seen in severe cases. In the diffuse type, the ascending aorta is small and inconspicuous.

Echocardiography

Real-time echocardiography demonstrates (1) supravalvular narrowing of the ascending aorta (Fig 16–42), (2) concentric left ventricular hypertrophy, and (3) supravalvular pulmonary stenosis when it coexists. Doppler interrogation is more difficult in this lesion, although a gradient may be documented by the modified Bernoulli equation (see above).

Angiocardiography

Biplane supravalvular aortography following retrograde aortic catheterization in the long-axis projection is preferred. Angiographic findings include (1) supravalvular aortic narrowing, (2) diffuse hypoplasia of the ascending aorta (Fig 16–43), (3) aortic insufficiency (15%), (4) coarctation (15%), and (5) stenosis of brachiocephalic and abnormal aortic branches at their origin. The descending thoracic and abdominal aorta may show either hypoplasia or stenotic areas and should be evaluated, as should

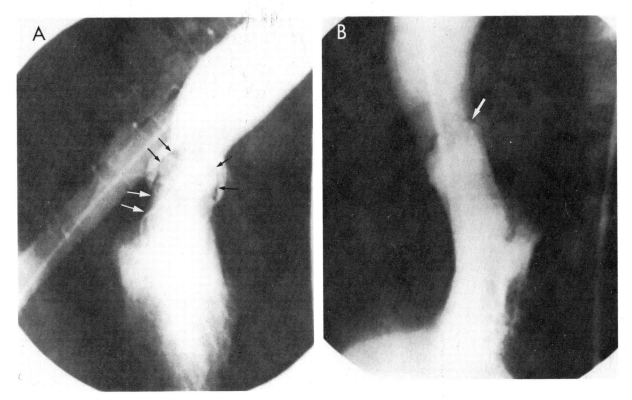

FIG 16–40.
Aortic stenosis. AP **(A)** and lateral **(B)** long-axis left ventriculograms show characteristic doming and thickening of the aortic valve leaflets *(arrows)*. Note the clear definition and elongation of the left ventricular outflow tract in these projections. The straight segment of the superior interventricular septum is nicely identified on the frontal projection *(white arrows)*.

the pulmonary artery, because of their frequent (50%) involvement (see Fig 18–8).

Magnetic Resonance Imaging

MRI is an excellent modality to evaluate patients with SAS syndrome enabling recognition of SAS and peripheral pulmonary stenosis in multiple planes (Fig 16–44). It is also useful in the postoperative patient.

Prognosis

The prognosis is fairly poor. Surgical intervention is necessary in severe cases and may necessitate a ventriculoaortic bypass. Complications include aortic aneurysms and infective endocarditis.

MUSCULAR SUBAORTIC STENOSIS (HYPERTROPHIC OBSTRUCTIVE CARDIOMYOPATHY)

Muscular subaortic stenosis, or hypertrophic obstructive cardiomyopathy, is a form of obstructive cardiomyopathy with asymmetric hypertrophy of the septal portion of the left ventricular outflow tract. Muscular subaortic stenosis has also been referred to as asymmetric septal hypertrophy, obstructive cardiomyopathy, and idiopathic hypertrophic subaortic stenosis (IHSS).

Incidence

Familial occurrence is seen in 25% to 35% of patients. Spontaneous occurrence accounts for 65% to 75% of cases. An autosomal dominant inheritance pattern with a high degree of penetrance has been reported. Sexual incidence is equal. Hypertrophic cardiomyopathy may also be associated with Turner and Noonan syndromes and Friedreich ataxia. Infants of diabetic mothers may have a reversible form of hypertrophic cardiomyopathy.

Pathophysiology

Pathologic findings include (1) disproportionate hypertrophy of the interventricular septum when compared with the left ventricular wall, (2) fibrous

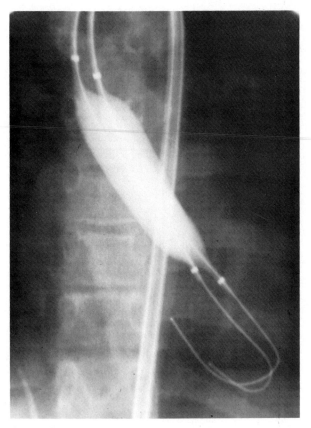

FIG 16–41.
Balloon angioplasty in aortic stenosis. Retrograde bifemoral artery introduction of balloon catheters passing into the left ventricle with complete obliteration of the AS waist deformity, a dramatic decrease in the aortic gradient, and only minor postangioplasty aortic insufficiency observed with an aortic root injection.

plaque formation of the left ventricular outflow tract, (3) left ventricular hypertrophy, and (4) thickening of the anterior leaflet of the mitral valve. Physiologic changes relate to systolic anterior motion (SAM) of the anterior mitral valve leaflet against the hypertrophied ventricular septum producing left ventricular outflow obstruction. Failure of mitral leaflet apposition during systole may result in mitral regurgitation.

Clinical Manifestations

Symptoms usually appear in the older child, but may not develop until the third or fourth decade. These include dyspnea, fatigue, angina, and occasionally, sudden death. Murmurs are difficult to hear and are of a systolic ejection type.

Chest Roentgenography

Mild cardiomegaly of a left ventricular configuration is present in the majority of older children or adult patients. In the later stages of the disease, left atrial enlargement and pulmonary venous congestion may be seen. In severe cases in the young child, massive cardiomegaly will occasionally be present. The differential diagnosis includes cardiomyopathies and carditis.

Echocardiography

Real-time two-dimensional echocardiography clearly defines the asymmetric thickening of the interventricular septum as well as the abnormal orientation of the anterior mitral valve leaflet into the left ventricular outflow tract in midsystole (Fig 16–45).

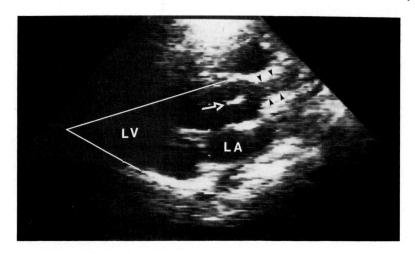

FIG 16–42.
Supravalvular aortic stenosis. A long-axis real-time echocardiogram defines normal-sized aortic sinuses of Valsalva, with the closed aortic valve producing a linear central echo density *(arrow)* leading directly into a strikingly narrowed ascending aorta *(arrowheads)*. LV, left ventricle; *LA*, left atrium.

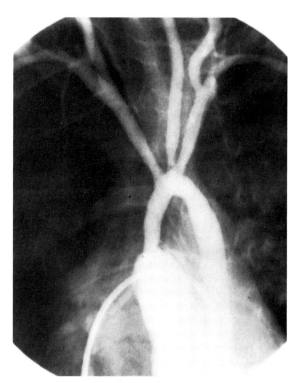

FIG 16–43.
Supravalvular aortic stenosis. An AP projection of a left ventriculogram in an LAO projection shows a normal left ventricular outflow tract and sinuses of Valsalva with immediate narrowing and hypoplasia of the entire ascending aorta and aortic arch. Stenoses at the point of origins of the brachiocephalic vessel are also identified.

These findings are similarly documented with M-mode echocardiography showing (1) a septal–left ventricular posterior wall ratio of greater than 1.3:1, (2) premature closure of the aortic valve, and (3) anterior midsystolic motion of the anterior mitral valve leaflet.

Angiocardiography

Biplane long-axis cineangiocardiography with biventricular injection optimally identifies the asymmetric septal hypertrophy. Other findings include (1) SAM of the mitral valve against the ventricular septum producing left ventricular outflow obstruction, (2) mitral regurgitation, and (3) left ventricular hypertrophy (Fig 16–46). MRI may be helpful in the differential diagnosis of intramural fibroma.

Prognosis

The prognosis is poor in symptomatic patients, with a 15% 5-year mortality and 35% 10-year mortality. Surgical resection of the muscular septum in the subaortic region is indicated for patients with severe gradients not controlled medically (propranolol).

SUBVALVULAR AORTIC STENOSIS (EXCLUDING IHSS)

Subvalvular AS (excluding IHSS) affects approximately 13% of all patients with left ventricular outflow obstruction (see Table 15–1).

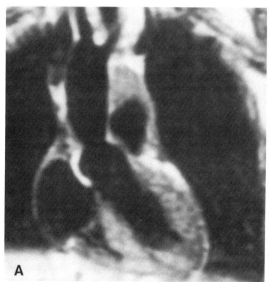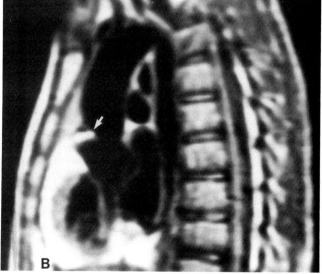

FIG 16–44.
A 13-year-old with supravalvular aortic stenosis (SAS). **A,** coronal 5-mm and **B,** sagittal 5-mm spin-echo MR images demonstrate SAS with a thick diaphragm *(arrow)* just above the aortic sinuses.

Also noted is a right aortic arch with aberrant origin of the left subclavian artery.

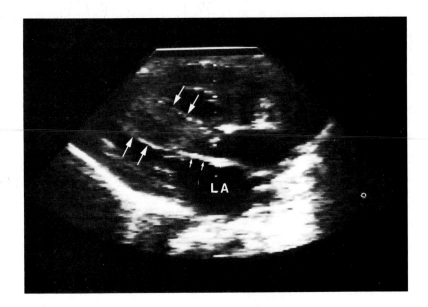

FIG 16–45.
Asymmetric septal hypertrophy. A long-axis two-dimensional echocardiogram shows striking thickening of the interventricular septum *(large arrows)* that is producing significant subaortic ob-

struction. The anterior mitral valve leaflet *(small arrows)* comes into direct contact with this grossly enlarged septum in diastole.

Pathophysiology

Lesions seen include (1) a thin subvalvular membrane, (2) a somewhat thicker fibromuscular ring approximately 1 cm below the valve, and (3), rarely, a fibromuscular subaortic tunnel. Subvalvular AS may be associated with a VSD and occasionally with an AV canal or a single ventricle. Subvalvular aortic stenosis is an integral part of the Shone anomaly

(parachute mitral valve, supravalvular stenosing ring of the left atrium, subaortic stenosis, and co-arctation of the aorta). Other acquired effects of this lesion include (1) secondary aortic insufficiency related to thickening and deformity of the aortic valve secondary to proximal turbulent flow, post-stenotic dilatation of the ascending aorta when the subvalvular membrane is in immediate proximity to the aortic valve or in the presence of aortic

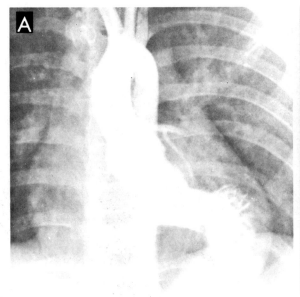

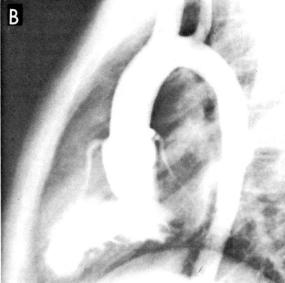

FIG 16–46.
Obstructive cardiomyopathy. Selective AP **(A)** and lateral **(B)** left ventriculograms during left ventricular systole demonstrate prominence of the interventricular septum; the left ventricular outflow

tract becomes narrowed and obstructed. The systolic anterior motion of the anterior leaflet of the mitral valve may be appreciated in the lateral view with cineangiography.

regurgitation, and concentric left ventricular hypertrophy.

Clinical Manifestations

Clinical symptoms are mild until a later age when signs of left ventricular failure with dyspnea, syncope, and tachypnea may ensue. Subvalvular AS is much more common in the male and has a 6:1 male preponderance. If other congenital heart lesions are present, symptoms may occur earlier that are related to those lesions.

Chest Roentgenography

A pattern of left ventricular hypertrophy is seen in the older child. Later manifestations, if stenosis is severe, are left ventricular dilatation and failure. Chest roentgenographic findings are usually normal in the infant and young child. Poststenotic dilatation of the ascending aorta usually will not be seen unless aortic regurgitation has developed. Differential diagnostic considerations are mainly those of other left heart obstruction lesions, endocardial fibroelastosis, and cardiomyopathies.

Echocardiography

Two-dimensional real-time echocardiography readily identifies the discrete membranous (Fig 16–47) as well as fibromuscular and tunnel-type subaortic lesions. Other findings include systolic preclosure of the aortic valve and systolic flutter of the leaflets.

Angiocardiography

Biplane long-axis angiocardiography is ideal for visualization and evaluation of the various types of subvalvular AS. The thin, membranous type may be difficult to visualize unless the membrane is demonstrated tangential to the central roentgen beam (Fig 16–48). Other lesions that should be evaluated with angiography include (1) mitral regurgitation and stenosis, (2) associated septal defects, and (3) aortic valve abnormality (i.e., insufficiency).

Prognosis

The prognosis is good with surgical resection of the discrete membranous subvalvular lesion. Success with attempted correction of the fibromuscular or tunnel lesions is poor from a direct approach. Occasionally an apical left ventricular–aortic conduit (see Fig 21–19) may be necessary in these lesions with severe obstruction. Progressive hypertrophy, a continued gradient, and mitral and aortic valve dysfunction are common complications.

COARCTATION OF THE AORTA

Coarctation of the aorta is classified into: (1) juxtaductal and its variants and (2) postductal (adult) types. The juxtaductal type, usually seen in infants

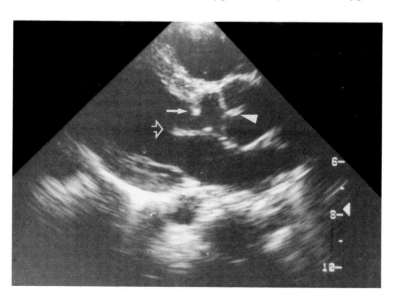

FIG 16–47.
Membranous subaortic stenosis. A long-axis parasternal real-time echocardiogram demonstrates a linear echogenic structure projecting posteriorly from the superior interventricular septum that represents a discrete membranous subaortic stenosis *(arrow)*. The anterior mitral valve leaflet *(open arrowhead)* and closed aortic leaflets *(closed arrowhead)* can be seen (compare with Fig 16–3,B).

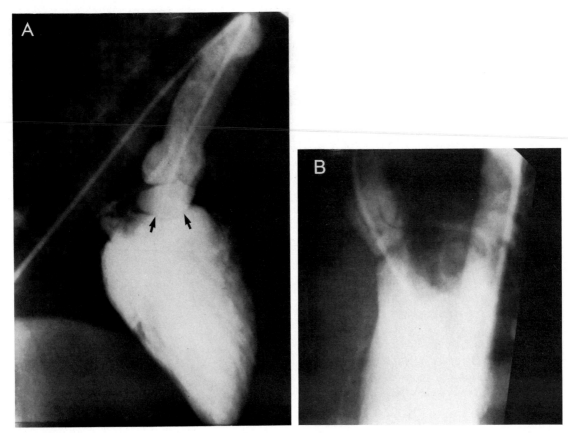

FIG 16–48.
Subvalvular aortic stenosis. AP **(A)** and lateral **(B)** long-axis left ventriculograms show a discrete subaortic membrane *(arrows)* approximately 1 cm below the aortic valve leaflets.

and small children, typically has hypoplasia of the transverse arch and aortic isthmus. In juxtaductal coarctation the ductus is astride the area of coarctation. In adults or children with postductal coarctation, the lesion is distal to the ductus arteriosus/ligamentum arteriosum.

Incidence

Coarctation accounts for approximately 5% of CHD; males predominate 2:1 without significant familial occurrence (see Table 15–1). Associated anomalies are frequent. They include (1) PDA (66%); (2) VSD (33%); and (3) other lesions including transposition of the great vessels, ASD, mitral stenosis or regurgitation, endocardial fibroelastosis, AV canal, and common ventricle. A bicuspid aortic valve is common. Other noncardiac conditions include respiratory distress syndrome (RDS), prematurity, tracheoesophageal fistula, and Turner syndrome. Coarctation also may be seen with various syndrome complexes (see Chapter 18 for discussion of cardiac abnormalities associated with syndromes and chromosomal aberrations).

Pathophysiology

Upper extremity hypertension is invariably present, probably relating to combined mechanical and renal factors. The mechanical process is compensated by development of collateral blood flow with enlargement of intercostal, superior epigastric, and mediastinal vessels. Intercostal artery dilatation and pulsation produce secondary rib notching. Left ventricular hypertrophy is proportionate to the degree of aortic obstruction.

Clinical Manifestations

Infants with coarctation, particularly when associated with left-to-right shunts, i.e., VSD or PDA, present with dramatic signs of CHF, usually in the first month of life, typically at 10 to 14 days of age. Clinical symptoms include dyspnea, poor feeding, tachycardia, and peripheral cyanosis. The murmur is variable in infants but, when heard, is similar to that in the older child. Differential blood pressures in the lower limbs are noted in two thirds of patients, but they are less dramatic when the child is in severe CHF.

Clinical signs of failure are rare in children over 1 year of age, and the diagnosis usually relates to findings of an incidental murmur, hypertension, or the recognition of abnormalities on chest roentgenograms. The murmur is a soft systolic ejection type that is heard best posteriorly in the left paravertebral area. Blood pressure discrepancies are readily identified. Additional murmurs related to associated lesions may be present.

Chest Roentgenography

Infants present with (1) moderate to marked cardiomegaly with a nonspecific configuration, (2) pulmonary venous congestion and failure (see Fig 15–1), and (3) poststenotic dilatation of the descending aorta of variable prominence. CHF presenting between the first and fourth weeks strongly suggests coarctation. Differentiation from an interrupted aortic arch is difficult.

Older patients (over 1 year) usually have normal heart size to mild cardiomegaly, the latter with a left ventricular configuration. Rib notching (see Table 15–8) is the hallmark of this condition and is usually seen after 5 years but occasionally is present in the first few years of life (see Fig 15–12). The third, fourth, and fifth ribs are usually involved posteriorly but notching may be seen in the third through ninth ribs. Poststenotic dilatation of the aorta below the coarctation will usually occur, and a figure-3 sign related to the dilatation of the left subclavian artery above and the poststenotic aortic segment below (see Fig 15–9,A) is frequently evident. The imprint of the aorta on the adjacent barium-filled esophagus

is known as the E sign (see Fig 15–9,B). Dilatation of the ascending aorta and brachiocephalic vessels is frequently observed. Retrosternal enlargement of the internal mammary arteries may be seen in the lateral chest radiograph. True coarctation must be differentiated from pseudocoarctation.

Echocardiography

Two-dimensional echocardiography from the suprasternal notch or subxiphoid projection may directly visualize the area of aortic narrowing and poststenotic dilatation of the aorta (Fig 16–49). Unfortunately, the adjacent lung sometimes interferes with optimal visualization. Doppler interrogation of the aorta below the coarctation may show an altered amplitude and wave pattern related to the coarctation effect. A gradient across the coarctation may be calculated by use of the modified Bernoulli equation (see Chapter 15, Section 2, under Echocardiography). Additional M-mode or two-dimensional findings include a bicuspid aortic valve and concentric left ventricular hypertrophy.

Angiocardiography

Long-axis biplane left ventriculography usually will not only adequately identify any intracardiac defect of significance but will also visualize the various forms of coarctation (Fig 16–50). The entire arch should be closely evaluated for degrees of hypoplasia. The bicuspid aortic valve can be visualized on left ventricular or aortic root injections. Delayed films will demonstrate collateral flow to the descend-

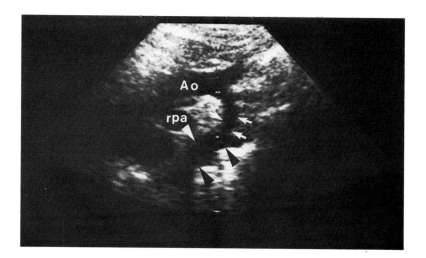

FIG 16–49.
Coarctation of the aorta. Suprasternal real-time echocardiogram defining a prominent ascending aorta (*Ao*) and innominate artery, with a hypoplastic transverse aortic arch *(arrows)* extending into an area of poststenotic dilatation of the thoracic aorta *(arrowheads)*. The right pulmonary artery *(rpa)* projects centrally within the aortic arch.

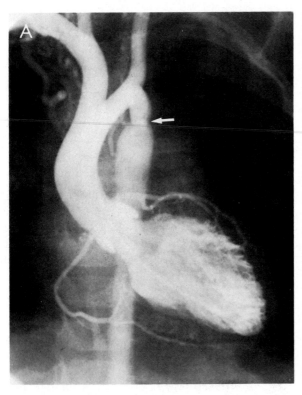

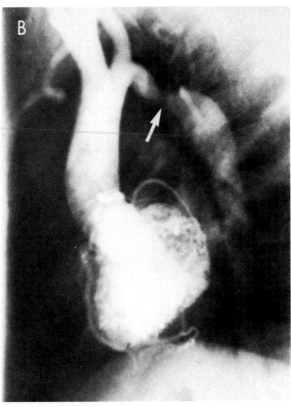

FIG 16–50.
Coarctation of the aorta. AP **(A)** and lateral **(B)** long-axis left ventriculograms demonstrate mild hypoplasia of the aortic isthmus with a focal area of coarctation *(arrow)* and moderate poststenotic dilatation distal to the coarctation site. Prominent internal mammary and collateral vessels are seen on the right. Note the absence of the left subclavian artery that has originated from the site of coarctation and filled on late films by vertebral artery steal.

ing aorta (Fig 16–51). Occasionally, ascending aortography will be necessary to better visualize the arch and site of coarctation. In the infant, angiocardiography may be accomplished by right heart catheterization with a balloon catheter through the foramen ovale and into the left ventricle. Retrograde aortic catheterization is usually needed in older patients and may be preferable if balloon angioplasty is being considered as a therapeutic measure.

Magnetic Resonance Imaging

MRI, particularly with cardiac and respiratory gating, will nicely identify the lesion in all children. The sagittal or sagittal oblique projection will clearly visualize the entire aortic arch and coarctation (Fig 16–52).

Prognosis

The prognosis is good in older patients with isolated lesions with either surgical resection or balloon angioplasty. Operative mortality in infants, especially with complex lesions, hypoplasia of the arch, or major defects, is high and ranges to 40%. Aneurysms or pseudoaneurysms may develop after either operative repair or balloon angioplasty (Fig 16–53). Recurrent coarctation, more common in small children after operation, is suggested by persistence or redevelopment of rib notching (Fig 16–54), and may be treated by balloon angioplasty. Mesenteric ischemia and hyperreactive hypertension may complicate operative repair of coarctation in all age groups.

AORTIC ARCH INTERRUPTION

Aortic arch interruption (AAI) is characterized by discontinuity of the arch between the proximal ascending aorta and the distal descending aorta. AAI differs from atresia of the aortic arch in that complete discontinuity exists between the aortic arch and the descending aorta. A fibrous remnant connects the ascending and descending aorta in aortic arch atresia. AAI is classified by the site of arch interruption and subclassified by the origin of the right subclavian artery: I, interruption distal to the

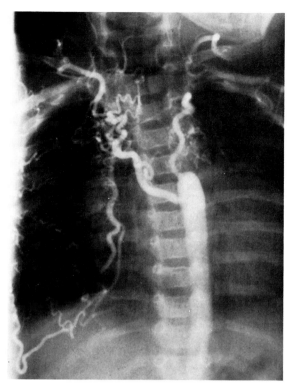

FIG 16–51.
Coarctation of the aorta. Collateral blood flow through direct mediastinal collateral, internal mammary, long thoracic, and intercostal arteries into the posterior intercostal arteries filling the thoracic aorta distal to the site of coarctation.

left subclavian artery (42%); II, interruption between the left carotid artery and the left subclavian artery (53%); and III, interruption between the innominate artery and the left carotid artery (5%). The right subclavian artery may arise from the innominate artery, the descending aorta, or the right pulmonary artery.

Pathophysiology

The pathophysiology is similar to that seen in severe coarctation. Associated defects are common, with 95% having PDA and 80% having VSDs. Other commonly associated malformations include truncus arteriosus and aorticopulmonary window.

Clinical Manifestations

Clinical signs and symptoms are basically similar to those in severe infantile coarctation with early development of CHF.

Chest Roentgenography

Chest roentgenograms show moderate cardiomegaly with a nonspecific silhouette and changes of pulmonary venous hypertension (Fig 16–55). Increased

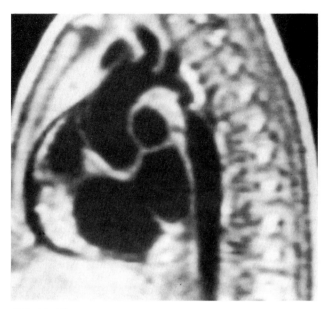

FIG 16–52.
Coarctation of the aorta. Sagittal oblique 3-mm spin-echo MRI (LAO equivalent) demonstrates the thoracic aorta in its entirety and depicts well the aortic isthmus and coarctation in this 1-year-old girl.

pulmonary flow related to associated left-to-right shunt may also be evident in older infants. The trachea may show an unusual straight vertical orientation without the usual deviation related to the aortic arch. Rib notching in older children is dependent on

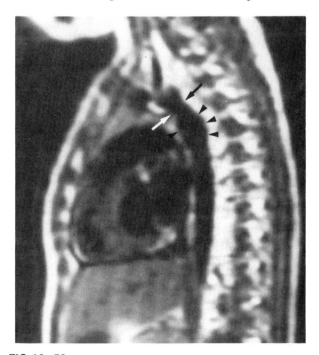

FIG 16–53.
Aneurysm after a balloon angioplasty. Respiratory- and cardiac-gated, sagittal T1-weighted MRI shows mild narrowing of the distal aortic arch *(arrows)* at the coarctation repair site with an aneurysm of the adjacent proximal thoracic aorta *(arrowheads).*

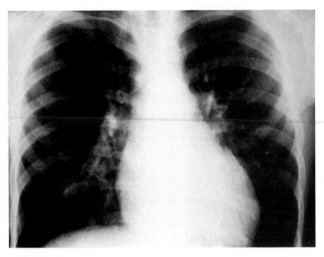

FIG 16–54.
An 8½-year-old girl with recoarctation. Chest radiograph demonstrates left rib deformities from previous thoracotomy at age 2 weeks, dilatation and deformity of the left-sided descending aorta, and right lateral rib notching. As the left subclavian artery was utilized during neonatal coarctation repair, no left-sided rib notching is seen.

the site of interruption: bilateral (I), right-sided (II, III), or left-sided (I) with aberrant right subclavian artery (see Table 15–8).

Echocardiography

Real-time echocardiography demonstrates the straight ascending aorta and continuation directly

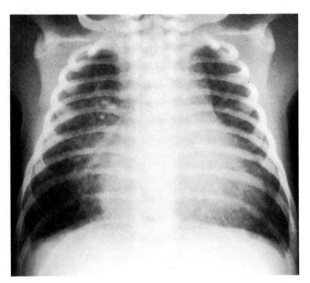

FIG 16–55.
Interrupted aortic arch in a 1-week-old infant with moderate cardiomegaly and severe congestive failure. The trachea tends to be relatively midline, although difficult to identify; no aortic arch structures are evident.

into the brachiocephalic vessels without a typical rounded-arch configuration. A large patent ductus typically joins the pulmonary artery into the descending thoracic aorta and mimics an aortic arch. The frequent VSDs may also be identified in various locations.

Angiocardiography

Biplane, long-axis, left ventriculography or ascending aortography demonstrates the straight ascending aorta with direct continuation in the brachiocephalic vessels and absence of the aortic arch (Fig 16–56). Pulmonary arteriography shows the large patent ductus continuing into the descending thoracic aorta. Intracardiac defects include (1) membranous and supracristal VSDs, (2) subaortic stenosis, and (3) a bicuspid aortic valve.

Prognosis

The overall prognosis is fair with operative correction related to use of a conduit across the aortic arch or use of the left subclavian artery. When associated intracardiac shunts are present, pulmonary artery banding for palliation, prior to later total repair, may be required.

PSEUDOCOARCTATION OF THE AORTA

Pseudocoarctation is characterized by elongation and kinking of the aortic arch at the ligamentum arteriosum without a focal area of narrowing or pressure gradient. A bicuspid aortic valve, PDA, and subaortic stenosis may also be present. The abnormality is often noted as an incidental finding on chest roentgenograms although occasionally it may produce a soft turbulent flow murmur. Blood pressures are equal in the arms and legs.

Chest Roentgenography

An abnormally prominent aortic arch projecting somewhat high and to the left may raise the question of coarctation or an aortic or ductal aneurysm. The elongated arch with kinking is often best visualized in the lateral chest roentgenogram. Real-time echocardiography and Doppler interrogation may be able to adequately evaluate the arch and establish a diagnosis. Otherwise, catheterization and angiography or MRI (Fig 16–57) is needed to rule out a true lesion with a minor gradient.

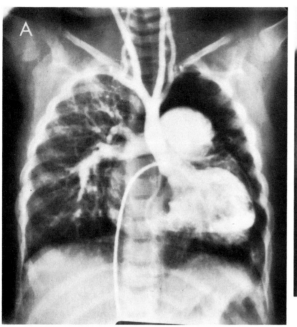

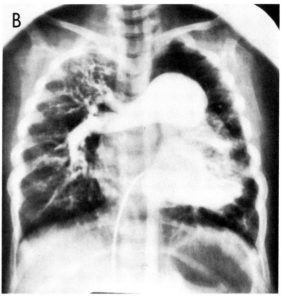

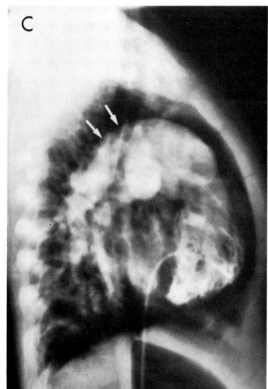

FIG 16–56.
Interrupted aortic arch. **A,** an AP left ventriculogram shows a characteristic treelike branching of the brachiocephalic vessels with an absence of the transverse aortic arch and very little visualization of the descending thoracic aorta. A left-to-right shunt through a VSD produces moderate visualization of the enlarged pulmonary vessels. AP **(B)** and lateral **(C)** right ventriculograms show the continuation of the enlarged main pulmonary artery into the descending thoracic aorta through the large PDA *(arrows)*. Some minor right-to-left shunting through the VSD produces faint opacification of the left heart and brachiocephalic vessels. (From Roberts WC, et al: *Circulation* 1962; 26:39. Used by permission.)

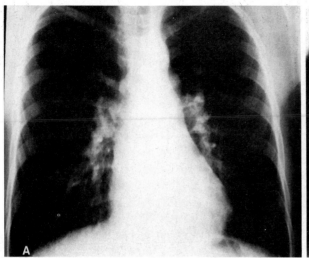
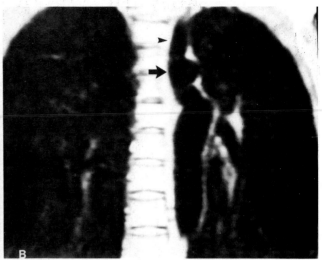

FIG 16–57.

Pseudocoarctation in a 15-year-old boy after VSD and subaortic stenosis repair. **A,** chest radiograph demonstrates abnormal dilatation of the proximal descending aorta. No rib notching is present.

B, coronal MR scan demonstrates pseudocoarctation with dilatation of the proximal descending aorta. *Arrowhead,* left subclavian artery; *arrow,* aortic arch.

ENDOCARDIAL FIBROELASTOSIS

Endocardial fibroelastosis is classified in relation to chamber involvement, valvular involvement, and whether or not there is associated CHD.

Incidence

Endocardial fibroelastosis is present in approximately 1% of all patients with CHD (see Table 15–1). Left ventricular involvement is the most common (98%), while right and left heart involvement is seen in approximately 16%. With left ventricular involvement, 60% have left atrial involvement. Twenty-five percent of cases are isolated, while 75% have associated CHD. Valvular involvement may be seen in approximately 50% of patients (aortic and mitral valve).

A fairly high incidence of familial involvement has been documented as well as the previously noted frequent association with CHD. Besides an intrinsic basic congenital etiology, other suggested etiologic factors include intrauterine infection and premature intrauterine closure of the foramen ovale.

Pathophysiology

Since endocardial fibroelastosis is commonly associated with congenital heart defects, most physiologic manifestations relate to the primary process. Coarctation, a patent ductus, and aortic atresia are the most common associated lesions. Pathologically, the endocardium is a thickened pearly-white layer cov-

ering the entire left ventricular wall with increased stiffness of the ventricle. Increased elastic and fibrous tissues with small round-cell infiltration can also be identified on histologic examination.

Clinical Manifestations

Symptoms usually develop in the first month of life that are related to CHF with dyspnea, tachypnea, irritability, and mild cyanosis. These symptoms may relate to myocardial dysfunction or to the effects of the associated lesions, i.e., aortic atresia or stenosis and coarctation.

Chest Roentgenography

Moderate to marked cardiomegaly with left heart dilatation and CHF are commonly seen at the time of presentation (Fig 16–58). Left lower lobe atelectasis is common from left atrial enlargement compressing the left mainstem bronchus. Arch abnormalities may be noted if associated with coarctation. Primary differential considerations are (1) acute myocarditis, (2) anomalous origin of the left coronary artery, and (3) other forms of cardiomyopathy.

Echocardiography

Real-time and M-mode echocardiography demonstrate dilatation of the left ventricle and outflow tract without hypertrophy and with poor left ventricular function (Fig 16–59). Other associated cardiac lesions may also be identified.

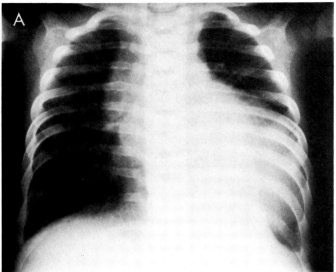
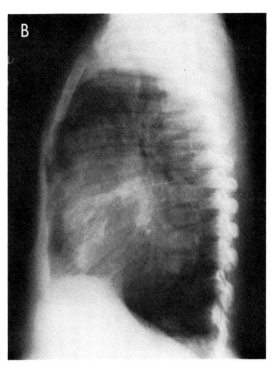

FIG 16–58.
Endocardial fibroelastosis. AP **(A)** and lateral. **(B)** chest roentgenograms show marked cardiomegaly with striking left ventricular dilatation, congestive heart failure, and left lower lobe atelectasis. The lateral view shows displacement and narrowing of the left mainstem bronchus.

Angiocardiography

Left ventricular long-axis angiocardiography usually demonstrates a dilated left ventricle with poor left ventricular function, often associated with mitral regurgitation. This examination may also confirm AS, coarctation, VSD, and PDA if present. Aortic root injection or selective coronary angiography may be important in excluding an anomalous origin of the left coronary artery as a differential diagnosis.

Prognosis

The prognosis is fair with aggressive digitalis treatment. Without cardiomegaly, an 80% survival rate

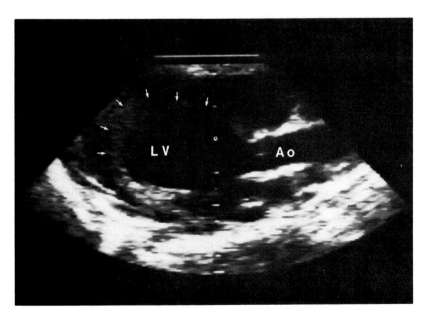

FIG 16–59.
Endocardial fibroelastosis. A long-axis echocardiogram demonstrates marked left ventricular enlargement. Real-time and M-mode studies (not shown) showed markedly diminished left ventricular contractility.

can be expected. The survival rate is lower if marked cardiomegaly is present or there are other associated lesions.

REFERENCES

Pulmonary Valvular Stenosis With Intact Ventricular Septum

Burrows PE, Benson LN, Smallhorn JS, et al: Angiographic features associated with percutaneous balloon valvotomy for pulmonary valve stenosis. *Cardiovasc Intervent Radiol* 1988; 11:111.

Castaneda-Zuñiga WR, Formanek A, et al: Radiologic diagnosis of different types of pulmonary stenosis. *Cardiovasc Radiol* 1978; 1:45.

Elliott LP: Right ventriculography in pulmonary valve stenosis, in Elliott LP (ed): *Cardiac Imaging in Infants, Children, and Adults.* Philadelphia, JB Lippincott, 1991, p 241.

Elliott LP, Schiebler GL: Pathophysiology and roentgenographic findings in pulmonary valve stenosis, in Elliott LP (ed): *Cardiac Imaging in Infants, Children, and Adults.* Philadelphia, JB Lippincott, 1991, p 235.

Fellows KE, Martin EC, Rosenthal A: Angiocardiography of obstructing muscular bands of the right ventricle. *Am J Roentgenol* 1977; 128:249.

Freedom RM, Culham JAG, Moes CAF: *Angiocardiography of Congenital Heart Disease.* New York, Macmillan, 1984.

Jaffe RB: Pulmonary valve stenosis: Echocardiography, in Elliott LP (ed): *Cardiac Imaging in Infants, Children, and Adults.* Philadelphia, JB Lippincott, 1991, p 239.

Nugent EW, Freedom RM, Nora JJ, et al: Clinical course in pulmonary stenosis. *Circulation* 1977; 56:1.

Park JH, Yoon YS, Yeon KM, et al: Percutaneous pulmonary valvuloplasty with a double-balloon technique. *Radiology* 1987; 164:715.

Shapira M, Heidelberger K, Behrendt DM, et al: The pulmonary vasculature in pulmonary valvular stenosis. *Am J Cardiol* 1980; 45:450.

White RI Jr, Mitchell SE, Kan J: Interventional procedures in congenital heart disease. *Cardiovasc Intervent Radiol* 1986; 9:286.

Valvular Aortic Stenosis

Bisset GS III, Meyer RA: Obstructive left heart lesions. *Semin Roentgenol* 1985; 20:247.

Broderick TW, Higgins CB, Guthaner DF, et al: Critical aortic stenosis in neonates. *Radiology* 1978; 129:393.

Edmunds LH, Wagner HR, Heymann MA: Aortic valvulotomy in neonates. *Circulation* 1980; 61:421.

Fowles RE, Martin RP, Abrams JM: Two-dimensional echocardiographic features of bicuspid aortic valve. *Chest* 1979; 75:434.

Freedom RM, Culham JAG, Moes CAF: *Angiocardiography of Congenital Heart Disease.* New York, Macmillan, 1984, p 369.

Roberts WC: The congenitally bicuspid aortic valve: A study of 85 autopsied cases. *Am J Cardiol* 1970; 26:72.

White RI Jr, Mitchell SE, Kan J: Interventional procedures in congenital heart disease. *Cardiovasc Intervent Radiol* 1986; 9:286.

Supravalvular Aortic Stenosis

Bolen JL, Popp RL, French JW: Echocardiographic features of supravalvular aortic stenosis. *Circulation* 1975; 52:817.

Keane JF, Fellows KE, LaFarge CG, et al: The surgical management of discrete and diffuse supravalvular aortic stenosis. *Circulation* 1975; 52:817.

Kurlander GJ, Petry EL, Taybi H, et al: Supravalvular aortic stenosis: Roentgen analysis of 27 cases. *Am J Roentgenol* 1966; 98:782.

Nasrallah AT, Nihill M: Supravalvular aortic stenosis. Echocardiographic features. *Br Heart J* 1975; 37:662.

Sheikh KH, Adams DB, Kisslo J: Echo-Doppler evaluation of aortic valve stenosis, in Elliott LP (ed): *Cardiac Imaging in Infants, Children, and Adults.* Philadelphia, JB Lippincott, 1991, p 254.

White RD: Magnetic resonance imaging of aortic valve stenosis, in Elliott LP (ed): *Cardiac Imaging in Infants, Children, and Adults.* Philadelphia, JB Lippincott, 1991, p 261.

Muscular Subaortic Stenosis

Hagaman JF, Wolfe C, Craige E: Early aortic valve closure and combined idiopathic hypertrophic subaortic stenosis and discrete subaortic stenosis. *Am J Cardiol* 1980; 45:1083.

Maron BJ: Cardiomyopathies, in Adams FH, Emmanouilides GC, Riemenschneider TA (eds): *Heart Disease in Infants, Children, and Adolescents.* Baltimore, Williams & Wilkins, 1989.

Martin RP, Radowski H, French JW, et al: Idiopathic hypertrophic subaortic stenosis viewed by wide angle phased array echocardiography. *Circulation* 1979; 59:1206.

Redwood DR, Scherer JL, Epstein SE: Biventricular cineangiography in the evaluation of patients with asymmetric septal hypertrophy. *Circulation* 1974; 49:1116.

Riggs T, Hirschfeld SS, Rajai H: Pediatric spectrum of dynamic left ventricular obstruction. *Am Heart J* 1980; 99:301.

Subvalvular Aortic Stenosis (Excluding IHSS)

Berry TE, Azia KU, Paul MH: Echocardiographic assessment of discrete subaortic stenosis in childhood. *Am J Cardiol* 1979; 43:957.

Freedom RM, Culham JAG, Moes CAF: *Angiocardiography of Congenital Heart Disease.* New York, Macmillan, 1984, p 389.

Katz NM, Buckley MJ, Liberthson RR: Discrete membranous subaortic stenosis. *Circulation* 1977; 56:1034.

Kelley JJ, Higgins CB, Kirkpatrick SE: Axial left ventriculography with discrete subaortic stenosis. *Radiology* 1980; 135:77.

Krueger SK, French JW, Forder AD, et al: Echocardiography in discrete subaortic stenosis. *Circulation* 1979; 59:506.

Shone JD, Sellers RD, Anderson RC, et al: The developmental complex of "parachute mitral valve," supravalvular ring of the left atrium, subaortic stenosis and coarctation of the aorta. *Am J Cardiol* 1963; 11:714.

White RI Jr, Mitchell SE, Kan J: Interventional procedures in congenital heart disease. *Cardiovasc Intervent Radiol* 1986; 9:286.

Coarctation of the Aorta, Aortic Arch Interruption, and Pseudocoarctation of the Aorta

Babbit DB, Cassidy GE, Godard JE: Rib notching in aortic coarctation during infancy and childhood. *Radiology* 1974; 110:169.

Bank ER, Aise AM, Rocchini AP, et al: Coarctation of the aorta in children undergoing angioplasty: Pretreatment and posttreatment MR imaging. *Radiology* 1987; 162:235–240.

Bisset GS III, Meyer RA: Obstructive left heart lesions. *Semin Roentgenol* 1985; 20:244.

Burrows PE: Magnetic resonance imaging of the aorta in children. *Semin Ultrasound CT MR* 1990; 11:221.

Dungan WT, Char F, Gerald BE, et al: Pseudocoarctation of the aorta in childhood. *Am J Dis Child* 1970; 119:401.

Freedom RM, Bain HH, Esplugas E, et al: Ventricular septal defect in interruption of aortic arch. *Am J Cardiol* 1977; 39:572.

Freedom RM, Culham JAG, Moes CAF: *Angiocardiography of Congenital Heart Disease.* New York, Macmillan, 1984, p 464.

Higgins CB, French JW, Silverman JF, et al: Interruption of the aortic arch: Preoperative and postoperative clinical hemodynamic and angiographic features. *Am J Cardiol* 1977; 36:563.

Hoeffel JC, Henry M, Mentre B, et al: Pseudocoarctation or congenital kinking of the aorta: Radiological considerations. *Am Heart J* 1975; 89:429.

Jaffe RB: Complete interruption of the aortic arch. I. Characteristic radiographic findings in 21 patients. *Circulation* 1975; 52:714.

Jaffe RB: Complete interruption of the aortic arch. II. Characteristic angiographic features with emphasis on collateral circulation to the descending aorta. *Circulation* 1976; 53:161.

Jaffe RB: Radiographic manifestations of congenital anomalies of the aortic arch. *Radiol Clin North Am* 1991; 29:319.

Liberthson RR, Pennington DG, Jacobs JL, et al: Coarctation of the aorta: Review of 234 patients and clarification of management problems. *Am J Cardiol* 1979; 43:835.

Martin EC, Strafford MA, Gersony W: Initial detection of coarctation of the aorta: An opportunity for the radiologist. *Am J Roentgenol* 1981; 137:1015.

Moes CAF, Freedom RM: Aortic arch interruption with truncus arteriosus or aorticopulmonary septal defect. *Am J Roentgenol* 1980; 135:1011.

Neye-Bock S, Fellows KE: Aortic arch interruption in infancy: Radio- and angiographic features. *Am J Roentgenol* 1980; 135:1005.

Sahn DJ, Allen HD, McDonald G, et al: Real-time cross-sectional echocardiographic diagnosis of coarctation of the aorta: Prospective study of echocardiographic-angiographic correlations. *Circulation* 1977; 56:762.

Stern J, Lander P, Palayew MJ: Coarctation of the aorta: Additional signs. *J Can Assoc Radiol* 1979; 30:40.

von Schulthess GK, Higashino SM, Higgins SS, et al: Coarctation of the aorta: MR imaging. *Radiology* 1986; 158:469–474.

White RI Jr, Mitchell SE, Kan J: Interventional procedures in congenital heart disease. *Cardiovasc Intervent Radiol* 1986; 9:286.

Endocardial Fibroelastosis

Freedom RM, Culham JAG, Moes CAF: *Angiocardiography of Congenital Heart Disease.* New York, Macmillan, 1984, p 358.

Hunter AS, Keay AJ: Primary endocardial fibroelastosis: An inherited condition. *Arch Dis Child* 1973; 48:66.

Keith JD, Rose V, Manning JA: Endocardial fibroelastosis, in Keith JD, Rowe RD, Vlad P (eds): *Heart Disease in Infancy and Childhood.* New York, Macmillan, 1978, p 941.

Manning JA, Sellers FJ, Bynum R, et al: Medical management of clinical endocardial fibroelastosis. *Circulation* 1974; 19:60.

SECTION 3

Cyanotic Congenital Heart Disease With Increased Pulmonary Blood Flow (Admixture Shunts)

COMPLETE TRANSPOSITION OF THE GREAT ARTERIES

Complete or dextrotransposition of the great arteries (d-TGA) is the most common form of cyanotic CHD with increased pulmonary flow and accounts for 5% to 9% of CHD (see Table 15–1). The prognosis is extremely poor without early palliation (Rashkind balloon atrial septostomy) or corrective surgery with Mustard, Senning, or great-vessel-switch procedures. Many variations of transposition are present and are more completely reviewed in works by Van Praagh and others. In isolated d-TGA, the aorta is transposed anteriorly and to the right and originates from the right ventricle, with the pulmonary artery posteriorly positioned and originating from the left ventricle.

Incidence

The incidence is 1 in 4,000 live births. The male to female ratio is 2 to 3:1. Infants of diabetic mothers have a significantly increased risk of d-TGA.

Pathophysiology

A completely separate pulmonary and systemic vascular circuit is present that is incompatible with life without other associated shunts. Mixing occurs through a VSD, PDA, ASD, or patent foramen ovale. Approximately 70% of patients with d-TGA will have an intact ventricular septum and no left ventricular outflow obstruction. The two most commonly associated major lesions are VSD and left ventricular outflow tract obstruction typically coexisting with a VSD. The causes of left ventricular outflow tract obstruction in complete or dextrotransposition of the great arteries are listed in Table 16–2.

Clinical Manifestations

Cyanosis presents at birth and is more severe in patients without VSD. Cyanosis, acidosis, and congestive failure are the primary early manifestations and are exaggerated by closure of a patent ductus. Auscultation reveals no murmur or a very soft innocent-sounding murmur. When other lesions are present, murmurs related to these lesions may be heard (i.e., VSD, pulmonary stenosis, etc.).

Chest Roentgenography

Roentgenographic findings are variable and are primarily related to the presence or absence of PVS. Findings include (1) hyperinflation of the lungs and depression of the diaphragm, (2) a narrow base of the heart, (3) an "egg-shaped" or "egg-on-side" cardiac configuration, (4) thymic atrophy, and (5) mild cardiomegaly (see Figs 15–5 and 16–60). Pulmonary flow is normal in the neonate until pulmonary vascular resistance decreases; then, pulmonary flow typically is increased unless left ventricular outflow tract obstruction or PVS is present. If pulmonary hypertension, left ventricular outflow tract obstruction, or closure of the atrial septostomy has occurred, congestive failure is frequent, particularly in patients with a VSD. Differential diagnoses include truncus arteriosus with normal or increased flow; when d-TGA is associated with PVS, tetralogy of Fallot and tricuspid atresia must be excluded.

TABLE 16–2.

Causes of Left Ventricular Outflow Tract Obstruction in Complete or Dextrotransposition of the Great Arteries

Pulmonary valvular stenosis
Subvalvular obstruction
Fibrous diaphragm
Fibromuscular tunnel
Malalignment and posterior displacement of infundibular septum
Aneurysm of the membranous septum
Dynamic septal-mitral opposition
Abnormal or accessory mitral valve tissue
Abnormal mitral chordal attachments
Herniation of tricuspid valve tissue through VSD

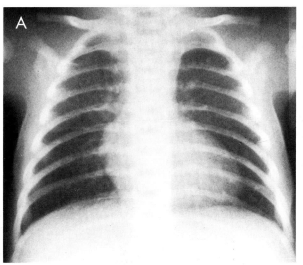
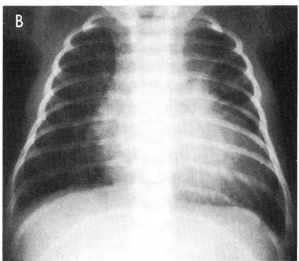

FIG 16–60.

Transposition of the great arteries (TGA). **A,** an AP roentgenogram in a 3-week-old infant shows an egg-shaped cardiac silhouette, flat pulmonary artery segment secondary to its transposed position posterior to the aortic root, and only mild evidence of increased pulmonary vasculature and cardiomegaly. Involution of the thymus and depression of the diaphragm indicate continued hypoxia after the Rashkind balloon atrial septostomy. **B,** the same patient at 1 year of age. Note the progressive cardiomegaly with an abnormal silhouette and a much greater degree of admixture shunt (see Fig 15–5).

Echocardiography

Real-time echocardiography easily identifies the abnormal position of the aorta and pulmonary artery (Fig 16–61). Other associated valvular and septal defects and arch abnormalities are readily identified. The pulmonary valve and subvalvular area should be evaluated closely because of their frequent involvement. Coronary artery origins should also be determined. Doppler may be helpful in identifying intracardiac and ductal shunts.

Angiocardiography and Catheterization

Right heart ventriculography demonstrates a large trabeculated right ventricle in a normal position giving rise to a smooth-walled infundibulum and transposed aortic valve and root. With the presence of a VSD, a right-to-left ventricular shunt will be noted. The aortic arch is on the left except when associated with PVS in which case a right arch may be seen in 75% of patients. The right ventricle may be hypoplastic (poor prognosis).

Long-axis left ventriculography usually shows a normal-sized left ventricle, although frequently it is compressed by the large right ventricle. The left ventricle gives origin to the pulmonary artery (Fig 16–62, *A* and *B*). The pulmonary valve and subvalvular area must be closely evaluated for stenosis (Fig 16–63; Table 16–2). Pulmonary valve and anterior mitral leaflet continuity must be established to dif-ferentiate d-TGA from double-outlet right ventricle (see Fig 15–13,B). An aortogram to visualize the coronary arteries should be performed with balloon occlusion of the ascending aorta (Berman angiographic catheter) if an arterial-switch operation is planned. Filming in the AP projection should be performed with caudal-cranial angulation of 40 to 45 degrees ("laid-back" aortogram) supplemented with the lateral projection. Many coronary artery anomalies are present with d-TGA and are well illustrated by Mandell et al. and Mayer et al.

A balloon atrial septostomy must be performed early in the course of catheterization, frequently before angiography if a supporting echocardiogram is diagnostic of d-TGA. This improves atrial level mixing and oxygenation and allows for safer, further cardiac catheterization.

Prognosis

Survival rates of 70% to 80% can be expected to the age of 2 years after balloon atrial septostomy or other operative procedure (pulmonary artery banding). When utilizing a Mustard or Senning procedure, normal physiologic blood flow by intra-atrial shunting can be accomplished. An arterial switch and transplantation of the coronary arteries (Jatene procedure) is the preferred reparative operation in the absence of left ventricular outflow tract obstruction. Postoperative complications include supravalvular narrowing of the pulmonary artery (see Fig

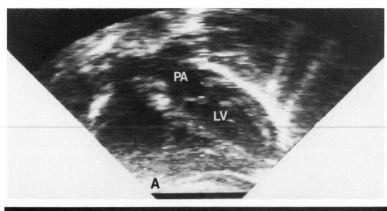

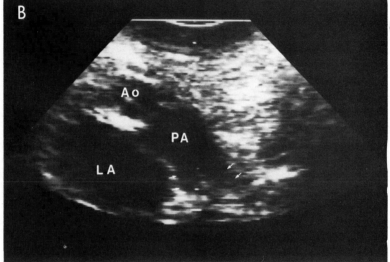

FIG 16–61.
Dextrotransposition of the great arteries (d-TGA). **A,** a subxiphoid two-dimensional echocardiogram shows a large main pulmonary artery *(PA)* with right and left pulmonary arteries originating poste- riorly from the left ventricle *(LV)*. **B,** a short-axis view shows the or- igin of the aorta *(Ao)* anteriorly and to the right of the pulmonary artery *(PA)*. *LA,* left atrium.

21–14,A and B) or aortic and left ventricular isch- emia from coronary artery obstruction (see Fig 15–30). (See discussion of operative procedures and complications, Chapter 21). The prognosis is always worse when associated with a VSD and PVS.

SINGLE VENTRICLE

Single ventricle (common ventricle, univentricular heart, cor triloculare biatriatum) can be defined as a heart containing one ventricular chamber receiving blood through both the mitral and tricuspid valves or, frequently, a common AV valve. The great ves- sels are commonly transposed with complications of pulmonic or systemic outflow obstructions.

Incidence

A single ventricle constitutes approximately 1.5% of CHD (see Table 15–1) and is slightly more common in males. It is found in 1 in 6,500 live births.

Pathophysiology

A single left ventricle usually has d-TGA or cor- rected transposition (l-TGA). Other types include a single right ventricle and an undifferentiated ventri- cle. An outlet chamber may or may not exist and be associated with either bulboventricular or valvular stenosis, or both. Asplenia syndrome often is present.

Clinical Manifestations

Early cyanosis and congestive failure are common, with the degree of cyanosis depending in part on the degree of pulmonary outflow obstruction. A pansystolic murmur is frequent with an associated hyperactive heart.

Chest Roentgenography

Roentgenographic manifestations primarily relate to the great vessel orientation. A single ventricle

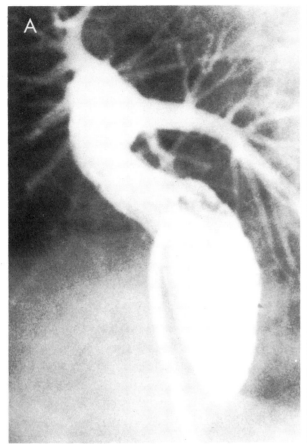 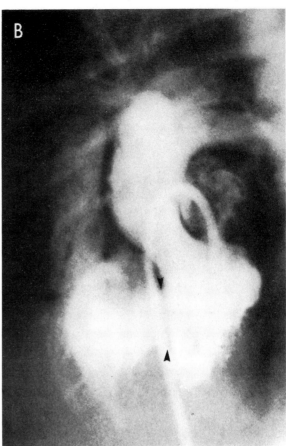

FIG 16–62.
TGA. **A,** a long-axis left ventriculogram shows a transposed pulmonary artery with normal mitral-pulmonary valve continuity and no evidence of pulmonary stenosis. **B,** a similar left ventriculogram shows a moderate muscular VSD *(arrowheads)* (see Fig 15–13, *B*).

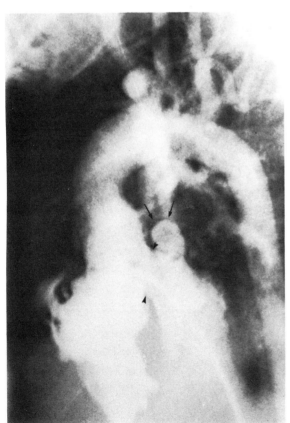

FIG 16–63.
Dextrotransposition of the great arteries with pulmonary obstruction. A long-axis left ventriculogram shows transposed aorta and pulmonary artery, a large VSD *(arrowheads)* with left-to-right shunting, and severe PVS with doming of the thickened pulmonary leaflets *(black arrows)*.

with dextrotransposition simulates findings of conventional transposition of the great vessels. With corrected transposition, the aorta is often border-forming in the upper left heart margin. Pulmonary flow is increased in the absence of pulmonary outflow obstruction. Cardiomegaly is usually noted unless pulmonary outflow obstruction is present.

Echocardiography

Real-time echocardiography is particularly valuable in this condition for differentiating TGA with a VSD from a single ventricle with transposition. A ventricular septum will not be evident, and two AV valves are usually seen (Fig 16–64). When a common AV valve exists, this can be readily visualized. The aorta and pulmonary artery relations are easily defined and d- and l-TGA differentiated.

Angiocardiography

Biplane long-axis angiocardiography should be performed with a large bolus injection (2 mL/kg) with a high flow rate. Ventricular chamber shape, number of AV valves, outflow chamber position, and great vessel relations all must be evaluated (Fig 16–65). Pulmonary and aortic outflow obstructions may exist along with the occasional presence of coarctation.

Magnetic Resonance Imaging

MRI is an ideal modality to determine the segmental anatomy and evaluate the central pulmonary arteries before the Fontan procedure. MRI may also differentiate single ventricle with d-TGA from d-TGA with large VSD (Fig 16–66). MRI in the coronal plane often demonstrates well the bulboventricular foramen and outlet chamber (Fig 16–67).

Prognosis

Palliative surgery, i.e., pulmonary artery banding, may be helpful in the neonate when large pulmonary shunts exist. Systemic-pulmonary shunting will be needed in the presence of PVS. Reconstructive procedures include a Fontan procedure, occasionally ventricular septation, and rarely a Damus procedure to bypass subaortic or aortic valve obstruction (see Chapter 21).

CORRECTED TRANSPOSITION OF THE GREAT ARTERIES

Corrected TGA is characterized by ventricular inversion and levotransposition resulting in discordant AV and ventriculoarterial connections (see Chapter 18). In the uncomplicated type, systemic venous return passes from the right atrium through the mitral valve into a morphologic left ventricle and then to the posterior and medially positioned pulmonary ar-

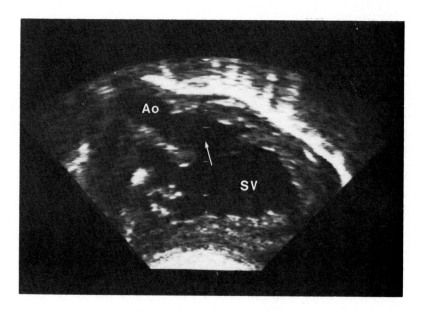

FIG 16–64.
Common ventricle with TGA. A two-dimensional subxiphoid parasternal echocardiogram shows changes secondary to a single ventricle (SV), with a well-defined infundibular chamber giving rise to the levotransposed aorta (Ao). The arrow denotes the bulboventricular foramen. Two separate AV valves were also apparent in other projections (not shown).

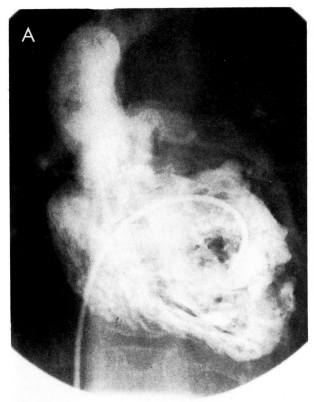

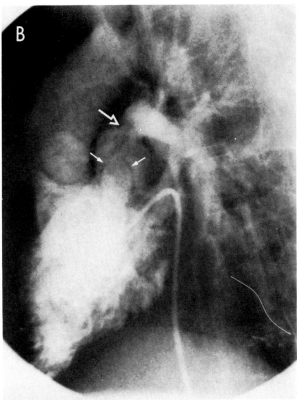

FIG 16–65.
Common ventricle with TGA and PVS. AP **(A)** and lateral **(B)** ventriculograms show the large, moderately trabeculated common ventricle giving rise to transposed great arteries. PVS *(arrows)* and a pulmonary artery band *(open arrow)* are present. The right aortic arch is also evident.

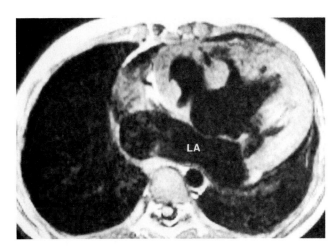

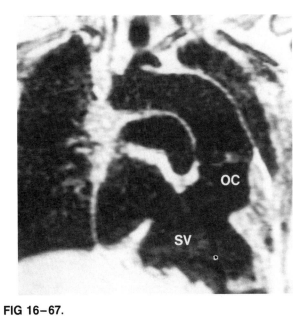

FIG 16–66.
Common single ventricle. Axial spin-echo MR image at the level of the left atrium *(LA)* demonstrates the mitral valve and single ventricle. Axial images at a lower level demonstrated a small tricuspid valve.

FIG 16–67.
Single ventricle with levotransposition and pulmonary valve atresia. Coronal MR image demonstrates the venous atrium, single ventricle *(SV)*, bulboventricular foramen leading to the outlet chamber *(OC)*, and the levotransposed aorta. The pulmonary artery and atretic valve are seen medial to the aorta (see Fig 19–11).

tery. Pulmonary venous return is to the normally positioned left atrium, and then through the tricuspid valve to the systemic morphologic right ventricle and out the levotransposed aorta. In this state blood flows in a physiologic manner.

Unfortunately, only 1% of patients with l-TGA are without other significant intracardiac defects. Frequently associated anomalies singly or in combination are (1) VSD; (2) PVS or subvalvular stenosis; (3) abnormalities of the systemic AV (tricuspid) valve, including the Ebstein malformation with regurgitation; and (4) disturbances of the AV conduction system predisposing to complete or partial heart block. Dextroversion and abnormalities in situs may be present with l-TGA (see Chapter 18). Corrected transposition of the great arteries may also be present with single ventricle (see Single Ventricle above and Fig 16–67).

Incidence

Corrected transposition of the great arteries constitutes 1% of CHD (see Table 15–1). It is slightly more common in males and occurs in 1 in 13,000 live births. Occasionally, other variations in visceral and atrial situs occur.

Pathophysiology

Ninety-five percent of patients have atrial-visceral situs solitus. The ventricles are inverted with the morphologic right ventricle on the left and the morphologic left ventricle on the right (the levo-form of ventricular loop development). This inverted ventricular relationship with atrial situs solitus produces AV discordance. The great vessels are transposed with the aorta anteriorly to the left and the pulmonary artery arising posteriorly from the inverted medially positioned right ventricle. There is mitral-pulmonary continuity. With the tricuspid valve related to the systemic ventricle, tricuspid incompetence may occur (20%). Inversion of the coronary arteries accompanies the ventricular inversion.

Clinical Manifestations

Clinical presentation relates to the intracardiac lesions. With large intracardiac shunts, patients commonly present with CHF, whereas those patients with PVS are commonly cyanotic. Murmurs exist in 60% of patients and relate to associated intracardiac lesions.

Chest Roentgenography

The characteristic configuration of l-TGA is abnormal fullness in the mid- and upper left heart border, which produces a gentle slope that is straight to convex in relation to the levotransposed position of the ascending aorta (Fig 16–68,A). Other variable findings include (1) absence of a defined main pulmonary artery segment, (2) increased pulmonary blood flow in the absence of pulmonary outflow obstruction, (3) a high position of the right pulmonary artery, and occasionally (4) dextroversion with situs solitus or levocardia with situs inversus. Primary differential diagnostic considerations are other forms of transposition, single ventricle, and truncus arteriosus.

Echocardiography

Real-time echocardiography is particularly helpful in this condition in which definition of the great vessel relationships, ventricular septal anatomy, and orientation of the plane of the ventricular septum are critical (Fig 16–68, B and C). Mitral-pulmonary continuity is appreciated with either real-time or M-mode studies.

Angiocardiography

AP and lateral biplane angiocardiography and angled projections are necessary for optimal anatomical evaluation. The ventricles are usually side by side and their morphology must be studied in detail. The morphologic left ventricle in its medial position gives rise to the pulmonary artery (Fig 16–69,A and B). The pulmonary valve and subvalvular area must be closely examined for stenosis, in which case right-to-left shunting through the VSD can usually be seen. A ventriculogram of the systemic ventricle shows morphologic characteristics of a trabeculated right ventricle giving rise to the levotransposed aorta with the aortic valve in a relatively cephalic position (Fig 16–69,C). With associated VSD, physiologic left-to-right shunting will be apparent. Other variable findings include AV valve regurgitation, tricuspid valve dysplasia, Ebstein malformation, aneurysm of the membranous septum, and a right aortic arch.

Prognosis

The prognosis depends mainly on the severity of associated malformations. CHF and heart block are

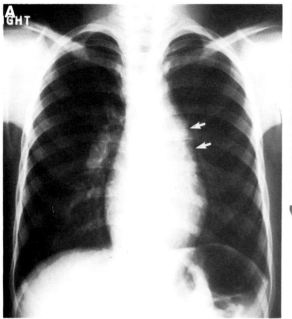

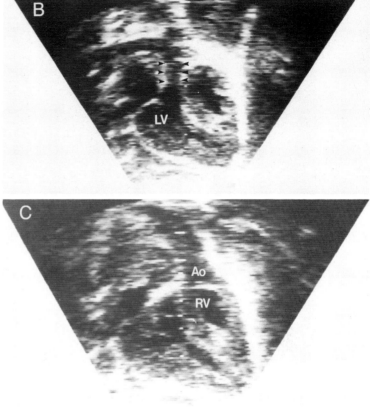

FIG 16–68.
Corrected transposition of the great arteries (I-TGA). **A,** characteristic convex mid-upper left heart border related to transposition of the ascending aorta anteriorly and to the left. This represents the relatively rare patient without intrinsic congenital malformations. Most patients have PVS, VSD (or a common ventricle), abnormalities of the systemic AV valve, and conduction disturbances. **B,** two-dimensional echocardiogram in the subcostal projection demonstrates origin of the medially positioned pulmonary artery *(arrowheads)* from the right-sided morphologic left ventricle *(LV).* **C,** two-dimensional echocardiogram in the subcostal projection in a plane slightly anterior to **B** demonstrates origin of the levotransposed aorta *(Ao)* from the left-sided morphologic right ventricle *(RV).* (**B** and **C** from Jaffe RB: Corrected transposition with ventricular septal defect—echocardiography, in Elliott LP (ed): *Cardiac Imaging in Infants, Children, and Adults.* Philadelphia, JB Lippincott, 1991, p 634. Used by permission.)

common, necessitating a pacemaker. Pulmonary artery banding is necessary when associated with a single ventricle, and systemic-to-pulmonary shunts are necessary when the pulmonary outflow obstruction is severe.

TOTAL ANOMALOUS PULMONARY VENOUS RETURN (TAPVR)

TAPVR indicates total pulmonary venous drainage to the systemic venous circulation.

Incidence

TAPVR accounts for 1% to 2% of CHD (see Table 15–1). The male-to-female ratio is approximately 2:1. TAPVR is of four types: (1) supracardiac (50%); (2) cardiac (30%); (3) infracardiac (15%); and (4) mixed (5%). These types may be further subdivided into obstructed and nonobstructed categories, with 50% to 66% being obstructed. The infracardiac type

is always obstructed. TAPVR is almost always present in asplenia syndrome.

Pathophysiology

The pathophysiologic state depends on (1) the quantity of pulmonary flow and resistance, (2) pulmonary venous obstruction, (3) the size of the obligatory ASD, (4) the presence of a PDA, and (5) right ventricular compliance. With high pulmonary flow and good mixing, cyanosis is mild and symptoms minimal until CHF ensues. With pulmonary venous obstruction, cyanosis is severe, and early death is common without operative correction.

Clinical Manifestations

Infants with obstructed TAPVR always present with severe cyanosis, marked dyspnea, hepatomegaly, and no or insignificant-sounding murmurs. Patients without pulmonary venous obstruction show equiv-

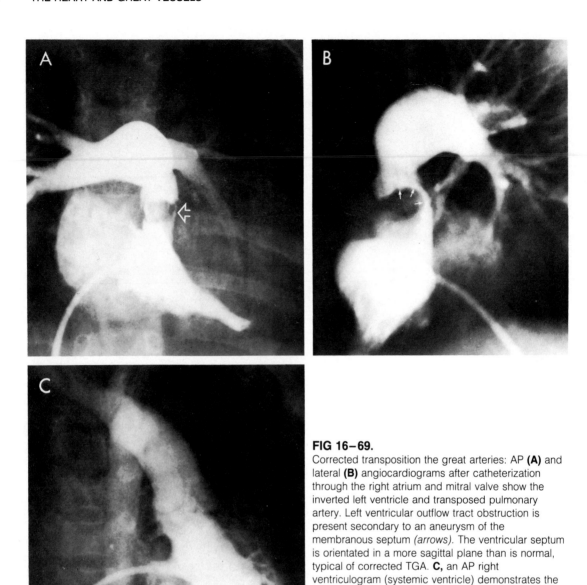

FIG 16–69.
Corrected transposition the great arteries: AP **(A)** and lateral **(B)** angiocardiograms after catheterization through the right atrium and mitral valve show the inverted left ventricle and transposed pulmonary artery. Left ventricular outflow tract obstruction is present secondary to an aneurysm of the membranous septum *(arrows)*. The ventricular septum is orientated in a more sagittal plane than is normal, typical of corrected TGA. **C,** an AP right ventriculogram (systemic ventricle) demonstrates the inverted right ventricular position lateral to the venous ventricle giving rise to the levotransposed aortic root.

ocal cyanosis, tachypnea, dyspnea, poor feeding, hepatomegaly, failure to thrive, and CHF. Other findings include a gallop rhythm, a loud first heart sound, and a split second sound.

Roentgenography

TAPVR With Obstruction
Roentgenographic features are (1) normal cardiac configuration and size, (2) pulmonary venous congestion or edema, or both, (3) thymic atrophy, (4) depression of the diaphragm, and (5) occasional

pleural effusion (Fig 16–70). The primary differential diagnosis is diffuse interstitial pulmonary disease including pulmonary lymphangiectasia.

TAPVR Without Obstruction
Common roentgenographic features include (1) cardiomegaly with right atrial and right ventricular enlargement, (2) an enlarged main pulmonary artery, (3) increased pulmonary flow, and (4) occasional CHF. The primary differential diagnoses are other large left-to-right and admixture shunts.

In the older patient with a nonobstructed sup-

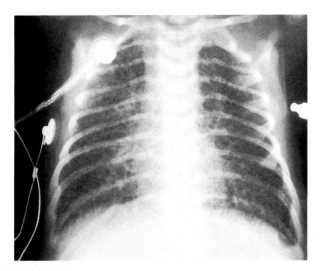

FIG 16–70.
Obstructive supracardiac total anomalous pulmonary venous return (TAPVR): An AP chest roentgenogram in this newborn shows a characteristic pattern of pulmonary venous congestion, a small cardiac silhouette, thymic involution, and hyperinflation. An identical pattern would also be seen with the infracardiac type of TAPVR.

racardiac-type anomalous venous return, characteristic enlargement of the left vertical vein and right SVC produces the so-called snowman or figure-8 cardiac silhouette (Fig 16–71). Other variations in anomalous drainage may produce focal enlargement of the azygos vein, dilatation of the right SVC (Fig 16–72), or visualization of abnormal veins directed toward the superior right hilum. The esophagogram may also show an abnormal identation of the anterior wall in the upper- to midatrial level, again related to the common pulmonary vein (Fig 16–73).

Echocardiography

Real-time echocardiography can commonly track the anomalous pulmonary venous drainage to its aberrant drainage site (Fig 16–74). Other findings include (1) enlargement of the right atrium and tricuspid annulus and right ventricle, (2) paradoxical septal motion in the nonobstructive types, and (3) evidence of pulmonary hypertension. ASDs and PDA (when present) are similarly detected.

Angiocardiography

Because of the large number of complex variations in cases of anomalous pulmonary venous return, angiocardiography is still the best method for a complete evaluation. Biplane AP and lateral cineangiography is performed by injecting contrast material into the main pulmonary artery or, selectively, into the right or left pulmonary artery (Fig 16–75). Balloon occlusion of a PDA may be necessary to im-

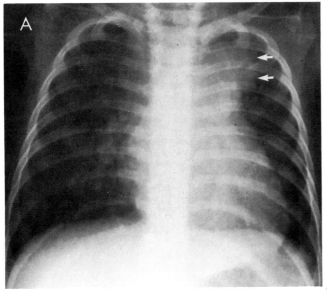

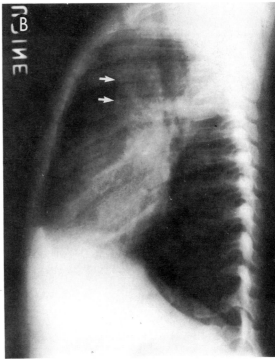

FIG 16–71.
Supracardiac TAPVR to the left vertical vein (snowman): AP **(A)** and lateral **(B)** chest roentgenograms in a 5-month-old infant. The snowman cardiac silhouette is already evident, with relative aneurysmal dilatation of the left vertical vein in **A** *(arrows)*. Increased pulmonary flow and hyperinflation of the lungs are characteristic of this cyanotic condition. On the lateral film **(B)**, a band of increased density *(arrows)* anterior to the trachea represents the dilated left vertical vein and right SVC.

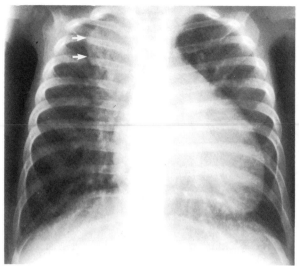

FIG 16–72.
TAPVR to the right SVC: an AP chest roentgenogram shows aneurysmal dilatation of the SVC *(arrows)*. Cardiomegaly with a right ventricular configuration and increased pulmonary blood flow is present.

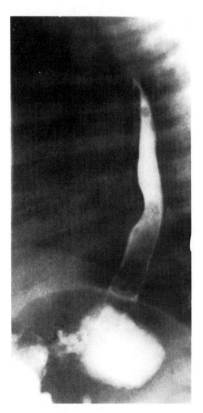

FIG 16–73.
TAPVR. A lateral esophagogram spot film shows a focal indentation on the anterior surface of the esophagus just below the carina at the level of the left atrium that is secondary to the anomalous pulmonary venous confluence of TAPVR. A large coronary sinus secondary to an anomalous pulmonary venous return could produce the same findings.

prove pulmonary artery filling (Figs 16–76 and 16–77). Not only is it necessary to determine the anatomical type of anomalous venous return but also the coexistence of pulmonary venous obstruction. At times, the catheter can be introduced up the SVC to the innominate and vertical vein, with retrograde injection into the pulmonary venous confluence better demonstrating the anatomical malformation (Fig 16–78). Patients with intracardiac anomalous return to the coronary sinus may show a striking aneurysmal dilatation of the distal coronary sinus.

Magnetic Resonance Imaging

Axial and coronal MRI are useful in the evaluation of unusual forms of TAPVR. The operative anastomosis between the common pulmonary vein and left atrium may be defined clearly by axial MRI and the areas of stenosis identified.

Prognosis

Symptoms may be ameliorated by Rashkind balloon septostomy improving mixing at the atrial level. Early operation is mandatory, especially in TAPVR with obstruction and to avoid pulmonary hypertension.

COR TRIATRIATUM AND OTHER ANOMALIES OF THE PULMONARY VEINS

Cor triatriatum reflects the failure to incorporate the common pulmonary veins into the posterior left atrial wall. This produces a membrane with variable obstruction separating the accessory chamber receiving the pulmonary veins from the left atrium. Collateral flow through a persisting left vertical vein is common, bypassing the obstruction and creating pathophysiologic findings similar to supracardiac TAPVR. Varying degrees of pulmonary venous obstruction relate to the size of the orifice in the membrane.

Roentgenographic findings are mainly those arising from pulmonary venous congestion. The diagnosis may be established with echocardiography, angiocardiography (Fig 16–79), MRI, or cine–computed tomography (cine-CT). Other variations in drainage occur in this condition, including anomalous drainage into the right atrium or coronary sinus. Primary differential considerations are congenital supravalvular mitral ring and congenital mitral stenosis.

Other rare forms of pulmonary venous anomalies include atresia of the common pulmonary vein

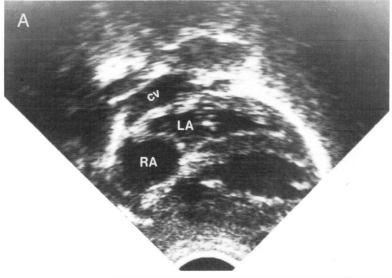

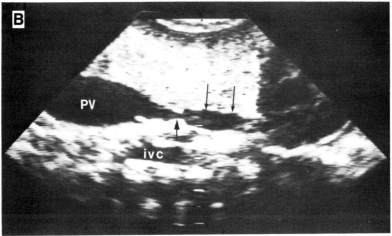

FIG 16–74.
A, TAPVR to the left vertical vein. Subcostal projection at the level of the right atrium *(RA)* and left atrium *(LA)*. The right and left pulmonary veins enter into the common pulmonary vein *(CV)* posterior to the left atrium rather than into the left atrium. Other imaging planes from the suprasternal notch, not illustrated, demonstrate the continuation of the common pulmonary vein into the left vertical vein and the left innominate vein. The ASD is not visualized in the image illustrated. (From Jaffe RB: Total anomalous pulmonary venous connection—echocardiography in Elliott LP (ed): *Cardiac Imaging in Infants, Children, and Adults.* Philadelphia, JB Lippincott, 1991, p 671. Used by permission.) **B,** real-time echocardiogram shows changes related to infradiaphragmatic pulmonary venous return. The common venous channel *(arrows)* extends below the diaphragm, with an area of venous stenosis *(large arrow)* at its junction with the portal vein *(PV)* (*ivc,* inferior vena cava).

and stenosis of the individual pulmonary veins (unilateral or bilateral).

TRUNCUS ARTERIOSUS (PERSISTENT TRUNCUS ARTERIOSUS, TRUNCUS ARTERIOSUS COMMUNUS, AND COMMON AORTICOPULMONARY TRUNK)

Truncus arteriosus is an anomaly characterized by a single vessel arising from the ventricles, overriding a VSD, and supplying the systemic, pulmonary, and coronary circulations. Only one semilunar valve is present. Embryologically, truncus arteriosus represents a failure of the truncus arteriosus to divide into a completely separate ascending aorta and pulmonary artery.

Classification

Many classifications have been developed, but probably the most widely utilized was that of Collette and Edwards, which categorizes truncus arteriosus as (1) type I (50%), where a single pulmonary trunk arises from the common truncal vessel branching into right and left pulmonary arteries; (2) type II (30%), where right and left pulmonary arteries arise

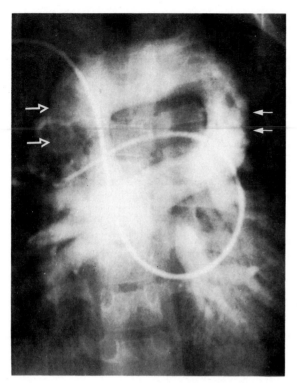

FIG 16–75.
Supracardiac TAPVR. A late venous angiogram after a right pulmonary artery injection shows the characteristic anomalous pulmonary venous drainage secondary to nonobstructed supracardiac TAPVR. The left vertical vein is dilated and bulges laterally *(arrows)* along with the dilatation of the innominate vein and SVC *(open arrows)*.

close together from the posterior wall of the truncal vessel; (3) type III, where the right and left pulmonary arteries arise from either side of the common trunk; and (4) type IV, where no pulmonary arteries arise from the ascending trunk but the lungs are supplied by systemic bronchial or pulmonary vessels. Some authors (Van Praagh) think that the last-named category is not a true example of truncus arteriosus and should be classified with pulmonary atresia. Many other classifications and variations have been described.

Incidence

The reported incidence is approximately 1% of CHD, with an occurrence in 1 in 11,000 live births (see Table 15–1). Other associated malformations include interruption of the aortic arch, a hypoplastic aortic isthmus, coarctation, and PDA. It may occur with DiGeorge syndrome. Unilateral absence of a pulmonary artery has been reported in 12% of patients (Mair et al.). Truncal valve stenosis and insufficiency, and anomalies of the coronary arteries may also be present.

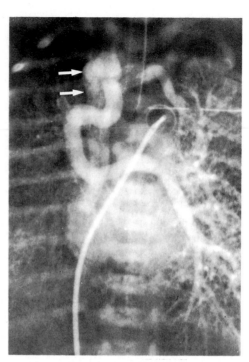

FIG 16–76.
Mixed supracardiac TAPVR. A late pulmonary venous angiogram after a left pulmonary artery injection shows circuitous venous drainage predominantly to the SVC *(arrows)*, with the left upper lobe draining anomalously through the innominate vein.

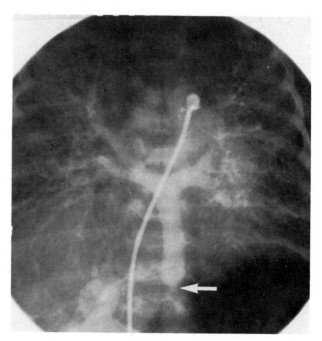

FIG 16–77.
Infracardiac TAPVR. A late pulmonary venous angiocardiogram after main pulmonary artery injection with balloon catheter occlusion of a PDA demonstrates classic findings of infracardiac TAPVR. Note the stenosis of the common pulmonary vein at its junction with the portal system *(arrow)* (see Fig 16–74,B).

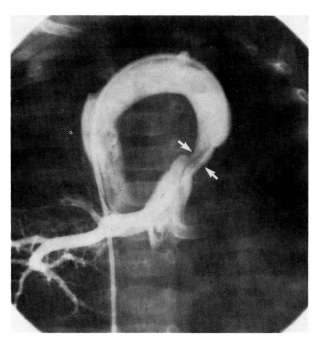

FIG 16–78.
Supracardiac TAPVR with obstruction. Pulmonary venous angiogram following retrograde catheterization of the SVC, innominate vein, and left vertical vein. Note the point of narrowing and obstruction *(arrows)* caused by compression of this venous channel between the left main pulmonary artery and left mainstem bronchus or by intrinsic stenosis.

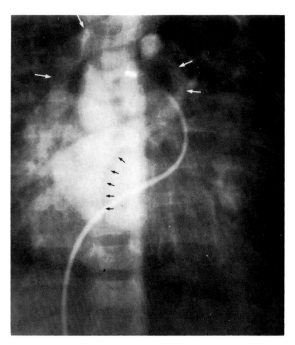

FIG 16–79.
Cor triatriatum. A late pulmonary venous angiogram shows a fenestrated membrane *(black arrows)* dividing the left atrium, with collateral venous drainage to the left vertical vein *(white arrows)* and subsequent visualization of the innominate vein and SVC. The roentgenographic patterns of cor triatriatum may resemble those of nonobstructed or obstructed TAPVR, depending upon septal defects and other patent venous collateral channels.

Pathophysiology

The pathophysiologic process relates to increased pulmonary flow with an admixture of systemic and pulmonary blood. Complications include pulmonary hypertension, increased pulmonary vascular resistance, and truncal valve insufficiency. The truncal valve is usually tricuspid (66%), with the remainder being either bicuspid or quadricuspid valves. In rare cases, stenosis at the origin of the pulmonary arteries may be present, produce decreased pulmonary flow, and exaggerate the cyanosis. Hypoxemia may lead to myocardial ischemia and poor function.

Clinical Manifestations

Most patients present early in life with cyanosis, failure to thrive, dyspnea, and CHF. The heart is enlarged with a prominent second sound that is usually single. An apical systolic ejection click and soft pansystolic or ejection murmur is heard in most patients.

Chest Roentgenography

Common chest roentgenographic findings include (1) moderate cardiomegaly, (2) a narrow base of the heart, (3) a high cephalic origin of the left pulmonary artery, (4) a right aortic arch (in 25%–33% of patients), (5) increased pulmonary blood flow, (6) a depressed diaphragm, and (7) thymic atrophy (Fig 16–80). The primary differential diagnosis is d-TGA. In a small second group of patients, pulmonary flow is decreased because of pulmonary artery stenosis or increased pulmonary resistance.

Echocardiography

Real-time echocardiography readily identifies (1) a large single truncal vessel overriding (2) a large VSD, and (3) a large echogenic truncal valve with fibrous continuity with the anterior leaflet of the mitral valve. The main pulmonary artery in type I can usually be identified by its origin from the truncal vessel (Fig 16–81).

Angiography

Large volume (2 mL/kg) biplane AP and lateral cineangiography should be performed by injecting contrast into the proximal truncal vessel or main pulmonary artery in type I lesions (Fig 16–82). Sup-

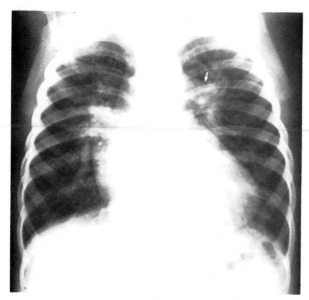

FIG 16–80.
Truncus arteriosus, type I, in a 1-year-old infant with classic high cephalic origin of the left pulmonary artery *(arrow)* and relative vertical descent of the left lower lobe pulmonary artery. A prominent left aortic arch (although a right aortic arch is present in one third of patients) and moderate cardiomegaly are evident. The main pulmonary artery segment is flat, the pulmonary vasculature increased, and the lungs hyperexpanded secondary to hypoxia.

plementation with oblique views may be necessary, particularly in differentiating types II and III from type I when a short main pulmonary artery segment exists. Ventriculography, although rarely necessary, will demonstrate the conal VSD. The aortic arch, coronary arteries, and truncal valve should be closely evaluated because of frequently associated

variations. The recognition of separate pulmonary and aortic valves permit differentiation of an aortico-pulmonary window from truncus arteriosus type I.

Prognosis

Primary repair is usually performed in infancy with VSD closure and placement of a valved conduit between the right ventricle and pulmonary arteries (Rastelli procedure). Postoperative complications include calcification of the valve and/or conduit with obstruction (see Figs 21–28 and 21–29). Balloon valvuloplasty and conduit replacement may be necessary (see Chapter 21).

DOUBLE-OUTLET RIGHT VENTRICLE

A double-outlet right ventricle (DORV) is characterized by the origin of both great vessels predominantly from the right ventricle, and by bilateral muscular infundibula, and absence of AV–semilunar valve continuity. A VSD is invariably present and may be classified as: (1) subaortic, (2) subpulmonic, (3) doubly committed, or (4) noncommitted (remote). The great vessel relations are variable but most commonly seen are side-by-side great vessels with the aorta to the right of the pulmonary artery (Taussig-Bing malformation) and the aorta anterior to the right of the pulmonary artery. PVS is frequently present, especially when the VSD is subaortic. DORV can occur with dextro-, meso-, or levocardia, and may be associated with asplenia syndrome.

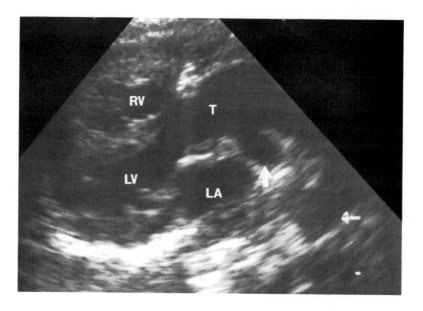

FIG 16–81.
Truncus arteriosus. Two-dimensional long-axis echocardiogram shows the large truncal vessel *(T)* overriding the large VSD. A large pulmonary vessel arises posteriorly from the truncal vessel *(arrow)*. RV, right ventricle; LV, left ventricle; LA, left atrium.

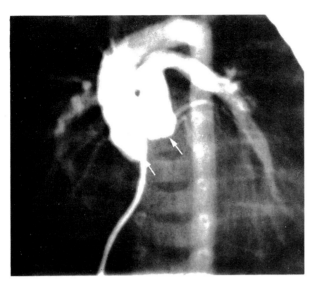

FIG 16–82.
Truncus arteriosus, type I. Injection into the truncal root shows the large truncal valve (arrows) and simultaneous filling of a short main pulmonary artery segment and aortic arch. The origin of both pulmonary arteries is high, particularly the left, and there is symmetric flow to both lungs.

Incidence

DORV constitutes 1% to 3% of all CHD (see Table 15–1). Associated lesions include coarctation or an interrupted aortic arch. The male-female ratio is approximately 2:1.

Pathophysiology

This lesion represents an admixture shunt with increased pulmonary blood flow. Patients with Taussig-Bing malformation with subpulmonic VSD have pathophysiologic findings similar to those of complete transposition.

Clinical Manifestations

Symptoms depend on the type of lesion present as well as the size of the pulmonary shunt and commitment of the VSD. Mild to marked cyanosis may be present. Without PVS, clinical findings are similar to a VSD. With PVS, clinical findings simulate the tetralogy of Fallot. Those patients with subpulmonic VSD without PVS present early with cyanosis and mimic transposition of the great vessels. Without PVS, CHF is frequent.

Chest Roentgenography

Chest roentgenographic features correlate closely with the presence or absence of PVS or aortic arch obstruction. Without pulmonary obstruction, find-

ings include (1) moderate cardiomegaly (right ventricular configuration), (2) large convex main pulmonary artery, (3) increased pulmonary blood flow, (4) thymic atrophy, and (5) a depressed diaphragm with hyperinflation of the lung. Early congestive failure suggests coarctation or an interrupted aortic arch.

With PVS, findings are (1) mild cardiomegaly with a right ventricular configuration, (2) a concave main pulmonary artery, (3) diminished pulmonary blood flow, and (4) a left aortic arch. If visceral heterotaxia is evident, cardiosplenic syndrome, especially asplenia, should be considered.

Echocardiography

Real-time echocardiography demonstrates (1) side-by-side transposition of the great vessels with the aorta usually anterior and to the right, (2) overriding of the aortic root in relation to the ventricular septum, (3) a VSD, (4) subpulmonic and subaortic stenosis when present, and (5) absent fibrous continuity of the semilunar and AV valves (Fig 16–83). Differential diagnoses are primarily tetralogy of Fallot and d-TGA with VSD.

Angiocardiography

Biplane right and left ventricular injections are necessary with filming in the AP and lateral, long-axis, and four-chamber projections to identify all anatomical abnormalities. Aortic root injections may also be needed. The VSD must be well visualized and its commitment to the great vessels adequately demonstrated (Fig 16–84). The semilunar valves, subpulmonic area, and aortic arch may all show anomalies requiring evaluation. Typically the aortic and pulmonary valves are at the same cephalocaudal position. The diagnosis of DORV is dependent on identification of more than half of each great vessel originating from the morphologic right ventricle.

Magnetic Resonance Imaging

MRI is very helpful, especially in the axial plane and occasionally in the coronal plane, for localization and relations of the VSD to the great vessels (Fig 16–85).

Prognosis

Total correction is the primary goal but early palliative procedures may be necessary including Rashkind balloon atrial septostomy and systemic–pulmonary artery shunting when associated with pulmonary obstruction. Definitive repair requires closure of the

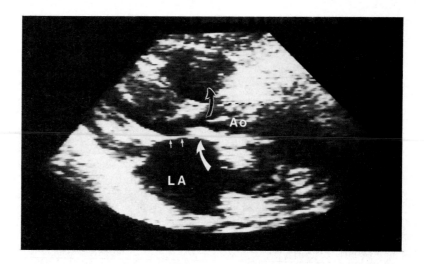

FIG 16–83.
Double-outlet right ventricle (DORV) echocardiogram. A long-axis view demonstrates an aortic root (Ao) overriding the interventricular septum and separated from the mitral valve (small arrows) by a segment of conal musculature (curved arrow). A supracristal VSD is present (black arrow). The discontinuity of the mitral valve from the semilunar valve is critical in this diagnosis and is better seen with the total real-time examination.

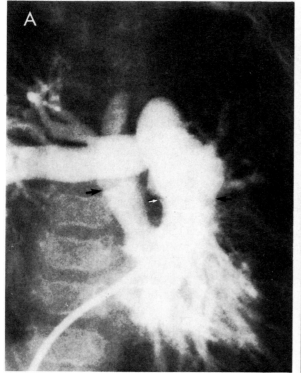

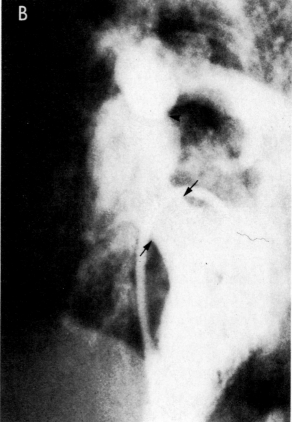

FIG 16–84.
DORV. **A,** an AP cineangiocardiogram shows the aortic and pulmonary valves (arrows) at the same relative cephalocaudal position. Subaortic conal musculature narrows the aortic outflow tract. **B,** DORV, Taussig-Bing variety. A left ventriculogram (lateral long-axis) shows the supracristal VSD (arrows) opening into the subpulmonic outflow tract (Taussig-Bing type). A pulmonary artery band (arrowhead) is present, with the aorta and pulmonary artery directly superimposed in the lateral view.

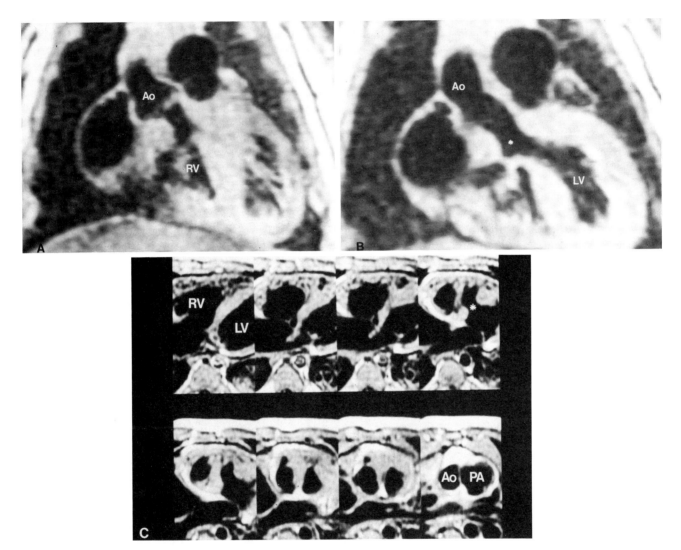

FIG 16–85.
DORV and subaortic VSD in a 7-week-old infant. **A,** coronal 3-mm spin-echo MR image demonstrates origin of the aorta *(Ao)* from the right ventricle *(RV)* with mild subaortic narrowing from conal musculature. An additional coronal image 6 mm anterior to **A** demonstrated the origin of the pulmonary artery from the right ventricle. **B,** a coronal 3-mm spin-echo MR image, 3 mm posterior to **A,** demonstrates that the only egress of blood from the left ventricle *(LV)* is through the subaortic VSD (*) into the aorta *(Ao).* **C,** an 8-month-old infant with DORV with subpulmonic VSD (Taussig-Bing malformation): composite axial 3-mm spin-echo MR images, inferosuperior, demonstrate the left ventricle *(LV)* and subpulmonic VSD (*). The great vessels are side by side with the pulmonary artery *(PA)* to the right of the aorta *(Ao).* More superior images demonstrated the bifurcation of the pulmonary artery and a pulmonary artery band in satisfactory position. *RV,* right ventricle.

VSD and placement of internal and external conduits to establish physiologic blood flow between the left ventricle and aorta and right ventricle and pulmonary artery (see Chapter 21; Fig 21–27). Some patients with associated lesions may require an arterial-switch procedure, Damus procedure, or Fontan procedure and these are discussed in Chapter 21. Mortality remains moderate, particularly for patients with PVS and aortic arch malformations.

DOUBLE-OUTLET LEFT VENTRICLE

A double-outlet left ventricle (DOLV) is an extremely rare malformation characterized by both great vessels arising entirely or predominantly from the anatomical left ventricle and overriding, to a varying degree, an associated VSD. There is normal aortic–anterior mitral valve leaflet continuity. Associated defects include subpulmonic and subaortic obstruction. The great vessels have a variable relation with the aorta, most commonly to the right of the pulmonary artery. Clinically and radiologically, this condition closely simulates tetralogy of Fallot and other forms of TGA, depending upon the presence or absence of pulmonary obstruction.

Chest Roentgenography

Radiologic manifestations are nonspecific and relate predominantly to the presence or absence of PVS. In the latter case, the findings are similar to tetralogy of Fallot with a normal heart size and decreased pulmonary flow. Without PVS, moderate cardiomegaly and increased pulmonary blood flow are evident. Primary differential considerations in this setting are (1) truncus arteriosus, (2) TGA, and (3) TAPVR.

Echocardiography

Echocardiography demonstrates the abnormal origin of the pulmonary artery from the left ventricle, normal aortic-mitral continuity, and VSD.

Angiocardiography

Biplane AP and lateral and axial left ventricular angiocardiography demonstrates (1) the abnormal origin of the pulmonary artery from the left ventricle, (2) the VSD defect, and (3) aortic–anterior mitral valve leaflet continuity. The ventricular septum must be profiled to determine the origin of both great vessels entirely or predominantly from the left ventricle.

Prognosis

Surgical correction is feasible with an external conduit from the right ventricle to the pulmonary arteries (Rastelli procedure) and closure of the VSD. A Fontan procedure may be necessary if the right ventricle is hypoplastic.

REFERENCES

Complete Transposition of the Great Arteries

Alpert BS, Bloom KR, Olley PM, et al: Echocardiographic evaluation of right ventricular function in complete transposition of the great arteries: Angiographic correlates. *Am J Cardiol* 1979; 44:270.

Carey LS, Elliott LP: Complete transposition of the great vessels: Roentgenographic findings. *Am J Roentgenol* 1974; 91:529.

Castaneda AR, Trusler GA, Paul MH, et al: The early results of treatment of simple transposition in the current era. *J Thorac Cardiovasc Surg* 1988; 95:14–28.

Chrispin A, Small P, Rutter N, et al: Echoplanar imaging of normal and abnormal connections of the heart and great arteries. *Pediatr Radiol* 1986; 16:289.

Didier D, Higgins CB, Fisher MR, et al: Congenital heart disease: Gated MR imaging of 72 patients. *Radiology* 1986; 158:227.

Freedom RM, Culham JAG, Moes CAF: *Angiocardiography of Congenital Heart Disease.* New York, Macmillan, 1984, p 514.

Jaffe RB, Orsmond GS, Veasy LG: Inadvertent ligation of the left pulmonary artery. *Radiology* 1986; 161: 355–357.

Kidd BSL: Complete transposition of the great arteries, in Keith JD, Rowe RD, Vlad P (eds): *Heart Disease in Infancy and Childhood,* ed 3. New York, Macmillan, 1978, p 590.

Mandell VS, Lock JE, Mayer JE, et al: The "laid-back" aortogram: An improved angiographic view for demonstration of coronary arteries in transposition of the great arteries. *Am J Cardiol* 1990; 65:1379–1383.

Mayer Jr., JE, Sanders SP, Jonas RA, et al: Coronary artery pattern and outcome of arterial switch operation for transposition of the great arteries. *Circulation* 1990; 82(suppl 4):4-139–4-145.

Shapiro SR, Potter BM: Transposition of the great arteries. *Semin Roentgenol* 1985; 20:110.

Soulen RL, Donner R, Capitanio M: Postoperative evaluation of complex congenital heart disease by magnetic resonance imaging. *Radiographics* 1987; 7:975.

Tonkin LD, Sansa M, Elliott LP, et al: Recognition of developing left ventricular outflow tract obstruction in complete transposition of the great arteries. *Radiology* 1980; 134:53.

Unger FM, Cavanaugh DJ, Johnson GF, et al: Radiologic and real-time echocardiographic evaluation of the cyanotic newborn. *Radiographics* 1986; 6:603.

Van Praagh R: Transposition of the great arteries. II: Transposition clarified. *Am J Cardiol* 1971; 28:739.

Single Ventricle

Didier D, Higgins CB, Fisher MR, et al: Congenital heart disease: Gated MR imaging in 72 patients. *Radiology* 1986; 158:227.

Elliott LP: Angiography in single ventricle or univentricular heart in Elliott LP (ed): *Cardiac Imaging in Infants, Children, and Adults*. Philadelphia, JB Lippincott, 1991, p 688.

Elliott LP: Pathophysiology and roentgenologic findings in single ventricle or univentricular heart, in Elliott LP (ed): *Cardiac Imaging in Infants, Children, and Adults*. Philadelphia, JB Lippincott, 1991, p 675.

Freedom RM, Culham JAG, Moes CAF: *Angiocardiography of Congenital Heart Disease*. New York, Macmillan, 1984, p 593.

Keeton BR, Macartney FJ, Rees PG, et al: Univentricular heart of right ventricular type with double or common inlet. *Circulation* 1979; 59:403.

Kidd BSL: Single ventricle, in Keith JD, Rowe RD, Vlad P (eds): *Heart Disease in Infancy and Childhood*. New York, Macmillan, 1978, p 408.

Macartney FJ, Partridge JB, Scott O, et al: Common or single ventricle: An angiocardiographic and hemodynamic study of 42 patients. *Circulation* 1976; 53:543.

Seward JB, Tajik AJ, Hagler DJ, et al: Echocardiogram in common (single) ventricle: Angiographic-anatomic correlation. *Am J Cardiol* 1977; 39:217.

Shinebourne EA, Lau K, Calcaterra G, et al: Univentricular heart of right ventricular type: Clinical, angiographic and electrocardiographic features. *Am J Cardiol* 1980; 46:439.

Soto B, Bertranou EG, Bream PR, et al: Angiographic study of univentricular heart of the right ventricular type. *Circulation* 1979; 60:1325.

Swischuk LE: Single ventricle. *Semin Roentgenol* 1985; 20:130.

White RD, Higgins CB: Evaluation of single ventricle using magnetic resonance imaging, in Elliott LP (ed): *Cardiac Imaging in Infants, Children, and Adults*. Philadelphia, JB Lippincott Co, 1991, p 685.

Corrected Transposition of the Great Arteries

Bream PR, Elliott LP, Bargeron LM: Plain film findings of anatomically corrected malposition: Its association with juxtaposition of the atrial appendages and right aortic arch. *Radiology* 1978; 126:589.

Freedom RM, Culham JAG, Moes CAF: *Angiocardiography of Congenital Heart Disease*. New York, Macmillan, 1984, p 536.

Guit GL, Bluemm R, Rohmer J, et al: Levotransposition of the aorta: Identification of segmental cardiac anatomy using MR imaging. *Radiology* 1986; 161:673–679.

Kidd BSL: Congenitally corrected transposition of the great arteries, in Keith JD, Rowe RD, Flad P (eds): *Heart Disease in Infancy and Childhood*, ed 3. New York, Macmillan, 1978, p 615.

Krongrad E, Ellis K, Steeg CN, et al: Subpulmonic obstruction in congenitally corrected transposition of the great arteries due to ventricular membranous septal aneurysm. *Circulation* 1976; 54:179.

Ruttenberg HD: Corrected transposition of the great arteries, in Moss AJ, Adams FH, Emmanouilides GC (eds): *Heart Disease in Infants, Children and Adolescents*, ed 2. Baltimore, Williams & Wilkins, 1977, p 338.

White RD: Magnetic resonance imaging of corrected transposition, in Elliott LP (ed): *Cardiac Imaging in Infants, Children, and Adults*. Philadelphia, JB Lippincott, 1991, p 635.

Total Anomalous Pulmonary Venous Return

Budorick NE, McDonald V, Flisak ME, et al: The pulmonary veins. *Semin Roentgenol* 1989; 24:127–140.

Cathman GE, Nadas AS: Total anomalous pulmonary venous connection: Clinical and physiological observations in 75 pediatric patients. *Circulation* 1970; 42:143.

Freedom RM, Culham JAG, Moes CAF: *Angiocardiography of Congenital Heart Disease*. New York, Macmillan, 1984. p 274.

Haworth SG, Reid L, Simon G: Radiologic features of the heart and lungs in total anomalous pulmonary venous return in early infancy. *Clin Radiol* 1977; 28:561.

Moes CAF, Freedom RM, Burrows PE: Anomalous pulmonary venous connections. *Semin Roentgenol* 1985; 20:134.

Paster SP, Swenson RE, Yabek SM: Total anomalous pulmonary venous connection: Report of 10 cases and review of the literature. *Pediatr Radiol* 1977; 6:132.

Sahn DJ, Allen JD, Lange LW, et al: Cross-sectional echocardiographic diagnosis of sites of total anomalous pulmonary venous drainage. *Circulation* 1979; 60:1317.

Turley K, Tucker WY, Ullyot DJ, et al: Total anomalous pulmonary venous connection in infancy: Influence of age and type of lesion. *Am J Cardiol* 1980; 45:92.

Unger FM, Cavanaugh DJ, Johnson GF, et al: Radiological and real-time echocardiographic evaluation of the cyanotic newborn. *Radiographics* 1986; 6:603.

Weaver MD, Chen JTT, Anderson PAW, et al: Total anomalous pulmonary venous connection to the left vertical vein. *Radiology* 1976; 118:679.

Cor Triatriatum and Other Anomalies of the Pulmonary Veins

Bisset GS III, Kirks DR, Strife JL, et al: Cor triatriatum: Diagnosis by MR imaging *Am J Roentgenol* 1987; 149:567.

Canedo MI, Strefadouros MA, Frank MJ, et al: Echocardiographic features of cor triatriatum. *Am J Cardiol* 1977; 40:615.

Jolles H, Henry DA, Rupp SB: General case of the day—Cardiac MR of cor triatriatum. *Radiographics* 1988; 8:1227–1231.

MacMillan RM, Rees MR, Maranhao V, et al: Cinecomputed tomography of cor triatriatum. *J Comput Assist Tomogr* 1986; 10:124.

Marin-Garica J, Tandon R, Lucxas RV Jr, et al: Cor triatriatum: Study of 20 cases. *Am J Cardiol* 1975; 35:59.

Soulen RL, Donner R, Capitanio M: Postoperative evaluation of complex congenital heart disease by magnetic resonance imaging. *Radiographics* 1987; 7:975.

Van der Horst RL, Gotsman MS: Cor triatriatum: Angiographic diagnosis by retrograde catheterization of the dorsal accessory chamber. *Br J Radiol* 1971; 44:273.

Truncus Arteriosus

Calder L, Van Praagh R, Van Praagh S, et al: Truncus arteriosus communis: Clinical angiocardiographic and pathologic findings in 100 patients. *Am Heart J* 1976; 92:23.

Collett RW, Edwards JE: Persistent truncus arteriosus: Classification according to anatomic types. *Surg Clin North Am* 1949; 29:1245.

Crupi G, Macartney FJ, Anderson RH: Persistent truncus arteriosus: A study of 66 autopsy cases with special reference to definition and morphogenesis. *Am J Cardiol* 1977; 40:569.

Freedom RM, Culham JAG, Moes CAF: *Angiocardiography of Congenital Heart Disease.* New York, Macmillan, 1984, p 437.

Hernanz-Schulman M, Fellows KE: Persistent truncus arteriosus: Pathologic, diagnostic and therapeutic considerations. *Semin Roentgenol* 1985; 20:121.

Mair DD, Ritter DG, Danielson GK, et al: Truncus ateriosus with unilateral absence of a pulmonary artery. Criteria for operability and surgical results. *Circulation* 1977; 55:642–647.

Moes CAF, Freedom RM: Aortic arch interruption with truncus arteriosus or aorticopulmonary septal defect. *Am J Roentgenol* 1980; 135:1011.

Nath PH, Zollikofer CL, Castaneda-Zuñiga WR, et al: Persistent truncus arteriosus associated with interruption of the aortic arch. *Br J Radiol* 1980; 53:853.

Rossiter SJ, Silverman JF, Shumway NE: Pattern of pulmonary arterial supply in patients with truncus arteriosus. *J Thorac Cardiovasc Surg* 1978; 75:74.

Van Praagh R: Classification of truncus arteriosus communis (TAC). *Am Heart J* 1976; 92:129.

White RD: Magnetic resonance imaging of truncus arteriosus in Elliott LP (ed): *Cardiac Imaging in Infants, Children, and Adults.* Philadelphia, JB Lippincott, 1991, p 700.

Double-Outlet Left Ventricle

Bharati S, Leve M, Stewart R, et al: The morphologic spectrum of double outlet left ventricle and its surgical significance. *Circulation* 1978; 58:558.

Brandt TWT, Calder AL, Barratt-Boyes BG, et al: Double outlet left ventricle. Morphologic cineangiographic diagnosis and surgical treatment. *Am J Cardiol* 1976; 38:897.

Conti V, Adams F, Mulder DG: Double outlet left ventricle. *Ann Thorac Surg* 1974; 18:402.

Freedom RM, Culham JAG, Moes CAF: *Angiocardiography of Congestive Heart Disease.* New York, Macmillan, 1984, p 588.

Double-Outlet Right Ventricle

Adkins EW, Martin TE, Alexander JA, Knauf DG, Victorica BE: MR in double-outlet right ventricle. *Am J Roentgenol* 1989; 152:128–130.

DiSessa TG, Hagan AD, Pope C, et al: Two-dimensional echocardiographic characteristics of double outlet right ventricle. *Am J Cardiol* 1979; 44:1146.

Freedom RM, Culham JAG, Moes CAF: *Angiocardiography of Congenital Heart Disease.* New York, Macmillan, 1984, p 555.

Hagler DJ, Tajik AJ, Seward JB, et al: Double outlet right ventricle: Wide angle two-dimensional echocardiographic observations. *Circulation* 1981; 63:419.

Hallerman FJ, Kincaid OW, Ritter DG, et al: Angiocardiographic findings in origin of both great arteries from the right ventricle. *Am J Roentgenol* 1970, 66.

Lincoln C, Anderson RH, Shinebourne EA, et al: Double outlet right ventricle with malposition of the aorta. *Br Heart J* 1975; 37:453.

Mayo JR, Robertson D, Sommerhoff B, et al: MR imaging of double outlet ventricle. *J Comput Assist Tomogr* 1990; 14:336–339.

Muster AJ, Bharati S, Azia KU, et al: Taussig-Bing anomaly with straddling mitral valve. *J Thorac Cardiovasc Surg* 1979; 77:832.

Sondheimer HM, Freedom RM, Olley PM: Double outlet right ventricle: spectrum and prognosis. *Am J Cardiol* 1977; 89:709–714.

Sridaromonp S, Ritter DG, Feldt RH, et al: Double outlet right ventricle: Anatomic and angiographic correlation. *Mayo Clin Proc* 1978; 53:555.

Yoo S-J, Lim T-H, Park I-S, et al: MR anatomy of ventricular septal defect in double-outlet right ventricle with situs solitus and atrioventricular concordance. *Radiology* 1991; 181:501–505.

Zamora R, Moller JH, Edwards JC: Double outlet right ventricle: Anatomic types and associated anomalies. *Chest* 1975; 68:672.

SECTION 4

Cyanotic Congenital Heart Disease With Decreased Pulmonary Flow

TETRALOGY OF FALLOT

The tetralogy of Fallot (TOF) classically consists of (1) a large defect in the anterior portion of the ventricular septum, (2) obstruction of the right ventricular outflow tract, (3) overriding of the aortic root above the VSD, and (4) right ventricular hypertrophy. Right ventricular obstruction may relate to infundibular or pulmonary valve stenosis. One must identify normal aortic–mitral valve fibrous continuity and underdevelopment or malalignment of the subpulmonic conus. These areas are important in distinguishing other forms of cyanotic CHD such as DORV with PVS and transposition of the great vessels with PVS. TOF is the most common (10%) form of cyanotic CHD (see Table 17–1).

Pathophysiology

Pathophysiologic and clinical manifestations are extremely variable and related to the degree of right ventricular outflow obstruction. Infundibular and associated valvular stenosis are common (40%). Other less common malformations include high infundibular stenosis with valvular PVS or diffuse hypoplasia of the infundibular tract. Other associated anomalies include (1) a right aortic arch (25%); (2) peripheral PVS; (3) complete fibrous atresia of the main pulmonary artery (pseudotruncus); (4) fibrous atresia of the left pulmonary artery; (5) coronary artery anomalies, particularly the origin of the left anterior descending coronary artery from the right coronary artery and single coronary artery (5%–10%); (6) bicuspid aortic valve; (7) PDA; (8) PAPVR; (9) ASD or AV canal, or both; and (10) a persistent left SVC.

Clinical Manifestations

Cyanosis relates to the severity of right heart obstruction; infants are rarely cyanotic at birth, except those with pulmonary atresia. Ninety percent of patients become cyanotic by 6 months of age. Failure is rarely seen. Dyspnea is an early clinical manifestation, and paroxysmal dyspneic spells produce typi-

cal "blue spells." Clubbing is a late manifestation. Heart murmurs are striking, related to a loud ejection murmur along the left sternal edge due to right ventricular obstruction. The first component of the second heart sound in the pulmonary area is loud; the second component is soft and delayed. A continuous murmur indicates (1) a persistent PDA or (2) large systemic–pulmonary artery collaterals. Complications include thromboembolic disease and brain abscesses from right-to-left intracardiac shunting.

Chest Roentgenography

Radiologic findings in TOF are extremely variable depending upon the degree of right heart obstruction and right-to-left shunting. In the infant with a balanced physiologic state with little right-to-left shunting, the chest roentgenographic findings may appear normal. A right aortic arch may be the only clue to the presence of TOF (25%) (see Table 15–5). In older children, the typical "boot-shaped heart" develops with (1) a prominent elevated right ventricular apex, (2) a concave main pulmonary artery segment, (3) decreased hilar and central pulmonary vessels, (4) hyperexpanded hyperlucent lungs, (5) thymic atrophy, and (6) a right aortic arch (see Figs 15–4, 16–86, and 16–89,A). Other less frequent roentgenographic manifestations include (1) prominent systemic-pulmonary collaterals producing pulmonary vascular disorganization or abnormal indentation upon the esophagus on esophagrams (see Fig 16–89,B); (2) unilateral absence of the pulmonary artery, usually the left one; and (3) rib notching due to collateral vessels.

Echocardiography

M-mode, two-dimensional (Fig 16–87) and Doppler echocardiograms demonstrate (1) overriding of the aortic root above (2) a VSD, (3) normal aortic-mitral continuity, (4) an enlarged aortic root and right aortic arch in approximately 25% of patients, (5) small pulmonary arteries, (6) a narrowed right ventricular

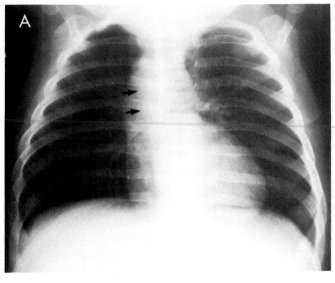
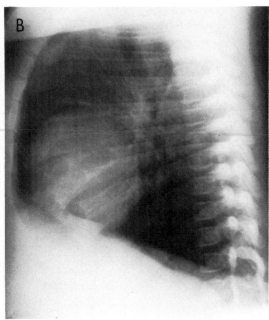

FIG 16–86.
Tetralogy of Fallot. AP **(A)** and lateral **(B)** chest roentgenograms show hyperlucent lungs with diminished central hilar pulmonary vessels in both the AP and lateral views. The main pulmonary artery segment is flat to concave, and a prominent right aortic arch and descending thoracic aorta *(arrows)* are evident. Thymic involution and hyperinflation are characteristic of cyanosis and stress in this 5-month old infant (see Fig 15–4).

outflow tract, (7) valvular PVS, and (8) right ventricular hypertrophy.

Angiocardiography

Angiocardiography is important for evaluating (1) the infundibular, valvular, and main pulmonary artery anatomy; (2) the entire ventricular septum for the possibility of multiple defects; (3) the AV valve relationships because of known associated AV canals, (4) the coronary arteries, and (5) aortic arch and brachiocephalic vessel anatomy. A biplane right ventriculogram in the sitting-up projection or other angulated projections (see Garcia-Medina et al.) evaluates (1) the outflow tract and (2) pulmonary artery anatomy (Fig 16–88). The biplane long-axis left ventriculogram evaluates (1) the VSD and (2) the mitral-aortic relations. A long-axis aortic root injection

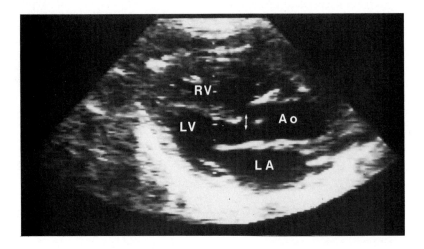

FIG 16–87.
Tetralogy of Fallot. A long-axis two-dimensional echocardiogram shows the aortic root *(Ao)* overriding the ventricular septum and VSD *(arrows)* and normal fibrous aortic-mitral continuity. *RV,* right ventricle; *LV,* left ventricle; *LA,* left atrium.

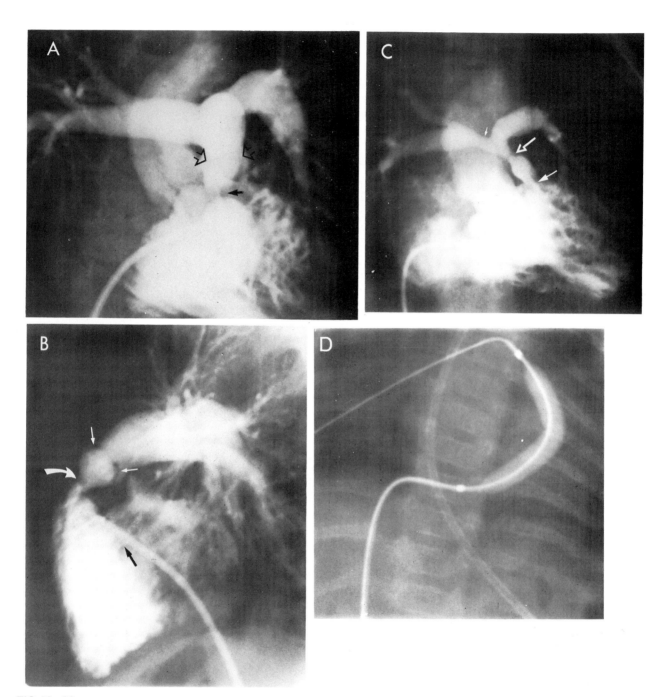

FIG 16–88.

Tetralogy of Fallot. **A,** an AP sitting-up right ventriculogram demonstrates marked infundibular stenosis *(black arrow)*, PVS *(open arrow)* with mild narrowing of the left pulmonary artery projecting behind the main pulmonary artery, right ventricular hypertrophy, and right-to-left shunting into a large aorta. **B,** a lateral view in the same patient shows the infundibular and valvular pulmonary stenoses *(white arrows)* and the VSD with right-to-left shunting *(black arrow)*. **C,** a sitting-up right ventriculogram shows severe infundibular ste-

nosis *(white arrow)*, a dysplastic stenotic pulmonary valve *(open arrow)*, and peripheral stenosis of the main and right pulmonary artery *(small white arrow)*. Right ventricular hypertrophy and moderate right-to-left shunting are present. **D,** balloon angioplasty of the pulmonary valve in a 1-month-old with tetralogy of Fallot: a minimal residual waist is noted at the valve annulus with associated angulation of the balloon catheter.

is important for evaluating the coronary arteries, in particular, the left anterior descending branch, which frequently is anomalous.

In patients with pulmonary atresia, the central pulmonary artery anatomy must be evaluated either through (1) an aortogram (Fig 16–89,C) or injection of systemic-pulmonary artery collaterals or a PDA, (2) a pulmonary venous wedge angiogram produc-

ing retrograde flow into the pulmonary artery confluence, or (3) MRI.

Magnetic Resonance Imaging

Axial MRI of the central pulmonary arteries has become a common imaging procedure in patients before and after operation (see Chapter 17 for a discus-

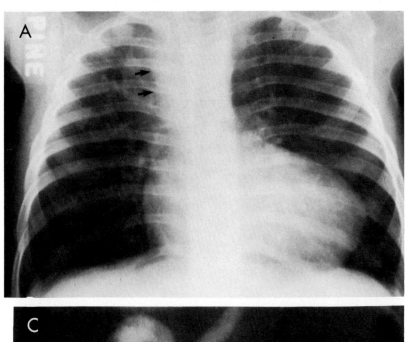

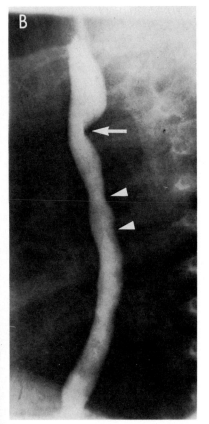

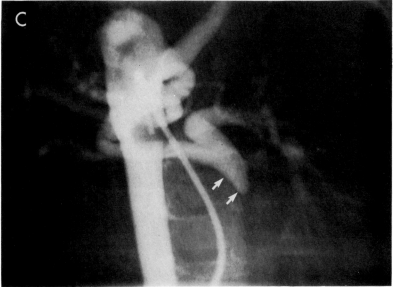

FIG 16–89.

Pulmonary atresia and VSD—pseudotruncus. **A,** an AP chest roentgenogram shows a prominent right aortic arch *(arrows)* and boot-shaped cardiac silhouette, with a concave pulmonary artery and disordered pulmonary vessels particularly evident in the right upper lobe. **B,** a lateral esophagogram shows abnormal retroesophageal vascular impressions. The most proximal impression *(arrow)* is an aberrant left subclavian artery from the right aortic arch, while the more caudal undulations *(arrowheads)* are pressure effects of the systemic pulmonary artery collaterals arising from the thoracic aorta. **C,** a sitting-up thoracic aortogram shows systemic thoracic pulmonary artery collaterals with retrograde filling of a small main pulmonary artery and annulus *(arrows)*. The demonstrated confluence and patency of these vessels make surgical correction feasible.

sion of MRI). Thin-section axial images can depict pulmonary arteries not clearly defined by angiography (see Fig 15–28).

Prognosis

The long-term prognosis is good. The severely cyanotic patient needs an early modified Blalock-Taussig shunt (see Chapter 21). Prostaglandin E is useful in maintaining a patent ductus until surgical procedures can be performed in the severely cyanotic patient with pulmonary atresia. Propranolol may ameliorate symptoms by decreasing right ventricular outflow tract obstruction. Definitive surgery is postponed beyond the newborn period. Balloon angioplasy may temporarily relieve pulmonary obstruction (see Fig 16–88, *D*).

TETRALOGY OF FALLOT WITH ABSENCE OF THE PULMONARY VALVE

TOF with absent or rudimentary pulmonary valve tissue is a rare variation associated with massive dilatation of the main, right, or left pulmonary arteries, individually or severally. Besides the usual TOF anomalies, ASD, tricuspid atresia, PDA, DORV, and AV canal may also be present. Rarely, congenital absence of the pulmonary valve may occur as an isolated lesion.

Others may present with either volume overload symptoms and congestive failure or cyanosis related to right-to-left shunts. Pulmonary distress related to the external compression of the trachea or bronchi by the massively dilated pulmonary arteries is not uncommon and may be associated with tracheobronchomalacia. Symptoms may suggest respiratory tract obstruction as seen with arch anomalies or pulmonary artery sling.

Chest Roentgenography

Roentgenographic manifestations include (1) moderate to marked cardiomegaly, (2) a striking prominence of the proximal pulmonary arteries, (3) decreased peripheral pulmonary vasculature, (4) tracheal compression, and (5) air trapping (general or unilateral) (see Figs 15–11 and 16–90,A and B).

Echocardiography

Echocardiography shows some of the findings described in the tetralogy of Fallot and, in addition, the striking enlargement of the pulmonary artery; dilation of the right ventricle and a dysplastic appearance of the pulmonary annulus are evident. Doppler studies confirm the massive pulmonary insufficiency.

Angiocardiography

Angiographic evaluation is basically similar to that described for tetralogy of Fallot. Right-sided ventriculography using larger amounts of contrast is necessary to adequately demonstrate the massively dilated right ventricle and pulmonary vessels. Typically the pulmonary annulus is stenotic and insufficient with rudimentary valve tissue, and there is little, if any, infundibular narrowing. The VSD may be seen with either left or right ventriculography (Fig 16–90, C and D).

TRICUSPID ATRESIA

Tricuspid atresia is characterized by (1) a complete absence of the right AV valve, (2) ASD, (3) VSD, and (4) hypoplasia of the right ventricle. Frequent associated abnormalities include (1) valvular or subvalvular PVS, (2) TGA, (3) a right aortic arch (see Table 15–5), (4) dextrocardia, (5) TAPVR, and (6) unilateral absence of the pulmonary artery. A right aortic arch is much more common if transposition and PVS are associated anomalies. Tricuspid atresia constitutes 2% to 3% of CHD (see Table 15–1).

Pathophysiology

Tricuspid atresia produces an area of fibrosis in the floor of the right atrium, frequently with an area of depression or umbilication. An obligatory right-to-left shunt occurs through a stretched foramen ovale or ASD. The left ventricle enlarges and becomes hypertrophic. Type I tricuspid atresia (70%) has normal arterial relations and is subdivided into those with pulmonary atresia and an absent right ventricle (73%), those with a hypoplastic pulmonary artery with a small right ventricle and VSD (13%), and those with a large VSD with no PVS (13%). Type II (25%) features associated d-TGA, and is subdivided into lesions with or without pulmonary stenosis. Type III (5%) represents associated l-TGA with ventricular inversion and atresia of the left AV (tricuspid valve).

Clinical Manifestations

Cyanosis, relative to the right-to-left shunt and the degree of right ventricular outflow obstruction, is moderate to severe in 85% to 90% of patients. The

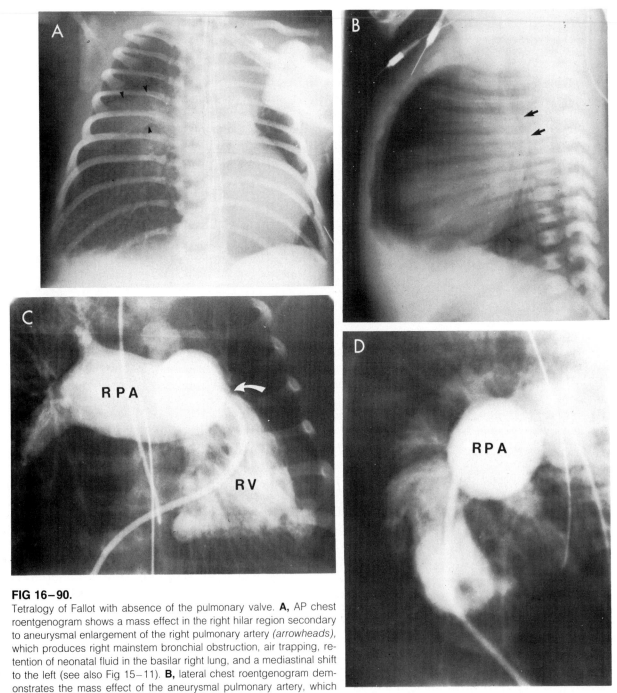

FIG 16—90.
Tetralogy of Fallot with absence of the pulmonary valve. **A,** AP chest
roentgenogram shows a mass effect in the right hilar region secondary
to aneurysmal enlargement of the right pulmonary artery *(arrowheads),*
which produces right mainstem bronchial obstruction, air trapping, retention of neonatal fluid in the basilar right lung, and a mediastinal shift
to the left (see also Fig 15—11). **B,** lateral chest roentgenogram demonstrates the mass effect of the aneurysmal pulmonary artery, which
produces striking narrowing of the central tracheobronchial airway *(arrows)* at the level of the carina. **C** and **D,** AP and lateral
pulmonary arteriograms demonstrate the aneurysmal dilatation primarily involving the right pulmonary artery with evidence of pulmonary regurgitation through a dysplastic pulmonary valve *(arrow)*. There is faint visualization of the aorta secondary to right-to-left
shunting and a VSD.

rare patient with a large VSD and no PVS exhibits mild cyanosis. Spontaneous closure of the VSD or development of PVS produces progressive cyanosis.

Other manifestations include (1) dyspnea, (2) jugular pulsations related to atrial contractions, and (3) a loud ejection murmur along the left sternal border. Congestive failure occurs in those rare instances with a large VSD and increased pulmonary blood flow.

Chest Roentgenography

Characteristic findings include (1) normal heart size or mild cardiomegaly, (2) decreased pulmonary vascularity, (3) hyperlucent lungs with diaphragmatic depression, (4) a concave main pulmonary artery segment (Fig 16–91), and (5) a right aortic arch (9%–25%). Five percent of patients show increased pulmonary blood flow and moderate to marked cardiomegaly with a prominent main pulmonary artery.

Other rare findings include (1) a juxtaposed atrial appendage (particularly with associated TGA) (Fig 16–92) and (2) dilated venae cavae.

Echocardiography

Two-dimensional echocardiography will demonstrate (1) tricuspid atresia, (2) a small right ventricle, (3) VSD, (4) great-vessel relations, and (5) ASD (Fig

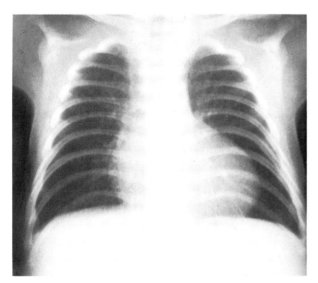

FIG 16–91.
Tricuspid atresia. An AP chest roentgenogram shows hyperlucent lungs with deficient central pulmonary vasculature secondary to a right-to-left shunt. Mild cardiomegaly and a concave main pulmonary artery segment are present. Thymic atrophy is consistent with hypoxia and a relatively inconspicuous aortic arch. These findings closely simulate those seen in tetralogy of Fallot.

16–93). Doppler evaluation will show a right-to-left shunt at the atrial level and a left-to-right shunt through the VSD as well as failure of flow through the tricuspid valve area.

Angiocardiography

Injection of contrast medium into the SVC or right atrium shows sequential flow from the right atrium to the left atrium to the left ventricle. Frequently the small right ventricle and pulmonary artery will subsequently be seen along with filling of the aortic root. Early in the sequence, a triangular nonopacified area caudad to the right atrium can be seen related to the nonopacified hypoplastic right ventricle (Fig 16–94). Biplane long-axis left ventriculography better defines the (1) enlarged left ventricle, (2) VSD, (3) hypoplastic right ventricle, and (4) pulmonary artery and obstructive lesions. The right aortic arch, if present, and the great-vessel relations in those patients with transposition are best seen with left ventriculography.

Prognosis

A palliative measure to increase the pulmonary flow, i.e., a modified Blalock-Taussig shunt, will produce considerable palliation. Later more long-term palliative procedures can be performed that are related to caval pulmonary (Glenn procedure) or atrial atriopulmonary shunting (Fontan procedure) (see Chapter 21).

PULMONARY ATRESIA WITH AN INTACT VENTRICULAR SEPTUM (HYPOPLASTIC RIGHT HEART SYNDROME)

This malformation is characterized by (1) pulmonary atresia, (2) hypoplasia of the right ventricle, and (3) hypoplasia of the tricuspid valve annulus. Occasionally, in patients with tricuspid insufficiency (20%), there will be marked enlargement of the right atrium and right ventricle. The incidence of hypoplastic right heart syndrome is between 1% and 2% (see Table 15–1).

Pathophysiology

With complete right heart obstruction, an obligatory right-to-left shunt occurs at the atrial level through a stretched foramen ovale or true ASD. Cyanosis is present, with severity depending upon the size of the associated patent ductus. The pathophysiology is similar to that in patients with tricuspid atresia.

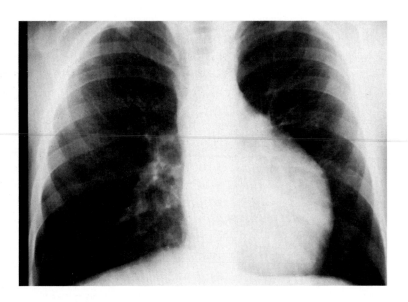

FIG 16–92.
Tricuspid atresia, complete transposition, and juxtaposition of the atrial appendages in a 13-year-old boy. Frontal chest radiograph demonstrates the characteristic cardiac configuration of this mal- formation with an inconspicuous right atrial contour and an abnor- mal convex upper left heart margin from juxtaposition of the right and left atrial appendages.

The aortic arch is invariably on the left, and visceral atrial situs solitus is the rule.

Clinical Manifestations

Typical clinical findings include (1) cyanosis, (2) tachypnea, (3) hepatomegaly, (4) peripheral edema, (5) gallop rhythm, and (6) murmurs from tricuspid regurgitation or a PDA. Congestive failure may oc- cur with a large patent ductus.

Chest Roentgenography

Radiologic manifestations correlate with the compe- tency of the tricuspid valve. With a competent tri- cuspid valve, the roentgenographic manifestations include (1) normal heart size or mild cardiomegaly, and (2) decreased pulmonary blood flow, unless the patient is receiving prostaglandin therapy (Fig 16–95). In patients with significant tricuspid insuffi- ciency, cardiomegaly with marked enlargement of the right atrium is present. The pulmonary blood flow may be increased in those rare patients with a large patent ductus after neonatal pulmonary vascu- lar resistance decreases.

Echocardiography

Real-time two-dimensional echocardiography dem- onstrates: (1) an abnormally thickened, atretic pul- monary valve, (2) a small pulmonary annulus, (3) a hypertrophic small right ventricle, (4) an enlarged right atrium, and (5) an ASD or a large foramen ovale (Fig 16–96). Doppler interrogation is impor- tant and demonstrates a right-to-left atrial shunt, ab- sence of a VSD, and no forward or retrograde flow through the pulmonary valve. With tricuspid insuffi- ciency, Doppler evaluation similarly confirms this defect, and real-time study shows an enlarged right atrium and right ventricle.

Angiocardiography

With a competent tricuspid valve, biplane right ven- triculography with a small amount of contrast me- dium (Fig 16–97) will demonstrate (1) right ventricu- lar hypertrophy and hypoplasia; (2) atresia of the pulmonary valve, usually with an adequate in- fundibulum; (3) competency of the tricuspid valve; and (4) occasional retrograde filling of the coronary arteries from right ventricular sinusoids. If tricuspid insufficiency exists, large-volume injection will be necessary to evaluate right ventricular size and the severity of tricuspid regurgitation. Long-axis left ventriculography will visualize the normal conflu- ence of the pulmonary vessels through either a patent ductus or, rarely, collateral systemic-pulmo- nary flow. The primary differential consideration is that of Ebstein anomaly in those patients with tricus- pid insufficiency. These patients will have pulmo- nary insufficiency seen on aortography with flow through the PDA, pulmonary artery, and then into the right ventricle.

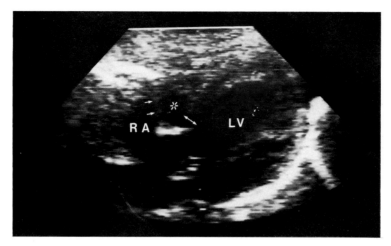

FIG 16–93.
Tricuspid atresia. Subxiphoid real-time echocardiogram shows an atretic tricuspid valve *(arrows)* with a hypoplastic right ventricle (*) and VSD *(double-headed arrow)*.

Prognosis

Prostaglandin E can maintain the patency of a patent ductus and produce adequate pulmonary flow. Palliation with a modified Blalock-Taussig shunt will maintain adequate pulmonary flow. Pulmonary valvulotomy (Brock procedure) is usually performed at the same time to stimulate further development of the hypoplastic right ventricle. If the right ventricle remains hypoplastic, a Fontan procedure may be performed (see Chapter 21.)

AORTIC ATRESIA (HYPOPLASTIC LEFT HEART SYNDROME)

Aortic atresia is characterized by hypoplasia of the entire left heart including (1) the ascending aorta, (2) the aortic annulus, (3) the left ventricle, (4) the mitral valve, and (5) the left atrium. Critical AS is included in this category by some authors. Approximately 1% of all CHD involves the aortic atresia complex, although it represents approximately 9% of structural defects recognized in the newborn infant (see Table 15–1).

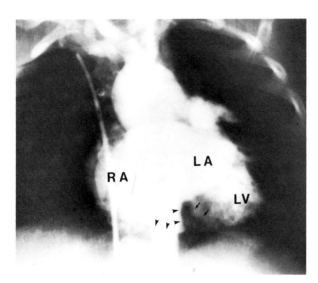

FIG 16–94.
Tricuspid atresia. Angiocardiogram with right atrial–SVC injection shows effects of the right-to-left shunt at the atrial level, with contrast filling the right atrium *(RA),* left atrium *(LA),* and left ventricle *(LV).* The triangular lucent chamber, outlined by *arrows* and *arrowheads,* represents the incompletely opacified hypoplastic right ventricle. *Arrowheads* also demarcate the atretic tricuspid valve.

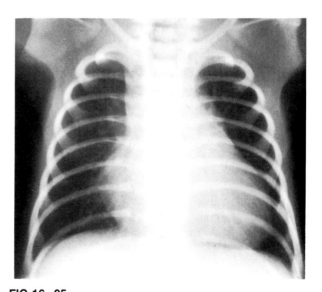

FIG 16–95.
Hypoplastic right heart syndrome secondary to pulmonary atresia. AP chest roentgenogram shows moderate cardiomegaly, diminished pulmonary flow with hyperlucent lungs, relatively inconspicuous pulmonary vessels, and a prominent aortic arch.

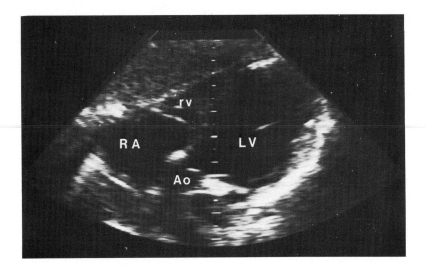

FIG 16–96.
Hypoplastic right heart syndrome. A two-dimensional subxiphoid echocardiogram shows the small hypoplastic, hypertrophic right ventricle *(rv)*. Tricuspid valve motion may be limited and simulate tricuspid atresia; however, a VSD cannot be identified. *RA*, right atrium; *LV*, left ventricle; *Ao*, aortic root.

Pathophysiology

Pathologic manifestations include (1) a hypertrophic or hypoplastic left ventricle, (2) usually small aortic sinuses of Valsalva, (3) a small aortic annulus and ascending aorta, (4) normal but small coronary arteries, (5) a small mitral valve annulus or atresia (25%), and (6) PDA. Occasionally, a true ASD or VSD may be present.

All pulmonary and systemic circulation depends on the right ventricle, resulting in right heart enlargement and hypertrophy. Systemic flow depends on pulmonary venous blood returning to the right heart at the atrial level and subsequently flowing from right to left through the PDA with filling of both the aortic arch and brachiocephalic vessels and descending aorta. Failure and death relate to myocardial ischemia secondary to restrictive coronary flow or poor arteriovenous mixing.

Clinical Manifestations

CHF usually develops in the first few hours. Tachypnea is present from birth and cyanosis within the first

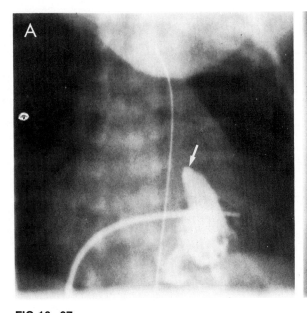

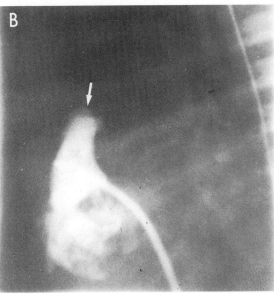

FIG 16–97.
Hypoplastic right heart syndrome. AP **(A)** and lateral **(B)** right ventriculograms demonstrate pulmonary atresia *(arrows)* with a hypoplastic right ventricle and intact ventricular septum.

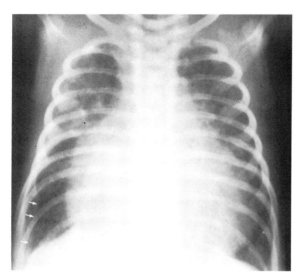

FIG 16–98.
Hypoplastic left heart syndrome. AP chest roentgenogram of a 2-day-old infant shows moderate cardiomegaly, severe pulmonary venous congestion with interstitial fluid, and areas of atelectasis or edema. Depression of the diaphragm is secondary to hypoxia. There is minimal fluid in the right major fissure *(arrows)*.

24 to 48 hours. Other clinical findings include tachycardia, hepatomegaly, gallop rhythm, rales, poor peripheral pulses, and murmurs in 50% of patients.

Chest Roentgenography

Roentgenographic findings include (1) moderate to marked cardiomegaly, (2) a globular cardiac silhouette suggesting combined chamber enlargement, (3) pulmonary venous congestion with interstitial fluid lines or pleural fluid, (4) hyperinflation, and (5) thymic atrophy (Fig 16–98).

Differential considerations include (1) critical AS, (2) mitral atresia, (3) severe coarctation or interrupted aortic arch, and (4) cardiomyopathy, such as in endocardial fibroelastosis and infants of diabetic mothers.

Echocardiography

Real-time echocardiography shows (1) a diminutive ascending aorta with an aortic root diameter of less than 5 mm; (2) a small, thick-walled left ventricle; (3) a small mitral valve annulus with restricted leaflet motion; and (4) a dilated right heart, pulmonary artery, and large patent ductus (Fig 16–99).

Angiocardiography

Echocardiography usually confirms the diagnosis, although if operative intervention is considered, angiography is necessary. Retrograde aortography, usually performed through an umbilical artery catheter, will show (1) retrograde flow into the ascending aorta, (2) a small hypoplastic ascending aorta, and (3) retrograde filling of small coronary arteries (Fig 16–100). The absence of antegrade washout through the aortic valve confirms atresia. Transient left-to-right shunting through the patent ductus occasionally is observed. In the lateral view, the relative posterior position of the left anterior descending coronary artery implies the diminutive size of the left ventricle.

Prognosis

This lesion is universally fatal, with 80% dying within the first week. Heart transplantation or a

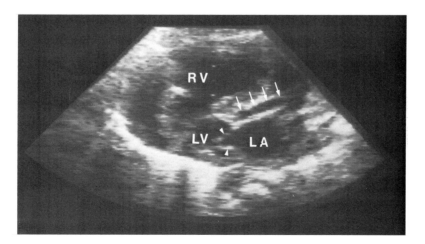

FIG 16–99.
Hypoplastic left heart syndrome. Long-axis two-dimensional echocardiogram shows a hypoplastic ascending aorta *(arrows)*, a hypoplastic left ventricle *(LV)*, and a large right ventricle *(RV)*. Arrowheads outline a hypoplastic mitral valve. *LA*, left atrium.

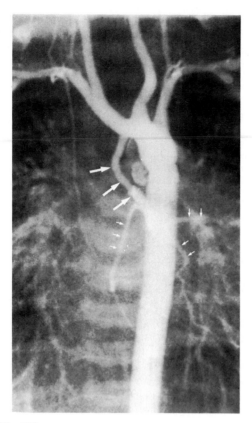

FIG 16–100.
Hypoplastic left heart syndrome. A retrograde aortogram was performed after aortic catheterization through the umbilical artery. Retrograde filling of the entire ascending aorta demonstrates the severe hypoplasia *(large arrows)*, and there is retrograde filling into the coronary arteries *(small arrows)*. Left-to-right shunting also occurs through a patent ductus, with contrast visible in peripheral pulmonary artery branches.

staged Norwood procedure are alternative forms of therapy but have high mortality (see Chapter 21).

EBSTEIN ANOMALY OF THE TRICUSPID VALVE

Ebstein anomaly is characterized by a malformed, redundant, and dysplastic tricuspid valve displaced downward into the right ventricle. This partitions the right ventricle into an atrialized upper segment and an apical outflow chamber. The lesion is extremely variable and is usually associated with tricuspid insufficiency. Ebstein anomaly may occur also in patients with ventricular inversion related to l-TGA. The Ebstein malformation constitutes less than 1% of all CHD.

Pathophysiology

Because of the displaced tricuspid valve, and the associated tricuspid insufficiency and relative compe-

tency of the foramen ovale, the right atrium is usually markedly enlarged. The atrialized segment of the right ventricle is thin and the pulmonary conus segment is hypertrophied. Associated anomalies include (1) pulmonary stenosis or atresia, (2) PDA, and (3) VSD. Right-to-left shunting produces some degree of cyanosis and relates to the patency of the foramen ovale.

Clinical Manifestations

Cyanosis occurs in 75% of patients, more often in the neonatal period or in later childhood. Other clinical findings include (1) dyspnea, (2) systolic murmur related to tricuspid insufficiency, and (3) a loud first heart sound and split second heart sound. Electrocardiographic changes may be quite helpful including a right bundle-branch block, a large T wave, a prolonged PR interval, and low-voltage QRS segments. Patients also may present with Wolff-Parkinson-White syndrome and tachyarrhythmias.

Chest Roentgenography

Radiographs are extremely variable. Typically, in the cyanotic neonate, one sees (1) marked cardiomegaly, primarily related to striking right atrial enlargement, with a globular cardiac silhouette, and (2) decreased pulmonary blood flow (Fig 16–101). In older children without cyanosis, marked variability exists with (1) mild to moderate cardiomegaly related to

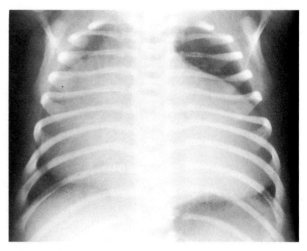

FIG 16–101.
Ebstein malformation of the tricuspid valve in a neonate with marked cardiomegaly related to massive dilatation of the right atrium. Right-to-left shunting occurs through the foramen ovale or ASD. Compression atelectasis of the left lower lobe is evident along with decreased pulmonary vasculature. Similar findings may be seen with tricuspid insufficiency associated with pulmonary atresia.

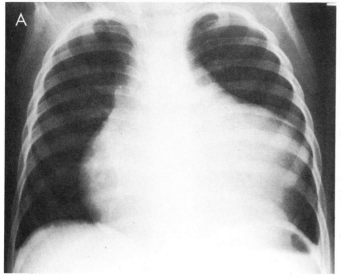

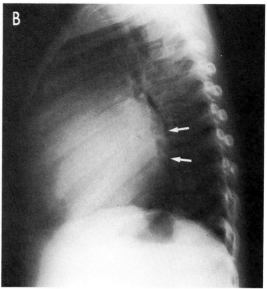

FIG 16–102.
Ebstein anomaly. AP **(A)** and lateral **(B)** chest roentgenograms in a 2-year-old with moderate cardiomegaly. although the right atrial dilatation is less striking than in Figure 16–101. In the lateral view, the enlarged right atrium produces a prominent posterior cardiac margin *(arrows)*. The pulmonary vasculature is only mildly decreased with a limited right-to-left shunt.

right atrial enlargement and (2) normal pulmonary blood flow (Fig 16–102).

Differential considerations include (1) primary tricuspid insufficiency, (2) tricuspid insufficiency related to pulmonary atresia, and (3) Uhl anomaly of the right ventricle.

Echocardiography

Two-dimensional echocardiography in the four-chamber view readily identifies (1) the displaced tricuspid valve with the septal and posterior leaflets adherent to the right ventricular wall, (2) the dys-plastic nature of the tricuspid valve with a large, redundant anterior leaflet originating from the tricuspid annulus, and (3) marked enlargement of the right atrium (Fig 16–103). M-mode studies show delayed closure of the tricuspid valve in relation to the mitral valve. Doppler ultrasound readily identifies tricuspid regurgitation (see Fig 15–20).

Angiography

AP and lateral right ventriculograms characterize the malformation with (1) the displaced tricuspid valve in relation to the tricuspid annulus, which is local-

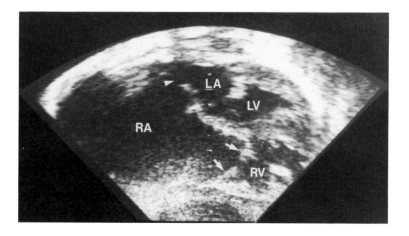

FIG 16–103.
Ebstein anomaly. Two-dimensional echocardiogram in a subxiphoid projection shows massive enlargement of the right atrium *(RA)*, with the tricuspid valve *(arrows)* displaced caudad into the right ventricle *(RV)* to create a large atrialized component of the right ventricle. The *arrowhead* designates an ASD. *LA,* left atrium; *LV,* left ventricle.

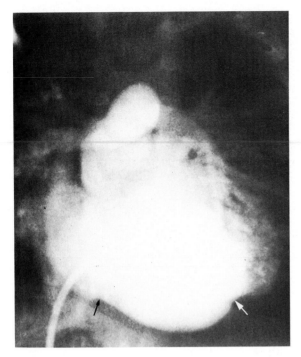

FIG 16–104.
Ebstein anomaly. AP cine–right atriogram shows the characteristic changes of Ebstein anomaly, with the true tricuspid annulus evident at the first notch along the lower right heart border *(black arrow)*, the displaced tricuspid leaflet producing a second notch *(white arrow)* further to the patient's left, and the smooth-walled atrialized segment of the right ventricle occupying the area between these arrows. The main pulmonary artery is displaced medially.

ized by the position of the right coronary artery; (2) caudad bulging of the atrialized portion of the right ventricle; (3) secondary notch in the midinferior ventricular margin related to the displaced tricuspid leaflet; (4) tricuspid insufficiency; and (5) right atrial enlargement (Fig 16–104). Right-to-left shunting may be seen at the atrial level. Primary differential considerations include tricuspid insufficiency as a primary lesion or secondary to pulmonary atresia. The displaced tricuspid valve will not be identified in these conditions. Pulmonary atresia can be differentiated by the demonstration of pulmonary insufficiency in patients with Ebstein anomaly on aortography. This occurs from retrograde filling of the pulmonary arteries through a PDA.

Magnetic Resonance Imaging

MRI readily demonstrates the abnormal tricuspid valve and right atrial and ventricular morphology.

Prognosis

The prognosis in the symptomatic neonate or infant is poor, with 50% mortality by the end of the first month. Patients presenting later usually do well for many years and may be aided by palliative procedures, including the Glenn operation or Blalock-Taussig shunting if associated with PVS. Other procedures attempting to utilize functional components of the right ventricle have also been performed such as plication of the tricuspid valve with associated ASD closure.

REFERENCES

Tetralogy of Fallot

Becker S, Hoeffel JC, Worms AM, et al: Angiographic appearance of tetralogy of Fallot: 100 cases. *Ann Radiol (Paris)* 1980; 23:23.

Calder AL, Brandt TW, Barratt-Boyes BG, et al: Variants of tetralogy of Fallot with absent pulmonary valve leaflets and origin of one pulmonary artery from the ascending aorta. *Am J Cardiol* 1980; 46:106.

Davis GD, Fulton RE, Ritter DG, et al: Congenital pulmonary atresia with ventricular septal defect: Angiographic and surgical correlates. *Radiology* 1978; 128:133.

Didier D, Higgins CB, Fisher MR, et al: Congenital heart disease: Gated MR imaging in 72 patients. *Radiology* 1986; 158:227.

Diethelm E, Soto B, Nath PH, et al: Pulmonary vascularity in patients with pulmonary atresia and ventricular septal defect. *Radiography* 1985; 5:243.

Dunnigan A, Oldham HN, Benson DW: Absent pulmonary valve syndrome in infancy: Surgery reconsidered. *Am J Cardiol* 1981; 48:117.

Fellows KE, Freed MD, Keane JR, et al: Results of routine preoperative coronary angiography in tetralogy of Fallot. *Circulation* 1975; 51:561.

Fellows KE, Smith J, Keane JF: Preoperative angiocardiography in infants with tetralogy of Fallot. *Am J Cardiol* 1981; 47:1279.

Freedom RM, Culham JAG, Moes CAF: *Angiocardiography of Congenital Heart Disease.* New York, Macmillan, 1984, p 173.

Garcia-Medina V, Bass J, Braunlin E, et al: A useful projection for demonstrating the bifurcation of the pulmonary artery. *Pediatr Cardiol* 1990; 11:147–149.

Mirowitz SA, Gutierrez FR, Canter CE, et al: Tetralogy of Fallot: MR findings. *Radiology* 1989; 171:207–212.

Nagai Y, Komatsu Y, Nakamura K, et al: Echocardiographic findings of congenital absence of the pulmonary valve with tetralogy of Fallot. *Chest* 1979; 75:481.

Nath PH, Soto B, Bini RM, et al: Tetralogy of Fallot with atrioventricular canal: An angiographic study. *J Thorac Cardiovasc Surg* 1984; 87:421.

Singh SP, Rigby ML, Astley R: Demonstration of pulmonary arteries by contrast injection into pulmonary veins. *Br Heart J* 1978; 40:55.

Soto B, Pacifico AD, Luna RF, et al: Radiographic study of congenital pulmonary atresia with ventricular septal defect. *Am J Roentgenol* 1977; 129:1027.

Soto B, Pacifico A, Seballos R, et al: Tetralogy of Fallot: An angiographic-pathologic correlative study. *Circulation* 1981; 64:558.

Soulen RL, Donner R, Capitanio M: Postoperative evaluation of complex congenital heart disease by magnetic resonance imaging. *Radiographics* 1987; 7:975.

Strife JL: Tetralogy of Fallot. *Semin Roentgenol* 1985; 20:160.

Unger FM, Cavanaugh DJ, Johnson GF, et al: Radiologic and real-time echocardiographic evaluation of the cyanotic newborn. *Radiographics* 1986; 6:603.

Tricuspid Atresia

Freedom RM, Culham JAG, Moes CAF: *Angiocardiography of Congenital Heart Disease.* New York, Macmillan, 1984, p 82.

LaCorte MA, Dick M, Schur G, et al: Left ventricular function in tricuspid atresia: Angiographic analysis in 28 patients. *Circulation* 1975; 52:996.

Silverman NH, Payot M, Stanger P: Simulated tricuspid valve echoes in tricuspid atresia. *Am Heart J* 1978; 95:761.

Tandon R, Edwards JE: Tricuspid atresia: A re-evaluation and classification. *J Thorac Cardiovasc Surg* 1974; 67:530.

Unger FM, Cavanaugh DJ, Johnson GF, et al: Radiologic real-time echocardiographic evaluation of the cyanotic newborn. *Radiographics* 1986; 6:603.

Weinberg PM: Anatomy of tricuspid atresia and its relevance to current forms of surgical therapy. *Ann Thorac Surg* 1980; 29:306.

Pulmonary Atresia With an Intact Ventricular Septum (Hypoplastic Right Heart Syndrome)

Bharati S, McCallister HA, Chiemmongkoltip P, et al: Congenital pulmonary atresia with tricuspid insufficiency: Morphologic study. *Am J Cardiol* 1977; 40:70.

Freedom RM, Culham JAG, Moes CAF: Differentiation of functional and structural pulmonary atresia: Role of aortography. *Am J Cardiol* 1978; 41:914.

Freedom RM, Culham JAG, Moes CAF: *Angiocardiography of Congenital Heart Disease.* New York, Macmillan, 1984, p 231.

Freedom RM, Moes CAF: The hypoplastic right heart complex. *Semin Roentgenol* 1980; 20:169.

Jacobstein MD, Fletcher B, Goldstein S, Riemenschneider TA: Magnetic resonance imaging in patients with hypoplastic right heart syndrome. *Am Heart J* 1985; 110:154–158.

Lewis DS, Amitai N, Sincha A, et al: Echocardiographic diagnosis of pulmonary atresia with intact ventricular septum. *Am Heart J* 1979; 97:82.

Patel RG, Freedom RM, Moes CAF, et al: Right ventricular volume determinations in 18 patients with pulmonary atresia and intact ventricular septum. *Circulation* 1980; 61:428.

Rowe RD, Freedom RM, Mehrizi A: *The Neonate With Congenital Heart Disease.* Philadelphia, WB Saunders, 1981, p 330.

Unger FM, Cavanaugh DJ, Johnson GF, et al: Radiologic real-time echocardiographic evaluation of the cyanotic newborn. *Radiographics* 1986; 6:603.

Van Praagh R, Ando M, Van Praagh S, et al: Pulmonary atresia: Anatomic considerations, in Kidd BSL, Rowe RD (eds): *The Child With Congenital Heart Disease After Surgery.* Mt Kisco, NY, Futura Publishing, 1976, p 103.

Aortic Atresia (Hypoplastic Left Heart Syndrome)

Bass JL, BenSchachar G, Edwards JE: Comparison of M-mode echocardiography and pathologic findings in the hypoplastic left heart syndrome. *Am J Cardiol* 1980; 45:79.

Farooki ZQ, Henry JG, Green EW: Echocardiographic spectrum of the hypoplastic left heart syndrome: Clinicopathologic correlation in 19 newborns. *Am J Cardiol* 1976; 38:337.

Freedom RM, Culham JAG, Moes CAF, et al: Selective aortic root angiography in the hypoplastic left heart syndrome. *Eur J Cardiol* 1976; 4:25.

Freedom RM, Culham JAG, Moes CAF: *Angiocardiography of Congenital Heart Disease.* New York, Macmillan, 1984, p 339.

Norwood WI, Kirkin JK, Sanders SP: Hypoplastic left heart syndrome: Experience with palliative surgery. *Am Cardiol* 1980; 45:87.

Roberts WC, Perry LW, Chandra RS, et al: Aortic valve atresia: New classification based on necropsy study of 73 cases. *Am J Cardiol* 1976; 37:753.

Unger FM, Cavanaugh DJ, Johnson GF, et al: Radiologic real-time echocardiographic evaluation of the cyanotic newborn. *Radiographics* 1986; 6:603.

Ebstein Anomaly of the Tricuspid Valve

Anderson KR, Lie JT: Pathologic anatomy of Ebstein's anomaly of the heart revisited. *Am J Cardiol* 1978; 41:739.

Deutsch V, Wexler L, Blieden LC, et al: Ebstein's anomaly of the tricuspid valve: Critical review of roentgen features and additional angiographic signs. *Am J Roentgenol* 1975; 125:395.

Freedom RM, Culham JAG, Moes CAF: *Angiocardiography of Congenital Heart Disease.* New York, Macmillan, 1984, p 111.

Hirschlau JJ, Sahn KD, Hagan AD, et al: Cross-sectional echocardiographic features of Ebstein's anomaly of the tricuspid valve. *Am J Cardiol* 1977; 40:400.

Kambe T, Ichimiya S, Toguchi M, et al: Apex and subxiphoid approaches to Ebstein's anomaly of the tricuspid valve. *Am Heart J* 1980; 100:53.

Link KM, Herrera MA, D'Souza VJ, et al: MR imaging of Ebstein's anomaly: Results in four cases. *Am J Roentgenol* 1988; 150:363.

Pernot C, Hoeffel JC, Henry M, et al: Congenital tricuspid insufficiency. *Cardiovasc Radiol* 1978; 1:37.

Takayasu S, Obunai Y, Kono S: Clinical classification of Ebstein's anomaly. *Am Heart J* 1978; 95:154.

Tao MS, Partridge J, Radford D: The plain chest radiograph in uncomplicated Ebstein's disease. *Clin Radiol* 1986; 37:551.

17

Vascular Rings and Great Vessel Anomalies

AORTIC ARCH ANOMALIES

Anomalies of the great vessels, e.g., an anomalous right subclavian artery, are frequently incidental findings, although other lesions tend to produce significant signs of tracheal, bronchial, or esophageal compression. Anomalies of the great vessels are frequently identified on plain films or esophagograms. The frequency of arch anomalies varies from 0.5% to 3.0%, depending on the inclusion of various anomalies.

Pathophysiology

With use of the hypothetical double arch system described by Edwards (Fig 17–1), the development of the normal aortic arch and all other anomalous malformations can be explained by the failure of differ-

ent segments of the right fourth dorsal arch to regress normally. In the normal development of the left aortic arch, complete regression of the right fourth dorsal aortic segment occurs between the origin of the right subclavian artery and the upper left descending aorta. The anomaly created by a similar regression on the left side produces the more typical right aortic arch with mirror-image branching of the brachiocephalic vessels characteristically seen in congenital heart disease (CHD) (tetralogy of Fallot). When both segments of the arch remain open, a functioning double aortic arch results.

Clinical Manifestations

Important clinical manifestations, usually dating from birth, include: (1) wheezing, (2) stridulous

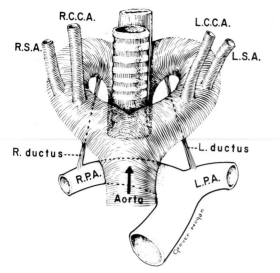

FIG 17–1.
A diagram of the Edwards hypothetical double aortic arch system shows bilateral aortic arches and bilateral ductus arteriosus. *RSA*, right subclavian artery; *RCCA*, right common carotid artery; *LSA*, left subclavian artery; *LCCA*, left common carotid artery; *RPA*, right pulmonary artery; *LPA*, left pulmonary artery. (From Shuford WH, Sybers RG, Weens HS: *Am J Roentgenol* 1972; 116:126. Used by permission.)

breathing that is constant but exacerbated by crying, (3) tachypnea, (4) dyspnea or cyanosis, and (5) dysphagia. Symptoms usually become evident between 3 weeks and 2 years and are evident in 75% to 90% of patients with significant anomalies.

Evaluation of Vascular Rings

The suggested workup of a suspected vascular ring anomaly is listed in Figure 17–2.

Chest Roentgenography

Chest roentgenograms that penetrate the mediastinum well will frequently show the abnormal indentation or deviation of the trachea that results from a prominent right aortic arch segment (Fig 17–3). This finding, in the absence of cyanotic CHD, implies a vascular ring until proved otherwise. A high-kilovoltage anteroposterior (AP) film with added filtration of the tracheal airway (Fig 17–4), or chest fluoroscopy of the trachea, and esophagography can confirm the abnormal tracheal and esophageal indentations caused by the prominent arch segments on the right of the trachea and posterior to the esophagus. Some surgeons feel comfortable when utilizing this limited evaluation to proceed with the operation, while others prefer additional evaluations with ultrasound, angiography, cine–computed tomography (cine-CT), and magnetic resonance imaging (MRI).

In most institutions MRI is now the preferred modality for the definitive evaluation of vascular rings. If aortography is utilized for the evaluation of arch anomalies, biplane AP and lateral or long-axis views are usually sufficient. For pulmonary sling, the sitting-up AP and lateral projections are optimal.

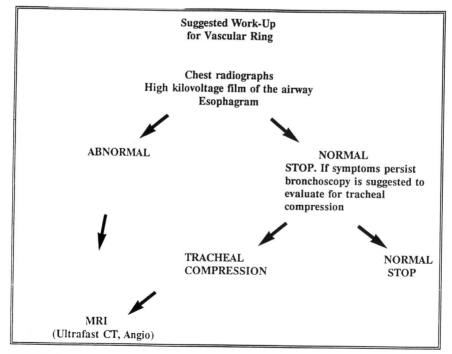

FIG 17–2.
Suggested workup for vascular ring.

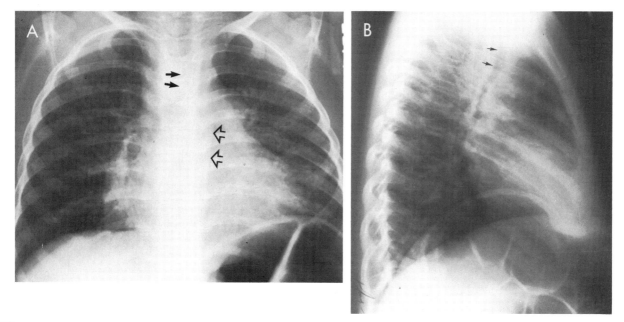

FIG 17–3.
Vascular ring–double aortic arch with left arch atresia. **A,** an AP chest roentgenogram in 3-year-old with chronic respiratory disease demonstrates a right aortic arch displacing the trachea to the left *(arrows)* with a left-sided descending thoracic aorta *(open arrows)* (see Fig 17–12). There is scattered pneumonic or atelectatic pulmonary disease in the perihilar and right middle lobe area. **B,** a lateral view shows anterior bulging of the trachea *(small black arrows)* that is consistent with a large retrotracheal vascular structure or other mass.

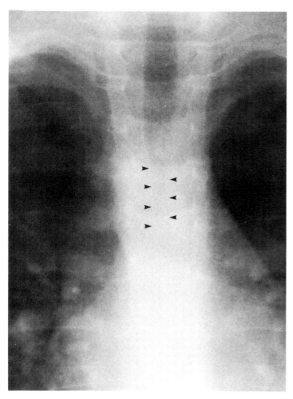

FIG 17–4.
High-kilovoltage peak film made with added filtration to better define the tracheobronchial airway. A prominent right aortic arch narrows the trachea and pushes the right tracheal wall medially *(arrowheads)*. Similar findings on the left, although less evident, are related to a double aortic arch.

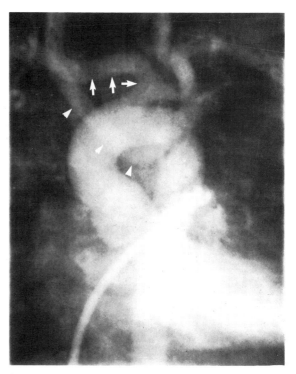

FIG 17–5.
An angiocardiogram in an infant with chronic respiratory distress shows leftward origin of the right common carotid artery to the left of the trachea *(arrows)* and an aberrant retroesophageal right subclavian artery *(arrowheads)*. The pretracheal and retroesophageal course of these vessels respectively may be a more significant contributing cause of respiratory distress than either lesion alone.

Echocardiography

Two-dimensional echocardiography will usually identify a double aortic arch or right aortic arch anomaly. A complete evaluation of brachiocephalic vessels and associated fibrous bands related to interruption of the left arch component may be difficult.

Left Aortic Arch

Aberrant Origin of the Right Subclavian Artery

This anomaly, in which the right subclavian artery is the most distal brachiocephalic vessel, is a common anomaly generally thought to be an incidental finding occurring in approximately 0.5% of normal autopsies. The vessel runs a typical oblique course retroesophageally upward and to the right. Rarely, it courses between the trachea and esophagus and frequently coexists with CHD. If present distal to a coarctation, only unilateral left-sided rib notching is present. It may be a rare cause of tracheal compression when combined with a bicarotid truncus, or tortuous right common carotid artery (Fig 17–5).

An esophagogram shows a typical oblique defect in the AP projection that starts on the left at the T3–4 level, proceeds cephalad to the right at a 60- to 70-degree angle, and terminates at T2–3. In the lateral view, a small posterior and oblique impression on the esophagus can be seen as the vessel passes in its oblique course (Fig 17–6).

Left Aortic Arch With Right Descending Aorta

This uncommon malformation is characterized by a left aortic arch arising from the ascending aorta and passing to the left of the trachea, and a retroesophageal transverse arch passing behind the esophagus and then continuing as a right descending aorta. If associated with an aberrant right subclavian artery arising as the fourth branch of the aortic arch, and a right ligamentum arteriosum, a vascular ring may be formed. The malformation may be recognized on a chest radiograph by a left aortic arch deviating the trachea to the right, and by the right descending aorta (Fig 17–7,A). An esophagogram will demonstrate a large oblique posterior esophageal impression passing downward from cephalic left to caudad

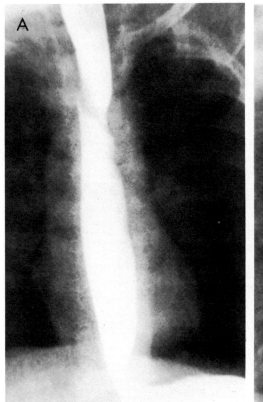

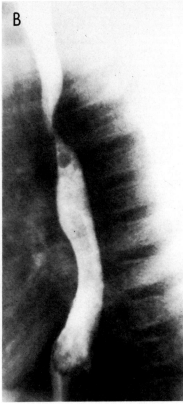

FIG 17–6.
Aberrant right subclavian artery. AP **(A)** and lateral **(B)** esophagograms show the characteristic posterior esophageal oblique defect progressing from the caudal left side to the cephalic right side.

This lesion by itself is usually considered an incidental finding and not related to airway or esophageal obstruction.

right. The malformation can be confirmed by angiography (Fig 17–7,B) or MRI.

Left Cervical Aortic Arch

A left cervical aortic arch is characterized by an aortic arch extending abnormally high in the upper mediastinum–low cervical region on the left side. A left cervical arch is less common than a right cervical arch. The branching of the aortic arch vessels is variable. The common carotid arteries may arise normally from the cervical arch, or there may be separate origins of the internal and external carotid arteries. Patients with a left cervical arch may present with a pulsatile left supraclavicular mass that may be mistaken for an aneurysm, or symptoms of a vascular ring. On the chest radiograph, upper mediastinal widening may be present, with the left cervical arch displacing the trachea to the right and anteriorly. As the cervical arch passes posteriorly behind the esophagus to descend on the right side, it may produce a large oblique esophageal impression passing from cephalic left to caudad right. The malformation can be confirmed by angiography or MRI.

Innominate Artery Compression Syndrome

Anterior tracheal compression by the innominate artery may rarely cause symptoms of respiratory obstruction. Infants may present with frequent respiratory infections, stridor, respiratory arrest, and are frequently misdiagnosed as having tracheomalacia. The malformation usually is recognized in symptomatic patients during bronchoscopy when a pulsatile impression is seen on the anterior wall of the trachea, approximately 1 to 2 cm above the carina. A lateral chest radiograph may show anterior tracheal compression (Fig 17–8,A), but is nondiagnostic. An esophagogram, if performed, is normal and serves only to exclude more common vascular rings. MRI can confirm the findings noted at bronchoscopy (Fig 17–8,B and C).

Tracheal Compression by the Left Aortic Arch With Right Lung Agenesis

Anterior tracheal compression may occur by a normal left aortic arch in patients with right lung agenesis and dextroposition. As the displaced ascending aorta passes from right to left, the trachea is compressed anteriorly. This anatomical relationship produces obstruction similar to that seen with the innominate artery compression syndrome. Posterior displacement of the trachea with anterior compression may be seen on the lateral chest radiograph, on high-kilovoltage films of the neck with added filtration or fluoroscopy, and is confirmed with bronchoscopy or MRI, or both.

Double Aortic Arch

This anomaly can be categorized as (1) a complete functioning double aortic arch and (2) a double aor-

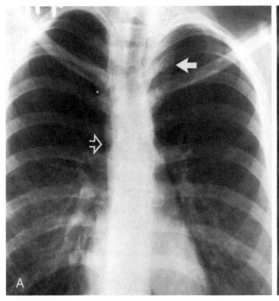
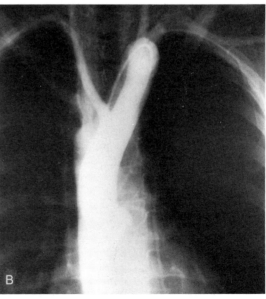

FIG 17–7.
An 18-year-old woman with left aortic arch and right descending aorta. **A,** chest radiograph demonstrates a left superior mediastinal density *(closed arrow)* representing the ascending aorta and arch, and right paraspinal density *(open arrow)* of the right descending aorta. The trachea is minimally displaced to the right. **B,** aortogram, frontal projection, demonstrates the left ascending aorta high in the left superior mediastinum, a retroesophageal transverse arch, and right descending aorta.

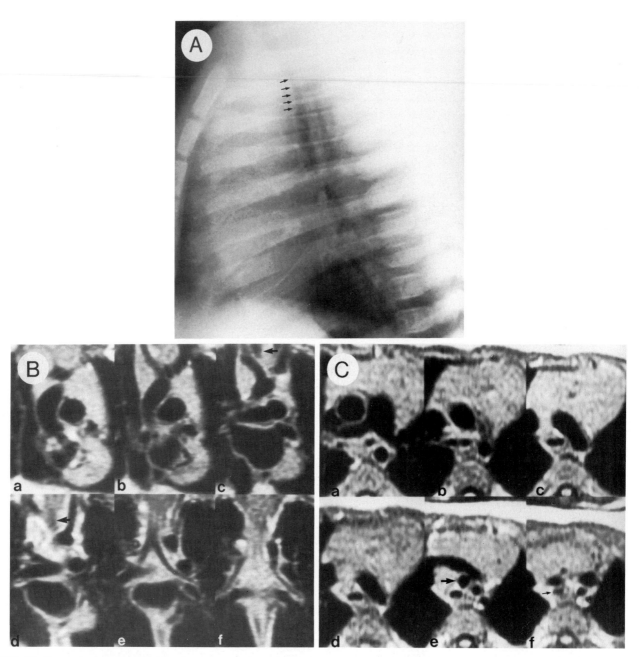

FIG 17–8.
Innominate artery compression syndrome in a 2-month-old infant with respiratory distress. At bronchoscopy, "total collapse of the tracheal wall just above the carina by an oblique coursing vessel compressing the anterior tracheal wall" was seen. **A,** lateral chest film demonstrates anterior tracheal compression *(arrows).* **B,** composite coronal interleaved 3-mm spin-echo images (anteroposterior): *(a)* the ascending aorta and pulmonary artery are seen; *(b)* the origin of the right innominate artery is partially visualized; *(c)* the origin and oblique course of the right innominate artery over the trachea *(arrow)* are well seen; *(d)* the origin of the left common carotid artery is seen. Note also the compressed trachea *(arrow); (e)* tracheal bifurcation. Note the compression of the trachea just above the carina; *(f)* the right and left lower lobe bronchi and left

pulmonary artery are seen. **C,** composite axial interleaved 3-mm images (inferosuperior): *(a)* the ascending aorta, left descending aorta, main pulmonary artery, and right and left bronchi are seen; *(b)* the proximal right and left bronchi and the inferior margin of the aortic arch are seen; *(c)* the aortic arch and proximal right and left bronchi are seen; *(d)* the superior margin of the aortic arch and tracheal bifurcation are seen; *(e)* the origin of the right innominate *(arrow),* left common carotid, and left subclavian arteries is seen. The left innominate vein is anterior to the left innominate artery; *(f)* the trachea *(arrow)* is markedly compressed by the innominate artery as it passes anteriorly and to the right. (From Jaffe RB: *Semin Ultrasound CT MR* 1990; 11:219. Used by permission.)

tic arch with interruption of the left arch at varying positions with fibrous continuity of the interrupted segment. A double arch is the most common cause of a symptomatic vascular ring in infants and young children.

Functioning Double Aortic Arch

A complete (functional) double aortic arch represents persistence of both the right and left aortic arches. Two vessels arise from the ascending aorta and course dorsal, one on each side of the trachea and esophagus, to join posteriorly, usually into a left descending aorta. The left arch is anterior and the right arch is posterior. Occasionally, with a descending right thoracic aorta, these arch relationships are reversed. In the usual course, the right arch is larger. This anomaly of the aortic arch is usually isolated without CHD.

Chest Roentgenography. Chest roentgenographic diagnosis is difficult in the infant. In the older child the pattern simulates a right aortic arch, although occasionally, in the lateral view, AP narrowing of the trachea may be observed. Pulmonary dis-

ease is frequently coexistent (see Fig 17–3). A high-kilovoltage film with added filtration in the frontal projection of the tracheal airway will demonstrate the trachea to the left, and may show distal narrowing (see Fig 17–4).

Esophagography provides more definitive information and shows typical indentations on the lateral and posterior aspects of the esophagus. Typically, with the larger right posterior segment, a prominent indentation is observed on the right side and posterior aspect of the esophagus. The left arch produces a less striking esophageal indentation that is usually somewhat more caudad when seen in the AP view (Fig 17–9,A). The posterior esophageal impression is frequently horizontal and more prominent (Fig 17–9,B) than is the typical aberrant right subclavian artery with a left aortic arch.

Magnetic Resonance Imaging and Angiocardiography. While some surgeons and clinicians do not believe further evaluation is necessary, MRI in the coronal and axial planes (Fig 17–10) or aortography (Fig 17–11) does provide more definitive preoperative information concerning patency, relative size,

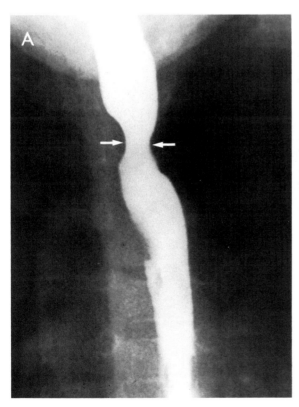
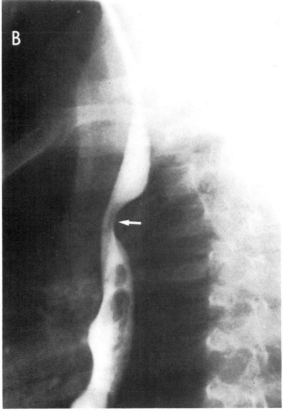

FIG 17–9.
Double aortic arch. AP **(A)** and lateral **(B)** esophagograms demonstrate prominent indentations on both the right and left sides of the esophagus in the AP projection *(arrows)* as well as a large transverse defect in the posterior portion of the esophagus *(arrow)* in the lateral view.

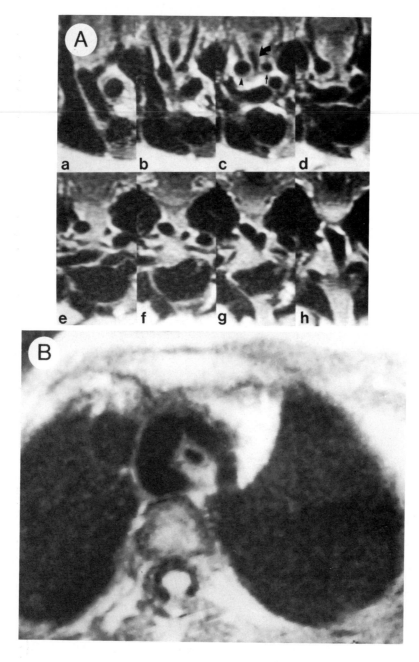

FIG 17–10.
Double aortic arch with both arches patent. **A,** composite coronal interleaved 3-mm spin-echo images (anteroposterior) in a 16-month-old boy with symptoms of a vascular ring: *(a)* the ascending aorta bifurcates into right and left arches; *(b)* the right arch gives origin to the right common carotid, the left arch to the left common carotid; *(c)* the right arch *(arrowhead)* is larger than the left arch *(small arrow)*. Note the narrowed trachea *(curved arrow)* as it passes between the two arches; *(d)* the right arch gives origin to the right subclavian and vertebral arteries, and the left arch gives origin to the left subclavian and vertebral arteries; *(e–g)* the arches pass posteriorly to join together in *(g)*; *(h)* the aorta de-

scends just to the left of midline. **(From Jaffe RB:** *Semin Ultrasound CT MR* 1990; 11:208. Used by permission.) **B,** a 5-year-old girl with double aortic arch: this axial 5-mm spin-echo image demonstrates the dominant right arch and smaller left aortic arch encircling the trachea. As the right arch passes posteriorly to join the left arch to form a left descending thoracic aorta, there is a tendency to a right posterior arch and left anterior arch. **(Courtesy of Jerald Kuhn, Children's Hospital of Buffalo, N.Y. From Cohen MD, Edwards MK:** *Magnetic Resonance Imaging of Children.* **New York, Decker, 1990. Used by permission.)**

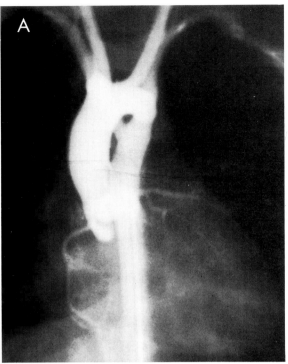
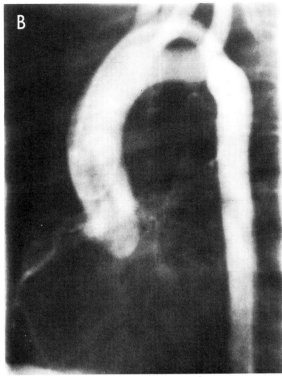

FIG 17–11.
Double aortic arch. AP **(A)** and lateral **(B)** retrograde aortograms. The catheter passes through the smaller right posterior arch into the ascending aorta; each right and left branch gives rise to the appropriate brachiocephalic vessels. At the time of the examination, the catheter was also passed through the anterior left-sided aortic arch and documented the patency of both limbs.

and relations. Angiograms in the AP and lateral or long-axis projections are preferred. Treatment relates to the severity of symptoms.

Double Aortic Arch With Partial Atresia of the Left Arch

This anomaly in arch development results from regression of varying segments of the left aortic arch with fibrous continuity of the segments completing the vascular ring (Fig 17–12,A, C, and E). Patients have many of the roentgenographic manifestations seen with double aortic arch. This anomaly is more common than a true simple right aortic arch except in those cases with mirror-image branching and cyanotic CHD. The most common variations in this category are those with atresia between the left common carotid and left subclavian arteries (Fig 17–12,E) or distal to the left subclavian artery (Fig 17–12,A and C). An aortic diverticulum may be present and adds significantly to the posterior esophageal impression.

Chest Roentgenography. Chest roentgenograms show a prominent right aortic arch segment in the AP projection (Figs 17–3 and 17–13). Esophagograms show impressions on both sides of the esophagus, although predominantly on the right,

and a prominent indentation on the posterior esophageal wall (Fig 17–14). The descending aorta is more often right-sided. Angiography (Fig 17–15) or MRI demonstrates a lack of patency of the left aortic arch with a left innominate artery and, frequently, an aortic diverticulum at the junction of the right arch and upper descending aorta in subtype 1 (Fig 17–12,A). Patients with atresia between the left common carotid and left subclavian arteries (subtype 3) will show separate origins of the left common carotid artery from the ascending aorta, and the left subclavian artery from the aortic diverticulum (Figs 17–12,E and 17–16).

Right Aortic Arch

A right aortic arch has many similarities to a double arch with left arch atresia. The malformations result from interruption of the segments of the left aortic arch in relation to the great vessel origins.

Right Aortic Arch With Mirror-Image Branching

The most common variation of right aortic arch is mirror-image branching of the major brachiocephalic vessels. A right aortic arch with mirror-image

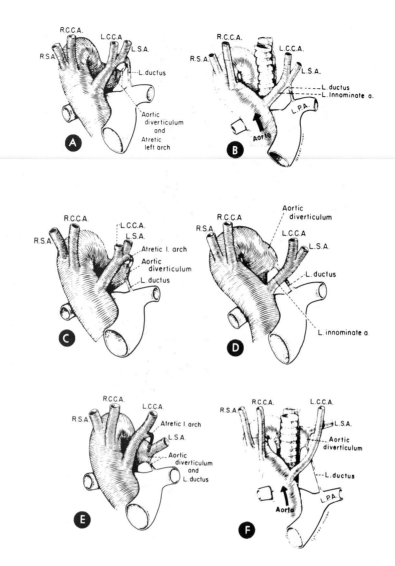

FIG 17–12.
Double aortic arch with left arch atresia, subtypes 1, 2, and 3 *(left column)*, and their respective right aortic arch counterparts *(right column)*. **A,** subtype 1. **B,** Mirror-image branching, no vascular ring. **C,** subtype 2. **D,** mirror-image branching, rare type. **E,** subtype 3. **F,** aberrant left subclavian artery. The anatomical differ- ence between the double-arch malformation and its right arch counterpart is the persistence of an atretic segment in the double arch anomaly. (From Shuford WH, Sybers RG, Weens HS: *Am J Roentgenol* 1972; 116:137. Used by permission.)

branching is not a true vascular ring inasmuch as the ligamentum arteriosum arises from the anteriorly positioned left innominate artery and descends to the left pulmonary artery without creation of a true vascular ring (see Fig 17–12). This anomaly is com- monly associated with cyanotic CHD: tetralogy of Fallot, truncus arteriosus, tricuspid atresia, and transposition of the great arteries (TGA) with pul- monary valvular stenosis (PVS) (see Table 15–5). Rarely, a right aortic arch with mirror-image branch- ing may cause a vascular ring if the ligamentum ar- teriosum extends from the left pulmonary artery to an aortic diverticulum of the right-sided upper de- scending aorta (see Fig 17–12,D). A lateral esopha- gogram will show a large retroesophageal impres- sion from the aortic diverticulum and ligamentum arteriosum.

Right Aortic Arch With Aberrant Left Subclavian Artery

A right aortic arch with aberrant origin of the left subclavian artery is a common cause of a vascular ring in infants and children. The distal portion of the rudimentary left arch may persist as a diverticulum giving origin to the left subclavian artery (see Fig 17–12,F). Since the ligamentum arteriosum typically attaches to the aortic diverticulum or left subclavian artery, a true vascular ring is created.

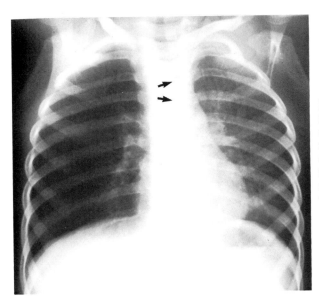

FIG 17–13.
Double aortic arch with left arch atresia in an AP expiratory chest roentgenogram in 2-year-old with chronic respiratory distress. Air trapping in the right lung is evident along with a prominent right aortic arch and striking deviation of the trachea to the left *(arrows)*. Air trapping is a relatively rare complication of aortic vascular rings, with right mainstem bronchial obstruction secondary to a double aortic arch with atresia of the left arch, subtype 3-E (see Fig 17–12).

Chest radiographs show typical changes of a right aortic arch deviating the trachea to the left, and the azygos vein to the right. On the esophagogram the aortic diverticulum and aberrant left subclavian artery produce a large retroesophageal impression. The aberrant left subclavian artery may also produce an impression running obliquely from caudal right to cephalad left. MRI (Fig 17–17) or angiography will delineate the vascular anatomy (see Fig 17–12,F).

Right Aortic Arch With Left Descending Aorta (Circumflex Aorta)

This malformation, considered by some to be a form of double aortic arch with left atresia, is characterized by a right aortic arch, retroesophageal segment, and left descending aorta, and is a mirror image of the left aortic arch with right descending aorta. When associated with an aberrant left subclavian artery, which frequently arises from an aortic diverticulum with stenosis at its origin, and a tight ligamentum arteriosum, a symptomatic vascular ring is formed. On radiographic study one may visualize a right aortic arch, distal tracheal displacement to the left, left descending aorta, and large posterior and oblique impressions on the esophagogram by the retroesophageal segment of the aorta. The malformation can be confirmed by aortography (Fig 17–18) or MRI.

Right Cervical Aortic Arch

A right cervical aortic arch occurs when there is abnormal cephalic migration of the aortic arch into the supraclavicular and neck region. A right cervical arch is more common than a left cervical arch. The branching of the aortic arch vessels is variable. The common carotid arteries may arise normally from the cervical arch or there may be separate origins of both internal and external carotid arteries. The position of the brachiocephalic vessels and ligamentum arteriosum determines which patients are symptomatic from a vascular ring. Clinically a pulsatile mass may be present in the supraclavicular region, with or without symptoms of a vascular ring. Radiographic findings include (Fig 17–19,A): (1) right superior mediastinal widening, (2) tracheal displacement to the left and anteriorly, (3) a large oblique impression on the esophagogram from cephalic right to caudad left, and (4) a left descending aorta. The malformations can be confirmed by MRI or angiography (Fig 17–19,B). Operation is indicated in patients with symptoms of a vascular ring.

Right Aortic Arch With Isolation of the Left Subclavian Artery

A final variation of a right aortic arch is isolation of the left subclavian artery attached by a functioning or nonfunctioning ductus arteriosus to the left pulmonary artery. This is not a true vascular ring and is of primary interest because of the clinical variation created in the brachiocephalic pulses and, occasionally, subsequent subclavian steal syndrome. The anomaly is frequently associated with CHD.

ABERRANT LEFT PULMONARY ARTERY (PULMONARY SLING)

When the left sixth aortic arch fails to develop normally or becomes obliterated and the left pulmonary

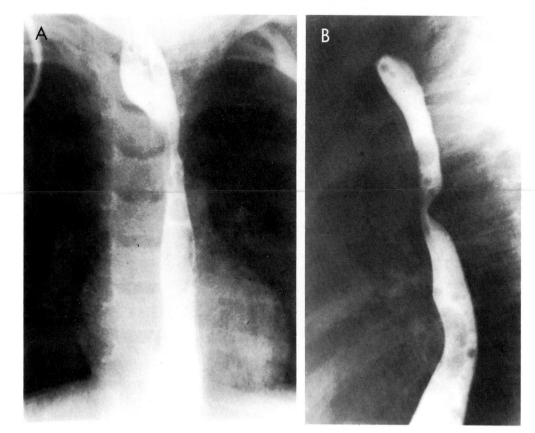

FIG 17–14.
Double aortic arch with atresia of the left arch. AP **(A)** and lateral **(B)** esophagogram spot films show a prominent impression on the right and a posterior esophageal transverse indentation in the lat-eral view. There is associated evidence of narrowing and compression of the trachea near the carina.

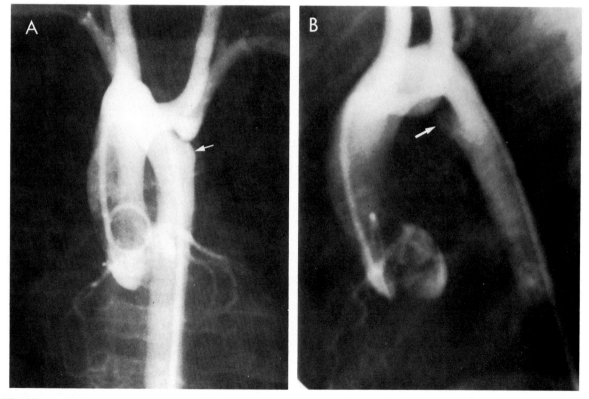

FIG 17–15.
Double aortic arch with left arch atresia. AP **(A)** and lateral **(B)** retrograde aortograms show atresia distal to the origin of both left-sided brachiocephalic vessels. The vascular ring is completed by the residual fibrous segment and the ligamentum arteriosum. Aortic diverticulum is indicated by an *arrow* (see Fig 17–12).

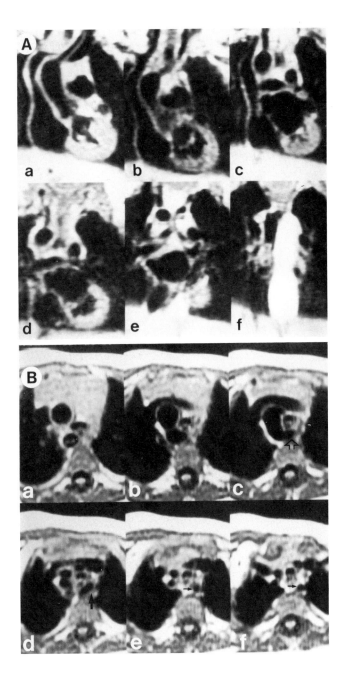

FIG 17–16.
A 3-month-old infant with symptoms of a vascular ring secondary to a double aortic arch with left arch atresia between the left common carotid and left subclavian arteries (subtype 3). An esophagogram demonstrated bilateral esophageal impressions suggestive of a double aortic arch, similar to Figure 17–9,A. **A,** composite coronal interleaved 3-mm spin-echo images (anteroposterior): *(a and b)* the ascending aorta gives origin to the left common carotid artery; *(c)* the right aortic arch gives origin to the right common carotid artery; *(d)* the right subclavian artery arises from the right aortic arch; *(e and f)* the origin of the left subclavian artery from the aortic diverticulum is seen; gastroesophageal reflux of formula also is noted. This branching pattern cannot be differentiated from right aortic arch with aberrant left subclavian artery. **B,** composite axial interleaved 3-mm images (inferosuperior): *(a)* seen are the ascending aorta, right descending aorta, and tracheal bifurcation; *(b*

and *c)* seen is the right aortic arch. The aortic diverticulum *(arrow)* is seen in *(c); (d)* as the left subclavian artery *(arrow)* arises from the aortic diverticulum, it appears tethered anteriorly. The left common carotid artery is seen anterior to the trachea and posterior to the left innominate vein; *(e and f)* the left subclavian artery *(arrow)* then returns to its normal position. The origins of the right common carotid and right subclavian arteries are seen in *(e)*. While this branching pattern cannot be differentiated from a right aortic arch with aberrant left subclavian artery, the course of the left subclavian artery as it appears tethered anteriorly, plus the AP esophagogram, suggested a double aortic arch with left arch atresia between the left common carotid and left subclavian arteries (subtype 3). This was confirmed at operation. **(From Jaffe RB:** *Semin Ultrasound CT MR* 1990; 11:211. **Used by permission.)**

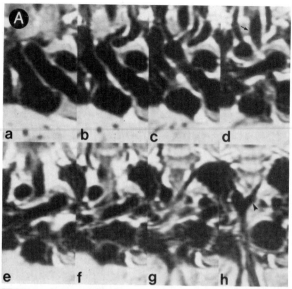

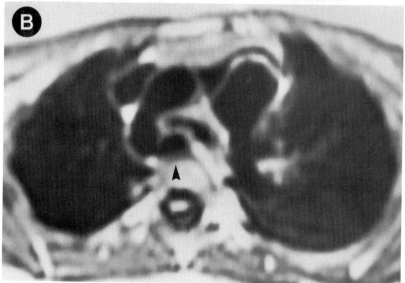

FIG 17–17.

A 4-year-old boy with symptoms of vascular ring secondary to a right aortic arch with aberrant left subclavian artery. **A,** composite coronal interleaved 3-mm spin-echo images (anteroposterior): *(a)* left ventricular outflow tract and ascending aorta are seen between the superior vena cava and right atrium and pulmonary artery; *(b)* origin of the left common carotid artery is partially visualized. The left innominate vein is just lateral to the left common carotid artery; *(c)* the origin of the left common carotid and right common carotid arteries is seen; *(d)* the origin of the right common carotid artery

from the right aortic arch is better visualized. Note that the trachea *(arrow)* is deviated to the left; *(e–g)* the right aortic arch passes posteriorly and gives origin to the right subclavian and right vertebral arteries in *(g)*. Part of the left subclavian artery is also noted; *(h)* the left subclavian artery arises from the aortic diverticulum *(arrowhead)* originating from the posterior right aortic arch. **B,** axial 3-mm image confirms the right aortic arch with posterior aortic diverticulum *(arrowhead)*. (From Jaffe RB: *Semin Ultrasound CT MR* 1990; 11:212. Used by permission.)

artery subsequently fails to develop, the left lung's arterial supply is derived from an anomalous vessel originating from the right pulmonary artery. This aberrant left pulmonary artery passes between the trachea and esophagus and produces a vascular sling or ring (Fig 17–20). It is frequently accompanied by significant hypoplasia or dysplasia of the trachea and main bronchi. These structures are dis-

placed to the left and compressed by the aberrant vessel to produce tracheobronchomalacia or intrinsic cartilaginous malformation.

Clinical Manifestations

Stridor, wheezing, and dyspnea progressing to frank cyanosis develop shortly after birth. Symp-

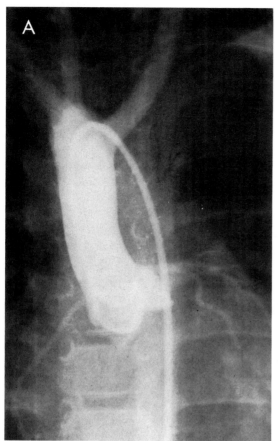
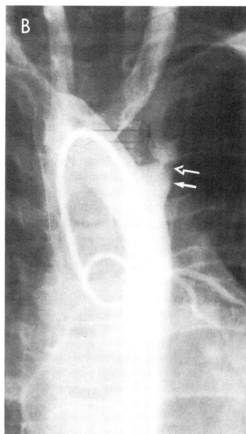

FIG 17–18.
A 5-year-old girl with symptoms of a vascular ring secondary to a right aortic arch with left descending aorta (circumflex aorta). **A,** AP aortogram demonstrates a right aortic arch with sequential origin of the left common carotid, right common carotid, and right subclavian arteries. **B,** the aorta passes behind the esophagus to descend on the left. The left subclavian artery arises from a small diverticulum *(arrow)* with stenosis at its origin *(open arrow)*. At operation the left ligamentum arteriosum completed the vascular ring. This arch anomaly may also be considered as a form of double aortic arch with left arch atresia.

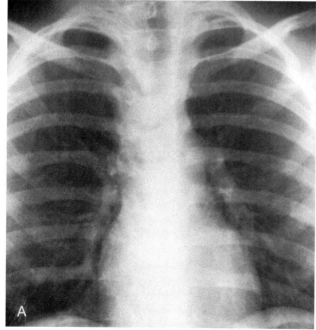
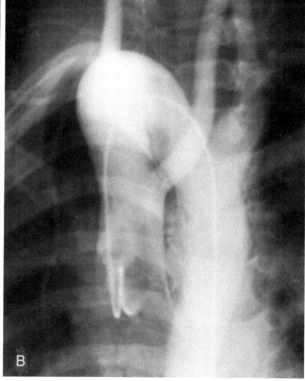
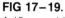

FIG 17–19.
A 13-year-old boy with a pulsatile right supraclavicular mass secondary to a right cervical aortic arch. **A,** chest radiograph demonstrates tracheal displacement to the left and a right supraclavicular mass at the upper margin of the film. The descending aorta is not visualized. **B,** aortogram (shallow left anterior oblique projection) confirms a right cervical aortic arch.

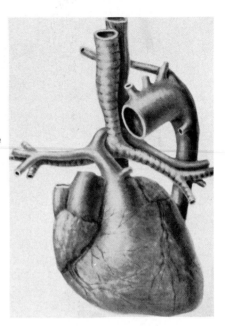

FIG 17–20.
Pulmonary artery sling. Diagram of anomalous origin of the left pulmonary artery from the right pulmonary artery, showing its retrograde course between the trachea and esophagus. Note the hypoplasia of the distal trachea, often representing an intrinsic malformation with complete cartilaginous rings that may extend into the right and left mainstem bronchi. This tracheal malformation is one of the most serious aspects of this anomaly.

toms tend to be more severe than with other types of vascular rings. Significant unilateral bronchial obstruction of the right lung may occur.

Chest Roentgenography

When the anomalous vessel obstructs the right mainstem bronchus, trapped fetal fluid in the right lung is seen in the newborn. In neonates and infants, a hyperlucent right lung is usually seen (Fig 17–21). The left hilum is usually low, and

the mainstem bronchi may show a horizontal "inverted T-shaped" pattern. Branching to the upper and lower lobes tends to originate at a more peripheral level. Anterior bowing of the trachea at the carina may be seen on the lateral chest film (Fig 17–22,A).

Esophagography characteristically identifies an indentation on the anterior wall of the esophagus at the level of the carina, and the trachea is anteriorly displaced from the esophagus at this level (Fig 17–22,B). Occasionally, the esophagogram may

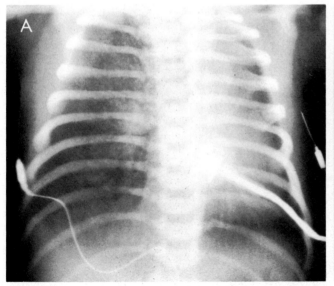
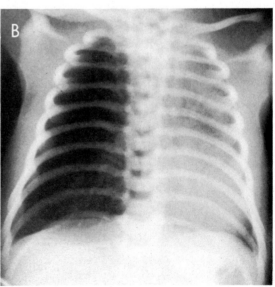

FIG 17–21.
Pulmonary artery sling. **A,** an AP chest film of a neonate aged 6 hours shows unilateral retained fetal fluid, increased lung volume, and hazy ill-defined parenchymal densities secondary to right mainstem bronchial obstruction. **B,** a follow-up film at the age of 6 days shows resorption of the fetal lung fluid now producing a unilateral hyperlucent lung secondary to air trapping.

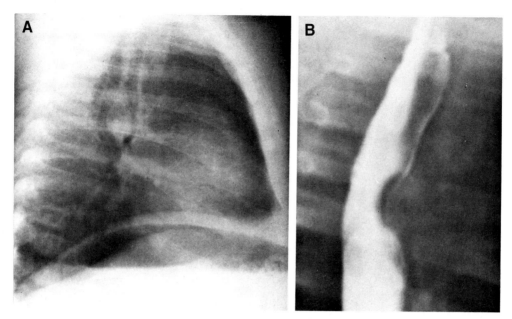

FIG 17–22.
Pulmonary artery sling. A lateral chest roentgentogram **(A)** and lateral esophagogram **(B)** show the anomalous left pulmonary artery between the air-filled trachea and esophagus on the lateral chest film and a focal nodular indentation on the anterior portion of the esophagus at the level of the carina. This esophageal indentation is similar to that noted with total anomalous pulmonary venous return because of the venous confluence. However, the latter is usually in a more caudal position.

show normal anatomy. Bronchoscopy is recommended to evaluate the tracheobronchial tree for extrinsic pulsatile compression effects as well as underlying tracheobronchomalacia (see Fig 17–2).

Echocardiography
Real-time studies will fail to demonstrate a normal pulmonary artery bifurcation (moustache appearance). Instead, the left pulmonary artery is seen to originate from the right pulmonary artery and course back to the left lung (Fig 17–23).

Magnetic Resonance Imaging and Angiography
Pulmonary arteriography or MRI confirms the diagnosis. Biplane studies in the sitting-up position are recommended (Fig 17–24) at pulmonary arteriography. Thin-section MRI in the axial plane demonstrates the aberrant course of the left pulmonary ar-

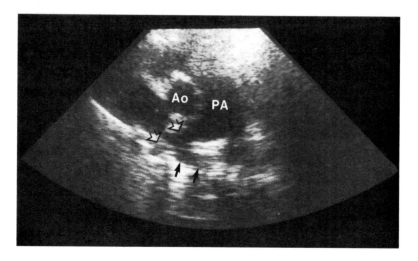

FIG 17–23.
Pulmonary artery sling. Short-axis real-time echocardiogram at the level of the aortic root (Ao) and main pulmonary artery (PA) shows the large main and right pulmonary artery (open arrows) giving rise to the left pulmonary artery (black arrows), which deviates back to the left.

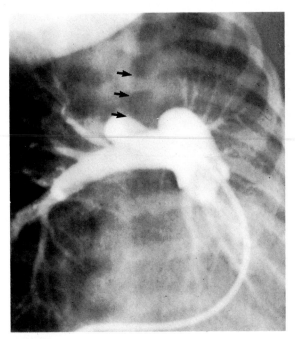

FIG 17–24.
Pulmonary artery sling. A sitting-up AP pulmonary arteriogram demonstrates the left pulmonary artery ascending just to the right of the trachea *(arrows)* and then traveling posteriorly and caudad to branch normally to the left lung.

tery, tracheal compression, and hyperinflation of the right lung (Fig 17–25).

Prognosis

The prognosis is guarded even with surgical correction because of the underlying frequent tracheal hy-

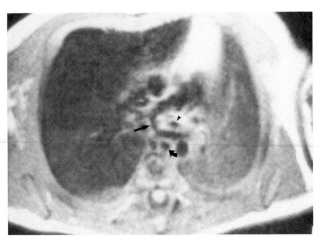

FIG 17–25.
A 5-day-old infant with pulmonary sling. Axial MR image demonstrates aberrant origin of the left pulmonary artery (LPA) *(straight arrow)* from the right pulmonary artery. The LPA passes posterior to the trachea *(arrowhead)* and anterior to the esophagus *(curved arrow)* to enter the left lung. Hyperinflation of the right lung is also present. **(Courtesy of Shashikant Sane.)**

poplasia or tracheobronchomalacia. At the time of vascular surgery, the surgeon should be prepared for reconstructive procedures of the tracheobronchial tree.

CONGENITAL ANOMALIES OF THE PULMONARY ARTERIES

Congenital anomalies of the pulmonary arteries are seen as isolated lesions, in many forms of CHD, and frequently in syndrome complexes. The central pul-

TABLE 17–1.
Congenital Anomalies of the Pulmonary Arteries

1. Hypoplastic pulmonary artery with and without anomalous pulmonary venous return
   a. Scimitar syndrome—with anomalous pulmonary venous return to the inferior vena cava (IVC) (Fig 15–7)
   b. Tetralogy of Fallot—without anomalous pulmonary venous return
   c. Pulmonary hypoplasia
2. Unilateral absence of a pulmonary artery
   a. As an isolated lesion—pulmonary aplasia or hypoplasia
   b. With a patent ductus arteriosus—especially with an absent right pulmonary artery
   c. With tetralogy of Fallot—especially with an absent left pulmonary artery
3. Anomalous origin of the left pulmonary artery from the right pulmonary artery (pulmonary sling) (Figs 17–20, through 17–25)
4. Direct connection of the right pulmonary artery to the left atrium
5. Peripheral pulmonary artery stenosis
   a. Idiopathic
   b. Rubella (Fig 15–14)
   c. Supravalvular aortic stenosis syndrome (Fig 18–8)
   d. Takayasu arteritis
   e. Tetralogy of Fallot (Fig 16–88)
   f. Arteriohepatic dysplasia (Alagille syndrome)
   g. Cutis laxa
   h. Ehlers-Danlos syndrome

6. Absence of pulmonary artery origin from the heart
   a. Pulmonary atresia
   b. Truncus arteriosus (Fig 16–82)
   c. Ductal origin of pulmonary artery(s)
   d. Systemic–pulmonary artery collaterals (Figs 16–89 and 21–31,A)
   e. Coronary collaterals to the lung
7. Anomalous origin of one pulmonary artery from the ascending aorta
   a. Anomalous origin of the right pulmonary artery from the ascending aorta (hemitruncus arteriosus) (Fig 16–24)
   b. Anomalous origin of the left pulmonary artery from the ascending aorta—with tetralogy of Fallot
8. Pulmonary arteriovenous malformations
   a. Classic discrete pulmonary arteriovenous fistula
   b. Pulmonary telangiectasia
   c. Hereditary hemorrhagic telangiectasia (Osler-Rendu-Weber syndrome)

monary arteries develop from the sixth brachial arches, while the peripheral pulmonary arteries develop from the splanchnic plexus of the lungs. Table 17–1 presents a useful classification of congenital anomalies of the pulmonary arteries. More details of frequent pulmonary artery anomalies are found in Chapter 7 and elsewhere in Part III.

REFERENCES

Aortic Arch Anomalies

Dominiguez R, Oh KS, Dorst JP, et al: Left aortic arch with right descending aorta. *Am J Roentgenol* 1978; 130:917.

Edwards JE: Anomalies of the derivatives of the aortic arch system. *Med Clin North Am* 1948; 32:925.

Freedom RM, Culham JAG, Moes CAF: *Angiocardiography of Congenital Heart Disease.* New York, Macmillan, 1984, p 487.

Garti IJ, Aygen MM, Levy MJ: Double aortic arch anomalies: Diagnosis by countercurrent right brachial arteriography. *Am J Roentgenol* 1979; 133:251.

Jaffe RB: Magnetic resonance imaging of vascular rings. *Semin Ultrasound CT MR* 1990; 11:206.

Jaffe RB: Radiographic manifestations of congenital anomalies of the aortic arch. *Radiol Clin North Am* 1991; 29:319.

Knight L, Edwards JE: Right aortic arch types and associated cardiac anomalies. *Circulation* 1974; 50:1047.

McCormick TL, Kuhns LR: Tracheal compression by a normal aorta associated with right lung agenesis. *Radiology* 1979; 120:659–660.

McLoughlin MJ, Weisbrod B, Weis DJ, et al: Computed tomography in congenital anomalies of the aortic arch and great vessels. *Radiology* 1981; 138:399.

Nath PH, Castaneda-Zuñiga WR, Zoilikofer C, et al: Isolation of subclavian artery. *Am J Roentgenol* 1981; 137:683.

Predey TA, McDonald V, Demos TC, et al: CT of congenital anomalies of the aortic arch. *Semin Roentgenol* 1989; 24:96–111.

Shuford WH, Sybers RG: *The Aortic Arch and Its Malformations.* Springfield, Ill, Charles C Thomas, 1974.

Spindolo-Franco H, Fish BG: Abnormalities of the aortic arch and pulmonary arteries—vascular rings and slings, in Elliott LP (ed): *Cardiac Imaging in Infants, Children, and Adults.* Philadelphia, JB Lippincott, 1991, p 344.

Aberrant Left Pulmonary Artery

Berdon WE, Baker DH: Vascular anomalies and the infant lung: Rings, slings and other things. *Semin Roentgenol* 1972; 7:39.

Berdon WE, Baker DH, Wung JT, et al: Complete cartilage-ring tracheal stenosis associated with anomalous left pulmonary artery: The ring-sling complex. *Radiology* 1984; 152:57–64.

Corbett DB, Washington JE: Respiratory obstruction in the newborn and excessive pulmonary fluid. *Am J Roentgenol* 1971; 112:18.

Gumbiner CH, Mullins CE, McNamara DG: Pulmonary artery sling. *Am J Cardiol* 1980; 45:311.

Jaffe RB: Magnetic resonance imaging of vascular rings. *Semin Ultrasound CT MR* 1990; 11:206–220.

Spindolo-Franco H, Fish BG: Abnormalities of the aortic arch and pulmonary arteries—vascular rings and slings, in Elliott LP (ed): *Cardiac Imaging in Infants, Children, and Adults.* Philadelphia, JB Lippincott, 1991, p 34.

Tonkin IL, Elliott LP, Bargeron LM Jr: Concomitant axial cineangiography and barium esophagography in the evaluation of vascular rings. *Radiology* 1980; 135:69.

Williams RG, Jaffe RB, Condon VR: Unusual features of pulmonary sling. *Am J Roentgenol* 1979; 133:1065.

Congenital Anomalies of the Pulmonary Arteries

Abe T, Kuribayashi R, Sato M, et al: Direct communication of the right pulmonary artery with the left atrium. *J Thorac Cardiovasc Surg* 1972; 62:38–44.

Bahler RC, Carson P, Traks E, et al: Absent right pulmonary artery. *Am J Med* 1969; 46:64–71.

Boijsen E, Kozuka T: Angiographic demonstration of systemic arterial supply in abnormal pulmonary circulation. *Am J Roentgenol* 1969; 106:70–80.

Currarino G, Willis KW, Johnson AF Jr, et al: Pulmonary telangiectasia. *Am J Roentgenol* 1976; 127:775–779.

Dines DE, Arms RA, Bernatz PE, et al: Pulmonary arteriovenous fistulas. *Mayo Clin Proc* 1974; 49:460–465.

Ellis K: Developmental abnormalities in the systemic blood supply to the lungs. *Am J Roentgenol* 1991; 156:669–679.

Freedom RM, Culham JAG, Moes CAF: Anomalies of pulmonary arteries, in Freedom RM, Culham JAG, Moes CF (eds): *Angiocardiography of Congenital Heart Disease.* New York, Macmillan, 1984, p 254.

Freedom RM, Culham JAG, Moes CAF: Hemitruncus arteriosus (anomalous origin of one pulmonary artery from the ascending aorta) in Freedom RM, Culham JAG, Moes CF (eds): *Angiocardiography of Congenital Heart Disease.* New York, Macmillan, 1984, p 453.

Gomes AS: MR imaging of congenital anomalies of the thoracic aorta and pulmonary arteries. *Radiol Clin North Am* 1989; 27:1171.

Higgins CB, Wexler L: Clinical and angiographic features of pulmonary arteriovenous fistulas in children. *Radiology* 1976; 119:171–175.

Julsrud PR: Magnetic resonance imaging of the pulmonary arteries and veins. *Semin Ultrasound CT MR* 1990; 11:184–205.

Keane JF, Maltz D, Bernhard WF, et al: Anomalous origin of one pulmonary artery from the ascending aorta. *Circulation* 1974; 50:588–594.

Keiffer SA, Amplatz K, Anderson RC, et al: Proximal interruption of a pulmonary artery. *Am J Roentgenol* 1965; 95:592–597.

Kleinman PK: Pleural telangiectasia and absence of a pulmonary artery. *Radiology* 1979; 132:281–284.

Krause DW, Kuehn HJ, Sellers RD, et al: Roentgen sign associated with an aberrant vessel connecting right main pulmonary artery to left atrium. *Radiology* 1974; 111:177–178.

Lynch DA, Higgins CB: MR imaging of unilateral pulmonary artery anomalies. *J Comput Assist Tomogr* 1990; 14:187.

Oh KS, Bender TM, Bowen A, et al: Plain radiographic, nuclear medicine and angiographic observations of hepatogenic pulmonary angiodysplasia. *Pediatr Radiol* 1983; 13:111.

Panicek DM, Heitzman ER, Randall PA, et al: The continuum of pulmonary development anomalies. *Radiographics* 1987; 7:747–772.

Rosenfield NS, Kelley MJ, Jensen PS, et al: Arteriohepatic dysplasia: Radiologic features of a new syndrome. *Am J Roentgenol* 1980; 1135:1217–1223.

Spindola-Franco H, Fish BG: Abnormalities of the aortic arch and pulmonary arteries—vascular rings and slings in Elliott LP (ed): *Cardiac Imaging in Infants, Children, and Adults.* Philadelphia, JB Lippincott, 1991, p 344.

Weintraub RA, Fabian CE, Adams DF: Ectopic origin of one pulmonary artery from the ascending aorta. *Radiology* 1966; 86:666–676.

White RI Jr, Mitchell SE, Barth KH, et al: Angioarchitecture of pulmonary arteriovenous malformations. *Am J Roentgenol* 1983; 140:681–686.

18

Cardiac Malposition, Cardiosplenic Syndromes, and Chromosomal Anomalies

CARDIAC MALPOSITIONS

The evaluation of cardiac malpositions and cardiac-visceral discordance is very complex and difficult. Approaching these conditions by utilizing a systematic, segmental approach with familiar anatomical terminology helps to simplify the evaluation of these patients. Analysis must include (1) atrial positions, (2) atrioventricular (AV) relations and connections, and (3) ventricular–great vessel relations and connections. Segmental relations can be deduced from the knowledge of cardiac-visceral relations; the basic configuration of the cardiac silhouette; and electrocardiographic, echocardiographic, and angiocardiographic evaluations (Table 18–1).

Definitions

Dextrocardia implies a cardiac silhouette predominantly to the right of the spine (Fig 18–1) without implication of intracardiac disturbance or atrial, ventricular, or great-vessel relations. Primary dextrocardia (dextroversion) relates to primary visceral cardiac development, while secondary dextrocardia (dextroposition) relates to thoracic or abdominal malformations.

In *levocardia* the cardiac silhouette is on the left without implication of internal cardiac structure.

Situs solitus (totalis) indicates "normal" visceral-cardiac relations with the cardiac apex, aortic arch, and stomach bubble on the left. The liver, inferior vena cava, and right atrial structures are on the right.

Situs inversus (totalis) indicates the mirror-image development of both the visceral and cardiac anatomy. This relation has only a slight increase in congenital heart disease (CHD).

Situs inversus viscerum (visceral situs inversus) indicates mirror-image development of the abdominal viscera and, for practical purposes, the cardiac atria. When accompanied by AV discordance (see below), a high incidence of CHD is expected.

In *visceral heterotaxia (ambiguous viscera)* numerous patients, particularly those with the asplenia or polysplenia syndrome, have an indeterminate configuration of viscera in which the liver tends to be horizontal and the stomach midline or on either the right or left side. Such cases are accompanied by multiple visceral and cardiac anomalies.

Inversion indicates the mirror-image or reversed positioning of anatomical structures. It applies to all portions of the segmental anatomy of the heart: atria, ventricles, and great vessels. A patient with a right-sided cardiac silhouette may have either inverted or noninverted ventricular anatomy just like a patient with levocardia.

AV concordance indicates that the right atrium is appropriately related to the right ventricle with similar relations in the left heart.

AV discordance indicates that the right atrium is anatomically related to the left ventricle and, similarly, the left atrium to the right ventricle.

TABLE 18–1.

Working Approach to Cardiac and Visceral Malpositions*

  I. Exclude cardiac malposition secondary to extracardiac abnormalities, e.g., hypoplastic lung.
  II. Evaluate for visceral heterotaxia secondary to asplenia or polysplenia
    1. Tracheobronchial tree for symmetry
    2. Pulmonary arteries for unilaterality or symmetry
    3. Lobation of the lung
    4. Hepatic symmetry—horizontal liver
    5. Position of the stomach
    6. Is the IVC present or is there azygos continuation of the IVC indicative of polysplenia?
  III. Determine cardiac and visceral relationships. Almost always the left atrium is on the side of the stomach.
    1. Normal visceral situs
      a. Dextrocardia—high incidence of CHD, particularly l-TGA with VSD and PVS
      b. Levocardia—no malposition; 1% incidence of CHD
    2. Visceral situs inversus
      a. Dextrocardia—1%–2% incidence of CHD
      b. Levocardia—almost 100% incidence of CHD, particularly forms of transposition

*IVC = inferior vena cava; CHD = congenital heart disease; l-TGA = corrected transposition of the great arteries; PVS = pulmonary valvular stenosis; VSD = ventricular septal defect.

Ventricular inversion indicates "normal" situs solitus with normally related great vessels, viscera, atria, and a levo-loop ventricle or inverted (mirror-image) ventricular position.

Ventricular noninversion is indicative of atrial-visceral situs solitus with dextro-loop ventricular development and normally related great vessels.

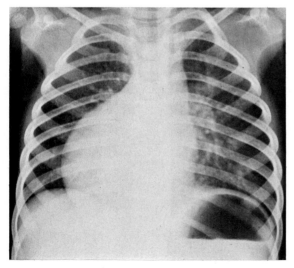

FIG 18–1.

Dextrocardia with visceral situs solitus (cardiac-visceral discordance) without intrinsic organic heart disease. This is a rare combination; most patients with cardiac-visceral discordance have significant CHD.

Segmental Considerations

This approach includes the evaluation of the atrial-visceral relations, atrial–systemic venous connections, AV connections, ventricular relations, and great-vessel relations and connections. Any specific segment in this normal anatomical sequence may be interrupted. A simplified approach to cardiac and visceral malpositions is summarized in Table 18–1.

Atriovisceral (Splenic) Relations

Atrial situs can usually be ascertained by evaluation of the abdominal viscera. A high correlation of normal atrial situs exists when the stomach bubble can be identified on the left with a normal right liver silhouette, a right eparterial bronchus, and a normal right-sided inferior vena cava (IVC). *Atrial situs inversus* is indicated by the reversal of any or all of the aforementioned. *Indeterminate atrial situs*, or common atrium, is suggested by visceral heterotaxia, bilateral bilobed or trilobed lungs, or bilateral symmetric hyparterial or eparterial bronchi. It is also suggested by gastrointestinal malrotation, biliary malformations or atresia, and interruption of the hepatic or subhepatic segment of the IVC with azygos continuation. With the last-named group of indeterminate situs malformations, a high incidence of cardiosplenic syndromes is likely.

Atrial Relations and Systemic Venous Connection

Normal atrial relations and systemic venous connection can be presumed with normal visceral laterality. Angiographically, the right atrium is characterized by a broad-based triangular right atrial appendage with a wide orifice. The left atrium projects to the left of the right atrium and is characterized by a large crescent-shaped atrial appendage projecting anterosuperolaterally with a small orifice. The superior vena cava (SVC) connections are less constant, and bilateral SVCs are frequent even with situs solitus. The left system usually connects with the coronary sinus. With visceral situs inversus, mirror-image positioning of the atrial chambers and venous connections are anticipated. With visceral heterotaxia (ambiguous viscera) atrial positions cannot be adequately determined, and frequently a common atrium and anomalies in systemic venous connection are present.

Asplenia syndrome exhibits bilateral right-sidedness of abdominal and pulmonary viscera with two right atrial appendages present and, frequently, two SVCs draining into the common atrium. The IVC may enter the atrium on the right or midline. The abdominal aorta and IVC are frequently on the same side.

Polysplenia syndrome is characterized by bilateral left-sidedness with a common atrium frequently demonstrating two left atrial appendages. The IVC is interrupted in the hepatic or subhepatic segment and continues to empty through the azygos system either on the right or through the left SVC. In the absence of visceral heterotaxia, visceral atrial discordance is extremely unusual.

Ventricular Relations and Localizations

In normal development, as the heart tube bulges forward, it initially bends to the right (dextro-loop) and then progresses to migrate toward the left. Such development places the bulbus cordis (future right ventricle) to the right and the more distal developing bulboventricular loop (left ventricle) to the left in appropriate juxtaposition to the right and left atria. This alignment creates what is generally referred to as ventricular noninversion and AV concordance. The developing heart tube may bend to the left in its initial stage and produce a mirror-image pattern or inverted ventricular position, which produces AV discordance with the right atrium related to the left ventricle and the left atrium to the right ventricle. With ventricular inversion there is inversion of the associated AV valve. This does not have any implication with respect to the direction of the apex to the right or left in the inverted ventricular alignment. Ventricular localization can usually be determined with echocardiography or angiocardiography. Angiographically and anatomically, the right ventricle is normally triangular with a coarse trabecular pattern, a prominent moderator band, and a septal band of the crista. A slightly elongated infundibular outflow tract with a smooth wall is characteristic. The left ventricle has a smooth wall and elongated oval configuration, fine minor sinus portion trabeculation, and a relatively short infundibular or subaortic outflow segment. There is fibrous continuity of the posterior aortic annulus with the anterior leaflet of the mitral valve.

With ventricular inversion and AV discordance, as may be seen in patients with situs solitus and corrected transposition of the great vessels, the elongated, cone-shaped left ventricle projects medially and anteriorly, with the interventricular septum fairly vertically or sagitally oriented. Mitral-semilunar (pulmonary) valve continuity may still be noted. A high recess can usually be seen in the anterosuperior aspect of the ventricle. The right ventricle then projects to the left and superiorly. It is frequently bulbous to triangular in shape. There is discontinu-

ity of the aortic semilunar and AV valve. The infundibulum is somewhat shortened and poorly formed, and the crista presents on the posterior ventricular-infundibular wall. With a normal dextroloop, noninversion of the coronary arteries is seen, while with a levo-loop, coronary arteries are inverted. With ventricular inversions and complex CHD, anomalies in the development of the subaortic and subpulmonic conus are frequently seen.

Great Arteries

Normally, the pulmonary artery connected to the right ventricle is positioned anteriorly and to the left, while the aorta connected to the left ventricle is positioned posteriorly and to the right. These vessels cross in the supracardiac area. Malposition of the great vessels is indicated whenever this anatomical relationship does not exist. *Transposition* describes the reversal of the anteroposterior (AP) relations of the great arteries. Most commonly, one considers transposition of the great vessels when the aorta arises from the right ventricle and the pulmonary artery from the left ventricle. *Dextro-* and *levo*-positions refer to the relationships of the aorta to the pulmonary artery. In the usual complete transposition, the aorta is anterior and to the right (dextrotransposition). Less commonly, the aorta is transposed anteriorly and to the left (levo-transposition). This latter malposition is usually associated with ventricular inversion or single ventricle. Other forms of great vessel malposition may exist with double-outlet right or left ventricle when both great vessels arise directly from one of the ventricular chambers. When only one great vessel or common arterial trunk is present, the vessel often arises centrally from the base of the ventricles, as in truncus arteriosus or pulmonary atresia with ventricular septal defect (VSD).

Ventricular–great-vessel relationships are often suggested on conventional chest roentgenograms. Normal relations exist when the ascending aorta can be visualized in the right superior mediastinum with the aortic arch evident on the left and a main pulmonary artery producing a convex configuration of the mid-upper left heart border. Since great-vessel–ventricular discordance occurs only with complex CHD, the demonstration of this normal relation tends to imply normal anatomical relations or milder forms of heart disease. Transposition is possible if the pulmonary artery segment is not visualized as a focal convexity and the ascending aorta cannot be seen. The latter is frequently difficult to see in the young infant. If there is an unusual long, convex margin of the mid- and upper left heart border, levotransposition of the great vessels and associated ventricular inversion or a single ventricle is suggested. These conclusions from plain films depend on the visualization of abnormal, decreased to increased, pulmonary flow, and the presence of normal visceral situs.

With these definitions of segmental anatomy, it is possible to describe the various combined malformations regardless of whether there is dextrocardia or levocardia. Situs may be designated as solitus, s; inversus, i; ambiguous, a. The cardiac loop and ventricular relations may be designated as d (dextro) for normal and l (levo) for left, and x may be used to indicate indeterminate. The relations of the semilunar valves and great arteries may be listed as normal solitus, s; dextrotransposition, d; and levotransposition, l. Malpositions of the great vessels with the aortic valve directed anteriorly to the pulmonary valve may be indicated as "a" and the inverted relation as "i." Then, listing the segments in the direction of blood flow produces a normal cardiac segmental symbolic relationship of s, d, s. Complete transposition of the great arteries with situs solitus would be symbolized by s, d, d. A similar anomaly with situs inversus would be i, l, l, etc. With this method it is easier to describe the segmental relations and the internal anatomy more adequately than with descriptive terminology. In some of the more common lesions, it is still simpler, because of common usage, to describe the lesions (e.g., tetralogy of Fallot, dextrotransposition of the great arteries (d-TGA), and so forth).

CHD with situs solitus and levocardia is relatively rare, probably less than 1% of all cases. With situs inversus totalis and dextrocardia, CHD remains rare, although its incidence may increase to 2%. The lesions are basically those seen with situs solitus. With visceral situs solitus and dextrocardia, however, the incidence of CHD increases dramatically to between 75% and 85%, and with visceral and atrial situs inversus and levocardia, CHD is almost always present. Complex CHD with some form of transposition of the great vessels is the rule in the last two categories. Mesocardia, a mild form of cardiac malrotation and malposition, may be seen with situs inversus, situs solitus, or situs ambiguous. Heart disease is also frequent with mesocardia, although indeterminate in severity and frequency.

CARDIOSPLENIC SYNDROMES (IVEMARK SYNDROME)

The cardiosplenic syndromes are the most common congenital anomalies associated with situs problems. These anomalies are suggested when visceral heterotaxia (situs ambiguous) is present with either levocardia or dextrocardia. These syndromes are characterized by (1) asplenia or polysplenia, (2) complex CHD, and (3) visceral heterotaxia (Table 18–2). All abnormalities may be visualized well on magnetic resonance imaging (MRI) (Fig 18–2,A–D).

Asplenia constitutes from 1% to 3% of CHD. The teratogenic insult occurs between the 30th and 40th days of gestation. The condition is characterized by (1) asplenia, (2) CHD, (3) liver symmetry, (4) gastrointestinal malformations, and (5) bilateral trilobed lungs with eparterial bronchi (Fig 18–3). Other occasional anomalies include (1) tracheoesophageal fistula, (2) imperforate anus, (3) biliary atresia, and (4) genitourinary anomalies. Cardiac abnormalities include (1) cardiac malposition (dextrocardia or mesocardia), (2) anomalous systemic venous return or bi-

TABLE 18–2.

Cardiosplenic Syndromes

Asplenia	Polysplenia
Congenital heart disease	Renal anomalies
Dextro- or levo-transposition of the great arteries	Congenital heart disease
Common ventricles, common atria	Atrial septal defect, common atrium
Pulmonary atresia or stenosis	Interrupted inferior vena cava with
Total anomalous pulmonary venous return with obstruction	azygos continuation
Atrioventricular canal	Other left-to-right shunts
Bilateral superior vena cava	
Agenesis of the spleen	Bilateral superior vena cava
Bilateral trilobed lungs	Multiple spleens
Bilateral eparterial bronchi	Bilateral bilobed lungs
Bilateral right pulmonary arteries	Bilateral hyparterial bronchi
Visceral heterotaxia	Bilateral left pulmonary arteries
Gastrointestinal anomalies	Visceral heterotaxia
Malrotation	Biliary atresia (absent gallbladder)
Microgastria	Malrotation

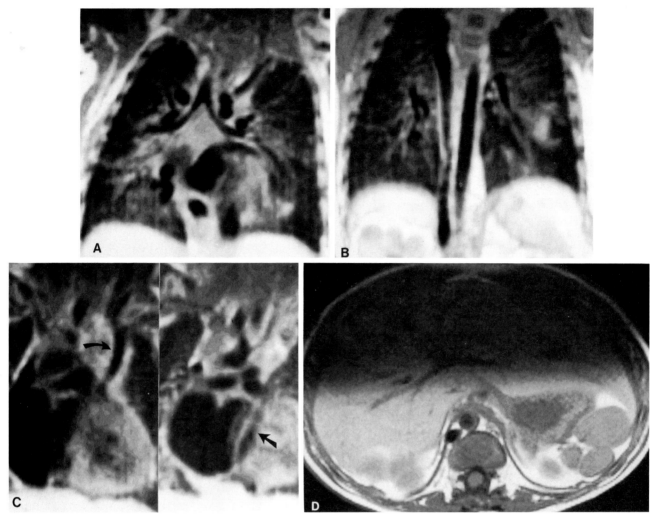

FIG 18–2.
Newborn infant with polysplenia syndrome. **A,** coronal 3-mm spin-echo MR image demonstrates a symmetric tracheobronchial tree with bilateral hyparterial bronchi (bilateral left-sidedness). **B,** coronal 3-mm spin-echo image demonstrates azygos continuation of the inferior vena cava with an enlarged azygos vein to the right of the spine. A portion of the left descending thoracic aorta is also vi-

sualized. **C,** composite axial 3-mm images demonstrate a left superior vena cava *(left, curved arrow)* emptying into the coronary sinus *(right, arrow).* **D,** axial 5-mm spin-echo image confirms the presence of multiple spleens. There is partial visualization of the transverse liver.

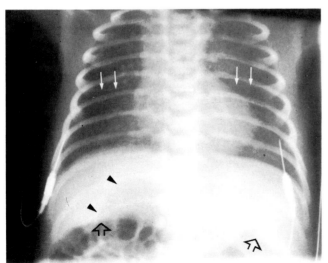

FIG 18–3.
Asplenia syndrome. Characteristic changes of bilateral right-sidedness with symmetry of the tracheobronchial tree, bilateral minor fissures *(white arrows),* visceral heterotaxia with the stomach to the right of the spine *(arrowheads),* and a horizontal liver configuration *(open arrows)* are present.

lateral SVC, (3) abdominal aorta-IVC juxtaposition, (4) total anomalous pulmonary venous return (TAPVR) (frequently the infracardiac type) (Fig 18–3), (5) TGA, (6) common AV valves, (7) pulmonary or subpulmonary stenosis, and (8) common ventricle or large VSD.

Polysplenia is characterized by (1) multiple spleens (Fig 18–2,D), (2) visceral heterotaxia, and (3) CHD. Additional characteristic findings include (1) bilateral hyparterial bronchi (Fig 18–2,A), (2) bilobed lungs, and (3) prominent azygos vein secondary to azygos continuation of the IVC (Figs 18–2,B and 18–4). Cardiac abnormalities include (1) cardiac malposition, (2) anomalous systemic venous return or interruption of the renal subhepatic segment of the IVC, (3) bilateral SVC (Fig 18–2,C), (4) ASD or AV canal, (5) VSD, and (6) partial anomalous venous return.

CHROMOSOMAL ANOMALIES AND SYNDROMES

Less than 0.5% of live births have chromosomal aberrations, and 1 in 7,000 infants show some chromosomal defect. Heart disease in these patients is moderate and approaches 100% in some of the trisomies.

Trisomy 21 (Down Syndrome)

The incidence of this disorder is 1 in 600 to 700 live births and is higher with increased maternal age.

CHD occurs in 40% to 70% of patients. Common defects include (1) AV canal, (see Fig 16–13) (2) atrial septal defect (ASD), (3) VSD, and (4) patent ductus arteriosus (PDA). Almost all forms of congenital cardiac malformations have been described. Noncardiac roentgenographic findings include: (1) 11 pairs of ribs, (2) malsegmentation of the sternum, (3) abnormal configuration of the pelvis, and (4) duodenal stenosis or atresia.

Trisomy 18 (E Syndrome)

The incidence is 1 in 4,000 live births and increases with maternal age. CHD occurs in 90% to 100% of affected infants. Common defects include: (1) VSD, (2) PDA, and (3) ASD.

Trisomy 13 (D Syndrome)

The incidence is 1 in 7,000 to 14,000 live births. CHD is found in approximately 80% of cases. Common defects include: (1) VSD and (2) double-outlet right ventricle.

Turner Syndrome (X Monosomy) and Noonan Syndrome

This syndrome is characterized by web neck, cubitus valgus, short stature, shield chest, and lymph-

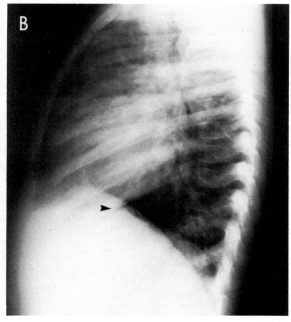

FIG 18–4.
Polysplenia syndrome. AP **(A)** and lateral **(B)** chest roentgenograms demonstrate cardiac-visceral discordance (right-sided stomach) and interruption of the hepatic segment of the inferior vena cava *(arrowhead)*, producing an acute angle between the cardiac silhouette and diaphragm. The dilated azygos vein is not well seen. Note the persistent left superior vena cava *(black arrowheads)* and increased pulmonary vasculature related to an atrioventricular canal.

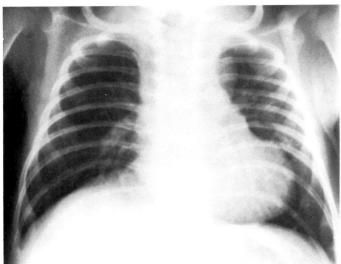

FIG 18–5.
Marfan syndrome. AP chest roentgenogram shows dilatation of the ascending aorta, aortic arch, and descending thoracic aorta. Mild cardiomegaly is related to aortic and mitral insufficiency. Scoliosis and pectus excavatum have not yet developed.

edema. CHD is present in 25% to 66% of patients; coarctation is the most common lesion (70%). Noonan syndrome has many similar clinical and cardiac findings except for a greater incidence of pulmonary valvular stenosis and hypertrophic cardiomyopathy.

Klinefelter Syndrome (XXY Anomaly)

This is characterized by atrophic male genitalia, a eunuchoid appearance, and mental retardation. CHD occurs in 10%. Common defects include: (1) tetralogy of Fallot, (2) ASD, (3) VSD, and (4) tricuspid atresia.

Marfan Syndrome (Arachnodactyly, Dolichostenomelia)

This condition is an autosomal dominant disorder of connective tissue, primarily elastic tissues. Clinical manifestations include (1) long limbs, (2) muscle atrophy, and (3) hyperextendable joints. Cardiac malformations primarily relate to (1) cystic medial necrosis of the ascending aorta, which may progress to aortic dissection (Fig 18–5); (2) aneurysmal dilatation of the ascending aorta and sinus of Valsalva; (3) aortic insufficiency; (4) mitral valve prolapse and insufficiency; and (5) pulmonary artery dilatation. Symptoms of heart failure, usually related to valvular insufficiencies, develop in childhood or in young adulthood.

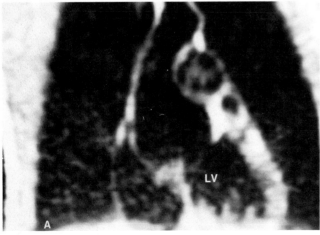
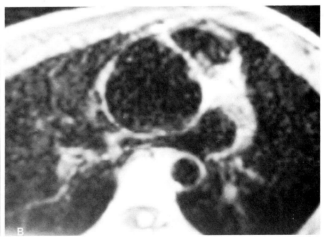

FIG 18–6.
Cystic medial necrosis in a 16-year-old boy with Marfan syndrome. **A,** coronal 10-mm spin-echo MR image demonstrates characteristic features of the cystic medial necrosis with marked dilatation of the aortic sinuses and proximal ascending aorta. *LV,* left ventricle.

B, axial 10-mm spin-echo image demonstrates compression of the right pulmonary artery by the dilated aortic sinuses and ascending aorta. The left descending thoracic aorta is normal in size.

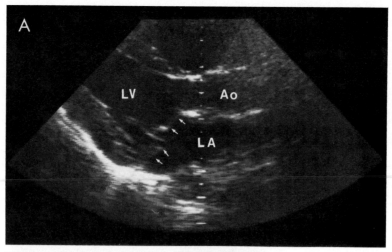

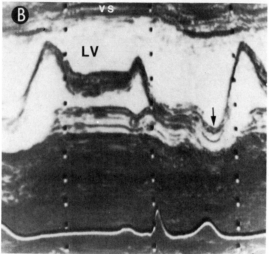

FIG 18–7.
Mitral valve prolapse. **A,** a real-time long-axis echocardiogram shows the mitral valve leaflets *(arrows)* bulging cephalically into the left atrium *(LA)* instead of assuming a more cone-shaped configuration toward the left ventricular *(LV)* cavity *(Ao,* aortic root). **B,** an M-mode echocardiogram shows a hammock-shaped configuration *(arrow)* of the closed mitral valve leaflets bulging posteriorly instead of assuming a straight, anteriorly sloping configuration.

FIG 18–8.
Peripheral pulmonary stenosis. An AP sitting-up right ventriculogram shows severe supravalvular pulmonary stenosis *(large arrow)* and diffuse involvement of the right and left main pulmonary arteries *(small arrow).*

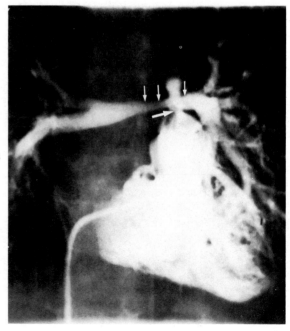

TABLE 18–3.

Syndromes With Cardiac Lesions

Syndrome	Lesion
Ellis-van Creveld syndrome	ASD (single atrium) and VSD
Ehlers-Danlos syndrome	ASD, AV canal, and tetralogy of Fallot
Osteogenesis imperfecta	Aneurysmal dilatation of the great vessels and valvular insufficiency
Holt-Oram syndrome	ASD, VSD
Williams syndrome (supravalvular aortic stenosis) (idiopathic hypercalcemia)	Supravalvular aortic stenosis and peripheral pulmonary artery stenosis (Fig 18–8)
Trisomy 22	Multiple forms of CHD (50%)
Cat-eye syndrome (47 XX/XY)	TAPVR, tetralogy of Fallot, tricuspid atresia, ASD, or VSD
Deletion syndromes (cri du chat, Wolf, carp mouth, etc.)	Moderate incidence, various CHDs
Fetal alcohol syndrome	VSD
Asplenia/polysplenia	See discussion under Cardiosplenic Syndromes
Uhl anomaly	Thinning and enlargement of the right ventricle with right heart failure
Arteriohepatic dysplasia (Alagille syndrome)	Pulmonary stenosis (PS), valvular/peripheral, VSD, ASD, PDA, and coarctation
Cardioauditory syndromes	PS
Cardiofacial syndrome (Cayler syndrome)	VSD, PDA, tetralogy of Fallot, right aortic arch
CHARGE* association	Miscellaneous CHD
DiGeorge syndrome	Interrupted aortic arch, truncus, tetralogy of Fallot
Floppy valve syndrome	Mitral and aortic valve involvement with insufficiency
Kawasaki syndrome	See Chapter 19
Lutembacher syndrome	ASD with mitral valve stenosis
Mucolipidosis III	Valvular heart disease and myocardial failure
Mucopolysaccharidosis	Myocardial infiltration and failure (see Chapter 19)
Neurofibromatosis	Abnormalities of the aorta and major branches, renovascular hypertension
Oculoauriculovertebral dysplasia (Goldenhar syndrome)	Tetralogy of Fallot, ASD, VSD, coarctation
Rubella syndrome	PDA, peripheral pulmonary stenosis, pulmonary artery hypoplasia (see Fig. 15–14)
Shone syndrome	Parachute mitral valve, subaortic stenoses, coarctation, supravalvular left atrial ring
Takayasu arteritis	Large-vessel arterial obstruction, aortic and mitral insufficiency
Thoracoabdominal wall defect (Ravitch syndrome)	Dextroposition, pericardial defects with abdominal organ herniation, VSD, ASD, PS and tetralogy of Fallot, and ventricular diverticula
VATER* association	VSD, PDA, tetralogy of Fallot, single ventricle
Velocardiofacial syndrome	VSD

*ASD = atrial septal defect; CHARGE = coloboma, heart disease, atresia of choanae, retarded growth and development, genital hypoplasia, and ear anomalies or deafness; PDA = patent ductus arteriosus; VATER = vertebral defects, imperforate anus, tracheoesophageal fistula, and radial and renal dysplasia; VSD = ventricular septal defect.

Cardiac and aortic involvement can usually be confirmed with echocardiography, particularly in the evaluation of the ascending aorta and sinuses of Valsalva. MRI is the preferred modality for serial evaluation of patients with cystic medial necrosis to evaluate changes in aortic size and development of dissection (Fig 18–6). Doppler ultrasound can recognize aortic and mitral insufficiency. Mitral valve pro-

lapse can be appreciated either with real-time or M-mode studies (Fig 18–7).

Other syndromes and their most common cardiac lesions are listed on Table 18–3. Many other rare syndromes with associated cardiac malformations are known but are too numerous to mention here.

REFERENCES

Cardiac Malpositions

Attie F, Soni J, Ovseyeviz J, et al: Angiographic studies of atrial ventricular discordance. *Circulation* 1980; 62:407.

Bharati S, Leve M: Positional variants of the heart and its component chambers. *Circulation* 1979; 59:886.

Brandt PWT, Calder AL: Cardiac connections: The segmental approach to radiologic diagnosis in congenital heart disease. *Curr Probl Diagn Radiol* 1977; 7:1.

Carusco G, Becker AE: How to determine atrial situs. Considerations initiated by three cases of absent spleen with a discordant anatomy between bronchi and spleen. *Br Heart J* 1979; 41:559.

Elliott LP: An angiocardiographic and plain film approach to complex congenital heart disease. Classification and simplified nomenclature. *Curr Probl Cardiol* 1978; 3:1.

Freedom RM, Culham JAG, Moes CAF: *Angiocardiography of Congenital Heart Disease.* New York, Macmillan, 1984, p 17.

Shinebourne EA, Macartney FJ, Anderson RH: Sequential chamber localization—logical approach to diagnosis in congenital heart disease. *Br Heart J* 1976; 38:327.

Squaracia U, Ritter DG, Kincaid OW: Dextrocardia: Angiocardiographic study and classification. *Am J Cardiol* 1973; 32:965.

Stanger P, Rudolph AM, Edwards JE: Cardiac malposition. A review based on study of 65 necropsied specimens. *Circulation* 1977; 56:159.

Tonkin IL, Kelley MJ, Bream PR, et al: The frontal chest film as a method of suspecting transposition complexes. *Circulation* 1976; 53:1016.

Tynan MJ, Becker AE, Macartney FJ, et al: Nomenclatures and classification of congenital heart disease. *Br Heart J* 1979; 41:544.

Van Praagh R: Terminology of congenital heart disease: Glossary and commentary. *Circulation* 1977; 56:139.

Van Praagh R: Importance of segmental situs in the diagnosis of congenital heart disease. *Semin Roentgenol* 1985; 20:254.

Winer-Muram HT, Tonkin ILD: The spectrum of heterotaxic syndromes. *Radiol Clin North Am* 1989; 27:1147.

Cardiosplenic Syndromes

Buirski G, Jordan SC, Joffe HS, et al: Superior vena caval abnormalities: Their occurrence rate, associated cardiac abnormalities and angiographic classification in a pediatric population with congenital heart disease. *Clin Radiol* 1986; 37:131.

Freedom RM, Culham JAG, Moes CAF: *Angiocardiography of Congenital Heart Disease.* New York, Macmillan, 1984, p 643.

Freedom RM, Fellows KE Jr: Radiographic visceral patterns in asplenia syndrome. *Radiology* 1973; 106:387.

Jelinek JS, Stuart PL, Done SL, et al: MRI of polysplenia syndrome. *Magn Reson Imaging* 1989; 7:681.

Randall PA, Moller JH, Amplatz K: The spleen and congenital heart disease. *Am J Roentgenol* 1973; 119:551.

Rose V, Izukawa T, Moes CAF: Syndromes of asplenia and polysplenia. A review of the cardiac and noncardiac malformations with special reference to diagnosis and prognosis. *Br Heart J* 1975; 37:840.

Ruttenberg HD: Corrected transposition of the great arteries: Splenic syndromes (asplenia, polysplenia), in Moss AJ, Adams FH, Emmanouilides GC (eds): *Heart Disease in Infants, Children and Adolescents.* Baltimore, Williams & Wilkins, 1977, p 338.

Soto B, Pacifico AD, Souza AS Jr, et al: Identification of thoracic isomerism from the plain chest radiograph. *Am J Roentgenol* 1978; 131:995.

Van Praagh R: Importance of segmental situs in the diagnosis of congenital heart disease. *Semin Roentgenol* 1985; 20:254.

Winer-Muram HT, Tonkin ILD: The spectrum of heterotaxic syndromes. *Radiol Clin North Am* 1989; 27:1147.

Chromosomal Anomalies and Syndromes

Cole RB: Noonan's syndrome: A historical perspective. *Pediatrics* 1980; 66:468.

Come PC, Kulkley GH, McKusick VA, et al: Echocardiographic recognition of silent aortic root dilatation in Marfan's syndrome. *Chest* 1977; 72:789.

Freedom RM, Gerald PS: Congenital heart disease and the cat eye syndrome. *Am J Dis Child* 1973; 126:16.

Kaufman RL, et al: Variable expression of the Holt-Oram syndrome. *Am J Dis Child* 1974; 127:21.

Lin AE, Perloff JK: Upper limb malformations associated with congenital heart disease. *Am J Cardiol* 1985; 55:1576.

O'Brien KM: Congenital syndrome with congenital heart disease. *Semin Roentgenol* 1985; 20:104.

Petitalot JP, Chaix AF, Barraine R: Echocardiographic follow-up in Marfan's syndrome: Mitral, tricuspid, and aortic valve prolapse with calcification of patient foramen ovale. *J Clin Ultrasound* 1986; 14:707.

Rosenthal A: Cardiovascular malformations in Klinefelter's syndrome: Report of 3 cases. *J Pediatr* 1972; 80:471.

Sandor GGS, Smith DF, MacLeod PM: Cardiac malformations in the fetal alcohol syndrome. *J Pediatr* 1981; 93:771.

Smith DW, Jones KL: *Recognizable Patterns of Human Malformation,* ed 3. Philadelphia, WB Saunders, 1982.

19

Acquired Heart Disease

SECTION 1

Myocardial Diseases (Cardiomyopathy)

RHEUMATIC FEVER AND RHEUMATIC HEART DISEASE

Rheumatic fever is a clinical syndrome that follows a small percentage of group A β-hemolytic streptococcal infections. It is characterized by carditis, arthritis, chorea, subcutaneous nodules, and occasionally erythema marginatum. Late complications include significant residual rheumatic valvular heart disease. It remains a common disease in Third World countries, and a recent significant resurgence of cases in the United States has been reported. Both sexes are equally affected, with the onset of disease usually between the ages of 5 and 10 years.

Rheumatic fever follows infection by 10 to 21 days and is probably related to an autoimmune reaction. Certain children are more susceptible than others, and there is a significantly increased chance of sibling involvement or involvement of closely associated children.

Clinical Manifestations

Major manifestations (Jones criteria) include arthritis (75%), carditis (pericardium, myocardium, or endocardium), chorea, subcutaneous nodules, and erythema marginatum. Minor manifestations include fever, elevated erythrocyte sedimentation rate, prolonged PR interval, and arthralgia. A positive C-reactive protein test reaction and evidence of a preceding streptococcal infection, by antibody or culture confirmation, support the diagnosis.

Chest Roentgenography

In the acute phase, chest roentgenographic findings may be normal or show pericardial or cardiac enlargement and congestive heart failure (CHF). Interstitial and alveolar edema, and pleural and occasionally pericardial effusions, may be seen on chest radiographs. In chronic rheumatic valvular disease, focal chamber enlargement, particularly involving the left ventricle and left atrium, is frequent. With aortic insufficiency, general fullness of the entire left heart that is secondary to enlargement of both the left atrium and left ventricle is seen. These chamber enlargements can also be confirmed by the relative relations of the left ventricle and atrium as projected in the lateral roentgenogram. Left atrial enlargement secondary to mitral valve involvement is characterized by an enlarged left atrial appendage producing a focal bulge along the mid-upper left heart border (Fig 19–1). This is unlike the more generalized left atrial enlargement seen with other causes of mitral regurgitation or generalized left heart dilatation.

Echocardiography

Two-dimensional and color Doppler evaluation is important in the determination of atrial and ventricular size, ventricular function, and valvular abnormalities (Fig 19–2). Color Doppler studies, in particular, readily evaluate aortic and mitral valve insufficiencies as well as associated stenosis (see Fig 15–17).

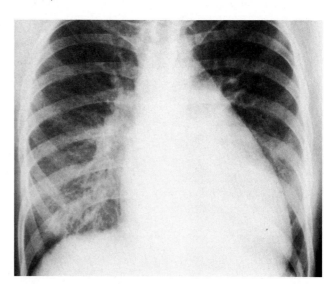

FIG 19–1.
A 13-year-old girl with acute rheumatic fever: frontal chest radiograph demonstrates pulmonary venous hypertension with interstitial edema, and well-defined Kerley B lines. Cardiomegaly is present with moderate left atrial and left ventricular enlargement from mitral regurgitation. The large left atrial appendage produces an abnormal convexity along the left heart margin below the main pulmonary artery.

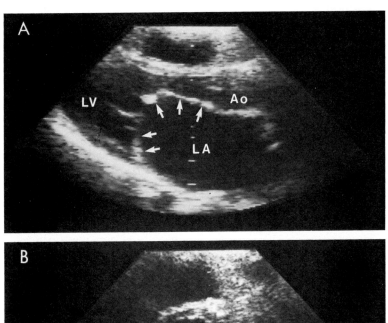

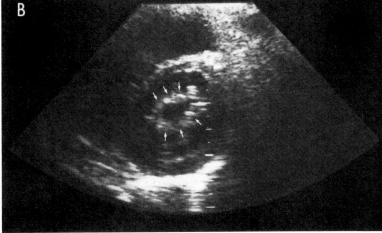

FIG 19–2.
Mitral stenosis secondary to rheumatic heart disease. Real-time long-axis **(A)** and short-axis **(B)** echocardiograms show the doming and thickening of the mitral valve leaflets *(arrows)*. Note the large left atrium *(LA)* in the long-axis projection and small fish-mouthed configuration, marginal increased echogenicity *(small arrows)*, and restricted opening of the mitral valve in the short-axis view. *LV,* left ventricle; *Ao,* aortic root.

INFECTIVE CARDIOMYOPATHIES

Infective cardiomyopathies include fairly common bacterial infectious agents and coxsackievirus (Fig 19–3) along with unusual infections such as that caused by *Trypanosoma cruzi* (Chagas disease) and diphtheria. An acute illness with dyspnea, tachypnea, and congestive failure are characteristic.

COLLAGEN-VASCULAR DISEASE

Collagen-vascular diseases, including juvenile rheumatoid arthritis, periarteritis nodosa, systemic lupus erythematosus, dermatomyositis, and scleroderma, may all present with significant cardiac involvement. They all affect the connective tissue system, probably on an autoimmune basis, with fibrinoid degeneration and proliferation.

Periarteritis Nodosa

This condition is characterized by polyarteritis involving the small- and medium-sized vessels with clinical features of arthralgia, weakness, malaise, and pain. The kidneys are typically involved. Cardiac involvement is less common and secondary to coronary arteritis. Congestive failure is then seen, and pericarditis may occur. Angiography of small- and medium-sized arteries, including the coronary arteries, may demonstrate small aneurysms.

Systemic Lupus Erythematosus

This condition is characterized by an erythematous skin rash but otherwise has many characteristics similar to periarteritis nodosa. Pericarditis is some-

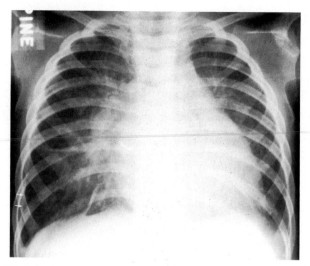

FIG 19–3.
Viral myocarditis. Severe venous congestion with interstitial Kerley lines in the bases, fissural fluid *(arrows)*, and moderate cardiomegaly are present.

what more common and frequently associated with endocarditis and valvular involvement.

Dermatomyositis

Systemic manifestations are similar to those seen in the previously discussed collagen-vascular diseases; however, involvement of muscles and cutaneous tissues is more common, while cardiac and pericardial involvement is rare (10%).

Scleroderma

While exceedingly rare in childhood, when present, cardiac manifestations are frequent (50%). Other frequently involved areas include the cutaneous and subcutaneous tissues and, less frequently, the esophagus, musculature, and blood vessels.

CARDIOMYOPATHY SECONDARY TO METABOLIC DISEASES

Glycogen Storage Disease (Pompe Disease)

This rare autosomal recessive condition is secondary to a lack of acid α-1,4-glucosidase and produces a typical infiltrative, congestive cardiomyopathy. Clinical manifestations appear between 2 and 6 months and include anorexia, failure to thrive, dyspnea, tachypnea, weakness, hepatomegaly, macroglossia, and congestive failure. The Pompe type of glycogen storage disease with predominant cardiac involve-

ment must be differentiated from von Gierke disease and other forms of storage disease (Fig 19–4). Left ventricular outflow tract obstruction and marked myocardial thickening without dilatation may be seen on echocardiography and angiocardiography.

Mucopolysaccharidosis

A rare metabolic inherited disorder secondary to deficiencies in lysosomal enzymes, mucopolysaccharidosis leads to the abnormal storage of mucopolysaccharides. Cardiac involvement occurs in 50% of patients and produces primarily aortic and mitral insufficiency, although primary myocardial involvement may occur; all lead to CHF. Other manifestations include skeletal deformities, corneal opacities, and mental retardation.

THYROID DISORDERS

Hyperthyroidism

Hyperthyroidism is a high output state with tachycardia, irritability, sweating, tremors, and a bounding pulse. CHF is rare, but atrial fibrillation may be present. There may be mild to moderate cardiomegaly and rarely CHF.

Hypothyroidism

Cardiac manifestations are less likely than with hyperthyroidism. When present, they are those of

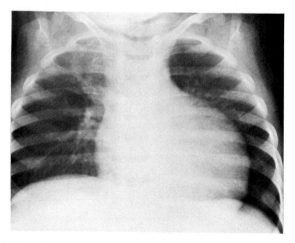

FIG 19–4.
Glycogen storage disease of the heart (Pompe disease) in a 16-month-old girl with moderate cardiomegaly and globular cardiac silhouette. A right upper lobe atelectatic-pneumonic density is also evident. The ventricular walls were grossly thickened rather than dilated.

nonspecific cardiac enlargement and occasionally congestive failure.

CARDIOMYOPATHY SECONDARY TO NEUROMUSCULAR DISEASES

Friedreich Ataxia

Friedreich ataxia is a rare hereditary neurologic disorder with cardiac involvement secondary to hypertrophy of the muscle fibers of the cardiac chambers and associated round-cell infiltration. While neurologic manifestations such as gait disturbance usually precede cardiac manifestations, cardiovascular disease may be the presenting manifestation in 10% of cases. Cardiac manifestations include coronary artery stenosis, myocardial fibrosis, and hypertrophic cardiomyopathy, with left ventricular outflow tract obstruction.

Progressive Muscular Dystrophy

Progressive muscular dystrophy is a rare hereditary muscular disorder with relatively rare cardiac involvement. Left ventricular hypertrophy may develop early in the disease and lead to generalized cardiac enlargement and congestive failure. The Duchenne type is most commonly seen in boys in early childhood with progressive fatigability, difficulty in rising owing to muscular weakness, and a waddling gait.

HYPERTROPHIC CARDIOMYOPATHY (ASYMMETRIC SEPTAL HYPERTROPHY)

The genetic form of hypertrophic cardiomyopathy was discussed in Chapter 16. Hypertrophic cardiomyopathy may also be seen with Turner and Noonan syndrome, Friedreich ataxia, leopard syndrome, and in infants of diabetic mothers. Hypertrophy of the ventricular septum exceeding the thickness of the posterior left ventricular wall, and left ventricular outflow tract and, rarely, right ventricular outflow tract obstruction may be seen on echocardiography and angiography. Cardiac disease in infants of diabetic mothers is discussed below.

CARDIAC DISEASE IN INFANTS OF DIABETIC OR PREDIABETIC MOTHERS

Infants of diabetic or prediabetic mothers frequently exhibit cardiovascular problems including (1) asymmetric septal hypertrophy (hypertrophic obstructive cardiomyopathy) with left ventricular outflow tract obstruction, (2) cardiomegaly with a poorly functioning heart because of intrinsic cardiomyopathy that is possibly secondary to hypoxia or hypoglycemia, or both, and (3) other intrinsic congenital cardiac malformations. Other manifestations include involvements of the genitourinary, nervous, gastrointestinal, and pulmonary systems. Combined system involvement constitutes the Vater syndrome (see Table 18–3).

Asymmetric septal hypertrophy occurs in this condition, as in the genetic form of hypertrophic cardiomyopathy with hypertrophy of the muscle bundles involved in the upper two thirds of the ventricular septum. There may be some degree of involvement of the adjacent anterior and posterior free walls of the right and left ventricles. Unlike the genetic form of hypertrophic cardiomyopathy, the septal hypertrophy resolves within the first year of life. Intrinsic congenital heart disease (CHD) occurs in approximately 4% with ventricular septal defect (VSD), transposition of the great vessels, and coarctation being the most common lesions.

Chest Roentgenography

Cardiomegaly, CHF, and respiratory distress syndrome (RDS) are common chest film findings. Increased subcutaneous fat, especially along the lateral chest wall, may be helpful in suggesting the diagnosis (Fig 19–5).

Echocardiography

Asymmetric septal hypertrophy shows disproportionate thickening of the mid- to upper portion of the ventricular septum and, to some extent, the free anterior and posterior left ventricular walls, with a septal-posterior wall ratio greater than 1.3:1. Narrowing of the left ventricular outflow tract may be seen with systolic anterior motion of the mitral valve and midsystolic preclosure or flutter of the aortic valve until septal thickness resolves to normal. Other intrinsic congenital heart lesions may also be identified. Cardiac dilatation and function may also be evaluated.

Angiocardiography

Septal thickening can be demonstrated with biventricular injection in the long axial projection. Left ventricular and, rarely, right ventricular outflow tract obstruction also may be seen.

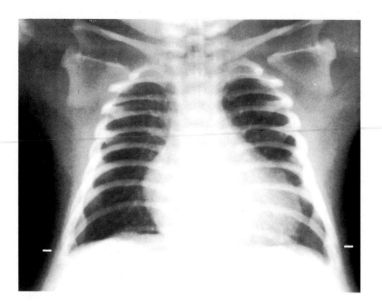

FIG 19–5.
Infant of a diabetic mother. An AP chest roentgenogram shows characteristic increased subcutaneous fat along the lateral chest walls bilaterally *(white bars)* with a combined right and left thick-ness greater than 8 mm. There is mild cardiomegaly with a non-specific cardiac silhouette but with evidence of asymmetric septal hypertrophy on echocardiography (see Fig 16–45).

OTHER CARDIOMYOPATHIES

Endocardial fibroelastosis (EFE) may occur as a primary disease with a high incidence of familial involvement, or secondary to CHD, particularly when associated with left ventricular outflow tract obstruction. Primary EFE has been discussed in Chapter 16. Ninety-five percent of patients with primary EFE have ventricular dilatation. Rarely, the left ventricle may be normal or small in size and these patients have impaired ventricular filling on hemodynamic study, and mild to moderate reduction in left ventricular contractility.

Persistence of spongy myocardium is a rare myocardial disorder characterized by the persistence of excessively prominent ventricular trabeculations and deep intertrabecular recesses. It may occur as a primary form of CHF (isolated noncompaction of left ventricular myocardium) or accompany other forms of CHD, particularly those with right or left ventricular outflow tract obstruction. Two-dimensional echocardiography and angiography demonstrate unusually fine trabeculations and multiple myocardial recesses.

Other rare forms of cardiomyopathy may include histiocytoid cardiomyopathy of infancy characterized by intractable supraventricular or ventricular tachydysrhythmia, hypereosinophilic syndrome with features of restrictive cardiomyopathy and mural thrombi, and right ventricular dysplasia (Uhl anomaly) with marked right ventricular thinning and ventricular tachydysrhythmias.

HIGH OUTPUT STATES

Anemias

Chronic severe anemia is an important cause of cardiomegaly and CHF. Most commonly observed in thalassemia major and sickle cell anemia, chronic anemia leads to high output and generalized enlargement of all cardiac chambers. Clinical features of anemia include pallor, lassitude, and specific features related to the specific anemia type. CHF not only relates to volume overload but to myocardial hypoxia secondary to an inadequate coronary oxygen content. Typical features of cardiomegaly and CHF are common (Fig 19–6).

Arteriovenous Malformations

Large arteriovenous malformations or fistulas present with high output failure and cardiomegaly. Most commonly these malformations are cerebral, but they may occur in the liver, other viscera, or the extremities. Marked cardiomegaly is the rule. In spite of marked cardiomegaly, congestive failure is less conspicuous than with other forms of marked heart enlargement (Fig 19–7,A and B). Enlargement of the aorta may be appreciated, and with cerebral malformations, the brachiocephalic vessels may also be enlarged. Real-time ultrasound is helpful not only in evaluating the size of the heart and vascular structures but also in actual demonstration of the arteriovenous malformation in the head, liver, or other organs (Fig 19–7,C).

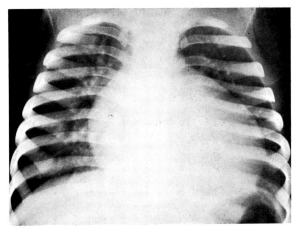

FIG 19–6.
Generalized cardiac dilatation secondary to long-standing anemia with a hemoglobin level of 3.2 g/100 mL. Cardiac dilatation is slow to develop with anemia and persists for a considerable period after correction of the anemia.

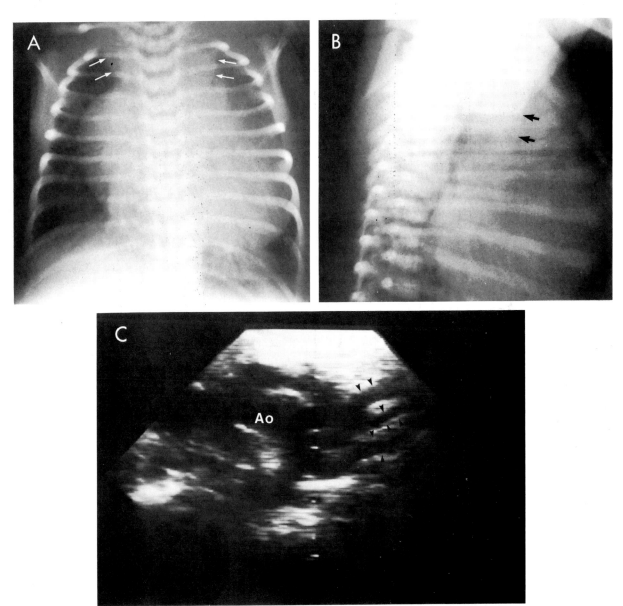

FIG 19–7.
Cerebral arteriovenous malformation. AP **(A)** and lateral **(B)** chest roentgenograms in a neonate show marked cardiomegaly out of proportion to the degree of congestive failure. Widening of the superior mediastinum *(arrows)* is secondary to dilatation of the ascending aorta and brachiocephalic vessels. Compression left lower lobe atelectasis is present in the retrocardiac area. **C,** a real-time echocardiogram confirms a large aorta *(Ao)* and brachiocephalic vessels *(arrowheads)*. The echoencephalogram visualized a large vein of Galen aneurysm (not shown).

Angiography, computed tomography (CT) or cine-CT, or magnetic resonance imaging (MRI) will further identify the malformation.

Chorioangioma of the Placenta

Chorioangioma is the most common benign tumor of the placenta. This hemangiomatous neoplasm results in arteriovenous shunting between the umbilical artery and vein. This may produce a syndrome of polyhydramnios, fetal hypoxia, and high output cardiac state with cardiomegaly and CHF in the neonate. Echocardiography will demonstrate dilatation of the inferior vena cava, cardiac chambers, and thoracic and abdominal aorta secondary to the arteriovenous shunting in utero.

Twin-Twin Transfusion Syndrome

In twin-twin transfusion syndrome there is an intrauterine discrepancy in blood volume between twins. One twin suffers from polycythemia, the other from anemia, at birth. The donor twin is anemic with cardiomegaly and occasionally congestive failure and hydrops. The recipient twin is polycythemic and also may show cardiomegaly, and congestive failure (neonatal plethora syndrome).

REFERENCES

Rheumatic Fever and Rheumatic Heart Disease
Hirschfeld SS, Kaimal PK: Echocardiographic evaluation of acquired valvular diseases of the heart. *Semin Roentgenol* 1979; 14:116.

Schieken RM, Kerber RE: Echocardiographic abnormalities in acute rheumatic fever. *Am J Cardiol* 1976; 38:458.

Veasy LG, Wiedmeier SE, Orsmond GS, et al: Resurgence of rheumatic fever in the intermountain United States. *N Engl J Med* 1987; 316:421.

Collagen-Vascular Disease
Eggebrecht RF, Kleiger RE: Echocardiographic patterns in scleroderma. *Chest* 1977; 71:47.

Ghafour AS, Gutgesell HP: Echocardiographic evaluation of left ventricular function in children with congestive cardiomyopathy. *Am J Cardiol* 1979; 44:1332.

Maron BJ: Cardiomyopathies, in Adams FH, Emmanouilides GC, Riemenschneider TA (eds): *Heart Disease in Infants, Children, and Adolescents.* Baltimore, Williams & Wilkins, 1989.

Paget SA, Bulkley GH, Grauer LF, et al: Mitral valve disease in systemic lupus erythematosus: A cause of severe congestive heart failure reversed by valve replacement. *Am J Med* 1975; 59:134.

Steiner RE: The roentgen features of the cardiomyopathies. *Semin Roentgenol* 1969; 4:311.

Cardiomyopathy Secondary to Metabolic Diseases
Johnson GL, Vine DL, Cottrill GM, et al: Echocardiographic mitral valve deformity in the mucopolysaccharidoses. *Pediatrics* 1981; 67:401.

Rees A, Elbl F, Minhas K, et al: Echocardiographic evidence of outflow tract obstruction in Pompe's disease (glycogen storage disease of the heart). *Am J Cardiol* 1976; 37:1103.

Renteria VG, Ferrans VJ, Roberts WC: The heart in Hurler syndrome. *Am J Cardiol* 1976; 38:487.

Schieken RM, Kerber RE, Ionasescu VV, et al: Cardiac manifestations of the mucopolysaccharidoses. *Circulation* 1975; 52:700.

Thyroid Disorders
Farrehi C, Mitchell M, Fawcett DM: Heart failure in congenital thyrotoxicosis. *Pediatrics* 1968; 37:640.

Cardiomyopathy Secondary to Neuromuscular Diseases
Boehm TM, Dickerson RB, Glasser SP: Hypertrophic subaortic stenosis occurring in a patient with Friedreich's ataxia. *Am J Med Sci* 1970; 260:279.

Freedom RM, Culham JAG, Moes CAF: Anomalies of the coronary arteries, in Freedom RM, Culham JAG, Moes CAF (eds): *Angiocardiography of Congenital Heart Disease.* New York, Macmillan, 1984, p 407.

Perloff JK: Cardiomyopathy associated with heredofamilial neuromyopathic disease. *Mod Concepts Cardiovasc Dis* 1971; 40:23.

Ruschhaupt DG, Thilenius OG, Cassels DE: Friedreich's ataxia associated with hypertrophic subaortic stenosis. *Am Heart J* 1972; 84:95.

Walton JN, Gardner-Medwin D: Progressive muscular dystrophy and the myotonic disorders, in Walton JN (ed): *Disorders of Voluntary Muscles,* ed 3. London, Churchill Livingstone, 1974, p 561.

Hypertrophic Cardiomyopathy (Asymmetric Septal Hypertrophy)
Baltaxe HA, Levin AR, Ehlers KH, et al: The appearance of the left ventricle in Noonan's syndrome. *Radiology* 1973; 109:155–159.

Ellis K: Use of angiocardiography in cardiomyopathies, in Elliott LP (ed): *Cardiac Imaging in Infants, Children, and Adults.* Philadelphia, JB Lippincott, 1991, p 477.

Gottlieb S, Meltzer RS: Echocardiography in cardiomyopathies, in Elliott LP (ed): *Cardiac Imaging in Infants, Children, and Adults.* Philadelphia, JB Lippincott, 1991, p 468.

Cardiac Disease in Infants of Diabetic or Prediabetic Mothers

Dunn V, Condon VR, Nixon GW, et al: Infants of diabetic mothers: Radiographic manifestations. *Am J Roentgenol* 1981; 137:123.

Gutgesell HP, Speer ME, Rosenberg HS: Characterization of the cardiomyopathy in infants of diabetic mothers. *Circulation* 1980; 61:441.

Maron GJ, Tajik AJ, Ruttenberg HD, et al: Echocardiographic abnormalities in infants of diabetic mothers. *Circulation* 1982; 65:7.

Wolfe RR, Way GL: Cardiomyopathies in infants of diabetic mothers. *Johns Hopkins Med J* 1977; 140:177.

High Output States

Clarke CT, Geoh TH, Blackwood A, et al: Massive pulmonary arteriovenous fistula in the newborn. *Br Heart J* 1976; 38:1092.

Cubberley DA, Jaffe RB, Nixon GW: Sonographic demonstration of galenic arteriovenous malformations in the neonate. *Am J Neuroradiol* 1982; 3:435.

Holden AM, Fyler DC, Shillito J Jr, et al: Congestive heart failure from intracranial arteriovenous fistula in infancy. Clinical and physiologic considerations in eight cases. *Pediatrics* 1972; 49:30.

Lindsay J Jr, Meshel JC, Patterson RH: The cardiovascular manifestations of sickle cell disease. *Arch Intern Med* 1974; 133:643.

Sapire CW, Casta A, Donner RM, et al: Dilatation of the ascending aorta: A radiological and echocardiographic diagnostic sign in arteriovenous malformations in neonates and young infants. *Am J Cardiol* 1979; 44:493.

Swischuk LE, Crowe JE, Mewborne EG: Large vein of Galen aneurysm in the neonate: A constellation of diagnostic chest and neck radiologic findings. *Pediatr Radiol* 1977; 6:4.

Tonkin ILD: Placental chorioangioma: Rare cause of congestive heart failure and hydrops fetalis in the newborn. *Am J Roentgenol* 1980; 134:181–183.

SECTION 2

Valvular Diseases

BACTERIAL ENDOCARDITIS

Bacterial endocarditis is a rare but serious cardiac disease of childhood. It may be classified as (1) acute, (2) subacute, or (3) chronic. In acute or subacute forms in patients under 2 years of age, the disease affects one or more normal heart valves in the absence of underlying heart disease. In patients over 2 years of age, endocarditis is usually superimposed on CHD. Streptococcal infection is the most common etiologic agent; staphylococcal infection is second, but is the prevalent organism with intravenous drug abusers and in tricuspid endocarditis.

Clinical Manifestations

Fever, malaise, anemia, pallor, and sepsis are common. Hematuria and petechiae indicate embolic phenomena.

Chest Roentgenography

Cardiomegaly and CHF are common (Fig 19–8). Abnormalities in the silhouette may indicate underlying CHD. With right heart involvement, parenchymal pulmonary lesions related to septic emboli are frequent.

Other Imaging

Echocardiography will demonstrate echogenic masses attached to the valves or walls of the heart (Fig 19–9). Underlying cardiac disease may also be recognized along with a degree of myocardial dysfunction. Mycotic aneurysms may develop when infections involve the great arteries or a patent ductus (Fig 19–10). Prompt diagnosis by CT or cine-CT, digital subtraction angiography, or MRI is critical in this life-threatening process (Fig 19–11).

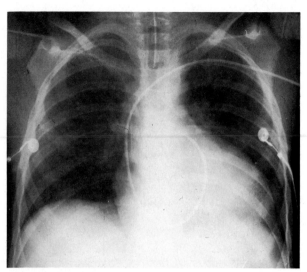

FIG 19–8.
Bacterial endocarditis. AP supine chest roentgenogram in a patient with bacterial endocarditis superimposed upon congenital aortic valve disease. Gross cardiomegaly and left heart dilatation with mild congestive failure are present. A Swan-Ganz catheter is in the main pulmonary artery, and a central venous line is in the superior vena cava.

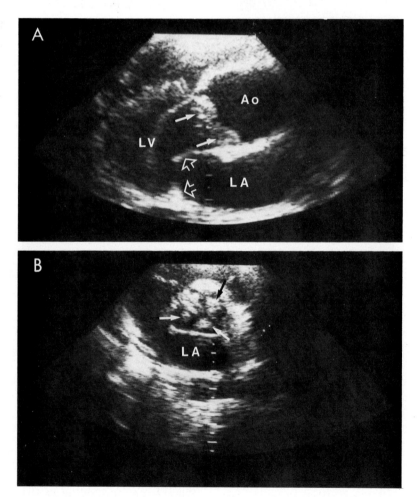

FIG 19–9.
Bacterial endocarditis. Long-axis **(A)** and short-axis **(B)** echocardiograms at the level of the aortic root show the echogenic vegetations attached to all three aortic valve cusps *(arrows)*. Dilatation of the ascending aorta is related to the preexisting valvular aortic stenosis. Echogenic mitral valves *(open arrows)* with limited opening of the anterior mitral leaflet indicate mitral stenosis.

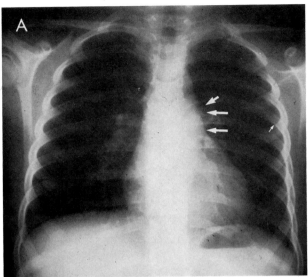
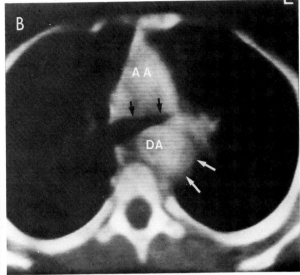

FIG 19–10.
Mycotic aneurysm. **A,** coarctation of the aorta with secondary mycotic aneurysm involving the poststenotic segment of the thoracic aorta. A fusiform paravertebral mass projects into the retrocardiac space *(arrows)*. Minor rib notching is also evident *(small arrows)* with mild cardiomegaly. **B,** a dynamic contrast-enhanced CT scan at the level of the carina and left mainstem bronchus *(black arrows)* demonstrates a contrast-filled mycotic aneurysm extending posteriorly into the paravertebral area with a relative fusiform configuration *(white arrows)*. AA, ascending aorta; DA, descending aorta.

MITRAL VALVE PROLAPSE

Mitral valve prolapse refers to the posterior protrusion of mitral valve tissue beyond the boundary of the mitral annulus during systole. One or both mitral valve leaflets may be involved, and mitral insufficiency varies from minor to severe.

Mitral valve prolapse is probably a congenital malformation occurring as a familial condition and is occasionally associated with myxomatous mitral

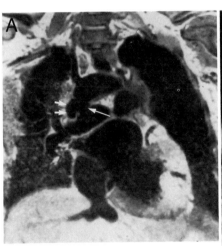
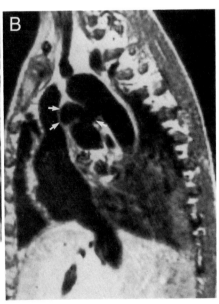

FIG 19–11.
MRI of mycotic aneurysm after Potts anastomosis between the right descending aorta and right pulmonary artery. Coronal **(A)** and sagittal **(B)** cardiac-gated spin-echo images demonstrate a mycotic aneurysm *(arrows)* extending anterolaterally from the Potts anastomosis (same patient as in Figure 16–67).

valve degeneration and CHD (ostium secundum atrial septal defect). It may occur as a complication of acquired heart disease, e.g., ischemic heart disease, bacterial endocarditis, Marfan syndrome, mucopolysaccharidosis.

Clinical Manifestations

Clinical findings include apical midsystolic or late systolic murmurs and nonejection clicks, ventricular and supraventricular arrhythmia, and occasionally, severe myocardial ischemia and CHF.

Chest Roentgenography

Findings vary from normal to minor left atrial enlargement. On rare occasions, with severe myocardial ischemia, left ventricular dilatation is present. CHF occurs most often with complicated acquired varieties.

Echocardiography

Anterior and posterior mitral valve leaflet prolapse may be seen with real time and M-mode studies (see Fig 18–8). Color Doppler examination may help to quantitate the severity of mitral regurgitation.

Angiocardiography

The left ventriculogram, in the long-axis projection, demonstrates "billowing" of the leaflets posteriorly into the left atrial annulus to varying degrees. Some scalloping and irregularity of the prolapsed tissue may also be evident.

Prognosis

The prognosis in isolated (congenital) mitral valve prolapse is good. In acquired or degenerative cases or with associated intrinsic cardiac malformation, progressive insufficiency and cardiac dysfunction are expected.

CONGENITAL TRICUSPID REGURGITATION

This is a rare congenital anomaly presenting in the newborn with right heart failure, marked cardiomegaly, and cyanosis. Congenital tricuspid regurgitation may be secondary to: (1) Ebstein malformation (see Figs 16–101 and 16–102), (2) tricuspid valve

dysplasia, (3) pulmonary atresia with intact septum, and (4) anoxic states with myocardial ischemia.

Clinical Manifestations

Tachycardia, pansystolic murmur with a gallop rhythm, and cyanosis are common.

Chest Roentgenography

Marked cardiac enlargement (wall-to-wall heart) nearly obscures the lungs. Pulmonary blood flow appears diminished with small central pulmonary vessels owing to right-to-left interatrial shunting.

Echocardiography

Echocardiogram demonstrates marked right heart enlargement. Doppler evaluation confirms the tricuspid regurgitation (see Fig 15–18) as well as right-to-left shunting at the atrial level. Other intrinsic congenital heart lesions may also be demonstrated, e.g., pulmonary atresia.

Angiocardiography

Right ventriculography demonstrates marked enlargement of the right ventricle, right atrium, tricuspid regurgitation, and right-to-left shunting at the atrial level. There is frequently no filling of the pulmonary artery, and the differential diagnosis of pulmonary atresia with tricuspid insufficiency must be resolved. Since a patent ductus is usually present, a retrograde aortogram will fill the ductus and pulmonary artery, demonstrate pulmonary regurgitation, and thus rule out pulmonary atresia. Pulmonary regurgitation may also be evaluated by Doppler ultrasound.

CONGENITAL AORTIC INSUFFICIENCY

This rare congenital lesion produces cardiomegaly with left ventricular dilatation, dilatation of the ascending and descending aorta (Fig 19–12), and occasionally CHF. Doppler echocardiography will demonstrate aortic insufficiency and left ventricular dilatation. Aortography can confirm the diagnosis and differentiate other lesions simulating congenital aor-

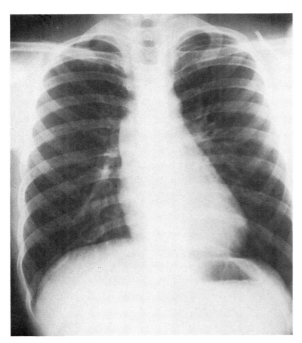

FIG 19–12.
Congenital aortic stenosis and insufficiency. There is moderate dilatation of the ascending aorta, aortic arch, and descending thoracic aorta. Mild left ventricular dilatation is present.

tic insufficiency, e.g., an aortico–left ventricular tunnel or a ruptured sinus of Valsalva aneurysm.

CONGENITAL MITRAL REGURGITATION

Congenital mitral regurgitation may be a primary malformation or part of a complex CHD. The abnormality primarily results from malformation of the valve or tensor apparatus, papillary muscle abnormality, or a ruptured chorda. It has been reported with corrected transposition of the great arteries (systemic atrioventricular valve), single ventricle, atrioventricular canal, Hurler syndrome, homocystinuria, Marfan syndrome, myocarditis and myocardiopathy, mitral valve prolapse, and anomalous origin of the left coronary artery.

Imaging

Chest roentgenography demonstrates marked cardiomegaly with left ventricular and left atrial enlargement. Venous congestion may be present. Doppler and real-time echocardiography demonstrate mitral regurgitation as well as some of the associated valvular defects and underlying cardiac problems. Left ventricular angiography will confirm and grade the mitral regurgitation as well as evaluate associated lesions.

REFERENCES

Bacterial Endocarditis

Berger M, Delfin LA, Jelveh M, et al: Two-dimensional echocardiographic findings in right sided infective endocarditis. *Circulation* 1980; 61:855.

Ellis K, Jaffe C, Malm JR, et al: Infective endocarditis: Roentgenographic considerations. *Radiol Clin North Am* 1973; 11:415.

Jaffe RB, Condon VR: Mycotic aneurysms of the pulmonary artery and aorta. *Radiology* 1975; 116:291–298.

Martin RP, Meltzer RS, Chia BL, et al: Clinical utility of two-dimensional echocardiography in infective endocarditis. *Am J Cardiol* 1980; 46:379.

Melvin ET, Berger M, Lutzker LG, et al: Noninvasive methods for detection of valve vegetations in infective endocarditis. *Am J Cardiol* 1981; 47:271.

Rubenson DS, Tucker CR, Stinson EB, et al: The use of echocardiography in diagnosing culture-negative endocarditis. *Circulation* 1981; 64:641.

Talano JV, Menlman DJ: Two-dimensional echocardiography in infective endocarditis. *Semin Ultrasound CT MR* 1981; 2:149.

Mitral Valve Prolapse

Hickey AJ, Wolfers J, Wilcken DEL: Mitral valve prolapse. *Med J Aust* 1981; 1:31.

Jerasaty RM: Mitral valve prolapse: Click syndrome. *Prog Cardiovasc Dis* 1973; 15:623.

Kittredge RD, Shimonura S, Cameron A, et al: Prolapsing mitral valve leaflets: Cineangiographic demonstration. *Am J Roentgenol* 1970; 109:84.

Krivokapich J, Child JS, Dadourian BJ: Reassessment of echocardiographic criteria for diagnosis of mitral valve prolapse. *Am J Cardiol* 1988; 61:131–135.

Congenital Tricuspid Regurgitation, Aortic Insufficiency, and Mitral Regurgitation

Berman W Jr, Whiteman V, Stanger P, et al: Congenital tricuspid incompetency simulating pulmonary atresia with intact ventricular septum: A report of two cases. *Am Heart J* 1978; 96:655.

Bucciarelli RL, Nelson RN, Egan EA II: Transient tricuspid insufficiency of the newborn: A form of myocardial dysfunction in stressed newborns. *Pediatrics* 1977; 59:330.

Chan CC, Morganroth J: Tricuspid regurgitation and tricuspid prolapse demonstrated with contrast cross-section echocardiography. *Am J Cardiol* 1980; 46:983.

Freedom RM, Culham JAG, Moes CAF: Differentiation of functional and structural pulmonary atresia: Role of aortography. *Am J Cardiol* 1978; 41:914.

Meltzer RS, Hoogenhuyze DV, Surruys PW, et al: Diagnosis of tricuspid regurgitation by contrast echocardiography. *Circulation* 1981; 63:1093.

SECTION 3

Coronary Artery Disease and Anomalies

MUCOCUTANEOUS LYMPH NODE SYNDROME (KAWASAKI DISEASE)

Kawasaki disease is characterized by an acute illness with fever, conjunctivitis, edema of the hands and feet, and an erythematous rash on the trunk, palms, and soles. Red, dry mucous membranes, fissures about the mouth, lymphadenopathy, leukocytosis, and an elevated erythrocyte sedimentation rate are also common.

Clinical Cardiac Manifestations

In the acute phase, little evidence of cardiac involvement is identified. Later, coronary thromboarteritis leads to aneurysmal dilatation of the coronary arteries, coronary thrombosis, left ventricular ischemia and dysfunction, myocardial infarction, and rarely, death.

Chest Roentgenograms

Acutely, the heart appears normal. Later, with coronary arteritis, cardiomegaly and CHF may be seen.

Echocardiography

Aneurysmal dilatation of the proximal coronary arteries may be identified (Fig 19–13) in the later

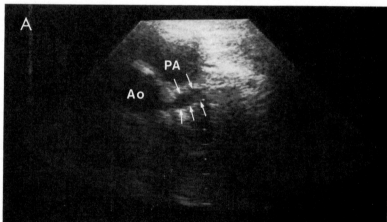

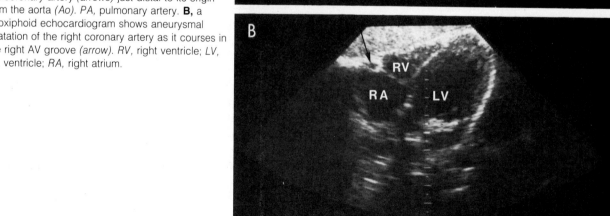

FIG 19–13.
Kawasaki disease. **A,** a short-axis echocardiogram at the aortic root shows aneurysmal dilatation of the left coronary artery *(arrows)* just distal to its origin from the aorta *(Ao)*. PA, pulmonary artery. **B,** a subxiphoid echocardiogram shows aneurysmal dilatation of the right coronary artery as it courses in the right AV groove *(arrow)*. RV, right ventricle; *LV,* left ventricle; *RA,* right atrium.

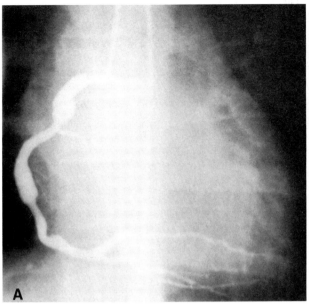

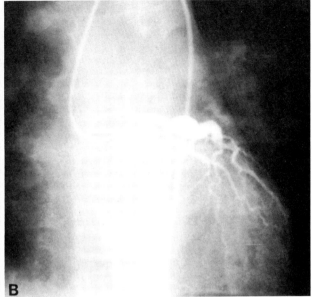

FIG 19–14.
A 10-year-old girl with mucocutaneous lymph node syndrome (Kawasaki disease): selective right **(A)** and left **(B)** coronary angiograms in the frontal projection demonstrate multiple fusiform and saccular aneurysms of the proximal and mid–right coronary artery and proximal left anterior descending coronary artery. A follow-up angiogram 1 year later was unchanged.

stages of the illness in 15% to 20% of patients. Cardiac dysfunction may also be determined.

Angiocardiography

Aortography and coronary arteriography may occasionally be necessary to define the extent of coronary artery involvement in patients with left ventricular dysfunction (Fig 19–14).

Prognosis

The prognosis is good with aspirin and gamma globulin therapy.

CORONARY CALCINOSIS (IDIOPATHIC HYPERCALCEMIA OF INFANCY)

This condition indicates a rare generalized vascular abnormality with calcification of the internal elastic lamina that is associated with fibrosis and proliferation of the medium-sized arteries. Myocardial ischemia, infarction, and death may ensue. Clinical presentation is from birth to 2 years. Clinical signs include (1) dyspnea, (2) tachycardia, (3) pallor, (4) weakness, (5) respiratory distress, and (6) poor feeding. Chest roentgenography demonstrates generalized cardiomegaly and CHF. Calcification may be seen in the brachiocephalic, brachial, or subclavian arteries. Coronary calcification may be seen, particularly with chest fluoroscopy.

ATHEROSCLEROSIS

This is a relatively rare lesion of infancy and childhood and is particularly related to patients with familial hypercholesterolemia or familial type II hyperlipoproteinemia. Cardiomegaly and CHF secondary to myocardial ischemia may be seen.

MISCELLANEOUS

Many other congenital malformations of coronary arteries may be seen and are usually associated with CHD (see Chapter 17). Coronary artery anatomy is important in surgical planning, particularly in patients with tetralogy of Fallot and in transposition where arterial-switch procedures are being contemplated. Angiography with biplane studies, either with aortic root or selective coronary arteriography, is indicated in either anteroposterior (AP), lateral, or long-axis projections, with cranial-caudad angulation, if needed, to facilitate the planning.

REFERENCES

Andersen GE, Friss-Hansen B: Neonatal diagnosis of familial type II hyperlipoproteinemia. *Pediatrics* 1976; 52:2.

Bisset GS III, Strife JL, McCloskey J: MR imaging of coronary artery aneurysms in a child with Kawasaki disease. *Am J Roentgenol* 1989; 152:805–807.

Bloch A, Dinsmore RE, Lees RS: Coronary arteriographic findings in type II and type IV hyperlipoproteinemia. *Lancet* 1976; 1:928.

Frey EE, Matherne GP, Mahoney LT, et al: Coronary artery aneurysms due to Kawasaki disease: Diagnosis with ultrafast CT. *Radiology* 1988; 167:725–726.

Fujiwara T, Fujiwara H, Ueda T, et al: Comparison of macroscopic, postmortem, angiographic and two-dimensional echocardiographic findings of coronary aneurysm in children with Kawasaki disease. *Am J Cardiol* 1986; 57:761–764.

Hewitt I, Yu JS, Kozlowski K, et al: Generalized arterial

obstruction in the newborn with calcification. *Aust Paediatr J* 1977; 13:239.

Kuribayashi S, Ootaki M, Tsuji M, et al: Coronary angiographic abnormalities in mucocutaneous lymph node syndrome: Acute findings and long-term follow-up. *Radiology* 1989; 172:629–633.

Lussier-Lazaroff J, Fletcher BD: Idiopathic infantile arterial calcification: Roentgen diagnosis of a rare cause of coronary artery occlusion. *Pediatr Radiol* 1973; 1:224.

Onouchi Z, Simazu S, Kiyosawa N, et al: Aneurysms of the coronary arteries in Kawasaki disease: An angiographic study of 30 cases. *Circulation* 1982; 66:1.

Takahashi MT, Mason W, Lewis AB: Regression of coronary aneurysms in patients with Kawasaki syndrome. *Circulation* 1987; 75:387–394.

SECTION 4

Pericardial Disease

CONGENITAL ABSENCE OF THE PERICARDIUM

Congenital absence of the pericardium is probably secondary to early atrophy of the left duct of Cuvier, which is responsible for the blood supply to the embryonic pleuropericardial membrane. In normal individuals, this membrane forms the left pericardium. The right duct of Cuvier forms the superior vena cava, almost always ensuring adequate nutrition to the right pleuropericardial membrane.

Congenital absence of the left pericardium, either partial or total, accounts for the great majority of cases. Congenital isolated right-sided pericardial defects, total pericardial absence, and diaphragmatic pericardial defects are rare. Total absence of the left pericardium is the most common defect, accounting for approximately 70% of patients. Approximately 30% of patients have associated congenital anomalies of the heart and lung, including patent ductus arteriosus, atrial septal defect, tetralogy of Fallot, and pulmonary sequestration.

Patients may present with chest pain, systolic murmurs, usually heard along the left sternal border or in the pulmonary area, and an abnormal point of maximal cardiac impulse, usually seen in patients with complete absence of the left pericardium. Although usually considered a benign condition, congenital pericardial defects are potentially serious in

that death may occur from herniation and strangulation of the heart.

Chest radiographs in patients with partial or small left-sided pericardial defects demonstrate the heart to be in normal position, but the configuration is abnormal except for those cases without extension of the left atrial appendage outside the confines of the defect. The abnormality consists of varying degrees of prominence or enlargement in the vicinity of the left atrial appendage along the left upper heart border (Fig 19–15,A). A partial pericardial defect can be confirmed when gas enters the pericardial sac secondary to a diagnostic left pneumothorax, or by visualization of the left atrial appendage extending through the pericardial defect on CT or MRI examination (Fig 19–15,B and C).

In patients with complete absence of the left pericardium, the chest radiograph demonstrates the heart to be displaced to the left with concomitant clockwise rotation so that the left border of the heart is formed by the right ventricle. Characteristically, the trachea is midline. Varying degrees of prominence of the main pulmonary artery along the left upper heart border are noted. There may be separation between the aortic arch and the pulmonary artery with interposition of a segment of lung between the aorta and pulmonary artery, and also between the inferior border of the heart and the left hemidia-

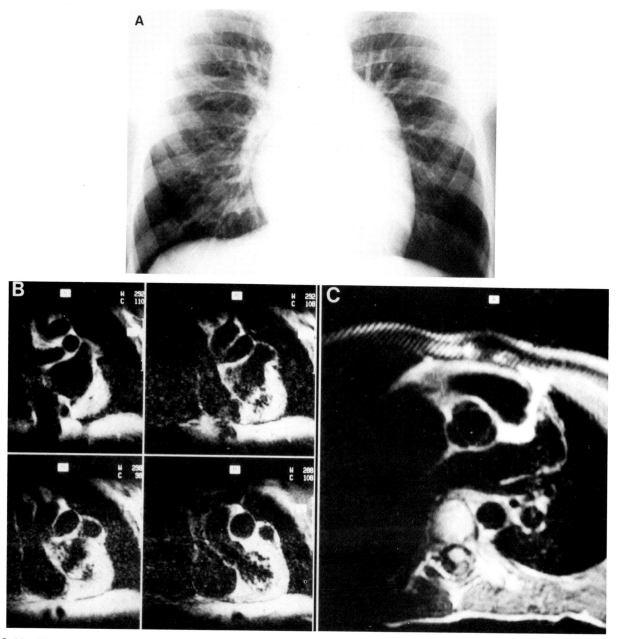

FIG 19–15.
A 9-year-old boy with congenital partial absence of the left pericardium. **A,** chest radiograph demonstrates abnormal prominence of the left atrial appendage (LAA) along the upper left heart margin. **B,** coronal interleaved 5-mm MRIs (posteroanterior) confirm herniation of the LAA through a partial defect in the left pericardium. **C,** axial oblique MRI through the left atrium and atrial appendage demonstrates herniation of the LAA through the pericardial defect. The tricuspid aortic valve in its systolic position also is well seen.

phragm. Unusual prominence of the left atrial appendage may be noted along the left heart margin (Fig 19–16). Fluoroscopy may demonstrate abnormal mobility of the heart during contraction, and unusually prominent pulsations of the left atrial appendage.

In patients with partial right-sided pericardial defects, the chest radiograph may demonstrate an abnormal bulge along the right upper heart border in the vicinity of the superior vena cava from protrusion of a part of the right atrium through the defect. A part of the right upper lobe may also herniate into the pericardial sac.

The chest radiograph in patients with surgical defects of the pericardium may simulate the radiographic findings described above in patients with complete or partial absence of the left pericardium.

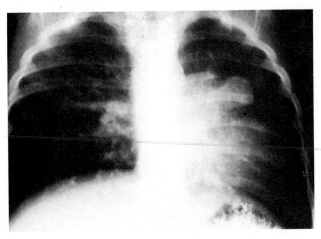

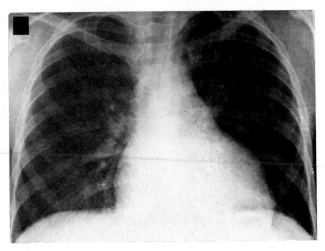

FIG 19–16.
A 10-month-old boy with congenital complete absence of the left pericardium discovered incidentally at fluoroscopy. Rotation of the heart into the left chest with striking prominence of the left atrial appendage (LAA) is seen. Lung is interposed between the heart and left diaphragm. Prominent pulsations of the LAA were evident at fluoroscopy.

FIG 19–17.
Traumatic hemopericardium in an 8-year-old boy who fell onto a metal pipe. AP chest film shows an enlarged pericardial-cardiac silhouette with a globular water-bottle configuration. Pericardiocentesis yielded 850 mL of bloody fluid; and at surgery a 1-cm tear was found at the base of the aorta, with blood oozing directly into the pericardial cavity. **(Courtesy of Dr. George Veasy, Salt Lake City.)**

PERICARDITIS

Pericarditis represents the inflammatory response of the pericardium to a variety of insults including acute rheumatic fever, bacterial and viral infections, trauma (Fig 19–17), and rheumatoid and idiopathic factors. It is relatively rare in children.

Clinical Manifestations

Fever is usually present with infectious pericarditis. Dyspnea and precordial pain may be seen with any causative factor. Physical findings include a friction rub and diminished heart tones.

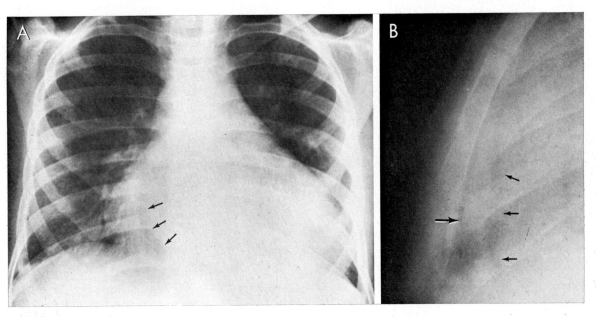

FIG 19–18.
Pericardial effusion demonstrated by an epicardial fat shadow in an 11-year-old boy with acute rheumatic pancarditis. **A,** an AP chest film shows a large cardiac-pericardial silhouette with a curvilinear radiolucent line paralleling the true cardiac silhouette in the right cardiophrenic angle *(arrows).* **B,** in a lateral roentgenogram, extrapericardial fat produces a linear substernal radiolucency *(large arrow)* and a second linear radiolucency *(small arrows)* indicating epicardial fat; the water density between these fat lines indicates pericardial effusion.

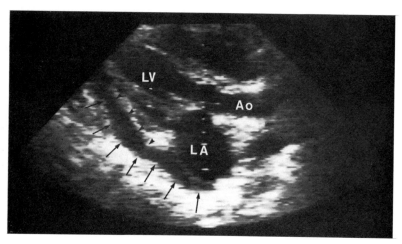

FIG 19–19.
Pericardial effusion. A real-time echocardiogram demonstrates a sonolucent area between the posterior left ventricular wall *(arrow-* *heads)* and the pericardium *(arrows)* that is characteristic of pericardial effusion.

Chest Roentgenography

An enlarged pericardial-cardiac silhouette is usually evident, with differentiation of primary cardiomegaly always difficult. The classic roentgenographic manifestation is a globular or pear-shaped cardiomediastinal silhouette (Figs 19–17 and 19–18,A). The contour of the heart is smoother than normal; the margins are filled out, and the cardiac chambers and great vessel contours may be obliterated. The lower cardiac margin next to the diaphragm may form a more acute angle than normal, and the cardiac sil- houette changes significantly from the supine to the upright position. Fluoroscopy may demonstrate diminished cardiac pulsations, but this can be misleading and is also seen in patients with dilated hearts. Visualization of the epicardial fat as a lucent line deep to the outer border of the enlarged pericardial-cardiac silhouette may confirm the diagnosis. The line frequently appears in the retrosternal space in the lateral chest film or along the left heart border in the posteroanterior (PA) projection (Fig 19–18,B). Fluoroscopy may be more sensitive than chest films are in demonstrating this finding.

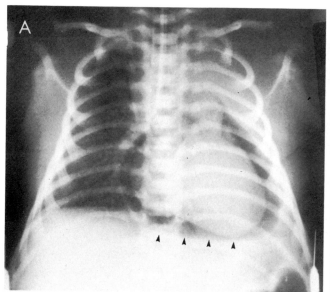
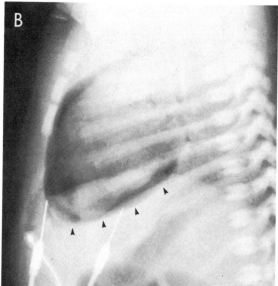

FIG 19–20.
Pneumopericardium. AP **(A)** and lateral **(B)** chest roentgenograms in a premature infant show a radiolucent zone around the cardiac silhouette with a characteristic well-defined continuation between the lower cardiac margin and the diaphragm *(arrowheads).* Note the endotracheal tube in the right mainstem bronchus and the left lung atelectasis.

Echocardiography

Real-time echocardiography is the primary imaging modality in the diagnosis of pericardial effusion. A linear sonolucent area will be seen around the heart, particularly in the posterior left ventricular region. A lucent space larger than 2 mm indicates significant pericardial effusion (Fig 19–19). Caution should be exercised in differentiating pericardial from pleural effusions.

OTHER FORMS OF PERICARDIAL ABNORMALITY

Constrictive-Restrictive Pericarditis

This disease is usually the sequela of prior inflammatory pericarditis. With thickening of the pericardium and adhesions, cardiac function is altered by restriction of diastolic filling. The cardiac silhouette may be normal with poor contractility at fluoroscopy; calcifications occasionally are noted. Dilatation of the superior and inferior venae cavae, pericardial thickening, and flattening of the right atrial contour may be seen with angiography, cine-CT, and MRI.

Pneumopericardium

This rare pericardial process is usually seen in the premature infant undergoing assisted ventilation. Roentgenographic findings are those of a continuous layer of air around the heart and particularly across the anterior mediastinal diaphragmatic surface. The air in the pericardial space will not ascend over the region of the great vessels, which differentiates it from a pneumomediastinum (Fig 19–20).

REFERENCES

Bergmann H Jr, Leisch F, Schutzenberger W, et al: Diagnosis of pericardial effusion by means of one- and two-dimensional echocardiography. *Ultraschall Med* 1981; 2:25.

Doppman JL, Rienmuller R, Lissner J, et al: Computed tomography in constrictive pericardial disease. *J Comput Assist Tomogr* 1981; 5:1.

Glover LBB, Barcia A, Reeves TJ: Congenital absence of the pericardium: A review of the literature with demonstration of a previously unreported fluoroscopic finding. *Am J Roentgenol* 1969; 106:542–549.

Haaz WS, Mintz GS, Kotler MN, et al: Two dimensional echocardiographic recognition of the descending aorta: Value in differentiating pericardial from pleural effusions. *Am J Cardiol* 1980; 46:739.

Lichtenberg GS, Meltzer RS: Echocardiography in pericardial disease, in Elliott LP (ed): *Cardiac Imaging in Infants, Children, and Adults*. Philadelphia, JB Lippincott, 1991, p 390.

Lloyd EA, Curcio CA: Lymphoma of the heart as an unusual cause of pericardial effusion. *S Afr Med J* 1980; 58:937.

Miller SW: Imaging pericardial disease. *Radiol Clin North Am* 1989; 27–1113.

Moncada R, Demos TC, Posniak HV, et al: Computed tomography of pericardial heart disease, in Elliott LP (ed): *Cardiac Imaging in Infants, Children, and Adults*. Philadelphia, JB Lippincott, 1991, p 396.

Olson MC, Posniak HV, McDonald V, et al: Computed tomography and magnetic resonance imaging of the pericardium. *Radiographics* 1989; 9:633–649.

Soulen RL, Stark DD, Higgins CB: Magnetic resonance imaging of constrictive pericardial disease. *Am J Cardiol* 1985; 55:480–484.

Stanford W: Computed tomography and ultrafast computed tomography in pericardial disease, in Elliott LP (ed): *Cardiac Imaging in Infants, Children, and Adults*. Philadelphia, JB Lippincott, 1991, p 415.

White RD, Zisch RJ: Magnetic resonance imaging of pericardial disease and paracardiac and intracardiac masses, in Elliott LP (ed): *Cardiac Imaging in Infants, Children, and Adults*. Philadelphia, JB Lippincott, 1991, p 420.

20

Cardiac Tumors and Arrhythmias

CARDIAC TUMORS

Cardiac tumors in infancy and childhood are rare. They may be either (1) intrinsic to the heart and pericardium or (2) metastatic. *Intracavitary tumors* usually present with sudden dyspnea, failure, cyanosis, shock, or bizarre central nervous system manifestations from embolization. *Intramural lesions* more often produce signs related to inflow or outflow obstruction or ventricular or supraventricular arrhythmias. Pericardial tumors may be asymptomatic until they impinge upon cardiac chambers or create significant tamponade.

Intrinsic Tumors

Eighty percent of cardiac tumors in children are intrinsic tumors. *Rhabdomyoma* is the most common and appears between 6 months and 5 years of age. It is generally a small tumor with a circumscribed mass projecting into the ventricular cavity (Fig 20–1). Most patients have tuberous sclerosis (50%) and may have multiple myocardial tumors. *Intramural fibroma* is the next most common intrinsic tumor and presents as a single large tumor mass in the myocardium usually of the left ventricle or ventricular septum (Figs 20–2 and 20–3); these lesions may be calcified. *Myxomas* are rare and usually occur in the left atrium and produce symptoms related to mitral valve obstruction. Primary sarcomas may occur and frequently metastasize.

Pericardial tumors (20% of all cardiac tumors) include teratoma, fibroma, lipoma, angioma, leiomyoma, and lymphangioma. They may be an incidental finding, although they frequently produce pericardial effusions with occasional secondary tamponade. The differential diagnosis includes other masses in the mediastinum, e.g., teratoma, lymphoma.

Metastatic Tumors

Metastatic tumors are rare and usually arise from leukemia or lymphoma, neuroblastoma, hepatoblastoma, Wilms tumor, or Ewing tumor. Involvement may be by direct extension from intra-abdominal organs via the inferior vena cava or be bloodborne.

Chest Roentgenography

Findings are markedly variable depending upon the type and location of the tumor. Dilatation related to cardiac dysfunction or obstruction is frequently present. With pericardial tumors, effusion is the rule, with the cardiac silhouette either that of effusion or an abnormal cardiac contour.

Echocardiography

Two-dimensional echocardiography usually can define the mass and determine its intracavitary, intramural, or pericardial relations (see Fig 20–2). Involvement of the valves and chambers is readily appreciated and Doppler ultrasound can evaluate valvular dysfunction.

Other Imaging Procedures

Magnetic resonance imaging (MRI) represents the definitive imaging modality to further define pericardial, myocardial, endocardial, or intracavitary relations (see Fig 20–3). Angiocardiography can ade-

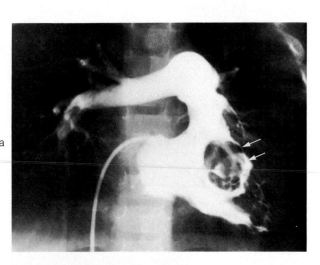

FIG 20–1.
Rhabdomyoma. A right ventriculogram demonstrates a round filling defect projecting into the right ventricular cavity *(arrows)* secondary to a rhabdomyoma in a child with tuberous sclerosis.

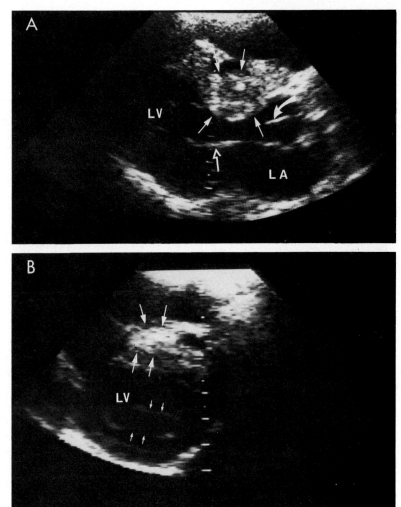

FIG 20–2.
Intracardiac fibroma. Long-axis **(A)** and short-axis **(B)** real-time echocardiograms demonstrate an echogenic round mass lying within the interventricular septum *(arrows)* just below the aortic valve *(curved arrow)*. Histologically, this was a benign fibroma; however, resection was incomplete, and recurrence developed. The mitral valve is designated by the *open arrow* and *small arrows. LV,* left ventricle; *LA,* left atrium.

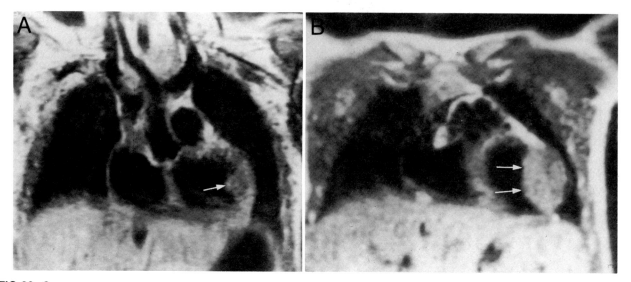

FIG 20–3.
Intramural fibroma viewed by MRI. Anterior **(A)** and posterior **(B)** serial coronal cardiac-gated T1-weighted images of the left ventri- cle show a moderately large intramural fibroma of the left ventricu- lar apex *(arrows).*

quately demonstrate the intracavitary and endocar- dial lesions (see Fig 20–1). Simultaneous long-axis biventricular injections are particularly useful with septal tumors.

ARRHYTHMIAS

Rhythm disturbances are rare in infants and children although reasonably common (1%–2%) during late pregnancy when fetal monitoring is utilized. Su- praventricular premature beats are the most com- mon dysrhythmia. Many of the cardiac rhythm dis- turbances are transitory and benign.

Paroxysmal supraventricular tachycardia may occur in utero or in the postnatal period. In utero, it is one of the causes for neonatal hydrops and congestive failure. In the child, if this condition persists, cardio- megaly will ensue and pulmonary edema may be seen on chest roentgenograms (Fig 20–4). The heart rate usually ranges from 140 to 240 beats per minute. In the absence of underlying congenital heart dis- ease, the prognosis is good.

Persistent atrial tachycardia is a fairly common postnatal condition. It may occur secondary to Wolff-Parkinson-White syndrome and be associated with the Ebstein malformation of the tricuspid valve. If atrial tachycardia persists, clinical failure may oc- cur with palpitations, shortness of breath, and de- velopment of cardiomegaly and congestive failure.

Atrial flutter, atrial fibrillation, and *paroxysmal ven- tricular tachycardia* are relatively rare forms of ar- rhythmia. Clinical findings are related to the heart rate and duration of arrhythmia. Persisting arrhyth- mia leads to cardiomegaly and congestive failure.

Complete heart block may be congenital and occur as an isolated finding or accompany various forms of congenital heart disease, particularly corrected trans- position of the great vessels. It is most often second- ary to heart surgery. The heart rate is usually around 60 beats per minute, but when it approaches 40, syncope, respiratory distress, dyspnea, and cy- anosis may become evident. Chest radiographs show mild cardiomegaly, mild aortic dilatation and, occasionally, venous congestion related to the large stroke volume in these patients. A film made during a period of atrioventricular dyssynchrony may show

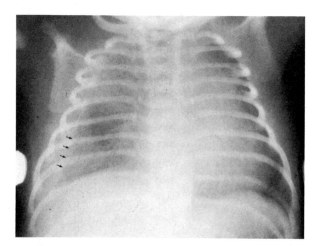

FIG 20–4.
Intrauterine paroxysmal atrial tachycardia. An AP chest roentgeno- gram in a newborn with tachypnea demonstrates moderate right pleural effusion *(arrows)*, cardiomegaly, and congestive heart fail- ure.

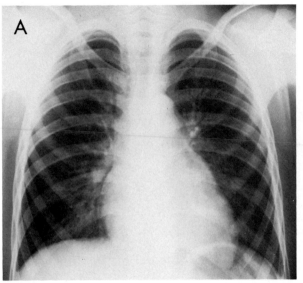
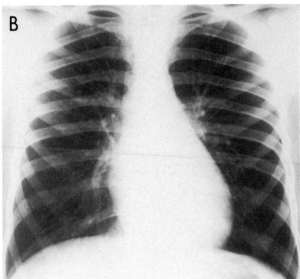

FIG 20–5.
Complete congenital heart block. PA chest roentgenograms (**A** and **B**) made within a few minutes of one another show a pattern of cardiomegaly and venous congestion secondary to atrioventricular dissociation and effects of a large stroke volume that changes to a totally normal appearance of the heart and lungs on the second film (**B**). (From Jaffe RB, Sherman SA, Condon VR, et al: *Radiology* 1976; 121:434. Used by permission.)

a transient pattern of pulmonary congestion when the left atrium contracts simultaneously with left ventricular contraction against the closed mitral valve (Fig 20–5). Primary congenital heart block rarely needs treatment. If recurrent syncopal episodes occur, epicardial or transvenous pacemaker insertion may be necessary.

REFERENCES

Cardiac Tumors

Barberger-Gateau P, Pacquet M, Desaulniers D, et al: Fibrolipoma of the mitral valve in a child: Clinical and echocardiographic features. *Circulation* 1978; 58:955.

Casolo F, Biasi S, Galzarini L, et al: MRI as an adjunct to echocardiography for the diagnostic imaging of cardiac masses. *Eur J Radiol* 1988; 8:226.

Chadraratna PAN, Aronow WS, Wong D: Echocardiography of intracardiac and extracardiac tumors. *Semin Ultrasound CT MR* 1981; 2:143.

Cornalba G, Dore R: Cardiac tumor associated with tuberous sclerosis. *J Comput Assist Tomogr* 1985; 9:809.

de Ruiz M, Potter JL, Stavinoha J, et al: Real-time ultrasound diagnosis of cardiac fibroma in a neonate. *J Ultrasound Med* 1985; 4:367.

Higgins CB, Lipton MJ: Computed tomographic and magnetic resonance imaging of cardiac and paracardiac tumors, in Elliott LP (ed): *Cardiac Imaging in Infants, Children, and Adults.* Philadelphia, JB Lippincott, 1991, p 490.

Hoadley SD, Wallace RL, Miller JF, et al: Prenatal diagnosis of cardiac tumors presenting as an arrhythmia. *J Clin Ultrasound* 1986; 14:639.

Houser S, Forges N, Stewart S: Rhabdomyoma of the heart: A diagnostic and therapeutic challenge. *Ann Thorac Surg* 1980; 29:373.

Lund JT, Ehman RL, Julsrud PR, et al: Cardiac masses: Assessment by MR imaging. *Am J Roentgenol* 1989; 152:469.

Reisner SA, Meltzer RS: Echocardiography in cardiac tumors, in Elliott LP (ed): *Cardiac Imaging in Infants, Children, and Adults.* Philadelphia, JB Lippincott Co, 1991, p 487.

Rienmuller R, Tiling R: Evaluation of paracardiac and intracardiac masses in children. *Semin Ultrasound CT MR* 1990; 11:246–250.

Stanford W, Abu-Yousef M, Smith W: Intracardiac tumor (rhabdomyoma) diagnosed by in utero ultrasound: Case report. *J Clin Ultrasound* 1987; 15:337.

Stanford W, Rooholamini SA, Galvin JR: Ultrafast computed tomography for the detection of intracardiac thrombi and tumors, in Elliott LP (ed): *Cardiac Imaging in Infants, Children, and Adults.* Philadelphia, JB Lippincott, 1991, p 494.

Arrhythmias

Farooki ZQ, Green WW: Multifocal atrial tachycardia in two neonates. *Br Heart J* 1977; 39:872.

Gonge HM, Wladimiroff JW, Noordam MJ, et al: Fetal cardiac arrhythmias and their effect on volume blood flow in descending aorta of human fetus. *JCU* 1986; 14:607.

Higgins CB, Higgins SS, Kelley MJ, et al: Heart failure in the neonate due to extreme abnormalities of heart rate: Clinical and radiographic features. *Am J Roentgenol* 1980; 134:359.

Jaffe RB, Sherman SA, Condon VR, et al: Congenital complete heart block. *Radiology* 1976; 121:434.

McCue CM, Mantakas ME, Tingelstad JB, et al: Congenital heart block in newborns of mothers with connective heart disease. *Circulation* 1977; 56:82.

21

Cardiac Operations and Interventional Procedures

Evaluation of the postoperative chest radiograph
Common cardiac operations
Interventional catheterization procedures

EVALUATION OF THE POSTOPERATIVE CHEST RADIOGRAPH

After cardiac operation, serial chest radiographs enable the pediatric radiologist to accurately monitor the patient's condition. When compared with preoperative radiographs, a small decrease in heart size is frequently seen immediately after operation, secondary to hypovolemia, but is transitory. Large increases in heart size after operation are suggestive of inadequate drainage of the pericardial space and development of pericardial effusion. Mediastinal widening typically is seen after median sternotomy, and gradually resolves in 1 to 2 weeks, but progressive widening in mediastinal contour from preoperative radiographs imply continued mediastinal hemorrhage necessitating treatment. Small pleural effusions after a thoracotomy are common, but moderate to large effusions indicate continued bleeding and inadequate chest drainage. Moderate to large pleural effusions are commonly seen in patients following the Fontan procedure complicated by low output. Persistent pleural effusions are suggestive of chylothorax, and may follow inadvertent severance of the thoracic duct or from elevated superior vena cava pressures as may be seen in patients with Glenn shunts or superior vena cava obstruction after the Mustard procedure (Fig 21–1). They may disappear after the patient has been placed on a low fat diet, but often clear only after ligation of the thoracic duct.

Subsegmental and segmental atelectasis is seen in almost all patients following operation, particu-

larly in the left lower lobe, especially in patients with large ventricular septal defect and others with left atrial enlargement narrowing the left mainstem bronchus. Pulmonary edema may develop unilaterally or bilaterally following systemic–pulmonary artery shunts (Fig 21–2), but should resolve in several days on diuretic therapy. Persistent pulmonary edema may be indicative of pulmonary venous obstruction as may be seen in patients after repair of total anomalous pulmonary venous drainage, or baffle obstruction after the Mustard procedure for transposition. It also may be an indication of persisting systemic outflow obstruction or poor myocardial function, as may be seen in patients with anoxia or sepsis. Disseminated airspace disease indicative of pulmonary hemorrhage may occur in patients with sepsis, shock, and disseminated intravascular coagulation. Elevation of a hemidiaphragm after operation is indicative of phrenic nerve injury. Fluoroscopy or ultrasonography will reveal paradoxical movement during inspiration. Patients that fail extubation should also be evaluated for phrenic nerve injury that may not be recognized with the patient intubated and ventilated.

COMMON CARDIAC OPERATIONS

Tables 21–1 and 21–2 describe and illustrate common cardiac operations—palliative cardiac operations and operative repair, respectively. The procedure, its description and the radiologic findings and complications are discussed and illustrated.

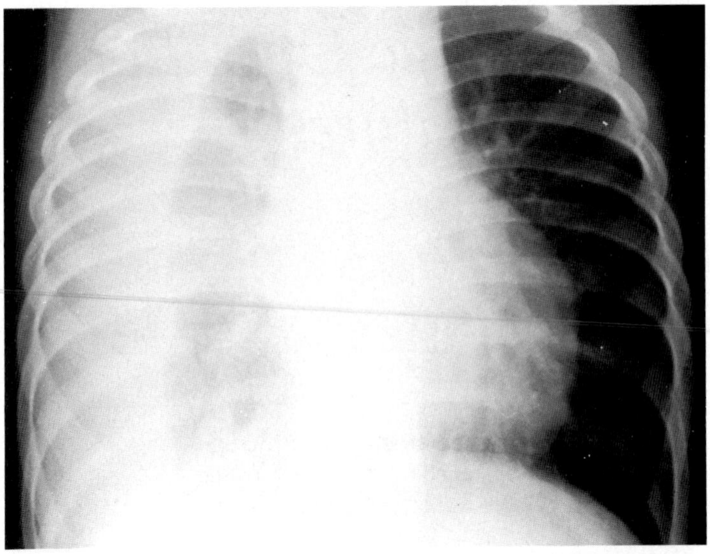

FIG 21–1.
A 1½-year-old boy with superior vena cava obstruction 1 year after a Mustard procedure for transposition. Right lateral decubitus chest radiograph demonstrates a large right chylothorax (see also Fig 21–21).

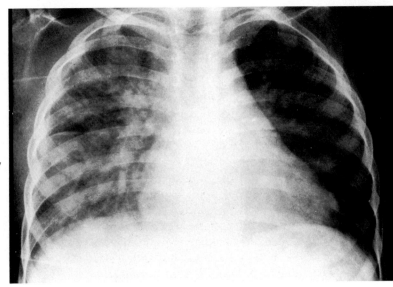

FIG 21–2.
Unilateral pulmonary edema in a neonate after Waterston-Cooley anastomosis for tetralogy of Fallot. Chest radiograph several hours after operation demonstrates unilateral right pulmonary edema and small right pleural effusion.

TABLE 21–1.

Palliative Cardiac Operations

Procedure	Description	Radiologic Findings and Complications
Procedures to increase pulmonary blood flow		
Venous		
Glenn shunt	Superior vena cava (SVC)–pulmonary artery (PA) shunt. May use right SVC–right PA or left SVC–left PA. Performed as a palliative procedure in tricuspid atresia and other forms of cyanotic heart disease, usually as a staging procedure prior to a Fontan anastomosis. Performed by dividing the PA, and ligating the proximal portion. The distal PA is anastomosed end to side with the SVC. The SVC is ligated on the cardiac side of the anastomosis directing the SVC flow into the ipsilateral PA (Fig 21–3). Rarely, flow can be augmented to the lung by creation of an arteriovenous fistula in the ipsilateral axilla, thus increasing SVC flow.	Late complications include anastomotic narrowing, SVC syndrome, thrombotic occlusion of the ipsilateral PAs, and pulmonary arteriovenous malformations with intrapulmonary right-to-left shunting (Fig 21–4). Increased SVC pressure may result in collateral flow, particularly through the azygos vein effectively decreasing pulmonary blood flow (Fig 21–5). Operative ligation or coil occlusion of these collateral vessels may be necessary to increase SVC blood flow (see Fig 21–33).

Bidirectional Glenn shunt (Abram modification)	Right or left SVC-PA anastomosis. Similar to above, but the proximal PA is not ligated. SVC flow is directed to both pulmonary arteries (Fig 21–6). Similar to Fontan procedure, but only directs SVC flow to the pulmonary arteries. Inferior vena cava blood flow remains intracardiac.	Similar to Glenn shunt.
Arterial		
Blalock-Taussig shunt	Subclavian artery–PA shunt. This systemic-PA shunt is used for palliation of cyanotic heart disease, especially tetralogy of Fallot (TOF). The subclavian artery is divided, preferably on the side of the innominate artery. The proximal portion is anastomosed end to side to the ipsilateral PA. The distal stump of the subclavian is ligated. One of the advantages of this procedure is that the size and length of the subclavian artery limit flow and usually prevent development of pulmonary hypertension. After the operation radiologic findings may include ipsilateral elevation and enlargement of the PA, increased pulmonary blood flow on the side of the shunt, and unilateral rib notching.	Complications include kinking of the subclavian artery, anastomotic narrowing (see Fig 15–27 and Fig 21–7), and elevation and kinking of the PA. Retrograde propagation of thrombus to involve a carotid artery may be seen. Mediastinal and intercostal collaterals supply circulation to the arm. Rarely, a withered arm may result from ligation of the subclavian artery (Fig 21–8). Pulmonary hypertension is rare after the procedure.
Modified Blalock-Taussig shunt	Similar to standard Blalock-Taussig shunt, except that the subclavian artery is not divided, but rather a synthetic graft is anastomosed side to side to the subclavian and ipsilateral PA (Fig 21–9).	Radiographic findings and complications are similar to the Blalock-Taussig shunt except that rib notching should not be present. If the synthetic conduit is too short it may cause kinking of the subclavian/PA.
Central shunt	Systemic-PA shunt used for palliation of cyanotic congenital heart disease utilizing a synthetic 4–5-mm-diameter graft between the ascending aorta and the PA.	Complications include increased pulmonary blood flow and pulmonary hypertension if the shunt is too large. Anastomotic narrowing/kinking may also be seen decreasing effective PA blood flow.
Potts anastomosis	Systemic-PA shunt created by a side-to-side anastomosis between the descending aorta and ipsilateral PA. This is an extrapericardial shunt and is rarely performed in patients with cyanotic heart disease because of the potential development of pulmonary hypertension, and considerable difficulty in dismantling the shunt during later operative repair.	Like the Waterston-Cooley shunt, the anastomosis must be of proper size; if too large, pulmonary hypertension may develop; if too small, there will be insufficient flow to the lungs. A mycotic aneurysm at the anastomotic site is a rare complication (Fig 19–11).
Waterston-Cooley anastomosis	Systemic-PA shunt formed by side-to-side anastomosis of the ascending aorta to the right PA. This palliative procedure for cyanotic congenital heart disease is rarely performed because of the potential development of pulmonary hypertension (Fig 21–10).	Following operation, unilateral pulmonary edema can develop, but is usually transient (see Fig 21–2). The common complication of this anastomosis is the development of pulmonary hypertension, particularly in the right lung, frequently accompanied by obstruction of flow to the left PA (Fig 21–11).
Procedure to decrease pulmonary blood flow		
Pulmonary artery band	Palliative procedure to decrease pulmonary arterial blood flow in patients with large left-to-right shunts protecting the PAs from systemic pressures and resultant pulmonary hypertension. Synthetic material is placed around the main PA just above the pulmonary valve and the band is gradually tightened to constrict the main PA and decrease the pulmonary arterial pressures to approximately one-half systemic pressure in the newborn. When definitive operative repair is performed at a later date, the pulmonary band can be removed and, if necessary, reconstructive surgery performed on the main PA.	If metallic staples have been used to tighten the band, they are visible often as a series of parallel staples in the region of the main PA (Fig 21–12). Angiography in patients with PA band typically show thickening of the pulmonary valve leaflets, nodularity along the edges of the valve leaflets, doming of the pulmonary valve during systole, and poststenotic dilatation of the PA distal to the band. Calcification may develop in the main PA, but a calcified aneurysm of the main PA is rare. Distal migration of the PA band may produce significant obstruction of the proximal right and left pulmonary arteries (Fig 21–13). Subaortic stenosis may also develop following pulmonary artery band in patients with ventricular septal defect, and in patients with single ventricle or univentricular hearts with narrowing of the bulboventricular foramen.

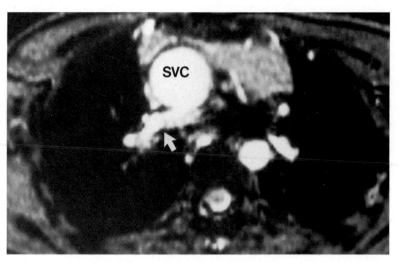

FIG 21–3.
Glenn shunt in a 7-year-old girl with pulmonary atresia. Axial gradient-recalled cine-MRI demonstrates a patent Glenn anastomosis between the superior vena cava *(SVC)* and right pulmonary artery *(arrow)*.

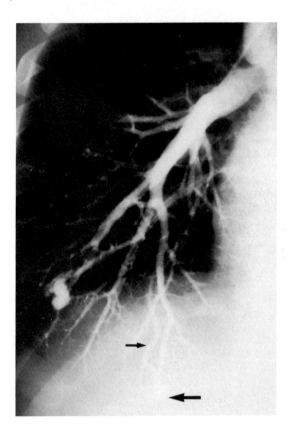

FIG 21–4.
A 19-year-old boy with Glenn shunt for tricuspid atresia. Right pulmonary angiogram following catheter passage from the arm across the Glenn shunt demonstrates two small pulmonary arteriovenous malformations (AVM) in the right lower lung. The smallest AVM behind the diaphragm *(large arrow)* has early venous opacification *(small arrow)* similar to the larger AVM.

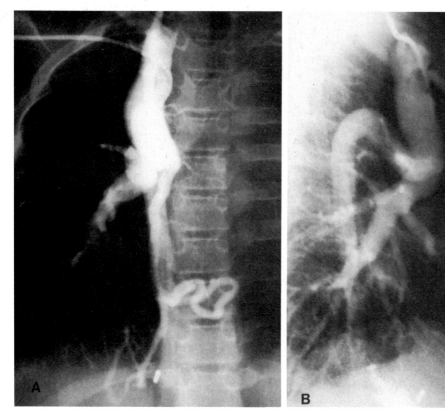

FIG 21–5.
A 10-year-old girl with Glenn anastomosis for tricuspid atresia at age 5 months. Frontal **(A)** and lateral **(B)** angiograms after superior vena cava injection demonstrate a patent Glenn anastomosis but collateral flow down the enlarged azygos vein and right internal mammary vein decreases pulmonary blood flow. The patient underwent ligation of the azygos and right internal mammary veins.

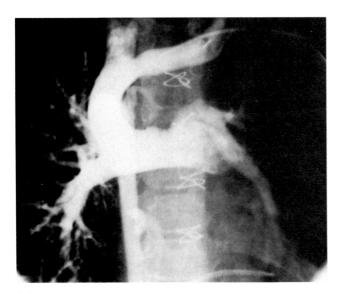

FIG 21–6.
Bidirectional Glenn shunt. Superior vena cava injection in the frontal projection demonstrates a patent bidirectional Glenn shunt with opacification of both right and left pulmonary arteries. Collateral flow, however, down the azygos system effectively decreases pulmonary blood flow. The patient underwent coil occlusion of the azygos vein (see Fig 21–33).

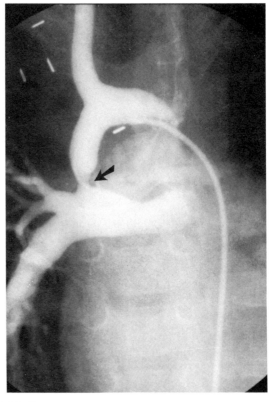

FIG 21–7.
Stenotic right Blalock-Taussig shunt for tetralogy of Fallot with left aortic arch. The right subclavian artery is stenotic at the anastomosis with the right pulmonary artery *(arrow)*.

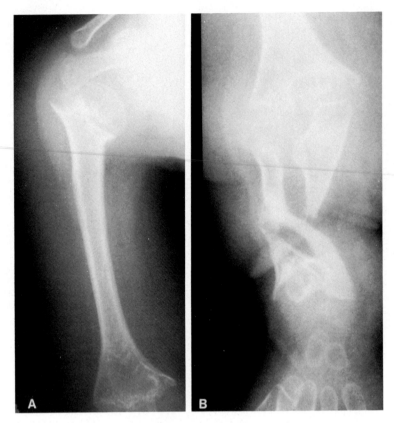

FIG 21–8.
Withered right arm after right Blalock-Taussig shunt as a neonate. **A,** right humerus: ischemic changes of the proximal and distal metaphyses are noted. **B,** right forearm: severe ischemic changes of the radius and ulna are noted.

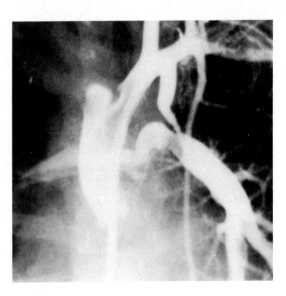

FIG 21–9.
Stenotic modified left Blalock-Taussig shunt in a 1½-year-old girl with tetralogy of Fallot. Injection of contrast medium into the left innominate artery arising from the right aortic arch demonstrates the modified left Blalock-Taussig shunt with stenosis at its anastomosis with the left pulmonary artery.

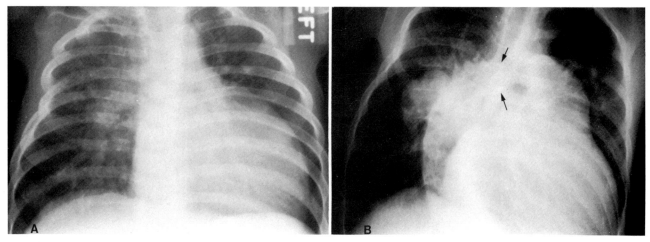

FIG 21-10.
Waterston-Cooley procedure for tricuspid atresia with development of pulmonary arterial hypertension. **A,** chest radiograph 1 year after Waterston-Cooley anastomosis for tricuspid atresia demonstrates differential pulmonary blood flow, increased to the right lung, and normal to the left lung. Changes related to a right thoracotomy and cardiomegaly with left ventricular dilatation also are seen. **B,** chest radiograph 13½ years after Waterston-Cooley anastomosis demonstrates severe changes of pulmonary arterial hypertension in the right lung with calcification *(arrows)* of the markedly enlarged right pulmonary artery. Peripheral attenuation of the distal right pulmonary artery, thoracic scoliosis, and normal pulmonary flow to the left lung secondary to proximal left pulmonary artery obstruction also are noted.

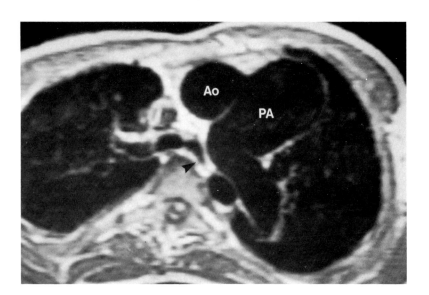

FIG 21-11.
Waterston-Cooley anastomosis with pulmonary hypertension. A 20-year-old with pulmonic atresia after having a Waterston-Cooley shunt as an infant. Axial 5-mm spin-echo MRI demonstrates the Waterston-Cooley shunt between the ascending aorta *(Ao)* and pulmonary artery *(PA)* with aneurysmal dilatation of the central pulmonary artery and left pulmonary artery. The right pulmonary artery was not visualized. Note compression and posterior displacement of the left mainstem bronchus *(arrowhead)* and descending aorta by the aneurysmally dilated left pulmonary artery.

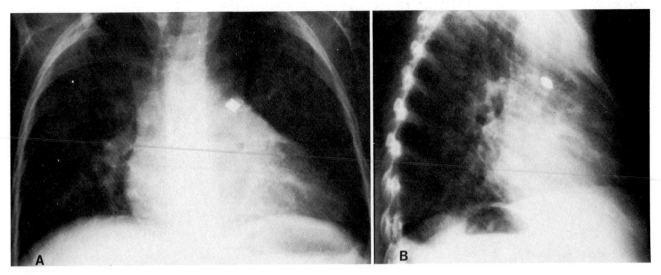

FIG 21–12.
A 3-year-old girl with pulmonary artery band for membranous and muscular ventricular septal defects (VSDs). Frontal **(A)** and lateral **(B)** chest radiographs demonstrate multiple parallel staples in the region of the main pulmonary artery. These staples have been placed to gradually tighten the synthetic pulmonary artery band around the pulmonary artery to decrease the pulmonary arterial pressures to approximately one-half systemic pressure.

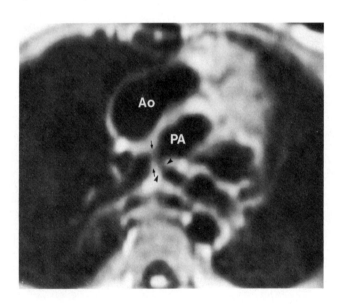

FIG 21–13.
Distal migration of the pulmonary artery band (axial 3-mm spin-echo MRI). In this 1-year-old patient with single ventricle and dextrotransposition, the pulmonary artery band has migrated distally with marked stenosis of the proximal right *(arrows)* and proximal left *(arrowheads)* pulmonary artery. *Ao,* anterior aorta; *PA,* posterior pulmonary artery.

TABLE 21-2.

Operative Repair

Procedures	Description	Radiologic Findings and Complications
Arterial switch (Jatene procedure)	Definitive repair of complete transposition of the great vessels. The aorta and pulmonary arteries (PAs) are divided above the valves and the great vessels switched. The coronary arteries are removed from the aorta with a button of tissue and are reimplanted into the neoaorta.	Complications include supravalvular pulmonary stenosis (most common) (Fig 21–14) at the anastomotic site, supravalvular aortic stenosis, and myocardial ischemia secondary to kinking of the coronary arteries or obstruction at the ostia. (see Fig 15–30). Following operation, the neoaorta may obstruct the proximal PA.
Blalock-Hanlon	Operative removal of the atrial septum. Performed as a palliative procedure to improve atrial mixing in patients with complex cyanotic congenital heart disease.	Complications are rare with this procedure.
Brock procedure	Relief of right ventricular outflow obstruction performed blindly via a right ventriculotomy. The stenotic or atretic pulmonary valve is fractured and infundibular tissue can be excised to relieve subvalvular obstruction.	Complications include false passage and inadvertent damage to the adjacent posterior aortic valve.
Damus-Stansel-Kaye (Damus) procedure	Palliative procedure for certain types of complex cyanotic congenital heart disease with systemic outflow tract obstruction, particularly univentricular heart with obstructive bulboventricular foramen, forms of double-outlet right ventricle, complete transposition with subaortic stenosis, and forms of hypoplastic left heart syndrome. The procedure involves division of the PA and anastomosis of the proximal portion to the ascending aorta. This procedure effectively bypasses systemic outflow tract obstruction. Operations performed concurrently with the Damus procedure include Fontan anastomosis, Rastelli conduits, or systemic-PA shunts to provide pulmonary blood flow.	Moderately high operative mortality largely related to the serious complex cyanotic congenital heart disease. The pulmonary valve may become insufficient because of distortion.
Fontan procedure	Palliative atrial-pulmonary anastomosis for treatment of cyanotic congenital heart disease, particularly tricuspid atresia, forms of single ventricle, and hypoplastic left heart syndrome. Originally described by Fontan and Bidet for treatment of tricuspid atresia utilizing a technique of interposing a valved conduit between the right atrium (RA) and left PA, inserting a valve into the inferior vena cava, closing the atrial septal defect, and performing a superior vena cava–right PA shunt (Glenn anastomosis). Currently most commonly performed is closure of the atrial septal defect and direct placement of a valveless conduit between the RA and PA (Fig 21–15). Less commonly a valved conduit between the RA and PA is used.	Complications include atrial arrhythmias, low cardiac output, and obstruction of the prosthetic valve/conduit. Intrapulmonary arteriovenous shunting has been demonstrated with ^{99m}Tc-labeled macroaggregated albumin, but microscopic arteriovenous malformations have not been demonstrated angiographically as have been described with the Glenn procedure.
Fenestrated Fontan procedure	Similar to Fontan procedure but with creation of a small 4-mm fenestration to allow right-to-left interatrial shunting and temporary decompression of the right heart (Fig 21–16,A). After repeat catheterization and a trial of balloon occlusion of the fenestration, the small defect may be closed with an occlusion device (Fig 21–16,B) or operation.	
Modified Fontan procedure	Modification of Fontan procedure utilized for palliation of tricuspid atresia. The right ventricle is enlarged and subpulmonic obstruction relieved, and a valved conduit or aortic homograft placed from the RA to the right ventricular outflow tract (Figs 21–17,A and 21–18,B and C). In these patients pulmonary flow is right ventricular–dependent, an improvement over the standard Fontan procedure in which pulmonary flow is right atrial–dependent.	Complications are similar to those described for the Fontan procedure. Additional complications include obstruction of the conduit by the free intraventricular septum and sternal compression (Figs 21–17,B and 21–18,A).

(Continued on page 21-13.)

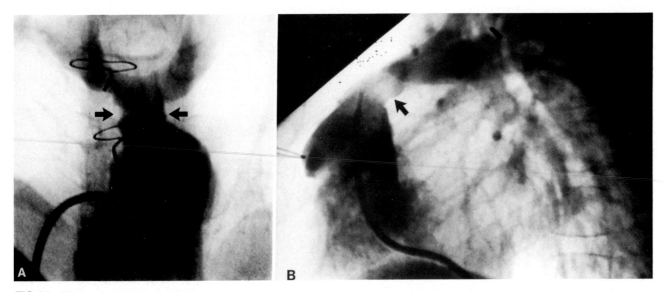

FIG 21–14.
Peripheral pulmonary artery stenosis following arterial switch for transposition. Frontal **(A)** and lateral **(B)** digital angiograms following right ventricular injection demonstrate mild peripheral pulmo-nary artery stenosis at the anastomotic site *(arrows)* in this 7-year-old following arterial switch for transposition.

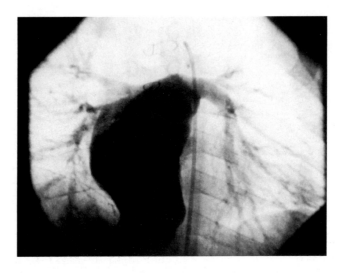

FIG 21–15.
Fontan procedure in a 16-year-old boy with single ventricle and levotransposition. Frontal digital angiogram after injection of contrast medium into the inferior vena cava–right atrial junction opac-ifies the right atrium and its anastomosis with the pulmonary artery. A pigtail catheter is present in the left descending thoracic aorta.

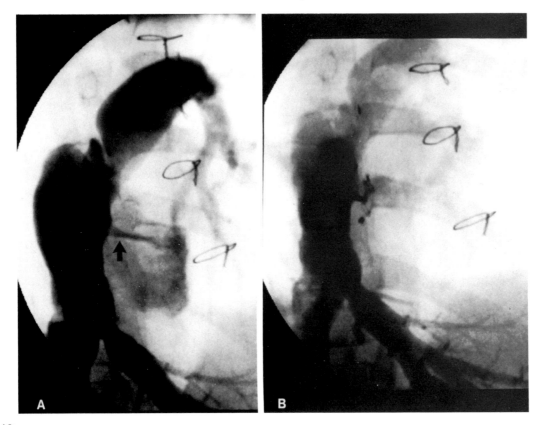

FIG 21–16.
Catheter closure of a fenestrated Fontan procedure in a 4½ year old boy with right Glenn anastomosis, and fenestrated Fontan procedure for palliation of single ventricle. **A,** digital angiogram in the shallow right anterior oblique projection during right atrial injection demonstrates the Fontan anastomosis to the left pulmonary artery and right-to-left shunt flow *(arrow)* into the left atrium through the surgically created 4-mm fenestration. **B,** repeat digital angiogram in the shallow right anterior oblique projection after catheter closure with an experimental clamshell occlusion device demonstrates a very small residual shunt into the left atrium that should close spontaneously. One side of the occlusion device is in the Fontan anastomosis, the other in the left atrium.

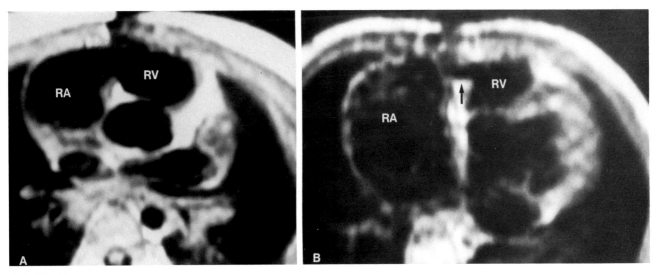

FIG 21–17.
Modified Fontan procedure. **A,** 7-year-old girl with tricuspid atresia after a right atrial–right ventricular outflow tract conduit. Axial 5-mm spin-echo MRI in end diastole shows wide patency of the conduit between the right atrium *(RA)* and right ventricular outflow tract *(RV)*. **B,** 9-year-old boy with tricuspid atresia after a right atrial–right ventricular outflow conduit. Axial 5-mm spin-echo MRI at end diastole demonstrates narrowing of the conduit between the enlarged right atrium *(RA)* and right ventricular outflow tract *(RV)* by the medial free wall of the right ventricle *(arrow)*.

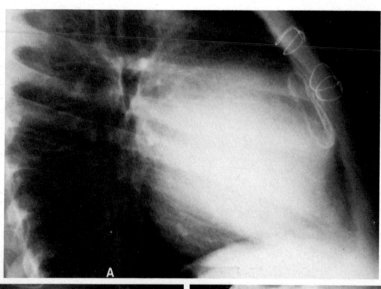

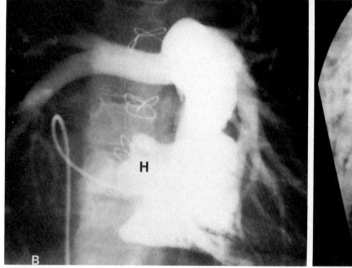

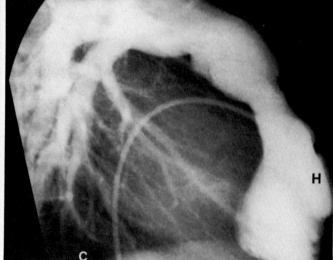

FIG 21–18.
Modified Fontan procedure. **A,** lateral chest radiograph demonstrates calcification and compression of the aortic homograft placed from the right atrium to the right ventricular outflow tract in this patient with tricuspid atresia. Frontal **(B)** and lateral **(C)** right ventricular angiograms after catheter passage through the aortic homograft into the right ventricle demonstrate the aortic homograft *(H)* and mild hypoplasia of the right ventricle.

TABLE 21–2 (cont.).

Operative Repair

Procedures	Description	Radiologic Findings and Complications
Left ventricular apical-to-aortic conduit	Palliative procedure to bypass left ventricular outflow tract obstruction. A valved conduit is placed from the left ventricular apex to the abdominal aorta (Fig 21–19).	Complications include prosthetic valve/conduit obstruction and subsequent development of left ventricular outflow obstruction and failure. Following operation, anterior or medial impression on the gastric fundus and narrowing of the distal esophagus may be seen. Rarely, dysphagia and gastric erosion may occur (Bickers et al.).
Mustard procedure	Palliative repair of complete transposition of the great vessels. The atrial septum is excised and a pericardial or Dacron baffle is then sewn in place to direct superior and inferior vena cava flow through the mitral valve into the left ventricle which supplies the pulmonary circulation (Fig 21–20,A and B). The pulmonary venous return is directed through the tricuspid valve into the right ventricle which supplies the systemic circulation (Fig 21–20,C and D).	Common complications include systemic venous obstruction, pulmonary venous obstruction, and right ventricular (systemic) failure. Baffle obstruction may occur early due to compression of the left atrium by extracardiac clot, or late due to scarring, tethering, or incorrect positioning of the baffle. A baffle leak may result in intra-atrial shunting (Fig 21–21). Systemic venous obstruction, particularly of the superior vena cava, is a late complication in 6% of cases and may cause symptoms of syncope, chylothorax (see Figs 21–1 and 21–21). superior vena cava syndrome, and communicating hydrocephalus. Dilatation of the azygos/hemiazygos veins is an indication of systemic venous baffle obstruction (see Figs 21–22,A and 21–23). Pulmonary venous obstruction occurs as a late complication in approximately 4% of patients and is characterized by pulmonary venous hypertension and development of interstitial and alveolar pulmonary edema (Fig 21–24).
Norwood procedure	Palliative staged procedure for hypoplastic left heart syndrome, still in evolution. In stage I, the main PA is transected and an incision is made into the diminutive ascending aorta, aortic arch, and descending aorta. The hypoplastic aorta is enlarged with a homograft and anastomosed to the proximal PA. The patent ductus arteriosus is ligated and an atrial septectomy performed. The distal main pulmonary artery is oversewn, and a Blalock-Taussig or central shunt placed to the pulmonary arteries. In stage II, performed around 6–12 mo, a bidirectional Glenn anastomosis is placed, and the Blalock-Taussig or central shunt ligated (Fig 21–25). Stage III, performed by 2 yr, is a conversion of the Glenn anastomosis to a Fontan procedure (completion Fontan).	This procedure is associated with high morbidity and mortality. Obstruction at multiple levels, particularly the anastomosed PAs by the neoaorta and distal aorta, may be seen.
Pericardial and Dacron patch graft	Placement of pericardial and Dacron graft to operatively enlarge the right ventricular outflow tract, particularly in patients with tetralogy of Fallot. A right ventriculotomy is made, and the infundibular musculature resected. A piece of Dacron is placed across the operative incision to enlarge the right ventricular outflow tract, and if necessary can be extended across the pulmonary annulus and main PA to the PA bifurcation to enlarge a hypoplastic main PA. Currently, Dacron is placed over the right ventricular outflow tract and pericardium over the PAs.	Following operation the originally inconspicuous right ventricular outflow tract and PA become more prominent and with time show increasing convexity in this region. This prominence of the right ventricular outflow tract is normal and should not be called an aneurysm. Occasionally, calcification can be seen along the margins of the pericardial and Dacron patch graft. Rarely, postoperative aneurysms of the right ventricular outflow tract can develop, particularly in patients with persistent right ventricular outflow obstruction, residual left-to-right shunts, and significant pulmonary regurgitation (Fig 21–26).
Intracardiac conduit	Intracardiac baffle, popularized by Rastelli, placed to establish continuity between the left ventricle and aorta (Fig 21–27,A) or rarely the PA. Performed usually in patients with double-outlet right ventricle and forms of transposition, particularly transposition with ventricular septal defect (VSD) and subpulmonic stenosis. Usually accompanied by an extracardiac conduit from the right ventricle to the PAs (Fig 21–27,B and C), or an arterial switch in patients with forms of transposition when the baffle has been placed to direct left ventricular blood flow to the PA.	The most common complication following this operation is residual obstruction between the left ventricle and aorta, either at the level of the VSD, or from redundancy or incorrect placement of the intracardiac baffle. When the VSD must be enlarged during placement of the baffle, complete heart block may result necessitating a pacemaker.

(Continued on page 21-20.)

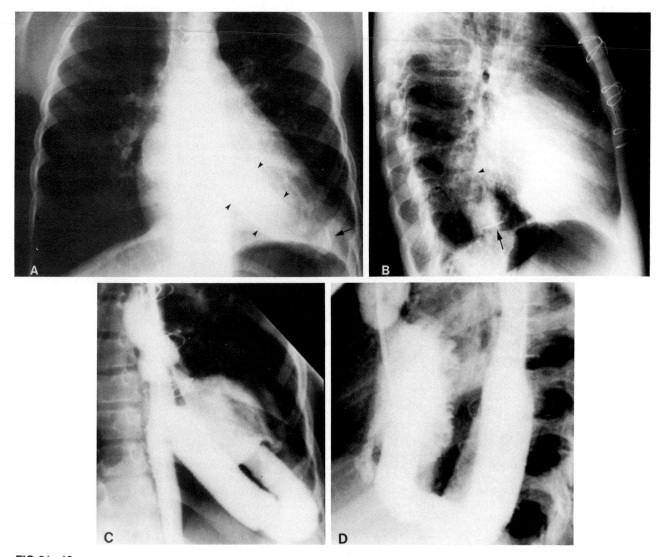

FIG 21–19.
Left ventricular apical-to-aortic conduit. Frontal **(A)** and lateral **(B)** chest radiographs demonstrate a valved *(arrow)* conduit *(arrowheads)* from the left ventricular apex to the thoracic aorta in this 13-year-old girl with severe subaortic obstruction that could not be re-lieved with two earlier operations. Right anterior oblique **(C)** and left anterior oblique **(D)** left ventricular angiograms demonstrate the valved conduit from the left ventricular apex to the thoracic aorta. Subaortic obstruction is present.

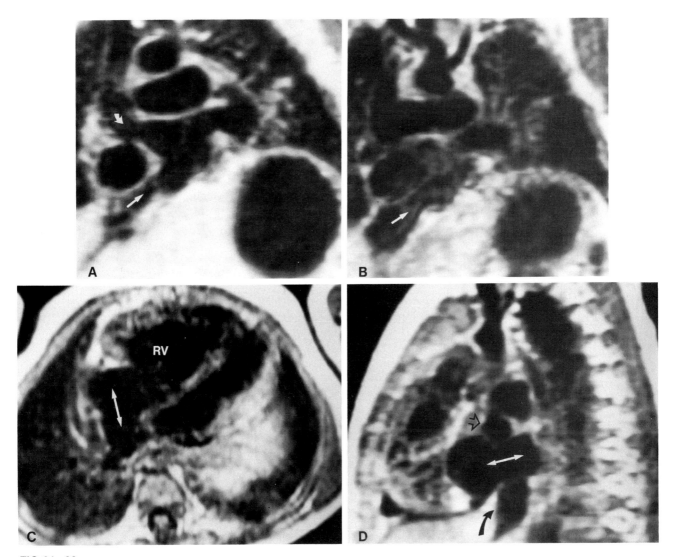

FIG 21–20.
Mustard procedure for complete transposition. **A,** coronal 5-mm spin-echo MRI demonstrates the systemic venous limb of the atrial baffle in this 1-year-old boy. The superior vena cava *(curved arrow)* enters the superior aspect and the inferior vena cava *(straight arrow)* enters the lower aspect of the systemic venous limb. Elevation of the left hemidiaphragm secondary to phrenic nerve injury is noted above the gas-filled stomach. **B,** coronal 5-mm spin-echo MRI of a slightly different level better demonstrates entrance of the inferior vena cava into the inferior aspect *(arrow)* of the systemic venous limb. Intraluminal echoes are consistent with slow venous flow. **C,** axial 3-mm spin-echo MRI reveals wide patency of the pulmonary venous limb of the atrial baffle *(arrows)*. *RV,* right ventricle. **D,** sagittal 5-mm spin-echo MRI shows wide patency of the pulmonary venous limb of the atrial baffle *(closed arrows)*. The systemic venous limb of the atrial baffle receiving the superior vena cava *(open arrow)* and inferior vena cava *(closed arrow)* are also seen.

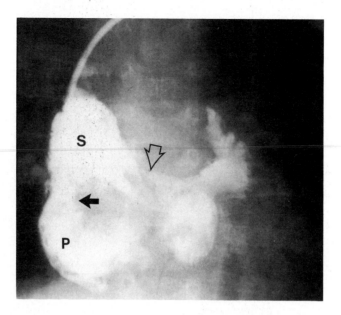

FIG 21–21.

Mustard procedure for complete transposition with systemic venous obstruction and chylothorax. The chest radiograph is illustrated in Figure 21–1. Frontal angiogram following injection of contrast into the superior aspect of the systemic venous limb of the atrial baffle (S) demonstrates severe obstruction of flow (open arrow) in this portion of the atrial baffle. A baffle leak (closed arrow) into the pulmonary venous limb of the atrial baffle (P) is also present.

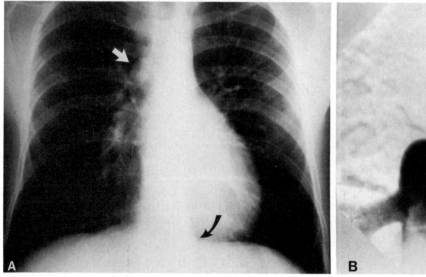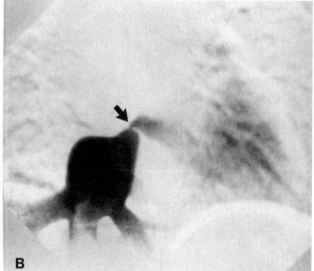

FIG 21–22.

Mustard procedure for transposition with systemic venous obstruction. **A,** chest radiograph demonstrates dilatation of the azygos vein (white arrow) and hemiazygos vein (black arrow) indicating collateral flow from systemic venous obstruction. **B,** frontal digital angiogram following injection into the inferior vena cava demonstrates severe obstruction in the inferior aspect of the systemic venous limb of the atrial baffle (arrow). An injection into the superior vena cava also demonstrated obstruction of the superior aspect of the systemic venous limb of the atrial baffle similar to Figure 21–21.

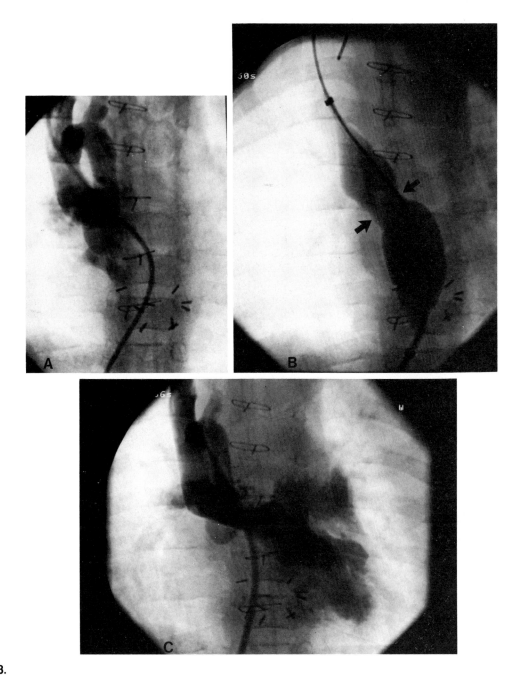

FIG 21–23.
Mustard procedure for transposition with systemic venous obstruction, alleviated by balloon angioplasty. **A,** in this patient with superior vena cava syndrome secondary to systemic venous obstruction following the Mustard procedure, the catheter has been passed from the inferior vena cava across the inferior aspect into the superior aspect of the systemic venous limb of the atrial baffle and then into the superior vena cava. Frontal digital angiogram demonstrates complete obstruction of flow in the superior aspect of the systemic venous limb. Collateral flow through the azygos vein is seen. **B,** during balloon angioplasty of the superior aspect of the systemic venous limb, a waist is seen at the site of obstruction *(arrows)* with the balloon inflated to 20 mm. **C,** repeat frontal digital angiogram after balloon angioplasty now demonstrates patency across the superior aspect of the systemic venous limb with filling of the left ventricle.

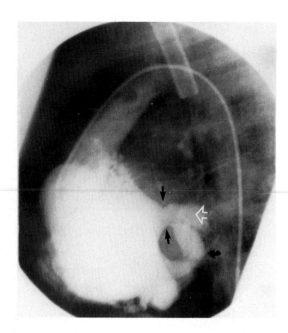

FIG 21–24.
Pulmonary venous obstruction after a Mustard procedure for transposition. This lateral cineangiocardiogram was made after a retrograde catheter passage across the aortic valve and through the right ventricle and tricuspid valve into the distal portion of the pulmonary venous limb of the atrial baffle. Some retrograde flow of contrast into the proximal portion of the pulmonary venous limb of the atrial baffle *(open arrow)* outlines severe obstruction *(closed arrows)* in the midportion of the pulmonary venous limb. There is also retrograde opacification of the coronary sinus *(curved arrow);* this is not of significance.

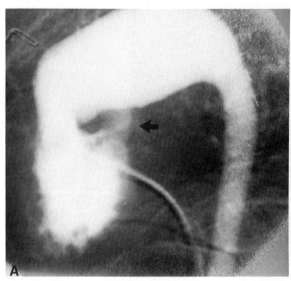 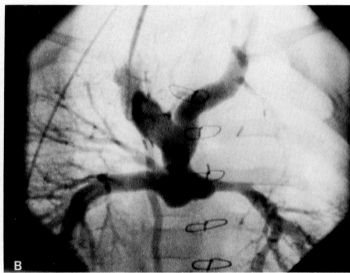

FIG 21–25.
Norwood procedure, stage II, in a 1-year-old boy with hypoplastic left heart syndrome. **A,** lateral digital right ventricular angiogram opacifies the large homograft connecting the main pulmonary artery with the descending aorta. There is early opacification of the hypoplastic aorta *(arrow)* via its anastomosis with the pulmonary artery–descending aorta conduit. **B,** AP digital angiogram after catheterization of the right internal jugular vein and injection of contrast medium into the right innominate vein opacifies the right and left innominate veins and bidirectional Glenn shunt with opacification of the pulmonary arteries. The left pulmonary artery shows proximal narrowing, and nonfilling of the left upper lobe. Collateral flow through the right and left internal mammary veins is also seen.

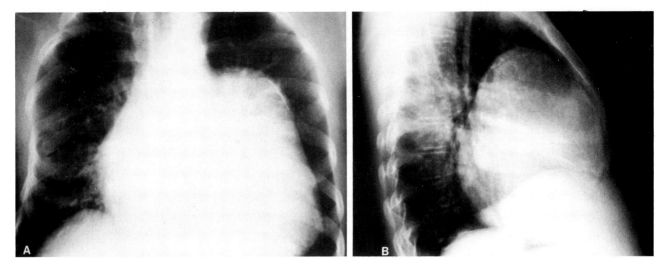

FIG 21–26.
Tetralogy of Fallot repair with aneurysmal dilatation of the right ventricular outflow tract patch. Frontal **(A)** and lateral **(B)** chest radiographs demonstrate aneurysmal dilatation of the right ventricular outflow tract patch with marginal calcification. Moderate cardiomegaly is present secondary to severe pulmonary regurgitation with right ventricular dilatation.

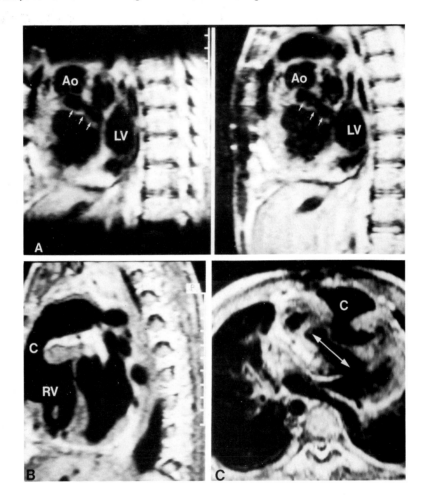

FIG 21–27.
Repair of double-outlet right ventricle with transposition utilizing an intracardiac and extracardiac conduit. **A,** sagittal 3-mm adjacent spin-echo MRIs demonstrate the intracardiac conduit and VSD *(arrows)* establishing continuity between the left ventricle *(LV)* and transposed aorta *(Ao)*. Posterior to the aorta is the pulmonary artery which has been ligated just above the valve. **B,** sagittal 3-mm spin-echo MRI demonstrates the extracardiac conduit *(C)* establishing continuity between the right ventricle *(RV)* and pulmonary arteries. The ventricular septum and left ventricle are posterior to the right ventricle. **C,** axial 3-mm spin-echo MRI demonstrates the patent intracardiac conduit *(arrows)* between the left ventricle and aorta, and external cardiac conduit *(C)* between the right ventricle and pulmonary artery.

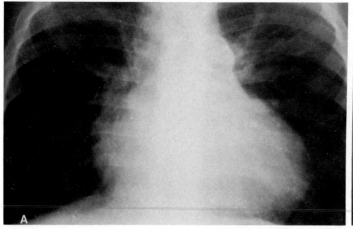
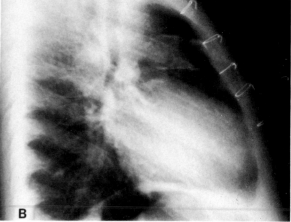

FIG 21–28.

Truncus arteriosus repair utilizing an extracardiac conduit. Frontal **(A)** and lateral **(B)** chest radiographs demonstrate calcification of the extracardiac conduit between the right ventricle and pulmo-nary arteries in this 3-year-old patient following repair of truncus ar-teriosus.

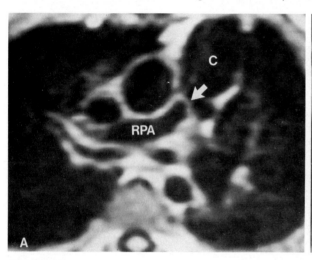
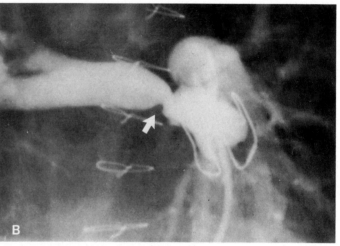

FIG 21–29.

Truncus arteriosus repair utilizing an extracardiac conduit with anastomotic stenosis. **A,** axial 3-mm spin-echo MRI demonstrates anastomotic obstruction *(arrow)* between the extracardiac conduit *(C)* and right pulmonary artery *(RPA)*. **B,** frontal pulmonary artery angiogram with injection of contrast into the conduit just distal to the prosthetic valve confirms the anastomotic narrowing *(arrow)* of the proximal right pulmonary artery.

TABLE 21–2   (cont.).

Operative Repair

Procedures	Description	Radiologic Findings and Complications
Extracardiac conduit	Extracardiac conduit, originally designed by Rastelli, is placement of an external conduit between the right ventricle and PAs during operative repair of patients with tetralogy of Fallot with pulmonary atresia, truncus arteriosus, and forms of double-outlet right ventricle (Fig 21–27,B and C). Either a homograft aortic valve with segment of ascending aorta or a Dacron conduit with porcine aortic valve is used.	Following operation, calcification of the conduit/prosthetic valve may be seen and is a clue to the development of conduit obstruction (Fig 21–28). Postoperative obstruction may occur at the proximal or distal anastomotic sites (Fig 21–29), at the level of the prosthetic valve, or within the conduit related to a neointimal fibrotic peel.
Senning procedure	Palliative repair for patients with complete transposition of the great vessels. This procedure is similar to a Mustard procedure directing superior and inferior venae cavae flow through the mitral valve into the left ventricle, and pulmonary venous flow through the right tricuspid valve into the right ventricle.	The operation has a lower incidence of systemic or pulmonary venous obstruction than the Mustard procedure.
Subclavian flap	Utilization of the proximal left subclavian artery for coarctation repair. The left subclavian artery is ligated distal to the vertebral artery, and the proximal portion of the subclavian artery utilized to enlarge the aortic isthmus and site of coarctation during coarctation repair.	Anastomotic narrowing is the primary complication. The left arm is supplied by mediastinal and intercostal collaterals.

INTERVENTIONAL CATHETERIZATION PROCEDURES

In the past 25 years, beginning with Rashkind balloon atrial septostomy in 1966, catheters have been utilized with increasing frequency to perform therapeutic procedures within the heart. During the past decade, the development of balloon catheters has resulted in significant advancement in intracardiac therapeutic procedures (Table 21–3). Atrial septostomies can now be performed with balloon or blade catheters. During the past decade balloon catheters have been utilized to dilate valves (balloon valvuloplasty) and efficaciously treat patients with congenital pulmonary valve (see Figs 16–37 and 16–88,D) or aortic valve stenosis (see Fig 16–41), rheumatic mitral stenosis, and bioprosthetic valve stenosis. Balloon catheters also have been utilized to dilate vessels (balloon angioplasty) to treat coarctation (see Fig 16–53), stenosis following coarctation repair, peripheral pulmonary artery stenosis (Fig 21–30), pulmonary venous stenosis, and patients with baffle obstruction of the superior or inferior vena cava (see Fig 21–23). It occasionally proves efficacious in the treatment of anastomotic narrowing in patients with Blalock-Taussig shunts. In certain patients balloon catheters are indicated in the treatment of membranous subaortic stenosis. Occlusion devices are being developed and are in the investigational stage for the closure of atrial (see Fig 16–12). and ventricular septal defects (see Fig 16–7), and patent ductus arteriosus (see Fig 16–20). Coil occlusion is useful

TABLE 21–3.

Interventional Catheterization Procedures

Atrial septostomy
  Balloon
  Blade
Valve dilatation (balloon valvuloplasty)
  Pulmonary valve stenosis (Figs 16–37, 16–88,D)
  Aortic valve stenosis (Fig 16–41)
  Rheumatic mitral valve stenosis
  Bioprosthetic "pulmonary" valve stenosis
Vessel dilatation (balloon angioplasty)
  Coarctation (Fig 16–53)
  Peripheral pulmonary artery stenosis (Fig 21–30)
  Pulmonary venous stenosis
  Atrial baffle obstruction of the superior or inferior vena cava (Fig 21–23)
  Systemic–pulmonary artery shunts
Miscellaneous
  Subaortic stenosis
Vascular stents
  Venous
  Arterial
Occlusion devices
  Atrial septal defect (Fig 16–12)
  Ventricular septal defect (Fig 16–7)
  Patent ductus arteriosus (Fig 16–20)
  Systemic–pulmonary artery collaterals (Fig 21–31)
  Systemic–pulmonary artery shunts (Fig 21–32)
  Venous collaterals (Fig 21–33)
  Aberrant arteries (Fig 16–32)
  Pulmonary artioevenous malformations
Foreign body retrieval (Fig 21–35)

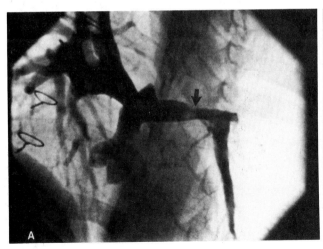 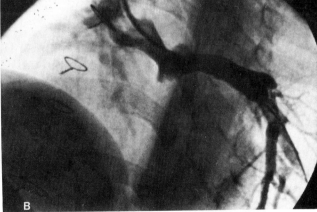

FIG 21–30.
Balloon angioplasty of peripheral pulmonary artery stenosis. **A,** digital pulmonary angiogram in the axial left anterior oblique projection following catheter passage down the superior vena cava into the pulmonary artery in this patient with bidirectional Glenn procedure demonstrates peripheral left pulmonary artery stenosis at the site of previous left pulmonary artery repair *(arrow).* **B,** repeat digital pulmonary angiogram following balloon angioplasty with an 8-mm, then a 12-mm balloon demonstrates complete relief of the left pulmonary artery obstruction.

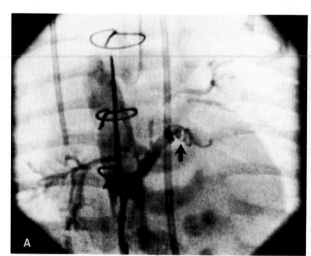

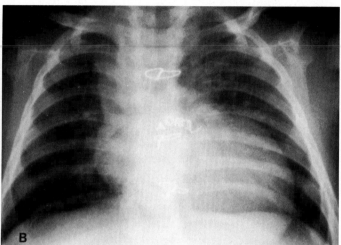

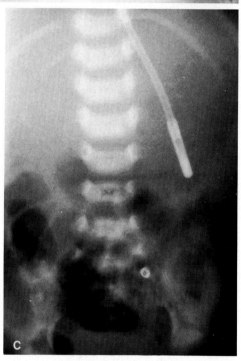

FIG 21–31.
Coil occlusion of systemic-pulmonary collaterals in a neonate with pulmonary atresia.
A, frontal digital aortogram demonstrates coil occlusion *(arrow)* of a systemic–pulmonary artery collateral to the left lung arising from the right descending aorta. **B,** chest radiograph demonstrates multiple vertebral anomalies, right ventricular enlargement, absence of the main pulmonary artery segment, right aortic arch, and coil occlusion of the systemic–pulmonary artery collateral to the left lung. **C,** abdominal radiograph demonstrates a "lost" occlusion coil shown angiographically to be in the left external iliac artery.

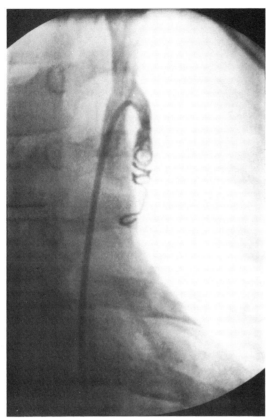

FIG 21–32.
Coil embolization of a left Blalock-Taussig shunt. Digital angiogram following injection in the proximal left Blalock-Taussig shunt confirms occlusion of the shunt after placement of a Gianturco coil.

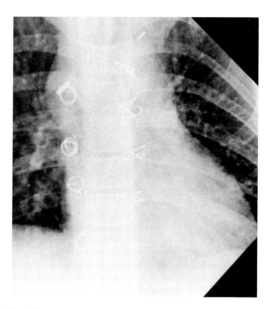

FIG 21–33.
Coil occlusion of the azygos vein (same patient as in Figure 21–6). In this patient with bidirectional Glenn shunt, coil occlusion of the azygos vein has been performed at multiple levels to prevent collateral flow through the azygos system bypassing the Glenn shunt.

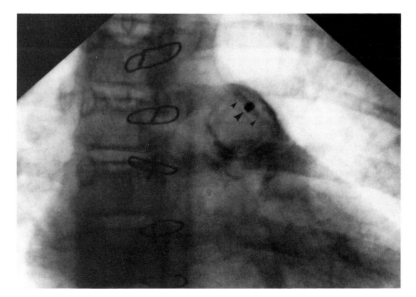

FIG 21–34.
Digital spot radiograph demonstrates a broken balloon *(small arrowheads)* and catheter fragment *(large arrowhead)* lodged in the calcified extracardiac conduit following attempted balloon angioplasty of the prosthetic valve in this patient after repair of truncus arteriosus.

FIG 21–35.
Catheter retrieval of broken right atrial line. **A,** lateral chest radiograph demonstrates a right atrial line fractured just below the skin during attempted removal 4 days after tetralogy of Fallot repair. **B,** fluoroscopic spot film in the frontal projection demonstrates the wire snare in position adjacent to the end of the right atrial catheter fragment. **C,** the snare has been retracted into the guiding catheter around the end of the catheter fragment. The guiding catheter, snare, and catheter fragment were withdrawn as a unit through a 6F sheath in the right femoral vein.

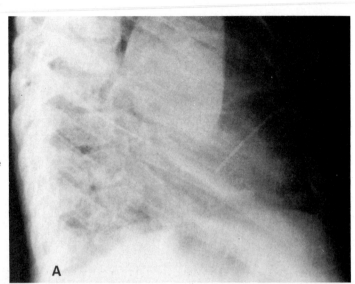

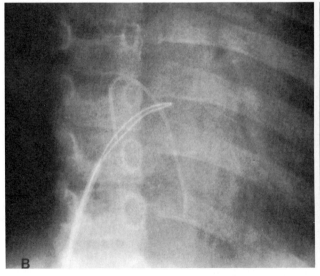

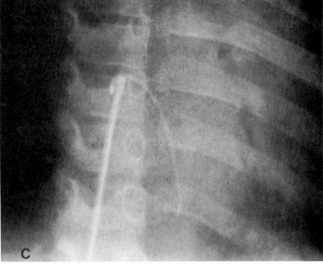

for the embolic closure of systemic–pulmonary artery collaterals (Fig 21–31,A and B), systemic–pulmonary artery shunts (Fig 21–32), venous collaterals (Fig 21–33), aberrant arteries (see Fig 16–32), and pulmonary arteriovenous malformations. Rigid metallic vascular stents are being developed for long-term therapy of arterial and venous obstruction in the superior and inferior venae cavae, pulmonary arteries, and peripheral arteries. Common complications that may result from interventional procedures include "lost" occlusion coils (Fig 21–31,C) and "lost" balloons or balloon fragments (Fig 21–34). Catheter retrieval of intravascular foreign bodies has been used to remove broken fragments of indwelling catheters that have become severed, and embolized distally (Fig 21–35). Many of these procedures are discussed further in Chapters 16 and 21.

Acknowledgments

The author gratefully acknowledges the dedicated work of the Primary Children's Medical Center Medical Imaging staff and our clinical colleagues, without whose help Part III would not have been possible. Dr. Barbara S. Reid wrote the section on nuclear cardiology and Dr. Victoria E. Judd wrote the sections on fetal echocardiography and electrocardiography. Dr. Rex Deitz assisted in the cardiac operation section. Two-dimensional and color-flow echocardiograms were obtained by our ultrasonographers Laura Newren, Joyce Lukken, Amanda Horne, Alice Olsen, and Britt Lewis. Technical assistance in magnetic resonance imaging was provided by Colette Madsen, Shari Combe, Mickey Falkner, and Greg Fenstermaker. Technical assistance in angiocardiography and digital angiography was provided by Cheryl Fitzgerald, Matthew Judd, and Laurie Coburn. Outstanding secretarial support for this manuscript was provided by Valorie Kemp and Margaret Farrell, whose long hours and dedication greatly assisted the authors in the preparation of these chapters.

REFERENCES

Common Cardiac Operations

Ascuitto RJ, Ross-Ascuitto NT, Markowitz RI, et al: Aneurysms of the right ventricular outflow tract after tetralogy of Fallot repair: Role of radiology. *Radiology* 1988; 167:115–119.

Bailey WW, Kirklin JW, Bargeron LM Jr, et al: Late results with synthetic valved external conduits from venous ventricle to pulmonary arteries. *Circulation* 1977; 56(suppl 2):2-73–2-79.

Bargeron LM Jr, Karp RB, Barcia A, et al: Late deterioration of patients after superior vena cava to right pulmonary artery anastomosis. *Am J Cardiol* 1972; 30:211–216.

Berman MA, Barash PS, Hellenbrand WE, et al: Late development of severe pulmonary venous obstruction following the Mustard operation. *Cardiovasc Surg* 1976; 56:2-91–2-94.

Bickers GH, Williams SM, Harned RK, et al: Gastroesophageal deformities of left ventricular-abdominal aortic conduit. *Am J Roentgenol* 1982; 138:867–869.

Boruchow IB, Bartley TD, Elliott LP, et al: Late superior vena cava syndrome after superior vena cava-right pulmonary artery anastomosis. *N Engl J Med* 1969; 281:646–650.

Bridges ND, Jonas RA, Mayer JE, et al: Bidirectional cavopulmonary anastomosis as interim palliation for high-risk Fontan candidates. *Circulation* 1990; 82(suppl 4):170–176.

Bridges ND, Lock JE, Castaneda AR: Baffle fenestration with subsequent transcatheter closure: Modification of the Fontan operation for patients at increased risk. *Circulation* 1990; 82:1681–1689.

Bull C, de Leval MR, Stark J, et al: Use of subpulmonary ventricular chamber in the Fontan circulation. *J Thorac Cardiovasc Surg* 1983; 85:21–31.

Castaneda AR, Trusler GA, Paul MH, et al: The early results of treatment of simple transposition in the current era. *J Thorac Cardiovasc Surg* 1988; 95:14–28.

Ceithami EL, Puga FJ, Danielson GK, et al: Results of the Damus-Stansel-Kaye procedure for transposition of the great arteries and for double-outlet right ventricle with subpulmonary ventricular septal defect. *Ann Thorac Surg* 1984; 38:433–437.

Clark RA, Colley DP, Siedlecki E: Late complications at repair site of operated coarctation of aorta. *Am J Roentgenol* 1979; 133:1071–1075.

Clouthier A, Ash JM, Smallhorn JF, et al: Abnormal distribution of pulmonary blood flow after the Glenn shunt or Fontan procedure: Risk of development of arteriovenous fistulae. *Circulation* 1985; 72:471–479.

Di Donato RM, Wernovsky G, Walsh EP, et al: Results of the arterial switch operation for transposition of the great arteries with ventricular septal defect. *Circulation* 1989; 80:1689–1705.

Driscoll DJ, Nihill MR, Vargo TA, et al: Late development of pulmonary venous obstruction following Mustard's operation using a Dacron baffle. *Circulation* 1977; 55:484–488.

Ellis K: Postoperative roentgen evaluation of total correction of tetralogy of Fallot. *Circulation* 1973; 47:1335–1348.

Engle MA, Diaz S: Long-term results of surgery for congenital heart disease: I. Surgery of specific anomalies. *Circulation* 1982; 65:415–419.

Engle MA, Diaz S: Long-term results of surgery for congenital heart disease: II. Surgery of specific anomalies (continued), surgical procedures and devices, and surgical techniques. *Circulation* 1982; 65:634–638.

Formanek G, Hunt C, Castaneda A, et al: Thickening of pulmonary valve leaflets following pulmonary artery banding. *Radiology* 1971; 98:75–78.

Freed MD, Rosenthal A, Pauth WH Jr, et al: Development of subaortic stenosis after pulmonary artery banding. *Circulation* 1973; 47–48 (suppl 3):3-7–3-110.

Freedom RM, Benson LN, Smallhorn JF, et al: Subaortic stenosis, the univentricular heart, and banding of the pulmonary artery: An analysis of the courses of 43 patients with univentricular heart palliated by pulmonary artery banding. *Circulation* 1986; 73:758–764.

Freedom RM, Culham JAG, Olley PM, et al: Anatomic correction of transposition of the great arteries: Pre- and postoperative cardiac catheterization, with angiocardiography in five patients. *Circulation* 1981; 63:905–914.

George BL, Laks H, Klitzner TS, et al: Results of the Senning procedure in infants with simple and complex transposition of the great arteries. *Am J Cardiol* 1987; 59:426–430.

Girod DA, Fontan F, Deville C, et al: Long-term results after the Fontan operation for tricuspid atresia. *Circulation* 1987; 75:605–610.

Gutierrez F, Mirowitz S, Canter C: Magnetic resonance imaging in the evaluation of postoperative congenital heart disease. *Semin Ultrasound CT MR* 1990; 11:234–245.

Higgins CB, Reinke RT: Postoperative chylothorax in children with congenital heart disease. *Radiology* 1976; 119:409–413.

Hipona FA, Paredes S, Lerona PT: Roentgenologic analysis of common postoperative problems in congenital heart disease. *Radiol Clin North Am* 1971; 9:229–251.

Hoeffel JC, Henry M, Worms AM, et al: Results of catheterization after banding of the pulmonary artery: Observations on 27 cases. *Ann Radiol* 1973; 16:463–470.

Hoeffel JC, Pernot C, Worms AM, et al: Calcified aneurysm of the main pulmonary artery: A complication of banding. *Radiology* 1974; 113:167–168.

Kersting-Sommerhoff BA, Seelos KC, Hardy C, et al: Evaluation of surgical procedures for cyanotic congenital heart disease by using MR imaging. *Am J Roentgenol* 1990; 155:259–266.

Lang P, Norwood WI: Hemodynamic assessment after palliative surgery for hypoplastic left heart syndrome. *Circulation* 1983; 68:204–208.

Litwin SB, Fellows K: Systemic to pulmonary arterial shunts for patients with cyanotic congenital heart disease: Current status. *Pediatr Radiol* 1973; 1:41–46.

Marbarber JP, Sandza JG Jr, Hartmann AF Jr, et al: Blalock-Taussig anastomosis. *Cardiovasc Surg* 1977; 58:I74–I77.

McFaul RC, Tajik AJ, Mair DD, et al: Development of pulmonary arteriovenous shunt after superior vena cava–right pulmonary artery (Glenn) anastomosis. *Circulation* 1977; 55:212–216.

Mullins CE: Pediatric and congenital therapeutic cardiac catheterization. *Circulation* 1989; 79:1153–1159.

Norman JC, Nihill MR, Cooley DA: Valved apico-aortic composite conduits for left ventricular outflow tract obstructions. *Am J Cardiol* 1980; 45:1265–1271.

Pitlick P, French J, Guthaner D, et al: Results of intraventricular baffle procedure for ventricular septal defect and double outlet right ventricle or d-transposition of the great arteries. *Am J Cardiol* 1981; 47:307–314.

Rizk G, Moller JH, Amplatz K: The angiographic appearance of the heart following the Mustard procedure. *Radiology* 1973; 106:269–273.

Sidi D, Planche C, Kachaner J, et al: Anatomic correction of simple transposition of the great arteries in 50 neonates. *Circulation* 1987; 75:429–435.

Rocchini AP, Rosenthal A, Castaneda AR, et al: Subaortic obstruction after the use of an intracardiac baffle to tunnel the left ventricle to the aorta. *Circulation* 1976; 54:957–960.

Ross EM, McIntosh CL, Roberts WC: "Massive" calcification of a right ventricular outflow parietal pericardial patch in tetralogy of Fallot. *Am J Cardiol* 1984; 54:691–692.

Trusler GA, Williams WG, Cohen AJ, et al: The cavopulmonary shunt. *Circulation* 1990; (suppl 4):4-131–4-138.

Waldman JD, Lamberti JJ, George L, et al: Experience with Damus procedure. *Circulation* 1988; 78 (suppl 3):3-32–3-39.

Welch E, Zabaleta I, Fojaco R, et al: Aneurysms of the right ventricular outflow tract: A complication of aorta-main pulmonary (central) shunt. *Pediatr Cardiol* 1991; 12:229–232.

West PN, Hartmann AF Jr, Weldon CS: Long-term function of aortic homografts as the right ventricular outflow tract. *Circulation* 1977; 56 (suppl 2):2-66–2-72.

Yacoub MH, Bernhard A, Radley-Smith R, et al: Supravalvular pulmonary stenosis after anatomic correction of transposition of the great arteries: Cases and prevention. *Circulation* 1982; 66 (suppl 1):1-193–1-202.

Interventional Catheterization Procedures

Lock JE, Cockerman JT, Keane JF, et al: Transcatheter umbrella closure of congenital heart defects. *Circulation* 1987; 75:593–599.

Lock JE, Block PC, McKay RG, et al: Transcatheter closure of ventricular septal defects. *Circulation* 1988; 78:361–368.

Lois JF, Gomes AS, Smith DC, et al: Systemic-to-pulmonary collateral vessels and shunts: Treatment with embolization. *Radiology* 1988; 169:671–676.

Medellin GJ, Di Sessa TG, Tonkin ILD: Interventional catheterization in congenital heart disease. *Radiol Clin North Am* 1989; 27:1223.

Mullins CE: Pediatric and congenital therapeutic cardiac catheterization. *Circulation* 1989; 79:1153–1159.

O'Laughlin MP, Perry SB, Lock JE, et al: Use of endovascular stents in congenital heart disease. *Circulation* 1991; 83:1923–1939.

Rocchini AP: Transcatheter closure of atrial septal defects. *Circulation* 1990; 82:1044–1045.

Rome JJ, Keane JF, Perry SB, et al: Double-umbrella closure of atrial defects. *Circulation* 1990; 82:751–785.

PART 4

The Abdomen and Gastrointestinal Tract

BRUCE R. PARKER

Abdominal Wall and Peritoneal Cavity

The abdomen extends from the diaphragm superiorly to the pelvis inferiorly and includes both the intraperitoneal and extraperitoneal structures. The advent of cross-sectional imaging has made knowledge of abdominal anatomy and embryology even more important than was true earlier.

SECTION 1

Introduction to the Abdominal Wall

NORMAL ANATOMY

The diaphragm forms the roof of the abdomen. Its anatomy and development are discussed in Chapter 6. The posterior abdominal wall comprises the spine, the paraspinous muscles, and the tissues superficial to them. The posterior wall structures are discussed in Chapter 2. The remainder of the abdomen includes the abdominal wall and retroperitoneal and pelvic structures, discussed in this section, and the extraperitoneal organs which are discussed in Part V.

From superficial to deep, the anterior abdominal wall is comprised of the skin, superficial fascia (the Camper and Scarpa layers), subcutaneous fat, muscles, transverse fascia (the Gallaudet or innominate fascia), properitoneal fat, and the peritoneum. The paired rectus muscles run cephalocaudad in the midline. The paired anterolateral muscle groups include the external and internal oblique muscles and the transverse abdominal muscle (Fig 22–1). The aponeuroses of the external oblique muscles carry downward and medially to cover the front of the abdomen from the xiphoid to the pubis. At the lateral margins of the rectus muscles, the aponeuroses split to form the spigelian fascia which forms the anterior and posterior rectus sheaths. The sheaths join in the midline forming the linea alba which separates the two rectus muscles by up to 6 mm.

The lowermost portion of the aponeurosis of the external oblique muscle ends in a thickened free border, the inguinal ligament, which runs from the anterior superior iliac spine to the pubic tubercle. The subcutaneous (or external) inguinal ring is an opening in the aponeurosis of the external oblique muscle between the inguinal ligament inferiorly and the

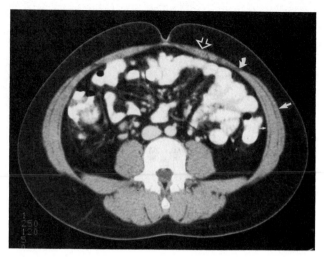

FIG 22–1.
CT scan at the level of the umbilicus in an obese 11-year-old boy demonstrates the abdominal musculature to good advantage. The external oblique muscle *(solid white straight arrow)* and the transverse abdominal muscle *(small white arrow)* are seen on either side of the internal oblique muscle. The aponeurosis of the external oblique muscle becomes the spigelian fascia *(curved white arrow)* which splits to form the anterior and posterior sheaths of the rectus abdominus muscle *(open arrow)*.

tendinous portion superiorly. The spermatic cord in males or the round ligament in females passes through the inguinal canal.

DEVELOPMENT OF THE ANTERIOR ABDOMINAL WALL, PERITONEAL CAVITY, AND MIDGUT

The embryologic development of the anterior abdominal wall is intimately associated with that of the midgut. The early embryonic abdominal cavity is open to the extraembryonic coelom, and its laterally placed walls consist of ectoderm and mesoderm without blood vessels, muscles, or nerves. These lateral margins fold inward as do a cephalic and a caudal fold, all of which are necessary for normal closure of the anterior abdominal wall. During the sixth week, the mesoderm of the paraspinous myotomes migrates laterally and ventrally, its leading edge differentiating into the widely separated rectus muscles. Meanwhile, the main mass of the mesoderm forms the oblique and transverse muscles. The two rectus muscles are approximated beginning at the cranial and caudal ends, becoming completely fused by the 12th week at the linea alba, except for the umbilical ring.

The midgut is that part of the intestinal tract supplied by the superior mesenteric artery. It extends from the second portion of the duodenum to the transverse colon, most commonly in its mid- to distal portion. Initially, the embryonic gut is a straight tube with the superior mesenteric artery in its dorsal mesentery. Ventrally, the midgut communicates with the yolk sac via the vitelline duct (yolk stalk).

At the beginning of the sixth week, the elongating intestinal tube buckles ventrally through the umbilical cord into the extraembryonic coelom (Fig 22–2,A). The vitelline duct is the lead point for this umbilical herniation of the midgut. The portion of the midgut cephalad to the vitelline duct grows rapidly, forming the many loops of the small intestine. The caudal limb grows rather more slowly with the development of the cecal diverticulum being the most important feature at this stage.

Within the umbilical cord, the midgut rotates 90 degrees counterclockwise around the axis of the superior mesenteric artery (Fig 22–2,B). During the tenth week, the intestines return rapidly to the intraembryonic coelom, now the embryonic peritoneal cavity, rotating another 180 degrees as they do (Fig 22–2,C). The cecum is last to return, coming to rest initially in the right upper quadrant and then descending to the right lower quadrant as the ascending colon elongates (Fig 22–2,D).

Initially, the entire midgut is on a dorsal mesentery, but as the duodenum, the cecum, and the ascending colon are pressed against the posterior abdominal wall, their portions of the dorsal mesentery fuse with the posterior peritoneum, making these structures retroperitoneal. The dorsal mesentery of the small bowel, then, is a fan-shaped structure fixed along a linear attachment from the duodenojejunal junction to the ileocolic junction.

As the anterior abdominal wall closes, the umbilical cord is left open containing its three blood vessels, the omphalomesenteric (vitelline) duct, and allantois (Fig 22–3). The omphalomesenteric duct runs from the future distal ileum to the extraembryonic coelom. The allantois is a vestigial structure in the human extending from the portion of the embryonic cloaca that will become the bladder dome to a blind end inside the umbilical cord. The omphalomesenteric duct normally involutes while the allantois persists as the urachus or median umbilical ligament.

The 4-week embryo has a curve in its intraembryonic coelom which represents the future pericardial cavity, while its lateral limbs represent the future pleural and peritoneal cavities. This cavity is open to the extraembryonic coelom. By the end of the fourth week, recognizable pericardial and peritoneal cavities are present connected by two small

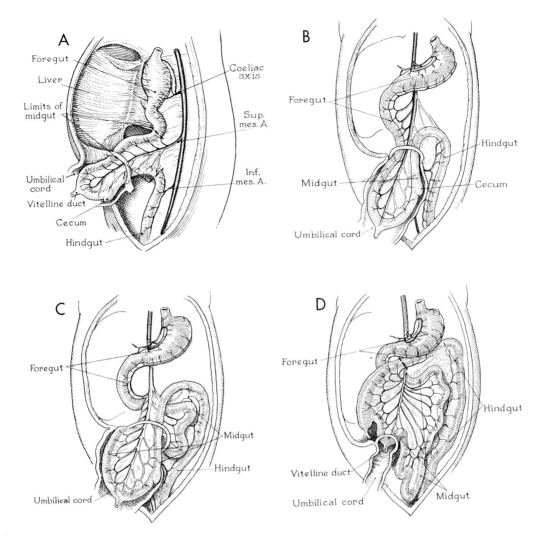

FIG 22–2.
Normal fetal rotation of the midgut in successive stages. **A,** lateral view, 5th fetal week. The foregut, hindgut, and midgut are suspended from the posterior wall in the common dorsal mesentery. Part of the midgut and superior mesenteric artery protrude into the umbilical cord and form a physiologic umbilical hernia. The foregut derives its blood supply from the celiac axis, the midgut from the superior mesenteric artery, and the hindgut from the inferior mesenteric artery. **B,** frontal view, 8th fetal week. The midgut has rotated 90 degrees counterclockwise so that the prearterial segment now lies on the right and the postarterial segment on the left. External rotation is complete. **C,** frontal view, 10th fetal week. The midgut is returning to the abdominal cavity and is undergoing internal rotation. Note that the proximal end of the midgut returns first and that it passes to the right and behind the superior mesenteric artery. Succeeding loops are then packed into the left upper abdominal quadrant and later into the right side and lower portions of the abdomen. **D,** at about the 11th fetal week, all of the midgut has returned to the abdominal cavity and has rotated an additional 180 degrees counterclockwise from its position in **B** and a total of 270 degrees from its original position shown in **A.** The process of rotation is now complete, and the mesenteries are then fixed onto the posterior wall of the abdomen in the areas indicated in *stipple.* In the case of failure of rotation or incomplete rotation, the cecum and small intestine remain in their early fetal patterns, and more important, the stage of fixation is missed. Without its anchorage to the posterior abdominal wall, the malplaced midgut is prone to twist around the superior mesenteric artery on a narrow mesenteric pedicle to form a volvulus. The volvulus usually impinges on the third portion of the duodenum and causes complete or incomplete obstruction at this level (Modified from Golden R: *Radiologic Examination of the Small Intestine.* Philadelphia, JB Lippincott, 1945.)

pericardioperitoneal canals. Ultimately, the lung buds grow into these canals and the pleural cavity is separated from the pericardial cavity by the cranial pleuropericardial membranes and from the peritoneal cavity by the caudal pleuroperitoneal membranes. These latter membranes fuse with the dorsal mesentery of the esophagus and with the septum transversum, the future diaphragm, to complete the separation of the thoracic cavities from the abdominal cavity. These cavities have a parietal wall lined by mesothelium derived from the somatic mesoderm which will become the peritoneum. The developing

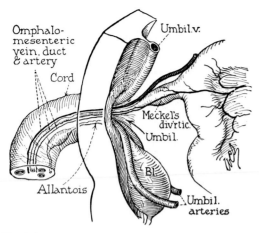

FIG 22–3.
Omphalomesenteric vessels and duct and the allantoic stalk. Persistence of the duct gives rise to a wide variety of malformations including Meckel diverticulum. Persistence of the allantoic stalk causes various urachal deformities. (From an original drawing by Thomas S. Cullen.)

peritoneal cavity has a protrusion known as the processus vaginalis which extends through the inguinal ring. It is normally obliterated before birth, but its persistence may lead to inguinal hernias. The visceral lining is derived from the splanchnic meso-

derm. Of interest with respect to the relative incidence of right- and left-sided Bochdalek hernias is that the right pleuropericardial canal normally closes before the left one. Normal closure is effected before the intestines return to the coelomic cavity. If there is persistence of a patent canal at this time, the returning intestines may pass into the thorax, often taking the stomach and spleen with them on the left and the liver on the right.

REFERENCES

DiSantis DJ, Siegel MJ, Katz ME: Simplified approach to umbilical remnant abnormalities. *Radiographics* 1991; 11:59.

Duhamel B: Embryology of exomphalos and allied malformations. *Arch Dis Child* 1963; 38:142.

Gray SW, Skandalakis JE: *Embryology for Surgeons.* Philadelphia, WB Saunders, 1972.

Hutchin P: Somatic anomalies of the umbilicus and anterior abdominal wall. *Surg Gynecol Obstet* 1965; 120:1075.

Moore KL: *The Developing Human,* ed 4. Philadelphia, WB Saunders, 1988.

SECTION 2

Abdominal Wall Abnormalities

HERNIAS

Diaphragmatic Hernias

Herniation of abdominal contents can occur superiorly into the thorax, inferiorly through the femoral and inguinal canals, anteriorly through abdominal wall defects or the umbilical ring, and, very rarely, posteriorly through defects in the musculature. Diaphragmatic hernias are discussed more fully in Chapters 6, 25, and 52. Herniation of the stomach through the esophageal hiatus is the most common of these. A sliding hiatus hernia in which the esophagogastric junction is above the hiatus is the most frequently occurring. A paraesophageal hernia occurs when the gastric fundus and proximal body herniate into the chest leaving the esophagogastric

junction in near-normal position (see Figs 25–38, 25–43,D, and 25–44,C).

Hernias may occur posteriorly and laterally through patent pleuroperitoneal canals, also known as the *foramina of Bochdalek.* Bochdalek hernias usually occur during fetal development and present in the newborn (see Chapter 52), but delayed Bochdalek hernias in older children are being reported with increasing frequency (Fig 22–4). In the newborn, the hernias are more commonly left-sided, but the opposite is true in patients with delayed appearance. Berman et al. reported 26 patients with Bochdalek hernias diagnosed more than 8 weeks after

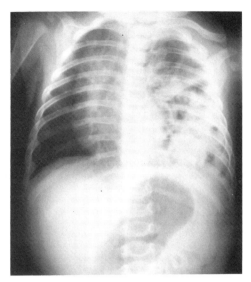

FIG 22–4.
Delayed presentation of Bochdalek hernia in a 5-month-old infant with 3 weeks of respiratory distress. Prior well-baby visits had demonstrated no abnormality. Following surgical repair, no significant pulmonary hypoplasia was identified.

birth. Misdiagnosis had occurred in 16 of the patients. Only one third of the patients had pulmonary hypoplasia, consistent with a later onset of the herniation than is true of those patients diagnosed at birth. A rare variant is herniation of abdominal contents into the pericardium through an incompletely closed pericardioperitoneal canal. The diagnosis of

Bochdalek hernia is usually made by clinical means and plain film radiography in which loops of bowel can be seen in a hemithorax with corresponding displacement of the mediastinum to the contralateral side. If the diagnosis is in doubt, ultrasound (US) can identify peristalsis of loops of bowel in the thorax or contrast studies can definitely document the herniation of the intestines.

The *foramen of Morgagni* is an anterior and medial diaphragmatic defect through which hernias occur less commonly in children than in adults. Small hernias are difficult to diagnose on plain film since the most common structure to herniate through the foramen is the transverse mesocolon which appears as a solid mass in the cardiophrenic angle. The liver commonly herniates through the foramen in young children (Fig 22–5). If bowel, usually transverse colon, herniates through the foramen, an air-filled structure may be seen in the same location. The hernias are more common on the right than left but may be bilateral. US, computed tomography (CT), and magnetic resonance (MR) have all been used to identify the contents of the hernia.

Groin and Pelvic Hernias

Indirect inguinal hernias are the most common form of inferior abdominal wall herniation. If the processus vaginalis remains open, bowel can herniate through

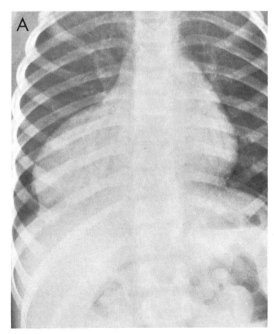

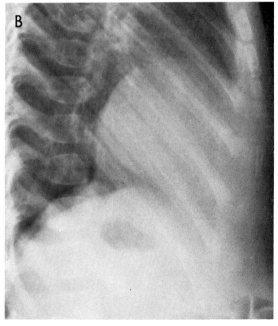

FIG 22–5.
Morgagni hernia in a 4-year-old girl in whom a chest radiograph was performed for symptoms of upper respiratory infection. Note the typical anterior position with a portion of the liver herniating through the foramen of Morgagni.

the inguinal ring into the scrotum in boys (Fig 22–6,A) or through the canal of Nuck into the labia majora in girls (Fig 22–6,B), the latter being relatively infrequent. Most inguinal hernias in children are asymptomatic, but incarceration or stangulation can lead to intestinal obstruction. A sliding hernia may cause sufficient bowel irritation to lead to ileus or even intermittent functional obstruction.

Inguinal hernias may be seen coincidentally on plain films, usually presenting as a loop of bowel in the scrotum. In cases where the loop is persistently fluid-filled, US can identify the intestinal wall surrounding the intraluminal fluid and may show small bubbles of air or peristalsis. These findings help differentiate a hernia from a hydrocele which results from imcomplete closure of the processus vaginalis. Contrast studies are rarely needed, but a small bowel series may demonstrate the herniated loop. Contrast enema with extensive reflux into the small intestine in infants with intestinal obstruction may show a pinched-off loop at the entrance to the inguinal canal. Contrast peritoneography (herniography) is rarely used any longer. Wechsler et al. have demonstrated the CT and MR appearance of inguinal hernias. These studies are rarely needed for diagnostic purposes in children, but the hernias may be incidental findings on studies performed for other reasons.

Direct inguinal hernias, those in which the hernia sac is medial to the epigastric vessels, are acquired rather than congenital and uncommon in children. *Femoral hernias* are also uncommon in the pediatric age group. The intestine herniates through the femoral ring and presents at the saphenous opening. Wechsler et al. have demonstrated the value of CT in differentiating femoral hernias from other abdominal wall masses which may have similar clinical presentations. *Hernias through the obturator foramen* typically occur in elderly women and are rarely, if ever, found in children. *Sciatic hernias* pass through the sciatic foramen into the buttock. Again, they are unusual in childhood but need to be included in the differential diagnosis of pelvic tumors which extend into the buttock such as rhabdomyosarcoma and endodermal sinus tumor.

Anterior Abdominal Wall Defects With Herniation

The majority of patients with anterior wall defects and herniation present in the newborn period and are discussed more thoroughly in Chapter 52. *Omphaloceles* occur in patients in whom the midgut does not return to the intraembryonic coelomic cavity by the tenth week. This leads to failure of infolding of the lateral abdominal walls. The gut appears outside the anterior abdominal wall in infants in the base of the umbilical cord and is surrounded by a translucent sac of peritoneum and amnion (Fig 22–7). With large defects, the liver may also partially herniate

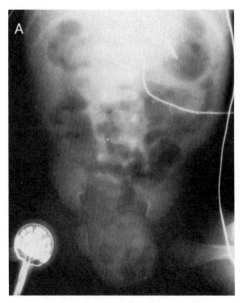
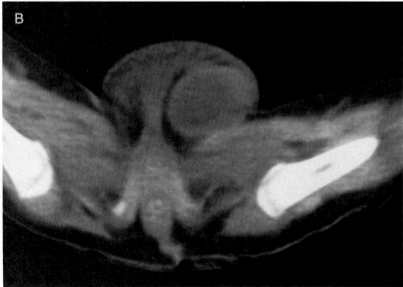

FIG 22–6.
A, AP view of the abdomen and pelvis in a newborn boy demonstrates an enlarged scrotum with multiple air-filled loops of intestine within it secondary to indirect inguinal hernia. **B,** CT scan through the groin in a 3-month-old girl with massive ascites and a palpable left inguinal hernia shows the hernia passing through the inguinal canal.

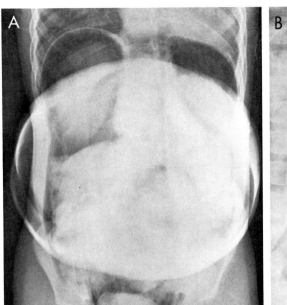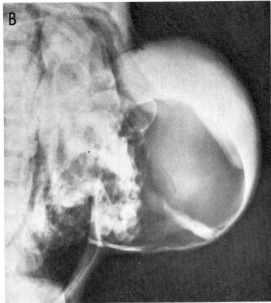

FIG 22-7.
Frontal **(A)** and lateral **(B)** views of the abdomen in a patient with omphalocele and pneumoperitoneum. Note that both loops of bowel and liver are included within the enclosed sac.

into the sac. When the cephalic fold as well as the lateral folds fails to develop, the result is *ectopia cordis* in which congenital heart disease and defects in the pericardium, diaphragm, abdominal wall, and sternum are associated (see Chapter 6). *Gastroschisis* is a paraumbilical herniation of unknown cause in newborns, half of the affected patients being prematures. Clinical differentiation from omphalocele can be made by noting the presence of a normal umbilical cord and the lack of a covering sac.

Umbilical hernias are common protrusions through the umbilical ring (Fig 22-8). The majority regress as the child grows and no diagnostic or therapeutic procedures are usually required. The hernia may rarely become incarcerated or strangulated, but the clinical diagnosis is obvious and imaging studies are not needed. The other abdominal wall hernias are rare in childhood. *Paraumbilical hernias* after infancy are unusual until adulthood. *Epigastric hernias* are defects in the linea alba between the xiphoid and umbilicus. *Spigelian hernias* are herniations through defects in the aponeurosis of the external oblique muscle and frequently are incarcerated and strangulated. CT is diagnostic in most cases as it is with epigastric hernias. *Cloacal exstrophy* results from failure of development of the caudal fold. *Prune-belly syndrome* is the result of failure of development of the anterior wall musculature (Fig 22-9). These last two entities are discussed in Part VII.

UMBILICAL REMNANT ABNORMALITIES

The omphalomesenteric or vitelline duct can remain open throughout its length or at either end or in its midportion (Fig 22-10). DiSantis et al. have defined the completely open duct as type 1, the open-ended as type 2, and the open midportion as type 3. In

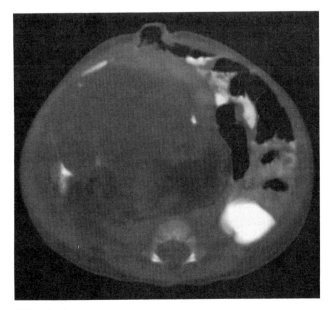

FIG 22-8.
Umbilical hernia in a 3-month-old girl with cystic teratoma. Although umbilical hernias are commonly seen spontaneously, there is an increased incidence in patients with abdominal masses.

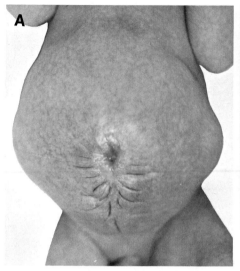

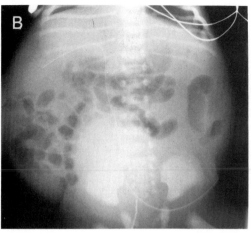

FIG 22–9.
A, photograph of a 5-week-old boy with prune-belly syndrome, congenital absence of the abdominal musculature. **B,** abdominal radiograph of a different patient with prune-belly syndrome dem-

onstrating flaccidity of the abdominal wall with marked dilatation of the bladder. An umbilical venous catheter has been misplaced in the right portal vein.

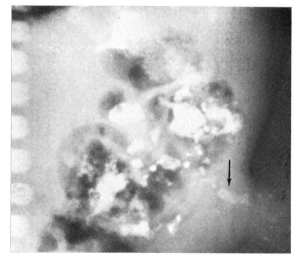

type 1, fecal material can pass through the open duct from the terminal ileum to the umbilicus (Fig 22–11). The opening at the umbilicus frequently can be probed and contrast material injected which passes directly into the ileum.

In type 2 open at the umbilical end, there is a fistulous tract from the umbilicus to the closed portion of the omphalomesentric duct. A nonfecal discharge may be found. Contrast injection reveals a blind-ending sinus tract. Type 2 open at the ileal end is a Meckel diverticulum. Type 3, a vitelline duct cyst open only in the midportion of the duct, is usually

FIG 22–10.
Congenital malformations that may result from persistence of the omphalomesenteric duct: *a,* persistent cord between the ileal wall and the closed umbilicus. *b,* cyst in this same cord. *c,* cyst anchored at the umbilical end of the cord but free at the ileal end. *d,* Meckel diverticulum attached to the closed umbilicus by a closed cord. *e,* everted mucocele of the umbilicus with the cord attachment to the ileal wall. *f,* fecal fistula open at both the umbilical and ileal ends. *g,* Meckel diverticulum open at the ileal end but blind at the umbilical end, which is unattached. *h,* intramural cystic diverticulum. *i,* local stenosis of the ileum at the site of the mouth of a persistent omphalomesenteric duct. (From Cullen TS: *Embryology, Anatomy and Diseases of the Umbilicus.* Philadelphia, WB Saunders, 1916. Used by permission.)

FIG 22–11.
Lateral film of the abdomen after an upper GI series demonstrates barium flowing from the ileum through a patent omphalomesenteric duct to the umbilicus and the anterior abdominal wall.

it is the most common congenital anomaly of the gastrointestinal (GI) tract, occurring in up to 4% of the population, according to autopsy studies. As an omphalomesenteric duct remnant, it projects from the antimesenteric side of the ileum anywhere from 16 to 80 cm proximal to the ileocecal valve, depending somewhat on age. Since the diverticulum represents an opening into the embryonic duct, it contains all four intestinal wall layers, making it a true diverticulum.

Most Meckel diverticula are asymptomatic and found incidentally on imaging studies or at surgery or autopsy. They can lead to intestinal obstruction by acting as a lead point for intussusception, inverting into the ileal lumen, or leading to small bowel volvulus around a persistent vitelline duct remnant leading from the diverticulum to the umbilicus. Since 15% of Meckel diverticula contain heterotopic gastric mucosa, affected patients may present with abdominal pain or GI hemorrhage secondary to peptic ulceration. Less commonly, the diverticula may include duodenal or jejunal mucosa or pancreatic tissue.

Patients with intestinal obstruction present with typical plain film findings (see Chapter 27). Barium studies may demonstrate the point of obstruction but the diverticulum or vitelline duct remnant is usually not seen. Itagaki et al. reported an ultrasonic "double target sign" in two patients with intussusception secondary to Meckel diverticulum. The two

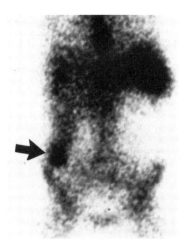

FIG 22–12.
Pertechnetate nuclear medicine scan of the abdomen in a patient with chronic anemia secondary to GI blood loss. Note the collection of radiopharmaceutical *(arrow)* in the right lower quadrant. Meckel diverticulum was demonstrated at surgery and contained gastric mucosa at histologic examination.

asymptomatic but can lead to ileal volvulus. Vitelline duct cysts of types 2 and 3 may be large enough to be identified on US and CT as subumbilical cystic masses.

Meckel diverticulum is not only the most commonly identified omphalomesenteric duct remnant,

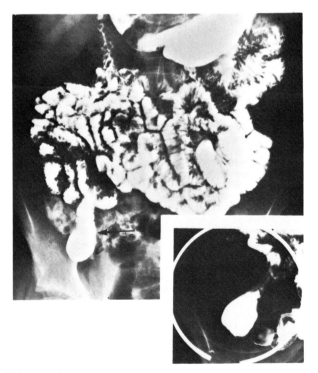

FIG 22–13.
Delayed abdominal film following upper GI series in a 9-year-old child with abdominal pain demonstrates filling of a Meckel diverticulum *(arrow)*. *Inset*, pressure spot film of the involved area.

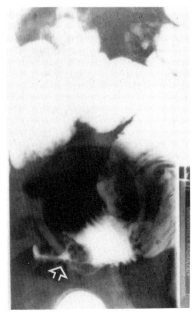

FIG 22–14.
Pressure spot film of a Meckel diverticulum in a patient with a history of GI bleeding demonstrates a characteristic peptic ulcer with a barium-filled niche and radiating folds *(arrow)*.

targets are adjacent to one another but of differing sizes.

Patients with symptoms suspicious of peptic disease of the diverticulum are best examined initially with technetium 99m pertechnetate imaging. Since the pertechnetate ion is secreted by gastric mucosa, the scan may show abnormal accumulation of radiopharmaceutical in the right midabdomen or right lower quadrant (Fig 22–12). False-positive scans may result from the presence of ectopic gastric mucosa in other parts of the intestinal tract. False-negative results may occur secondary to a variety of factors. The false-negative rate may be reduced by pretreating the patient with cimetidine and glucagon.

Contrast small-bowel series or enema may demonstrate a Meckel diverticulum (Figs 22–13 and 22–14), but the sensitivity is very low and routine barium studies are of little value. Angiography has been used to evaluate active GI bleeding from Meckel diverticulum and can be enhanced by the use of digital subtraction techniques. Routh et al. reported abnormal, irregular vessels supplied by an elongated, nonbranching ileal artery in two patients with Meckel diverticulum who had a history of GI bleeding but were not actively bleeding at the time of angiography. Arterial embolization in patients bleeding from Meckel diverticulum has been reported. CT may show evidence of Meckel diverticu-

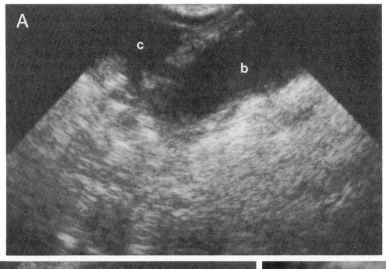

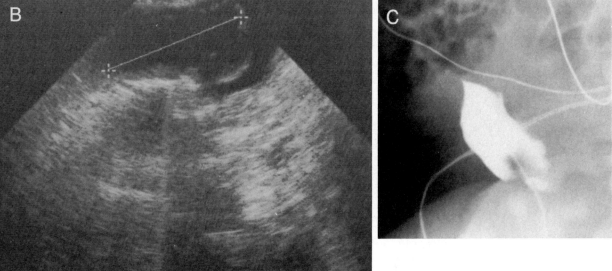

FIG 22–15.
A, longitudinal US demonstrates a fluid-filled tubular structure between the bladder *(b)* and a cystic structure *(c)* in the anterior abdominal wall. **B,** transverse scan at the level of the umbilicus demonstrates a cystic structure just deep to the umbilicus. At surgery, a urachal cyst directly connecting to the bladder was excised. **C,** cystogram in another patient demonstrates characteristic beaking of the anterosuperior aspect of the bladder caused by a patent proximal urachus. The remainder of the urachus from this point to the umbilicus is completely closed.

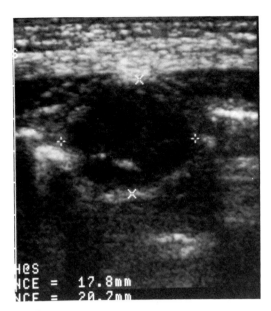

FIG 22–16.
Transverse sonogram at the level of the umbilicus demonstrates a hypoechoic structure just deep to the abdominal wall. When the transducer was placed on the abdomen, purulent material was expressed from the umbilicus. An infected urachal cyst was removed at surgery.

litis, but CT diagnosis of a diverticulum is more likely to be incidental. Giant Meckel diverticulum containing enteroliths may be seen on plain film, CT, or US.

The residuum of the embryonic allantois is known as the urachus. A fully patent urachus connects the bladder to the umbilicus, permitting urine to pass between them (Fig 22–15). The umbilical opening may be difficult to catheterize because of its small size but often the bladder can be filled in this way. Alternatively, a voiding cystourethrogram may demonstrate the connection. A urachal remnant patent only in its distal subumbilical portion may present with an umbilical discharge, especially when infected (Fig 22–16). They are most easily identified by US. When open at the proximal end, the patent urachus appears as an extension of the bladder, most commonly at its anterosuperior portion (Fig 22–15,C). Urachal lesions are discussed more fully in Parts V and VII.

REFERENCES

Hernias

Bair JH, Russ PD, Pretorius DM, et al: Fetal omphalocele and gastroschisis: A review of 24 cases. *Am J Roentgenol* 1986; 147:1047.

Balthazar EJ, Subramanyam BR, Megibow A: Spigelian hernia: CT and ultrasonography diagnosis. *Gastrointest Radiol* 1984; 9:81.

Berman L, Stringer D, Ein SH, et al: The late-presenting pediatric Bochdalek hernia: A 20-year review. *J Pediatr Surg* 1988; 23:735.

Currarino G: Incarcerated inguinal hernia in infants: Plain films and barium enema. *Pediatr Radiol* 1974; 2:247.

Franken EA Jr: Anomalies of the anterior abdominal wall: Classification and roentgenology. *Am J Roentgenol* 1971; 112:58.

Newman B, Davis PL: Sonographic and magnetic resonance imaging of an anterior diaphragmatic hernia. *Pediatr Radiol* 1989; 20:110.

Oh KS, Condon VR, Norst RP, et al: Peritoneographic demonstration of femoral hernia. *Radiology* 1978; 127:209.

Toyama WM: Combined congenital defects of the anterior abdominal wall, sternum, diaphragm, pericardium, and heart: A case report and review of the syndrome. *Pediatrics* 1972; 50:778.

Wechsler RJ, Kurtz AB, Needleman L, et al: Crosssectional imaging of abdominal wall hernias. *Am J Roentgenol* 1989; 153:517.

Umbilical remnant abnormalities

Aggarwal S, Kumar A, Nijhawans, et al: Bleeding Meckel's diverticulum demonstrated by digital subtraction angiography. *Pediatr Radiol* 1989; 19:438.

Cullen TS: *Embryology, Anatomy, and Diseases of the Umbilicus.* Philadelphia, WB Saunders, 1916.

Diamond RH, Rothstein RD, Aloni A: Role of cimetidine-enhanced technetium-99m pertechnetate imaging for visualizing Meckel's diverticulum. *J Nucl Med* 1991; 32:1422.

DiSantis DJ, Siegel MJ, Katz ME: Simplified approach to umbilical remnant abnormalities. *Radiographics* 1991; 11:59.

Grosfield JL, Franken EA: Intestinal obstruction in the neonate due to vitelline duct cysts. *Surg Gynecol Obstet* 1974; 138:527.

Itagaki A, Uchida M, Ueki K, et al: Double targets sign in ultrasonic diagnosis of intussuscepted Meckel diverticulum. *Pediatr Radiol* 1991; 21:148.

Lowman RM, Waters LL, Stanley HW: The roentgen aspects of the congenital anomalies in the umbilical region. *Am J Roentgenol* 1953; 70:883.

Okazaki M, Higashihara H, Yamasaki S, et al: Arterial embolization to control life-threatening hemorrhage from a Meckel's diverticulum. *Am J Roentgenol* 1990; 154.

Routh WD, Lawdahl RB, Lund E, et al: Meckel's diverticula: Angiographic diagnosis in patients with non-acute hemorrhage and negative scintigraphy. *Pediatr Radiol* 1990; 20:152.

Salomonowitz E, Wittich G, Hajek P, et al: Detection of intestinal diverticula by double-contrast small bowel enema: Differentiation from other intestinal diverticula. *Gastrointest Radiol* 1983: 8:271.

Sfakianakis GN, Haase GM: Abdominal scintigraphy for ectopic gastric mucosa: A retrospective analysis of 143 studies. *Am J Roentgenol* 1982; 138:7.

Torii Y, Hisatsune I, Imamura K, et al: Giant Meckel diverticulum containing enteroliths diagnosed by computed tomograpy and sonography. *Gastrointest Radiol* 1989; 14:167.

SECTION 3

The Peritoneal Cavity

The peritoneal cavity includes the GI viscera, the hepatobiliary structures, the spleen and pancreas, and the associated blood vessels, nerves, and supporting mesenteries. Diseases of these structures are discussed in the appropriate individual chapters.

Situs solitus refers to the intra-abdominal organs being in their normal positions with the liver in the right upper quadrant, the spleen and stomach in the left upper quadrant, and the cecum in the right lower quadrant. Abnormalities of abdominal situs are most intimately involved with splenic abnormalities and are best understood in relationship to splenic position and anomalies, as discussed in Chapter 24.

PNEUMOPERITONEUM

Free intraperitoneal air is most commonly a consequence of perforation of a hollow viscus. In the neonate, this occurs most frequently in babies with intestinal obstruction, necrotizing enterocolitis, or spontaneous gastric perforation of unknown cause. In children beyond the neonatal period, perforated peptic ulcers and inflammatory bowel disease may produce pneumoperitoneum. Pneumoperitoneum is rarely found with appendiceal perforation. Trauma, both accidental and nonaccidental, may cause pneumoperitoneum, as discussed in Chapter 30. Tension pneumomediastinum can dissect along the retroperitoneum and the subadventitial layer of the mesenteric vessels, rupturing freely into the peritoneal cavity. Its differentiation from perforated viscus is discussed below.

Pneumoperitoneum may be suspected clinically because of the history of an underlying disease which predisposes to bowel perforation, because of acute abdominal distention with increased tympany on physical examination, or it may be a fortuitous finding on imaging examinations of the chest or abdomen. Patients typically have pneumoperitoneum following abdominal surgery, although the free air clears more rapidly in children than in adults. Several studies have demonstrated clearing of free air in 68% to 90% of postoperative children by 24 hours but free air was seen normally 6 to 7 days postoperatively in 2% to 3% of Wiot's cases.

The diagnosis of pneumoperitoneum is most easily made on horizontal-beam plain films obtained to rule out free air or intestinal obstruction. Upright films show air collecting between the diaphragm and the liver on the right and between the diaphragm and the liver, spleen, stomach, and colon on the left (Fig 22–17). The intra-abdominal viscera fall away from the diaphragm in the upright position, making visualization of the free air relatively easy.

Young children and children too ill to sit or stand can be examined in the decubitus position or supine using horizontal-beam technique. The decubitus view should be obtained with the right side up

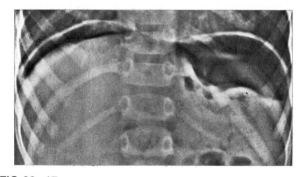

FIG 22–17.
Free intraperitoneal air on an upright examination of the abdomen in a 2-year-old boy with perforated gastric ulcer. Air is easily demonstrated between the diaphragm and the liver on the right and the spleen and stomach on the left.

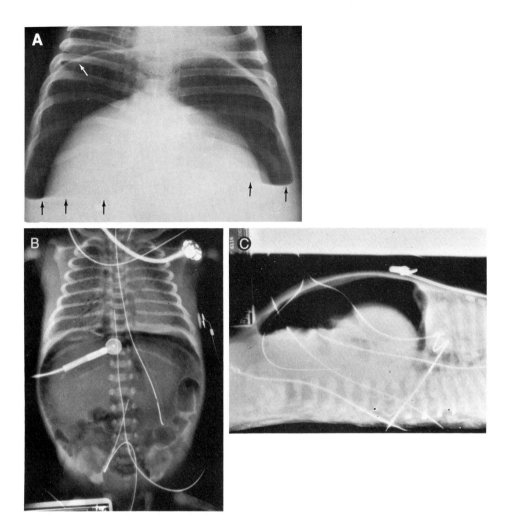

FIG 22–18.
A, massive amount of free air in the abdomen with air-fluid levels on an upright film in a patient with pyopneumoperitoneum. **B,** digitally enhanced AP view of the chest and abdomen in a newborn with pulmonary interstitial emphysema, pneumomediastinum, and pneumoperitoneum. There is a large amount of gas in the perito-neal cavity with a positive Rigler sign as well as decreased density of the liver compared with the extraperitoneal soft tissues. **C,** digitally enhanced cross-table lateral view of the same patient demonstrates large pneumoperitoneum without air-fluid levels, suggesting that the air has dissected into the peritoneum from the chest.

to allow the liver to fall away from the wall of the peritoneal cavity, permitting free air to be seen between the liver and the abdominal wall. Small amounts of free air may be difficult to distinguish from intraluminal air if the left-side-up decubitus view is obtained. On the horizontal-beam supine film, free air appears between the anterior surface of the liver and the anterior abdominal wall (Fig 22–18,C), but small amounts of free air may be more difficult to define than on the decubitus or upright view.

Horizontal-beam films are useful in the newborn to differentiate pneumoperitoneum caused by a perforated viscus from that caused by dissecting pneumomediastinum. The latter is usually suspected because of the history of assisted ventilation and the presence of pneumomediastinum on the chest radio-graph. A ruptured viscus permits both air and fluid to escape into the peritoneal cavity causing extraluminal air-fluid levels (Fig 22–18,A). Dissecting pneumomediastinum causes only air to dissect into the peritoneal space so no significant free air-fluid level is identified on horizontal-beam examination (Fig 22–18,C).

Pneumoperitoneum can be diagnosed on supine films as well. It is imperative to recognize the signs on supine films as a single kidney-ureter-bladder film (KUB) may be the only film requested if free air is not clinically suspected. A sufficiently large amount of free air can be seen as a large ovoid lucency overlying the abdominal contents (Fig 22–19,A). This has been called the "football sign" because of the similarity of its shape to a rugby ball. This lucency caused by the free air rising to an ante-

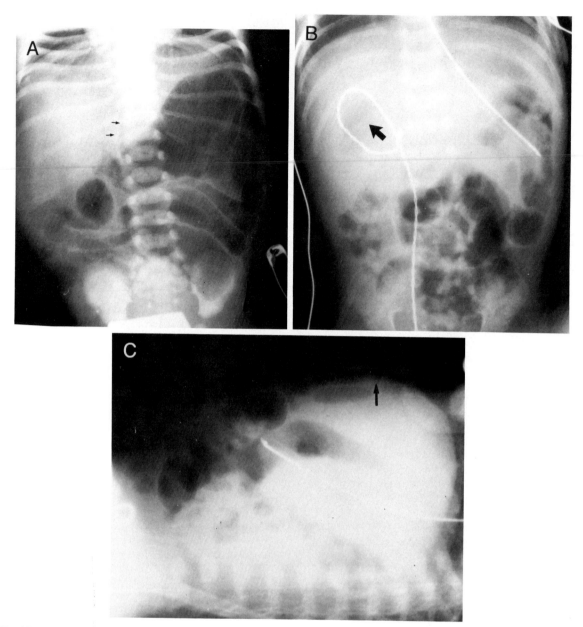

FIG 22–19.
A, supine view of the abdomen in an infant with perforated viscus. A large oval lucency overlies the entire abdomen, representing the "football sign." Both sides of the bowel wall can be seen in the left lower quadrant, representing the Rigler sign. The *arrows* demonstrate the very thin dense line of the falciform ligament which is outlined by air on both sides. **B,** supine view of the abdomen in an infant with necrotizing enterocolitis. A small collection of gas is noted in the Morison pouch, the hepatorenal recess *(arrow).* **C,** same patient in the supine position using horizontal-beam technique. Air is demonstrated between the liver and anterior abdominal wall *(arrow).*

rior position in the abdomen is most easily appreciated where it projects over the liver. The normal liver is the same radiographic density as the abdominal wall musculature. The overlying air on a supine film makes the liver look more lucent than the adjacent muscles. Smaller amounts of free air will cause a rounded lucent bubble to project over the midabdomen.

As the liver falls away from the anterior perito-

neal surface in the supine position, free air can dissect along both sides of the falciform ligament which is attached to the anterior abdominal wall. It appears as a very thin opaque line running vertically just to the right of the spine in a nonrotated film (Fig 22–19,A).

Pneumoperitoneum will give the bowel wall the appearance of an arciform line rather than its usual appearance of an arciform edge. This line is caused

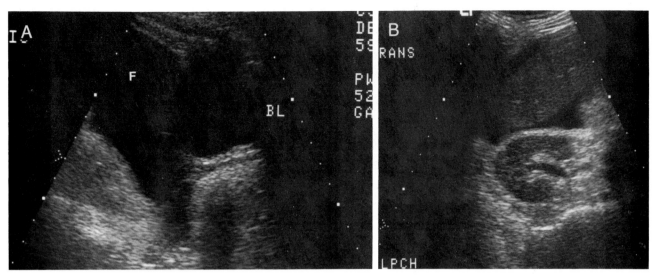

FIG 22–20.
A, transverse sonogram through the pelvis demonstrates a collection of free fluid *(F)* adjacent to the bladder *(BL).* **B,** transverse scan through the right upper quadrant demonstrates a small amount of free fluid collecting between the liver and kidney in the Morison pouch.

by the presence of air on both sides of the bowel wall and is known as the Rigler sign (see Figs 22–18B and 22–19,A). A pseudo-Rigler sign occurs when two loops of dilated bowel are adjacent to one another, but the finding is usually more focal than it is with a true Rigler sign. The line seen in the pseudo-Rigler is thicker than with free air because it represents a double thickness of bowel wall. This is not always a reliable differentiation, however, because the underlying disease causing perforation may lead to a thickened bowel wall.

Small amounts of free air may present on supine films only as localized collections in the right upper quadrant. According to Levine et al., linear collections represent air in the right subhepatic space while triangular collections are seen with air in the Morison pouch, the hepatorenal fossa. The linear lucency may represent air in the fissure of the ligamentum teres, as described by Cho and Baker. The collections are invariably medial in the right upper quadrant and are more likely to be seen in older children and adults than in infants, although Brill et al. described six newborns with necrotizing enterocolitis in whom air in the Morison pouch was the only compelling evidence of pneumoperitoneum (Fig 22–19,B and C). A less commonly seen sign of pneumoperitoneum is the "inverted-V" sign caused by air outlining the median umbilical folds in the pelvis.

ASCITES

A small amount of fluid is normally present in the peritoneal cavity and may be seen incidentally on cross-sectional imaging. Pathologic intraperitoneal fluid collections stem from a variety of causes and include blood, usually from trauma; urine secondary to rupture of an obstructed collecting system; pus in cases of peritonitis; bile from biliary tract rupture;

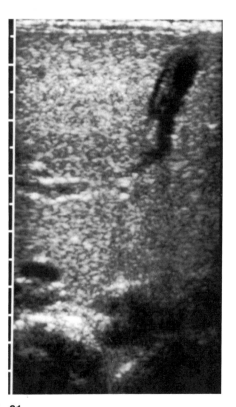

FIG 22–21.
Oblique sonogram through the liver demonstrates ascitic fluid in the fissure of the ligamentum teres. The ligament, the obliterated umbilical vein, can be seen within the fluid collection.

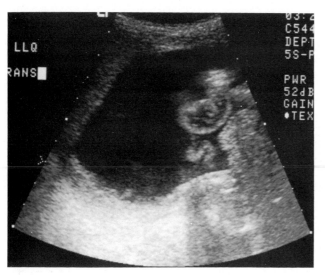

FIG 22–22.
Transverse sonogram through the left lower quadrant demonstrates a massive fluid collection outlining thick-walled loops of intestine in a patient with graft-versus-host disease following bone marrow transplantation.

and cerebrospinal fluid (CSF) in patients with ventriculoperitoneal shunts for treatment of hydrocephalus. Transudative ascites is most commonly found in patients with hepatobiliary disease, especially cirrhosis, heart failure, hypontremia, renal failure, peritonitis, and Budd-Chiari syndrome. Peritoneal metastases are less common in children than adults but, when present, usually cause an exudative ascites. Exudative ascites may also be seen with certain

intraperitoneal infections. Rupture of the GI tract results in fluid as well as air escaping into the peritoneal cavity.

Fluid can be found in a variety of intraperitoneal locations which may change rapidly with changes in patient position. The greater peritoneal cavity, the lesser sac, the Morison pouch, the paracolic gutters, the pelvis, and recesses formed by many of the peritoneal ligaments are all sites where fluid can collect (Fig 22–20). The larger the amount of fluid, the more likely the fluid is to be found throughout the abdomen. Typically, small amounts of ascites collect in the pelvis when the patient is supine. As the amount of fluid increases, it moves cephalad along the paracolic gutters into the subhepatic spaces and the Morison pouch. It can sometimes be identified in the fossa of the ligamentum teres (Fig 22–21). A sufficient volume of ascites eventually spreads through the peritoneal cavity, separating bowel loops, and into the mesenteric recesses (Fig 22–22). Loculated ascites is rare in children, although encysted collections of CSF may be seen when an abnormally positioned ventriculoperitoneal shunt tube has eroded the peritoneal lining (Fig 22–23).

Plain films are only sensitive to large amounts of intraperitoneal fluid (Fig 22–24). The bowel loops may appear centrally located with widened paracolic gutters, although this appearance may be simulated by fluid-filled colon. Separation of bowel loops may occur, but this can be simulated by large amounts of

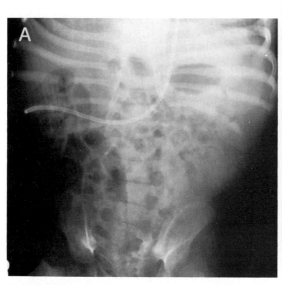

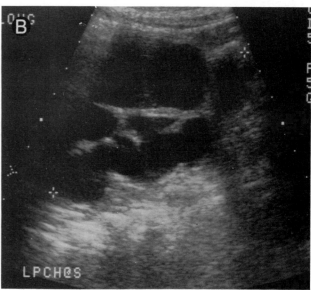

FIG 22–23.
A, supine view of the abdomen in a child with a large spina bifida and postsurgical repair of meningomyelocele demonstrates the tip of the ventriculoperitoneal shunt tube to be in the right midabdomen against the peritoneal wall. The tip of the tube did not move with changes in position or with time. **B,** longitudinal sonogram in the right midabdomen demonstrates a fluid collection immediately subjacent to the abdominal wall with fluid-filled loops of bowel deep to it. A CSF cyst was drained at surgery.

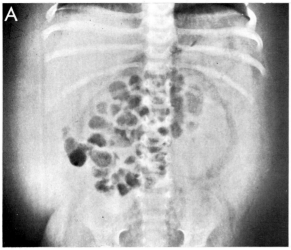

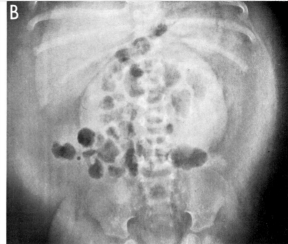

FIG 22–24.

AP views of the abdomen in a 16-month-old infant with nephrotic syndrome. **A,** abdominal distention is noted with numerous loops of gas-containing intestine floating in the center of the abdomen.

B, following the intravenous injection of contrast material, the opacified liver and kidneys can be seen, demonstrating the large amount of ascitic fluid present.

intraluminal fluid combined with relatively small amounts of intraluminal gas (Fig 22–25).

US is the most sensitive imaging modality for ascites, often visualizing even physiologic amounts of intraperitoneal fluid. Free fluid can be seen in the various peritoneal recesses and the pelvis and may cause apparent thickening of the gallbladder wall. Most transudates are echolucent collections. Complex fluid collections suggest blood, chyle, inflammatory cells, or peritoneal metastases (Fig 22–26). Ascites occasionally will pass through the esophageal hiatus or through patent pleuroperitoneal canals to present as intrathoracic fluid. CT is particularly useful in identifying the individual fluid-filled

spaces and gives useful diagnostic information if the ascites is secondary to an intraabdominal process. CT is not as sensitive to small volumes of fluid as is US.

ACUTE GENERALIZED PERITONITIS

Peritonitis is a diffuse inflammatory process usually of infectious etiology. The most common cause in children is ruptured appendix. Patients with inflammatory bowel disease may also develop peritonitis after rupture of the bowel. These entities are discussed more fully in Chapters 27 and 28. Chemical peritonitis can occur with bile leak and in patients

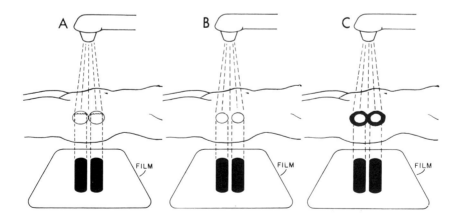

FIG 22–25.

Pseudoseparation of bowel loops. **A,** intraluminal fluid and gas simulate the appearance of bowel loop separation when there is more intraluminal fluid than gas. The x-ray beam "sees" the margin of the gas column rather than the margin of the bowel wall. **B,** true separation of bowel loops results from intraperitoneal fluid since

the x-ray beam sees only the gas within the bowel. **C,** thickened bowel wall simulates intraperitoneal fluid since the x-ray beam sees only the gas within the bowel. (**From Hoffman RB, Wankmuller R, Rigler LG et al:** *Radiology* **1966; 87:845. Used by permission.**)

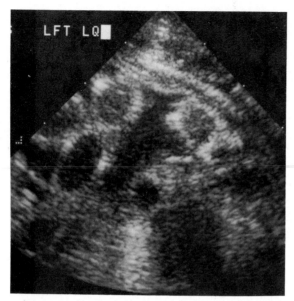

FIG 22–26.
Transverse sonogram through the left lower quadrant of a 1-year-old boy with disseminated intravascular coagulation and thrombocytopenia following surgery for congenital heart disease. There is a fluid collection separating multiple loops of bowel. However, the fluid is hypoechoic rather than anechoic which is the usual situation with ascites. Paracentesis revealed free fluid within the abdomen which had a high hematocrit.

with pancreatitis. Plain films in patients with peritonitis show a nonspecific adynamic ileus pattern with dilated bowel and multiple intraluminal air-fluid levels (Fig 22–27). The signs of associated ascites may be seen. In older children, the properitoneal fat plane may be obliterated.

Because of the ease of flow of fluid within the peritoneal cavity, abscesses may develop at sites distant from the perforation as well as in the immediate area, as discussed more fully in Chapters 27 and 28. The subhepatic and subphrenic areas are the most common distant sites for abscess formation. US will identify a focal collection of mixed echogenicity. CT shows a focal lesion with attenuation greater than clear fluid. The thickened walls of the abscess frequently enhance after the intravenous injection of contrast material. CT is particularly useful as a guide for percutaneous drainage of abscesses (see Chapter 27). Both gallium citrate– and indium-labeled white blood cells have been used as scintigraphic agents in the diagnosis of abscesses.

ABDOMINAL WALL AND PERITONEAL CALCIFICATION

Abdominal wall calcification is uncommon in infants and children. Calcification commonly follows subcu-

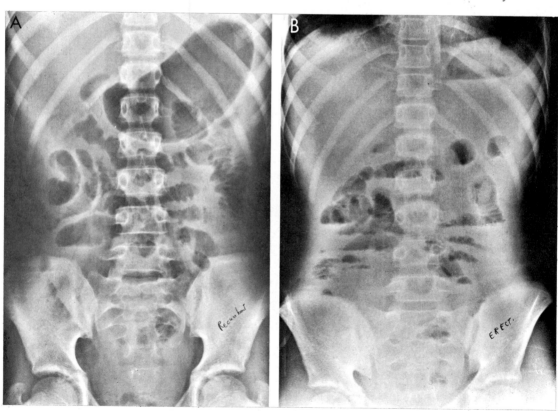

FIG 22–27.
Supine **(A)** and upright **(B)** views of the abdomen in a teen-age patient with purulent peritonitis. The gas-filled loops of small intestine are mildly dilated and separated from one another and multiple air-fluid levels can be seen throughout the small intestine.

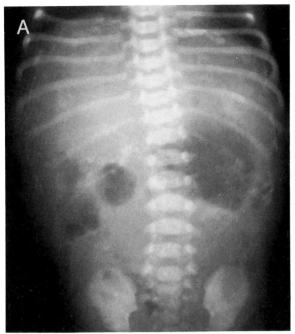

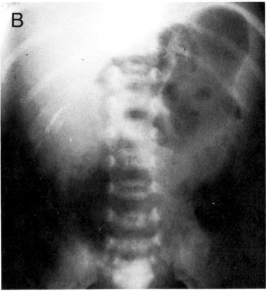

FIG 22–28.
A, a newborn with meconium peritonitis. Peritoneal calcifications are demonstrated throughout the abdomen, particularly in the upper half. **B,** meconium peritonitis in another patient. When small amounts of meconium calcify, it is usually along the inferior surface of the liver, as in this patient.

taneous fat necrosis in infants. Although some cases of fat necrosis are idiopathic, the majority are associated with neonatal sepsis. Patients with hypothermia, liver failure, and kidney failure may also undergo subcutaneous fat necrosis. Abdominal wall calcification in infants has also been described following subcutaneous emphysema and in a case of prune-belly syndrome.

In children, abdominal wall calcification may be seen in fibrodysplasia ossificans progressiva and myositis ossificans but these lesions are more common in the thoracic wall than the abdominal wall where they usually are posterior and paraspinous. Calcifications secondary to dermatomyositis are more likely to be in the extremities than the trunk but can be found in the abdominal wall. Subcutaneous hemangiomas may contain phleboliths.

The most common cause of peritoneal calcification in the neonate is meconium peritonitis (see Chapter 52). This occurs secondary to intrauterine intestinal perforation with meconium-induced chemical peritonitis (Fig 22–28). Meconium peritonitis is most frequently seen in association with small-bowel atresia which also occurs secondary to in utero intestinal perforation, but intestinal obstruction is not invariably present. Meconium peritonitis may also occur in neonates with cystic fibrosis. Peritoneal calcification in older children is quite rare. Intestinal perforation with subsequent peritonitis may cause calci-

fication. Tuberculous peritonitis may result in minimal to extensive calcification.

Most causes of intraabdominal calcification are related to specific organs and are discussed in the appropriate chapters.

REFERENCES

Pneumoperitoneum

Bray JF: The "inverted V" sign of pneumoperitoneum. *Radiology* 1984; 151:45.

Brill PW, Olson SR, Winchester P: Neonatal necrotizing enterocolitis: Air in Morison pouch. *Radiology* 1990; 174:469.

Cho KC, Baker SR: Air in the fissure for the ligamentum teres: new sign of intraperitoneal air on plain radiographs. *Radiology* 1991; 178;489.

Levine MS, Scheiner JD, Rubesin SE, et al: Diagnosis of pneumoperitoneum on supine abdominal radiographs. *Am J Roentgenol* 1991; 156:731.

Menuck L, Siemans PT: Penumoperitoneum: importance of right upper quadrant features. *Am J Roentgenol* 1980; 127:753.

Miller RE: Perforated viscus in infants: A new roentgen sign. *Radiology* 1960; 74:65.

Rigler LG: Spontaneous pneumoperitoneum: A roentgenologic sign found in the supine position. *Radiology* 1941; 37:604.

Wind ES, Pillari GP: Lucent liver in the newborn: a roentgenographic sign of pneumoperitoneum. *JAMA* 1977; 237:2218.

Wiot JF, Benton C, McAlister WH, et al. Postoperative pneumoperitoneum in children. *Radiology* 1967; 89:285.

Ascites and Acute Generalized Peritonitis

Churchill RJ: CT of intra-abdominal fluid collections. *Radiol Clin North Am* 1989; 27:653.

Colli A, Cocciolo M, Buccino G, et al: Thickening of the gallbladder wall in ascites. *JCU* 1991; 19:357.

Dinkel E, Lehnart R, Tröger J, et al: Sonographic evidence of intraperitoneal fluid: An experimental study and its clinical implications. *Pediatr Radiol* 1984; 14:299.

Grünebaum M, Ziv N, Kornreich L, et al: The sonographic signs of the peritoneal pseudocyst obstructing the ventriculo-peritoneal shunt in children. *Neuroradiology* 1988; 30:433.

Hoffman RB, Wankmuller R, Rigler LG: Pseudoseparation of bowel loops: a fallacious sign of intraperitoneal fluid. *Radiology* 1966; 87:845.

Meyers MA, Oliphant M, Berne AS, et al: The peritoneal ligaments and mesenteries: pathways of intraabdominal spread of disease. *Radiology* 1987; 163:593.

Newman B, Teele RL: Ascites in the fetus, neonate, and young child: emphasis on ultrasonographic evaluation. *Semin Ultrasound CT MR* 1984; 5:85.

Pandolfo I, Gaetta M, Scribano E, et al: Mediastinal pseudotumor due to passage of ascites through the esophageal hiatus. *Gastrointest Radiol* 1989; 14:209.

Abdominal Wall and Peritoneal Calcification

Blane CE, White SJ, Braunstein EM, et al: Pattern of calcification in childhood dermatomyositis. *Am J Roentgenol* 1984; 142:397.

Kirks DR, Taybi H: Prune-belly syndrome: an unusual cause of neonatal abdominal calcification. *Am J Roentgenol* 1975; 123:778.

Naidech HJ, Chawla HS: Soft-tissue calcification after subcutaneous emphysema in a neonate. *Am J Roentgenol* 1982; 139:374.

Taybi H: Thoracic and abdominal calcification in children: a review. *Perspect Radiol* 1989; 2:135.

23

The Hepatobiliary System

SECTION 1

Introduction to the Hepatobiliary System

NORMAL ANATOMY

The liver is the largest of the abdominal organs, occupying most of the right upper quadrant and extending across the midline. The liver is relatively larger in neonates and infants than it is in older children and adults. The right lobe is larger than the left, with the caudate and quadrate lobes being substantially smaller. The superior portion of the liver is in direct contact with the diaphragm. The posterior margin is in contact with the inferior vena cava (IVC), the right adrenal gland, and the distal esophagus. Inferiorly, the liver is in contact with the colon, the gallbladder, and the right kidney. The left lobe is in contact with the stomach. The visceral surface of the liver contains the porta hepatis with its vessels and biliary ducts. The two major intrahepatic biliary ducts join to form the common hepatic duct which is joined by the cystic duct coming from the

gallbladder to form the common bile duct. The common bile duct drains into the descending limb of the duodenum.

Cross-sectional imaging studies can identify the landmarks which divide the hepatic lobes from one another and into their respective segments. The right lobe is divided into anterior and posterior segments while the left lobe has medial and lateral segments. The interlobar and intersegmental fissures may contain sufficient fat to be identified on ultrasound (US), computed tomography (CT), and magnetic resonance (MR) imaging. Portions of the fissures also contain readily identifiable structures. The middle hepatic vein runs in the superior portion of the main interlobar fissure. The fissure for the round ligament, the obliterated umbilical vein, divides the segments of the left lobe. The right hepatic vein runs in part of the fissure separating the segments of the right lobe. Dodds et al. have defined the anatomy of the caudate lobe. Lafortune et al. have described the sonographic correlates of Couinaud's nomenclature for surgical anatomy of the hepatic segments. Nelson et al. have discussed the segmental anatomy of the liver on CT arterial portography and its relationship to hepatic surgical anatomy.

EMBRYOLOGY OF THE LIVER

The liver and biliary duct system, including the gallbladder, arise from the most caudal part of the foregut as a ventral bud early in the fourth week of embryonic life. This bud, known as the hepatic diverticulum, extends into the septum transversum, the future diaphragm. It divides into two parts as it grows between the layers of the ventral mesentery. The larger cranial part of the hepatic diverticulum develops into the liver. As well as giving rise to the hepatocytes, some of the proliferating endodermal cells also develop into the lining epithelium of the biliary system. The reticuloendothelial portions of the liver develop from the splanchnic mesenchyme of the septum transversum. The smaller caudal part of the hepatic diverticulum expands to form the gallbladder while its stalk becomes the cystic duct. The stalk which connects the cystic and hepatic ducts becomes the common bile duct connecting to the duodenum which also arises from the caudal foregut.

The liver grows very rapidly with the right lobe becoming the larger of the two initial lobes. The caudate and quadrate lobes are thought to develop as subdivisions of the right lobe, although this has been questioned by Dodds et al. who have suggested an alternative embryologic scheme for development of the caudate lobe. By the ninth week, the liver represents 10% of the embryo's weight primarily because of the hematopoietic function of the embryonic liver. Bile formation by hepatocytes begins during the 12th embryonic week. Bile pigments begin to develop in the 13th to 16th weeks. They enter the duodenum, giving the intraintestinal meconium its characteristic green color. The liver accounts for 5% of the newborn infant's weight.

The ventral mesentery is a double-layered membrane which gives rise to the gastrohepatic, hepatoduodenal, and falciform ligaments. The falciform ligament extends from the liver to the anterior abdominal wall. Its inferior free border contains the umbilical vein. The ventral mesentery also gives rise to the hepatic visceral peritoneum which fully covers the liver except for the bare area in contact with the diaphragm. This synopsis of liver embryology is taken from Moore.

HEPATOBILIARY IMAGING

Plain films play relatively little role in the evaluation of hepatobiliary diseases. Hepatomegaly is often identified on plain films, but liver size can be very difficult to evaluate since one must often rely on displacement of adjacent structures such as the colon or stomach to determine the actual margins of the liver. This is especially true in neonates and infants when there is insufficient fat around the hepatic capsule for identification. Cross-sectional imaging is a much more reliable way of determining liver size. Calcifications within the liver itself (Fig 23–1) or in the biliary system can be seen on plain films as can air in the portal venous system or biliary tree which may occur in some disease states (Fig 23–2). Profound fatty replacement of the liver may reduce its radiographic density, but cross-sectional imaging is much more sensitive to lesser degrees of fatty infiltration.

Ultrasound has been an extraordinarily useful tool in the evaluation of the liver and biliary system in children because it requires no conscious sedation or anesthesia and there is no ionizing radiation. Five-megahertz sector transducers are usually satisfactory for most children. A 3.5-MHz transducer may be necessary in older, larger children and adolescents. When the possibility of subcapsular disease, such as metastases, is being considered, a 5.0-MHz linear transducer is useful. The echogenicity of the liver should be homogeneous and uniform

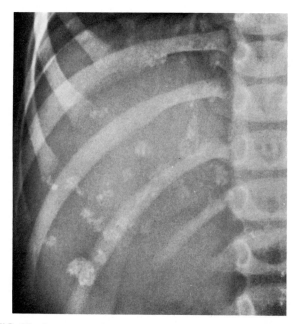

FIG 23–1.
Scattered calcifications in the liver of a boy 6 years of age with chronic granulomatous disease of childhood.

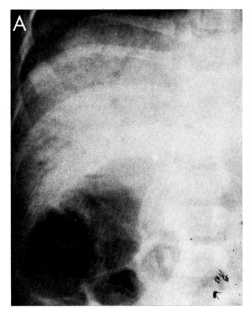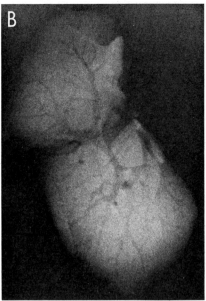

FIG 23–2.
Portal venous gas. **A,** radiolucent branching structures in the liver are best seen in the right hepatic lobe. Dilated bowel is also seen in this patient with necrotizing entercolitis. **B,** in a postmortem radiograph of the liver, gas in the venous radicles is seen in all parts of the liver. The radicles typically taper toward the edges of the liver. **(Courtesy of Dr. Bertram Levin, Chicago.)**

throughout. A complete examination requires evaluation of the hepatic parenchyma, the portal venous system, the hepatic veins, the hepatic arteries and intrahepatic bile ducts, the common bile duct, and the gallbladder. The upper limits for size of the common bile duct are 2 mm in the first year of life, 4 mm in older children, and 7 mm in adolescents and teenagers, according to Teele and Share. In neonates, however, the duct normally is difficult to identify and its easy visualization should raise the question of dilatation. Doppler US has been especially valuable in patients with portal hypertension and other vascular diseases. Doppler study is also useful in distinguishing the hepatic artery from the biliary ducts, a particular problem in neonates and infants, and has been useful in the evaluation of transplanted livers. Although the examination may be performed for suspected liver disease, full evaluation of the upper abdomen, including spleen, pancreas, and other upper abdominal organs and vascular structures should always be performed.

Nuclear medicine studies offer some physiologic as well as anatomical information. The Kupffer cells of the reticuloendothelial system of the liver and spleen take up technetium −99m sulfur colloid, permitting good anatomical definition of masses, including metastases, as well as information about the hepatic parenchyma in general. Singe photon emission tomography (SPECT) increases the sensitivity of

the procedure as well as improving the ability to evaluate, at least grossly, hepatic function. Biliary scanning has been especially useful in the attempt to differentiate neonatal hepatitis from congenital biliary atresia. The most commonly used agents are derivatives of iminodiacetic acid (IDA). These compounds are taken up by hepatocytes and secreted into the biliary ductules (Fig 23–3).

Computed tomography has added significantly to the evaluation of hepatobiliary disease, although it is used with less frequency in children than in adults. Because of the need for conscious sedation or anesthesia in young children and the exposure to ionizing radiation, CT has been most typically reserved for patients in whom a mass is either suspected or

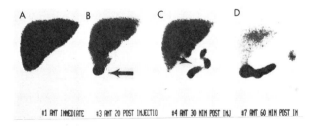

FIG 23–3.
Hepatobiliary scintigrams using ^{99m}Tc PIPIDA show immediate radionuclide uptake in the liver **(A).** On the 20- and 30-minute scans **(B and C),** radionuclide is seen in the small intestine *(arrows).* One hour after injection **(D),** radionuclide has cleared almost completely from the liver.

identified on US or nuclear medicine study. Better definition of cysts, tumors, metastases, and abscesses can be obtained with CT if the initial isotope study or sonogram is not definitive. CT is less often used for diffuse parenchymal liver disease, although fatty liver, hemachromatosis and hemosiderosis, and changes in parenchymal attenuation secondary to cirrhosis and fibrosis can readily be identified. Dynamic CT scanning is particularly useful in the evaluation of primary and metastatic tumors of the liver.

Similarly, *MR imaging* of the liver is usually reserved for patients with mass lesions which need better definition than can be obtained on US or nuclear medicine study. MR has an advantage over CT in that it does not use ionizing radiation and has multiplanar imaging capabilities. However, MR is certainly more costly and there is more of a problem with motion artifact in young children. Caron has reviewed the technical considerations in performing MR studies of the pediatric abdomen. Generally, the closest-fitting coil should be used to improve signal-to-noise ratio and improve resolution. Standard spin-echo sequences are most commonly used. Both T1- and T2-weighted sequences are useful for full evaluation. Gradient-recalled echo sequences are especially useful for evaluation of the vascular structures.

Endoscopic retrograde cholangiopancreatography (ERCP) is less frequently used in children than in adults. Nevertheless, the examination can be useful in certain congenital and acquired diseases of the biliary tree and pancreas. The examination is difficult to perform in younger children and is generally reserved for patients in the preadolescent age group at least. However, ERCPs can be performed even in infants, as reported by Guelrud et al. In some hands, *transhepatic cholangiography* is favored over ERCP. It has the advantage of showing the intrahepatic ducts to better advantage than is often possible with ERCP.

Arteriography is less commonly performed since the advent of cross-sectional imaging studies than it was previously, but there are some surgeons who still request a vascular study prior to tumor surgery, portosystemic venous anastomoses, or transplantation. Although the examination offers little further diagnostic information beyond that available from CT or MR, the hepatic and vascular anatomy are better defined. However, with increasing use of new MR sequences which demonstrate vascular anatomy to excellent advantage, the use of arteriography will continue to diminish as surgeons develop more trust in the anatomical efficacy of MR.

REFERENCES

Caron KH: Magnetic resonance imaging of the pediatric abdomen. *Semin Ultrasound CT MR* 1991; 12:448.

Dodds WJ, Erickson SJ, Taylor AJ, et al: Caudate lobe of the liver: Anatomy, embryology, and pathology. AJR 1990; 154:87.

Fisher MR, Woli SD, Hricak H, et al: Hepatic vascular anatomy on magnetic resonance imaging. AJR 1985; 144:739.

Guelrud M, Jaen D, Mendoza S, et al: ERCP in the diagnosis of extrahepatic biliary atresia. *Gastrointest Endosc* 1991; 37:522.

Lafortune M, Madore F, Patriquin H, et al: Segmental anatomy of the liver: A sonographic approach to the Couinaud nomenclature. *Radiology* 1991; 181:443.

Moore KL: *The Developing Human.* ed 4. Philadelphia, WB Saunders, 1988.

Mukai JK, Stack CM, Turner DA, et al: Imaging of surgically relevant hepatic vascular and segmental anatomy. Part 1: normal anatomy. AJR 1987; 149:287.

Nelson RC, Chezmar JL, Sugarbaker PM, et al: Preoperative localization of focal liver lesions to specific liver segments: Utility of CT during arterial portography. *Radiology* 1990; 176:89.

Parulekar SG: Ligaments and fissures of the liver: Sonographic anatomy. *Radiology* 1979; 130:409.

Teele RL, Share JC: Ultrasonography of the biliary tree in infants and children. *Appl Radiol* 1992; 21:15.

SECTION 2

Congenital Abnormalities

Agenesis of the liver is an uncommon abnormality which is being described with increasing frequency as a result of the increased use of cross-sectional imaging. Most commonly, the right lobe is absent with resulting compensatory hypertrophy of the left lobe of the liver and the caudate lobe. The gallbladder may be more posteriorly placed than in the normal situation. Associated congenital anomalies, especially those of the biliary tract, have been reported, as has portal hypertension. Most of the reported cases have been in adults in whom the differential diagnosis should include atrophy of the right lobe secondary to cirrhosis or tumor. In children, these latter diseases are unlikely to be the cause, and agenesis is the probable diagnosis when the right lobe cannot be identified. Agenesis of the left lobe has been reported less frequently. Lobar atrophy secondary to hepatic infarction has been described. The gallbladder may be congenitally absent, congenitally displaced, duplicated, or septated. Sonography and hepatobiliary imaging usually identify these rare abnormalities.

BILIARY ATRESIA AND NEONATAL HEPATITIS

These two entities each account for more than a third of cases of persistent jaundice in the neonatal period and are also discussed in Chapter 52. Less common causes include infection, metabolic diseases, hemolysis, and neonatal sepsis. Adrenal hemorrhage and a variety of drugs used in the neonatal period have also been described as causing jaundice in the newborn. Numerous other, even less common, causes of neonatal jaundice have been described.

Landing has suggested that biliary atresia and neonatal hepatitis may be differing manifestations of the same pathophysiologic process, one of fetal inflammatory cholangiopathy. In the form known as biliary atresia, variable parts of the biliary tree are completely obliterated. In the form known as neonatal hepatitis, the biliary tree remains patent, although there is substantial damage to the liver itself. Differentiating these two entities is critical because biliary atresia requires operative intervention while neonatal hepatitis is treated medically. Early diagnosis of biliary atresia is particularly important since the prognosis for long-term survival is markedly reduced if surgery is performed after 3 months of age. The diseases are so closely related that in up to one third of cases the diagnosis may not be correctly made, even by liver biopsy. Furuya et al. have described a paucity of interlobular bile ducts in a patient with neonatal hepatitis and cystic fibrosis.

Abdominal US is the recommended first imaging examination for neonates with pathologic jaundice. US may identify other anatomical causes for the patient's jaundice, such as choledochal cyst or stones. Generally, the gallbladder will be visualized and appear normal in up to 90% of patients with neonatal hepatitis. About 10% of patients with this disease may be so severely affected that the gallbladder is not seen on US. In most patients with biliary atresia, the gallbladder cannot be visualized. In about one fifth of cases, however, the gallbladder may be seen, although in many of these cases it may appear smaller than expected in the fasting infant. Nevertheless, because of this overlap, US by itself is not deemed sufficient by most authors to differentiate the two lesions, and other imaging evaluations are necessary.

Ikeda et al. have reported that serial US may be useful in the differentiation of neonatal hepatitis and biliary atresia when the gallbladder is visualized. According to these authors, postprandial contraction can be seen in patients with neonatal hepatitis but not in patients with biliary atresia. Weinberger et al., however, reported a case of biliary atresia with postprandial gallbladder contraction. Changes in the Doppler-assessed portal venous velocity have been described in patients with biliary atresia by Grunert et al. Wanek et al. have reported a correlation of decreased velocity with postoperative prognosis. Their patients with reduced portal venous velocity came to transplantation while the patients with normal velocity did well with portoenterostomy.

Radioisotope studies of the biliary tree are the most likely noninvasive imaging studies to be diagnostic (Fig 23–4). Evaluation of the blood pool phase, the hepatic phase, and the presence or absence of radioisotope in the gastrointestinal tract (GI) are all necessary in the proper evaluation of bil-

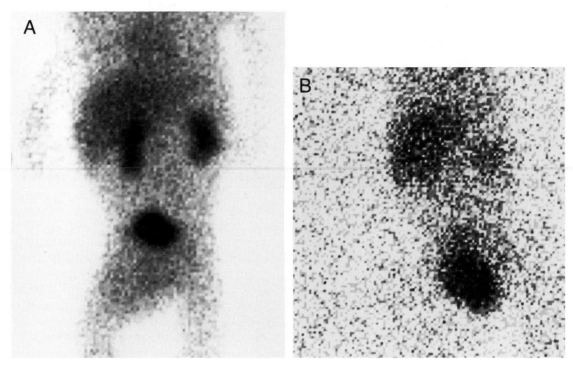

FIG 23–4.
Biliary atresia. **A,** 60 minutes following the injection of ^{99m}Tc HIDA, radioactivity is noted throughout the soft tissues with poor accumulation in the liver and most accumulation in the kidneys and bladder. There is no evidence of activity in the biliary tree or activity in the intestine. **B,** at 24 hours, there continues to be no evidence of intestinal activity.

iary atresia. If the early scans do not demonstrate isotopic activity in the GI tract, delayed scans, up to 24 hours, should be obtained. The presence of radioisotope in the GI tract excludes biliary atresia, but the absence of excretion of the radiopharmaceutical can be caused by other diseases. In fact, the most severe forms of neonatal hepatitis may cause sufficient liver damage to prevent amounts of isotope adequate for imaging purposes to be excreted into the GI tract.

When the diagnosis remains in doubt, other imaging studies may be necessary. Percutaneous cholecystocholangiography has been used by several centers, but is not widely performed. Since biliary atresia may affect only portions of the biliary tree, opacification of hepatic ducts as well as the common bile duct is necessary to exclude the diagnosis. Some patients have been brought to exploratory laparotomy. Since biopsy can be nondiagnostic, operative cholangiograms are usually performed in an attempt to identify the intrahepatic and extrahepatic portions of the biliary system (Fig 23–5). Guelrud et al. have described the use of ERCP in jaundiced neonates. Of 32 infants in whom ERCP was attempted, 30 had successful studies. These authors used their own prototypical duodenoscope for these studies. Untreated cases of biliary atresia may result in a rickets-like ap-

pearance in the bones. Fractures may also occur.

Approximately 10% of patients with biliary atresia have a syndrome which also includes polysplenia, azygos continuation of the IVC, preduodenal portal vein, hepatic arterial anomalies, and left-sided isomerism of the lungs. US can usually identify many portions of this syndrome, not only suggesting the correct diagnosis, but giving important preoperative information to the surgeon. Day et al. used CT postoperatively to define associated congenital and acquired abnormalities such as polysplenia and portal hypertension.

Treatment for neonatal hepatitis is medical unless there is such severe liver destruction that transplantation is necessary. Biliary atresia is treated by various forms of portoenterostomy, the Kasai procedure. The exact form of procedure used depends on the degree of obliteration of the biliary tree. The operation is successful in upward of 50% of patients when performed under the age of 3 months, but because of progressive obliteration of the bile ducts survival rates drop rapidly when surgery is performed after this age. Even those patients with good short-term to mid-term results may eventually develop cholangitis, cirrhosis, and portal hypertension. Ever more frequently, these patients are coming to liver transplantation.

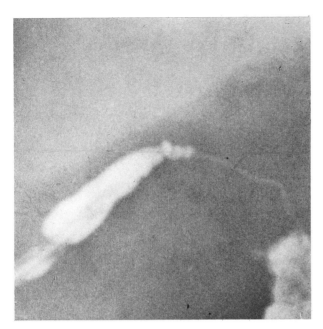

FIG 23–5.
Operative cholangiogram in a 4-month-old infant with persistent jaundice since birth. Contrast material injected into the contracted gallbladder enters the duodenum via a single duct. No hepatic ducts were identified on this examination or at surgery in this infant who had extrahepatic biliary atresia.

In the Kasai procedure, the porta hepatis is dissected and a loop of small intestine is brought up and anastomosed to the exposed draining biliary radicles. Initially, the bowel loop is brought out to the skin so a loopogram can be used to identify ret-

rograde filling of the bile ducts in cases of suspected failure of the procedure. More commonly, biliary scintigraphy is used to evaluate the patency of the portoenterostomy. Isotopic activity should appear in the bowel by 1 hour after administration. Patients may develop ascending cholangitis with cystic dilatation of the intrahepatic bile ducts and subsequent "bile lakes" secondary to stasis. These accumulations of bile are easily seen on US and can be drained percutaneously with variable results. Percutaneous transhepatic cholangiography has also been used to test the patency of the Kasai anastomosis.

Less common causes of persistent jaundice in the neonate include bile plug syndrome and choledocholithiasis. These entities are discussed in Chapter 52. Spontaneous rupture of the common duct may occur in older infants and young children as well as in newborns (Fig 23–6). Patients commonly present with bile ascites. Biliary scintigraphy demonstrates activity in the ascitic fluid. Cholangiography is the definitive diagnostic study.

ALAGILLE SYNDROME (ARTERIOHEPATIC DYSPLASIA)

Paucity and hypoplasia of interlobular bile ducts in association with other congenital abnormalities is known as the Alagille syndrome or arteriohepatic dysplasia. Alagille et al. have described five major components of this syndrome: (1) abnormal facies

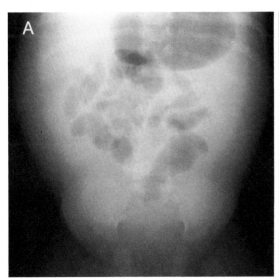

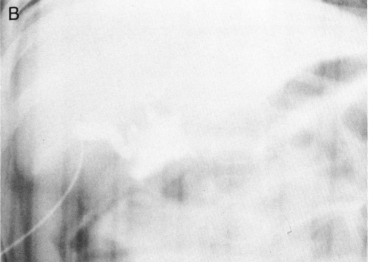

FIG 23–6.
Spontaneous rupture of the common bile duct. **A,** this 9-week-old girl presented with massive ascites. Kidney-ureter-bladder imaging (KUB) demonstrated evidence of fluid in the flanks with centrally placed loops of intestine. Paracentesis revealed biliary ascites. **B,** operative cholangiogram with injection of contrast material into a small gallbladder demonstrates some filling of the common bile duct and intrahepatic ducts with leak of contrast material from a spontaneous perforation of the common bile duct.

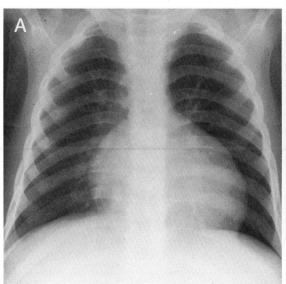
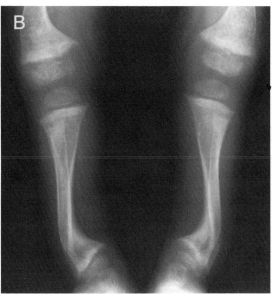

FIG 23–7.
Alagille syndrome. Patient with heart murmur and abnormal liver function tests. **A,** PA view of the chest demonstrates cardiac enlargement. Cardiac evaluation revealed pulmonic stenosis. **B,** ra- chitic changes in the metaphyses with undertubulation, osteopenia, and varus deformities of the distal femora and tibias. Liver biopsy revealed biliary duct hypoplasia compatible with Alagille syndrome.

(large forehead, small pointed chin, hypertelorism, poorly developed nasal bridge), (2) chronic cholestasis, (3) posterior embryotoxon, (4) butterfly vertebrae, and (5) pulmonary artery hypoplasia or stenosis (Fig 23–7). The last may be either isolated or associated with complex cardiac anomalies. Half of the cases will have four of these abnormalities, 30% will have all five features, and 15% will have three of the abnormalities. A number of other congenital abnormalities are seen less frequently, including caudal dysplasia. The bones may show significant osteoporosis with undertubulation.

Affected patients usually present in the neonatal period, although some present months to years later with cholestatic jaundice. The imaging characteristics in the newborn period are similar to those in biliary atresia, but the findings of other components of this syndrome should lead to the correct diagnosis. Patients presenting beyond the newborn period may have US findings suggestive of cirrhosis with an inhomogeneous echographic pattern and evidence of regenerating nodules. Typically, biliary imaging fails to show normal excretion of radioisotope into the GI tract. The definitive diagnosis is usually made by liver biopsy, at which time the intraoperative cholangiogram usually demonstrates patency of the extrahepatic biliary tree.

Most patients with Alagille syndrome die before the end of the third decade, but survival into the fifth decade has been reported. Hepatocellular carcinoma, as a complication of Alagille syndrome, has been reported in both children and adults.

Hypoplasia of the interlobular bile ducts without associated congenital anomalies has been described as well. The differentiation from biliary atresia can be made either by later age of presentation, hepatic wedge biopsy, or by demonstration of an intact extrahepatic biliary tree. Alagille et al. have described the characteristics of 80 patients with the syndromic form of interlobular bile duct hypoplasia and 31 cases of the nonsyndromic form.

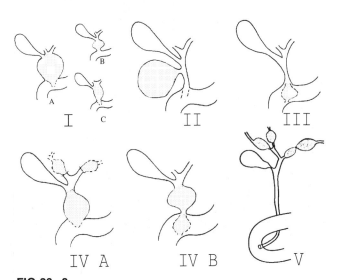

FIG 23–8.
Todani's classification of choledochal cysts. See text. (Modified from Crittenden SL, McKinley MJ: *Am J Gastroenterol* 1985; 80:643.)

CHOLEDOCHAL CYST

Choledochal cyst refers to dilatation of the common bile duct, which can be either saccular or fusiform. A frequently used classification is that of Alonson-Lej who described four types. Todani has modified the classification, describing five types with several subtypes (Fig 23–8). Gastroenterologists are increasingly accepting the Todani classification. The several types differ in etiology and pathogenesis as well as in appearance and presentation. The most common form, found in 80% to 90% of cases according to

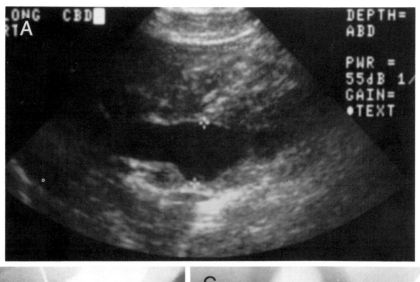

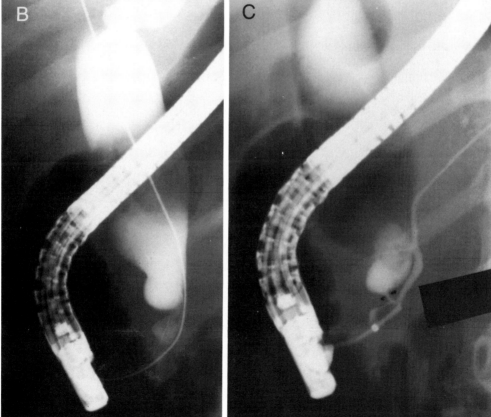

FIG 23–9.
Type I choledochal cyst. **A,** longitudinal sonogram of the right upper quadrant demonstrates marked dilatation of the common bile duct. **B,** endoscopic retrograde cholangiopancreatography (ERCP) demonstrates dilatation of the common bile duct. The intra-hepatic ducts were not visualized. **C,** the common bile duct is seen to drain into the pancreatic duct more than 2 cm proximal to the sphincter of Oddi.

Crittenden et al., is type I, consisting of dilatation of the common bile duct over a variable length and of varying degree (Fig 23–9). Todani divides type I into three subtypes. Babbitt et al. suggested that type I choledochal cyst is caused by an abnormal insertion of the common bile duct into the pancreatic duct proximal to the sphincter of Oddi (Fig 23–9C). This anomaly permits reflux of pancreatic enzymes into the common bile duct with subsequent inflammation and weakening of the wall. According to Rosenfield and Griscom, this pathogenetic mechanism may occur in 60% of patients. Wiedmeyer et al., however, have demonstrated this anomalous ductal connection to be present on ERCP in all eight of their patients, and other authors agree that the theory of Babbitt et al. is the most plausible for type I choledochal cyst. McHugh and Daneman described biliary duct dilatation in two patients with multiple GI atresias causing bile drainage into a closed loop. One case simulated a type I choledochal cyst.

Type II choledochal cyst consists of one or more diverticula of the common bile duct and is found in 2% of cases. Type III is a choledochocele, dilatation of the intraduodenal portion of the duct with both the common bile duct and pancreatic duct emptying into it, and is found in 1.5% to 5.0% of cases (Fig 23–10). Todani's type IVA is multiple intrahepatic and extrahepatic cysts and occurs in 19% of patients. Type IVB is multiple extrahepatic cysts and is rare. Todani's type V and Alonson-Lej's type IV are Caroli disease, which is discussed below. Type IVA of Todani may also represent a form of Caroli disease

but has also been called type I with intrahepatic involvement. Type I, the most frequently seen, is more common in girls than boys in Occidentals, but the sex ratio is equal in Asia. About 65% of all reported cases are from Japan.

Choledochal cyst may present in infancy with cholestatic jaundice and be clinically inseparable from neonatal hepatitis or biliary atresia. However, US and radionuclide studies usually suggest the correct diagnosis which can be confirmed, if necessary, on CT or contrast studies (Fig 23–11). In older children and young adults, the clinical presentation is quite variable. A characteristic triad of abdominal pain, obstructive jaundice, and fever has been reported, but only a minority of patients present with all three findings. According to Sherman et al. abdominal pain is the most characteristic presentation, with obstructive jaundice, fever, pale stools, hepatomegaly, palpable mass, and splenomegaly being other presenting features.

US is usually the first imaging study requested, since nearly all of the possible modes of presentation point to a hepatobiliary problem. The markedly dilated common bile duct in type I is readily discernible (Fig 23–9A). The gallbladder can usually be identified adjacent to the dilated common duct, and the cystic duct may also be seen. Most frequently, the intrahepatic ducts are normal, but varying degrees of dilatation have been described. Sludge or stones may be identified within the dilated duct (Fig 23–11B). Although the diagnosis of type I choledochal cyst can be made with a high degree of accu-

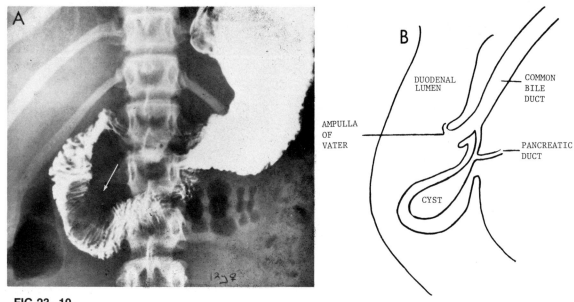

FIG 23–10.
Choledochocele in a 12-year-old girl with abdominal pain. **A,** large filling defect *(arrow)* in the duodenum caused by the choledochocele. **B,** drawing of findings at surgery.

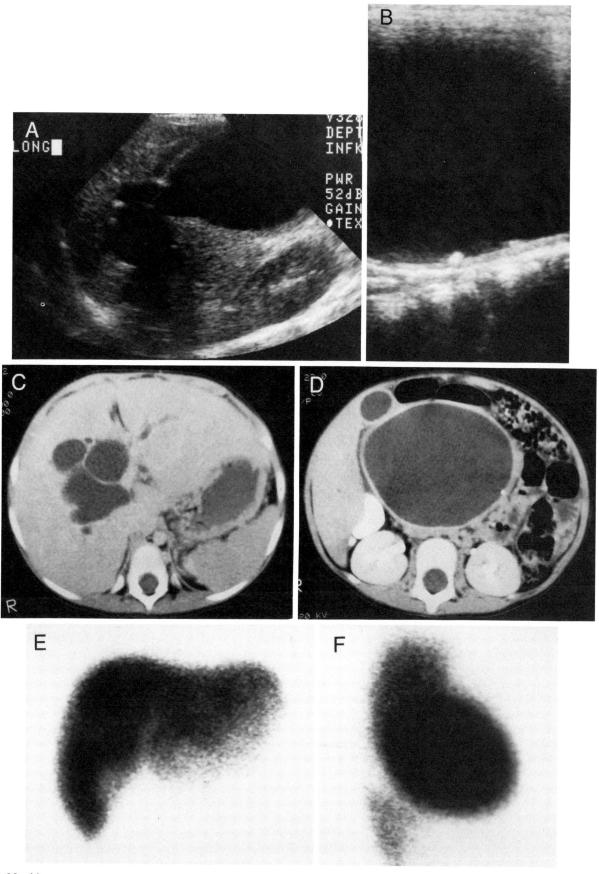

FIG 23–11.
Choledochal cyst. **A** and **B,** longitudinal and transverse sonograms demonstrate marked dilatation of the common bile duct. In the dependent portion of the cystic dilatation, a stone with posterior shadowing is identified. **C,** CT through the liver demonstrates marked dilatation of the common bile duct and hepatic ducts and lesser dilatation of the intrahepatic duct system. **D,** CT scan in a more inferior cut demonstrates massive cystic dilatation of the common bile duct with a calcified stone on the left. The gallbladder with a slightly thickened wall but normal-sized lumen is seen to the right and anterior to the cystic mass. **E** and **F,** 15-minute and 6-hour scintigrams following the injection of ^{99m}Tc IDA demonstrates heterogeneous activity in the left lobe of the liver with subsequent filling of a large cystic mass in the region of the porta hepatis.

racy on US, corroborating imaging studies are usually performed.

If the diagnosis cannot be made definitively, percutaneous transhepatic cholangiography and ERCP have been reported useful (see Fig 23–9). Wiedmeyer et al. successfully performed ERCP in eight patients with type I choledochal cyst and anomalous entry of the common bile duct into the pancreatic duct, six of whom also had ectasia of the common channel. Savader et al. prefer the transhepatic approach, which better delineates the intrahepatic ducts and has less chance of causing cholangitis than does ERCP. It is technically more difficult, however, especially in patients during the first few years of life.

CT will show the cyst to better advantage than US (Fig 23–11C and D), but does not demonstrate the ductal anatomy as well as cholangiography (Fig 23–12). Since this information is important to the surgeon, CT is of less value in the routine workup. However, it may be quite useful in evaluating intrahepatic cysts and evidence of infection, especially abscess formation. MR may show similar results. Upper GI series was commonly used for diagnosis prior to the advent of cross-sectional imaging because of the extrinsic pressure effect of the cyst on the duodenum but no longer plays a role in the evaluation of these patients.

Biliary scintigraphy may show the dilated common bile duct (Fig 23–11,E and F). Camponovo et al. reported the findings in 12 cases of proven choledochal cyst. The dilated duct was demonstrated within 1 hour in seven patients, on delayed scans in three patients, and not at all in two patients.

The most common complication of type I choledochal cyst is ascending cholangitis. Cirrhosis of the liver can occur with subsequent portal hypertension. Cyst rupture has been reported. There is a 20 times greater incidence of carcinoma of the biliary tree in patients with choledochal cyst. The risk is low in the first decade of life but increases with advancing age.

CAROLI DISEASE

Type IV (Alonson-Lej) or type V (Todani) choledochal cyst is segmental nonobstructive dilatation of the intrahepatic bile ducts. The cause of Caroli disease is unknown, but it is a developmental defect occurring during embryonic or fetal hepatogenesis. Least commonly, only intrahepatic biliary duct ectasia is present. More commonly, there is associated hepatic fibrosis and, in many instances, infantile polycystic renal disease. It may well represent one end of the spectrum of polycystic disease of the liver and kidneys discussed below.

Although the disease is present from birth, most

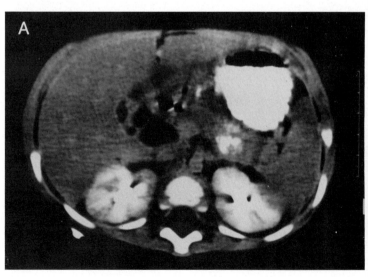
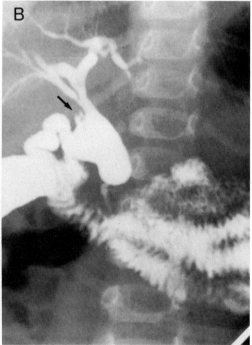

FIG 23–12.
Choledochal cyst. Patient with fever, leukocytosis, and right upper quadrant pain had a choledochal cyst demonstrated on US and CT **(A)**. Cholangiogram **(B)** demonstrates an area of walled-off perforation *(arrow)* and a markedly dilated common bile duct and hepatic ducts.

patients do not present until later in life when abdominal pain secondary to cholangitis usually brings them to medical attention. The abdominal pain may also be related to hepatic abscesses secondary to cholangitis or to biliary stones secondary to stasis. Patients with associated hepatic fibrosis may develop portal hypertension while those without hepatic fibrosis do not. Monolobar Caroli disease has been reported, 88% of the cases involving the left lobe.

Plain films are usually not revealing unless biliary stones are seen, and US is typically the first imaging study performed. In most patients, the ectatic ducts will be large enough to recognize on US (Fig 23–13). Recognition of the connection of the ectatic ducts with one another and the rest of the ductal system is critical in distinguishing Caroli disease from polycystic liver disease. The dilated ducts may give the appearance of surrounding the portal vein radicles, the "intraluminal portal vein sign" (Fig 23–13C). Toma et al. believe this sign to be pathognomonic for Caroli disease. Biliary sludge and calculi are common findings within the anechoic dilated ducts. Both the gallbladder and common bile duct may be enlarged. Marchal et al. have described intraluminal protrusions of the duct wall (see Fig 23–13C). If an abscess is present, one or more cysts will show mixed echogenicity rather than the anechogenicity of the uncomplicated cysts. The kidneys should be examined at the same time. They

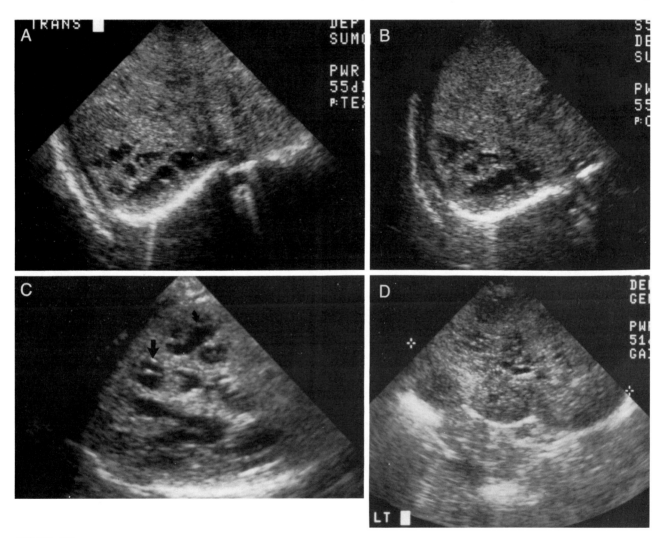

FIG 23–13.
Caroli disease in a patient wihth hepatic fibrosis and polycystic renal disease. **A,** transverse US scan of the liver demonstrates cystic structures in the posterior aspect of the right lobe. **B,** slightly more cephalad, several of the cystic structures can be seen communicating. There is heterogeneous increased echogenicity of the liver parenchyma compatible with hepatic fibrosis which was documented on liver biopsy. **C,** an "intraluminal portal vein" radicle *(straight arrow)* courses through the dilated duct. Intraluminal protrusions of the duct wall are also identified *(curved arrow)*. **D,** an enlarged lobulated kidney shows loss of corticomedullary differentiation.

may be normal, frankly polycystic, or, more commonly, show increased echogenicity, especially of the medullary portions (Fig 23–13*D*). Corticomedullary differentiation may be lost.

Hepatic scintigraphy may show multiple filling defects if the ducts are sufficiently dilated. The patients with hepatic fibrosis have hepatomegaly and, frequently, splenomegaly. Biliary imaging with ^{99m}Tc IDA compounds shows focal defects during the hepatic phase which gradually increase in activity as the radiopharmaceutical collects in the dilated ducts while the remainder of the liver shows decreased activity with time. Activity in the GI tract will be seen but it is frequently delayed because of bile stasis.

CT is an excellent way to show the extent of disease, especially the intrahepatic ductal ectasia. A "central dot" may be seen which corresponds to the intraluminal portal vein seen on sonography. If the ducts are only minimally dilated, the connections between them and the rest of the biliary tree may be more easily seen on CT than on US. If an abscess is present, the affected cyst will typically show higher attenuation than the others. The common duct and gallbladder typically are dilated. Cystic disease of the kidneys may be identified as will splenomegaly in those patients with hepatic fibrosis. A specific role for MR has not been defined.

Cholangiography, either transhepatic or ERCP, demonstrates dilated communicating cystic and tubular ductal ectasia with dilatation of the common duct and gallbladder. Stones and biliary sludge are usually identified. The relative merits of transhepatic studies and ERCP have been discussed by Savader et al. and by Wiedmeyer et al.

FIBROPOLYCYSTIC DISEASES

The intriguing association of polycystic renal disease with polycystic liver disease or congenital hepatic fibrosis has been recognized for a number of years. Several classification systems have been devised, each with its advantages and disadvantages. Summerfield et al. have suggested a new classification based on the clinical, imaging, and histologic features of 51 patients. These authors were struck by the overlap between several entities and have brought them together in a unified grouping. Of interest is that they include choledochal cysts and Caroli disease in this classification because of the overlap. For instance, there were 12 patients with hepatic fibrosis, 8 with Caroli disease, and 12 with both. One patient with choledochal cyst had the typical intrahepatic bile duct ectasia of Caroli disease

while another had associated congenital hepatic fibrosis. Two patients with infantile polycystic liver disease also had hepatic fibrosis and intrahepatic ductal ectasia, while 10 patients with adult polycystic liver disease did not. Further work is required to validate these authors' contentions, but they are achieving increasing acceptance.

Congenital hepatic fibrosis, with or without associated biliary duct ectasia, is an autosomal recessive inherited abnormality. The associated renal abnormalities are infantile and adult polycystic disease, renal dysplasia, and medullary cystic disease. Those patients who present in the newborn or infant period do so because of the severity of their renal disease upon which the course and prognosis depend. Those patients who present later in childhood or in adulthood have less renal involvement and frequently come to attention because of hepatomegaly or portal hypertension. Patients with hepatic fibrosis have surprisingly near-normal liver function studies.

Alvarez et al. have described the US characteristics of congenital hepatic fibrosis (Fig 23–14*A*). The liver is large. Splenomegaly may or may not be present, depending on the presence or absence of portal hypertension. The hepatic echogenicity is homogeneously or heterogeneously increased. With associated Caroli disease, there will be intrahepatic bile duct ectasia and dilatation of the gallbladder (see Fig 23–13). If portal hypertension is present, its characteristic imaging findings (see below) will be seen. Associated renal lesions can also be identified and should always be sought (Fig 23–14*B*). CT and MR imaging do not have a routine role in this disease but may be performed if complications are suspected or in the patient with portal hypertension of unknown cause. The findings are nonspecific with areas of heterogeneously increased and decreased attenuation on CT (Fig 23–14*C*) and of signal intensity on MR. These modalities may better define intrahepatic ductal ectasia and associated extrahepatic duct dilatation. The renal lesions are shown to good advantage.

Polycystic liver disease is divided into infantile and adult forms. The less common infantile type has an autosomal recessive inheritance. The more common adult form is autosomal dominant. The patients with the recessive form usually present early because of the severity of the associated polycystic renal disease. Patients with the dominant form present in adulthood with nephrogenic symptoms, although the findings are often found in asymptomatic children with a positive family history.

On US, the cysts are anechoic (Fig 23–15). Occasionally, one may see included echogenic debris if

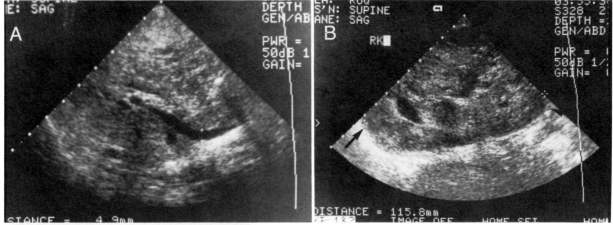

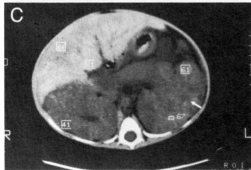

FIG 23–14.
Congenital hepatic fibrosis and polycystic kidneys in a 1-year-old girl with hypertension. **A,** US demonstrates a large echogenic liver. The cursors are at the margins of the portal vein. **B,** a renal sonogram shows an enlarged predominantly echogenic kidney *(arrows)* with loss of normal corticomedullary distinction. **C,** an unenhanced CT scan shows hepatomegaly and bilateral nephromegaly. The relatively hyperdense cortical areas show the radiating pattern of the dilated collecting tubules *(arrow).*

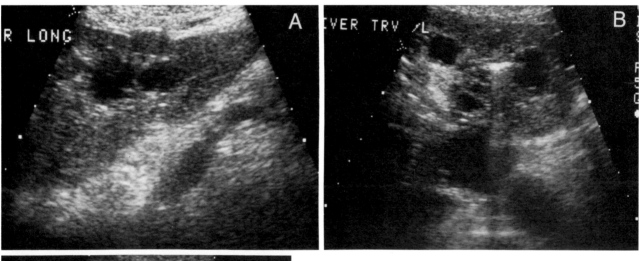

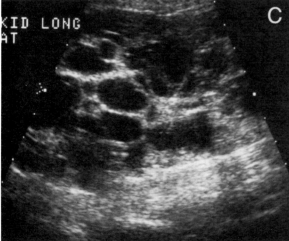

FIG 23–15.
Polycystic liver disease. **A** and **B,** longitudinal and transverse sonograms through the left hepatic lobe reveal multiple cysts. **C,** longitudinal sonogram through the left kidney demonstrates nephromegaly secondary to adult-type autosomal dominant polycystic kidney disease. (Courtesy of R. Brooke Jeffrey, Jr., M.D., Stanford, Calif.)

hemorrhage has occurred. On CT, the cysts are of lower attenuation than the surrounding parenchyma. They are usually of uniform attenuation, although of differing size, and are sharply demarcated from the surrounding parenchyma. On MR, the cysts will have characteristically decreased signal with T1-weighted and increased signal with T2-weighted spin-echo sequences, although Davis et al. have reported heterogeneous signal intensity within the cysts, presumably because of hemorrhages of varying ages.

Microhamartomas are a common incidental finding at pathologic examination of the liver. Summerfield et al. have noted an increased incidence of microhamartomas in patients with fibropolycystic disease of the liver. They are too small to see on imaging studies but may give rise to hepatobiliary carcinomas. There is an increased incidence of biliary duct and pancreatic cancer in patients with Caroli disease and choledochal cyst, a low incidence of hepatocellular carcinoma in congenital fibrosis, and almost no malignant complications in polycystic liver disease.

CONGENITAL SOLITARY CYSTS

Solitary cysts are uncommon in children, benign, and are usually found incidentally at imaging studies or surgery. They may be symptomatic when large, presenting as a palpable abdominal mass or with symptoms, including obstructive jaundice, related to mass effect on adjacent structures. Pliskin et al. have described an adult who developed a squamous cell carcinoma in a congenital cyst.

US is usually diagnostic, demonstrating an intrahepatic anechoic lesion sharply demarcated from the surrounding liver parenchyma (Fig 23–16). Rarely, a cyst may be exophytic and nuclear scintigraphy will be useful in differentiating it from cystic dilatation of the biliary tree. The cyst will appear as a photopenic area on the hepatic phase and show no increase in activity during the delayed scans. Both CT and MR will show the characteristics of a cyst. Neither study is indicated in the workup of a sonographically solitary cystic mass, but a cyst may be seen fortuitously when a patient is being studied for another indication.

GLYCOGEN STORAGE DISEASE

Although numerous metabolic diseases affect the liver, the abdominal imaging findings are generally meager and nondiagnostic. Glycogen deposition causes hepatomegaly and increased attenuation on

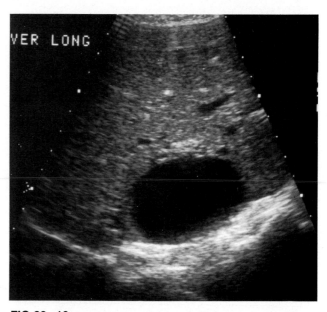

FIG 23–16.
Hepatic cyst. Longitudinal US scan reveals an asymptomatic simple cyst in the posterior portion of the right hepatic lobe which was identified as an incidental finding.

CT. The glycogen storage diseases, however, also cause fatty infiltration of the liver so the net effect is variable depending on the relative amounts of glycogen and fat present. Many of the metabolic disorders lead to cirrhosis or cholelithiasis and are discussed in Sections 4 and 6, respectively. Patients with type I glycogen storage disease may develop hepatic adenomas and hepatocellular carcinoma. These lesions are discussed in Section 7.

REFERENCES

Congenital Anomalies: Biliary Atresia, Neonatal Hepatitis, Alagille Syndrome
Abramson SJ, Berdon WE, Altman RP, et al: Biliary atresia and noncardiac polysplenic syndrome: US and surgical considerations. *Radiology* 1987; 163:377.

Adear H, Barki Y: Multiseptated gallbladder in a child: Incidental diagnosis on sonography. *Pediatr Radiol* 1990; 20:192.

Alagille D, Estrada A, Hadchouel M, et al: Syndromic paucity of interlobular bile ducts (Alagille syndrome or arteriohepatic dysplasia): Review of 80 cases. *J Pediatr* 1987; 110:195.

Alagille D, Odievre M, Gautier M, et al: Hepatic ductular hypoplasia associated with characteristic facies, vertebral malformations, retarded physical, mental and sexual developmental and cardiac murmur. *Pediatrics* 1975; 86:63.

Bekassy AN, Garwicz S, Wiebe T, et al: Hepatocellular

carcinoma associated with arteriohepatic dysplasia in a 4-year-old girl. *Med Pediatr Oncol* 1992; 20:78.

Brun P, Gauthier F, Boucher D, Brunelle F: Échographie et atrésie des voies biliaires chez l'enfant. *Ann Radiol (Paris)* 1985; 28:259.

Collay R, Anne F, de Vanssay de Blavous P, et al: Agénésie du lobe hépatique droit. *Ann Radiol (Paris)* 1990; 33:108.

Day DL, Mulcahy PF, Dehner LP, et al: Post-operative abdominal CT scanning in extrahepatic biliary atresia. *Pediatr Radiol* 1989; 19:379.

Demirci A, Diren HB, Selcuk MB: Computed tomography in agenesis of the right lobe of the liver. *Acta Radiol* 1990; 31:105.

Diaz MJ, Fowler W, Hnatow BJ: Congenital gallbladder duplication: preoperative diagnosis by ultrasonography. *Gastrointest Radiol* 1991; 16:198.

Furuya KN, Roberts EA, Canny GJ, et al: Neonatal hepatitis syndrome with paucity of interlobular bile ducts in cystic fibrosis. *J Pediatr Gastroenterol Nutr* 1991; 12:127.

Gerhold JP, Klingensmith WC III, Kuni CC, et al: Diagnosis of biliary atresia with radionuclide hepatobiliary imaging. *Radiology* 1983; 146:499.

Grunert D, Stier B, Schoning M: The portal system and hepatic artery in children with biliary atresia. I: Ultrasound and simple duplex ultrasound parameters. *Klin Pädiatr* 1990; 202:24.

Guelrud M, Jaen D, Mendoza S, et al: ERCP in the diagnosis of extrahepatic biliary atresia. *Gastrointest Endosc* 1991; 37:522.

Haaga JR, Morrison SC, County J, et al: Infarction of the left hepatic lobe in a neonate on serial CTs: Evolution of a pseudomass to atrophy. *Pediatr Radiol* 1991; 21:150.

Haller JO, Condon VR, Berdon WE, et al: Spontaneous perforation of the bile duct in children. *Radiology* 1989; 172:621.

Hardoff R, Hardoff D: Scintigraphic evaluation of septated hypokinetic gallbladder in a teenager. *Clin Nucl Med* 1990; 15:117.

Ikeda S, Sera Y, Akagi M: Serial ultrasonic examination to differentiate biliary atresia from neonatal hepatitis—special reference to changes in size of the gallbladder. *Eur J Pediatr* 1989; 148:396.

Ishii K, Matsuo S, Hirayama Y, et al: Intrahepatic biliary cysts after hepatic portoenterostomy in four children with biliary atresia. *Pediatr Radiol* 1989; 19:471.

Kakitsubata Y, Nakamura R, Mitsuo H, et al: Absence of the left lobe of the liver: US and CT appearance. *Gastrointest Radiol* 1991; 16:323.

Kanematsu M, Imaeda T, Yamawaki Y, et al: Agenesis of the right lobe of the liver: case report. *Gastrointest Radiol* 1991; 16:320.

Kasai M, Kimura S, Asakura Y, et al: Surgical treatment of biliary atresia. *J Pediatr Surg* 1968; 3:665.

Katayama H, Suruga K, Kurashige T, et al: Bone changes in congenital biliary atresia. Radiologic observation of 8 cases. *AJR* 1975; 124:107.

Kirks DR, Coleman RE, Filston HC, et al: An imaging approach to persistent neonatal jaundice. *AJR* 1984; 142:461.

Kocoshis SA, Cottrill CM, O'Connor WN, et al: Congenital heart disease, butterfly vertebrae and extrahepatic biliary atresia: A variant of arteriohepatic dysplasia? *J Pediatr* 1981; 99:436.

Landing BH: Considerations of the pathogenesis of neonatal hepatitis, biliary atresia, and choledochal cyst: The concept of infantile obstructive cholangiopathy. *Prog Pediatr Surg* 1974; 6:113.

Lilly JR, Karren FM: Contemporary surgery of biliary atresia. *Pediatr Clin North Am* 1985; 32:1233.

Majd M: ^{99m}Tc-IDA scintigraphy in the evaluation of neonatal jaundice. *Radiographics* 1983; 3:88.

Perez Becerra E, Fuster M, Fraga M, et al: Alagille's syndrome: A family case and its association with hepatocellular carcinoma. *Rev Clin Esp* 1991; 188:459.

Radin DR, Colletti PM, Ralls PW, et al: Agenesis of the right lobe of the liver. *Radiology* 1987; 164:639.

Rodriguez JI, Rivera T, Palacios J: Alagille syndrome associated with caudal dysplasia sequence. *Am J Med Genet* 1991; 40:61.

Rosenfield NS, Kelley MJ, Jensen PS, et al: Arteriohepatic dysplasia: radiologic features of a new syndrome. *AJR* 1980; 135:1217.

Sommerville DA, Marks M, Treves ST: Hepatobiliary scintigraphy in arteriohepatic dysplasia (Alagille's syndrome): A report of two cases. *Pediatr Radiol* 1988; 18:32.

Spivak W, Sarkar S, Winter D, et al: Diagnostic utility of hepatobiliary scintigraphy with ^{99m}Tc-DISIDA in neonatal cholestasis. *J Pediatr* 1985; 106:171.

Treem WR, Grant EE, Barth KH, et al: Ultrasound guided percutaneous cholecystocholangiography for early differentiation of cholestatic liver disease in infants. *J Pediatr Gastroenterol Nutr* 1988; 7:347.

Wanek EA, Horgan JG, Karrer FM, et al: Portal venous velocity in biliary atresia. *J Pediatr Surg* 1990, 25:146.

Weber TR, Grosfeld JL: Contemporary management of biliary atresia. *Surg Clin North Am* 1984; 61:1079.

Weinberger E, Blumhagen JD, Odell JM: Gallbladder contraction in biliary atresia. *AJR* 1987; 149:401.

Williamson SL, Seibert JJ, Butler HL, et al: Apparent gut excretion of Tc-99m-DISIDA in a case of extrahepatic biliary atresia. *Pediatr Radiol* 1986; 16:245.

Yamamoto S, Kojoh K, Saito J, et al: Computed tomography of congenital absence of the left lobe of the liver. *J Comput Assist Tomogr* 1988; 12:206.

Choledochal Cyst, Fibropolycystic Disease, and Other Congenital Abnormalities

Alexander MC, Haaga JR: MR imaging of a choledochal cyst. *J Comput Assist Tomogr* 1985; 9:357.

Alonson-Leg F, Reven WB, Pessagno DJ: Congenital Choledochal cyst, with a report of two, and analysis of 94 cases. *Int Abstr Surg* 1959; 108:1.

Alvarez F, Bernard O, Brunelle F, et al: Congenital hepatic fibrosis in children. *J Pediatr* 1981; 99:370.

Athey PA, Lauderman JA, King DE: Case report: massive congenital solitary nonparasitic cyst of the liver in infancy. *J Ultrasound Med* 1986:5:585.

Babbitt DP, Starshak RJ, Clemett AR: Choledochal cyst: a concept of etiology. *Am J Roentgenol* 1973; 119:57.

Boyle MJ, Doyle GD, McNulty JG: Monolobar Caroli's disease. *Am J Gastroenterol* 1989; 84:1437.

Camponovo E, Buck JL, Drane WE: Scintigraphic features of choledochal cyst. *J Nucl Med* 1989; 30:622.

Caroli J, Soupault R, Kossakowski J, et al: La dilatation polykystique congénitale des voies biliaires intrahépatiques. Essai de classification. *Sem Hop (Paris)* 1958; 34:488.

Chilton SJ, Cremin BJ: The spectrum of polycystic disease in children. *Pediatr Radiol* 1981; 11:9.

Clinkscales NB, Trigg LP, Poklepovic J: Obstructive jaundice secondary to benign hepatic cyst. *Radiology* 1985; 154:643.

Crittenden SL, McKinley MJ: Choledochal cyst—clinical features and classification. *Am J Gastroenterol* 1985; 80:643.

Davies CH, Stringer DA, Whyte H, et al: Congenital hepatic fibrosis with saccular dilatation of intrahepatic bile ducts and infantile polycystic kidneys. *Pediatr Radiol* 1986; 16:302.

Davis PL, Kanal E, Farnum GN, et al: MR imaging of multiple hepatic cysts in a patient with polycystic liver disease. *Magn Reson Imaging* 1987; 5:407.

Doppman JL, Cornblath M, Dwyer AJ, et al: Computed tomography of the liver and kidneys in glycogen storage disease. *J Comput Assist Tomogr* 1982; 6:67.

Jequier S, Capusten B, Guttman F, et al: Childhood choledochal cyst with intrahepatic enlarged cyst-like bile ducts. *J Can Assoc Radiol* 1984; 35:73.

Kangarloo H, Sarti DA, Sample WF, et al: Ultrasonic spectrum of choledochal cysts in children. *Pediatr Radiol* 1980; 9:15.

Marchal GJ, Desmet VJ, Proesmans WC, et al: Caroli disease: High-frequency US and pathologic findings. *Radiology* 1986; 158:507.

McHugh K, Daneman A: Multiple gastrointestinal atresias: Sonography of associated biliary abnormalities. *Pediatr Radiol* 1991; 21:355.

Moreno AJ, Parker AL, Spicer MJ, Brown TJ: Scintigraphic and radiographic findings in Caroli's disease. *Am J Gastroenterol* 1984; 79:299.

Nakanuma Y, Terada T, Ohta G, et al: Caroli disease in congenital hepatic fibrosis and infantile polycystic disease. *Liver* 1982; 2:346.

Padhy AK, Gopinath PG, Basu AK, et al: Hepatobiliary scintigraphy in congenital cystic dilatation of biliary tract. *Clin Nucl Med* 1985; 10:703.

Pliskin A, Cualing H, Stenger RJ: Primary squamous cell carcinoma originating in congenital cysts of the liver. Report of a case and review of the literature. *Arch Pathol Lab Med* 1992; 116:105.

Premkumar A, Berdon WE, Levy J, et al: The emergence of hepatic fibrosis and portal hypertension in infants and children with autosomal recessive polycystic kidney disease. Initial and follow-up sonographic and radiographic findings. *Pediatr Radiol* 1988; 18:123.

Rosenfield N, Griscom Nt: Choledochal cysts: Roentgenographic techniques. *Radiology* 1975; 114:113.

Savader SJ, Benenati JF, Venbrux AC, et al: Choledochal cysts: classification and cholangiographic appearance. AJR 1991; 156:327.

Sherman P, Kolster E, Davies C, et al: Choledochal cysts: Heterogeneity of clinical presentation. *J Pediatr Gastroenterol Nutr* 1986; 5:867.

Sood GK, Mahapatra JR, Khurana A, et al: Caroli disease: Computed tomographic diagnosis. *Gastrointest Radiol* 1991; 16:243.

Sty JR, Hubbard AM, Starshak RJ: Radionuclide hepatobiliary imaging in congenital biliary tract ectasia (Caroli disease). *Pediatr Radiol* 1982; 12:111.

Suarez F, Bernard O, Gauthier F, et al: Bilio-pancreatic common channel in children. Clinical, biological and radiological findings in 12 children. *Pediatr Radiol* 1987; 17:207.

Summerfield JA, Nagafuchi Y, Sherlock S, et al: Hepatobiliary fibropolycystic diseases. A clinical and histological review of 51 patients. *J Hepatol* 1986; 2:141.

Todani T, Watanabe Y, Narusue M: Congenital bile duct cyst. *Am J Surg* 1977; 134:263.

Toma P, Lucigrai G, Pelizza A: Sonographic patterns of Caroli's disease: report of 5 new cases. *J Clin Ultrasound* 1991; 19:155.

Voyles CR, Smadja C, Shands WC, et al: Carcinoma in choledochal cysts: age-related incidence. *Arch Surg* 1983; 118:986.

Wiedmeyer DA, Stewart ET, Dodds WJ, et al: Choledochal cyst: Findings on cholangiopancreatography with emphasis on ectasia of the common channel. AJR 1989; 153:969.

SECTION 3

Infections of the Liver

Viral hepatitis is the most common diffuse infection of the liver in otherwise healthy children. Parasites are more common worldwide but typically involve the biliary tree, as in ascariasis, or produce focal infections of the liver, as in echinococcosis or amebiasis. Immunocompromised patients are susceptible to fungal infections.

Viral hepatitis after the perinatal period is most commonly caused by the hepatitis A, hepatitis B, and hepatitis C viruses. A number of other viruses, including mumps, varicella-zoster, herpes simplex, cytomegalovirus (CMV), adenovirus, coxsackievirus, and Epstein-Barr, have been implicated as causative agents in childhood. Most affected patients have a short-lived acute disease with complete recovery. Complications include subacute and chronic active hepatitis, cirrhosis, and hepatocellular carcinoma of the liver. Chronic active hepatitis may also be of a noninfectious etiology.

Imaging studies are rarely necessary in the acute state. Hepatomegaly will be seen on any imaging study. US most commonly demonstrates a heterogeneous increase in echogenicity, but decreased echogenicity may be noted in highly edematous areas. Periportal edema may make the normally increased echoes of the small portal veins even more prominent. The wall of the gallbladder may appear thickened. Toppet et al. performed US on 58 children with hepatitis A, all of whom had lymphadenopathy in the porta hepatis. CT scans may show heterogeneous changes in attenuation mirroring the echographic changes, but more commonly are normal except for hepatomegaly. Hepatic scintigraphy also shows hepatomegaly and may show decreased heterogeneous uptake in the liver with increased uptake in the spleen and bone marrow in some patients.

Pyogenic infection with abscess formation after the neonatal period is most commonly found in immunocompromised patients. *Staphylococcus aureus* is the most common pathogen. Patients with chronic granulomatous disease of childhood, a syndrome of leukocyte dysfunction, or those who have had bone marrow transplantation are at high risk for pyogenic abscesses. Other susceptible patients are those on immunosuppressive chemotherapy, with congenital or acquired immunodeficiency states, or with other intra-abdominal infection such as appendicitis and inflammatory bowel disease. Port and Leonidas described a case of cat-scratch fever in which hepatic granulomas appeared as hypoechogenic lesions which were of low attenuation on unenhanced CT.

Most patients develop one or more discrete masses, most frequently in the posterior right lobe, which have reduced echogenicity but are rarely anechoic. Through transmission is usually present. They are typically surrounded by a ring of hypoechogenic liver edema. Rarely, there is so much internal debris that the abscess may appear hyperechoic. Fluid-fluid levels have been described, and septations may be seen. Contrast-enhanced CT scans show the abscess to have lower attenuation than the surrounding liver parenchyma (Fig 23–17). A contrast-enhanced high-attenuation "wall" is often seen surrounded by a low attenuation ring of edema. MR scans typically show low or nearly isointense signal on T1-weighted images with hyperintense signal on T2-weighted images. Contrast enhancement may demonstrate a hyperintense ring around the abscess with persistent low signal within the mass, differentiating it from a solid tumor. Hepatic scintigraphy shows a focal filling defect but is less sensitive than echography, CT, or MR.

Hematogenous spread of pyogenic organisms may result in small microabscesses each of which will show the imaging characteristics described above (Fig 23–18). Acute tuberculous abscess cannot be differentiated on imaging studies from other pyogenic infections. Resolved tuberculosis may result in diffuse hepatic calcification. Percutaneous abscess drainage under US or CT guidance has become a well-accepted therapeutic procedure (see Fig 23–17B). The techniques used are the same as those in adults, although conscious sedation may be necessary for children. Small abscesses may be drained acutely, while chronic drainage through a percutaneously placed indwelling catheter may be necessary for large lesions.

Fungal infection also occurs most frequently in immunocompromised patients. The most common offending organism is *Candida albicans*, but other ubiquitous fungi, such as the agents implicated in

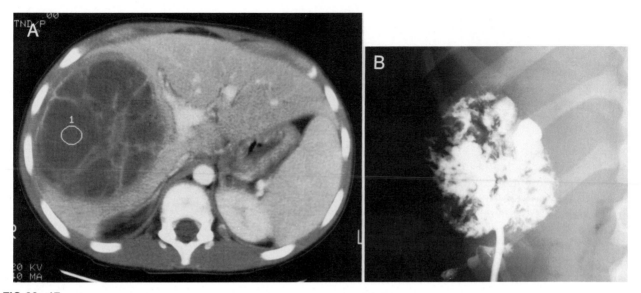

FIG 23–17.
Liver abscess. **A,** CT scan demonstrates a multiloculated, septated mass of decreased attenuation in the right lobe of the liver. There is increased attenuation of the septa. There is faintly seen edema between the abscess anteriorly and the enhanced normal liver. **B,** injection of contrast material following percutaneous drainage of this documented streptococcal abscess demonstrates the multiocular nature of the lesion with its irregularly marginated wall. (Courtesy of Robert Mindelzun, M.D., Stanford, Calif.)

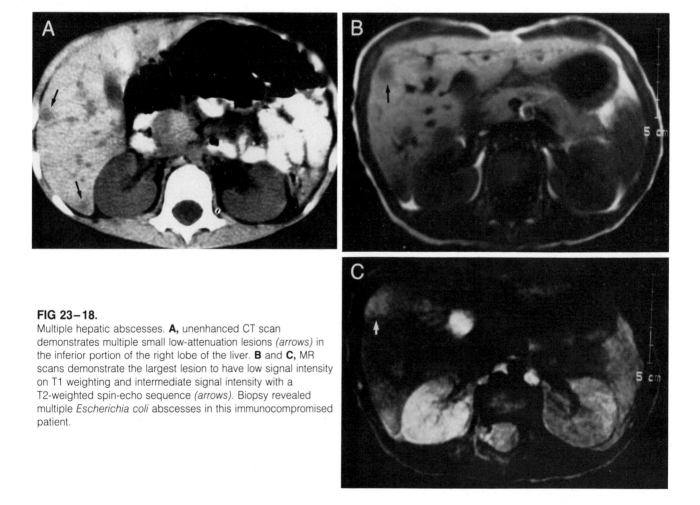

FIG 23–18.
Multiple hepatic abscesses. **A,** unenhanced CT scan demonstrates multiple small low-attenuation lesions *(arrows)* in the inferior portion of the right lobe of the liver. **B** and **C,** MR scans demonstrate the largest lesion to have low signal intensity on T1 weighting and intermediate signal intensity with a T2-weighted spin-echo sequence *(arrows)*. Biopsy revealed multiple *Escherichia coli* abscesses in this immunocompromised patient.

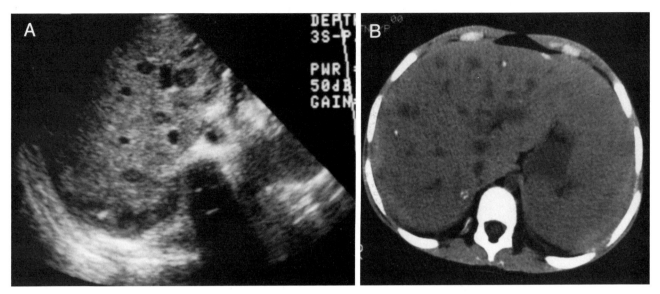

FIG 23–19.
Hepatic candidiasis. Transverse sonogram **(A)** and CT scan of the upper abdomen **(B)** demonstrates multiple "bull's-eye" lesions in the right lobe of the liver in an immunocompromised patient. The calcifications on the CT scan are presumed to represent sequelae of prior infection. Liver biopsy demonstrated candidiasis.

aspergillosis, histoplasmosis, coccidioidomycosis (in the endemic area), and nocardiosis, have been identified in fungal hepatitis. In cases of hepatic candidiasis, multiple small hypoechoic lesions are seen on US. Occasionally these lesions look like bull's eyes with a central hyperechoic area surrounded by an echolucent zone, an appearance thought to be specific for candidiasis (Fig 23–19). Pastakia et al. described a "wheel-within-wheel" appearance in which a hypoechoic center is surrounded by an echogenic zone which in turn is surrounded by a hyperechogenic zone.

Parasitic infestations are common worldwide with the offending organism varying from one endemic area to another. Ascariasis of the biliary tree is secondary to *Ascaris lumbricoides* infestation of the small intestine. The worms make their way into the biliary duct system, causing dilatation and pain. On imaging studies, the characteristic vermiform defects will be seen inside the dilated ducts. The worms are echogenic on US examination.

Echinococcosis (hydatid disease) is an infestation by the larval stage of the *Echinococcus* tapeworm. Of the forms found in humans, *E. granulosus* is more common than *E. multilocularis*. The disease is worldwide in distribution with the major endemic regions being the Middle East and Mediterranean nations, South America, and Australia. Beggs has reviewed the parasitologic, clinical, and radiologic aspects of *E. granulosus* infestation. The pathologic findings explain the findings on imaging studies. An echinococcal cyst has three layers surrounding clear transuda-

tive fluid. The rigid outer pericyst is formed by modified host cells. A middle, laminated membrane is acellular. The inner, or germinal, layer is thin and produces the laminated membrane and scolices which are the larval stage. The daughter cysts arise from the germinal membrane. The liver is the most involved organ, being affected in 75% of cases. The cysts may be single or multiple and may appear multilocular because of daughter cysts. The right lobe is most commonly involved. Superinfection usually occurs only after cyst rupture, since the intact middle layer is resistant to bacterial invasion.

Lewall and McCorkell have classified the sonographic findings of hepatic echinococeal cysts. Type I is a simple fluid-filled cyst which is anechoic with through transmission. In type IR, the germinal layer is seen as an undulating membrane secondary to rupture. Movable echogenic debris in the type I cysts, "echinococcal sand" representing detached scolices, helps differentiate them from simple cysts of the liver. Type II cysts contain daughter cysts whose walls are made up of only the inner and middle layers. Type III lesions are dead cysts, usually calcified and echogenic with shadowing. Lowell and McCorkell state that the natural progression of disease is from type I to type III.

CT can identify calcification in the cyst wall which may be too fine to see on plain films. The appearance of a split wall is secondary to separation of the laminated membrane from the germinal membrane. Increased echogenicity on US or increased attenuation on CT of the cyst fluid suggests bacterial superinfection. In these cases, the cyst is often less well defined and the wall may appear quite irregular and collapsed. MR imaging shows anatomical findings similar to those seen on CT with the fluid having long T1 and T2 relaxation times. A low-intensity rim may be seen, which Hoff et al. believe represents the pericyst and may be specific for echinococcus. Percutaneous drainage of echinococcal cysts has recently been successfully accomplished although surgical extirpation is still most frequently performed. Recent trials of medical therapy seem promising.

Not only is *E. multilocularis* less common than *E. granulosus*, it shows different imaging features, which were reviewed by Didier et al. Commonly seen patterns include irregular hepatomegaly, increased echogenicity, decreased CT attenuation,

multiple lesions, microcalcifications, and dilatation of intrahepatic bile ducts. These authors also describe involvement of parahepatic structures, portal hypertension, and involvement of the spleen, hepatic veins, and IVC.

Amebic abscesses caused by *Entamoeba histolytica* are most commonly solitary and are most frequently found in the right lobe of the liver. The infection is primarily intestinal with the liver involved secondary to spread via the portal vein. Amebic abscesses in children are most common under age 3 years and frequently are seen in the first year of life. On US, the lesions are seen peripherally in contact with the hepatic capsule. They are round or oval and hypoechoic with acoustic enhancement. An echogenic wall is not identified. Characteristically, homogeneous low-level echoes are seen throughout the le-

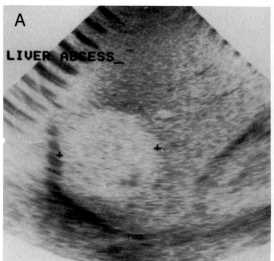

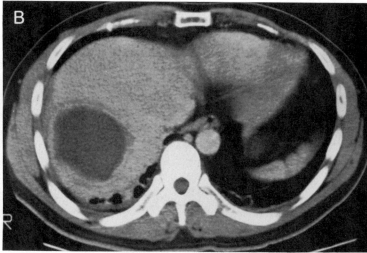

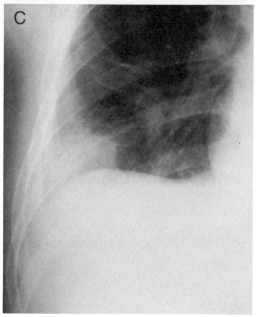

FIG 23–20.
Amebic abscess. **A,** sonogram demonstrates a hypoechogenic mass in the posterior aspect of the right lobe of the liver abutting the liver capsule. **B,** CT scan demonstrates a low-attenuation mass in the dome of the right lobe of the liver with a prominent "halo." The patient was subsequently found to have intestinal amebiasis. **C,** PA view of the chest demonstrates extension of the amebic process into the hemithorax. (Courtesy of Robert Mindelzun, M.D., Stanford, Calif.)

sion as the gain is increased. Oleszczuk-Raszbe et al. have reviewed the features differentiating pyogenic from amebic abscesses. Amebic abscesses are more likely to be better defined with a peripheral hypo-echogenic "halo" (Fig 23–20A). Pyogenic abscesses are less well defined and have central hypoechogenicity. The wall of the amebic abscess thickens with successful therapy as the echogenicity of the contents decreases.

Nuclear scintigraphy is more sensitive than US in the first 2 weeks of the disease, according to Katzenstein et al. The hepatic scan demonstrates a nonspecific photopenic mass lesion which may demonstrate rim enhancement. CT is not generally needed for diagnosis, but if performed will have an appearance similar to those described with pyogenic abscesses but with a low-attenuation halo (Fig 23–20B). Amebic abscesses are more commonly unilocular. Perforation through the diaphragm may occur (Fig 23–20C), as may intraperitoneal spread. Percutaneous aspiration in children is usually performed only if impending rupture is suspected clinically. Otherwise, patients generally do well with medical therapy.

REFERENCES

Beggs I: The radiology of hydatid disease. AJR 1985; 145:639.

Bernardino ME, Berkman WA, Plemmons M, et al: Percutaneous drainage of multiseptated hepatic abscess. *J Comput Assist Tomogr* 1984; 8:38.

Berry M, Bazaz R, Bhargava S: Amebic liver abscess: Sonographic diagnosis and management. *J Clin Ultrasound* 1986; 14:239.

Bezzi M, Teggi A, DeRosa F, et al: Abdominal hydatid disease: US findings during medical treatment. *Radiology* 1987; 162:91.

Callen PW, Filly RA, Marcus FS: Ultrasonography and computed tomography in the evaluation of hepatic microabscesses in the immunosuppressed patient. *Radiology* 1982; 136:433.

Cerri GG, Leite GJ, Simoes JB, et al: Ultrasonographic evaluation of ascaris in the biliary tract. *Radiology* 1983; 146:753.

Cremin BJ: Ultrasonic diagnosis of biliary ascariasis: "A bull's eye in the triple O". *Br J Radiol* 1982; 55:683.

Didier D, Weiler S, Rohmer P, et al: Hepatic alveolar echinococcosis: correlative US and CT study. *Radiology* 1985; 154:179.

Francis IR, Glazer GM, Amendola MA, et al: Hepatic abscesses in the immunocompromised patient: Role of CT in detection, diagnosis, management, and follow-up. *Gastrointest Radiol* 1986; 11:257.

Garel LA, Pariente DM, Nezelof C, et al: Liver involvement in chronic granulomatous disease: The role of ultrasound in diagnosis and treatment. *Radiology* 1984; 153:117.

Gerzof SG, Robbins AH, Birkett DH, et al: Percutaneous catheter drainage of abdominal abscesses guided by ultrasound and computed tomography. *N Engl J Med* 1981; 305:653.

Giorgio A, Amoroso P, Fico P, et al: Ultrasound evaluation of uncomplicated and complicated acute viral hepatitis. *J Clin Ultrasound* 1986; 14:675.

Grünebaum M, Ziv N, Kaplinsky C, et al: Liver candidiasis: The various sonographic patterns in the immunocompromised child. *Pediatr Radiol* 1991; 21:497.

Halvorsen RA, Korobkin M, Foster WL, et al: The variable CT appearance of hepatic abscesses. *Am J Roentgenol* 1984; 142:941.

Hayden CK, Toups M, Swischuk LE, et al: Sonographic features of hepatic amebiasis in childhood. *J Can Assoc Radiol* 1984; 35:279.

Hoff FL, Aisen AM, Walden ME, Glazer GM: MR imaging in hydatid disease of the liver. *Gastrointest Radiol* 1987; 12:39.

Katzenstein D, Rickerson V, Braude A: New concepts of amebic liver abscess derived from hepatic imaging, serodiagnosis, and hepatic enzymes in 67 consecutive cases in San Diego. *Medicine (Baltimore)* 1982; 61:237.

Khuroo MS, Zargar SA, Mahajan R, et al: Sonographic appearances in biliary ascariasis. *Gastroenterology* 1987; 93:267.

Khuroo MS, Zargar SA, Mahajan R: Echinococcus cysts in the liver: management with percutaneous drainage. *Radiology* 1991; 180:141.

Laurin S, Kande JV: Diagnosis of liver-spleen abscesses in children—with emphasis on ultrasound for the initial and follow up examinations. *Pediatr Radiol* 1984; 14:187.

Lewall DB, Bailey TM, McCorkell SJ: Echinococcal matrix: Computed tomographic, sonographic and pathologic correlation. *J Ultrasound Med* 1986; 5:33.

Lewall DB, McCorkell SJ: Hepatic echinococcal cysts: Sonographic appearance and classification. *Radiology* 1985; 155:773.

Lewall DB, McCorkell SJ: Rupture of echinococcal cysts: Diagnosis, classification and clinical implications. *AJR* 1986; 146:391.

Mathieu D, Vasile N, Fagniez PL, et al: Dynamic CT features of hepatic abscesses. *Radiology* 1985; 154:749.

Merton DF, Kirks DR: Amebic liver abscess in children: the role of diagnostic imaging. *AJR* 1984; 143:1325.

Miller JH, Greenfield LD, Wald BR: Candidiasis of the liver and spleen in childhood. *Radiology* 1982; 142:375.

Morris DL, Buckley J, Gregson R, et al: Magnetic resonance imaging in hydatid disease. *Clin Radiol* 1987; 38:141.

Mueller PR, Dawson SL, Ferrucci JT, et al: Hepatic echinococcal cyst: successful percutaneous drainage. *Radiology* 1985; 155:627.

Oleszczuk-Raske K, Cremin BJ, Fisher RM, et al: Ultrasonic features of pyogenic and amoebic hepatic abscesses. *Pediatr Radiol* 1989; 19:230.

Pastakia B, Shawker TH, Thaler M, et al: Hepatosplenic candidiasis: Wheels within wheels. *Radiology* 1988; 166:417.

Pineiro-Carrero VM, Andres JM: Morbidity and mortality in children with pyogenic liver abscess. *Am J Dis Child* 1989; 143:1424.

Port J, Leonidas JC: Granulomatous hepatitis in cat-scratch disease: Ultrasound and CT observations. *Pediatr Radiol* 1991; 21:598.

Radin DR, Ralls PW, Colletti PM, et al: CT of amebic liver abscess. *AJR* 1988; 150:1297.

Ralls PW: Sonography in the diagnosis and management of hepatic amebic abscess in children. *Pediatr Radiol* 1982; 12:239.

Ralls PW, Barnes PF, Johnson MB, et al: Treatment of hepatic amebic abscess: Rare need for percutaneous drainage. *Radiology* 1987; 165:805.

Ralls PW, Barnes PF, Radin DR, et al: Sonographic features of amebic and pyogenic liver abscesses: A blinded comparison. *AJR* 1987; 179:499.

Ralls PW, Colletti PM, Quinn MF, et al: Sonographic findings in hepatic amebic abscess. *Radiology* 1982; 145:123.

Remedios PA, Colletti PM, Ralls PW: Hepatic amebic abscess: cholescintigraphic rim enhancement. *Radiology* 1986; 160:395.

Schmiedl U, Paajanen J, Arakawa M, et al: MR imaging of liver abscesses: application of Gd-DTPA. *Magn Reson Imaging* 1988; 6:9.

Schulman A, Loxton AJ, Heydenrych JJ, et al: Sonographic diagnosis of biliary ascariasis. *AJR* 1982; 13:485.

Slovis TL, Haller JO, Cohen HL, et al: Complicated appendiceal inflammatory disease in children: Pylephlebitis and liver abscess. *Radiology* 1989; 171:823.

Stricof DD, Glazer GM, Amendola MA: Chronic granulomatous disease: Value of the newer imaging modalities. *Pediatr Radiol* 1984; 14:328.

Sty JR, Starshak RJ: Comparative imaging in the evaluation of hepatic abscesses in immunocompromised children. *J Clin Ultrasound* 1983; 11:11.

Terrier F, Becker CD, Triller JK: Morphologic aspects of hepatic abscesses at computed tomography and ultrasound. *Acta Radiol Diagn* 1983; 24:129.

Toppet V, Souyah H, Delplace O, et al: Lymph node enlargement as a sign of acute hepatitis A in children. *Pediatr Radiol* 1990; 20:249.

van Sonnenberg E, Mueller PR, Schiffman HR, et al: Intrahepatic amoebic abscesses: Indications for and results of percutaneous catheter drainage. *Radiology* 1985; 156:631.

Wall SD, Fisher MR, Amparo EG, et al: Magnetic resonance imaging in the evaluation of abscesses. *AJR* 1985; 144:1217.

SECTION 4

Diffuse Parenchymal Disease

There are a variety of diseases which cause diffuse imaging abnormalities throughout the liver. Although some of these diseases are of congenital origin, the hepatic manifestations are acquired as complications of the disease process or its treatment.

Cirrhosis of the liver is a diffuse disease in which the normal hepatic parenchyma is destroyed and replaced by fibrosis. The liver tissue regenerates in a focal nodular pattern. In the micronodular form, the nodules are 1 cm in diameter or smaller, whereas the macronodular form can have nodular diameters as large as 5 cm. Portal hypertension is a common finding, as discussed in Section 5. Cirrhosis is a secondary phenomenon that has been described in children with a variety of congenital and acquired diseases, including hepatitis, hepatic fibrosis, biliary atresia, cystic fibrosis, Budd-Chiari syndrome, and chronic biliary obstruction. Cirrhosis is also seen in a number of metabolic disorders, including alpha$_1$-antitrypsin deficiency, glycogen storage disease, galactosemia, tyrosinemia, and Wilson disease. Glass et al. described a patient with Gaucher disease in whom the hepatic CT scan showed a lobulated liver with decreased attenuation centrally which correlated well with autopsy-proven central liver necrosis. Portal hypertension was also present.

US examination of the cirrhotic liver shows the right lobe to be small (Fig 23–21). The caudate lobe and lateral segment of the left lobe are, in compensation, enlarged. The margins of the liver are irregular rather than smooth. Fatty infiltration of the liver causes increased echogenicity of the parenchyma while the fibrotic portions and regenerating nodules show reduced echogenicity. The intrahepatic vessels may be difficult to see because of compression by fibrosis. The gallbladder may be small, not seen, or have stones within it, depending on the primary disease leading to the cirrhosis. The findings of portal hypertension are often seen.

Hepatic scintigraphy shows a normal-sized or small liver with heterogeneous decreased uptake of the isotope-labeled colloid. Regenerating nodules show increased activity between areas of photopenic fibrosis. There is increased activity in the enlarged spleen and in the bone marrow (Fig 23–21,D). CT shows a small or normal-sized irregularly marginated liver (Fig 23–22) with decreased attenuation in areas of fatty infiltration and normal attenuation in

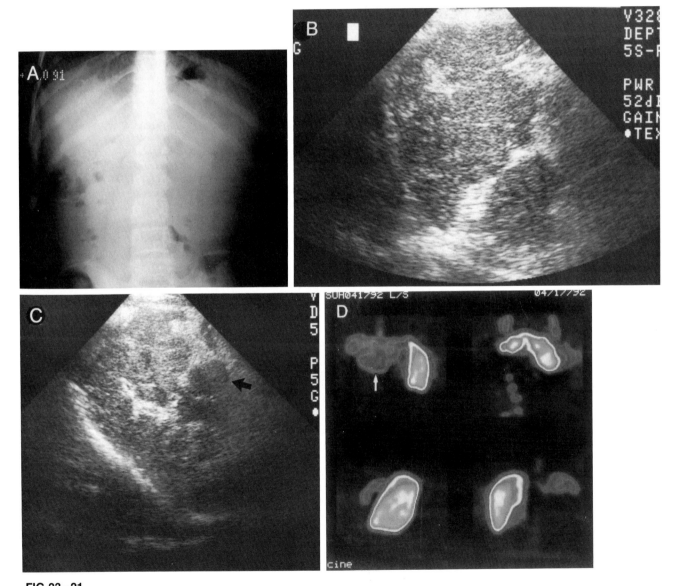

FIG 23–21.
Cirrhosis in a patient with cystic fibrosis. **A,** KUB demonstrates a small, shrunken liver in the right upper quadrant with marked splenomegaly on the left. **B** and **C,** transverse US scans of the right lobe of the liver at two different levels demonstrate mixed echogenicity with fatty replacement, a markedly lobular configuration to the small-volume liver, and regenerating nodules **C** *(arrow).* **D,** ^{99m}Tc colloid single photon emission tomography (SPECT) scan on a different patient *(clockwise from the top left:* anterior, right lateral, posterior, left lateral) demonstrates reduced activity in the liver with a relatively larger caudate lobe *(arrow).* Most activity is in the greatly enlarged spleen. (See also Plate 1 facing p. 950.) **(Courtesy of Michael L. Goris, M.D., Stanford, Calif.)**

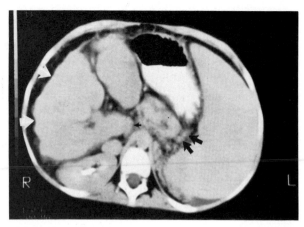

FIG 23–22.
Contrast-enhanced CT scan of an 11-year-old girl with cirrhosis and portal hypertension shows the small liver with nodular surface *(white arrows)* and caudate lobe hypertrophy *(small black arrow).* Venous collateral vessels are present in the hilum of the enlarged spleen *(large black arrows).*

areas of fibrosis and regenerating nodules. Contrast enhancement exaggerates the heterogeneity of attenuation. MR of the liver shows the anatomical abnormalities seen with US and CT. The signal intensity on spin-echo images is nonspecific and variable, depending on the degree of fatty infiltration and iron deposition. Regenerating nodules may be isointense with liver or show reduced signal intensity on T2-weighted images secondary to iron deposition. Gradient-recalied echo images are even more sensitive to the presence of iron, especially as the TE (echo time) is lengthened. Hepatocellular carcinoma com-

plicating cirrhosis is more common in adults than children. The differentiation of regenerating nodules from hepatocellular carcinoma may be difficult if the nodules are isointense with liver, but possible, for the T2-weighted signal may be decreased with nodules but increased with tumor.

Fatty infiltration of the liver is seen in diseases other than cirrhosis. Patients with endogenous Cushing syndrome or, more commonly, on steroid therapy, may develop diffuse fatty infiltration. Metabolic disorders such as familial hyperlipoproteinemia, glycogen storage disease, Wilson disease, and Reye syndrome may also cause diffuse fatty infiltration. The findings may also be present in patients on combination anticancer chemotherapy, on hyperalimentation, and with extreme malnutrition. On US, there is increased echogenicity of the liver parenchyma. Usually this is homogeneous but occasionally may be focal. On CT, there is often dramatic decreased attenuation of the liver parenchyma which becomes more pronounced after contrast enhancement (Fig 23–23). MR is not sensitive to diffuse fatty infiltration but may show increased signal on T1-weighted spin-echo imaging in areas of focal fatty infiltration.

Diffuse increased attenuation of the liver on CT scan is caused by *iron deposition in the liver* (Fig 23–24). In children, this is most commonly secondary to hemolytic anemia or to chronic repetitive transfusions as used in the treatment of thalassemia. US is usually unrevealing but MR findings are dramatic, with marked decrease in signal intensity on

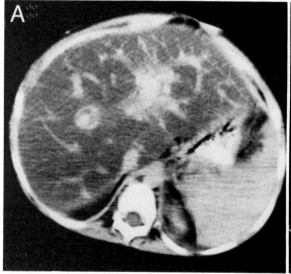

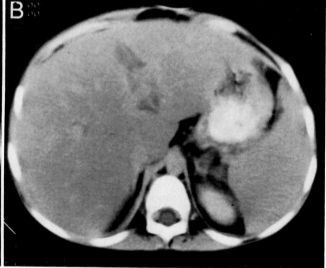

FIG 23–23.
Diffuse fatty infiltration of the liver in a 5-year-old boy 2 months after liver transplantation. **A,** enhanced CT scan shows low attenuation of both hepatic lobes and relative enhancement of hyperdense blood vessels. **B,** CT scan 8 days prior to clinical deterioration shows normal attenuation of the hepatic parenchyma.

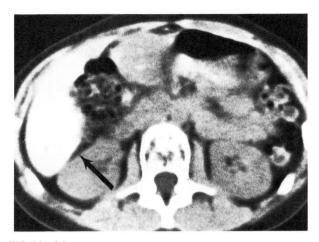

FIG 23–24.
An unenhanced CT scan of a 15-year-old girl with hemachromatosis shows the dense liver. The *arrow* overlies the right kidney.

T2-weighted images and, to a lesser degree, on T1-weighted images. As noted previously, glycogen storage disease may also cause increased attenuation on hepatic CT. Hernandez et al. found that the comparison of T1-weighted images of the liver with those of muscle was the best discriminator of iron overload. Spin-echo images were not able to quantitate iron overload satisfactorily. Although the MR signal of the liver is similar in hemachromatosis and hemosiderosis, Siegelman et al. demonstrated that patients with hemachromatosis had low signal intensity of the pancreas on T2-weighted spin-echo images, while four of five patients had normal splenic signal intensity. With iron overload, however, the spleen showed low-intensity signal in 14 of 14 patients while the pancreas had low signal in only 3 of 16. Thus, MR appears able to discriminate hemachromatosis from hemosiderosis.

REFERENCES

Baker MK, Schauwecker DS, Wenker JC, et al: Nuclear medicine evaluation of focal fatty infiltration of the liver. *Clin Nucl Med* 1986; 11:503.

Brasch RC, Wesbey GE, Gooding CA, et al: Magnetic resonance imaging of transfusional hemosiderosis complicating thalassaemia major. *Radiology* 1984; 150:767.

Daneman A, Matzinger MA, Martin DJ: Cirrhosis: An unusual pattern of enhancement on CT. *Pediatr Radiol* 1983; 13:162.

Doppman JL, Cornblath M, Dwyer AJ, et al: Computed tomography of the liver and kidneys in glycogen storage disease. *J Comput Assist Tomogr* 1982; 6:67.

Glass RBJ, Poznanski AK, Young S, et al: Gaucher disease of the liver: CT appearance. *Pediatr Radiol* 1987; 17:417.

Henschke CI, Goldman H, Teele RL: The hyperechogenic liver in children: Cause and sonographic appearance. *AJR* 1982; 138:841.

Hernandez RJ, Sarnaik SA, Lande I, et al: MR evaluation of liver iron overload. *J Comput Assist Tomogr* 1988; 12:91.

Macvicar D, Dicks-Mireaux C, Leonard JV, et al: Hepatic imaging with computed tomography of chronic tyrosinaemia type 1. *Br J Radiol* 1990; 63:605.

Murakami T, Kuroda C, Marukawa T, et al: Regenerating nodules in hepatic cirrhosis: MR findings with pathologic correlation. AJR 1990; 155:1227.

Ohtomo K, Itai Y, Ohtomo Y, et al: Regenerating nodules of liver cirrhosis: MR imaging with pathologic correlation. AJR 1990; 154:505.

Quinn SF, Gosink BB: Characteristic sonographic signs of hepatic fatty infiltration. AJR 1985; 145:753.

Siegelman ES, Mitchell DG, Rubin R, et al: Parenchymal versus reticuloendothelial iron overload in the liver: Distinction with MR imaging. *Radiology* 1991; 179:361.

Stark DD, Moseley ME, Bacon BR, et al: Magnetic resonance imaging and spectroscopy of hepatic iron overload. *Radiology* 1985; 154:137.

Weinreb JC, Cohen JM, Armstrong E, et al: Imaging the pediatric liver: MRI and CT. *AJR* 1986; 147:785.

SECTION 5

Abnormalities of Hepatic Vasculature

The normal arterial blood supply to the liver is variable. In 57% of patients, there is a single common hepatic artery which arises from the celiac axis in 90% of cases, from the superior mesenteric artery in 5%, and from other visceral branches of the aorta in 5%. In the 43% of patients with multiple origins of the hepatic arterial tree, the right hepatic artery arises from the superior mesenteric artery in half and the left hepatic artery, or more commonly the left lateral segmental artery, from the left gastric artery in most of the others. After giving rise to the gastroduodenal artery, the common hepatic artery becomes the proper hepatic artery, which divides into right and left trunks whose branches follow a segmental distribution.

The portal vein originates from the juncture of the superior mesenteric vein with the splenic vein. In the porta hepatis, the vein divides into right and left branches. Each branch further subdivides, following the same segmental distribution as the hepatic arteries and biliary ducts. The hepatic veins, however, are interlobar and intersegmental, running in the fissures which divide the lobes, the segments, and the subsegments. The venous branches join to form the three major hepatic veins. The middle and left hepatic veins most frequently form a common trunk just before entering the suprahepatic portion of the IVC. The right hepatic vein enters the suprahepatic IVC separately. The caudate lobe vein typically enters the intrahepatic portion of the IVC, as may small branches of the posterior segment of the right lobe.

Spontaneous portosystemic shunts have been described at various levels. Jabra and Taylor described an intrahepatic shunt in an infant diagnosed with color Doppler sonography. In the case of Mori et al., an enormous shunt between the portal and hepatic veins was associated with multiple coronary artery fistulas. Bellah et al. described a shunt from the portal vein to the suprahepatic vena cava while a patient reported by Rubin et al. had a shunt from the portal vein to the infrahepatic vena cava (Fig 23–25).

Congenital absence of the portal vein is rare.

Morse et al. described a patient with Goldenhar syndrome and absent portal vein. The patient subsequently developed hepatoblastoma. Preduodenal portal vein occurs when the inferior connection between the paired embryonic vitelline veins persists instead of undergoing normal atrophy. The anomaly is associated with biliary atresia and numerous small intestinal abnormalities, as described in Chapter 27. The preduodenal vein has been demonstrated by US, venography, and CT.

PORTAL HYPERTENSION

Portal hypertension can develop secondary to extrahepatic or intrahepatic causes. *Extrahepatic portal vein obstruction* is more common in children. The most frequent cause is idiopathic cavernous transformation of the portal vein, in which the occluded, usually atretic, portal vein is surrounded by serpiginous collateral vessels. Idiopathic cavernous transformation is probably secondary to portal vein thrombosis occurring years before clinical presentation. Neonatal omphalitis and umbilical vein catheterization have been suggested as causes of neonatal thrombosis but, most commonly, the cause is obscure. Other causes of extrahepatic portal hypertension include acute and subacute portal vein thrombosis in which the obstructed portal vein may still be seen even though cavernous transformation occurs, intrinsic portal vein webs, ascending mesenteric phlebitis, postoperative complications, and masses in the porta hepatis. The disease is usually silent until splenomegaly is noted or upper GI bleeding occurs. Liver function tests are typically normal.

Plain film findings are usually sparse except for splenomegaly. Paravertebral widening may be seen with large paraesophageal varices (see Fig 25–47) and the azygos vein may be dilated. Sonography shows splenomegaly and, occasionally, ascites, although the latter is more common with intrahepatic causes of portal hypertension, especially cirrhosis. The liver itself appears normal. The portal vein usually cannot be identified, but the serpiginous, tortuous collaterals are easily seen in the porta hepatis.

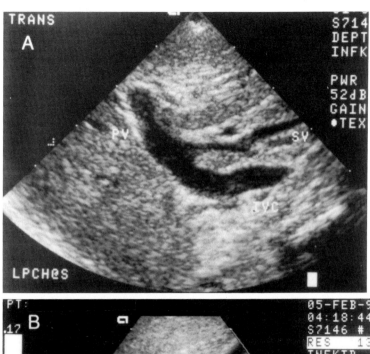

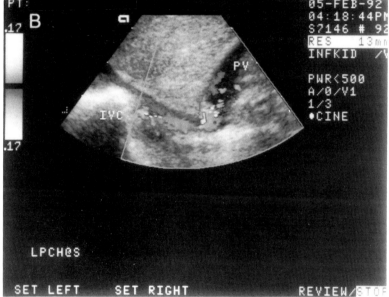

FIG 23–25.
A, transverse sonogram of the right mid-abdomen demonstrates the splenic vein draining into the portal vein which then drains directly into the subhepatic inferior vena cava (IVC). **B,** color Doppler examination of the portal vein and IVC demonstrates the venous flow directly from the portal vein into the IVC. No intrahepatic portal venous flow was demonstrated. (See also Plate 2 facing p. 951.)

Similar serpiginous vessels can be identified in the splenic hilum (Fig 23–26). Portosystemic collateral vessels can be identified with the coronary vein being the most frequently seen. Collaterals are frequently identified in the gastrohepatic ligament (see Fig 25–47) and can be seen adjacent to the esophagogastric junction. Other portosystemic pathways are more commonly seen with intrahepatic causes of portal vein obstruction, as noted below.

Brunelle et al. described thickening of the lesser omentum as a sign of portal venous hypertension in children. Patriquin et al. determined that the normal ratio of the thickness of the lesser omentum to the aortic diameter at the level of the crus of the diaphragm is less than 1.7. Ratios greater than 1.7 were seen in patients with portal hypertension, obesity, steroid therapy, and lymphadenopathy. Doppler US is useful to determine the character and direction of flow in collateral vessels. Hepatofugal flow and loss of normal respiratory pulsations on Doppler study are signs of portal hypertension.

On dynamic CT, the tortuous veins in the porta hepatis are easily seen and portosystemic collaterals are often identified. If a more acute thrombus is the

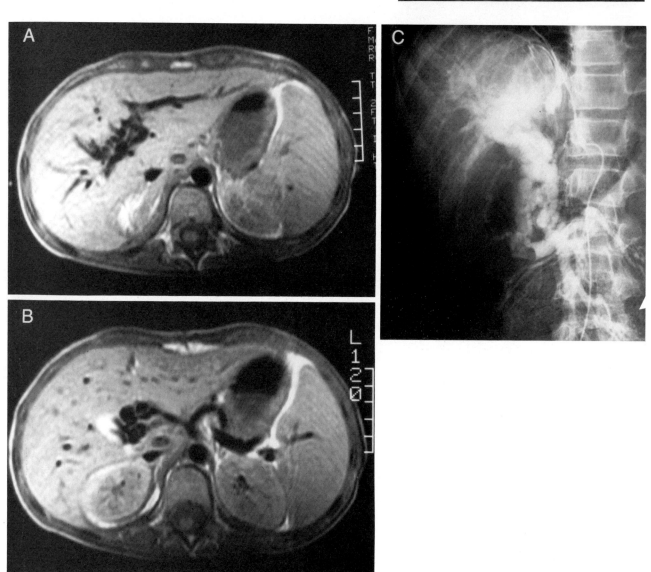

FIG 23-26.
Transverse sonogram through the spleen demonstrates dilated varices in the splenic hilum with minimal dilatation of intrasplenic vascular structures and heterogeneous echogenicity of the splenic parenchyma.

FIG 23-27.
Cavernous transformation of the portal vein with portal hypertension. **A** and **B,** axial MR scans through the porta hepatis demonstrate the portal cavernoma to excellent advantage. Note also the enlarged spleen and enlarged splenic vein. **C,** arterial portogram demonstrates the characteristic dilated tortuous vessels of a portal cavernoma.

cause of the portal hypertension, unenhanced scans may show the clot within the portal vein as a high-attenuation area. With contrast enhancement, the clot appears as a filling defect in the vein. Most MR studies of portal hypertension have been in adult patients with cirrhosis. With cavernous transformation, the tangled vessels in the porta can be identified (Fig 23–27), but the signal characteristics will vary with the presence, absence, and velocity of blood flow. Acute and subacute thrombosis of the portal vein can be identified but may be simulated by stagnant flow. Johnson et al. compared results of time-of-flight MR angiography (MRA) with arterial portography and endoscopy (see Fig 25–47,*D*). They concluded that MRA is a satisfactory technique for the identification of varices.

Arterial portography is less commonly utilized for diagnostic purposes than in the past, although usually obtained prior to portosystemic shunt surgery. Because of the variable origin of the hepatic arteries, injection of both celiac and superior mesenteric arteries is usually necessary. In the venous phase, the existing portosystemic collaterals are well seen, particularly those arising from the left gastric artery and coursing along the esophagus (Fig 23–28). Patency of the vessels to be shunted should be demonstrated.

The most common cause of *intrahepatic portal hypertension* is cirrhosis of the liver. Hepatitis and congenital hepatic fibrosis have also been implicated, as have a number of rare lesions. Portal vein thrombosis secondary to liver metastases has been described in as many as 8% of affected adults. Approximately one third of patients with hepatocellular carcinoma of the liver may also demonstrate portal thrombosis with secondary portal hypertension. Veno-occlusive disease of the liver (see below) and thrombosis of the hepatic veins or suprahepatic portion of the inferior vena cava (Budd-Chiari syndrome) may also lead to secondary portal hypertension.

The findings generally are similar to those described for extrahepatic portal hypertension, but there will also be symptoms, signs, and abnormal laboratory studies related to the underlying hepatic disease. In these cases, the portal vein is usually seen on imaging studies and may appear enlarged. Pulsed Doppler US is particularly useful in evaluating the flow characteristics within the portal vein, as well as within collaterals. Flow may be identified in the region of the ligamentum teres. This has been demonstrated to be in paraumbilical collaterals rather than in a "recanalized umbilical vein" as originally thought.

CT, in addition to the findings with extrahepatic portal hypertension noted above, will show the characteristics of the underlying disease process as well. With cirrhosis and posthepatitic states, the enlarged portal vein may also be demonstrated on CT. Varices may be more easily identified than they are in some cases of extrahepatic portal hypertension.

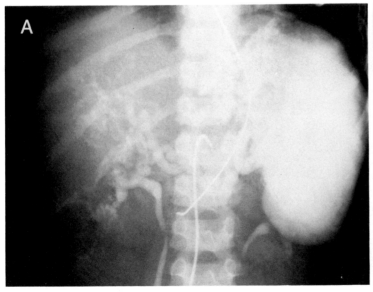
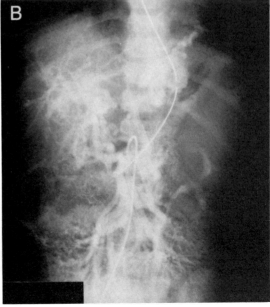

FIG 23–28.
Cavernous transformation of the portal vein. **A,** arterial portography demonstrates splenomegaly with early filling of a tortuous cavernoma. **B,** mesenteric arterial portogram demonstrates the portal cavernoma with numerous tortuous varices in the region of the esophagogastric junction.

There has been increasing interest in the use of MR in the evaluation of intrahepatic portal hypertension in adults. On MR imaging, the portal vein is usually well seen. However, slow or turbulent flow within the portal vein may cause increased signal intensity with T1-weighted images, simulating thrombosis. Second-echo proton-density images or T2-weighted spin-echo images will usually show decreased signal with turbulent flow and increased signal with a real thrombosis. MRA is better at demonstrating the flow characteristics within the portal vein and the collaterals. Torres et al. compared MR with angiography to determine the ability of the former to detect portal vein hemodynamics. Portal vein thrombosis was well demonstrated, but MR was not satisfactory in identifying the grading of blood flow in the portal vein, which can be done with angiography. Grade 1 is identified as good hepatopetal flow with visualization of peripheral vein branches. Grade 2 is fair hepatopetal flow with identification of tertiary portal vein branches. Grade 3 is poor hepatopetal flow with identification of only the main portal vein and its right and left branches. Grade 4 is hepatofugal flow. Of particular note is that Torres et al. were unable to identify grade 4 portal blood flow on MR. However, increasing use of new MRA sequences may make MR imaging more valuable preoperatively.

BUDD-CHIARI SYNDROME

Budd-Chiari syndrome is a rare disorder in children, developing after obstruction of the hepatic veins or the intrahepatic or suprahepatic portions of the IVC at a point where secondary hepatic vein obstruction occurs. In most instances, the etiology is not clear. Thrombosis can occur in a variety of hypercoagulable states, primary or secondary neoplasms, after trauma, or after liver transplantation. Obstruction secondary to congenital webs inside the hepatic veins or IVC has been reported. In children, hepatomegaly is usually the presenting characteristic of the acute form of the syndrome. In chronic Budd-Chiari syndrome, the typical findings of portal hypertension are usually present.

Sonography may demonstrate heterogeneous echogenicity of the liver. Areas of hypoechogenicity may be secondary to hemorrhagic infarction and necrosis. As these areas resolve, fibrosis and scarring may result in hyperechoic regions. The liver is generally large, with the caudate lobe being especially enlarged. Ascites may be identified. In chronic Budd-Chiari syndrome, the major hepatic veins may not be identified. More commonly, they can be seen, and color Doppler sonography is extremely useful in identifying the level of obstruction and the direction of flow in the portal venous system, hepatic veins, and IVC. With pulsed Doppler evaluation, markedly reduced or reversed flow in the hepatic veins and in the IVC may be seen. These findings, if present, are the most specific and sensitive for the imaging diagnosis of Budd-Chiari syndrome.

Hepatic scintigraphy discloses heterogeneous decreased activity throughout most of the liver with normal to increased activity in the caudate lobe which is not usually involved by the disease. Powell-Jackson et al. have shown these findings to be present in only 17% of the patients in their study.

CT is often less specific than one might expect, but typical features include hepatomegaly with an enlarged caudate lobe, thrombus in the hepatic veins, decreased caliber of the IVC, and ascites. Following contrast infusion, there is relatively greater enhancement of the caudate lobe with decreased enhancement peripherally. Intraluminal high-attenuation filling defects within the veins are virtually diagnostic of venous thrombosis. MR imaging shows findings comparable to those seen on CT scan. MRA, however, can show hepatic venous obstruction and collateral circulation, possibly as well as angiography and Doppler sonography. Although inferior vena cavography and retrograde hepatic venography have been considered the only truly sensitive imaging studies in the past, the combination of Doppler US and MRA is likely to replace them.

Lois et al. described an 8-year-old girl with Budd-Chiari syndrome secondary to membranous obstruction of the hepatic veins and a web in the IVC. The vessels were recanalized and dilated percutaneously via a transhepatic approach with prompt resolution of symptoms.

Hepatic veno-occlusive disease refers to obstruction of the hepatic venous system at the level of the central and sublobular veins. Most cases are secondary to toxicity from chemotherapy, hepatic radiation, or bone marrow transplantation, or from certain alkaloids. Less commonly, the disease may be seen in congenital immunodeficiency states and systemic lupus erythematosus. The only role of imaging techniques is to exclude Budd-Chiari syndrome by demonstrating the patency of the major hepatic veins and IVC. This can easily be accomplished by sonography. The definitive diagnosis requires biopsy and histologic examination of the liver.

REFERENCES

Alpern MB, Rubin JM, Williams DM, et al: Porta hepatis: Duplex Doppler US with angiographic correlation. *Radiology* 1987; 162:53.

Barton JW III, Keller MS: Liver transplantation for hepatoblastoma in a child with congenital absence of the portal vein. *Pediatr Radiol* 1989; 20:113.

Bellah RD, Hayek J, Teele RL: Anomalous portal venous connection to the suprahepatic vena cava: Sonographic demonstration. *Pediatr Radiol* 1989; 20:115.

Bolondi L, Gaiani S, Libassi S, et al: Diagnosis of Budd-Chiari syndrome by pulsed Doppler ultrasound. *Gastroenterology* 1991; 100:1324.

Boucher D, Brunelle F, Bernard O, et al: Ultrasonic demonstration of porto-caval anastomosis in portal hypertension in children. *Pediatr Radiol* 1985; 15:307.

Brunelle F, Alagille D, Pariente D, et al: Étude échographique de l'hypertension portal chez l'enfant. *Ann Radiol (Paris)* 1981; 24:121.

Brunelle F, Leblanc A, Chaumont P: Familial Budd-Chiari disease: angiographic study in two sisters. *Pediatr Radiol* 1981; 11:91.

Grant EG, Perrella R, Tessler FN, et al: Budd-Chiari syndrome: the The results of duplex and color Doppler imaging. *AJR* 1989; 152:377.

Hausdorf G: Sonography of caudal hepatic veins in children. Incidence, importance and relation to cranial hepatic veins. *Pediatr Radiol* 1984; 14:376.

Hosoki T, Chikazumi K, Tokunaga K, et al: Hepatic venous outflow obstruction: Evaluation with pulsed duplex sonography. *Radiology* 1989; 170:733.

Jabra AA, Taylor GA: Ultrasound diagnosis of congenital intrahepatic portosystemic venous shunt. *Pediatr Radiol* 1991; 21:529.

Johnson CD, Ehman RL, Rakela J, et al: MR angiography in portal hypertension: detection of varices and imaging techniques. *J Comput Assist Tomogr* 1991; 15:578.

Kriegshauser JS, Charboneau JW, Letendre L: Hepatic venocclusive disease after bone-marrow transplantation: Diagnosis with duplex sonography. *AJR* 1988; 150:289.

Lafortune M, Constantis A, Breton G, et al: The recanalized umbilical vein in portal hypertension: A myth. *AJR* 1985; 144:549.

Lois JF, Hartzman S, McGlade CT, et al: Budd-Chiari syndrome: Treatment with percutaneous transhepatic recanalization and dilation. *Radiology* 1989; 170:791.

Mathieu D, Vasile N, Dibie C, et al: Portal cavernoma: Dynamic CT features and transient differences in hepatic attenuation. *Radiology* 1985; 154:743.

Mathieu D, Vasile N, Gremier P: Portal thrombosis: Dynamic CT features and course. *Radiology* 1985; 154:737.

McCain AH, Bernardino ME, Sones PJ, et al: Varices from portal hypertension: Correlation of CT and angiography. *Radiology* 1985; 154:63.

McCarten KM, Teele RL: Preduodenal portal vein: Venography, ultrasonography, and review of the literature. *Ann Radiol (Paris)* 1978; 21:155.

Mori H, Hayaski K, Uetani M, et al: High-attenuation recent thrombus of the portal vein: CT demonstration and clinical significance. *Radiology* 1987; 163:353.

Mori K, Dohi T, Yamamoto H, et al: An enormous shunt between the portal and hepatic veins associated with multiple coronary artery fistulas. *Pediatr Radiol* 1990; 21:66.

Morse SS, Taylor KJW, Strauss EB, et al: Congenital absence of the portal vein in oculoauriculovertebral dysplasia (Goldenhar syndrome). *Pediatr Radiol* 1986; 16:437.

Moult PJA, Waite DW, Dick R: Posterior mediastinal venous masses in patients with portal hypertension. *Gut* 1975; 16:57.

Murphy FB, Steinberg HV, Shires GT, et al: The Budd-Chiari syndrome: A review. *AJR* 1986; 147:9.

Nelson RC, Lovett KE, Chezmar JL, et al: Comparison of pulsed Doppler sonography and angiography in patients with portal hypertension. *AJR* 1987; 149:77.

Odievre M, Chaumont P, Montagne JP, et al: Anomalies of the intrahepatic portal venous system in congenital hepatic fibrosis. *Radiology* 1977; 122:427.

Patriquin H, Lafortune M, Burns P, et al: The duplex Doppler examination of children and adults with portal hypertension: Technique and anatomy. *AJR* 1987; 149:71.

Patriquin H, Tessier G, Grignon A, et al: Lesser omental thickness in normal children: Baseline for detection of portal hypertension. *AJR* 1985; 145:693.

Powell-Jackson PR, Karani J, Erde RJ, et al: Ultrasound scanning and ^{99m}Tc sulphur colloid scintigraphy in diagnosis of Budd-Chiari syndrome. *Gut* 1986; 27:1502.

Ros PR, Viamonte M, Soila K, et al: Demonstration of cavernomatous transformation of the portal vein by magnetic resonance imaging. *Gastrointest Radiol* 1986; 11:90.

Rubin G, Parker BR, Garcia M, et al: Congenital shunt from the portal vein to the infrahepatic vena cava: clinical and imaging characteristics. Submitted for publication.

Sassoon C, Douillet P, Gronfalt AM, et al: Ultrasonographic diagnosis of portal cavernoma in children: A study of twelve cases. *Br J Radiol* 1980; 53:1047.

Stanley P: Budd-Chiari syndrome. *Radiology* 1989; 170:625.

Stark DD, Hahn PF, Trey C, et al: MRI of the Budd-Chiari syndrome. *AJR* 1986; 146:1141.

Torres WE, Gaylord GM, Whitmire L, et al: The correlation between MR and angiography in portal hypertension. *AJR* 1987; 148:1109.

Tsuda Y, Nishimura K, Kawakami S, et al: Preduodenal portal vein and anomalous continuation of inferior vena cava: CT findings. *J Comput Assist Tomogr* 1991; 15:585.

Vogelszang RL, Anschuetz SL, Gore RM: Budd-Chiari syndrome: CT observations. *Radiology* 1987; 163:329.

Wallace S: Primary liver tumors, in Parker BR, Castellino RA (eds): *Pediatric Oncologic Radiology,* St Louis, Mosby–Year Book, 1977.

Widrich WC, Srinivasan M, Semine MC, et al: Collateral pathways of the left gastric vein in portal hypertension. *AJR* 1984; 142:375.

Zirinsky K, Markisz JA, Rubenstein WA, et al: MR imaging of portal venous thrombosis: correlation with CT and sonography. *AJR* 1988; 150:283.

SECTION 6

Acquired Biliary Tract Disease

Cholelithiasis in children is uncommon. However, the diagnosis is being made with more frequency since the advent of real-time US. In addition, there are greater numbers of children being treated with therapeutic regimens that may lead to the development of gallstones. In infants, the use of total parenteral nutrition and certain diuretics have both been associated with cholelithiasis (Fig 23–29). Bilirubinate stones are most common. Chronic cholestasis probably plays a role in the pathophysiology. Infants with sepsis may also develop gallstones. Most stones in these patients resolve spontaneously. As noted previously, patients with congenital abnormalities of the biliary tree have a predisposition to the development of stones.

Although the majority of stones seen in older children are idiopathic, a number of underlying states have been associated with gallstones. Prominent among these are pancreatic abnormalities and intestinal problems which interfere with the normal enterohepatic circulation such as inflammatory bowel disease, cystic fibrosis, and the short-gut syn-

drome. Cystic fibrosis also produces cholelithiasis secondary to obstruction of the cystic duct by inspissated secretions. Patients with hemolytic anemia frequently develop bilirubinate stones. Gallstones have been reported following scoliosis surgery and cardiac surgery. Gallstones in infants and young children are usually asymptomatic. In older children, the symptoms are similar to those seen in adults with right upper quadrant colicky pain radiating to the shoulder and nausea and vomiting. However, a substantial percentage of older children with gallstones will be asymptomatic.

US is the primary imaging modality for the evaluation of cholelithiasis. Typical gallstones will be echogenic with prominent acoustic shadowing (Fig 23–30). Most stones will move with changes in patient position, and the routine examination usually includes examination in the upright or decubitus, or both positions, as well as in the supine position (Fig 23–31). Multiple gallstones may be seen, but the number of stones identified at sonography usually underestimates the number actually found at the

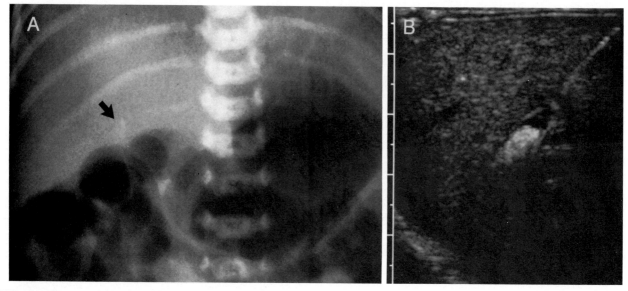

FIG 23–29.
Drug-induced cholelithiasis. **A,** coned-down view of the right upper quadrant in a 6-week-old infant treated with furosemide for chronic lung disease and congenital heart disease. **A,** calcification *(arrow)* is noted just above the hepatic flexure. **B,** longitudinal sonogram demonstrates multiple stones within the gallbladder causing prominent acoustic shadowing. The findings resolved without surgical intervention.

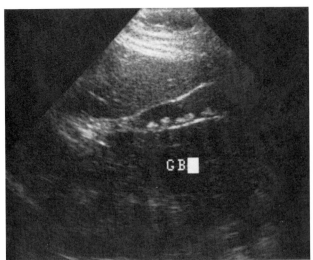

FIG 23–30.
Cholelithiasis. Longitudinal sonogram with the patient in the supine position demonstrates multiple echogenic densities in the gallbladder with acoustic shadowing in this 9-year-old patient, status post heart transplant and treatment with several cholelithogenic drugs and prolonged hyperalimentation.

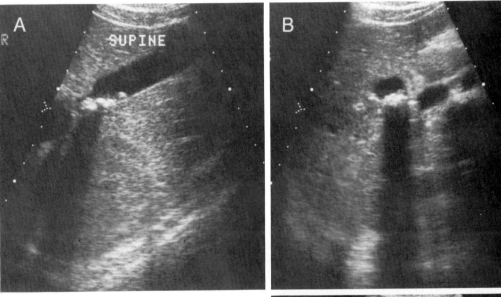

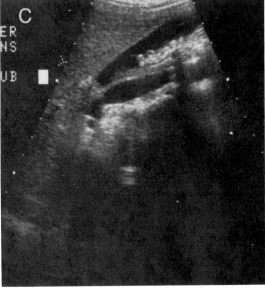

FIG 23–31.
Cholelithiasis in an 11-year-old boy with hereditary spherocytosis. **A** and **B,** longitudinal and transverse scans with the patient in the supine position demonstrate multiple echogenic foci near the neck of the gallbladder with prominent acoustic shadowing. **C,** with the patient in the decubitus position, the stones layer in the body of the gallbladder.

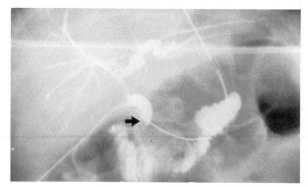

FIG 23–32.
Choledocholithiasis in a 6-month-old boy who had prolonged hyperalimentation and developed obstructive jaundice. Operative cholangiogram demonstrates a stone *(arrow)* in the distal common bile duct with dilatation of the proximal portion of the CBD.

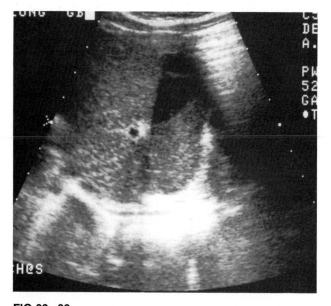

FIG 23–33.
Biliary sludge. Longitudinal sonogram through the gallbladder demonstrates nonshadowing echogenic material in the gallbladder with a concave meniscus typical of noncalculous biliary sludge.

time of surgical exploration. Collections of very small stones may not demonstrate acoustic shadowing and may mimic the appearance of biliary sludge in the gallbladder. The lack of acoustic shadowing in these cases makes differentiation difficult. However, the sludge is more likely to have a smooth outline, while multiple stones may have an irregular or roughened outline. Occasionally, if the bile within the gallbladder is of high density, the stones may seem to float on the surface, giving an apparent fluid level. Tumefactive sludge (see below) may mimic gallstones but the lack of acoustic shadowing usually leads to the correct diagnosis.

Stones are more likely to be symptomatic when

they pass into the cystic duct or the common bile duct (Fig 23–32). Sonography is less successful at demonstrating choledocholithiasis than it is in detecting cholelithiasis. Dilated extrahepatic bile ducts may be the only sign of an obstructing stone. In such cases, hepatobiliary scintigraphy is useful with delayed excretion of radiopharmaceutical into the GI tract. CT is occasionally used for direct imaging pur-

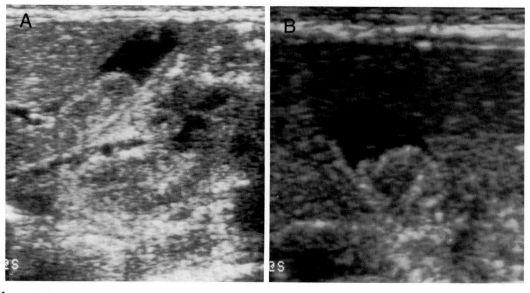

FIG 23–34.
Tumefactive sludge. Longitudinal **(A)** and transverse **(B)** sonograms demonstrate echogenic material within the gallbladder which has a convex margin and moves as a unit but has no shad-

owing. This is the typical appearance of a "sludge ball" or tumefactive sludge.

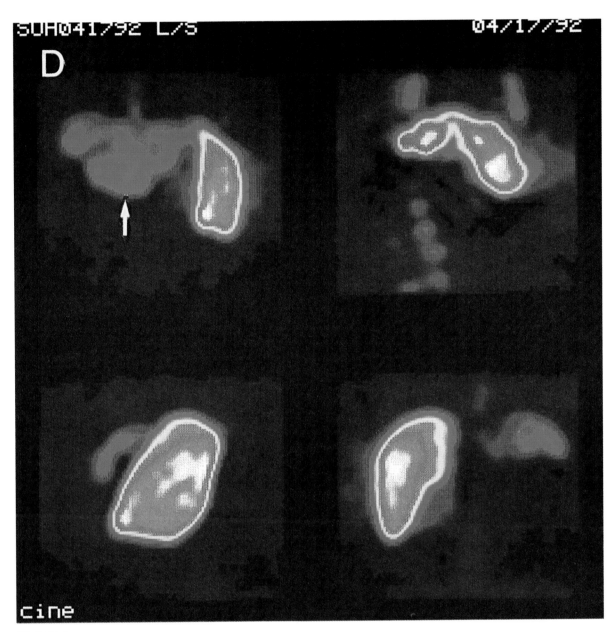

SOH041/92 L/S   04/17/92

D

cine

PLATE 1

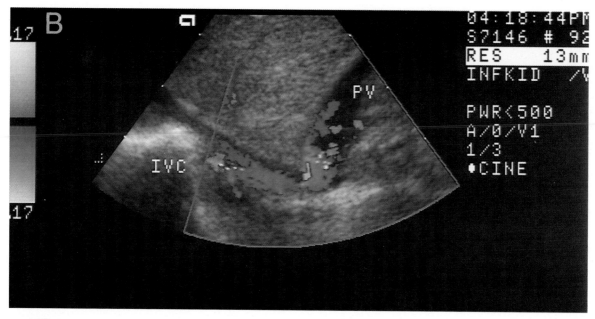

PLATE 2

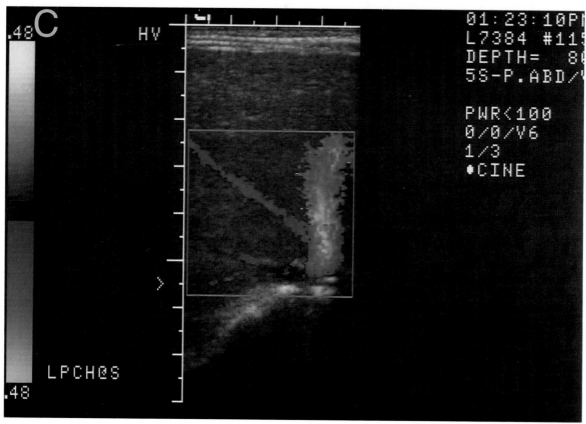

PLATE 3

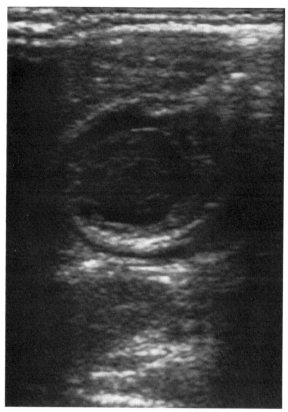

FIG 23-35.
Chronic cholecystitis. Transverse sonogram through the gallbladder demonstrates a markedly thickened, edematous gallbladder wall with echogenic material in the lumen. The patient had a history of chronic recurrent abdominal pain.

poses, but biliary stones are more commonly identified on CT as incidental findings. If a biliary tract stone is suspected but not seen on US, direct visualization by means of either percutaneous transhepatic cholangiography or by ERCP is generally accomplished. Stones are readily identified as nonopaque filling defects on these studies. Pariente et al. treated choledocholithiasis and the bile plug syndrome in ten infants by percutaneous placement of an angiographic catheter and subsequent removal of the obstructing material. Generally, however, nonoperative interventional treatment of cholelithiasis is rarely performed in children.

Biliary sludge is particulate matter within the bile, developing secondary to cholestasis. The sludge is formed predominantly of calcium bilirubinate particles and, depending on the underlying process, cholesterol crystals. On sonography, the sludge typically layers in the dependent portion and a fluid-fluid level may be seen (Fig 23–33). Occasionally, the sludge coalesces sufficiently to have the echographic appearance of a stone, so-called tumefactive sludge or sludge ball. Tumefactive sludge moves like a stone with changes in patient position, but does not demonstrate acoustic shadowing (Fig. 23–34). Biliary sludge does not cause symptoms and does not need treatment; it usually resolves with therapy of the underlying condition.

Only a small percentage of children with cholelithiasis will develop *cholecystitis*. Acalculous cholecystitis is infrequent in children. The sonographic findings of calculous cholecystitis and acalculous cholecystitis are similar except for the finding

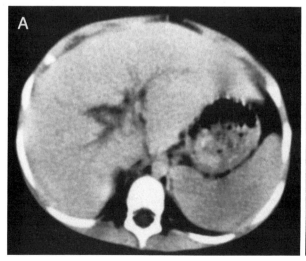

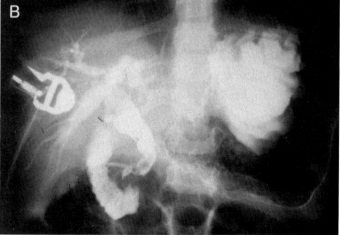

FIG 23-36.
This 4-year-old girl presented with symptoms of ascending cholangitis including fever, right upper quadrant pain, and jaundice. CT scan **(A)** demonstrated dilatation of the biliary ducts and common bile duct. Following successful treatment with antibiotics, surgical exploration demonstrated an obstructing intraductal cystic duplication of the common bile duct seen on cholangiogram **(B).**

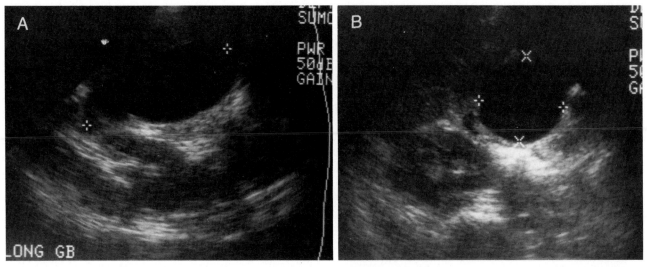

FIG 23–37.
Hydrops of the gallbladder. Longitudinal **(A)** and transverse **(B)** sonograms demonstrate a markedly enlarged gallbladder in a 3-year-old girl with Kawasaki disease. The hydrops resolved spontaneously as the patient's condition improved.

of gallstones in the former. Thickening of the gallbladder wall, distention of the gallbladder, pericholecystic fluid, biliary sludge, and edema of the gallbladder wall have all been described (Fig 23–35). These findings are nonspecific and, except for the presence of gallstones, may be seen in a variety of other entities, especially hepatitis. Other causes of thickening of the gallbladder wall include ascites, portal hypertension, hypoproteinemia, and congestive heart failure. Coughlin and Mann suggest that hepatobiliary imaging is underutilized in children with cholecystitis and report two cases in which they made the diagnosis with a ^{99m}Tc-labeled IDA derivative.

Ascending cholangitis is associated with biliary obstruction whether congenital or acquired (Fig 23–36). Although the patient may present with symptoms related to the cholangitis, appropriate therapy has to be directed to the underlying cause.

Sclerosing cholangitis is obliterative inflammatory fibrosis affecting the intrahepatic and extrahepatic biliary ducts. Sisto et al. reviewed 83 cases in childhood. Patients with inflammatory bowel disease, especially ulcerative colitis, accounted for 57% of the cases. Twenty-five percent were idiopathic, 15% in patients with Langerhans cell histiocytosis, and 10% in patients with disorders of the immune system. On sonography, nonspecific dilatation of the biliary system may be seen in association with thickening of the gallbladder wall. Stones may be identified in the gallbladder. CT findings are also nonspecific with focal dilatation of the biliary tree. With contrast enhancement, there may be increased attenuation of the ductal wall secondary to inflammatory changes. The definitive imaging study is cholangiography, either via the percutaneous transhepatic route or ERCP. The biliary tree is markedly irregular with areas of stricture and focal dilatation proximal to the strictures. Although occasionally segmental, the entire biliary tract is usually involved. Majoie et al. have developed a cholangiographic classification for primary sclerosing cholangitis which has yet to be tested for prognostic value.

Hydrops of the gallbladder is thought to be secondary to transient obstruction related to cholestasis. Hydrops is seen in the mucocutaneous lymph node syndrome (Kawasaki disease) (Fig 23–37) and has been associated with a multiplicity of infectious diseases including scarlet fever, leptospirosis, ascariasis, typhoid, and familial Mediterranean fever. Generalized sepsis and total parenteral nutrition have also been identified as sources of hydrops. Sonograms are striking with marked dilatation of the gallbladder. The wall thickness is usually normal. Sludge is seen in some cases. The biliary tree is otherwise normal, and the hydrops generally responds to conservative therapy. Sty et al. reported a case of gallbladder perforation in Kawasaki disease.

REFERENCES

Bradford BF, Reid BS, Weinstein BJ, et al: Ultrasonographic evaluation of the gallbladder in mucocutaneous lymph node syndrome. *Radiology* 1982; 142:381.

Brunelle F: Choledocholithiasis in children. *Semin Ultrasound CT MR* 1987; 8:118.

Callahan J, Haller JO, Cacciarelli AA, et al: Cholelithiasis in infants: Association with total parenteral nutrition and furosemide. *Radiology* 1982; 143:437.

Chinn DH, Miller EI, Piper N: Hemorrhagic cholecystitis. Sonographic and clinical presentation. *J Ultrasound Med* 1987; 6:313.

Classen M, Gotze H, Richter JH, et al: Primary sclerosing cholangitis in children. *J Pediatr Gastroenterol Nutr* 1987; 6:197.

Cohen EK, Stringer DA, Smith CR, et al: Hydrops of the gallbladder in typhoid fever as demonstrated by sonography. *J Clin Ultrasound* 1986; 14:633.

Colletti PM, Ralls PW, Siegel ME, et al: Acute cholecystitis: diagnosis with radionuclide angiography. *Radiology* 1987; 163:615.

Coughlin JR, Mann DA: Detection of acute cholecystitis in children. *J Can Assoc Radiol* 1990; 41:213.

Descos B, Bernard O, Brunelle F, et al: Pigment gallstones of the common bile duct in infancy. *Hepatology* 1984; 4:678.

El-Shafie M, Mah CL: Transient gallbladder distention in sick premature infants: the value of ultrasonography and radionuclide scintigraphy. *Pediatr Radiol* 1986; 16:468.

Fakhry J: Sonography of tumefactive biliary sludge. *AJR* 1982; 139:717.

Garel L, Lallemand D, Montagne J-P, et al: The changing aspects of cholelithiasis in children through a sonographic study. *Pediatr Radiol* 1981; 11:75.

Henschke CI, Teele RL: Cholelithiasis in children: Recent observations. *J Ultrasound Med* 1983; 2:481

Keller MS, Markle BM, Laffey PA, et al: Spontaneous resolution of cholelithiasis in infants. *Radiology* 1985; 157:345.

Kirks DR: Lithiasis due to interruption of the enterohepatic circulation of bile salts. *AJR* 1979; 133:383.

L'Heureux PR, Isenberg JN, Sharp HL, et al: Gallbladder disease in cystic fibrosis. *AJR* 1977; 128:953.

Lim JH, Ko YT, Kim SY. Ultrasound changes of the gallbladder wall in the cholecystitis: A sonographic-pathological correlation. *Clin Radiol* 1987; 38:389.

Little JM, Avramovic J: Gallstone formation after major abdominal surgery. *Lancet* 1991; 3375:1135.

Majoie CBLM, Reeders JWAJ, Sanders JB, et al: Primary sclerosing cholangitis: A modified classification of cholangiographic findings. *AJR* 1991; 157:495.

Matos C, Avni EF, van Gansbeke, et al: Total parenteral nutrition (TPN) and gallbladder diseases in neonates: Sonographic assessment. *J Ultrasound Med* 1987; 6:243.

Mirvis SE, Vainright JR, Nelson AW, et al: The diagnosis of acute acalculous cholecystitis: A comparison of sonography, scintigraphy, and CT. *AJR* 1986; 147:1171.

Neu J, Arvin A, Ariagno RL: Hydrops of the gallbladder. *Am J Dis Child* 1980; 134:891.

Palasciano G, Portincasa P, Vinciguerra V, et al: Gallstone prevalence and gallbladder volume in children and adolescents: An epidemiological ultrasonographic survey and relationship to body mass index. *Am J Gastroenterol* 1989; 84:1378.

Pariente D, Bernard O, Gauthier F, et al: Radiological treatment of common bile duct lithiasis in infancy. *Pediatr Radiol* 1989; 19:104.

Patriquin H, DePietro M, Barber FE, Teele RL: Sonography of thickened gallbladder wall: Causes in children. *AJR* 1983; 141:57.

Reif S, Sloven DG, Lebenthal E: Gallstones in children. Characterization by age, etiology, and outcome. *Am J Dis Child* 1991; 145:105.

Roca M, Sellier N, Mensire A, et al: Acute acalculous cholecystitis in *Salmonella* infection. Pediatr Radiol 1988; 18:421.

Samuels BI, Freitas JE, Bree RL, et al: A comparison of radionuclide hepatobiliary imaging and real time ultrasound for the detection of acute cholecystitis. *Radiology* 1983; 147:207.

Sisto A, Feldman P, Garel L, et al: Primary sclerosing cholangitis in children: study of five cases and review of the literature. *Pediatrics* 1987; 80:918.

Sty JR, Starshak RJ, Gorenstein L: Gallbladder perforation in a case of Kawasaki disease: Image correlation. *J Clin Ultrasound* 1987; 11:381.

Teele RL, Nussbaum AR, Wyly JB, et al: Cholelithiasis after spinal fusion for scoliosis in children. *J Pediatr* 1987; 111:857.

Williams HJ, Johnson KW: Cholelithiasis: A complication of cardiac valve surgery in children. *Pediatr Radiol* 1984; 14:146.

SECTION 7

Tumors and Tumorlike Conditions

Neoplasms of the liver are relatively rare in children. They account for about 2% of all childhood tumors. The malignant hepatic tumors are the tenth most common in childhood, but the third most common abdominal malignancy after Wilms tumor and neuroblastoma. Malignancies account for 64% of primary hepatobiliary tumors. Most clinically significant hepatic neoplasms present as asymptomatic palpable masses found by the parents or at routine physical examination. Differentiating benign from malignant hepatic masses on imaging studies has been actively studied. Boechat et al. showed both CT and MR to be excellent in differentiating benign from malignant tumors but less successful in discriminating between hepatocellular carcinoma, hepatoblastoma, and lymphoma. Rummeny et al., using T2-weighted spin-echo and phase-contrast MR sequences, correctly identified 87% of benign lesions.

BENIGN HEPATIC NEOPLASMS

Benign lesions account for 43% of primary liver neoplasms in children. Hemangiomas and hemangioendotheliomas, the mesenchymal vascular tumors, account for 50% of the benign tumors; mesenchymal hamartomas account for 22%, adenomas for 6%, focal nodular hyperplasia for 5%, and miscellaneous benign lesions, many of which are cystic in nature, account for 17%.

Cavernous hemangiomas are the most common of the benign hepatic tumors in adults. Because of occasional difficulties in distinguishing cavernous hemangiomas from other mesenchymal lesions, the overall incidence in children is not definitely known, but it may be significantly less than in adults. They are typically small and identified in children or adults incidentally on cross-sectional imaging studies performed for other reasons. Occasionally they are large, presenting in infancy as palpable masses or with high output congestive heart failure secondary to arteriovenous shunting through the tumor. Rarely, spontaneous rupture with massive hemoperitoneum occurs.

Much interest in definitive diagnosis of hemangiomas has resulted from the need to differentiate

them from hepatic metastases in adults. Although the same problem may obtain in children, metastases are much less common in the pediatric age group than in adults, in whom they are the most common hepatic malignancies. Children are also less likely than adults to have cirrhosis with regenerating nodules or focal nodular hyperplasia, other lesions which can be confused with hemangiomas. On sonograms, typical small hemangiomas are well circumscribed and hyperechoic compared with surrounding liver parenchyma (Fig 23–38). Acoustic shadowing may accompany larger lesions. Bree et al. believe this is secondary to hypervascularity. Very large lesions may be hyperechoic with a hypoechoic central area, possibly representing necrosis or fibrosis.

CT evaluation of small cavernous hemangiomas shows decreased attenuation on unenhanced scans. Calcification may be seen. With dynamic scanning, the lesion shows enhancement, beginning peripherally and progressing centrally. Prolonged enhancement, up to 20 to 30 minutes, may occur. The rim of the lesion may appear nodular or corrugated with papillary-like projections extending toward the center. The rim is especially bright after contrast enhancement. On MR, cavernous hemangiomas are of

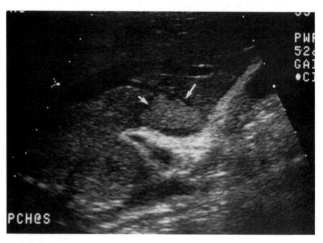

FIG 23–38.
Hepatic hemangioma. Longitudinal sonogram through the liver in a patient on hyperalimentation with abdominal pain demonstrates a focal area of increased echogenicity characteristic of benign cavernous hemangioma *(arrows)*. There is sludge in the gallbladder.

lower signal intensity than the adjacent liver on T1-weighted spin-echo images and of higher signal intensity on T2-weighted images. Contrast enhancement shows even brighter signal intensity on T2-weighted spin-echo images, especially at the periphery. The anatomical appearance is a homogeneous, rounded mass with sharply defined margins. Sulfur colloid scans are usually unrevealing or nonspecific, but SPECT scans using ^{99m}Tc-labeled red blood cells show normal to decreased flow associated with delayed blood pool activity. In a study comparing MR and red cell scans using SPECT, Birnbaum et al. found MR to have a sensitivity of 91% with an accuracy of 90%, while the nuclear medicine study had a sensitivity of 78% with 80% accuracy.

Large cavernous hemangiomas usually present in the first 6 months of life as an asymptomatic mass or with high output congestive heart failure. On sonography, there may be enlargement of the celiac axis and hepatic artery because of the increased arterial blood supply to the tumor. Similarly, the draining hepatic veins may be enlarged. The margins are usually lobulated as opposed to the smooth margins typically seen with smaller hemangiomas. Klein et al. noted that the presence of Doppler signal throughout the lesion is useful in differentiating these lesions from malignancy. On CT, the large tumors usually have a low-attenuation central area with peripheral enhancement following intravenous contrast injection. As with the small lesions, gradually increasing enhancement of the central portion may occur. Findings on isotope-labeled red blood cell scans and on MR scans are similar to those described for the smaller lesions. Angiography is less commonly performed than it was prior to the advent of cross-sectional imaging techniques. Irregular vessels arranged in an unorganized pattern with prolonged pooling of contrast material are frequently seen. The appearance is similar to that which may be found in hemangioendothelioma (see below) and even in malignancy. Embolization of the tumor can be accomplished. Fellows et al. have pointed out the importance of embolizing the frequently seen collateral vessels as well as the primary feeding vessels in order to achieve a good therapeutic effect.

Infantile hemangioendothelioma is much more likely to present as a symptomatic lesion than is cavernous hemangioma. Although there is a histologic difference between the two lesions, they may represent varying manifestations of etiologically similar entities. The most common presentation is a palpable abdominal mass, hepatomegaly, or diffuse abdominal distention. Congestive heart failure secondary to arteriovenous shunting has been reported but is less common than with giant hemangioma or arteriovenous malformations. In the series of Dachman, Lichtenstein et al. almost 20% of patients had associated hemangiomas of the skin.

The sonographic appearance of infantile hemangioendotheliomas is variable and nonspecific (Fig 23–39,B). The lesions may be either hyperechoic or hypoechoic. Dachman, Lichtenstein et al. describe one case which was cystic in appearance with no internal echoes. Most of the tumors are discrete on sonography, but a small percentage will be poorly delineated from the surrounding liver parenchyma.

On CT, hemangioendotheliomas demonstrate decreased attenuation compared with the normal liver parenchyma. The pattern may be homogeneous or heterogeneous. On unenhanced scans, as many as 40% of patients may demonstrate tumoral calcification. With intravenous contrast enhancement, there is a sharp increase in attenuation around the periphery of the mass with irregular increased enhancement throughout the lesion. With delayed scans, there is washout of the increased enhancement from the periphery of the lesion with progressive increase of enhancement in the central portion. Areas within the lesion that show no contrast enhancement may represent areas of necrosis or hemorrhage.

On spin-echo MR images, the central portion of the lesion is either isointense with the surrounding hepatic parenchyma or shows somewhat decreased signal intensity (Figs. 23–39D, and E). The rim may show minimally increased signal intensity. On T2-weighted images, the central portion of the lesion shows markedly increased signal intensity. The periphery also increases in signal intensity, but less so than the central portion. With MRA, enlarged feeding vessels may be identified.

Radionuclide studies are nonspecific but the blood pool studies may show increased activity corresponding with the large, high-flow feeding vessels. Angiography is less commonly used since the advent of enhanced CT scans and MRI, but demonstrates large major feeding vessels with decreased caliber of the aorta distal to their origin. Characteristically, there is prolonged pooling of contrast material within the mass (Fig 23–39,F). Internal arteriovenous shunting with large draining veins may be seen (Fig 23–39,C).

Mesenchymal hamartomas account for 22% of the benign liver tumors of childhood. They generally present in patients less than 2 years of age. As with most of the other tumors, an asymptomatic abdominal mass is usually the presenting complaint.

On US, mesenchymal hamartomas most typi-

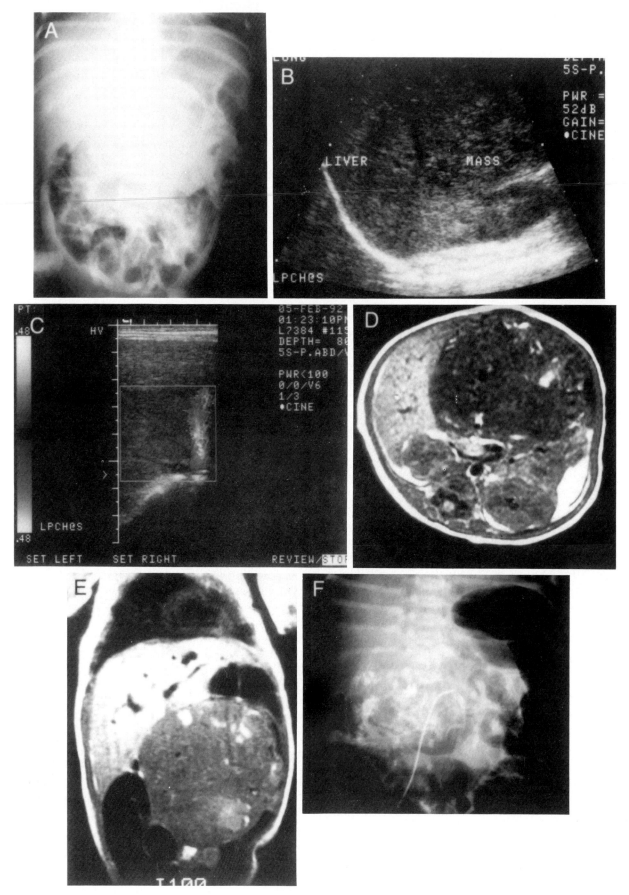

FIG 23–39.
Hemangioendothelioma. **A,** KUB in a 6-week-old boy demonstrates a large intraperitoneal mass displacing the gas-filled intestine. **B,** longitudinal sonogram demonstrates a mass in the left lobe of the liver which is of mildly heterogeneous echogenicity. **C,** Doppler examination of the hepatic veins demonstrates marked increased blood flow in the left hepatic vein compared with the middle and right hepatic veins. (See also Plate 3 facing p. 951.) **D** and **E,** axial and coronal MR scans using modified T1-weighted spin-echo technique demonstrate a large mass projecting from the left lobe of the liver. Multiple high signal areas within the mass are suggestive of pooled blood. **F,** late phase of an arteriogram demonstrates pooling of blood in dilated vascular spaces typical of infantile hemangioendothelioma.

cally demonstrate a multiseptated cystic mass (Fig 23–40,*A*). The cyst may be quite variable in size. Quite frequently, a single dominant cyst is seen. Occasionally, some echogenic material is seen within the cyst fluid secondary to blood. Less commonly, the hamartomas may appear solid on US with vascular findings like those of the other mesenchymally derived masses, hemangioma and hemangioendothelioma.

CT typically shows a multilocular cystic mass with septations of varying thickness. The noncystic components of the mass demonstrate enhancement with intravenous contrast material (Figs 23–40*B* and *C*). Roberts et al. described a 10-month-old infant with a mesenchymal hamartoma with characteristic sonographic and CT findings. MR showed a multiseptated mass with fluid-filled compartments and some displacement of intra-abdominal vessels.

Benign tumors of epithelial origin are less common in children than those of mesenchymal origin. *Focal nodular hyperplasia* (FNH) is unusual in children compared with adults. Occasionally, FNH may be found in patients with type I glycogen storage disease and has been reported following the Kasai procedure for biliary atresia. The lesion consists of hyperplastic hepatocytes with small bile ducts and lymphocytic infiltration. In most patients, the disease is asymptomatic and they usually present with hepatomegaly.

Sonographic evaluation demonstrates one or more masses which can be hypoechoic, hyperechoic, or isoechoic with the surrounding liver parenchyma. In about one third of cases, a small central scar may be seen. This corresponds with the histologically identifiable central collection of connective tissue, bile ducts, and blood vessels. Hepatic imaging with ^{99m}Tc-labeled sulfur colloid is extremely valuable in that one half to three fourths of all cases will show uptake of the radionuclide by Kupffer cells within the nodules.

On CT, the lesions are discrete and demonstrate homogeneous intense enhancement following the injection of iodinated contrast material. The central scar will be seen in up to 60% of lesions. With dynamic CT, the central scars may become especially enhanced, a characteristic of FNH. On MR, FNH may have a typical appearance. The lesions are homogeneous and isointense with the adjacent liver on all spin-echo sequences. The central scar, however, is usually hypointense on T1-weighted images and

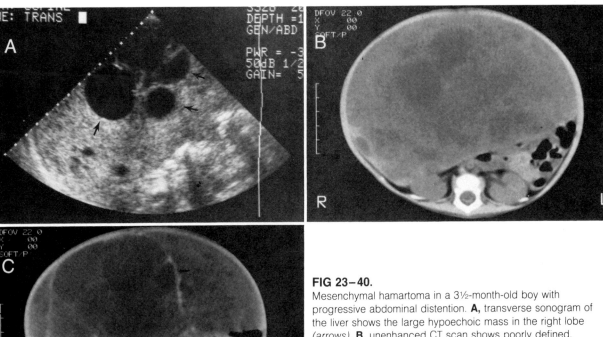

FIG 23–40.
Mesenchymal hamartoma in a 3½-month-old boy with progressive abdominal distention. **A,** transverse sonogram of the liver shows the large hypoechoic mass in the right lobe *(arrows).* **B,** unenhanced CT scan shows poorly defined, low-attenuation lesions. **C,** CT scan after contrast administration shows large hypovascular mass with enhancing septations.

hyperintense on T2-weighted images. The lesions of FNH appear poorly marginated on MR scans.

Hepatic adenomas are also more common in adults than in children but may be found in patients with type I and, less commonly, type VI glycogen storage disease. Like FNH, the US appearance may be hypoechoic, isoechoic, or hyperechoic. The hyperechoic lesions may appear to have a rim of lower echoge-

nicity, but the hypoechoic lesions have no well-defined wall. The adenomas do not take up labeled sulfur colloid and appear as photopenic defects on radioisotope liver scans.

CT demonstrates discrete lesions with homogeneous transient enhancement on dynamic studies (Figs 23–41,*A* and *B*). Some lesions will show lack of enhancement secondary to intratumoral hemor-

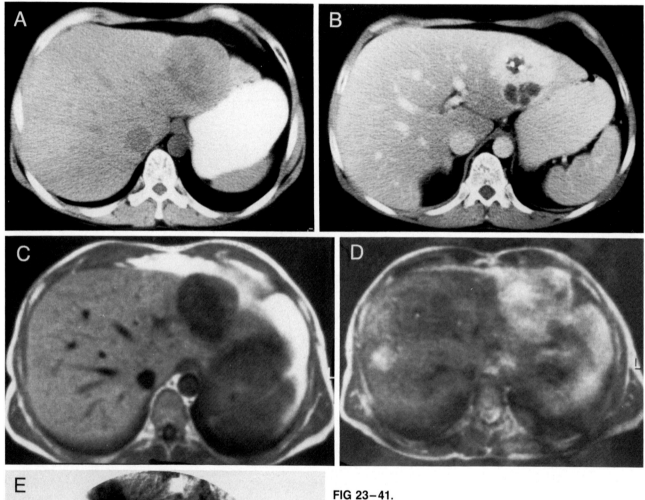

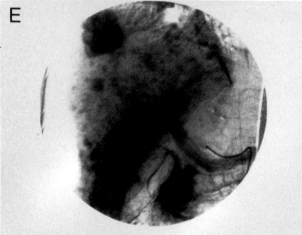

FIG 23–41.
Multiple hepatic adenomas in a patient with glycogen storage disease type I. **A,** unenhanced CT scan demonstrates a low-attenuation mass in the left lobe of the liver. The overall liver attenuation is higher than normal, compatible with glycogen storage disease type I. **B,** enhanced scan demonstrates increased attenuation of the lesion with low-attenuation areas within it suggesting hemorrhage or necrosis. **C,** axial T1-weighted spin-echo MR scan demonstrates low signal intensity within the large adenoma in the left lobe. **D,** axial T2-weighted scan demonstrates another lesion in the right lobe which was not appreciated on the prior imaging studies. **E,** digital subtraction angiography reveals multiple, highly vascular adenomas throughout the liver. (**Courtesy of Roger Jackman, M.D., Palo Alto, Calif.**)

rhage. On delayed scans, the lesions show only minimal increased attenuation compared with the surrounding liver parenchyma. On MR scans, the adenomas are usually hypointense or isointense with the surrounding liver on T1-weighted spin-echo images and may have a hypointense rim (Fig 23–41,*C*). On T2-weighted spin-echo images, the adenomas are usually of increased signal intensity compared with the liver parenchyma (Fig 23–41,*D*). The margins of the lesions are not well defined on MR, mimicking hepatocellular carcinoma. Even less commonly, the lesions may be isointense with surrounding liver simulating the MR appearance of FNH. The adenomas have a prolonged bright tumor stain on angiography (Fig 23–41,*E*).

Nodular regenerative hyperplasia of the liver is an underdiagnosed abnormality usually confused with FNH, regenerating nodules in cirrhosis, adenomas, or metastases. In the series reported by Dachman, Ros et al. 2 of 21 patients were children. The nodules are composed of cells resembling hepatocytes and are not associated with focal fibrosis. The nodules may bleed or cause portal hypertension from pressure on portal radicles. On sonography, the nodules are isoechoic but may have a hypoechoic center if hemorrhage has occurred. Sulfur colloid scintigraphy shows patchy uptake or areas of photopenia. On CT, the lesions are of lower attenuation than normal liver and do not enhance appreciably with intravenous contrast infusion. Arteriography may show vascular masses, but in most cases hepatic flow is poor because of associated portal hypertension.

Peliosis hepatis is a rare entity characterized by multiple small blood-filled spaces in the hepatic parenchyma. It has been associated with a variety of underlying diseases. In children, it has been most commonly found in association with the intake of androgens. More recent reports have associated it with type I glycogen storage disease, human immunodeficiency virus (HIV) infection, and oral contraceptives. Sonography shows decreased echogenicity. CT demonstrates low attenuation with contrast enhancement equal to or greater than normal liver.

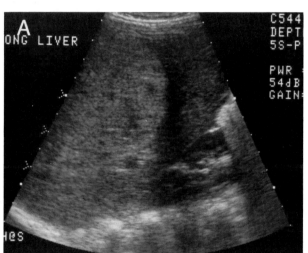

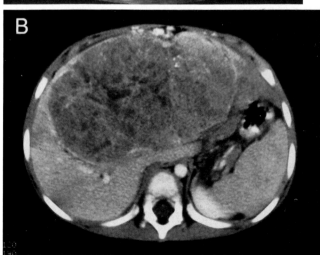

FIG 23–42.
Hepatoblastoma. **A,** longitudinal scan through the right lobe of the liver demonstrates a large heterogeneous echogenic mass abutting the relatively lower echogenic normal portion of the liver and the upper pole of the right kidney. **B,** contrast-enhanced CT scan through the mass demonstrates marked heterogeneity of attenuation with several areas of calcification identified. **C,** 1 month following initiation of chemotherapy, the mass is markedly shrunken with increasing areas of calcification. Following another month of chemotherapy, the mass was successfully removed surgically. **D,** in another patient, T1-weighted spin echo MR1 demonstrates a uniform low-intensity mass in the right lobe of the liver. **E,** T2-weighted image demonstrates the lobular nature of the mass, which has heterogeneously increased signal intensity.

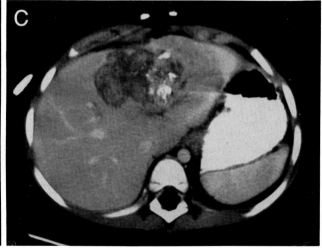

Angiography demonstrates delayed pooling of contrast without evidence of tumor vessels.

PRIMARY MALIGNANT HEPATOBILIARY TUMORS

The most common primary malignant tumor of the liver in children is hepatoblastoma, which accounts for 54% of cases. Hepatocellular carcinoma accounts for 35%, and carcinomas arising either from the liver or from the biliary tree account for 11%.

Hepatoblastoma usually presents as an asymptomatic abdominal mass in a child under 2 years of age. Patients with advanced tumors may present with anorexia, weight loss, vomiting, or abdominal pain. In rare cases of tumor rupture, the patient may present with an acute abdomen. There is a well-known relationship between hepatoblastoma and the Beckwith-Wiedemann syndrome and with hemihypertrophy. Hepatoblastoma has also been reported in patients born of mothers taking oral contraceptives and gonadotropins and in patients with the fetal alcohol syndrome. The tumor is most commonly found in the right hepatic lobe. Serum alpha-fetoprotein is usually elevated.

On plain films, hepatomegaly is identified and calcification is frequently seen. The most common sites of metastatic disease are the lungs, the local lymph nodes, and the brain. On sonography, the tumor demonstrates minimal increased echogenicity which is usually inhomogeneous (Fig 23–42,*A*). Occasionally, hypoechoic or even anechoic areas can be seen with necrosis or hemorrhage. At times, the calcifications are large enough to cause shadowing on US examination. Tumor infiltration and compression of the hepatic vessels can occur. Taylor et al. have demonstrated high-velocity flow with a frequency shift over 5-kHz using duplex Doppler sonography. The angiographic phase of hepatic scintigraphy demonstrates initial elevated activity in the tumor. Oshiro et al. reported homogeneous liver activity on hepatobiliary scan. On delayed scans, the area is typically photopenic, although Diament et al. have described a case of increased uptake of radiopharmaceutical, simulating the findings of focal nodular hyperplasia. On CT examination, the unenhanced scan demonstrates the tumor to have decreased attenuation with respect to the surrounding liver parenchyma. Rarely, the tumor is isodense and may not be well seen. Calcifications will be identified by CT in half of the patients (Fig 23–43). With intravenous contrast infusion, the normal liver parenchyma shows enhancement to a greater degree than the tu-

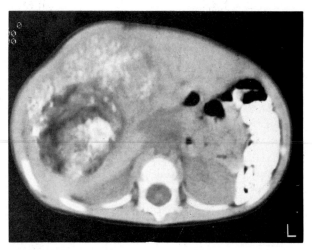

FIG 23–43.
Hepatoblastoma. Unenhanced CT scan demonstrates extensive amorphous calcification throughout the right lobe of the liver.

mor in most cases (Fig 23–42,*B* and *C*). Occasionally, tumors will show isointense enhancement with the normal liver parenchyma and sometimes will have increased enhancement.

On spin-echo MR images, the T1-weighted scans demonstrate decreased signal intensity of the tumor relative to surrounding liver parenchyma (see Fig 23–42,*D*). Occasionally, small hemorrhages are seen as increased signal intensity on the T1-weighted image. With T2-weighted images, the tumors show increased signal intensity which is usually inhomogeneous. The tumor may appear lobulated and have areas of fibrosis, both of which may show increased intensity with T2 weighting (see Fig 23–42,*E*). The hepatic vessels are generally well seen on spin-echo images but can be made even more strikingly apparent with MRA. Generally, MR gives sufficient information for preoperative evaluation. However, some surgeons still prefer to have an angiogram performed prior to surgery to demonstrate the vascular anatomy. The angiographic findings are characteristic of malignancy, but nonspecific, with tumor vessels and pooling frequently seen.

Hepatocellular carcinoma (Fig 23–44) typically occurs in children over age 4 years but may be seen in younger children. The association with cirrhosis is less common than it is in adults but may be seen in cases of hereditary tyrosinemia, biliary atresia, and chronic hepatitis. Alpha-fetoprotein will be elevated in 40% to 50% of patients with hepatocellular carcinoma.

The sonographic findings of hepatocellular carcinoma are much like those of hepatoblastoma described above. Miller and Greenspan described a "bull's-eye" echographic appearance. As with hepa-

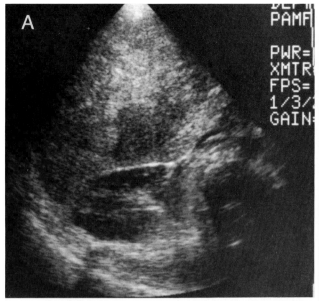

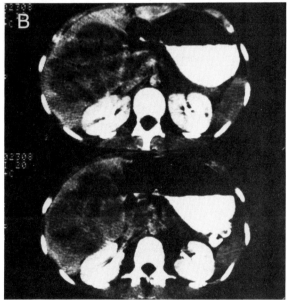

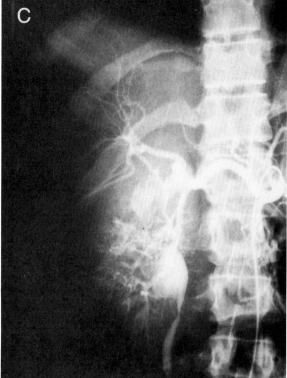

FIG 23–44.
Fibrolamellar hepatocellular carcinoma. **A,** sonogram through the inferior portion of the right lower lobe demonstrates a mass of slightly increased heterogeneous echogenicity anterior to the right kidney. **B,** contrast-enhanced CT scan demonstrates a large mass in the right lobe of the liver which has lower attenuation than the surrounding enhanced normal parenchyma. **C,** hepatic arteriogram demonstrates a minor degree of neovascularity in the inferior portion of the right lobe. At surgery, the entire right lobe was involved with tumor.

toblastoma, tumor infiltration of adjacent vessels can be readily identified. Doppler studies demonstrate increased size of the portal vein and increased velocity of blood flow.

On CT examination, the tumor may be a solitary mass, a large mass with smaller satellite lesions, or may diffusely involve the liver. On unenhanced scans, the tumor is typically of lower attenuation than the surrounding liver but may be isodense. There is usually a well-defined circumferential zone of decreased attenuation. Calcification is seen in up to 10% of cases.

Following intravenous contrast injection, enhancement can be quite intense, but heterogeneous. Vascular channels are identified on dynamic scan-

ning, and invasion of the portal vein, IVC, hepatic veins, and hepatic arteries may be seen. Intrinsic arterial-portal shunting may lead to transiently increased attenuation of the uninvolved lobes and prolonged portal vein enhancement. Although the margins are typically well defined, this is not a universal finding. If the tumor arises in a patient with underlying cirrhotic change, the differentiation from regenerating nodules may be difficult.

On spin-echo MR images, hepatocellular carcinoma is typically of lower signal intensity than normal tissue on T1-weighted images and of higher signal intensity on T2-weighted images. If a fibrous pseudocapsule is present, a low signal will be seen around the tumor. Displacement and invasion of the hepatic vessels can be seen to good advantage. Although spin-echo images are most typically obtained, Finn et al. report that short T1 inversion recovery (STIR) sequences demonstrate the tumor to better advantage and are more apt to show associated lymph node metastases.

A histologic variation of hepatocellular carcinoma is the fibrolamellar subtype which is typically seen in adolescents and young women. The imaging characteristics are generally similar to those described for other forms of hepatocellular carcinoma, but calcifications may be seen in as many as 35% to 40% of patients on unenhanced CT scans. Following intravenous administration of contrast, the enhanced scans usually look similar to those of other types of hepatocellular carcinoma. However, a small percentage of patients will show increased enhancement of the tumor similar to that seen with fibronodular hyperplasia and hepatic adenoma.

Undifferentiated embryonal sarcoma is a rare tumor of mesenchymal origin occurring in older children and young adults. Ros, Olmsted et al. have reviewed the radiologic and pathologic aspects of this tumor, which was most commonly known in the past as malignant mesenchymoma. Pathologically, the lesions can range from solid to primarily cystic and the imaging features correspond. Metastases

usually go to the lungs and skeleton. Sonography typically demonstrates a large intrahepatic mass which may be predominantly echogenic with small anechoic cystic, or predominantly cystic, areas with septations. The echogenic lesions may contain sufficient calcium to cause acoustic shadowing. CT demonstrates an intrahepatic mass that has lower attenuation values than the surrounding liver. Intralesional septations show increased attenuation. The tumor may be surrounded by a thin rim of tissue which enhances with intravenous contrast material and corresponds with the tumoral pseudocapsule seen on gross pathologic examination. With angiography, the masses are most commonly hypovascular, but may be hypervascular or avascular. Vessels are typically displaced and arteriovenous shunting with pooling of contrast material is uncommon.

Rhabdomyosarcoma of the bile ducts is one of the rarest forms of this tumor of mesenchymal origin. When the tumor arises in one of the large bile ducts, it is usually of the gross appearance of sarcoma botryoides (Fig 23–45). It causes obstruction and jaundice. The tumor may also arise in an intrahepatic duct and is then little different from other intrahepatic malignancies on imaging studies (Fig 23–46). Geoffrey et al. have reviewed the sonographic and CT findings in biliary duct rhabdomyosarcomas. US

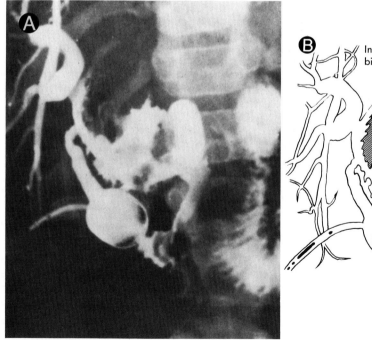

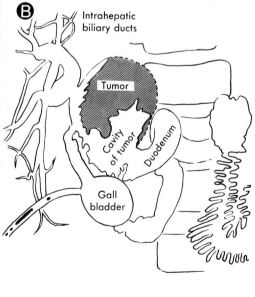

FIG 23–45.
Rhabdomyosarcoma of the common bile duct. **A,** cholangiogram demonstrates a large lobulated, ulcerated mass in the common bile duct adjacent to the sphincter of Oddi. The lobulations are typ-ical of sarcoma botryroides. **B,** drawing of findings. (From Lee FA: Rhabdomyosarcoma, in Parker BR, Castellino RA (eds): *Pediatric Oncologic Radiology.* St Louis, Mosby–Year Book, 1977.)

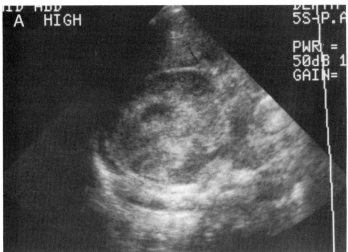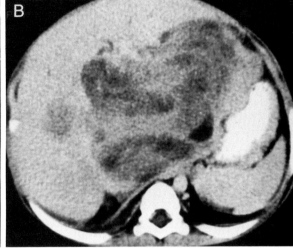

FIG 23–46.
Rhabdomyosarcoma arising from the intrahepatic biliary ducts. **A,** sonogram demonstrates a heterogeneous echogenic mass in the left lobe of the liver. **B,** CT scan demonstrates a diffuse lesion throughout the left lobe and portions of the right lobe of the liver that does not undergo contrast enhancement as much as the surrounding normal parenchyma.

typically identifies bile duct dilatation, if present. The mass tends to be hyperechoic but areas of hypoechogenicity secondary to necrosis or hemorrhage may be identified. Internal septa may be seen. On CT, the rhabdomyosarcoma is a low-attenuation lesion which demonstrates inhomogeneous enhancement following the infusion of intravenous contrast material. Verständig et al. have demonstrated the grapelike tumor cluster on CT and percutaneous transhepatic cholangiography. *Cholangiocarcinoma* may arise in preexisting choledochal cysts, but usually in adults.

HEPATIC METASTASES

Metastatic disease to the liver is most commonly from primary tumors arising in other abdominal organs. Wilms tumor and neuroblastoma are the two most common tumors metastasizing to the liver. Virtually any other solid tumor, other than those arising in the central nervous system, can metastasize to the liver. Lymphoma and leukemia are often considered metastatic lesions, but generally represent infiltration of the liver by systemic disease of multifocal origin.

Metastatic disease from neuroblastoma in infancy can simulate a primary liver tumor (Fig 23–47). Careful evaluation of the sites of origin of neuroblastoma should always be accomplished when a solid liver tumor is first discovered. Even though metastases to the liver from infantile neuroblastoma can be massive, the prognosis in children under the age of 1 year is still remarkably good. Beyond infancy, metastases are more likely to occur during the course of neoplastic disease than at presentation. As with infants, Wilms tumor and neuroblastoma are the most commonly metastasizing tumors to the liver in children older than 1 year of age.

Imaging studies of metastatic disease to the liver in children show results similar to those found in adults, depending to some degree on the nature of the primary tumor. Sonography typically identifies multiple discrete lesions, but numerous metastases, especially from neuroblastoma, may simulate a large heterogeneous mass. Most metastatic lesions are hypoechogenic. Neuroblastoma lesions may contain calcification and show acoustic shadowing. Large metastases from any tumor may undergo central necrosis or hemorrhage and show even lower areas of echogenicity within the center.

On CT, metastases are quite variable in appearance. The attenuation of metastases is usually lower than that of the surrounding liver and the difference is exaggerated with intravenous contrast enhancement. However, some tumors will cause metastatic lesions which are isodense with the surrounding liver parenchyma. Target-like concentric bands of variable attenuation may be seen with the lowest density being in the center in cases of tumor necrosis. Peripheral ring enhancement is frequent following contrast injection. The MR characteristics of liver metastases will depend to a large degree on the origin of the tumor. In general, there is lower signal intensity on T1 weighting and higher signal intensity on T2 weighting with respect to the normal liver parenchyma. Metastatic disease can be seen on radio-

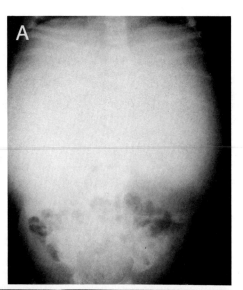

FIG 23–47.
Metastatic neuroblastoma. **A,** plain film of the abdomen in a 6-week-old girl with massive abdominal distention demonstrates a very large upper abdominal mass depressing the air-filled bowel inferiorly. **B** and **C,** longitudinal and transverse sonograms through the liver demonstrate a nodular liver with heterogeneous echogenicity. **D** and **E,** T1- and T2-weighted spin-echo MR scans demonstrate marked hepatomegaly, heterogeneous decreased signal intensity on T1-weighted and heterogeneous increased signal on T2-weighted images. The patient had no extra-abdominal metastatic lesions and the tumor had regressed almost completely 6 months after the initial studies.

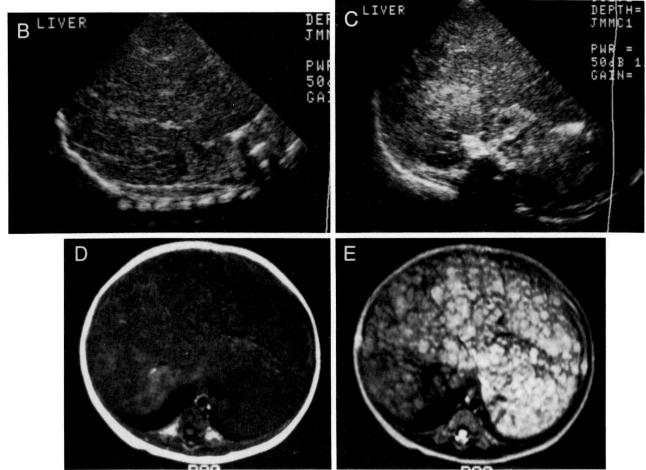

nuclide liver scans with multiple discrete photopenic areas or generalized decrease in activity. In general, the sensitivity of nuclear medicine studies is less than that of US, which is less than that of either CT or MR.

The distinction between metastatic disease and other hepatic masses is not always easy. Brody et al. reported a case of Wilms tumor in which hepatic metastases had the MR characteristics of cysts on spin-echo images. Brick et al. demonstrated small hepatic cysts on CT which had the appearance of solid lesions because of volume averaging. US was useful in differentiating these lesions from metastases and is a useful adjunct if the CT or MR appearance is not diagnostic. Goldberg et al. have demonstrated the greater value of ultrafast MR relative to that of standard MR in differentiating metastases from hemangiomas, a problem more commonly encountered in adults than in children.

REFERENCES

Abramson SJ, Barash FS, Seldin DW, et al: Transient focal liver scan defects in children receiving chemotherapy (pseudometastases). *Radiology* 1984; 150:701.

Abramson SJ, Lack EE, Teele RL: Benign vascular tumors of the liver in infants: sonographic appearance. AJR 1982; 138:629.

Adam A, Gibson RN, Soreide O, et al: The radiology of fibrolamellar hepatoma. *Clin Radiol* 1986; 37:355.

Atkinson GO Jr, Kodroff M, Sones PJ, et al: Focal nodular hyperplasia of the liver in children: A report of three new cases. *Radiology* 1980; 137:171.

Bates SM, Keller MS, Ramos IM, et al: Hepatoblastoma: Detection of tumor vascularity with duplex Doppler US. *Radiology* 1990; 176:505.

Birnbaum BA, Weinreb JC, Megibow AJ, et al: Definitive diagnosis of hepatic hemangiomas: MR imaging versus Tc-99m-labeled red blood cell SPECT. *Radiology* 1990; 176:95.

Boechat MI, Kangarloo H, Ortega J, et al: Primary liver tumors in children: comparison of CT and MR imaging. *Radiology* 1988; 169:727.

Bova JG, Dempsher CJ, Sepulveda G: Cholangiocarcinoma associated with type 2 choledochal cysts. *Gastrointest Radiol* 1983; 8:41.

Bree RL, Schwab RE, Glazer GM, et al: The varied appearances of hepatic cavernous hemangiomas with sonography, computed tomography, magnetic resonance imaging and scintigraphy. *Radiographics* 1987; 7:1153.

Brick SH, Hill MC, Lande IM: The mistaken or indeterminate CT diagnosis of hepatic metastases: The value of sonography. AJR 1987; 148:723.

Brodsky RI, Friedman AC, Maurer AM, et al: Hepatic cavernous hemangioma: Diagnosis with 99mTc-labelled red cells and single photon emission CT. AJR 1987; 148:125.

Brody AS, Seidel FG, Kuhn JP: Metasatic Wilms tumor to the liver with MR findings simulating cysts: Case report emphasizing need for integrated imaging. *Pediatr Radiol* 1989; 19:337.

Brunelle F, Chaumont P: Hepatic tumors in children: Ultrasonic differentiation of malignant from benign lesions. *Radiology* 1984; 150:695.

Brunelle F, Tammam S, Odievre M, et al: Liver adenomas in glycogen storage disease in children. Ultrasound and angiographic study. *Pediatr Radiol* 1984; 14:94.

Craig JR, Peters RL, Edmondson RL, et al: Fibrolamellar carcinoma of the liver: A tumour of adolescents and young adults with distinctive clinico-pathologic features. *Cancer* 1980; 46:372.

Dachman AH, Lichtenstein JE, Friedman AC, et al: Infantile hemangioendothelioma of the liver: A radiologic-pathologic-clinical correlation. AJR 1983; 140:1091.

Dachman AH, Pakter RL, Ros PR, et al: Hepatoblastoma: Radiologic-pathologic correlation in 50 cases. *Radiology* 1987; 164:15.

Dachman AH, Ros PR, Goodman ZD, et al: Nodular regenerative hyperplasia of the liver: Clinical and radiologic observations. AJR 1987; 148:717.

deCampo M, deCampo JF: Ultrasound of primary hepatic tumours in childhood. *Pediatr Radiol* 1988; 19:19.

Diament MJ, Parvey LS, Tonkin ILD, et al: Hepatoblastomas: Technetium sulfur colloid uptake simulating focal nodular hyperplasia. AJR 1982; 139:168.

Donovan AT, Wolverson MK, de Mello D, et al: Multicystic mesenchymal hamartoma of childhood: Computerized tomography and ultrasound characteristics. *Pediatr Radiol* 1981; 11:163.

Exelby PR, Filler RM, Grosfeld JL. Liver tumors in children in particular reference to hepatoblastoma and hepatocellular carcinoma: American Academy of Pediatrics Surgical Section Survey—1974. *J Pediatr Surg* 1975; 10:329.

Fellows KE, Hoffer FA, Markowitz RI, et al: Multiple collaterals to hepatic infantile hemangioendotheliomas and arteriovenous malformations: Effect on embolization. *Radiology* 1991; 181:813.

Ferrucci JT. MR imaging of the liver. Leo G. Rigler Lecture. AJR 1986; 147:1103.

Finn JP, Hall-Craggs MA, Dicks-Mireaux C, et al: Primary liver tumors in childhood: Assessment of resectability with high-field MR and comparison with CT. *Pediatr Radiol* 1990; 21:34.

Francis IR, Agha FP, Thompson NW, et al: Fibrolamellar hepatocarcinoma: Clinical, radiologic, and pathologic features. *Gastrointest Radiol* 1986; 11:67.

Freeny PC, Marks WM: Hepatic hemangioma: Dynamic bolus CT. AJR 1986; 147:711.

Friedburg H, Kauffmann GW, Bohn N, et al: Sonographic and computed tomographic features of embryonal rhabdomyosarcoma of the biliary tract. *Pediatr Radiol* 1984; 14:436.

Friedman AC, Lichtenstein JE, Goodman Z, et al: Fibrolamellar hepatocellular carcinoma. *Radiology* 1985; 157:583.

Geoffrey A, Couanet D, Montagne J-P, et al: Ultrasonography and computed tomography for diagnosis and follow-up of biliary duct rhabdomyosarcomas in children. *Pediatr Radiol* 1987; 17:127.

Gibney RG, Hendin AP, Cooperberg PL: Sonographically detected hepatic hemangiomas: Absence of change over time. AJR 1987; 149:953.

Giyanani VL, Meyers PC, Wolfson JJ: Mesenchymal hamartoma of the liver: Computed tomography and ultrasonography. *J Comput Assist Tomogr* 1986; 10:51.

Glazer GM, Aisen AM, Francis IR, et al: Hepatic cavernous hemangioma: Magnetic resonance imaging. *Radiology* 1985; 155:417.

Goldberg MA, Saini S, Hahn PF, et al: Differentiation between hemangiomas and metastases of the liver with ultrafast MR imaging: Preliminary results with T2 calculations. AJR 1991; 157:727.

Greenberg M, Filler RM: Hepatic tumors, in Pizzo PA, Poplack DG (eds): *Principles and Practice of Pediatric Oncology*. Philadelphia, JB Lippincott, 1989, pp 565–582.

Itai Y, Ohtomo K, Araki T, et al: Computed tomography and sonography of cavernous hemangioma of the liver. AJR 1983; 141:315.

Itai Y, Ohtomo K, Furui S, et al: Noninvasive diagnosis of small cavernous hemangioma of the liver: advantage of MRI. AJR 1985; 145:1195.

Itoh K, Nishimura K, Togashi K, et al: Hepatocellular carcinoma: MR imaging. *Radiology* 1987; 164:21.

Jennings CM, Merrill CR, Slater DN: Case report. The computed tomographic appearances of benign hepatic hamartoma. *Clin Radiol* 1987; 38:103.

Klein MA, Slovis TL, Chang CH, et al: Sonographic and Doppler features of infantile hepatic hemangiomas with pathologic correlation. *J Ultrasound Med* 1990; 9:619.

Li KC, Glazer GM, Quint LE, et al: Distinction of hepatic cavernous hemangioma from hepatic metastases with MR imaging. *Radiology* 1988; 169:409.

Lucaya J, Enriquez G, Amat L, et al: Computed tomography of infantile hepatic hemangioendothelioma. AJR 1985; 144:821.

Mathieu D, Bruneton JN, Drouillard J, et al: Hepatic adenomas and focal nodular hyperplasia: Dynamic CT study. *Radiology* 1986; 160:53.

Mattison GR, Glazer GM, Quint LE, et al: MR imaging of hepatic focal nodular hyperplasia: Characterization and distinction from primary malignant hepatic tumors. AJR 1987; 148:711.

Miller JH, Greenspan BS: Integrated imaging of hepatic tumors in childhood. *Radiology* 1985; 154:83.

Newman KD, Schisgall R, Reaman G, et al: Malignant mesenchymoma of the liver in children. *J Pediatr Surg* 1989; 24:781.

Ohtomo K, Itai Y, Hasizume K, et al: CT and MR appearance of focal nodular hyperplasia of the liver in children with biliary atresia. *Clin Radiol* 1991; 43:88.

Ohtomo K, Itai Y, Yoshikawa K, et al: Hepatic tumours: dynamic MR imaging. *Radiology* 1987; 163:27.

Oshiro K, Hanashiro Y, Shimabukuro K, et al: A hepatobiliary study with Tc-99m *N*-pyridoxyl-5-methyltryptophan (PMT) in a patient with hepatoblastoma. *Clin Nucl Med* 1991; 16:10.

Radin DR, Kanel GC: Peliosis hepatis in a patient with human immunodeficiency virus infection. AJR 1991; 156:91.

Reinig JW, Dwyer AJ, Miller DL, et al: Liver metastases: Detection with MR imaging at 0.5 and 1.5 T. *Radiology* 1989; 170:149.

Roberts EA, Liv P, Stringer D, et al: Mesenchymal hamartoma in a 10-month-old infant: Appearance by magnetic resonance imaging. *J Can Assoc Radiol* 1989; 40:219.

Ros PR, Goodman ZD, Ishak KG, et al: Mesenchymal hamartoma of the liver: Radiologic-pathologic correlation. *Radiology* 1986; 158:619.

Ros PR, Lubbers PR, Olmsted WW, et al: Hemangioma of the liver: Heterogeneous appearance of T2-weighted images. AJR 1987; 149:1167.

Ros PR, Olmsted WW, Dachman AH, et al: Undifferentiated (embryonal) sarcoma of the liver: radiologic-pathologic correlation. *Radiology* 1986; 161:141.

Rummeny E, Saini S, Wittenberg J, et al: MR imaging of liver neoplasmas. AJR 1989; 152:493.

Rummeny E, Weissleder R, Stark DD, et al: Primary liver tumors: diagnosis by MR imaging. AJR 1989; 152:63.

Ruymann FB, Raney RB Jr, Crist WM, et al: Rhabdomyosarcoma of the biliary tree in childhood; A report from the intergroup rhabdomyosarcoma study. *Cancer* 1985; 56:575.

Schiebler ML, Kressel HY, Saul SH, et al: MR imaging of focal nodular hyperplasia of the liver. *J Comput Assist Tomogr* 1987; 11:651.

Schmidt H, Ullrich K, von Lenglerke HJ, et al: Peliosis hepatis with type I glycogen storage disease. *J Inherited Metab Dis* 1991; 14:831.

Soyer P, Roche A, Levesque M, et al: CT of fibrolamellar hepatocellular carcinoma. *J Comput Assist Tomogr* 1991; 15:533.

Stanley P, Hall TR, Woolley MM, et al: Mesenchymal hamartomas of the liver in childhood: Sonographic and CT findings. AJR 1986; 147:1035.

Stark DD, Wittenberg J, Butch RJ, et al: Hepatic metastases: randomized controlled comparison of detection with MR imaging and CT. *Radiology* 1987; 165:399.

Taylor KJW, Ramos I, Morse SS, et al: Focal liver masses: differential diagnosis with pulsed Doppler US. *Radiology* 1987; 164:643.

Tonkin IL, Wrenn EL Jr, Hollabaugh RS: The continued value of angiography in planning surgical resection of benign and malignant hepatic tumors in children. *Pediatr Radiol* 1988; 18:35.

Tsukamoto Y, Nakata H, Kimoto T, et al: CT and angiography of peliosis hepatis. AJR 1984; 142:539.

Verständig A, Bar-Ziv J, Abu-Dalu KI, et al: Sarcoma botryoides of the common bile duct: Preoperative diagnosis by coronal CT and PTC. *Pediatr Radiol* 1991; 21:15-2.

Weinreb JC, Brateman L, Maravilla KR: Magnetic resonance imaging of hepatic lymphoma. AJR 1984; 143:1211.

Welch TJ, Sheedy PF II, Johnson CM, et al: Focal nodular hyperplasia and hepatic adenoma: Comparison of angiography, CT, US, and scintigraphy. *Radiology* 1985; 156:593.

Welch TJ, Sheedy PF II, Johnson CM, et al: Radiographic characteristics of benign liver tumours: Focal nodular hyperplasia and hepatic adenoma. *Radiographics* 1985; 5:673.

SECTION 8

Liver Transplantation

Liver transplantation in children is becoming a more commonly performed procedure, although still in a limited number of institutions. The most common disorders leading to liver transplantation are biliary atresia and metabolic diseases in which chronic liver failure, with or without cirrhosis, develops. Preoperative imaging studies play an important role in the assessment and diagnosis of the underlying liver disorder. Once the clinical decision to perform transplantation has been made, attention needs to be directed to the vascular anatomy. Initially, angiography was used in most patients, but duplex Doppler sonography is now the primary modality for evaluation of the hepatic and portal systems and the IVC. MR imaging is becoming more commonly used, and MRA appears to be the most sensitive imaging examination of all in the series of adult patients reported by Finn et al. Bisset et al. showed excellent correlation between sonography and MR for evaluation of size of the portal and hepatic veins. MR was more sensitive, however, in the detection of spontaneous portosystemic shunts in patients with portal hypertension.

Imaging studies are also critical in assessment of the transplanted liver. The most common complication is rejection, in which imaging studies are nonspecific, usually showing evidence of hepatomegaly with hepatic edema. Vascular complications, particularly hepatic artery or portal vein thrombosis, are well demonstrated by Doppler sonography. CT has been useful to show splenic infarction. The findings during infection of the transplanted liver are similar to those of rejection unless frank abscess formation has occurred. Pariente et al. have reviewed the biliary complications following liver transplantation. A combination of sonography and cholangiography identified the major lesions as bile duct dilatation and biloma formation after hepatic artery compro-mise and ductal dilatation secondary to complications of the biliary tree anastomosis. Percutaneous biliary drainage or balloon dilatation was frequently successful in relieving these complications.

REFERENCES

Bisset GS III, Strife JL, Balisteri WF: Evaluation of children for liver transplantation: value of MR imaging and sonography. *AJR* 1990; 155:351.

Dalen K, Day DL, Ascher NL, et al: Imaging of vascular complications after hepatic transplantation. *AJR* 1988; 150:1285.

Dominguez R, Young LW, Ledesma-Medina J, et al: Pediatric liver transplantation. Part II. Diagnostic imaging in postoperative management. *Radiology* 1985; 157:339.

Dupuy D, Costello P, Lewis D, et al: Abdominal CT findings after liver transplantation in 66 patients. *AJR* 1991; 156:1167.

Finn JP, Edelman RR, Jenkins RL, et al: Liver transplantation: MR angiography with surgical validation. *Radiology* 1991; 179:265.

Hoffer FA, Teele RL, Lillehei CW, et al: Infected bilomas and hepatic artery thrombosis in infant recipients of liver transplants: Interventional radiology and medical therapy as an alternative to retransplantation. *Radiology* 1988; 169:435.

Ledesma-Medina J, Dominguez R, Bowen AD, et al: Pediatric liver transplantation. Part I. Standardization of preoperative diagnostic imaging. *Radiology* 1985; 157:335.

Lehar SC, Zajko AB, Koneru B, et al: Splenic infarction complicating pediatric liver transplantation: Incidence and CT appearance. *J Comput Assist Tomogr* 1990; 14:362.

Pariente D, Bihet MH, Tammam S, et al: Biliary complications after transplantation in children: Role of imaging modalities. *Pediatr Radiol* 1991; 21:175.

Shaw BW Jr, Wood RP, Kaufman SS, et al: Review: liver transplantation therapy for children: Part 2. *J Pediatr Gastroenterol Nutr* 1988; 7:797.

24

The Spleen and Pancreas

In association with the hepatobiliary system, the spleen and pancreas are often considered among the accessory organs of digestion. Their physiologic functions, however, are quite different from one another, and the two organs are dealt with separately in this chapter.

SECTION 1

The Spleen

The spleen is more properly considered a lymphatic organ than an organ of digestion. In fact, the spleen is the largest of the body's lymphatic structures.

SPLENIC ANATOMY AND EMBRYOLOGY

Situated in the left upper quadrant, the spleen normally lies between the stomach and the diaphragm. It has two surfaces. The superolateral surface approximates the diaphragm which separates it from the ninth, tenth, and eleventh ribs and the inferior left lung and pleura. The visceral surface has a renal portion in relation to the superior pole of the left kidney and to the left adrenal gland. The gastric portion is in contact with the posterior wall of the stomach and the tail of the pancreas. The splenic hilum is a depression along the medial surface through which pass the splenic artery and vein and the splenic nerves. The inferior pole of the spleen abuts the splenic flexure of the colon. The spleen is maintained in its normal position by two ligaments formed by peritoneal folds. The phrenicosplenic ligament contains the major splenic vessels. The gastrosplenic ligament runs between the spleen and stomach and contains the short gastric and gastroepiploic arteries. The splenic vein courses rightward from the portal vein. In the adult, the spleen is comparable in length to the kidney.

The spleen appears in the fifth week of embryonic life as a localized thickening of the mesoderm in the dorsal mesogastrium above the pancreatic tail.

As the stomach rotates its greater curvature to the left, the spleen is carried with it into the left upper quadrant. The gastrosplenic ligament is derived from the residuum of the dorsal mesogastrium. The primary function of the embryonic spleen is erythropoiesis which is maximal in the mid–second trimester and subsequently diminishes.

IMAGING THE SPLEEN

Plain films may demonstrate the spleen in the left upper quadrant, displacing the stomach laterally and colon inferiorly. The spleen may be obscured when large amounts of gas are present in the gastrointestinal tract.

The spleen is easily identified on abdominal sonograms. It has a homogeneous sonographic texture. The splenic hilar vessels are usually well seen but intrasplenic vessels typically are not. Rosenberg et al. measured normal spleen length in children during quiet respiration. Using coronal scans, they measured the spleen and correlated the results with age, height, and weight. The upper limit of normal was 6.0 cm at 3 months, 6.5 cm at 6 months, 7.0 cm at 12 months, 8.0 cm at 2 years, 9.0 cm at 4 years, 9.5 cm at 6 years, 10.0 cm at 8 years, 11.0 cm at 10 years, and 11.5 cm at 12 years. The upper limit of normal at 15 years of age and older was 12.0 cm for girls and 13.0 cm for boys (Fig 24–1). As a general rule, the tip of the spleen should not extend below the inferior pole of the left kidney (Fig 24–2).

The normal spleen on computed tomography (CT) has a higher attenuation than the liver. Uni-

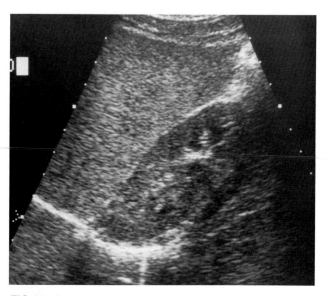

FIG 24–2.
Splenomegaly in a 9-year-old boy with hereditary spherocytosis. The inferior tip of the spleen projects below the lower pole of the left kidney.

form increase in attenuation occurs following the administration of intravenous contrast agents. The splenic vein is well demonstrated on dynamic scans and can usually be followed across the abdomen to its juncture with the superior mesenteric vein, forming the portal vein (Fig 24–3). The splenic artery can also be seen on dynamic scans. Since the artery is less tortuous in children than in adults, it frequently can be identified throughout much of its course.

The spleen on T1-weighted spin-echo magnetic resonance (MR) images has lower signal intensity than does the liver and slightly greater signal inten-

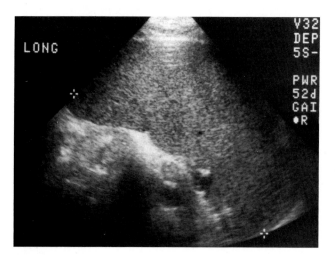

FIG 24–1.
Splenomegaly in a 14-year-old boy with acute myelogenous leukemia. Longitudinal sonogram demonstrates the splenic length to be 185 mm. Upper limit of normal at this age is 130 mm according to Rosenberg et al.

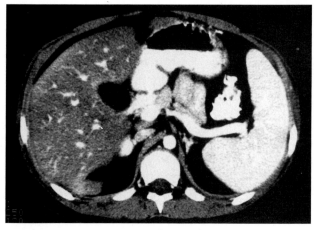

FIG 24–3.
Normal spleen in an obese 11-year-old boy on CT scan photographed at narrow window settings after intravenous contrast enhancement. There is uniform enhancement of the spleen and excellent visualization of the splenic vein.

sity than muscle. On T2-weighted images, the spleen has higher signal intensity than the liver. The major splenic vessels are well demonstrated because of the characteristic signal void of flowing blood.

Technetium 99m–labeled sulfur colloid is picked up by the spleen's reticuloendothelial system, permitting its visualization. Isotopic splenic scanning is useful for the identification of splenic ectopia, polysplenia, and asplenia, as well as numerous disease states as described below. Angiography is rarely used for intrasplenic diseases, but arterial portography for evaluation of the portal venous system demonstrates the spleen to good advantage.

CONGENITAL ANOMALIES

The most common congenital anomaly of the spleen is the presence of one or more *accessory spleens*, or spleniculi. They occur in 10% to 15% of the normal population and usually are found incidentally at autopsy or on imaging studies. They are six or less in number and most commonly are located in the splenic hilum, in association with the splenic vessels, or in the gastrosplenic ligament. They can be found, however, virtually anywhere in the abdomen. They rarely exceed 2 cm in diameter and are most frequently confused with splenic hilar or para-

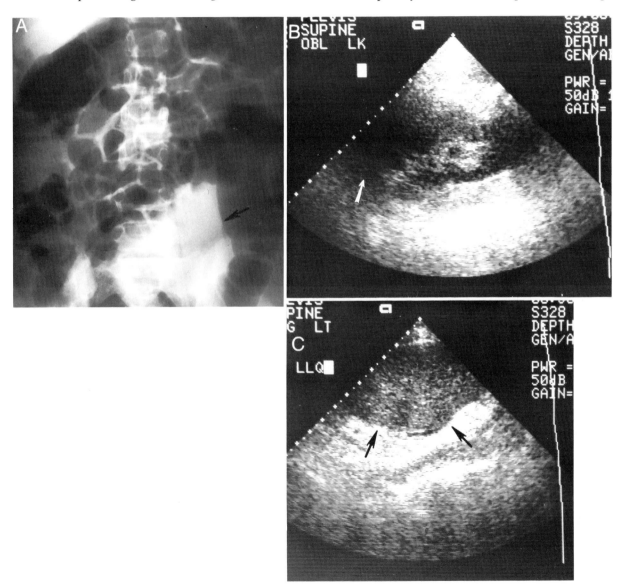

FIG 24–4.
Wandering spleen in a 10-year-old girl with a left lower quadrant mass and abdominal pain. **A,** abdominal radiograph demonstrates a left lower quadrant mass *(arrow)*. **B,** sonogram of the left upper quadrant demonstrates lack of splenic tissue *(arrow)* adjacent to the upper pole of the left kidney. **C,** sonogram of the mass in the left lower quadrant demonstrates echogenic splenic tissue *(arrows)*. Torsion of the spleen was found at surgery.

pancreatic lymph nodes. They can be identified frequently on ultrasound (US) or CT, but the definitive imaging study is ^{99m}Tc sulfur colloid liver-spleen scans.

Normally, the residuum of the dorsal mesogastrium fuses with the posterior peritoneum, helping keep the spleen in its normal position. When this fusion does not take place, the dorsal mesogastrium may persist as a long mesentery allowing the spleen to be displaced, the so-called *wandering spleen* (Fig 24–4). The most common location for these ectopic spleens is the left lower quadrant. They may present as asymptomatic masses and can be readily identified by US, CT, or sulfur colloid scan. Typically, no splenic tissue can be identified in the left upper quadrant, but a small accessory spleen may remain in the normal anatomical location. The wandering spleen may undergo torsion, causing severe pain secondary to ischemia. The twisted spleen has no uptake on radionuclide scan, no contrast enhance-

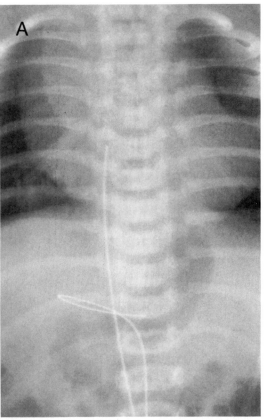

FIG 24–5.
Asplenia syndrome in a newborn with double outlet right ventricle. **A,** plain film demonstrates symmetric mainstem bronchi, midline liver, left-sided stomach, and a right-sided aorta containing an umbilical artery catheter. The umbilical venous catheter is coiled in the portal vein. **B,** transverse sonogram demonstrates the aorta *(A)* to be right-sided with the inferior vena cava (IVC) *(C)* to its right. *KID,* kidney. **C,** transverse sonogram at a more cephalad level demonstrates the midline liver and the IVC *(C)* crossing anterior to the aorta *(A).* No splenic tissue could be identified.

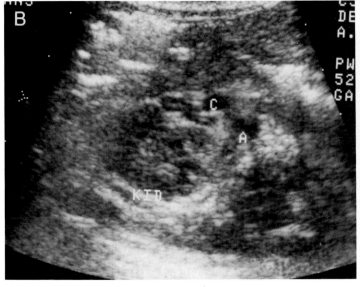

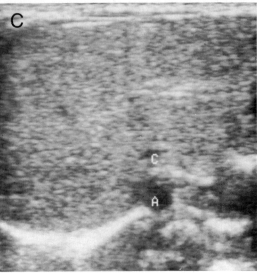

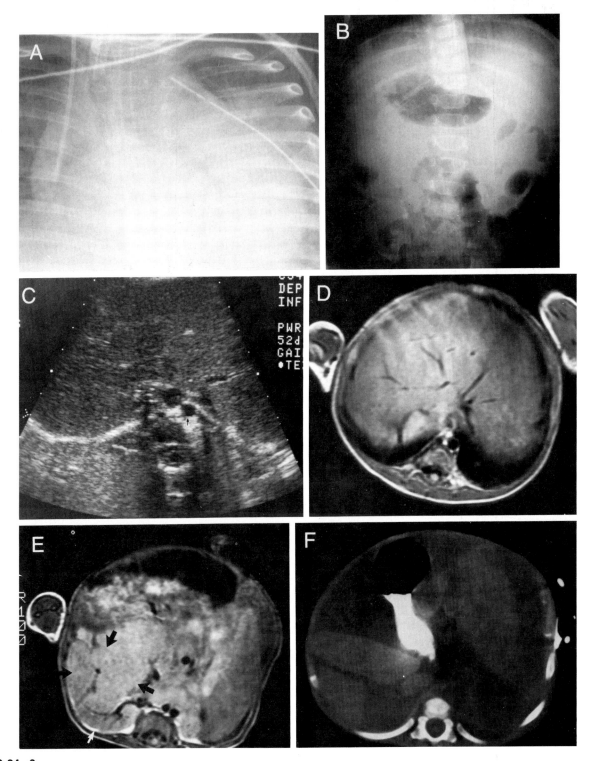

FIG 24–6.
Polysplenia syndrome in a 3-month-old girl with biliary atresia and no evidence of heart disease. **A,** chest radiograph performed following liver transplantation demonstrates the symmetric bronchi to good advantage because of the patient's postoperative pulmonary edema. **B,** preoperative kidney, ureter, bladder (KUB) film demonstrates a right-sided stomach and near-symmetric liver. **C,** transverse sonogram through the upper abdomen demonstrates a midline liver. The azygos vein *(arrow)* is enlarged because of azygos continuation of an interrupted IVC. **D,** MR scan through the upper abdomen, performed to map out vascular anatomy, demonstrates the midline liver. The gallbladder was not identified. **E,** MR through the midabdomen demonstrates multiple splenules *(black arrows)* and the lower pole of the right kidney *(white arrow).* **F,** postoperative CT scan after development of ascites demonstrates multiple spenules on the right and the transplanted liver on the left. Five splenules were identified at surgery.

ment on CT, and shows no flow on duplex Doppler sonography.

The *splenogonadal syndrome* is a rare anomaly in which a portion of the splenic anlage fuses with primitive left gonadal tissue in the first trimester. A normal spleen develops in the left upper quadrant. When a persistent cord of splenic or fibrous tissue connects the spleen with the left testis or epididymis, cryptorchidism usually results. Connection to the left ovary or mesovarium does not result in ovarian ectopia.

Abnormal visceroatrial situs is an intriguing set of entities in which the spleen plays a prominent role. The normal visceroatrial anatomy is known as situs solitus. Situs inversus refers to mirror-image visceroatrial anatomy. Patients with situs inversus are frequently asymptomatic although there is a slightly higher incidence of congenital heart disease. Another group of patients with interesting combinations of congenital anomalies have situs ambiguus (visceral heterotaxia). This last population is divided into two major groups, one with asplenia and one with polysplenia.

Patients with *asplenia* have right-sided isomerism (Fig 24–5). The spleen is absent, the liver appears to have two mirror-image right lobes with a midline gallbladder, and two trilobed lungs with eparterial (right-sided) mainstem bronchi are present in the thorax. Midgut malrotation is usually present and the stomach may be either right- or left-sided. The inferior vena cava (IVC) and aorta may lie on the same side of the spine. The IVC, then, crosses the midline anterior to the aorta to enter the atrium. Variable congenital cardiac lesions are present. The portal vein may pass anterior to the pancreas and duodenum.

Patients with *polysplenia* have left-sided isomerism (Fig 24–6). Multiple splenules are present. The liver is again midline, but the gallbladder may be hypoplastic or absent. Bilateral bilobed lungs with hyparterial (left-sided) bronchi are present as is complex congenital heart disease, often with common atrium and anomalous pulmonary venous return below the diaphragm. Interruption of the IVC with azygos continuation is common. The aorta and IVC may be on the same side. Preduodenal portal vein is common, especially in those patients with biliary atresia. Midgut malrotation and variable stomach position may be seen. Commonly associated congenital anomalies include biliary atresia, duodenal atresia, anal atresia, and tracheoesophageal fistula. A short pancreas has been described secondary to failure of development of the dorsal pancreatic bud (see below). Rare anomalies include central nervous system (CNS) malformations,

palatal abnormalities, and a congenitally absent left adrenal gland.

Tonkin and Tonkin and Hernanz-Schulman et al. have demonstrated the usefulness of noninvasive imaging in correctly identifying the major anomalies of asplenia and polysplenia syndromes. Combinations of US, CT, MR, and radionuclide liver-spleen scans are sufficiently sensitive to demonstrate the above-described anomalies and to preclude the need for angiography.

Splenomegaly in Congenital Disorders

An enlarged spleen is a common concomitant of a variety of congenital diseases in childhood. Patients with portal hypertension from a number of causes, including biliary atresia (see Chapter 23), have congestive splenomegaly. The hemolytic anemias frequently cause splenomegaly with hereditary spherocytosis, hereditary elliptocytosis, and thalassemia being the most common. The imaging findings are nonspecific unless there is evidence of extramedullary hematopoiesis or infarcts, both of which are more common in affected adults than in children. The former causes focal areas of increased echogenicity in the spleen while the latter present as focal areas of decreased echogenicity. Sickle cell anemia initially leads to splenomegaly followed by splenic atrophy secondary to multiple infarcts (Fig 24–7). In some cases, iron deposition will result in increased attenuation of the spleen on CT examination and decreased signal intensity on MR scans. The storage diseases generally cause nonspecific splenomegaly, but Gaucher disease may lead to splenic abnormalities on US. Hill et al, described focal hypoechoic collections of Gaucher cells as the most commonly seen pattern. The focal collec-

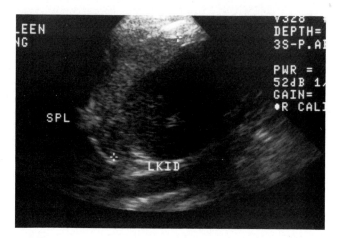

FIG 24–7.
Splenic atrophy in an 8-year-old girl with sickle cell anemia. The spleen *(SPL)* measured 6 cm in length. *LKID,* left kidney.

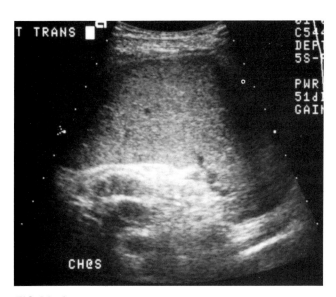

FIG 24–8.
Splenomegaly in a 9-year-old girl with cavernous transformation of the portal vein. Compared with Figures 24–1 and 24–2, the spleen has a heterogeneous echo pattern with enlarged intrasplenic vessels secondary to portal hypertension.

tions may occasionally be hyperechoic secondary to fibrosis.

ACQUIRED ABNORMALITIES

Splenomegaly can be found in a variety of acquired disorders, including infection and neoplasms, as dis-

cussed below. Acquired causes of portal hypertension, such as cavernous transformation of the portal vein and secondary cirrhosis of the liver, in patients with cystic fibrosis, may present with splenomegaly as may patients with extrahepatic hematopoiesis (Fig 24–8). Imaging studies of the spleen are nonspecific, but other findings, such as varices, may lead to the correct diagnosis. *Infectious disease* involving the spleen is most commonly seen in immunocompromised patients. Microabscesses are most commonly seen, especially with fungal infection such as candidiasis (Fig 24–9). If large enough, the microabscesses may be seen on sonograms, but CT may be necessary when the lesions are very small. Larger, solitary abscesses may also occur with candidiasis. They may be seen as hypoechoic areas on US and as low-attenuation areas on CT. In rare circumstances, calcification may be seen on unenhanced CT examination. Cox et al. reported splenic abscesses in cat-scratch fever. US showed multiple small, poorly defined nodules which coalesced into an abscess with mixed echogenicity, finally resolving into a calcified granuloma. Viral infections, including infectious mononucleosis, are more likely to cause nonspecific splenomegaly because of the diffuse infiltrative nature of the disease process or because of reactive hyperplasia of the spleen's reticuloendothelial tissue. Echinococcal cysts may be found in the spleen. Plain films may show calcification of the cyst wall. The cysts are generally anechoic, although one echogenic

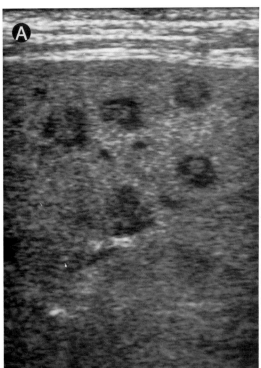

FIG 24–9.
Splenic candidiasis in a teen-aged boy following bone marrow transplantation. **A,** transverse sonogram of the enlarged spleen demonstrates the characteristic "target lesions" of *Candida* microabscesses. **B,** CT scan demonstrates numerous microabscesses in the spleen as well as larger abscesses in both spleen and liver.

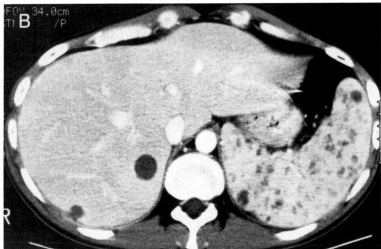

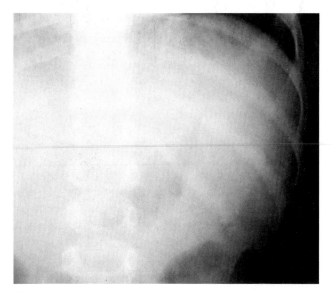

FIG 24–10.
Splenic calcifications in an 18-month-old boy with chronic granulomatous disease of childhood.

lesion was identified by Franquet et al. CT shows a focal lesion of lower attenuation than the surrounding splenic tissue that does not enhance after contrast administration. Tuberculosis, histoplasmosis, and coccidioidomycosis may produce multiple splenic granulomas, almost always associated with diffuse organ involvement secondary to hematogenous spread. Splenic granulomas may be found in patients with chronic granulomatous disease of childhood, appearing as calcifications on plain film and ill-defined hypoechogenic nodules on US (Fig 24–10).

Benign neoplasms of the spleen are most commonly cystic in nature. Primary splenic cysts may be (1) epithelial-lined such as epidermoid, dermoid, or transitional cell cysts, or (2) endothelial-lined such as lymphangiomas and hemangiomas. Acquired cysts may be infectious, usually due to *Echinococcus*, or posttraumatic. Epidermoid cysts are the most common noninfectious focal space-occupying lesions of the spleen (Fig 24–11). They are frequently large enough to appear on plain films as a left upper

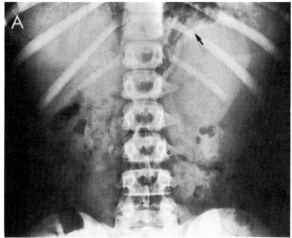

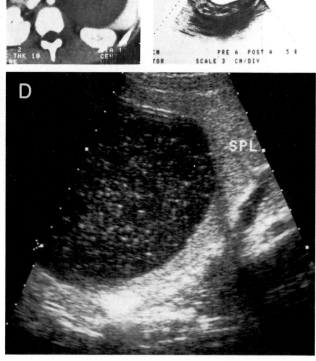

FIG 24–11.
Epidermoid cyst of the spleen in an asymptomatic 12-year-old girl. **A,** plain film shows a left upper quadrant mass displacing the stomach. **B,** CT shows the mass to be homogeneous with attenuation values equal to water. **C,** transverse sonogram demonstrates the mass to be anechoic (courtesy of Dr. E. Afshani, Buffalo). **D,** sonogram in another patient demonstrates echogenic lipid droplets within an epidermoid cyst. *SPL,* spleen.

quadrant mass displacing the stomach and colon. A rim of calcification may be seen. On sonograms, the cysts are characteristically anechoic and sharply demarcated from the surrounding normal splenic tissue. Internal fat droplets may cause the cyst to be hypoechoic rather than anechoic (Fig 24–11,*D*). Liver-spleen scintigraphy demonstrates a focal photopenic defect. Familial occurrence of an epidermoid cyst has been reported. Lymphangiomas are rare in children. They may cause multiple splenic cystic lesions. On sonography, they are most commonly septated and anechoic but may occasionally be hypoechoic because of floating debris. Acquired non-neoplastic cysts may occur after trauma or intrasplenic hemorrhage. The most common solid benign tumor of the spleen in children is *hamartoma*. They are most commonly echogenic, although cystic hamartomas have been reported. They may have radiopharmaceutical uptake at scintigraphic examination greater than that in the surrounding normal spleen. *Splenic hemangiomas* are usually small and associated with hemangiomas elsewhere. They may occasionally be large and associated with hypersplenism, thrombocytopenia, and consumption coagulopathy—the Kasabach-Merritt syndrome. The lesions are predominantly echogenic but may contain cystic spaces which suggest the correct diagnosis.

Malignant neoplasms of the spleen are usually metastatic or related to multifocal neoplastic disorders such as leukemia and lymphoma. Acute *lymphocytic leukemia* is the most common neoplastic disease in children and the patients usually have splenomegaly secondary to diffuse infiltration of the spleen. The other childhood leukemias also result in splenomegaly (see Fig 24–1). Chronic myelogenous leukemia is rare in children but is frequently accompanied by massive splenomegaly. Imaging studies of the spleen are rarely performed in children with leukemia since the diagnosis is made by other means, and the results of splenic imaging have no impact on the staging or prognosis. Sonograms demonstrate an enlarged spleen with heterogeneous echogenicity. Non-Hodgkin lymphoma often has a similar appearance but may also have focal lesions large enough to be seen on sonograms as ill-defined hypoechogenic areas, especially in patients with high-grade malignancy at histologic examination. On CT, they are low-attenuation lesions which do not show enhancement appreciably with intravenous contrast administration. Hodgkin disease may also cause diffuse splenic infiltration that may not be detectable on imaging studies, but is more likely than non-Hodgkin lymphoma to result in focal splenic masses (Fig

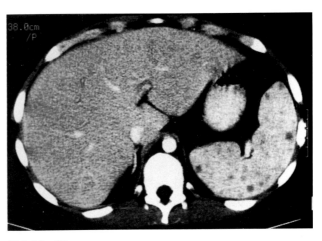

FIG 24–12.
Splenic Hodgkin disease in a 14-year-old boy. CT scan performed as part of staging evaluation demonstrates numerous low-attenuation lesions throughout the spleen. Splenic body revealed typical lesions of Hodgkin's disease.

24–12). Since splenic involvement may be the only subdiaphragmatic site, its detection is important for staging and prognosis. False-negative sonograms, CTs, and MRs are common because the imaging tissue characteristics of the Hodgkin disease lesions are similar to those of normal spleen when the organ is diffusely infiltrated with disease that is only microscopically detectable. Focal lesions may appear on sonograms and CT similar to those of non-Hodgkin lymphoma as described above. Splenic metastases from solid tumors are less common with childhood tumors than they are with those in adults. They may be single or multiple and frequently do not cause splenomegaly. US may show hypoechogenicity, hyperechogenicity, or a mixed pattern. Target lesions have been described in adults.

REFERENCES

The Spleen

Imaging the Spleen

Adler DD, Glazer GM, Aisen AM: MRI of the spleen: Normal appearance and findings in sickle-cell anemia. *AJR* 1986; 147:843.

Dittrich M, Milde S, Dinkel E, et al: Sonographic biometry of liver and spleen size in childhood. *Pediatr Radiol* 1983; 13:206.

Koga T, Morikawa Y: Ultrasonographic determination of the splenic size and its clinical usefulness in various liver diseases. *Radiology* 1975; 115:157.

Markisz JA, Treves ST, Davis RT: Normal hepatic and splenic size in children: Scintigraphic determination. *Pediatr Radiol* 1987; 17:273.

Mirowitz SA, Brown JJ, Lee JKT, et al: Dynamic gadolinium-enhanced MR imaging of the spleen: Normal enhancement patterns and evaluation of splenic lesions. *Radiology* 1991; 179:681.

Rosenberg HK, Markowitz RI, Kolberg H, et al: Normal splenic size in infants and children: sonographic measurement. AJR 1991; 157:119.

Vick CW, Hartenberg MA, Allen HA, et al: Abdominal pseudotumor caused by gastric displacement of the spleen: Sonographic demonstration. *Pediatr Radiol* 1985; 15:253.

Congenital Anomalies

Abramson SJ, Berdon WE, Altman RP, et al: Biliary atresia and noncardiac polysplenic syndrome: US and surgical considerations. *Radiology* 1987; 163:377.

Bollinger B, Lorentzen T: Torsion of a wandering spleen: ultrasonographic findings. *JCU* 1990; 18:510.

Dodds WJ, Taylor AJ, Erickson SJ, et al: Radiologic imaging of splenic anomalies. AJR 1990; 155:805.

Groshar D, Israel A, Barzilai A, et al: The value of scintigraphy in evaluation of a wandering spleen. *Clin Nucl Med* 1986; 11:42.

Hadar H, Gadoth N, Herskovitz P, et al: Short pancreas in polysplenia syndrome. *Acta Radiol* 1991; 32:299.

Herman TE, Siegel MJ: CT of acute spleen torsion in children with wandering spleen. AJR 1991; 156:151.

Herman TE, Siegel MJ: Polysplenia syndrome with congenital short pancreas. AJR 1991; 156:799.

Hernanz-Schulman M, Ambrosino MM, Genieser NB, et al: Current evaluation of the patient with abnormal visceroatrial situs. AJR 1990; 154:797.

Hill SC, Reinig JW, Barranger JA, et al: Gaucher disease: sonographic appearance of the spleen. *Radiology* 1986; 160:631.

Mandell GA, Heyman S, Alavi A, et al: A case of microgastria in association with splenic-gonadal fusion. *Pediatr Radiol* 1983; 13:95.

McLean GK, Alavi A, Ziegler MM, et al: Splenic-gonadal fusion: identification by radionuclide scanning. *J Pediatr Surg* 1981; 16(4 suppl 1):649.

Nemcek AA, Miller FH, Fitzgerald SW: Acute torsion of a wandering spleen: diagnosis by CT and duplex Doppler and color flow sonography. AJR 1991; 157:307.

Phillips GWL, Hemingway AP. Wandering spleen. *Br J Radiol* 1987; 60:188.

Setiawan H, Harrell RS, Perret RS: Ectopic spleen: A sonographic diagnosis. *Pediatr Radiol* 1982; 12:152.

Shiels WE II, Johnson JF, Stephenson SR, et al: Chronic torsion of the wandering spleen. *Pediatr Radiol* 1989; 19:465.

Subramanyam BR, Balthazar EJ, Horii SC: Sonography of the accessory spleen. AJR 1984; 143:47.

Tonkin ILD, Tonkin AK: Visceroatrial situs abnormalities:

sonographic and computed tomographic appearance. AJR 1982; 138:509.

Walther MM, Trulock TS, Finnerty DP, et al: Splenic gonadal fusion. *Urology* 1988; 32:521.

Winer-Muram HT, Tonkin IL: The spectrum of heterotaxic syndromes. *Radiol Clin North Am* 1989; 27:1147.

Acquired Abnormalities

Balthazar EJ, Hilton S, Naidich D, et al: CT of splenic and perisplenic abnormalities in septic patients. AJR 1985; 144:53.

Bartley DL, Hughes WT, Parvey LS, et al: Computed tomography of hepatic and splenic fungal abscesses in leukemic children. *Pediatr Infect Dis* 1982; 1:317.

Bradley MJ, Metreweli C: Ultrasound appearances of extramedullary hematopoiesis in the liver and spleen. *Br J Radiol* 1990; 63:816.

Cornaglia-Ferraris P, Perlino GF, Barabino A, et al: Cystic lymphangioma of the spleen. Report of CT scan findings. *Pediatr Radiol* 1982; 12:94.

Cox F, Perlman S, Sathyanarayana: Splenic abscesses in cat scratch disease: Sonographic diagnosis and follow-up. *JCU* 1989; 17:511.

Dachman AH, Ros PR, Murari JP, et al: Nonparasitic splenic cysts: A report of 52 cases with radiologic-pathologic correlation. AJR 1986; 147:537.

Daneman A, Martin DJ: Congenital epithelial splenic cysts in children: Emphasis on sonographic appearances and some unusual features. *Pediatr Radiol* 1982; 12:119.

Duddy MJ, Calder CJ: Cystic hemangioma of the spleen: Findings on ultrasound and computed tomography. *Br J Radiol* 1989; 62:180.

Franquet T, Montes M, Lecumberri FJ: Hydatid disease of the spleen: imaging findings in nine patients. AJR 1990; 154:525.

Goerg C, Schwerk WB, Goerg K, et al: Sonographic patterns of the affected spleen in malignant lymphoma. *JCU* 1990; 18:569.

Goerg C, Schwerk WB, Goerg K: Sonography of focal lesions of the spleen. AJR 1991; 156:949.

Gore RM, Shkolnik A: Abdominal manifestations of pediatric leukemias: Sonographic assessment. *Radiology* 1982; 143:207.

Hahn PF, Weissleder R, Stark DD, et al: MR imaging of focal splenic tumors. AJR 1988; 150:823.

Harris RD, Simpson W: MRI of splenic hemangioma associated with thrombocytopenia. *Gastrointest Radiol* 1989; 14:308.

Johnson MA, Cooperberg PL, Boisvert J, et al: Spontaneous splenic rupture in infectious mononucleosis: Sonographic diagnosis and follow-up. AJR 1981; 136:111.

Keidl CM, Chusid MJ: Splenic abscesses in childhood. *Pediatr Infect Dis J* 1989; 8:368.

King DJ, Dawson AA, Bayliss AP: The value of ultrasonic

scanning of the spleen in lymphoma. *Clin Radiol* 1985; 36:473.

Kuykendall JD, Shanser JD, Sumner TE, et al: Multimodal approach to diagnosis of hamartoma of the spleen. *Pediatr Radiol* 1977; 5:239.

Magid D, Fishman EK, Siegelman SS: Computed tomography of the spleen and liver in sickle cell disease. *AJR* 1984; 143:245.

Miller JH, Greenfield LD, Wald BR: Candidiasis of the liver and spleen in childhood. *Radiology* 1982; 142:375.

Okada J, Yoshikawa K, Uno K, et al: Increased activity on radiocolloid scintigraphy in splenic hamartoma. *Clin Nucl Med* 1990; 15:112.

Orduna M, Gonzalez de Orbe G, Gordillo MI, et al: Chronic granulomatous disease of childhood. Report of two cases with unusual involvement of the gastric antrum and spleen. *Eur J Radiol* 1989; 9:67.

Pastakia B, Shawker TH, Thaler M, et al: Hepatosplenic

candidiasis: wheels within wheels. *Radiology* 1988; 166:417.

Pawar S, Kay CJ, Gonzalez R, et al: Sonography of splenic abscess. *AJR* 1982; 138:259.

Rao BK, AuBuchon J, Lieberman LM, et al: Cystic lymphangioma of the spleen: a radiologic-pathologic correlation. *Radiology* 1981; 141:781.

Rose SC, Kumpe DA, Manco-Johnson ML: Radiographic appearance of diffuse splenic hemangiomatosis. *Gastrointest Radiol* 1986; 11:342.

Siniluto T, Paivansalo M, Lahde S: Ultrasonography of splenic metastases. *Acta Radiol* 1989; 30:463.

Strijk SP, Wagener DJ, Bogman MJ, et al: The spleen in Hodgkin disease; diagnostic value of CT. *Radiology* 1985; 154:753.

Younger KA, Hall CM: Epidermoid cyst of the spleen: A case report and review of the literature. *Br J Radiol* 1990; 63:652.

SECTION 2

The Pancreas

The pancreas contains both exocrine and endocrine glandular tissue. The exocrine functions are directed toward digestion with secretions exiting through the pancreatic duct into the duodenum. The islets of Langerhans are the endocrine tissues containing several types of hormone-producing cells.

ANATOMY AND EMBRYOLOGY

The pancreas lies transversely in the midabdomen. It is divided into head, body, and tail (Fig 24–13). The head is in the right midabdomen situated in the curve of the duodenum. At the junction of the inferior and left borders of the pancreatic head is a prolongation called the uncinate process. The anterior surface of the head is in contact with the transverse colon, the gastroduodenal artery, and several loops of small intestine. The anterior surface of the uncinate process is in contact with the superior mesenteric artery and vein. The posterior surface of the head is adjacent to the IVC, the common bile duct, the renal veins, and the aorta.

The body of the pancreas is in contact with the

stomach anterosuperiorly. Its posterior portion abuts the aorta, splenic vein, left kidney and adrenal gland, and the origin of the superior mesenteric artery. The small intestine lies inferior to the body. The tail is narrower in adults than the head or body and lies in the phrenicolienal ligament in contact with the gastric surface of the spleen and the splenic flexure of the colon.

The pancreas arises from two anlagen. The dorsal part develops from a diverticulum of the dorsal aspect of the duodenum caudal to the hepatic diverticulum. It grows upward and backward into the dorsal mesogastrium, forming part of the head and the entire body and tail. The ventral pancreatic bud is a diverticulum from the primitive bile duct and forms part of the head and the uncinate process. The two portions fuse abut the sixth week of embryonic life. The duct from the dorsal bud becomes the accessory pancreatic duct while that from the ventral bud enlarges to become the main duct after it fuses with the distal two thirds of the dorsal duct. The opening of the accessory duct is often obliterated.

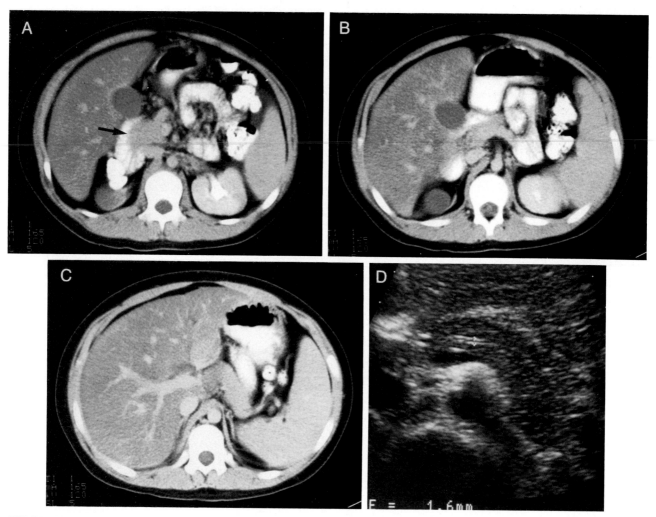

FIG 24–13.
Normal pancreas in an 11-year-old boy. **A,** the head of the pancreas *(arrow)* is slightly bulbous and is in contact with the contrast-filled duodenal sweep. **B,** the body of the pancreas is narrower than the head or tail and is seen anterior to the aorta from which the superior mesenteric artery is arising. **C,** the tail of the pancreas is thicker in children than in adults and extends to the spleen. **D,** transverse sonogram demonstrates the double track of a normal pancreatic duct.

IMAGING THE PANCREAS

The pancreas itself is not seen on plain films. Calcifications present in patients with chronic pancreatitis or cystic fibrosis (CF) may be identified on plain films of the abdomen (Fig 24–14). A pancreatic mass may be sufficiently large to displace adjacent gas-filled portions of the gastrointestinal tract.

Ultrasound usually provides good visualization of the pancreas in children since the relatively large left lobe of the liver can be used as an acoustic window. The pancreas is most easily seen if the stomach and duodenum are not dilated with gas. Several hours of fasting or decompression by nasogastric tube give optimal results. The body of the pancreas can be located anterior to the splenic vein. The tail is relatively larger in children than in adults and usually larger than the body. Siegel et al. have developed normal measurements of the pancreas according to age (Table 24–1). Ueda found that pancreatic size correlated best with body height but that there is sufficient individual variation that caution must be used in determining pancreaticomegaly. Teele and Share concluded that enlargement of the pancreas should be diagnosed when the anteroposterior (AP) dimension of the body is greater than 1.5 cm. The normal duct may be seen as a single- or double-track echogenic line anterior to the junction of the splenic and mesenteric veins (see Fig 24–13,D). There is a spectrum of pancreatic echogenicity relative to that of the liver, but in most children the pancreas is nearly isoechogenic with the liver. Walsh et al. report normally increased pancreatic echogenicity in neonates, especially prematures.

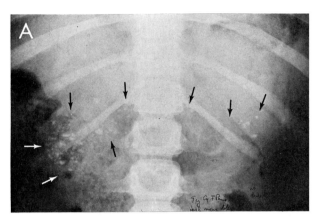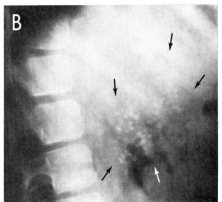

FIG 24–14.
Cystic fibrosis in a 9-year-old girl with multiple pancreatic calcifications seen in AP **(A)** and lateral **(B)** projections.

Computed tomography of the pancreas is much less frequently indicated than sonography but has value in certain diseases, especially tumors and pseudocysts with uncommon features. The pancreas is best visualized on CT during bolus injection of intravenous contrast material which readily identifies the adjacent vessels and with good gastrointestinal contrast to opacify the adjacent stomach and duodenum. The pancreas has lower attenuation than the liver both with and without intravenous contrast use. Since the pancreas in children is oblique to axial planes, multiple thin slices may be necessary for optimal visualization on CT.

Magnetic resonance imaging of the pancreas in children is more difficult than in adults because of adjacent gas-filled loops of intestine and motion artifact from peristalsis and respiration. The pancreas normally has signal intensity equal to that of liver on T1- and T2-weighted spin-echo images with mid–field strength magnets. Pancreatic images produced with high field strength magnets may have greater signal intensity than liver. To some degree, the signal will vary with age. Although normal children do not have as much intrapancreatic fat as adults, there is more fat in the pancreatic septa of postadolescent children than is found in preadoles-

cents. The value of MR of the pancreas is enhanced by the use of breath-holding techniques, generally not possible in younger children, fat suppression sequences, and contrast enhancement. Relatively few studies of these techniques are available in children, however.

Endoscopic retrograde cholangiopancreatography (ERCP) is useful in directly identifying the pancreatic duct. It is much less commonly performed in children than in adults. When ERCP is performed for evaluation of the common bile duct, a more common indication in children than pancreatic disease, the pancreatic duct is also visualized, and related or incidental abnormalities can be identified.

DEVELOPMENTAL AND HEREDITARY ABNORMALITIES

Pancreas divisum occurs when the dorsal and ventral ducts fail to fuse although the pancreas is otherwise anatomically normal. This anomaly has been described in 6% to 10% of adults undergoing ERCP; its true incidence is probably at the high end of this range. There may be a higher incidence of pancreatitis in patients with pancreas divisum although the most recent literature refutes this claim. Reports of CT examination of adults with pancreas divisum and pancreatitis demonstrate enlargement of both ducts in addition to the characteristic findings of pancreatitis (see below). Further enlargement of the duct can be provoked with pre-CT secretin stimulation. Increased thickness of the pancreatic head has been described. Zeman et al. reported that thin-section CT demonstrated the unfused ducts in 5 of 12 patients while two distinct pancreatic moieties separated by a fat cleft could be seen in 4 patients.

Congenital short pancreas occurs when the portion of the pancreas derived from the dorsal embryonic

TABLE 24–1.
Normal Sonographic Dimensions of the Pancreas in Childhood*

Age	Head†	Body†	Tail†
<1 mo	1.0 ± 0.4	0.6 ± 0.2	1.0 ± 0.4
1 mo–1 yr	1.5 ± 0.5	0.8 ± 0.3	1.2 ± 0.4
1–5 yr	1.7 ± 0.3	1.0 ± 0.2	1.8 ± 0.4
5–10 yr	1.6 ± 0.4	1.0 ± 0.3	1.8 ± 0.4
10–19 yr	2.0 ± 0.5	1.1 ± 0.3	2.0 ± 0.4

*Modified from Siegel MJ, Martin KW, Worthington JL: *Radiology* 1987; 165:15.
†Maximum anteroposterior dimension (cm) ± SD.

bud is absent and only that smaller portion derived from the ventral anlagen is present. The anomaly has been described in patients with the polysplenia syndrome. Only a globular pancreatic head can be identified on CT.

Ectopic pancreatic tissue is found most commonly in the stomach, duodenum, appendix, and in Meckel diverticulum. Ueda et al. described a noncommunicating gastric duplication cyst which contained ectopic pancreatic ducts and islets without acinae.

Annular pancreas in children is most frequently diagnosed at birth because of associated duodenal obstruction (see Chapter 52). However, in 50% of cases, the diagnosis is made beyond infancy. Several theories of embryonic dysgenesis have been put forth. Most suggest some form of rotational anomaly of the ventral bud, which may be bifid. The pancreatic annulus, the portion surrounding the duodenum, frequently has a separate duct entering the duodenum opposite the ampulla of Vater. Duodenal contents may reflux through this duct into the annulus. Forty percent of affected patients have associated duodenal stenosis or atresia; this is the group presenting in infancy. Many other associated abnormalities have been described, the most common being intestinal malrotation, tracheoesophageal fistulas, cardiac abnormalities, and anal atresia. These associated lesions are most common in patients who also have trisomy 21. Annular pancreas has also been described in the de Lange syndrome, with partial situs inversus, and as a cause of extrahepatic biliary obstruction. Pancreatitis affecting solely the annulus has been reported in adults.

Cystic fibrosis causes exocrine pancreatic insufficiency in 80% of affected patients. As is the case with the biliary ductules, the pancreatic ductules contain goblet cells which produce thickened mucus leading to obstruction. In young patients with CF, sonography shows pancreatic enlargement, but chronic obstruction ultimately results in shrinkage of the gland with increased echogenicity secondary to fatty infiltration and fibrosis (Fig 24–15). CT shows a shrunken pancreas with reduced attenuation secondary to fatty infiltration. Fibrosis without fatty infiltration is found infrequently. Unenhanced scans may show pancreatic calcifications. Ductal dilatation may be present and pancreatic cysts may be identified (Fig 24–16). In the MR study by Tham et al., 9 of 17 patients had an enlarged, lobulated pancreas with fatty infiltration, 5 had an atrophic pancreas with fatty infiltration, 1 had atrophy without fatty replacement, and 2 were normal. In a series of 18 patients who underwent MR, Murayama et al.

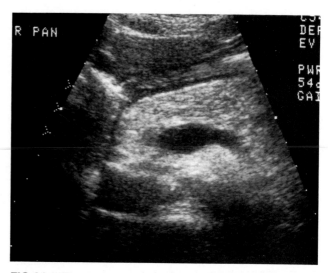

FIG 24–15.
Markedly echogenic pancreas in an 18-year-old woman with fatty infiltration of the pancreas secondary to cystic fibrosis.

found 12 with high signal intensity on T1-weighted spin-echo images indicative of fatty replacement, 3 with low signal intensity, and 3 normals. Their results corresponded well with the clinical stage.

Schwachman syndrome is an autosomal recessive disorder resulting in short stature, exocrine pancreatic insufficiency, a metaphyseal chondrodysplasia (see Chapter 44), and bone marrow dysfunction. Sonographic and CT evaluation of the pancreas demonstrates the same changes described above in patients with cystic fibrosis.

Von Hippel–Lindau syndrome is an autosomal dominant disorder characterized by hemangioblastomas of multiple organs, especially the retina and CNS, skin lesions, and cysts of numerous organs, including the pancreas. The pancreatic lesions are usually multiple (Fig 24–17). Mucinous cystadenomas of the pancreas have also been reported. The cysts are typically anechoic on US and have reduced attenuation on CT compared with the surrounding pancreatic tissue. Pancreatic calcifications can be seen on unenhanced CT scans. Adenocarcinoma occurs in affected adults. *Hereditary pancreatitis* is an autosomal dominant disease in which patients have recurrent episodes of pancreatitis. The findings are described below. *Beckwith-Wiedemann syndrome* is probably an autosomal dominant disorder and is characterized by visceromegaly, hemihypertrophy, and the development of malignant tumors in 10% to 15% of affected patients. Cross-sectional imaging studies may show nonspecific pancreatic enlargement. Patients may develop pancreatoblastoma or nesidioblastoma as discussed below under Pancreatic Neoplasms. *Congenital cysts* of the pancreas are

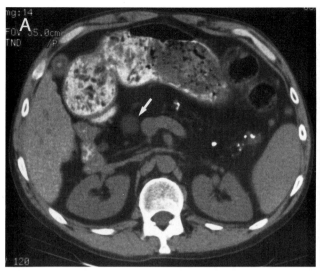
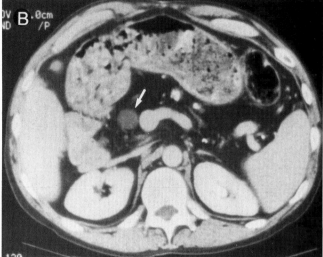

FIG 24–16.
Cystic fibrosis in a 19-year-old man with marked atrophy and fatty replacement of the pancreas. A large cyst *(arrow)* is present in the pancreatic head as seen on unenhanced **(A)** and enhanced **(B)** CT scans. Extensive mesenteric fat is seen secondary to steroid therapy in this patient who had a heart-lung transplant 6 months before this examination.

rare and often confused with omental or mesenteric cysts when large (Fig 24–18).

ACUTE PANCREATITIS

Acute pancreatitis is uncommon in childhood, possibly because the most frequently seen predisposing factors in adults, alcoholism and cholelithiasis, are rarely found in children. Weizman and Durie reported their experience in 61 children with acute pancreatitis. The most common etiology was multisystem disease including Reye syndrome, sepsis, shock, hemolytic-uremic syndrome, and viral infec-

tions. Mumps has been specifically implicated as an etiologic viral agent. Other causes included blunt trauma in 15%, congenital anatomical abnormalities in 10%, metabolic diseases in 10%, and drug toxicity in 3% of patients. No cause was identified in 25% of patients.

Anatomical abnormalities associated with pancreatitis include pancreas divisum (see above) and choledochal cyst. The latter may cause pancreatitis because of the abnormal insertion of the common bile duct into the pancreatic duct (see Chapter 23) which may permit reflux of bile into the pancreas. Associated metabolic disorders include hypercalce-

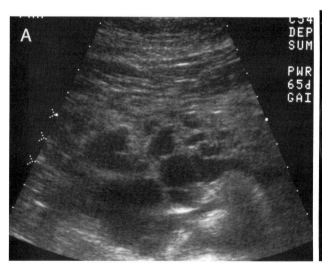
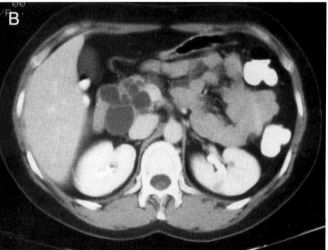

FIG 24–17.
Von Hippel-Lindau syndrome in a young woman caused multiple pancreatic cysts well demonstrated on sonography **(A)** and CT **(B).**

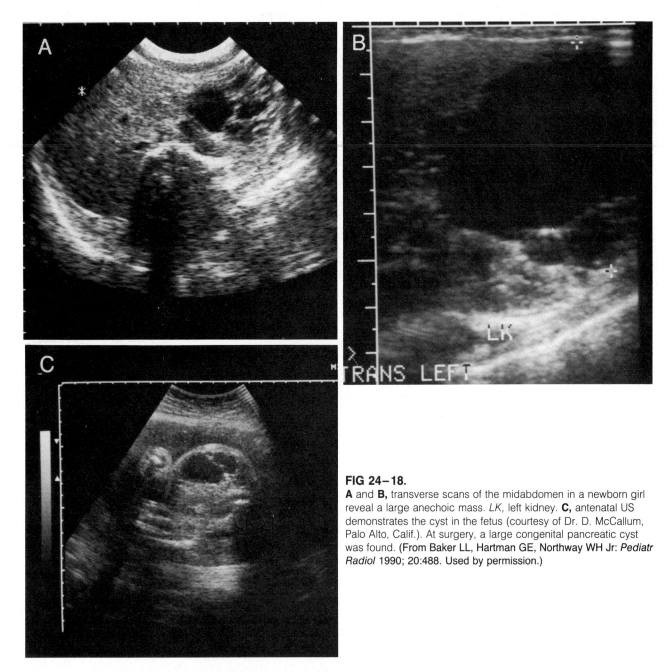

FIG 24–18.
A and **B,** transverse scans of the midabdomen in a newborn girl reveal a large anechoic mass. *LK,* left kidney. **C,** antenatal US demonstrates the cyst in the fetus (courtesy of Dr. D. McCallum, Palo Alto, Calif.). At surgery, a large congenital pancreatic cyst was found. (From Baker LL, Hartman GE, Northway WH Jr: *Pediatr Radiol* 1990; 20:488. Used by permission.)

mia, hyperlipidemia, and cystic fibrosis, while drugs implicated most frequently in the etiology are L-asparaginase, steroids, and acetaminophen. Lee et al. reported an increased incidence of biliary sludge in their adult patients with pancreatitis. They implicated the sludge as a probable cause of idiopathic acute pancreatitis in as many as 70% of affected patients.

Patients with nontraumatic acute pancreatitis typically present with abdominal pain, most frequently in the epigastrium. Nausea and vomiting are frequent companion symptoms. Elevation of serum concentrations of pancreatic enzymes (amylase, lipase, trypsinogen) is common, but not invariable,

so imaging studies may be useful in helping to confirm the diagnosis.

Plain film findings are nonspecific, but certain findings are suggestive. Reactive ileus of nearby gastrointestinal structures may lead to air-fluid levels in stomach and duodenum, focal dilatation of the duodenal sweep, and dilatation of the transverse colon ending abruptly at the splenic flexure. Left pleural effusion may occur. Although ascites is common, rarely is there an amount sufficient to appreciate on plain abdominal radiographs.

US is the imaging procedure of choice for evaluation of possible pancreatitis. Jeffrey has empha-

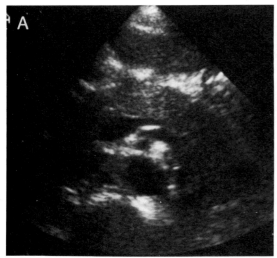
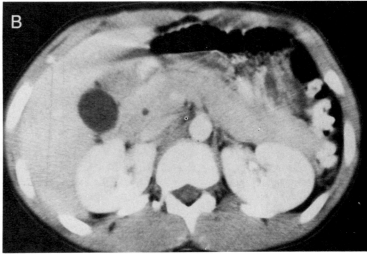

FIG 24–19.
A, transverse sonogram in an 11-year-old boy with idiopathic acute pancreatitis. The body of the pancreas is enlarged and mildly hypoechoic consistent with edema. **B,** CT scan confirms the swelling of the pancreas and demonstrates mild ductal dilatation in the pancreatic head.

sized the value of semierect and coronal scans as well as the standard scanning planes for optimal evaluation of the diseased pancreas. The edema that accompanies acute pancreatitis often results in a hypoechoic gland which is diffusely enlarged (Fig 24–19). A minority of affected patients will have increased pancreatic echogenicity (Fig 24–20,A) while some will have a normal-appearing pancreas. The pancreatic duct may be dilated but this is an inconstant finding, especially when the gland is markedly swollen, causing compression of the duct. Masses may be identified in the pancreas representing focal areas of fluid, hemorrhage, or phlegmon formation. The last is a focal inflammatory mass that is hypoechogenic. Ascites is usually identified.

The presence of acute fluid collections in the peripancreatic areas is useful evidence of acute pancreatitis. The most commonly involved areas are the lesser sac, anterior pararenal space, transverse mesocolon, and perirenal space. US is excellent at demonstrating these fluid collections. Fluid collections may be found as distant from the pancreas as the mediastinum and the inguinal regions. Fluid and inflammation may involve the adjacent splenic vein. Doppler examination is useful to rule out splenic vein thrombosis.

CT is not usually necessary for diagnosis although it may show pancreatic abnormalities to better advantage than US in difficult cases. The findings mirror those seen with US and include pancre-

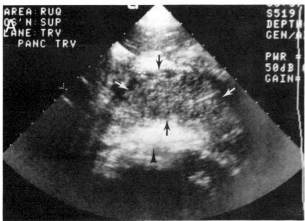
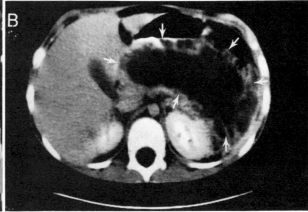

FIG 24–20.
Acute pancreatitis in a 7-year-old girl. **A,** transverse sonogram reveals a thickened pancreas *(arrows)* with a coarse hyperechoic pattern. **B,** CT scan 3 weeks later shows the large pseudocyst *(arrows)* which developed in the interim.

atic swelling, ductal dilatation, mass effect from phlegmon or hemorrhage, peripancreatic fluid collections, thickening of adjacent fascial planes, and ascites. Abscesses are particularly well delineated on CT. Balthazar et al. used dynamic CT scanning to evaluate necrosis in adults with acute pancreatitis. Necrosis was diagnosed when all or part of the gland did not show enhancement. Patients with necrosis had a higher rate of morbidity, mortality, and complications than those without necrosis. ERCP is excellent for examination of the pancreatic duct but is infrequently needed in children. It is a useful examination for evaluation of complicated or recurrent pancreatitis or in cases of unusual pseudocyst formation. The findings range from mild irregularity of the duct to ductal narrowing with acinar enlargement, which has been likened to a string of beads. Marked ductal ectasia is usually not seen in acute pancreatitis.

Pseudocyst formation is a potential complication of pancreatitis regardless of etiology (Fig 24–20,B). Although most pseudocysts are in the region of the pancreas itself (Fig 24–21), they may appear nearly anywhere in the abdomen and in the mediastinum (Figs 24–22 and 24–23). In adults, approximately 5% of patients with acute pancreatitis will develop pseudocysts. Although most pseudocysts resolve spontaneously, some will persist and require surgical intervention. Pseudocysts may be large enough to identify on plain films. They frequently cause a mass effect on adjacent structures, especially the stomach and duodenum, which may be identified on upper gastrointestinal studies performed for unexplained abdominal pain. Sonography is indicated

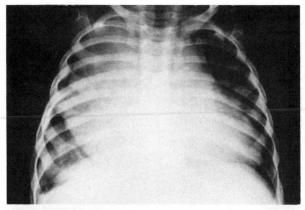
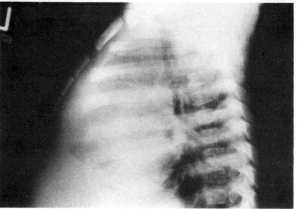

FIG 24–22.
Mediastinal pancreatic pseudocyst in a 10-month-old girl who presented with wheezing and tachypnea. (**Courtesy of Dr. S. Kirchner, Nashville.**)

when a pseudocyst is suspected. Pseudocysts are typically anechoic although some may contain debris. Their effect on adjacent organs may be identified on sonograms but is seen to better advantage with CT. ERCP usually shows the irregular ductal dilatation of chronic inflammation. Successful percutaneous drainage of pseudocysts has been achieved.

Skeletal changes, particularly bone marrow infarcts, have been long recognized as a complication of pancreatitis possibly related to increased levels of circulating lipase and to generalized enzymatic dysfunction of the pancreas. Plain films generally show late changes with characteristic medullary calcification. Haller et al. described MR findings which preceded radiographic findings in an adult.

CHRONIC PANCREATITIS

Chronic pancreatitis in children is even rarer than acute pancreatitis. Although it occurs as a sequela of the acute form, chronic pancreatitis can be found in association with other diseases. The findings in cystic fibrosis are discussed above. Familial hereditary

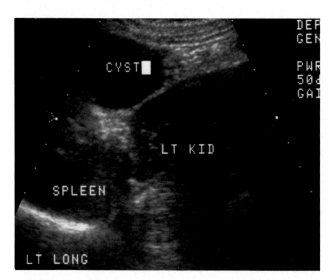

FIG 24–21.
Sonogram of a pancreatic pseudocyst in an adolescent girl demonstrates its intrapancreatic location adjacent to spleen and kidney.

pancreatitis is an autosomal dominant disease in which most patients present in childhood or during their teen-age years. Ductal dilatation (Fig 24–23,G), pseudocysts, and calcifications are the most commonly identified imaging abnormalities in chronic pancreatitis. Spencer et al. described a 2-year-old boy with abdominal pain and a large pancreatic hemorrhagic mass who was found to have chronic pancreatitis at surgery. Subsequent abdominal US of the patient's mother revealed pancreatic ductal dilatation and calcifications. Chronic fibrosing pancreatitis is characterized by bands of collagen enclosing normal acini. The result is a mass effect which simulates a tumor. Chronic pancreatitis may result in jaundice secondary to biliary duct stricture.

PANCREATIC NEOPLASMS

Pancreatic tumors, both benign and malignant, are very rare in childhood. Hormonally active tumors arise from the islet cells and may be benign or malignant. The B cells produce insulin; A cells produce glucagon; G cells, gastrin; D cells, somatostatin; and D_1 cells, vasoactive intestinal peptide (VIP) as well as secretin. Islet cell tumors are named after the hormone produced. Insulinoma is the most commonly found islet cell tumor in children. Gastrinomas may be found in children with Zollinger-Ellison syndrome. According to Grosfeld et al., 2 of 56 reported cases of VIP-producing tumors in children were islet cell tumors. Neurogenic tumors generated the hormone in the other patients. Glucagonomas and somatostatinomas have not been reported in children. Islet cell tumors may be found in association with tumors in other organs as part of the several multiple endocrine neoplasia (MEN) syndromes.

Patients with insulinoma present with hypoglycemia, typically manifested in children by erratic behavior and seizures. The symptoms are relieved by intravenous glucose administration and reproduced

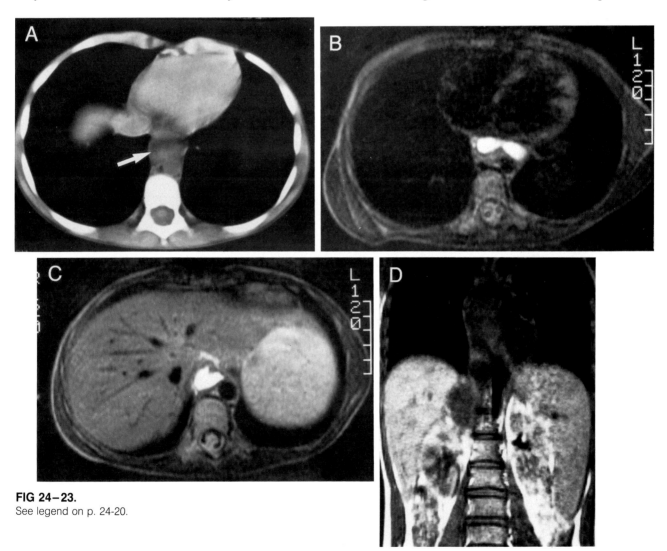

FIG 24–23.
See legend on p. 24-20.

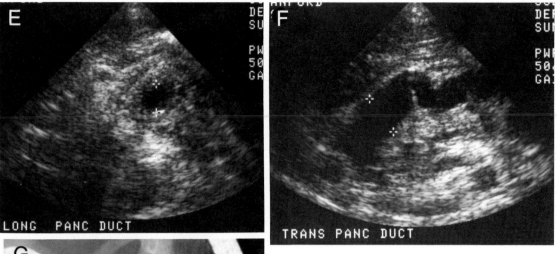

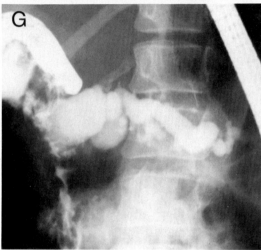

FIG 24–23 (cont.).
Mediastinal infiltration of a pancreatic pseudocyst. **A,** CT scan through the lower chest demonstrates a fluid-filled mass *(arrow)* anterior to the descending aorta. Axial T2-weighted MR scans through the lower mediastinum **(B)** and thoracoabdominal junction **(C)** demonstrate the fluid content of the mass. **D,** coronal T1-weighted MR scan demonstrates the low signal intensity mass extending from a position superior to the right kidney into the posterior mediastinum. Longitudinal **(E)** and transverse **(F)** sonograms of the midabdomen demonstrate marked dilatation of the pancreatic duct. **G,** ERCP demonstrates the dilated pancreatic duct characteristic of chronic pancreatitis.

with fasting under controlled circumstances. In Synn's series, only 3 of 12 pediatric patients with profound hypoglycemia had identifiable islet cell tumors. The others had islet cell hyperplasia or nesidioblastosis on histologic examination of specimens resulting from partial pancreatectomy. Islet cell tumors are round or oval and well circumscribed on sonography. They are hypoechoic but may have a hyperechoic rim, according to Rossi et al. Isoechoic and hyperechoic lesions have been described in children and young adults. They may be superficial or deep in the pancreas. CT can be useful since contrast enhancement may cause marked increased attenuation in the tumors. Since the tumors are hypervascular, arteriography may be necessary in high-risk patients in whom US and CT are nondiagnostic. Intraoperative US has been used successfully to locate functioning islet cell tumors in children. Brunelle et al. have performed transhepatic venous sampling in children with hyperinsulinism. Fifteen of 19 patients had elevated insulin levels when sampling of the portal, splenic, superior mesenteric, in-

ferior mesenteric, and pancreatic collateral veins was accomplished.

The exocrine tissues of the pancreas give rise to benign and malignant tumors which are hormonally inactive. Cystadenomas and adenocarcinoma of the pancreas occur in children and have even been described in infants. Bowlby described pancreatic adenocarcinoma in an adolescent male with Peutz-Jeghers syndrome. Giardiello et al. described a 100-fold increased risk of pancreatic adenocarcinoma in patients with this syndrome. The solid tumors are typically hyperechoic while the cystic lesions are anechoic or hypoechoic. Adenocarcinomas may have cystic or hemorrhagic areas resulting in mixed echogenicity. CT usually identifies a pancreatic mass of variable size often causing obstruction of the bile duct. Since the diagnosis of pancreatic carcinoma is so rare in children, only about 50 cases having been reported, imaging evaluation is often delayed, and metastases to lymph nodes and liver may be noted on CT. Rhabdomyosarcoma may arise primarily in the pancreas, as may lymphoma. Neuroblastoma has been reported in the pancreas secondary to direct extension.

Pancreatoblastoma arises from the pancreatic acinar cells usually in the head or tail of the gland. They represent persistence of the fetal anlage of the acinar cells. They are often large at presentation (up to 12 cm) with areas of central necrosis. US and CT findings are indistinguishable from adenocarcinoma. Stephenson et al. described the MR findings in a 2-year-old boy with pancreatoblastoma. T1-weighted spin-echo images showed low signal intensity while T2-weighted images had very high signal intensity. Although the findings were nonspecific, they suggested the malignant nature of the tumor and clearly excluded the kidney and adrenal glands as organs of origin.

REFERENCES

The Pancreas

Imaging the Pancreas

Allendorph M, Werlin SL, Geenen JE, et al: Endoscopic retrograde cholangiopancreatography in children. *J Pediatr* 1987; 110:206.

Herman TE, Siegel MJ: CT of the pancreas in children. AJR 1991; 157:375.

Lawson TL, Berland LL, Foley WD, et al: Ultrasonic visualization of the pancreatic duct. *Radiology* 1982; 144:865.

Siegel MJ, Martin KW, Worthington JL: Normal and abnormal pancreas in children: US studies. *Radiology* 1987; 165:15.

Teele RL, Share JC: *Ultrasonography of Infants and Children.* Philadelphia, WB Saunders. 1990, pp 389–404.

Ueda D: Sonographic measurement of the pancreas in children. *JCU* 1989; 17:417.

Walsh E, Cramer B, Pushpanthan C: Pancreatic echogenicity in premature and newborn infants. *Pediatr Radiol* 1990; 20:323.

Developmental and Hereditary Abnormalities

Baggott BB, Long WB: Annular pancreas as a cause of extrahepatic biliary obstruction. *Am J Gastroenterol* 1991; 86:224.

Baker LL, Hartman GE, Northway WH Jr: Sonographic detection of congenital pancreatic cysts in the newborn: Report of a case and review of the literature. *Pediatr Radiol* 1990; 20:488.

Choyke PL, Filling-Katz MR, Shawker TH, et al: Von Hippel-Lindau disease: Radiologic screening for visceral manifestations. *Radiology* 1990; 174:815.

Clavon M, Verain AL, Bigard MA: Cyst formation in gastroheterotopic pancreas: Report of two cases. *Radiology* 1988; 169:659.

Daneman A, Gaskin K, Martin DJ, et al: Pancreatic changes in cystic fibrosis: CT and sonographic appearances. AJR 1983; 141:653.

Hernanz-Schulman M, Teele RL, Perez-Atayde A, et al: Pancreatic cystosis in cystic fibrosis. *Radiology* 1986; 629.

Itoh Y, Hada T, Terano A, Itai Y, et al: Pancreatitis in the annulus of annular pancreas demonstrated by the combined use of computed tomography and endoscopic retrograde cholangiopancreatography. *Am J Gastroenterol* 1989; 84:961.

Kilman WJ, Berk RN: The spectrum of radiographic features of aberrant pancreatic rests involving the stomach. *Radiology* 1977; 123:291.

Lindstrom E, Ihse I: Computed tomography findings in pancreas divisum. *Acta Radiol* 1989; 30:609.

Lindstrom E, Ihse I: Dynamic CT scanning of pancreatic duct after secretin provocation in pancreas divisum. *Dig Dis Sci* 1990; 35:1371.

Liu P, Daneman A, Stringer DA, et al: Pancreatic cysts and calcification in cystic fibrosis. *J Can Assoc Radiol* 1986; 37:279.

Marsh TD, Farach L, Wood BP: Radiological case of the month. Obstructing annular pancreas. *Am J Dis Child* 1990; 144:505.

McHugo JM, McKeown C, Brown MT, et al: Ultrasound findings in children with cystic fibrosis. *Br J Radiol* 1987; 60:137.

Murayama S, Robinson AE, Mulvihill DM, et al: MR imaging of pancreas in cystic fibrosis. *Pediatr Radiol* 1990; 20:536.

Nguyen KT, Pace R, Groll A: CT appearance of annular pancreas: a case report. *J Can Assoc Radiol* 1989; 40:322.

Soulen MC, Zerhouni EA, Fishman EK, et al: Enlargement of the pancreatic head in patients with pancreas divisum. *Clin Imaging* 1989; 13:51.

Tham RTOT, Heyerman HGM, Falke THM, et al: Cystic fibrosis: MR imaging of the pancreas. *Radiology* 1991; 179:813.

Ueda D, Taketazu M, Itoh S, et al: A case of gastric duplication cyst with aberrant pancreas. *Pediatr Radiol* 1991; 21:379.

Willi UV, Reddish JM, Teele RL: Cystic fibrosis: Its characteristic appearance on abdominal sonography. AJR 1980; 134:1005.

Zeman RK, McVay LV, Silverman PM, et al: Pancreas divisum: thin-section CT. *Radiology* 1988; 169:395.

Acute and Chronic Pancreatitis

Albu E, Buiumsohn A, Lopez R, et al: Gallstone pancreatitis in adolescents. *J Pediatr Surg* 1987; 22:960.

Amundson GM, Towbin RB, Mueller DL, et al: Percutaneous transgastric drainage of the lesser sac in children. *Pediatr Radiol* 1990; 20:590.

Atkinson GO Jr, Wyly JB, Gay BB Jr, et al: Idiopathic fibrosing pancreatitis: A cause of obstructive jaundice in childhood. *Pediatr Radiol* 1988; 18:28.

Balthazar EJ, Robinson DL, Megibow AJ, et al: Acute pancreatitis: value of CT in establishing prognosis. *Radiology* 1990; 174:331.

Crombleholme TM, deLorimier AA, Adzick NS, et al: Mediastinal pancreatic pseudocysts in children. *J Pediatr Surg* 1990; 25:843.

Crombleholme TM, deLorimier AA, Way LW, et al: The modified Puestow procedure for chronic relapsing pancreatitis in children. *J Pediatr Surg* 1990; 25:749.

Fleischer AC, Parker P, Kirchner SG: Sonographic findings of pancreatitis in children. *Radiology* 1983; 146:151.

Ford EG, Hardin WD Jr, Mahour GH, et al: Pseudocysts of the pancreas in children. *Am Surg* 1990; 56:384.

Garel L, Brunelle F, Lallemand D, et al: Pseudocysts of the pancreas in children: Which cases require surgery? *Pediatr Radiol* 1983; 13:120.

Haller J, Greenway G, Resnick D, et al: Intraosseous fat necrosis associated with acute pancreatitis: MR imaging. *Radiology* 1989; 173:193.

Huntington DK, Hill MC, Steinberg W: Biliary tract dilatation in chronic pancreatitis: CT and sonographic findings. *Radiology* 1989; 172:47.

Jefferey RB Jr: Sonography in acute pancreatitis. *Radiol Clin North Am* 1989; 27:5.

Jeffrey RB Jr, Laing FC, Wing VW: Extrapancreatic spread of acute pancreatitis: New observations with real-time US. *Radiology* 1986; 159:707.

Lee SP, Nicholls JF, Park HZ: Biliary sludge as a cause of acute pancreatitis. *N Engl J Med* 1992; 326:589.

Millward SF, Breatnach E, Simpkins KC, et al: Do plain films of the chest and abdomen have a role in the diagnosis of acute pancreatitis? *Clin Radiol* 1983; 34:133.

Sadry F, Hausen H: Fatal pancreatitis secondary to iatrogenic intramural hematoma: A case report and review of the literature. *Gastrointest Radiol* 1990; 15:296.

Slovis TL, von Berg VJ, Mikelic V: Sonography in the diagnosis and management of pancreatic pseudocysts and effusions in childhood. *Radiology* 1980; 135:153.

Sonnenberg E, Wittich GR, Casola G, et al: Percutaneous drainage of infected and noninfected pancreatic pseudocysts: experience in 101 cases. *Radiology* 1989; 170:757.

Spencer JA, Lindsell DRM, Isaacs D: Hereditary pancreatitis: early ultrasound appearances. *Pediatr Radiol* 1990; 20:293.

Stoler J, Biller JA, Grand RJ: Pancreatitis in Kawasaki disease. *Am J Dis Child* 1987; 141:306.

Suarez F, Bernard O, Gauthier F, et al: Bilio-pancreatic common channel in children: Clinical, biological and radiological findings in 12 children. *Pediatr Radiol* 1987; 17:206.

Swischuk LE, Hayden CK Jr: Pararenal space hyperechogenicity in childhood pancreatitis. *Am J Roentgenol* 1985; 145:1085.

Weizman Z, Durie PR: Acute pancreatitis in childhood. *J Pediatr* 1988; 113:24.

Wheatley MJ, Coran AG: Obstructive jaundice secondary to chronic pancreatitis in children: Report of two cases and review of the literature. *Surgery* 1988; 104:863.

Ziegler DW, Long JA, Philippart AI, et al: Pancreatitis in childhood. *Ann Surg* 1988; 207:257.

Pancreatic Neoplasms

Bowlby LS: Pancreatic adenocarcinoma in an adolescent male with Peutz-Jeghers syndrome. *Hum Pathol* 1986; 17:97.

Brenner RW, Sank LI, Kerner MB, et al: Resection of a VIPoma of the pancreas in a 15-year-old girl. *J Pediatr Surg* 1986; 21:983.

Brunelle F, Negre V, Barth MO, et al: Pancreatic venous samplings in infants and children with primary hyperinsulinism. *Pediatr Radiol* 1989; 19:100.

Galiber AK, Reading CC, Charboneau JW: Localization of pancreatic insulinoma: comparison of pre- and intraoperative ultrasound with CT and angiography. *Radiology* 1988; 166:405.

Giardiello FM, Welsh SB, Hamilton SR, et al: Increased risk of cancer in the Peutz-Jeghers syndrome. *N Engl J Med* 1987; 316:1151.

Grant CS, Heerden J, Charboneau W: Insulinoma: the value of intraoperative ultrasonography. *Arch Surg* 1988; 123:843.

Grosfeld JL, Vane DW, Rescorla FJ, et al: Pancreatic tumors in childhood: Analysis of 13 cases. *J Pediatr Surg* 1990; 25:1057.

Hecht ST, Brasch RC, Styne DM: CT localization of occult secretory tumours in children. *Pediatr Radiol* 1982; 12:67.

Moynan RW, Neehout RC, Johnson TS: Pancreatic carcinoma in childhood. Case report and review. *J Pediatr* 1964; 65:711.

Robey G, Daneman A, Martin DJ: Pancreatic carcinoma in a neonate. *Pediatr Radiol* 1983; 13:284.

Rossi P, Allison DJ, Bezzi M: Endocrine tumors of the pancreas. *Radiol Clin North Am* 1989; 27:129.

Stephenson CA, Kletzel M, Seibert JJ, et al: Pancreatoblastoma: MR appearance. *J Comput Assist Tomogr* 1990; 14:492.

Sty JR, Wells RG: Other abdominal and pelvic masses in children. *Semin Roentgenol* 1988; 23:216.

Synn AY, Mulvihill SJ, Fonkalsrud EW: Surgical disorders of the pancreas in infancy and childhood. *Am J Surg* 1988; 156:201.

Telander RL, Charboneau JW, Haymond MW: Intraoperative ultrasonography of the pancreas in children. *J Pediatr Surg* 1986; 21:262.

Yakovac WC, Baker L, Hummeler K: Beta cell nesidioblastosis in idiopathic hypoglycemia of infancy. *J Pediatr* 1971; 79:226.

The Esophagus

SECTION 1

Normal Esophagus

NORMAL ANATOMY

The esophagus is a musculomembranous tubular structure extending from the distal hypopharynx at the level of the seventh cervical vertebra to the esophagogastric junction, normally at the level of the tenth thoracic vertebra. The caliber of the esophagus varies with peristaltic activity but is usually slightly narrower at both ends than during most of its intrathoracic course. Normal extrinsic impressions on the esophagus are caused by the aorta and the left main-stem bronchus. The esophagus frequently deviates slightly to the right at the level of the left atrium just before entering the esophageal hiatus of the diaphragm. The course and topographic relationships of the esophagus are shown in Figures 25–1 and 25–2.

METHODS OF EXAMINATION

Standard fluoroscopic and radiographic examination using opaque contrast media continue to be the primary imaging modalities used in evaluation of the esophagus. Radiation dose has been reduced by the use of videofluoroscopy instead of cinefluoroscopy and by the use of 100-mm and 105-mm spot-film cameras in place of standard spot-film devices and conventional film-screen combinations. Further dose reduction can be achieved by the use of digital fluoroscopy, but at substantially increased financial cost.

Infants and small children generally require immobilization for optimal results. Various commercial devices are available, but they may make patient rotation under the fluoroscope difficult. We have achieved excellent results by immobilizing the arms

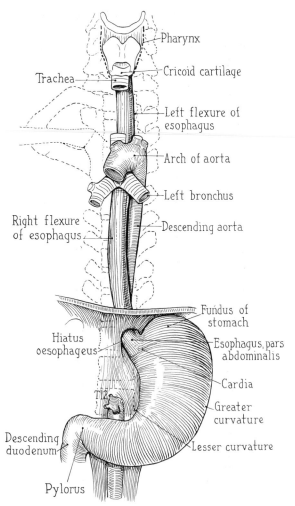

FIG 25–1.
Semischematic drawing of the normal esophagus shows its relation to the trachea, aorta, diaphragm, and stomach. (Modified from *Morris's Human Anatomy*, ed 10. New York, McGraw-Hill, 1943.)

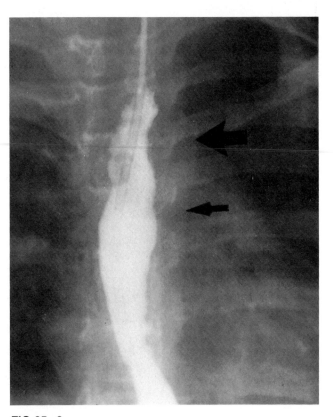

FIG 25–2.
Barium swallow demonstrates the impression of the aortic knob *(large arrow)* and the left main-stem bronchus *(small arrow)* on the barium-filled esophagus. These are normal impressions and are not to be confused with mediastinal abnormalities.

above the head with a soft towel and using a similar restraint for the lower extremities. Gonadal shielding is mandatory. A large lead shield on the fluoroscopic table also helps shield parents or personnel who may help in restraining the patient's lower extremities.

Barium suspensions are still the contrast media of choice unless esophageal perforation or tracheoesophageal fistula is suspected, or there is a high probability of aspiration. The typically small amounts of contrast medium aspirated secondary to unexpected swallowing dysfunction, reflux, and tracheoesophageal fistulas are usually cleared naturally from the normal airway with coughing. Nevertheless, careful fluoroscopic monitoring and small doses of oral contrast should be used at the initiation of the examination to preclude aspiration of significant amounts of contrast material. When barium is contraindicated, low-osmolar nonionic contrast media are safer than ionic media although substantially more expensive.

Evaluation of swallowing function should always be part of an esophageal imaging study. The infant should be fed by a bottle and nipple for this part of the study, and video-tape and spot-film images obtained in lateral projection (Fig 25–3). If the infant will not take barium from the nipple, a feeding tube can be inserted through the nipple into the baby's mouth and controlled injections made on the back of the tongue to initiate swallowing (Fig 25–4). If the patient does not ingest sufficient contrast material for evaluation of the esophagus distal to the base of the tongue, the remainder of the examination should be performed through a nasoesophageal tube. Generally, an 8F feeding tube is satisfactory. Smaller-caliber tubes do not permit rapid injection of sufficient volume. Video taping of the esophagus in anteroposterior (AP), lateral, and oblique projections should be performed. We further limit radiation by taking spot films only if an abnormality is identified.

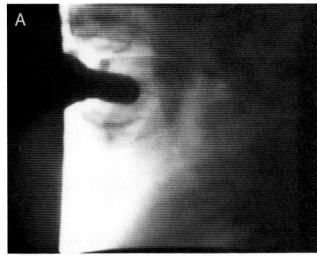

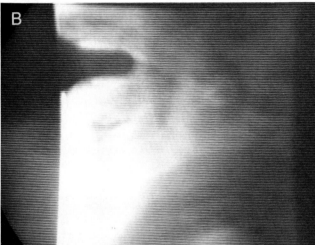

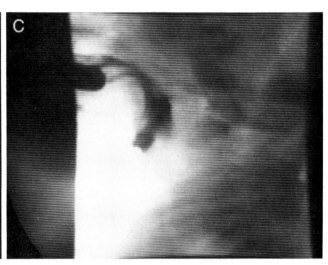

FIG 25–3.
Normal swallowing. **A,** as the nipple is inserted into the infant's mouth, the tongue and soft palate are relaxed and the nasopharynx open. **B,** at the initiation of suck, the tongue elevates, pushing the nipple to the roof of the mouth, and the soft palate elevates, closing off the nasopharynx. **C,** the initial swallow shows barium outlining the underside of the hard palate and soft palate, the posterior aspect of the base of the tongue, and entering the vallecula.

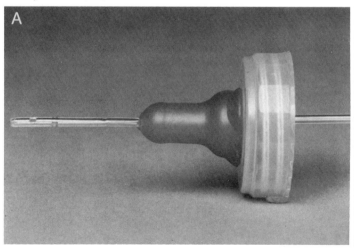

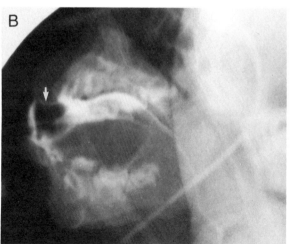

FIG 25–4.
A, No. 8 Silastic feeding tube is placed through a nipple so that a controlled injection can be made into the mouth and the swallowing mechanism observed. **B,** barium outlines the nipple *(arrow)* and the tube. (Modified from Poznanski A: *Radiology* 1969; 93:1106.)

Double contrast esophagography is difficult to perform in patients less than 8 years of age. Younger patients, even those who are otherwise cooperative, will usually let the gas escape by eructation before satisfactory films can be obtained. However, as demonstrated by Levine et al., the double contrast examination is most useful in patients with mucosal lesions, such as infectious esophagitis, which occur more commonly in older children (Fig 25–5). Unplanned double contrast esophagus studies frequently are obtained in infants who cry, swallow air, and eructate during the examination. Nuclear medicine and ultrasound (US) studies can be used to identify gastroesophageal reflux and are described in Section Five.

NORMAL ROENTGENOGRAPHIC APPEARANCE

Although radiologists have historically paid primary attention to anatomy, physiology, and pathologic conditions of the esophagus itself, the importance of pharyngeal and esophageal motility disorders requires an understanding of the anatomy and physiology of the pharynx as well. The three components of the pharynx are the nasopharynx, the oropharynx, and the hypopharynx (see Figs 5–1 and 5–2). The nasopharynx and oropharynx communicate through the velopharyngeal portal. Through a highly complex, coordinated neuromuscular mechanism, the portal closes during both speech and swallowing, although the specific neurologic pathways are different during these two physiologic functions. The hypopharynx extends from the velopharyngeal portal to the level of the larynx, including the epiglottis.

The oral phase of swallowing occurs when the patient chews and mixes food with saliva. This phase is very rapid during the injection of liquid contrast material, but the thrust of the tongue forward and superiorly can be seen. The bolus is transported quickly to the pharyngeal inlet along the dorsum of the tongue by extremely complicated peristaltic-like activity of the tongue muscles (see Fig 25–3,C).

During the pharyngeal phase of swallowing, numerous muscles contract in rapid progression to propel the bolus and elevate the soft palate, protecting the nasopharynx from reflux. The larynx and hyoid bone can be seen elevating secondary to the action of muscles which contract to seal off the oropharynx as the bolus is propelled into the cervical esophagus. The epiglottis concurrently seals off the trachea.

Over 50 different muscle groups contract during the oral and pharyngeal phases, but the esophageal

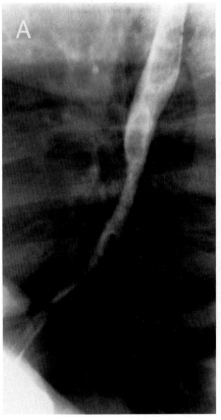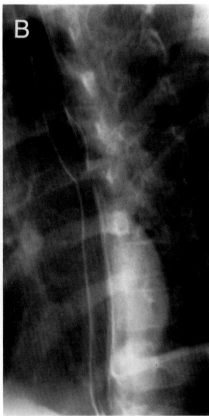

FIG 25–5.
Single **(A)** and double **(B)** contrast esophagogram in a 5-year-old boy six months after lye ingestion demonstrates narrowing of the mid-esophagus with distal aperistalsis. The mucosa is intact.

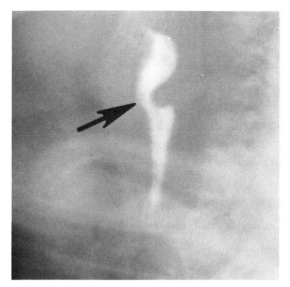

FIG 25–6.
Lateral view of a barium swallow demonstrates a normal posterior impression by the contracted cricopharyngeus muscle. This is a normal variant in a patient who had no swallowing difficulties.

phase of swallowing is relatively simpler. Distention of the cervical esophagus elicits peristalsis. The upper third of the esophagus has a striated muscle layer and effective peristalsis here is most dependent on medullary neural reflexes and the vagus

nerve. Peristalsis in the lower esophagus, with its smooth muscle layer, is independent of the central nervous system and relies predominantly on an intrinsic peristaltic mechanism which is modulated by vagus activity. Although this description is oversimplified, it does explain the variability of peristaltic activity in the upper and lower esophagus which can be seen in a variety of disease states.

The normal thoracic portion of the esophagus shows smooth primary stripping peristaltic waves during the passage of a single large bolus. Since each swallow elicits a new peristaltic wave, the normal peristaltic mechanism will appear interrupted during repetitive swallowing. Tertiary contractions are not seen in the normal infant and child. When older children are studied in the erect position, gravity plays an important role in the passage of contrast material.

On lateral view, the impression of the contracted cricopharyngeus muscle may be seen indenting the cervical esophagus posteriorly (Fig 25–6). Deviation by the aorta and the left atrium, as well as the impression by the left main-stem bronchus, is usually seen (see Fig 25–2).

The course of the esophagus may be affected by spinal and aortic abnormalities such as severe kyphoscoliosis and aortic ectasia. Aortic arch anoma-

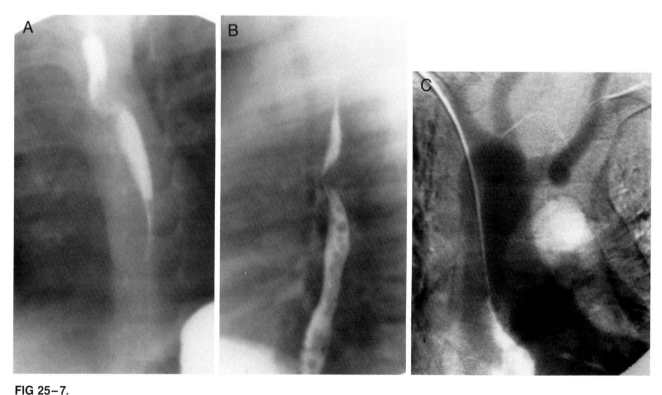

FIG 25–7.
A and **B,** double aortic arch with atrophy of the left arch and aberrant left subclavian artery demonstrates a characteristic posterior impression on the esophagus. **C,** intravenous digital subtraction angiography reveals the anomalous origin of the vessel.

lies (Fig 25–7) such as aberrant vessels, double aortic arch, and right aortic arch, will cause extrinsic effects on the lateral and posterior aspects of the esophagus and are discussed more fully in Chapter 17. Aberrant left pulmonary artery typically causes an anterior extrinsic compression defect (see Chapter 52).

REFERENCES

Belt T, Cohen MD: Metrizamide evaluation of the esophagus in infants. *Am J Roentgenol* 1984; 143:367.

Cohen MD: Choosing contrast media for the evaluation of the gastrointestinal tract of neonates and infants. *Radiology* 1987; 162:447.

Dodds WJ: The physiology of swallowing. *Dysphagia* 1989; 3:171.

Donner MW, Bosma JF, Robertson DL: Anatomy and physiology of the pharynx. *Gastrointest Radiol* 1985; 10:196.

Ginai AZ, Tenkate FJW, Ten Berg RGM, et al: Experimental evaluation of various available contrast agents for use in the upper gastrointestinal tract in case of suspected leakage: Effects on lungs. *Br J Radiol* 1984; 57:895.

Ginai AZ, Tenkate FJW, Ten Berg RGM, et al: Experimental evaluation of various available contrast agents for use in the upper gastrointestinal tract in case of suspected leakage: Effects on mediastinum. *Br J Radiol* 1985; 58:585.

Girdany BR: The esophagus in infancy: Congenital and acquired diseases. *Radiol Clin North Am* 1963; 1:557.

Girdany BR, Lee FA: X-ray examination of the gastrointestinal tract. *Pediatr Clin North Am* 1967; 14:3.

Jones B, Gayler BW, Donner MW: Pharynx and cervical esophagus, in Levine MS (ed): *Radiology of the Esophagus.* Philadelphia, WB Saunders, 1989, pp 311–336.

Kramer SS: Swallowing in children, in Jones B, Donner MW (eds): *Normal and Abnormal Swallowing: Imaging in Diagnosis and Therapy.* New York, Springler-Verlag, 1991, pp 173–188.

Levine MS, Rubesin SE, Ott DJ: Update on esophageal radiology. *Am J Roentgenol* 1990; 155:933.

McAlister WH, Askin FB: The effect of some contrast agents in the lung: an experimental study in the rat and dog. *Am J Roentgenol* 1983; 140:245.

McAlister WH, Siegel MJ: Fatal aspirations in infancy during gastrointestinal series. *Pediatr Radiol* 1984; 14:81.

Sauvegrain J: The technique of upper gastro-intestinal investigation in infants and children, in Kaufman HJ (ed): *Progress in Pediatric Radiology.* Basel, S Karger, 1969, pp 26–51.

SECTION 2

Disorders of Deglutition, the Velopharyngeal Portal, and Peristalsis

Most swallowing disorders in children are secondary to neurologic abnormalities of which cerebral palsy is the most common. Other neuromuscular disorders to be considered are brain-stem dysfunction, cranial nerve abnormalities, intracranial neoplasms, meningomyelocele, muscular dystrophy, and myasthenia gravis. Familial dysautonomia (Riley-Day syndrome) leads to autonomic dysfunction with esophageal dysmotility and frequent aspiration pneumonia. Disorders of the mouth and jaw such as micrognathia and macroglossia may also cause abnormal swallowing. Bulbar polio may be seen in patients who have not been properly immunized.

Depending on the specific neurologic defect, any or all components of the swallowing mechanism may be affected. Some severely damaged infants cannot suck and most of the barium drools out of the mouth. The tongue may not elevate to help initiate the swallowing mechanism. Abnormality of the neuromuscular mechanism elevating the soft palate may lead to reflux of contrast material into the nasopharynx with subsequent drooling and potential aspiration into the airway (Fig 25–8). Abnormalities of other muscle groups lead to defective function of the epiglottis and upper esophageal sphincter with aspiration into the airway being common.

Defective peristalsis may be found in patients with the above-mentioned neurologic disorders as

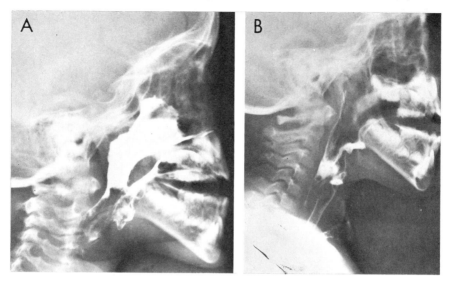

FIG 25–8.
A and **B,** marked reflux of swallowed barium into the nasopharynx secondary to neurogenic dysfunction of the muscles controlling the normal elevation of the soft palate.

well as in patients with connective tissue disorders and esophagitis. Patients with a history of repaired esophageal atresia frequently show abnormal peristalsis in the portion of the esophagus distal to the repair. Staiano et al. performed a manometric study demonstrating disordered motility in patients with colonic aganglionosis. Patients with disordered esophageal motility may show aperistalsis or hypoperistalsis with or without tertiary contractions (Fig 25–9). The latter are more common in cases of esophagitis, including those secondary to gastroesophageal reflux.

Specialized radiographic studies of deglutition in association with occupational therapists have been

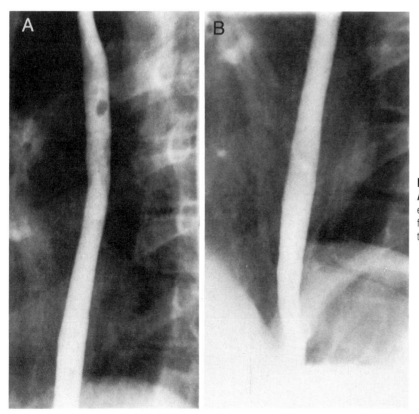

FIG 25–9.
A and **B,** "standing column" of barium in the esophagus of a patient who was aperistaltic following repair for esophageal atresia and tracheoesophageal fistula.

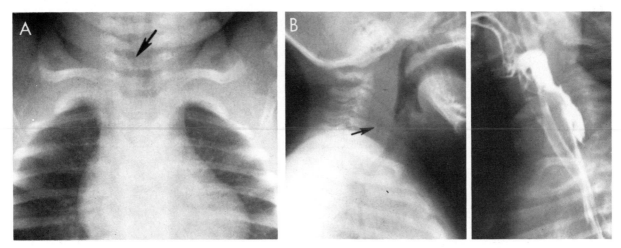

FIG 25–10.
Traumatic diverticulum of the pharynx in an infant 2 months of age who had a history of hematemesis and dysphagia. **A,** anteroposterior (AP) film of the thorax: the *arrow* shows a small collection of gas to the right of the trachea. **B,** lateral films with and without barium esophagogram; the *arrow* shows gas in the prevertebral soft tissues. The pseudodiverticulum is filled with barium and extends into the prevertebral soft tissues. The infant had had an apneic spell following which the father put his finger into the infant's mouth to pull the tongue forward and perforated the posterior portion of the pharynx.

popularized by the Johns Hopkins Swallowing Center. The patient is placed in the position in which he or she is usually fed. Contrast medium is mixed with increasingly thicker food mixtures from liquid barium to solid food mixed with barium. Video taping in the lateral projection allows evaluation of the patient's ability to handle differently textured foods and is of enormous value in planning appropriate diet.

Cricopharyngeal achalasia, failure of relaxation of the cricopharyngeus muscle, has been thought to be a primary cause of dysphagia. Most experts now agree that primary cricopharyngeal achalasia is probably uncommon. Secondary cricopharyngeal achalasia has been reported following trauma and in patients with autoimmune collagen disorders such as scleroderma and dermatomyositis. The results of studies from the Johns Hopkins Swallowing Center suggest that most cases of cricopharyngeal achalasia are secondary to gastroesophageal reflux (GER).

Direct pharyngeal trauma is an uncommon cause of disordered swallowing but may be seen after instrumentation, especially the passage of endotracheal, nasogastric, or orogastric tubes (Fig 25–10; see also Figs 52–15, 52–19). Disordered peristalsis may be seen in patients with obstructive lesions such as strictures and achalasia. Dysphagia with disordered esophageal motility may be seen in psychogenic disorders (globus hystericus) but many of these patients eventually have an organic lesion found. The diagnosis of psychogenic dysphagia should be made only after an exhaustive investigation, especially of the central nervous system, fails to make a diagnosis of an underlying organic disorder.

Retropharyngeal masses are rare causes of dysphagia. Hemangiomas, teratomas, lymphangiomas (cystic hygromas), and lymphomas may occur at different ages. Retropharyngeal abscesses (Fig 25–11) have other symptoms which usually lead to the cor-

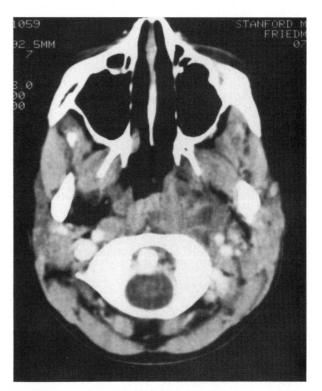

FIG 25–11.
Pharyngeal abscess in a 7-year-old girl with dysphagia, fever, and cervical lymphadenopathy. CT scan demonstrates a left parapharyngeal and prevertebral mass with a characteristic low-attenuation area in the middle.

rect diagnosis. Congenital pharyngeal diverticula are quite rare. Spinal anomalies may rarely cause dysphagia in children.

Scleroderma and mixed collagen disorders are rare in childhood, most frequently occurring in older adolescents and teenagers. Pharyngeal and cervical esophageal function is usually normal. Esophageal dysmotility typically begins at the level of the aortic arch where the esophageal muscle layer begins to change from striated to smooth muscle. Poor to absent primary peristalsis occurs in the distal two thirds of the esophagus. Resulting esophageal reflux, with or without esophagitis, may occur.

Dermatomyositis, on the other hand, primarily affects the striated muscle of the pharynx and upper esophagus. Dilatation of these structures frequently occurs as does reflux into the nasopharynx. The associated vasculitis may result in esophageal ulceration and perforation.

VELOPHARYNGEAL INCOMPETENCE

Disorders of the velopharyngeal portal are most commonly seen during evaluation of speech disorders. Although technically simple to perform, these studies are not part of the repertoire of most radiologists. They are most useful in patients being considered for cleft palate surgery and for those with speech disorders secondary to neurologic abnormalities. Because the muscles used in speech and swallowing are largely similar, useful information can be obtained from speech studies. The studies are feasible in most patients aged 5 years or older and can be performed in cooperative children as young as 3. The patient is placed in an upright lateral position. A small amount of barium is injected into the nose to coat the soft palate for easier visualization. Combined audio-video recording is obtained while the patient repeats a series of words and phrases de-

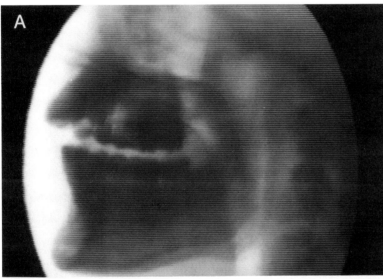

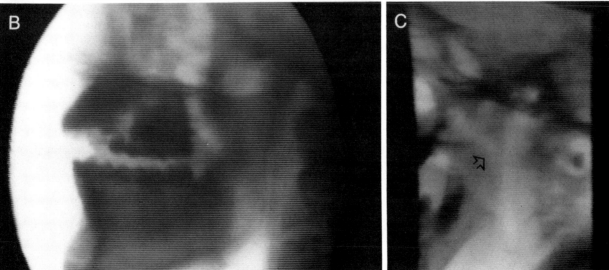

FIG 25–12.
Videofluorography during speech. **A,** during quiet breathing, the soft palate is relaxed and the nasopharyngeal air column is open. **B,** during phonation, the soft palate is elevated and extends posteriorly, completely closing off the nasopharyngeal air column. **C,** in a younger patient with severe nasal speech, the soft palate forms a normal right angle *(arrow)*, but does not close off the patent nasopharyngeal air column, leading to resonant speech.

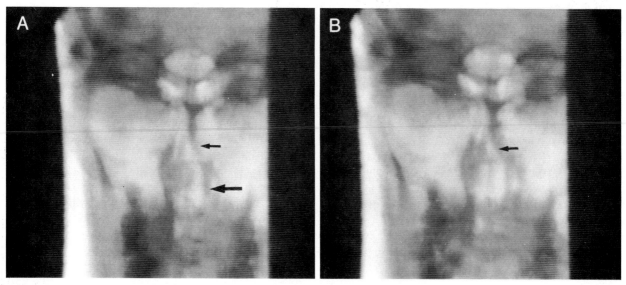

FIG 25–13.
Videofluorography in the modified Towne projection. **A,** during quiet breathing, the nasopharyngeal air column *(small arrow)* and the oropharyngeal air column *(large arrow)* are well demonstrated.

B, during speech, the nasopharyngeal air column *(arrow)* is reduced in diameter, but does not close completely in this patient with nasal speech.

signed to maximize function of the pharyngeal muscles. During speech, the soft palate should elevate, becoming nearly horizontal in its proximal two thirds (Fig 25–12). The distal one third remains roughly vertical and should make contact with the posterior pharyngeal wall throughout its course. The motion of the tongue can also be evaluated.

The procedure is then repeated with the patient's head in a modified Towne projection, allowing direct visualization of the oropharynx and nasopharynx (Fig 25–13). Skolnick and Cohn recommend doing this portion of the study with the patient prone, but we have found younger patients more tolerant of the procedure if kept in a sitting or standing position. The nasopharyngeal walls are seen to function during speech like the iris of a camera. In patients with velopharyngeal incompetence, failure of normal excursion of the soft palate and the muscular pharyngeal side walls is identified. A barium swallow completes the examination and is evaluated for nasopharyngeal reflux and fistulous communication between the oropharynx and nasopharynx. Speech studies have also proved quite valuable in the evaluation of patients following surgical repair of cleft palate. The study is quite useful in differentiating primary neuromuscular lesions, such as those seen in central nervous system disorders, from structural lesions, such as those in patients with craniofacial anomalies.

REFERENCES

Fisher SE, Painter M, Milmoe G: Swallowing disorders in infancy. *Pediatr Clin North Am* 1981; 28:845.

Gyepes MT, Linde LM: Familial dysautonomia: The mechanism of aspiration. *Radiology* 1968; 91:471.

Kramer SS: Special swallowing problems in children. *Gastrointest Radiol* 1985; 10:241.

Kramer SS: Radiologic examination of the swallowing impaired child. *Dysphagia* 1989; 3:117.

La Rossa D, Brown A, Cohen M, et al: Video-radiography of the velopharyngeal portal using the Towne's view. *J Maxillofac Surg* 1980; 8:203.

Skolnick ML: Video velopharyngography in patients with nasal speech, with emphasis on lateral pharyngeal motion in velopharyngeal closure. *Radiology* 1969; 93:747.

Skolnick ML, Cohn ER: *Videofluoroscopic Studies of Speech in Patients With Cleft Palate.* New York, Springer-Verlag, 1989.

Staiano A, Corazziari E, Andreotti MR, et al: Esophageal motility in children with Hirschsprung's disease. *Am J Dis Child* 1991; 145:310.

Stringer DA, Witzer MA: Velopharyngeal insufficiency on multiview videofluoroscopy: A comparison of projections. *Am J Roentgenol* 1986; 146:15.

Tuchman DN: Cough, choke, sputter: The evaluation of the child with dysfunctional swallowing. *Dysphagia* 1989; 3:111.

SECTION 3

Congenital Malformations

ESOPHAGEAL ATRESIA

Esophageal atresia, with or without tracheoesophageal fistula, is the most important congenital malformation of the esophagus. The varieties of esophageal atresia and tracheoesophageal fistula with their relative incidences are shown in Figure 25–14. The preoperative imaging evaluation of esophageal atresia and tracheoesophageal fistula is discussed in depth in Chapter 52. The preferred surgical repair of esophageal atresia is primary anastomosis of the proximal and distal pouches. When the atretic segment is too long, other approaches have been taken, including colonic interposition. Kleinman et al. described transgastrostomy balloon dilatation of the distal pouch under fluoroscopic control in three patients that enabled a primary anastomosis to be ac-

complished successfully which otherwise would not have been possible.

Most patients with isolated esophageal atresia and tracheoesophageal fistula do well following surgical repair. However, some patients have associated congenital malformations, upon which the ultimate prognosis of the patient depends. The VACTERL association is a mnemonic used to reflect the commonly associated, which are *v*ertebral,*a*nal atresia, *c*ardiac, *t*racheo*e*sophageal fistula, *r*enal, and *l*imb.

Nevertheless, complications following surgical treatment of esophageal atresia do occur and include recurrent fistula, esophageal stenosis, early leaking at the site of anastomosis, esophageal diverticula, and disordered esophageal motility from the site of anastomosis to the esophagogastric junction. Gil-

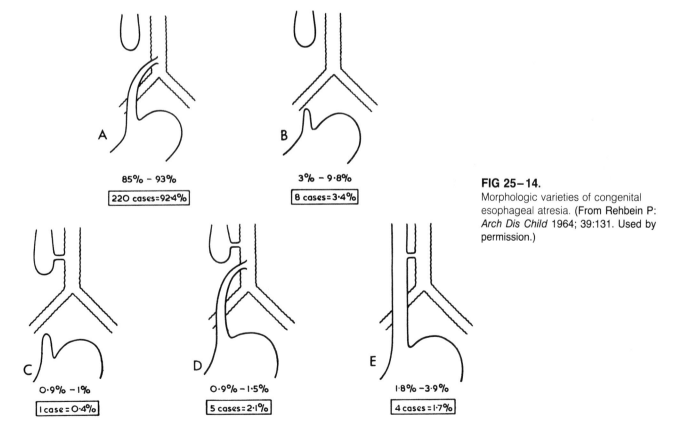

85% – 93%

220 cases=92·4%

3% – 9·8%

8 cases=3·4%

0·9% – 1%

1 case=0·4%

0·9% – 1·5%

5 cases=2·1%

1·8% –3·9%

4 cases=1·7%

FIG 25–14.

Morphologic varieties of congenital esophageal atresia. (From Rehbein P: *Arch Dis Child* 1964; 39:131. Used by permission.)

sanz et al. reported the occurrence of rib fusion and scoliosis as a long-term complication of thoracotomy for esophageal atresia. They suggest that this resulted from undiagnosed anastomotic leakage and mediastinitis.

Most typically, patients undergo gastrostomy at the time of surgical repair and no attempt is made at oral feedings until 1 to 2 weeks following surgery when edema has subsided and the esophagus is presumably patent. Prior to the institution of oral feedings, a contrast study of the esophagus should be performed. The site of anastomosis is readily identified (Fig 25–15). Although there is anatomical narrowing at the anastomotic site, contrast material normally flows readily past this area and the infants generally have no difficulty in tolerating oral liquid feedings.

The most commonly identified early complication of surgical repair is leakage at the site of anastomosis. Although these leaks typically close spontaneously, further surgical intervention may be necessary. An untreated postoperative fistula may lead to diverticulum formation (Fig 25–16). An apparent

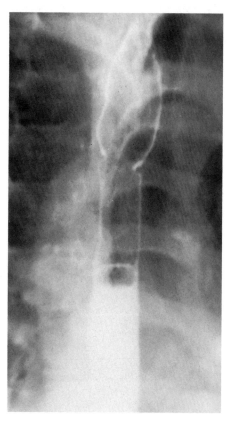

FIG 25–15.
Barium swallow following primary anastomosis of an esophageal atresia demonstrates slight narrowing at the anastomotic site. The patient was asymptomatic and had no difficulty swallowing either fluids or soft solid foods.

slight narrowing at the site of surgical anastomosis may persist for years, even though the patient has no functional problem. True stricture at the site of anastomosis usually leads to symptoms in the weeks following surgery. The dilated, fluid-filled proximal segment of the esophagus may impinge upon and narrow the tracheal lumen leading to cough and cyanosis. Griscom and Martin demonstrated a decrease in cross-sectional area of the trachea in patients with persistent respiratory symptoms 2 to 21 years after repair of esophageal atresia. Overfilling of the upper esophagus may lead to aspiration. Most patients respond to bougienage, and reoperation is infrequently necessary. Recurrent tracheoesophageal fistula may occur following surgery (Fig 25–17,B). These will typically be seen at the surgical site. Postoperative studies may also show a tracheoesophageal fistula that was not identified at the time of surgery. Typically these are proximal to the site of the anastomosis. If an actual stricture occurs at the site of surgical repair, solid food may become impacted (Fig 25–18). This is particularly true if the patient is fed hot dogs or similar foods which are difficult to chew completely. Certain dietary restrictions should be followed for several years following surgical repair of esophageal atresia. The most commonly identified abnormality following surgical repair of the esophagus is dysmotility. This finding is present in nearly all patients who have had esophageal atresia. Associated gastroesophageal reflux is very common in these patients and may lead to peptic esophagitis. This is likely the cause of the more distal esophageal strictures which can be seen in patients who have had a history of repaired esophageal atresia. Although hiatal hernia resulting from surgical traction on the lower esophageal segment following anastomosis has been reported, this is an unusual complication following surgery by trained pediatric surgeons.

Other cases of distal stenosis may represent true congenital narrowings if seen shortly after surgery (Fig 25–19). True congenital stenoses of the esophagus are probably less common than has been thought previously. Stenoses and lower esophageal webs probably represent variable manifestations of the same lesion. These congenital stenotic lesions are unlikely to be secondary to failure of proper vacuolization of the embryonically solid esophagus. They are often secondary to tracheoesophageal or gastric remnants (Fig 25–20). Fibromuscular thickening of the esophageal wall has been implicated in a number of cases of congenital stenosis. However, the question as to whether this could be a reaction to previous GER, no longer present, still needs to be

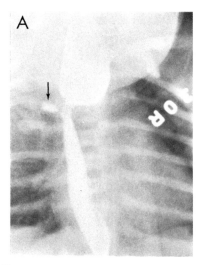
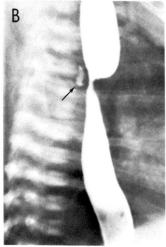
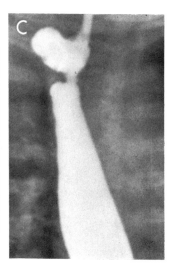

FIG 25–16.
Untreated postoperative fistula and diverticulum formation. A 3-week-old infant who has had repair of an esophageal atresia and tracheoesophageal fistula. **A,** AP and **B,** lateral spot films during fluoroscopy demonstrate a small leak of contrast material into the mediastinum. **C,** esophagogram 3 months later demonstrates a diverticulum at the level of the previously demonstrated mediastinal leakage.

considered. Anderson et al. reported a case of congenital esophageal stenosis secondary to a cartilage ring. Upper cervical esophageal webs are quite rare in children compared with the incidence in adults and are probably congenital in origin.

TRACHEOESOPHAGEAL FISTULAS

Congenital tracheoesophageal fistula without atresia is difficult to identify, both clinically and radiographically. These patients typically present with recurrent pneumonias either in infancy or later in childhood. Patients with unexplained chronic respiratory distress and recurrent pneumonia should always be considered at risk for the presence of a tracheoesophageal fistula, and radiographic examination is warranted.

Congenital tracheoesophageal fistula without atresia has commonly been called an H-fistula because of its appearance on esophagogram connecting the trachea and esophagus. However, the fistula typically runs cephalad from the esophagus to the

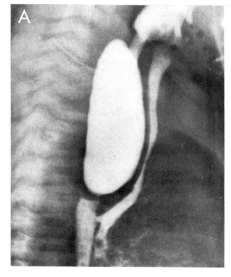
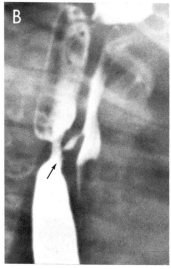

FIG 25–17.
Recurrent tracheoesophageal fistula. **A,** the proximal esophageal pouch is distended with contrast material and overflow aspiration fills the trachea. The trachea is compressed from behind by the dilated proximal portion of the esophagus and its lumen is narrowed. The fistula from trachea to distal esophagus is apparent. **B,** lateral esophagogram demonstrates a recurrent tracheoesophageal fistula *(arrow)* at the site of the original fistula. The fistula had been ligated but not divided.

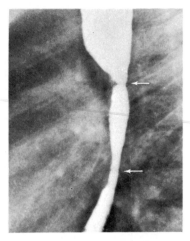

FIG 25–18.
Postoperative stricture. A patient 5 years of age who had had successful primary repair of esophageal atresia and tracheoesophageal fistula. The esophagus is narrow at the site of primary anastomosis *(upper arrow)*. At the junction of its middle and lower thirds *(lower arrow)*, the esophagus is narrow and does not distend normally. Boluses of food had become impacted at this level.

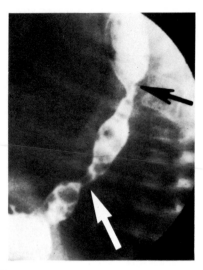

FIG 25–20.
Esophagogram demonstrates stenosis in the distal portion of the esophagus *(lower arrow)* secondary to tracheal remnants. The *upper arrow* identifies narrowing at the level of the primary esophageal anastomosis following repair of esophageal atresia. (Courtesy of Dr. E. Afshani, Buffalo, New York.)

trachea and looks more like an "N" (Fig 25–21). Large fistulas usually present very early in life and are relatively easy to see on esophagogram (Fig 25–22). More commonly, the fistulas are small, inconstantly patent, and may require repeated examinations to identify.

Horizontal-beam fluoroscopy, with the patient lying prone on the footboard with the fluoroscopic table in the upright position, is probably not neces-

sary in most cases. Certainly, such positioning is possible only in infancy. The examination, however, must be performed following passage of a naso-esophageal catheter. A major reason for inconstant patency of the fistula is that the normal esophageal mucosa is quite redundant and usually occludes the esophageal side of the fistula. Normal active swallowing may not distend the esophagus sufficiently

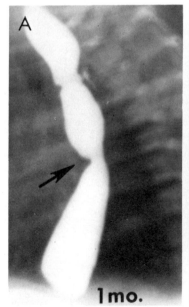

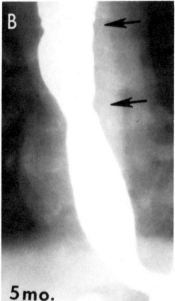

FIG 25–19.
Congenital esophageal stenosis in an infant with surgical repair of esophageal atresia and tracheoesophageal fistula. **A,** a small esophageal mediastinal leak at the anastomotic site is seen poste-riorly. The *arrow* demonstrates a fixed stenotic lesion distal to the site of the repair. **B,** persistent narrowing is seen 5 months later *(lower arrow).*

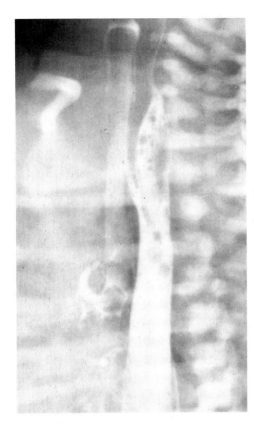

FIG 25–21.
Barium esophagogram demonstrates an N-fistula between the esophagus and trachea. Note that the fistula runs cephalad and obliquely anteriorly from the esophagus to the trachea.

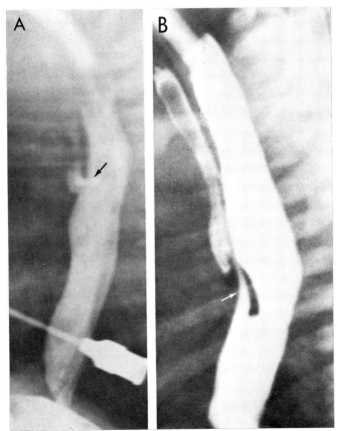

FIG 25–22.
Large congenital tracheoesophageal fistula without esophageal atresia. **A,** the *arrow* points to the fistulous tract extending anteriorly and cephalad toward the tracheal lumen. **B,** a lower tracheoesophageal fistula in a 7-day-old boy with imperforate anus.

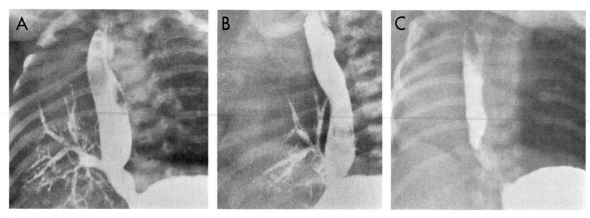

FIG 25–23.
Esophageal bronchus (esophageal lung). **A,** frontal and **B,** oblique films of the thorax of an infant 9 days of age show the right main bronchus originating from the distal end of the esophagus. **C,** the esophagus following right pneumonectomy.

to allow passage of contrast material into the fistula. The patient should be kept in the lateral recumbent position with the right side down. The examiner withdraws the catheter from the distal esophagus cephalad, forcefully injecting contrast material to distend the esophagus maximally under constant fluoroscopic monitoring. If a fistula is present, it will be seen in the lateral projection extending anteriorly and cephalad from the esophagus to the trachea. Slightly oblique views may be necessary to see its full course. Until a fistula is seen, the injection should continue until the catheter is withdrawn into the hypopharynx, but care must be taken not to allow contrast material to spill over into the trachea. The examination should be terminated as soon as a fistula is identified in order to minimize the amount of contrast material leaking into the airway.

Fistulas can be extremely difficult to identify and repetitive examinations may be necessary if the in-

dex of suspicion for the presence of a fistula is high. We have done as many as four esophagograms on patients before finally demonstrating a congenital tracheoesophageal fistula. Although there is a danger of spilling contrast material over into the airway with injection high in the cervical esophagus, it is important to examine this area, since many of the fistulas will occur at the level of the lower cervical or upper thoracic spine. Slow retraction of the catheter and careful fluoroscopic monitoring will prevent overflow into the trachea. Multiple fistulas without atresia have been reported, but are extraordinarily rare. Filston et al. have catheterized tracheoesophageal fistulas per ora, but this method is little used by others.

Rarely, the right main-stem bronchus originates from the esophagus resulting in an anomaly called esophagotrachea or esophageal bronchus (Fig 25–23). This anomaly leads to severe respiratory dis-

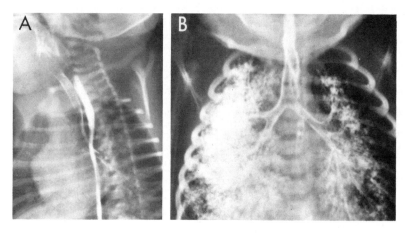

FIG 25–24.
Laryngoesophageal cleft in a 2-week-old infant. **A,** the oblique projection shows barium in the esophagus and in the trachea. **B,** at fluoroscopy, persistent flow of barium into the trachea and bronchi was seen at the level of the larynx. No neuromuscular abnormalities were identified. A small laryngoesophageal cleft was identified endoscopically.

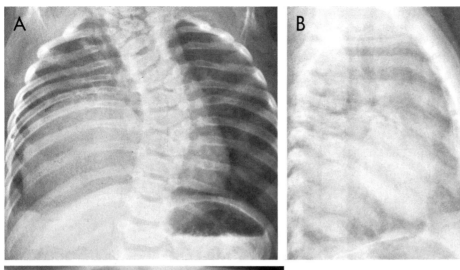

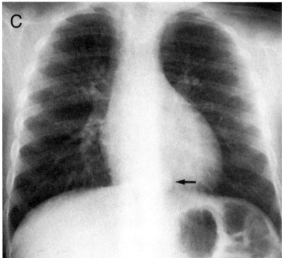

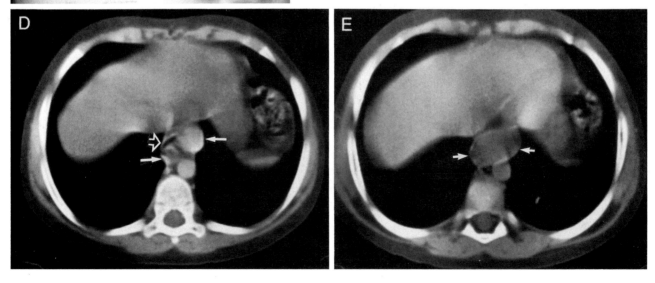

FIG 25–25.
Esophageal duplication. **A,** frontal and **B,** lateral projections of the chest demonstrate a large mass projecting into the right hemithorax. Multiple segmentation abnormalities of the spine are identified. **C,** PA film of a 3⁷/₁₂-year-old boy with leukemia and a mediastinal mass *(arrow).* **D,** and **E,** CT scans demonstrate a cystic mass *(solid arrow)* which does not communicate with the esophagus *(open arrow).* A noncommunicating esophageal duplication cyst was surgically excised.

tress with feeding and may be associated with esophageal atresia tracheoesophageal fistula, or both.

Laryngotracheoesophageal clefts are high fistulous communications between the hypopharynx and larynx. The cleft varies from a small communication between the larynx and esophagus to complete absence of the wall between esophagus and trachea—"persistent esophagotrachea." Patients with clefts present typically in infancy with respiratory distress during feeding. Stridor has been reported. Diagnosis is usually made by endoscopy or by contrast esophagogram (Fig 25–24). Wilkinson et al. reported a case of a complete cleft in which the diagnosis was made by demonstration of a common tracheal and esophageal lumen on computed tomography (CT). The lumen persisted inferiorly to the carina and hypoplasia of the right lung and cardiac dextroposition were also identified.

OTHER CONGENITAL MALFORMATIONS

Cysts and duplications are bronchopulmonary foregut malformations which arise from abnormalities of development, separation, and canalization of the embryonic foregut. The most anteriorly situated of these is the bronchogenic cyst, which is discussed in Chapters 14 and 51.

Enteric cysts, or gastroenteric cysts, arise from the posterior portion of the foregut and contain mucosa which, by histologic examination, is usually gastric or, occasionally, intestinal. Those cysts which also contain neural tissue are known as *neuroenteric cysts*. The latter have connections to the spinal canal and are invariably associated with vertebral anomalies of which the most commonly occurring are segmentation abnormalities. These congenital vertebral anomalies help differentiate neuroenteric cysts from other posterior mediastinal masses such as neuroblastoma. Plain films generally demonstrate a large posterior mediastinal mass, primarily in the right hemithorax, with associated vertebral abnormalities (Fig 25–25). US can confirm the cystic nature of the mass, but magnetic resonance (MR) or other imaging techniques for evaluation of the spinal canal should be obtained to identify associated intraspinal anomalies. Esophagograms will show displacement of the esophagus by the mass but no connection between the two structures. Those enteric cysts which contain gastric mucosa with acid and pepsin secretion can be identified by nuclear imaging. They may ulcerate or hemorrhage leading to draining sinuses in the thoracic wall, esophageal necrosis and perforation, and communication with other intrathoracic structures. Massive hemorrhage from ulceration has been reported.

True tubular duplications (Fig 25–25, *C, D,* and *E*) of the esophagus are even more rare than enteric cysts. They may communicate with the stomach or esophagus and be demonstrable on esophagogram. In the adult patient of Nakabara et al., a large duplication cyst ruptured directly into the esophagus. More commonly, they are asymptomatic or cause dysphagia because of their mass effect on the esophagus. Concomitant vertebral anomalies are not usually present. Hedlund and Bisset described an esophageal duplication cyst with an aberrant right subclavian artery which mimicked a vascular ring.

REFERENCES

Anderson LS, Shackelford GD, Mancilla-Jimenez R, et al: Cartilaginous esophageal ring: A cause of esophageal stenosis in infants and children. *Radiology* 1973; 108:665–666.

Aoki S, Machida T, Sasaki Y, et al: Enterogenous cyst of cervical spine: Clinical and radiological aspects (including CT and MR). *Neuroradiology* 1987; 29:291–293.

Briceno LI, Grases PJ, Gallego S: Tracheobronchial and pancreatic remnants causing esophageal stenosis. *J Pediatr Surg* 1981; 16:731.

Burroughs N, Leape LL: Laryngotracheoesophageal cleft: Report of a case successfully treated and review of the literature. *Pediatrics* 1974; 53:516.

Chang SH, Morrison L, Shaffner L, et al: Intrathoracic gastrogenic cysts and hemoptysis. *J Pediatr* 1976; 88:594.

Chitale AR: Gastric cysts of the mediastinum. *J Pediatr* 1969; 75:104.

Cumming WA, Reilly BJ: Fatigue aspiration. *Radiology* 1972; 105:387.

Dominguez R, Zarabi M, Oh KS, et al: Congenital oesophageal stenosis. *Clin Radiol* 1985; 36:263.

Dudley NE, Phelan PD: Respiratory complications in long-term survivors of oesophageal atresia. *Arch Dis Child* 1976; 51:279.

Filston HC, Rankin JS, Kirks DR: The diagnosis of primary and recurrent tracheoesophageal fistulas: Value of selective catheterization. *J Pediatr Surg* 1982; 17:144.

Fitch SJ, Tonkin ILD, Tonkin AK: Imaging of foregut duplication cysts. *Radiographics* 1986; 6:189–201.

Gilsanz V, Boechat IM, Birnberg FA, et al: Scoliosis after thoracotomy for esophageal atresia. *Am J Roentgenol* 1983; 141:457–460.

Griscom NT: Persistent esophagotrachea: The most severe degree of laryngotracheo-esophageal cleft. *Am J Roentgenol* 1966; 97:211–215.

Griscom NT, Martin TR: Trachea and esophagus after repair of esophageal atresia and distal fistula. *Pediatr Radiol* 1990; 20:447.

Hedlund GL, Bisset GS III: Esophageal duplication cyst and aberrant right subclavian artery mimicking a symptomatic vascular ring. *Pediatr Radiol* 1989; 19:543.

Hemalatha V, Batcup G, Brereton RJ, et al: Intrathoracic foregut cyst (foregut duplication) associated with esophageal atresia. *J Pediatr Surg* 1980; 15:178.

Hernandez RJ: Role of CT in the evaluation of children with foregut cysts. *Pediatr Radiol* 1987; 17:265–268.

Johnson JF, Sneoka BL, Mulligan ME, et al: Tracheoesophageal fistula: Diagnosis with CT. *Pediatr Radiol* 1985; 15:134–135.

Kamoi I, Nishitani H, Oshiumi Y, et al: Intrathoracic gastric cyst demonstrated by ^{99m}Tc pertechnetate scintigraphy. *Am J Roentgenol* 1980; 134:1081.

Kantrowitz LR, Pais MJ, Burnett K, et al: Intraspinal neurenteric cyst containing gastric mucosa: CT and MR findings. *Pediatr Radiol* 1986; 16:324–327.

Kirkpatrick JA, et al: The motor activity of the esophagus in association with esophageal atresia and tracheoesophageal fistula. *Am J Roentgenol* 1961; 86:884.

Kirks DR, Filston HC: The association of esophageal duplication cyst with esophageal atresia. *Pediatr Radiol* 1981; 11:214–216.

Kleinman PK, et al: Atretic esophagus: Transgastric balloon-assisted hydrostatic dilatation. *Radiology* 1989; 171:831.

Lacasse JE, Reilly BJ, Mancer K: Segmental esophageal trachea: A potentially fatal type of tracheal stenosis. *Am J Roentgenol* 1980; 134:829.

McCook TA, Felman AH: Retropharyngeal masses in infants and young children. *Am J Dis Child* 1979; 133:41.

Morgan CL, Grossman H, Leonidas J: Roentgenographic findings in a spectrum of uncommon tracheoesophageal anomalies. *Clin Radiol* 1979; 30:353–358.

Nakahara K, Fujii Y, Shinichiro M, et al: Acute symptoms due to a huge duplication cyst ruptured into the esophagus. *Ann Thorac Surg* 1990; 50:309.

Nakazato Y, Landing BH, Wells TR: Abnormal Auerbach plexus in the esophagus and stomach of patients with esophageal atresia and tracheoesophageal fistula. *J Pediatr Surg* 1986; 21:831.

Nakazato Y, Wells TR, Landing BH: Abnormal tracheal innervation in patients with esophageal atresia and tracheoesophageal fistula: Study of the intrinsic tracheal nerve plexuses by a microdissection technique. *J Pediatr Surg* 1986; 21:838.

Nishina T, Tsuchida Y, Saito S: Congenital esophageal stenosis due to tracheobronchial remnants and its associated anomalies. *J Pediatr Surg* 1981; 16:190.

Osman MZ, Girdany BR: Traumatic pseudodiverticulums of the pharynx in infants and children. *Ann Radiol* 1973; 16:143.

Parker AF, Christie DL, Cahill JL: Incidence and significance of gastroesophageal reflux following repair of esophageal atresia and tracheoesophageal fistula and the need for anti-reflux procedures. *J Pediatr Surg* 1979; 14:5.

Sheridan J, Hyde I: Oesophageal stenosis distal to oesophageal atresia. *Clin Radiol* 1990; 42:274.

Sieber WK, Girdany BR: Tracheo-esophageal fistula without esophageal atresia, congenital and recurrent. *Pediatrics* 1956; 18:935.

Stringer DA, Ein SH: Recurrent tracheo-esophageal fistula: A protocol for investigation. *Radiology* 1984; 151:637–641.

Stringer DA, Pablot SM, Mancer K: Grúntzig angioplasty dilatation of an esophageal stricture in an infant. *Pediatr Radiol* 1985; 15:424–426.

Superina RA, Ein SH, Humphreys RP: Cystic duplications of the esophagus and neurenteric cysts. *J Pediatr Surg* 1984; 19:527–530.

Thomason MA, Gay BB: Esophageal stenosis with esophageal atresia. *Pediatr Radiol* 1987; 17:197.

Toyohara T, Kaneko T, Araki H, et al: Giant epiphrenic diverticulum in a boy with Ehlers-Danlos syndrome. *Pediatr Radiol* 1989; 19:437.

Wilkinson AG, Mackenzie S, Hendry GMA: Complete laryngotracheoesophageal cleft: CT diagnosis and associated abnormalities. *Clin Radiol* 1990; 41:437.

SECTION 4

Acquired Esophageal Lesions

NONINFECTIVE ESOPHAGITIS

The most common cause of esophagitis in children is GER, which is discussed below. *Ingestion of caustic agents* is becoming less common as parents and other caregivers have become more cognizant of the dangers to children of careless storage of household agents. Nevertheless, the effects of caustic ingestion are still commonly seen and can be devastating. Acidic compounds typically affect the stomach while caustic esophagitis is secondary to alkalis, most commonly household lye compounds which are a mixture of sodium and potassium hydroxide. Burns of the mouth may not be seen or may be superficial since the time of contact is short. The upper esophagus is less likely to be affected than the middle or lower portions since transient cardiospasm may increase the time of contact between the agent and the lower esophageal mucosa.

Swelling of the epiglottis (Fig 25–26,*A*) indicates that the caustic agent has reached the hypopharynx and likely has been swallowed into the esophagus. Initial chest radiographs may reveal evidence of me-diastinitis with mediastinal widening and a dilated, gas-filled esophagus. Inflammation of the pharynx may cause disordered swallowing (Fig 25–26,*B*) with subsequent aspiration. Contrast esophagography is preferable to endoscopy since traumatic perforation may occur when a rigid endoscope is used. Spontaneous perforations may occur as may deep ulceration and tracheoesophageal fistulas. Therefore, the initial examination is preferably performed with low-osmolar, nonionic contrast material. If no perforation or fistula is seen, barium will provide better coating for thorough evaluation of the mucosa.

Mucosal irregularity, esophageal dysmotility, and ulceration may all be seen in the acute or sub-acute phase (Fig 25–27). Reactive fibrosis of the esophageal wall may cause the appearance of a stenotic rigid tube on fluoroscopy (Fig 25–28). Ultimately, esophageal stricture develops (Fig 25–29), necessitating esophagectomy and colonic interposition in the worst cases. Epithelial metaplasia (Barrett esophagus) may occur as may development of esophageal carcinoma in adulthood.

Epidermolysis bullosa dystrophica is a congenital

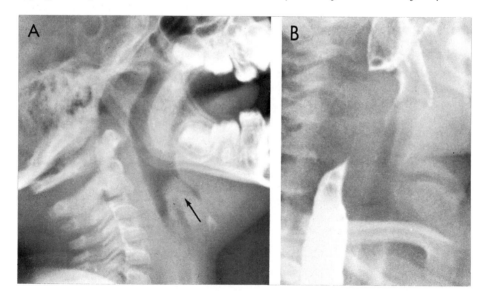

FIG 25–26.
A, lateral view of the nasopharynx demonstrates the epiglottis to be swollen *(arrow)* 20 hours after the injection of caustic material. **B,** barium swallow 2 weeks later demonstrates the proximal seg-ment of the cervical esophagus to be narrow with aspiration of contrast material into the trachea.

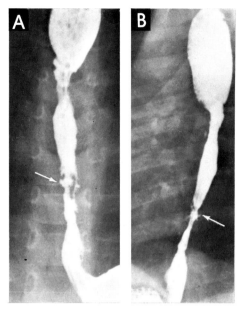

FIG 25–27.
Esophagograms in AP **(A)** and**(B)** lateral projections demonstrate multiple levels of narrowing, irregularity, and marginal ulcerations in a patient 6 weeks following ingestion of lye.

disease affecting squamous epithelium and causing esophagitis. The skin has numerous bullous lesions which are friable and easily abraded with sloughing of the skin even after the most minimal contact. These patients should not be restrained unless supervised by a dermatologist. Every effort must be made to have the child drink spontaneously as even the minimal trauma caused by a Silastic feeding tube may damage the esophageal epithelium. Loss of motility, mucosal irregularity, ulceration, and stenosis

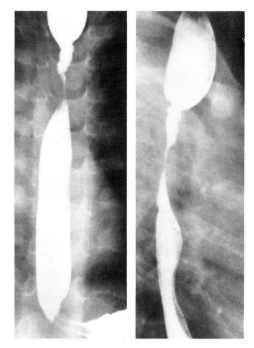

FIG 25–29.
Stricture of the esophagus in a 4-year-old boy 3 weeks after he had swallowed several tablets which contained anhydrous sodium hydroxide and copper sulfite.

may be found in these unfortunate children (Fig 25–30).

Crohn disease of the esophagus is rarely seen on imaging studies but is being described with increasing frequency by endoscopists. Ulceration and stricture are the most common findings. The same finding may be seen in *Behçet disease* which also may cause an ileocolitis resembling Crohn disease. The

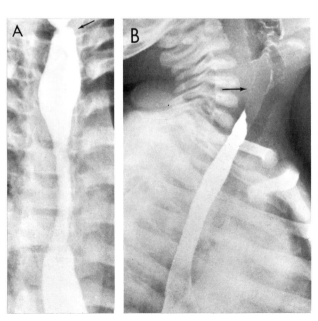

FIG 25–28.
A, AP esophagogram in a 7-year-old boy 5 years following ingestion of lye demonstrates narrowing of the midportion of the esophagus. The *arrow* demonstrates traumatic stricture of the esophagus secondary to multiple attempts at dilatation. **B,** lateral esophagram of the same patient shortly after ingestion of lye. Aspiration of barium into the proximal portion of the trachea and narrowing of the proximal portion of the esophagus are identified *(arrow).*

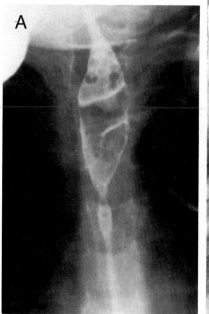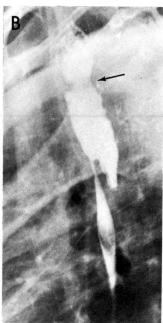

FIG 25–30.
Epidermolysis bullosa dystrophica. **A,** AP view of esophagogram demonstrates focal stricture formation in a 3-year-old girl. **B,** esophagogram in a different patient showing an annular stenosis just below the thoracic inlet *(arrow)*. Below this and posteriorly, a barium-filled pocket suggests an ulcer and submucosal abscess. (Courtesy of Dr. Melvin Becker, New York, N.Y.)

additional multisystem findings of Behçet disease affecting skin, mucous membranes, uvea, and central nervous system can differentiate these two entities, although they are not always present in children. Renner et al. reported three cases of *chronic granulomatous disease* of childhood with esophageal stricture caused by the primary disease rather than by opportunistic infection. McDonald et al. have described the esophageal lesions of *graft-versus-host disease* in patients who underwent bone marrow transplantation. Webs, ringlike narrowing, and smoothly tapering strictures may be seen on barium studies.

Radiation esophagitis from low-dose radiation therapy may be manifested by esophageal inflammation with resultant dysmotility, but rarely produces long-term effects. High-dose (above 25 Gy) radiation therapy is uncommonly used in young children but may lead to dysmotility, mucosal edema, superficial and deep ulceration, and stricture at any age. Similar findings have been described in patients exposed to a variety of chemotherapeutic agents, including antibiotics and quinidine as well as anticancer agents. The combined effects of radiation therapy and doxorubicin (Adriamycin) are especially likely to lead to esophagitis, as well as cardiac and other complications, because of their synergistic actions.

INFECTIVE ESOPHAGITIS

These lesions are usually secondary to opportunistic organisms and are seen in children who are immunocompromised as a result of congenital or acquired immunodeficiency syndromes or from immunosuppressive drugs. The most common infective agent is *Candida albicans (Monilia)* but viral agents such as cytomegalovirus (CMV) and herpes simplex virus may cause esophagitis by themselves or in conjunction with candidiasis. In adult patients with acquired immunodeficiency syndrome (AIDS), esophageal infection from human immunodeficiency virus (HIV) and from mycobacteria has been reported.

Double contrast examinations of the esophagus are more likely to be diagnostic than single contrast studies but these may be difficult to perform in young or uncooperative children. Dysmotility, elevated focal lesions (nodules or plaques), and mucosal edema are the common findings (Fig 25–31). Frank ulcers are more common with herpes and CMV esophagitis (Fig 25–32). Even if cultures are positive for *Monilia,* concomitant viral infection should be suspected if ulcers are seen. The characteristic "shaggy mucosa" of candidiasis is actually nonspecific and may be seen in the viral esophagitides as well.

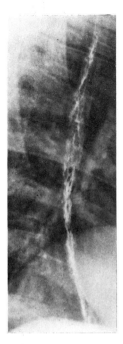

FIG 25–31.
Moniliasis. Esophagogram of a 15-year-old girl with aplastic anemia demonstrates marginal mucosal irregularities. The patient had documented moniliasis.

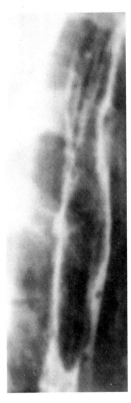

FIG 25–32.
Double contrast esophagogram in a leukemic patient severely immunocompromised by chemotherapy. Dysmotility, irregularity, inflammation, and small ulcers are seen. Esophagitis is due to combined candidiasis and cytomegalovirus infection.

DIVERTICULA

Diverticula of the esophagus proper are rare in children. Pulsion or pressure diverticula are herniations of the mucosa and submucosa through congenitally weak sites of the esophageal wall; little or none of the muscular layer is incorporated into the walls of such diverticula. Simple pressure diverticula are usually located above the clavicles and extend from a lateral wall of the esophagus posteriorly, where, after enlargement, they may displace the esophageal channel anteriorly and compress it. They are best seen in lateral and oblique projections, in which they appear as rounded pouches filled with barium; they fill quickly and empty relatively slowly. Traction diverticula are anterior or lateral projections of the esophageal lumen; their walls may be made up of mucosa alone; usually, however, all of the esophageal mural layers are present. They usually occur just below the tracheal bifurcation and almost always on the anterior wall. The traction is caused by the fibrous contraction of fibrotic lymph nodes and paraesophageal areolar tissue. Roentgenographically, they appear as triangular pouches that empty quickly. They are usually of little clinical importance except that they may be the sites of impaction and perforation of foreign bodies.

FOREIGN BODIES AND TRAUMA

Foreign bodies may be swallowed at any age. Even the youngest infants may be fed unusual articles by an obliging older sibling. Although the older child or parent may give a history of foreign body ingestion, young children often present with unexplained drooling, inability to swallow solids, or, less commonly, chest pain. Radiopaque foreign bodies are easily identified on plain films. Smooth objects, such as coins, the most commonly ingested foreign bodies, usually are seen at the thoracic inlet. Less commonly, they will stop at the level of the left mainstem bronchus or just above the esophagogastric junction. If coins are seen at other levels, underlying esophageal abnormalities should be considered. Sharp objects, pins being the most common, may present anywhere along the course of the esophagus if they penetrate the mucosa (Fig 25–33). Food, plastic and aluminum articles, and buttons are the most common nonopaque esophageal foreign bodies.

Plain films of the chest and neck should be the first imaging examination. Coins in the esophagus lie in the coronal plane (Fig 25–34) while those in the trachea lie in the sagittal plane, presumably because of the anatomy of the tracheal rings. Long-

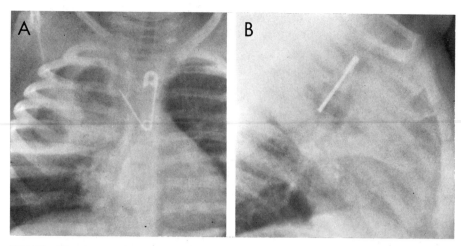

FIG 25–33.
The sharp point of an open safety pin projects through the wall of the esophagus **(A)** and produces inflammatory changes in the adjacent lung and pleura **(B).**

standing foreign bodies may have perforated, leading to pneumomediastinum or mediastinal mass. A foreign body such as incompletely chewed food may cause high-grade obstruction with air-fluid levels in the esophagus or a frothy appearance from mixed air and fluid. Impacted food most often occurs in patients who have underlying esophageal abnormalities.

Nonopaque foreign bodies may require esophagograms for diagnosis. Since the degree of potential obstruction is unknown before the examination, only a small amount of opaque material should be given initially. Spot films should be obtained in AP and lateral views. Contrast studies generally are not performed when an opaque foreign body is identified; however, they may be useful if there is concern about edema, stricture, or perforation. Currarino and Nikaidoh report four cases of foreign bodies in patients with vascular rings and suggest esophagograms be performed if there is clinical suspicion of such an anomaly. Herman and McAlister reported two cases of traumatic diverticula in patients with unsuspected foreign bodies.

The removal of esophageal foreign bodies by radiologists using Foley catheters is a highly contentious subject. The procedure was initially popularized by Campbell and colleagues who reported high success rates with no significant complications. Using their patient selection criteria and methods, many pediatric radiologists enjoyed great success with the procedure which reduced hospital time and financial cost to the patient manyfold. More recent reports, especially in the surgical literature, have raised doubts in the minds of many radiologists as to the wisdom of continuing to remove foreign bodies by this method. We continue to perform the procedure when requested to do so by our surgical colleagues after their—and our—careful evaluation, but we now appear to be in the minority. Nonopaque foreign bodies, identified on esophagogram, can also be removed by this method. In no instance should the procedure be attempted if an underlying esophageal abnormality is present or if edema or other potential complication is identified. In general, balloon-catheter removal is not recommended if the foreign body has been present for 24 hours or longer.

The other common cause of esophageal trauma is from placement of tubes and catheters which may perforate the pharynx or esophagus. Abrupt onset of

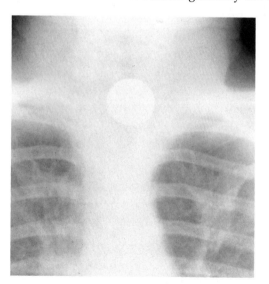

FIG 25–34.
AP view of the thorax demonstrates a coin lodged in the esophagus at the level of the thoracic inlet. Note that the coin lies in the coronal plane, whereas a coin lodged in the trachea would lie in the sagittal plane.

new respiratory symptoms, unusual catheter position, air in the soft tissues of the neck, chest, or mediastinum, and unexplained malfunction of the tube or catheter should lead one to suspect possible perforation. A traumatic pseudodiverticulum may result (see Fig 25–10). Perforation of the strictured esophagus secondary to dilatation therapy is a well-known complication of this procedure. If a contrast study is necessary after inconclusive plain film examination, low-osmolar, nonionic water-soluble contrast material should be used. Uncomplicated perforations usually resolve but strictures may occur.

Severe vomiting may lead to hematemesis, the *Mallory-Weiss syndrome.* Spontaneous esophageal rupture, the *Boerhaave syndrome,* may occur in infants presumably secondary to increased esophageal pressure from any one of several causes and present with hydropneumothorax. Both syndromes are extraordinarily rare in childhood.

REFERENCES

Amoury RA, Hrabovsky EE, Leonidas JC, et al: Tracheo-esophageal fistula after lye ingestion. *J Pediatr Surg* 1975; 10:273–276.

Appelvist P, Salmo M: Lye corrosion carcinoma of the esophagus. *Cancer* 1980; 45:2655.

Balthazar EJ, Megibow AJ, Hulnick D, et al: Cytomegalovirus esophagitis in AIDS: Radiographic features in 16 patients. *Am J Roentgenol* 1987; 149:919–923.

Becker MH, Swinyard CA: Epidermolysis bullosa dystrophica in children: Radiologic manifestations. *Radiology* 1968; 90:124.

Beer S, Avidan G, Viure E, et al: A foreign body in the oesophagus as a cause of respiratory distress. *Pediatr Radiol* 1982; 12:41–42.

Berdon WE: Editorial commentary on the manuscript entitled: Potential hazards of esophageal foreign body extraction, by CM Myer. *Pediatr Radiol* 1991; 21:99.

Campbell JB, Condon VR: Catheter removal of blunt esophageal foreign bodies in children: Survey of the Society for Pediatric Radiology. *Pediatr Radiol* 1989; 19:361.

Campbell JB, Davis WS: Catheter technique for extraction of blunt esophageal foreign bodies. *Radiology* 1973; 108:438–440.

Campbell JB, Quattromani FL, Foley LC: Foley catheter removal of blunt esophageal foreign bodies: Experience with 100 consecutive children. *Pediatr Radiol* 1983; 13:116.

Creteur V, Laufer I, Kressel HY, et al: Drug-induced esophagitis detected by double-contrast radiography. *Radiology* 1983; 147:365–368.

Currarino G, Nikaidoh H: Esophageal foreign bodies in children with vascular ring or aberrant right subclavian artery: Coincidence or causation? *Pediatr Radiol* 1991; 21:406.

Daunt N, Brodribb TR, Dickey JD: Oesophageal ulceration due to doxycycline. *Br J Radiol* 1985; 58:1209–1211.

Dubos JP, Bouchez MC, Kacet N, et al: Spontaneous rupture of the esophagus in the newborn. *Pediatr Radiol* 1986; 16:317–319.

Franken EA Jr: Caustic damage of the gastrointestinal tract: roentgen features. *Am J Roentgenol* 1973; 118:77–85.

Goodman P, Pinero SS, Rance RM, et al: Mycobacterial esophagitis in AIDS. *Gastrointest Radiol* 1989; 14:103.

Harell GS, Friedland GW, Daily WJ, et al: Neonatal Boerhaave's syndrome. *Radiology* 1970; 95:665–668.

Herman TE, McAlister WH: Esophageal diverticula in childhood associated with strictures from unsuspected foreign bodies of the esophagus. *Pediatr Radiol* 1991; 21:410.

Hillemeier C, Touloukian R, McCallum R, et al: Esophageal web: A previously unrecognized complication of epidermolysis bullosa dystrophica. *Pediatrics* 1981; 67:678–682.

Lallemand D, Huault G, Laboureau JP, et al: Laryngeal and oesophageal lesions in patients with herpetic disease. *Ann Radiol* 1974; 17:317–325.

Lepke RA, Libshitz HI: Radiation-induced injury of the esophagus. *Radiology* 1983; 148:375–378.

Levine MS: Radiology of esophagitis: A pattern approach. *Radiology* 1991; 179:1.

Levine MS, Laufer I, Kressel HY, et al: Herpes esophagitis. *Am J Roentgenol* 1981; 136:863–866.

Levine MS, Macones AJ Jr, Laufer I: *Candida* esophagitis: Accuracy of radiographic diagnosis. *Radiology* 1985; 154:581–587.

Lewicki AM, Moore JP: Esophageal moniliasis. *Am J Roentgenol* 1975; 125:218.

Matziner MA, Daneman A: Esophageal involvement in eosinophilic gastroenteritis. *Pediatr Radiol* 1983; 13:35–38.

Mauro MA, Parker LA, Hartley WS, et al: Epidermolysis bullosa: Radiographic findings in 16 cases. *Am J Roentgenol* 1987; 149:925–927.

McDonald GB, Sullivan KM, Plumley TF: Radiographic features of esophageal involvement in chronic graft-vs-host disease. *Am J Roentgenol* 1984; 142:501–506.

Myer CM: Potential hazards of esophageal foreign body extraction. *Pediatr Radiol* 1991; 21:97.

Renner WR, Johnson JF, Lichtenstein JE, et al: Esophageal inflammation and stricture: Complication of chronic granulomatous disease of childhood. *Radiology* 1991; 178:189.

Tischler JM, Helman CA: Crohn's disease of the esophagus. *J Can Assoc Radiol* 1984; 35:28–30.

Touloukian RJ, Beardsley GP, Ablow RC, et al: Traumatic perforation of the pharynx in the newborn. *Pediatrics* 1977; 59:1019–1022.

Vlymen WJ, Moskowitz PS: Roentgenographic manifestations of esophageal and intestinal involvement in Behcet's disease in children. *Pediatr Radiol* 1981; 10:193.

SECTION 5

Disorders at the Esophagogastric Junction

ANATOMY AND PHYSIOLOGY

Although the anatomy and physiology of the esophagogastric junction have been studied for decades, the mechanisms of normal and abnormal function, especially with respect to GER, are still incompletely understood. There is general agreement that the lower esophageal sphincter represents the true distal end of the esophagus and its most distal point is the true esophagogastric junction. This point may be radiographically identifiable on mucosal relief studies of the stomach (Fig 25–35), but may be difficult to identify during active swallowing studies. The lower esophageal sphincter is 3 to 4 cm long in adults, shorter in infants, and progresses toward its adult length throughout childhood.

The resting lower esophageal sphincter pressure is about 15 to 30 mm Hg higher than the resting pressure in the gastric fundus. During the initiation of swallowing, the intrasphincteric pressure drops rapidly, apparently mediated by the vagus nerve, to a level equal to fundal pressure. Thus, the pressure gradient between lower esophagus and stomach disappears during "dry swallowing," as occurs with a pacifier or thumb-sucking, as well as during true feedings. Additional antireflux activity is provided by the muscle of the esophageal hiatus of the diaphragm and by the membranous attachments of the lower esophagus to the diaphragm.

The intra-abdominal portion of the esophagus is probably relatively shorter in infants than in adults, but this varies with phases of respiration and swallowing and probably is not related to the pathophysiology of GER. The angle between the esophagus and stomach is less acute in infants than in adults. This may be a factor in permitting GER to occur even in normal infants.

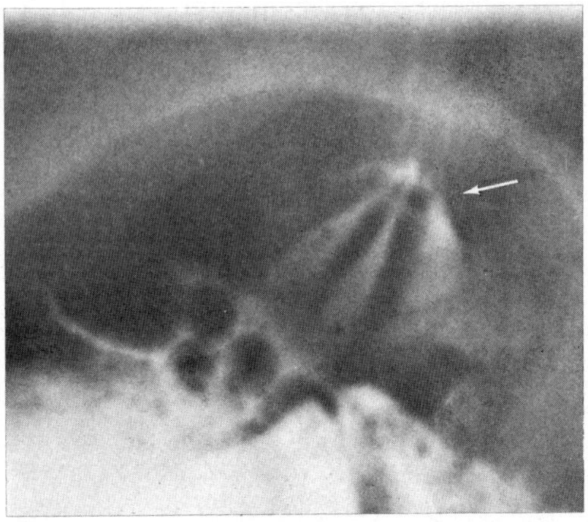

FIG 25–35.
Fluoroscopic spot film demonstrates the normal gastroesophageal junction. The *arrow* points to the convex margin of the "umbrella." The gastric folds diverge below. The parallel longitudinal esophageal folds are seen through the fundus above the margin of the umbrella.

GASTROESOPHAGEAL REFLUX

Anyone who has ever fed and burped an infant recognizes that gastroesophageal reflux occurs in virtually all normal babies. As with any physiologic mechanism, a wide range of normal can be seen. With GER, this varies from eructation with no vomiting of gastric contents to persistent "spitting-up" during and after feedings (Fig 25–36). Although sometimes alarming to parents, especially new ones, even persistent GER in otherwise healthy babies with normal weight gain is usually physiologic. If extreme, physiologic GER often responds to thickened feedings and maintenance of the semiupright posture, as in an infant seat. Spontaneous resolution of excessive spitting-up usually occurs by 9 months of age.

Pathologic GER may be difficult to differentiate from physiologic GER in the first weeks to months

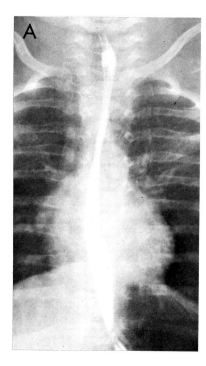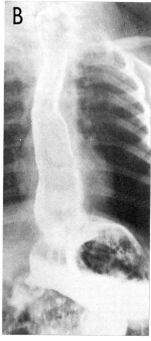

FIG 25–36.
A, esophagogram during swallowing demonstrates normal caliber of the esophagus. **B,** during eructation with massive gastroesophageal reflux, the caliber of the esophagus dilates enormously.

of life. However, progressively severe GER after 6 weeks of age may be the first sign of a truly abnormal state. Lack of response to simple dietary and postural therapy, especially if accompanied by deceleration of weight gain, may require evaluation for abnormal GER. Pathologic gastroesophageal reflux has been associated with failure to thrive, hematemesis, a variety of postural and neurologic disorders, torticollis, rumination, and sudden infant death syndrome. Chronic respiratory symptoms from aspiration into the upper airway and even into the lungs may occur. The incidence of pathologic GER is higher in patients with trisomy 21, cystic fibrosis, and organic brain disease, especially cerebral palsy.

The traditional imaging study for identification of GER has been the barium esophagogram. The examination should be a complete one with evaluation of swallowing, esophageal peristalsis, and other causes of vomiting such as gastric outlet obstruction. The total amount of barium given should be equivalent to a normal feeding volume. Since reflux is best identified with the patient in the supine position, sufficient barium must be given to reach the esophagogastric junction, which is anterior to most of the fundus. Insufficient barium may fill the dependent fundus and lead to reflux of air rather than contrast material (Fig 25–37). The examination should include intermittent fluoroscopy for 5 minutes. Some pediatric radiologists have suggested that three episodes of reflux to the level of the aortic arch within 5 minutes is pathologic. However, we have seen this much reflux in babies who are growing normally and are asymptomatic. The suggestion has been made that the only significant findings on barium swallow are continuous reflux, so-called chalasia, or signs of esophagitis.

Some radiologists advocate rolling the infant from side to side or increasing intra-abdominal pressure by external means. These maneuvers are nonphysiologic, however, and reflux elicited by them is of questionable significance. A pacifier may elicit reflux by stimulating constant swallowing. While not

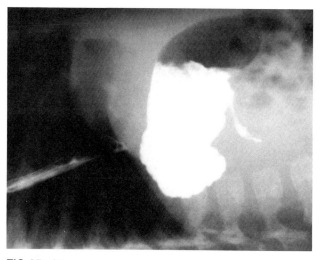

FIG 25–37.
Lateral cross-table view of the stomach demonstrates barium in dependent fundus, in the body, and in the distal esophagus. Note that insufficient barium would pool in the fundus below the esophagogastric junction and might lead to a false-negative reflux study.

strictly physiologic, the use of a pacifier simulates real-life conditions in a majority of infants. The pacifier has the additional advantage of reducing crying which has been shown to decrease GER.

Staging systems for GER have been developed. Typically, they differentiate between nonsignificant reflux, to the level of the aortic arch, and significant reflux above that level. Since there is virtually no correlation, however, between staging and clinical prognosis, few radiologists find staging useful. In fact, normal infants will fill the entire esophagus and pharynx without showing clinical evidence of abnormalities. If GER is seen, careful evaluation for reflux into the airway is important. Hiatal hernias are uncommonly identified (Fig 25–38).

Comparison with 24-hour intraesophageal pH probe monitoring, the standard against which all other tests for GER must be measured, shows disappointingly high rates of false-negative barium esophagograms. The one advantage that all imaging studies have over pH probe studies is that the latter may not record immediate postprandial GER since the milk or formula may partially neutralize the refluxing gastric acid. A chest film is frequently obtained at the initiation of a pH probe study to document the position of the probe, which should be at the level of the mid–left atrium (Fig 25–39).

Radionuclide studies for evaluation of GER are more sensitive than barium esophagograms, but they are commonly used in only a few centers with extensive experience. Food, milk, or formula containing the radionuclide is given orally following which immediate and delayed images are obtained (Fig 25–40,*A*). Semiquantitation is possible in addi-

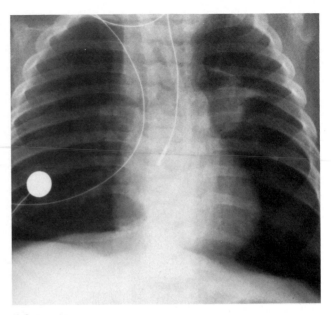

FIG 25–39.
AP view of the chest demonstrates proper position for pH probe placement with the tip of the probe approximately at the level of the mid–left atrium.

tion to the imaging studies. Concomitant gastric emptying studies (see Chapter 26) can also be performed.

US is the imaging examination which has shown the highest correlation with pH probe studies. Westra et al. reported 81% to 84% agreement between the two studies. Gomes and Menantreau described a US scoring system for GER which correlated well with results of pH probe studies and endoscopy. For US evaluation, the infant is supine and the area of the gastroesophageal junction identified. Water or dextrose solution is given orally or by tube in an amount equal to a normal feeding. Longitudinal imaging can identify fluid mixed with air bubbles refluxing into the distal esophagus (Fig 25–40,*B*). US, as well as being more accurate than barium esophagograms, has the additional advantage of not using ionizing radiation. This permits longer continuous monitoring than is possible with fluoroscopy. The disadvantages are that it is time-consuming and the esophagus may be difficult to identify in some children.

The most common complications of significant GER are failure to thrive, chronic and recurrent respiratory symptoms, and esophagitis. The imaging characteristics of reflux esophagitis are nonspecific, with dysmotility being the most common finding. This may vary from mild loss of normal primary stripping waves to tertiary contractions or aperistalsis. Frank ulceration can occur but is more common in adults with peptic esophagitis than in children. If

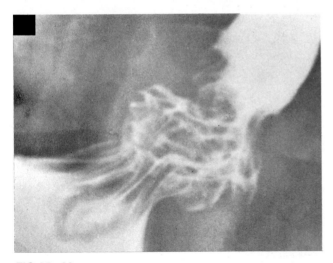

FIG 25–38.
Large hiatal hernia is identified in a mentally retarded boy with a history of vomiting and chronic blood loss. In addition to the hiatal hernia, marked gastroesophageal reflux was identified.

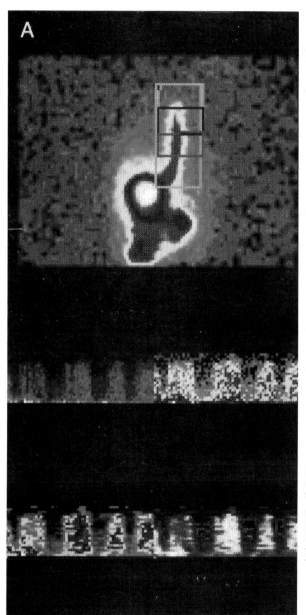

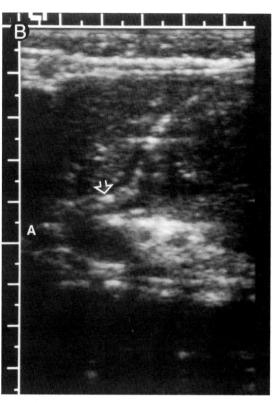

FIG 25–40.
Gastroesophageal reflux (GER). **A,** time-compressed image of
^{99m}Tc study for reflux, obtained over 5 minutes, demonstrates the
gastric fundus and prominent activity in the distal esophagus in a
patient with GER. (Courtesy of M.L. Goris, M.D., Stanford, Calif). **B,**
US of patient in the supine position demonstrates air bubbles and
fluid *(arrow)* in the esophagogastric junction during active GER.
The esophagus is identified anterior to the aorta *(A)*.

ulcers are present, they are typically in the lower
third of the esophagus near the esophagogastric
junction. Reflux esophagitis may lead to strictures,
most commonly in the midesophagus or lower third.
Barrett esophagus, with metaplasia of the esophageal epithelium, is less common than in adults and
in some cases is premalignant.

Pseudodiverticula are small intramural collections of barium which do not communicate with the
lumen as do mucosal ulcers. Less commonly seen in
children than in adults, they represent dilated excretory ducts of intramural mucous glands in patients
with reflux or peptic esophagitis. They are not typically seen adjacent to a stricture.

Although medical therapy may be satisfactory
for most cases of significant infantile GER, surgery
may be necessary for some infants with severe
symptoms, especially respiratory or profound failure
to thrive. Surgical antireflux procedures are commonly performed in brain-damaged children. The
most commonly used procedure is the Nissen fundoplication in which the upper fundus is wrapped
around the distal esophagus (Fig 25–41). The results
are variable, but long-term cessation of GER can be
accomplished in 60% to 70% of patients. If the wrap
is too tight, distal esophageal obstruction occurs; if
too loose, reflux may persist. In a small percentage
of patients, a hiatal hernia may develop (Fig 25–42).

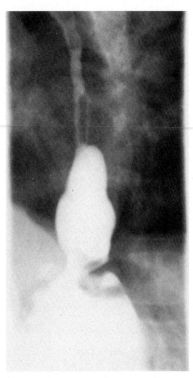

FIG 25–41.
Normal appearance of the gastroesophageal junction following Nissen fundoplication. Note the defect in the fundus caused by the wrap. Mild dilatation of the distal esophagus is commonly seen, especially early after surgery.

In extreme cases of esophagitis and stricture, esophagectomy with colonic interposition may be required.

HIATAL HERNIA

Small hiatal hernias may be seen with or without GER, may be transient, and may be of no clinical significance in the absence of GER (Fig 25–43). Larger hernias may be associated with symptoms, but are uncommon. Partial or complete intrathoracic stomach is rare but the findings on upper gastrointestinal (GI) series are dramatic (Fig 25–44). Paraesophageal hernias are very uncommon in children (see Fig 25–44).

ACHALASIA

Failure of relaxation of the lower esophageal sphincter, achalasia or cardiospasm, is rare in children although described even during infancy. There is often a deficiency of cells in the Auerbach plexus. Defective vagus nerve function or innervation is the most common pathophysiologic mechanism. Patients usually complain of dysphagia, chest pain, and symptoms related to lower esophageal obstruc-

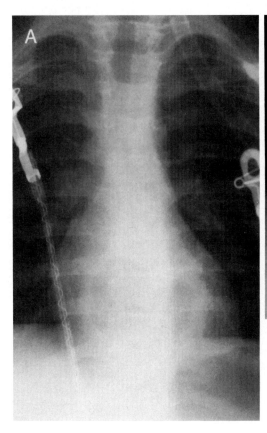

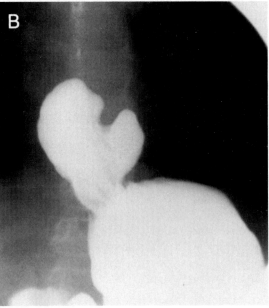

FIG 25–42.
Status post Nissen fundoplication. **A,** AP view of the chest demonstrates a large air-filled structure projected over the cardiac silhouette. **B,** esophagogram demonstrates herniation of the gastric fundus through the esophageal hiatus. The fundoplication is intact, and no gastroesophageal reflux was seen.

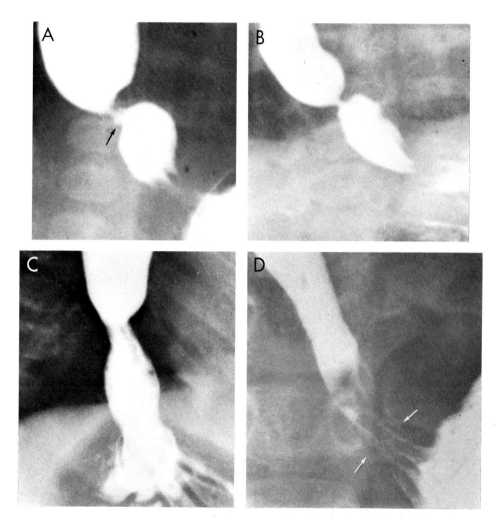

FIG 25–43.
Serial films of the gastroesophageal junction. **A,** at 3½ months of age, stricture and ulcer *(arrow)* of the distal segment of the esophagus and a small hiatal hernia are seen. **B,** at 5½ months, the ulcer is no longer present; the stricture persists. Gastrostomy had been performed. **C,** at 11 months, the hiatal hernia persists but the esophageal narrowing has diminished quite significantly. **D,** at 9 years, a small hiatal hernia remains *(arrows),* but the patient was asymptomatic.

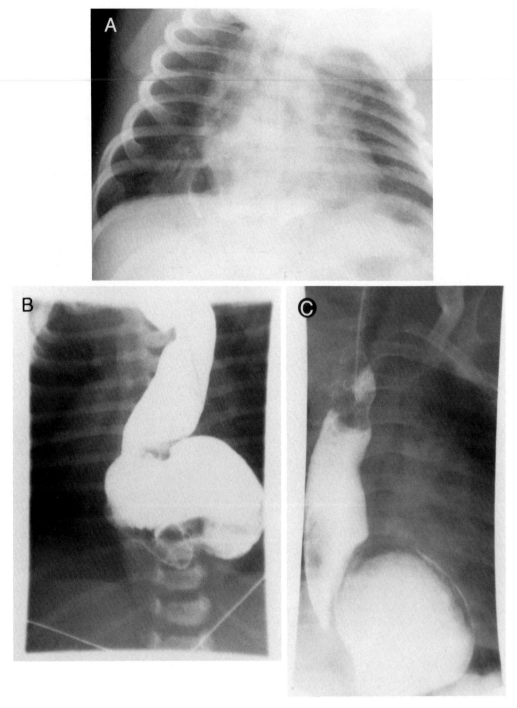

FIG 25–44.
A, AP view of the chest and **B,** esophagogram demonstrate a large intrathoracic stomach in a boy with marked symptoms of reflux and eructation. **C,** esophagogram on a different patient demonstrates a large paraesophageal hiatal hernia.

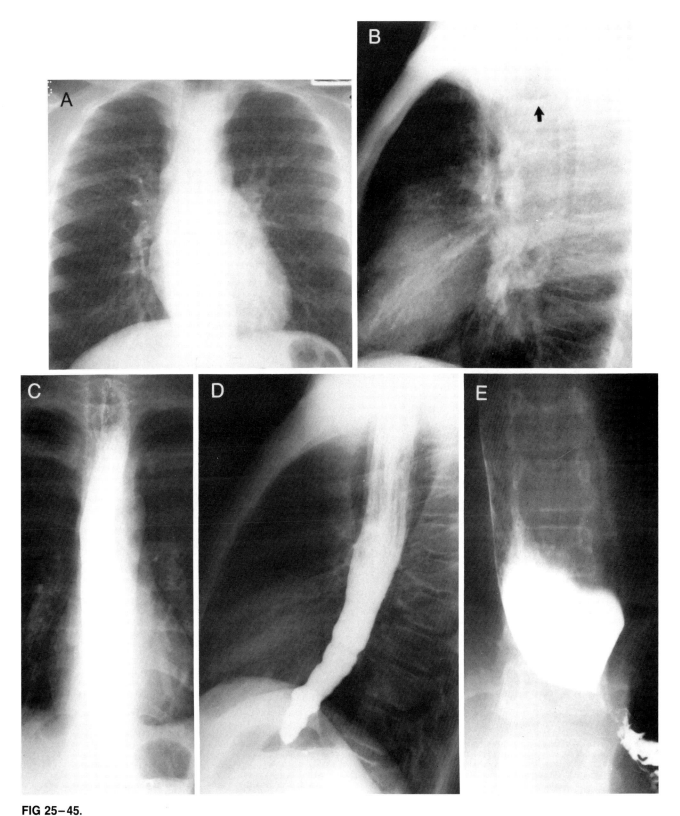

FIG 25–45.
Achalasia. **A,** frontal view of the chest demonstrates marked paravertebral widening secondary to dilated esophagus. **B,** lateral view of the chest demonstrates air-fluid level in the dilated esophagus *(arrow)*. **C,** frontal and **D,** lateral views of the esophagogram demonstrate marked dilatation with abrupt narrowing to a "beak" at the esophagogastric junction. **E,** spot film of the esophagogastric junction demonstrates the beak to better advantage.

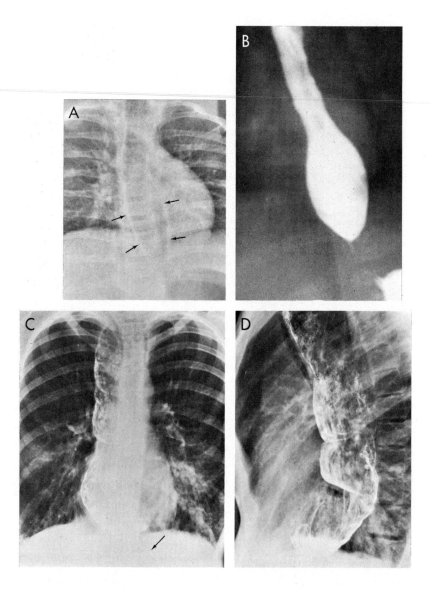

FIG 25–46.
Achalasia. **A,** frontal view of the chest demonstrates marked gaseous distention of the esophagus. **B,** esophagram on the same patient demonstrates markedly dilated esophagus with beak-like deformity at the esophagogastric junction. Endoscopy and manometry confirmed the diagnosis of achalasia. **C,** AP and **D,** lateral views of the chest of a 15-year-old girl with achalasia which has been symptomatic for at least 5 years. Chronic lung disease is identified and the markedly dilated esophagus is filled with retained swallowed material.

tion. In severe cases, regurgitation of undigested food is virtually diagnostic.

Although the definitive diagnosis is made by esophageal manometry, characteristic radiographic findings are typically seen. Upright chest radiographs may show an air-filled esophagus, often containing an air-fluid level (Fig 25–45). Esophagrams show normal swallowing and, frequently, normal peristalsis to the level of the aortic arch. Early cases may show vigorous but discoordinated peristaltic activity in the esophagus. A characteristic "beaking of the distal esophagus" (Figs 25–45 and 25–46) has been described. Ultimately, the esophagus may become completely atonic and remain markedly dilated, almost continuously filled with ingested material. We have seen one patient with Crohn disease of the esophagogastric junction mimicking achalasia.

REFERENCES

Ambrosino MM, Genieser NB, Banguru BS, et al: The syndrome of achalasia of the esophagus, ACTH insensitivity and alacrima. *Pediatr Radiol* 1986; 16:328–329.

Astley R, et al: A 20-year prospective follow-up of childhood hiatal hernia. *Br J Radiol* 1977; 50:400.

Berquist WE, Byrne WJ, Ament ME, et al: Achalasia: Diagnosis, management, and clinical courses in 16 children. *Pediatrics* 1983; 71:798–805.

Blane CE, Turnage RH, Oldham KT, et al: Long-term radiographic follow-up of the Nissen fundoplication in children. *Pediatr Radiol* 1989; 19:523.

Boix-Ochoa J, Lafuente JM, Gilvernet JM: Twenty-four hour esophageal pH monitoring in gastroesophageal reflux. *J Pediatr Surg* 1980; 15:74.

Bowen A'D: The vomiting infant: Recent advances and unsettled issues in imaging. *Radiol Clin North Am* 1988; 26:377–392.

Braun P, Nussle D, Roy CC, et al: Intramural diverticulosis of the esophagus in an eight-year-old boy. *Pediatr Radiol* 1978; 6:235–237.

Cleveland RH, Kushner DC, Schwartz AN: Gastroesophageal reflux in children: Results of a standardized fluoroscopic approach. *Am J Roentgenol* 1983; 141:53.

Darling DB, McCauley RGK, Leape LL, et al: The child with peptic esophagitis: A correlation of radiologic signs with esophageal pathology. *Radiology* 1982; 145:673.

Davies RP, Morris LL, Savage JP, et al: Gastroesophageal reflux: The role of imaging in diagnosis and management. *Australas Radiol* 1987; 31:157.

Euler AR, Ament ME: Detection of gastroesophageal reflux in the pediatric-age patient by esophageal intraluminal pH probe measurement (Tuttle test). *Pediatrics* 1977; 60:65.

Festen C: Paraesophageal hernia: A major complication of Nissen's fundoplication. *J Pediatr Surg* 1981; 16:496.

Gomes H, Menanteau B: Gastro-esophageal reflux: Comparative study between sonography and pH monitoring. *Pediatr Radiol* 1991; 21:168.

Harnsberger JK, Corey JJ, Johnson DG: Long-term follow-up of surgery for gastroesophageal reflux in infants and children. *J Pediatr* 1983; 102:505.

Heyman S: Esophageal scintigraphy (milk scans) in infants and children with esophageal reflux. *Radiology* 1982; 144:891.

Leape LL, Holder TM, Franklin JD, et al: Respiratory arrest in infants secondary to gastroesophageal reflux. *Pediatrics* 1977; 60:924–928.

Maclean AD, Houghton-Allen BW: Upper esophageal web in childhood. *Pediatr Radiol* 1975; 3:240–241.

Marshall JB, Kretschmar JM, Diaz-Arias AA: Gastroesophageal reflux as a pathogenic factor in the development of symptomatic lower esophageal rings. *Arch Intern Med* 1990; 150:1669.

McCauley RGK, Darling DB, Leonidas JC, et al: Gastroesophageal reflux in infants and children: A useful classification and reliable physiological technique for its demonstration. *Am J Roentgenol* 1978; 130:47–50.

McVeagh P, Howman-Giles R, Kemp A: Pulmonary aspiration studies by radionuclide milk scanning and barium swallow roentgenology. *Am J Dis Child* 1987; 141:917.

Peters ME, Crummy AB, Wojtowycz MM, et al: Intramural esophageal pseudodiverticulosis: A report in a child with a sixteen-year follow-up. *Pediatr Radiol* 1982; 12:262–263.

Piepsz A, Georges B, Perlmutter N, et al: Gastroesophageal scintiscanning in children. *Pediatr Radiol* 1981; 11:71–74.

Scott RB, O'Loughlin EV, Gall DG: Gastroesophageal reflux in patients with cystic fibrosis. *J Pediatr* 1985; 106:223–227.

Seibert JJ, Byrne WJ, Euler AR, et al: Gastroesophageal reflux—the acid test: Scintigraphy or the pH probe? *Am J Roentgenol* 1983; 140:1087–1090.

Starinsky R, Berlovitz J, Mores AJ, et al: Infantile achalasia. *Pediatr Radiol* 1984; 14:113–115.

Thoeni RF, Moss AA: The radiographic appearance of complications following Nissen fundoplication. *Radiology* 1979; 131:17.

Weaver JW, Kaude JV, Hamlin DJ: Webs of the lower esophagus: A complication of gastroesophageal reflux? *Am J Roentgenol* 1984; 142:289–292.

Wesley JR, Coran AG, Sarahan TM, et al: The need for evaluation of gastroesophageal reflux in brain-damaged children referred for feeding gastrostomy. *J Pediatr Surg* 1981; 16:866.

Westra SJ, Wolf BHM, Staalman CR: Ultrasound diagnosis of gastroesophageal reflux and hiatal hernia in infants and young children. *JCU* 1990; 18:477.

Winters C Jr, Spurling TJ, Chobanian SJ, et al: Barrett's esophagus: A prevalent, occult complication of gastroesophageal reflux disease. *Gastroenterology* 1987; 92:118.

Wolfson BJ, Allen JL, Panitch HB, et al: Lipid aspiration pneumonia due to gastroesophageal reflux: A complication of nasogastric lipid feedings. *Pediatr Radiol* 1989; 19:545.

Yulish BS, Rothstein FC, Halpin TC Jr: Radiographic findings in children and young adults with Barrett's esophagus. *Am J Roentgenol* 1987; 148:353–357.

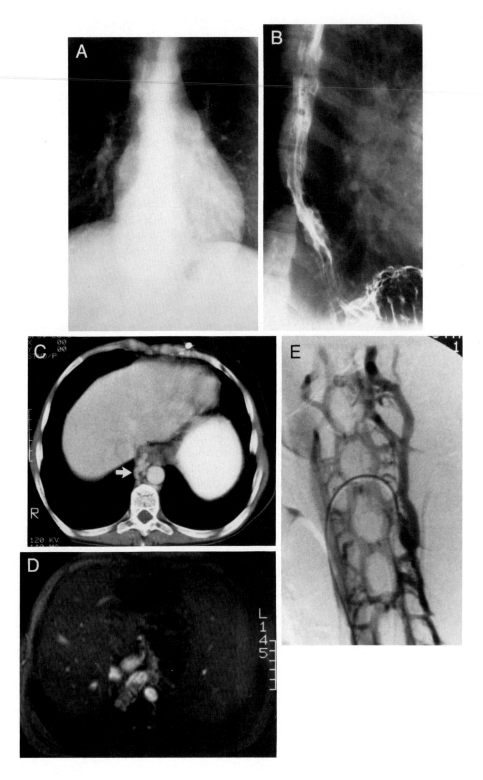

FIG 25–47.
Marked esophageal and paraesophageal collateral circulation in a 15-year-old girl with cavernous transformation of the portal vein. **A,** coned-down AP view of the chest reveals paravertebral widening at the level of the diaphragm. **B,** esophagogram demonstrates serpiginous filling defects in the distal esophagus and the gastric fundus consistent with varices. **C,** CT scan at the thoracoabdominal junction demonstrates multiple varices in the paraesophageal region *(arrow)*. **D,** MR scan using gradient-recalled echo sequence demonstrates right paraesophageal varices to good advantage. **E,** angiogram using digital subtraction technique demonstrates massive bilateral paravertebral collateral venous flow.

SECTION 6

Miscellaneous Abnormalities

ESOPHAGEAL VARICES

Esophageal varices are secondary to portal hypertension in children and are discussed more thoroughly in Chapter 23. The primary modality for identifying esophageal varices now is endoscopy rather than imaging studies. However, varices may be found in the evaluation of hematemesis or coincidentally when imaging studies are performed for other reasons. Rarely, paraesophageal varices cause sufficient irregularity of the esophagus so that they can be seen as paraspinous widening on chest radiographs (Fig 25–47,*A* and *B*). CT and MR may incidentally identify the varices when performed for other indications (Fig 25–47,*C* and *D*). US performed for evaluation of hepatic disease also may demonstrate varices incidentally. On barium esophagogram, the varices appear as serpiginous filling defects in the barium column (Fig 25–48). Barium paste gives better mucosal relief than liquid barium, but is not always found palatable by children. The primary treatment modality for esophageal varices, other than treatment of the underlying portal hypertension, is endoscopic sclerotherapy. Agha described acute complications following sclerotherapy, including mucosal ulceration, luminal narrowing, sinuses, fistulas, dissection, and perforation. Chronically, one may find strictures, mural defects, dysmotility, and obstruction.

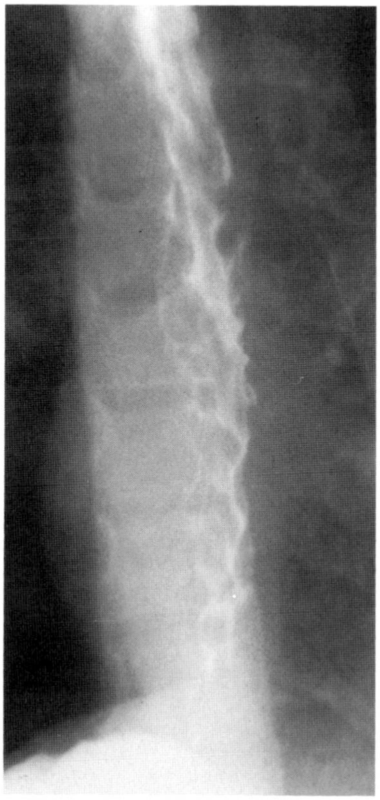

FIG 25–48.
Varices. Multiple serpiginous filling defects in the esophagus in a 7-year-old-girl with cavernous transformation of the portal vein and secondary portal venous hypertension.

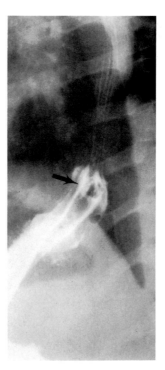

FIG 25–49.
Inflammatory gastroesophageal polyp presented as a filling defect in a 10-year-old boy with hiatal hernia. **(Courtesy of Dr. S. Kirschner, Nashville).**

NEOPLASMS

Esophageal tumors are extraordinarily rare in children and are usually benign. Hamartomas, leiomyomas, and hemangiomas have been reported. One of the most common pseudoneoplasms demonstrated is inflammatory polyps secondary to chronic GER and reflux (Fig 25–49). Carcinomas are even more rare and have been reported following caustic esophagitis and achalasia. Mediastinal tumors, such as lymphoma, teratoma, or neuroblastoma, may displace the esophagus but usually do not involve it primarily.

REFERENCES

Agha FP: The esophagus after endoscopic injection sclerotherapy: Acute and chronic changes. *Radiology* 1984; 153:37–42.

Isikawa T, Saeki M, Tsukune Y, et al: Detection of paraoesophageal varices by plain film. *Am J Roentgenol* 1985; 144:701–704.

Rose JD, Roberts GM, Smith PM: The radiological appearance of the esophagus after sclerotherapy for varices. *Clin Radiol* 1985; 36:355–358.

26

Stomach and Proximal Duodenum

SECTION 1

Normal Stomach and Duodenum

NORMAL ANATOMY

The stomach normally lies below the left hemidiaphragm and extends obliquely caudad and mediad to the pyloroduodenal flexure. Embryologically, the stomach begins as a straight tube which rotates clockwise 90 degrees around its long axis. The original posterior portion of the stomach becomes the left margin. Its differential growth is greater than the opposite side, resulting in a longer, greater curvature to the left and a shorter, lesser curvature to the right. The stomach is relatively fixed at its proximal end by the esophagogastric junction and at its distal end by the fixed retroperitoneal position of the first portion of the duodenum. Additionally, the stomach is attached to neighboring organs by four major peritoneal folds: the gastrophrenic, the gastrohepatic, the gastrosplenic, and the gastrocolic ligaments.

The stomach is divided into three portions. The fundus is the most bulbous portion and is that part superior to the esophagogastric junction. The body of the stomach is the portion bounded on either side by the greater and lesser curvatures, typically becoming slightly narrower in caliber as it reaches the distal portion. The gastric antrum and pylorus are the most distal portions of the stomach, having a slightly thicker wall than the fundus or body.

The normal shape, size, and position of the stomach are variable, depending on the volume of gastric content and the position, age, and body habitus of the individual. In infancy, the stomach appears high and transverse on contrast studies in most patients (Fig 26-1). The more longitudinal, J-shaped stomach is uncommonly seen in infants, but is characteristic in older children and adults (Fig 26-2). Although the appearance of the fundus and body may vary, the position and appearance of the pylorus are relatively similar from patient to patient.

The fundus and the greater curvature of the body normally exhibit marginal indentations caused by the normal folds in the mucosa, the gastric rugae. The pattern is inconstant, but rugal folds can usually be seen in most normal stomachs unless they are overdistended during barium examination. The mucosal contour is best evaluated with a small amount of contrast material spread over the surface. Double contrast studies of the stomach bring the mucosa into sharp relief, but cannot always be performed in

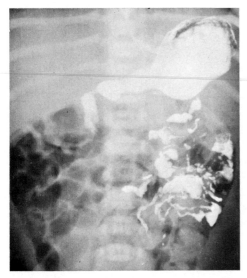

FIG 26–1.
Radiographic appearance of the normal stomach in early life. The stomach in this 6-day-old infant is high, conical in shape, and transverse. Rugal markings are not prominent.

young children. The rugae are least prominent in early infancy and become progressively more obvious in older patients.

Normal peristaltic waves can typically be seen even in neonates, although gastric motor activity increases with age. Normally, peristalsis is coordinated from the proximal to the distal stomach and is propulsive. The gastric antrum and pyloric region frequently demonstrate muscular spasm which in-

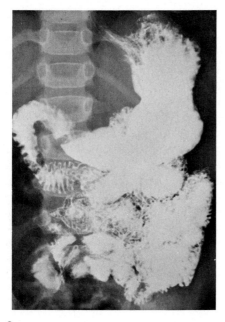

FIG 26–2.
The stomach in a 4-year-old boy is J-shaped with prominent rugal folds in the fundus.

terrupts the normal peristaltic propulsive waves (Fig 26–3). Gastric emptying time is far more variable in children than in adults, and this is particularly true in infants. Although maintenance of the supine position and gaseous distention of the stomach, which typically occurs in infants, may have a role in delayed gastric emptying, the effect of the delayed opening of the antrum and pylorus is probably most significant. It is not uncommon for a normal baby to have sufficient antropyloric spasm for contrast material to remain in the stomach for as long as 20 or 25 minutes before finally passing into the small intestine.

The duodenum, the most proximal portion of the small intestine, begins at the pyloroduodenal junction. The first portion of the duodenum begins at the pylorus and ends approximately at the neck of the gallbladder. It is almost completely covered by peritoneum, but is the only portion of the normal duodenum that is relatively mobile. The second or descending portion extends from the neck of the gallbladder and is in intimate contact with the head of the pancreas. The common bile duct enters its midportion. The third portion is once again horizontal and courses back to the left across the spine. Anteriorly, it is covered by peritoneum and is crossed by the superior mesenteric artery and vein. The fourth portion ascends along the left side of the aorta where it turns ventrally to become the jejunum at the level of the duodenojejunal flexure. The flexure is still retroperitoneal, keeping it fixed in the normal situation, and is further held in place by the ligament of Treitz. Of importance is that the proximal portion of the duodenum receives its blood supply from the celiac axis while the superior mesenteric artery supplies blood to the distal duodenum. Thus, while the stomach and first and second portions of the duodenum are derived from the embryonic foregut, most of the third and all of the fourth portion of the duodenum are of midgut origin and are often involved in midgut volvulus, which is discussed in Chapter 52.

EXAMINATION OF THE UPPER GASTROINTESTINAL TRACT

Contrast studies of the upper gastrointestinal tract under fluoroscopic control continue to be the standard examination for most abnormalities of the stomach and duodenum. Barium is the most commonly used contrast material. Water-soluble contrast is typically used for patients in whom an intestinal perforation is suspected. Although more expensive, low osmolar nonionic contrast material has largely

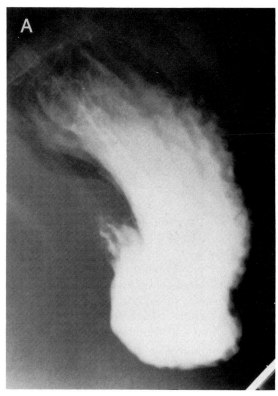

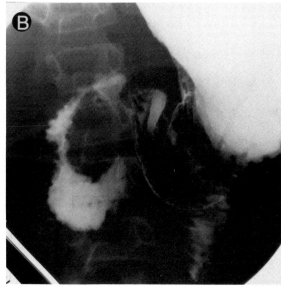

FIG 26–3.
Pyloric spasm. **A,** upper gastrointestinal tract series in a 7-year-old girl with crampy abdominal pain shows antropyloric spasm 30 minutes after barium ingestion. **B,** after parenteral administration of an anticholinergic agent there was easy passage of barium through an anatomically normal pylorus and duodenum.

replaced the older forms of water-soluble contrast media in the gastrointestinal tract when perforation is suspected. However, the higher osmolar contrast agents are still used occasionally for therapeutic purposes in infants with meconium ileus and in older patients with cystic fibrosis who have distal intestinal obstruction syndrome. The former is discussed more thoroughly in Chapter 52 and the latter in Chapter 27. The low osmolar nonionic contrast materials are sometimes used for patients with intestinal obstruction in whom it is desired to perform the examination by mouth. Again, this is predominantly in newborns, especially those who are suspected of having necrotizing enterocolitis or of having feeding intolerance secondary to strictures from previous necrotizing enterocolitis.

In patients who are old enough to cooperate, double contrast examinations are useful in many instances. In these cases, a higher-density barium is used and effervescent agents are administered to produce the double contrast. Double contrast studies are generally accepted as the upper gastrointestinal imaging examination of choice in adults. However, they require longer fluoroscopy times and a larger number of films than does the standard single contrast examination, and we do not use the double contrast examinations routinely on children. In fact, the examination in children should be tailored to the

specific clinical question to be answered in order to maintain the radiation exposure at the lowest possible levels. Intermittent fluoroscopy should always be used instead of constant fluoroscopy, careful collimation should be used, and photo spot-film cameras or digital fluoroscopy in place of standard film-screen combination spot films. Infants and young children, of necessity, are studied in the recumbent position. In older children, especially when double contrast studies are performed, the examination can be performed with a combination of recumbent and upright spot films.

Older children can be kept fasting overnight if the study is performed early in the morning. Children under 1 year of age have the potential for dehydration with this length of restriction, and we have found a 3-hour period sufficient to empty the normal stomach of foodstuffs. Infants who do have retained material in the stomach can be intubated and most of the retained material withdrawn satisfactorily. If aspiration through a tube is performed, the aspirate should be examined for the presence of bile or blood as a possible clue to the diagnosis of the infant's problem.

Most babies, having been kept fasting for 3 hours, will readily take barium from a bottle. The babies are generally more accepting of the bottle while they are in the supine position, even though

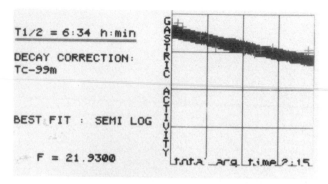

FIG 26–4.
(Same patient as in Fig 26–36.) Delayed gastric emptying after administration of ^{99m}Tc sulfur in formula. Half gastric emptying time was 6½ hours; normal is 60 to 90 minutes. (Courtesy of Michael L. Goris, M.D. Stanford, California)

this may introduce more air than if the babies are fed while in the prone position. The tube and nipple technique for examining swallowing is described in Chapter 25. Routine examination includes complete evaluation of the esophagus, the stomach, and the duodenum down to and including the duodenojejunal junction. We routinely use only spot films for the stomach and duodenum and take one overhead film at the end of the examination to visualize the proximal portion of the small intestine. Obviously, specific additional views will be necessary at times depending upon the results of the fluoroscopic examination. Since it is not necessary to include the pelvis in the radiographic field during upper gastrointestinal examination, it is imperative that gonadal shielding be used in all children.

Ultrasound (US) of the upper gastrointestinal tract is becoming more widely used. Findings are discussed under specific disease entities. Cohen et al. have pointed out the technical advantages gained by filling the stomach with fluid prior to US evaluation. Their technique is particularly critical when US is used for the detection of gastroesophageal reflux and quite useful in the evaluation for pyloric stenosis and other lesions at the gastric outlet. US evaluation of the duodenum is most useful in neonates and is discussed in Chapter 52.

Radionuclide gastric emptying studies are usually performed at the time of evaluation for gastroesophageal reflux. The infant is fed a liquid meal approximately the volume of a normal feeding. Technetium 99 sulfur colloid is typically added to the initial portion of the feeding with the dose based on the child's age and weight. The examination time varies by institution. Gelfand and Wagner suggest the increased accuracy of a 2-hour examination, while Miller studies the infants for 90 minutes. Miller gives the lower limit of normal gastric emptying as 45% at 60 minutes and 60% at 90 minutes (Fig 26–4).

As noted below, there are occasional reports of computed tomography (CT) and magnetic resonance (MR) findings in benign diseases of the stomach in the pediatric population. These are often incidental to the examination being performed for other reasons. Most authors agree that the only real utility of these expensive studies for gastric lesions in children is when malignancy is being considered in the differential diagnosis or when a proven malignancy is being staged.

REFERENCES

Cohen MD: Choosing contrast media for the evaluation of the gastrointestinal tract of neonates and infants. *Radiology* 1987; 162:447.

Cohen HL, Haller JO, Mester A, et al: Neonatal duodenum: Fluid-aided US examination. *Radiology* 1987; 164:805.

Gelfand MJ, Wagner GC: Gastric emptying in infants and children: Limited utility of 1-hour measurement. *Radiology* 1991; 178:379.

Miller J: Upper gastrointestinal tract evaluation with radionuclides in infants. *Radiology* 1991; 178:326.

Miller JH, Kemberling CR: Ultrasound of the pediatric gastrointestinal tract. *Semin Ultrasound CT MR* 1987; 8:349–365.

Stringer DA, Daneman A, Brunelle F, et al: Sonography of the normal and abnormal stomach (excluding hypertrophic pyloric stenosis) in children. *J Ultrasound Med* 1986; 5:183–188.

SECTION 2

Congenital Abnormalities

Congenital duplications of the stomach are rare. Large duplications are palpable on physical examination. Patients may also present with vomiting, hematemesis, and melena. Duplications arise most typically along the greater curvature of the stomach. When large, they may impinge on the gastric lumen and may be readily identified on barium study as an extraluminal mass (Fig 26–5). US may provide more specific information. The cyst is typically anechoic (Fig 26–6). The wall of the cyst, as reported by Moccia et al., may demonstrate a thin echogenic line representing the mucosa. Echogenic material within the cyst probably represents residua of hemorrhage or inspissated secretions. Rarely, the duplications may communicate with the lumen of the stomach or esophagus. Ueda et al. reported a case of gastric duplication in association with aberrant pancreas.

True congenital gastric *diverticula,* in which all elements of the gastric wall appear, represent incomplete duplications, and these can be seen when filled with barium. They are quite rare in children, are usually asymptomatic, and most occur near the esophagogastric junction. Intramural diverticula are seen typically in adults and arise near the gastric antrum. Girdany has described an 11-year-old girl with a large antral diverticulum causing partial gastric outlet obstruction (Fig 26–7).

Congenital microgastria with failure of rotation of the stomach is a rare anomaly in which fetal rotation of the stomach fails to occur and the greater and lesser curvatures do not develop. Also, there is no differentiation into fundus, body, antrum, and pyloric canal. The tiny tubular stomach remains in the midsagittal plane and is joined from above and behind at its summit by the esophagus (Fig 26–8). The duodenum projects directly ventrad from the pyloric end. The gastroesophageal junction is incompetent and gastroesophageal reflux is present. The esophagus is dilated and appears to take over the storage function of the inadequate stomach. Vomiting from birth, hematemesis, weight loss, and secondary anemia are the most common presenting features. Microgastria is often associated with asplenia. Polysplenia has also been reported, as have congenital

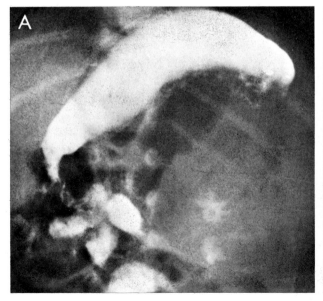
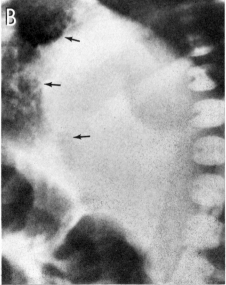

FIG 26–5.
Gastric duplication. **A,** in the AP projection, a large soft-tissue mass is seen deforming the greater curvature of the stomach and displacing it cephalad. **B,** on lateral examination, the stomach is seen to be displaced posteriorly by the large gastric duplication.

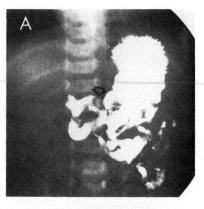
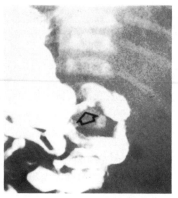

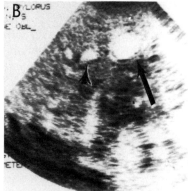

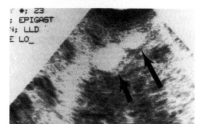

FIG 26–6.
Gastric duplication. **A,** upper GI series in a 3-day-old boy with a history of projectile vomiting. The narrowed pyloric channel *(arrows)* in frontal and prone oblique projections suggests an extrinsic pressure defect. **B,** transverse *(top)* and sagittal *(bottom)* sonograms demonstrate a fluid-filled cyst adjacent to the antrum *(arrow)* with a fluid-filled duodenal bulb *(arrowhead)* distal to it. On the sagittal sonogram, the *arrows* demonstrate the bilobed anechoic duplication cyst.

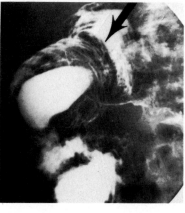
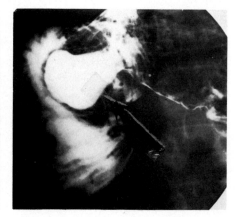

FIG 26–7.
Gastric diverticulum. On upper GI series, the coiled-spring appearance of intussusception is identified. On the right, the barium-filled diverticulum is seen to be featureless with the air-filled antrum proximal to it and the barium-filled duodenal sweep distal to it. The diverticulum originated at the gastroduodenal junction and was lined with gastric mucosa.

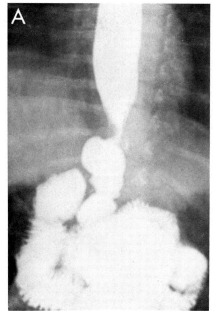
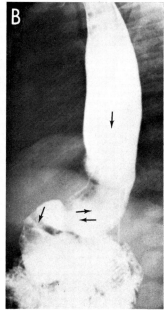

FIG 26–8.
Congenital microgastria with failure of rotation of the stomach in a
6-month-old infant. **A,** frontal and **B,** lateral projections demonstrate the stomach to be small and tubular in the midsagittal plane
of the abdomen. The cardia is incompetent; the dilated esophagus

serves as a storage organ *(top arrow)* and compensates for the inadequate stomach *(pair of lower arrows).* The first portion of the
duodenum comes directly off the pylorus and is directed ventrad
(left lower arrow).

heart disease and aganglionosis. Agastria, complete
lack of gastric development, is the most extreme
form of microgastria.

*Congenital pyloric and prepyloric atresia, stenosis,
and webs* are rare. They represent variations of the
same entity and vary anywhere from an intraluminal
diaphragm causing minimal obstruction to complete
discontinuity between the gastric antrum and the
pylorus or duodenum. The cause and pathogenesis
of these lesions is not known. Originally, it was
thought that there is failure of canalization of the
early fetal solid gastric epithelium, as is seen in
duodenal atresia, but more recently, the suggestion
has been made that the atresia, stenosis, or web may
be secondary to an intrauterine vascular accident as
it is the most common cause of jejunal and ileal atresia. Radiographically, the stomach is usually dilated.
With atresia, there may be no gas distal to the body
of the stomach. With stenosis and webs, there may
be varying degrees of gas seen. Epidermolysis
bullosa has been described in several cases of pyloric
atresia. Since the obstruction is complete, these patients typically present in the first hours or days after birth (see Chapter 52). Most congenital obstructive lesions of the proximal duodenum, such as atresia, stenosis, webs, and diaphragms, also present at
birth (see Chapter 52). Patients with stenosis of the
pylorus or with pyloric or duodenal webs may

present later in life, including adulthood (Fig 26–9).
Webs are more common than stenosis and are seen
on barium upper gastrointestinal (GI) series as circumferential thin filling defects in the antrum. The
pathogenesis may be multifactorial in the case of
gastric webs and those presenting at older ages may
be related to ulcer disease.

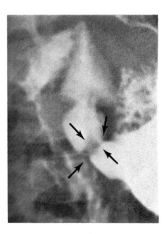

FIG 26–9.
Congenital incomplete prepyloric membrane in a 2-year-old girl
with nearly lifelong vomiting. The membrane caused an incomplete
pyloric obstruction, and in the upper GI series produces a transverse filling defect at the prepyloric level. At surgery, a membrane
with a central defect was found and removed. **(Courtesy of Dr. E.
Salzman, Denver.)**

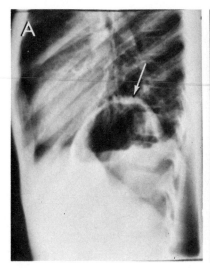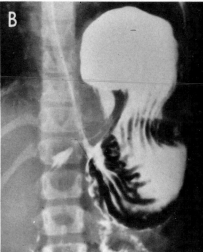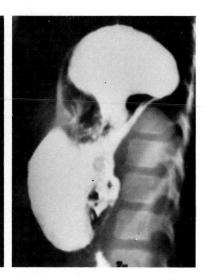

FIG 26–10.
Mesenteroaxial volvulus in a 7-year-old girl with abdominal pain and distention. **A,** on lateral chest examination, eventration of the diaphragm is demonstrated *(arrow)*. **B,** two films from the upper GI series demonstrate the gastroesophageal junction to be in a rela-

tively normal position. The gastric outlet in this instance lies superiorly and posteriorly. At surgery, the volvulus was easily reduced and the diaphragmatic eventration repaired. **(Courtesy of Dr. V. Condon, Salt Lake City.)**

Gastric volvulus is an uncommon condition of which two types have been described. As mentioned previously, the stomach is fixed by four ligaments which represent peritoneal folds. If the stomach is not fixed properly, it can rotate along an axis perpendicular to the long axis so that the pylorus comes to lie superiorly. This is known as mesenteroaxial volvulus and is associated with eventration of the left hemidiaphragm. There may be obstruction to both the gastric inlet and gastric outlet. Plain films

of the chest and abdomen show a large distended stomach below an elevated left hemidiaphragm (Fig 26–10). The stomach may also rotate around its long axis, a condition known as organoaxial volvulus. This is most commonly seen in association with large hiatus hernias, particularly of the paraesophageal type. Of the two types of gastric volvulus, the mesenteroaxial type represents a true emergency since the twist can compromise the blood supply to the stomach. Organoaxial volvulus is much less common and may, in fact, be chronic in nature. Upper GI series is usually necessary to make the diagnosis of organoaxial volvulus.

Ectopic pancreas (Fig 26–11) is an uncommon anomaly in which pancreatic tissue is found in the pyloric antrum or, less commonly, in the duodenum. Typically, there is a mound of tissue seen on upper GI series projecting into the barium-filled lumen. The mass is umbilicated and a central niche may be seen representing an attempt at duct formation.

FIG 26–11.
Aberrant pancreas. A rounded filling defect *(arrow)* is demonstrated along the inferior margin of the prepyloric antrum. In this case, the pathognomonic central umbilication is not identified.

REFERENCES

Agha FP, Gabriele OF, Abdulla FH: Complete gastric duplication. *Am J Roentgenol* 1981; 137:406.

Aintablian NH, Slim MS, Antoun BW: Congenital microgastria. *Pediatr Surg Int* 1987; 2:307.

Blank E, Chisholm AJ: Congenital microgastria: A case report with a 26 year follow-up. *Pediatrics* 1973; 51:1037–1041.

Bronsther B, Nadeau MR, Abrams MW: Congenital pyloric atresia: A report of three cases and review of the literature. *Surgery* 1971; 69:130–136.

Campbell JB, Rappaport LN, Skerket LB: Acute mesentero-axial volvulus of the stomach. *Radiology* 1972; 103:153–156.

Cremin BJ: Congenital pyloric antral membranes in infancy. *Radiology* 1969; 92:509–512.

DeGroot WG, Postumu R, Hunter AGW: Familial pyloric atresia associated with epidermolysis bullosa. *J Pediatr* 1978; 92:429–431.

Egelhoff JC, Bisset GS, Strife JL: Multiple enteric duplications in an infant. *Pediatr Radiol* 1986; 16:160–161.

Eklof O, Lassrich A, Stanley P, et al: Ectopic pancreas. *Pediatr Radiol* 1973; 1:24–27.

Felson B, Berkman YM, Hoyumpa AM: Gastric mucosal diaphragm. *Radiology* 1969; 92:513–517.

Flacks K, Stelman HH, Matsumoto PJH: Partial gastric diverticula. *Am J Roentgenol* 1965; 94:339–342.

Girdany BR: Peptic ulcer in childhood. *Pediatrics* 1953; 12:56.

Gorman B, Shaw DG: Congenital microgastria. *Br J Radiol* 1984; 57:260–262.

Hochberger O, Swoboda W: Congenital microgastria: a follow-up observation over six years. *Pediatr Radiol* 1974; 2:207–208.

Hulnick DH, Balthazar EJ: Gastric duplication cyst: GI series and CT correlation. *Gastrointest Radiol* 1987; 12:106–108.

Kangarloo H, Sample WF, Hansen G, et al: Ultrasonic evaluation of abdominal gastrointestinal tract duplication in children. *Radiology* 1979; 131:191–194.

Kilman WJ, Berk RN: The spectrum of radiographic features of aberrant pancreatic rests involving the stomach. *Radiology* 1977; 123:291–296.

Korber JS, Glasson MJ: Pyloric atresia associated with epidermolysis bullosa. *J Pediatr* 1977; 90:600–601.

Mandell GA, Heyman S, Alavi A, et al: A case of microgastria in association with splenic-gonadal fusion. *Pediatr Radiol* 1983; 13:95.

Moccia WA, Astacio JE, Kande JV: Ultrasonographic demonstration of gastric duplication in infancy. *Pediatr Radiol* 1981; 11:52.

Orense M, Garcia Hernandez JB, Celorio C, et al: Pyloric atresia associated with epidermolysis bullosa. *Pediatr Radiol* 1987; 17:435.

Shackelford G, McAlister WH, Brodeur AE, et al: Congenital microgastria. *Am J Roentgenol* 1973; 118:72–76.

Ueda D, Taketazu M, Itoh S, et al: Case of gastric duplication cyst with aberrant pancreas. *Pediatr Radiol* 1991; 21:379.

Wieczorek RL, Seidman I, Ranson JH, et al: Congenital duplication of the stomach: Case report and review of the English literature. *Am J Gastroenterol* 1984; 79:597–602.

Ziprkowski MN, Teele RL: Gastric volvulus in childhood. *Am J Roentgenol* 1979; 132:921–925.

SECTION 3

Acquired Disorders

HYPERTROPHIC PYLORIC STENOSIS

Hypertrophic pyloric stenosis (HPS) represents the most common cause of gastric outlet obstruction, either congenital or acquired. Although incidence figures vary from one country to another, approximately 1 in 500 liveborn children in the United States will develop pyloric stenosis. The age of the child at the onset of symptoms is usually 3 to 6 weeks with a range of 1 week to 3 months, but HPS has been described in the first week of life and occasionally in older children. The disease is unusual in premature infants. There is a positive family history in less than 5% of cases, but there is an increased incidence of pyloric stenosis in twin siblings of affected patients. Although the traditional history of the patient being a first-born male in the family is not always true, there is a definite male preponderance and first-borns do seem to be more affected than their younger siblings. In the United States, 80% to 85% of affected patients are males.

The cause of the disease is not known. The pathophysiology seems to be one of work hypertrophy of the circular muscle of the pylorus. This muscle becomes markedly hypertrophied as if under constant stimulation (Fig 26–12). Although a variety

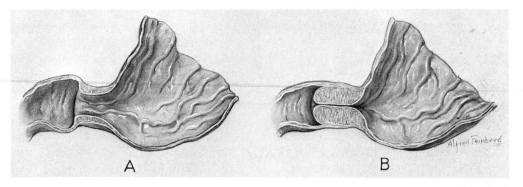

FIG 26–12.
The morbid anatomical changes in hypertrophic pyloric stenosis.
A, a normal stomach in a 4-week-old infant. Note that the pyloric
muscle is slightly thicker than that of the body of the stomach. **B,**
marked thickening of the pyloric muscle is noted secondary to hypertrophy of the circular layer. This thickened muscle is elongated,
projecting into the more proximal portion of the stomach. The pyloric canal is elongated and constricted. The pyloric muscle also
bulges into the base of the duodenal cap.

of theories as to the cause of this work hypertrophy
have been put forward, none has been proved.

Weiskittel et al, reported two cases of evolving
HPS in which normal US scans were followed 1 to 2
weeks later by US findings diagnostic of HPS. These
findings lend further credence to the belief that the
disease is acquired after birth and evolves over a
course of days to weeks. Latchaw et al. described
three older infants in whom classic pyloric stenosis
developed after prolonged transpyloric jejunal feeding tube placement.

The babies typically present with a history of
vomiting which is initially mild and is often interpreted as gastroesophageal reflux with excess "spitting-up." Careful history taking often reveals that
the vomiting started relatively early in life although
the child may not present for medical attention until
6 weeks of age or older. As the relative degree of obstruction increases, in the classic case the vomiting
ultimately becomes projectile. The projectile vomiting progresses rapidly and dehydration is common
when medical attention is not sought speedily. The
vomitus is not bile-stained. Approximately 5% of the
patients will be mildly jaundiced.

Physical examination is often diagnostic. Peristaltic waves may actually be seen on the abdominal
wall progressing from the left upper quadrant across
the epigastrium. The hypertrophied pyloric muscle
may be palpated in the midepigastrium by an experienced pediatric surgeon or pediatrician. If this is
the case, imaging studies may not be necessary, but
Forman et al. have questioned this approach. In
most countries, patients are treated with pyloromyotomy, although in Sweden there has been an extensive experience with successful nonsurgical therapy.

The approach to imaging studies has changed
dramatically over the last two decades. The imaging
examination of choice is now abdominal US if an experienced sonographer is available to perform the
study. We have had excellent success using 5-MHz
transducers. Gastric contents can interfere with the
examination, and we routinely place a nasogastric
tube and empty the stomach of air and foodstuffs.
The pylorus is frequently more easily seen if the
stomach is then filled with a dextrose-water solution
or other similar iso-osmolar fluid mixture. With the
patient in the supine position, the upper pole of the
right kidney is identified and the transducer moved
toward the xiphoid process. The examiner will usually identify the pylorus along this line. Images of
the pylorus should be obtained in both transverse
and longitudinal projections. Swischuk et al. have
pointed out the advantages of differing placements

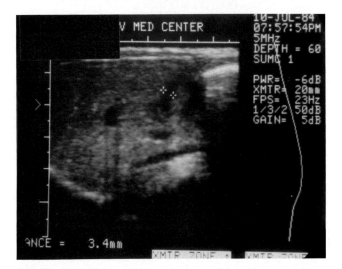

FIG 26–13.
Transverse US of the pylorus demonstrates thickened muscle,
measuring 3.4 mm. The characteristic findings of hypertrophic pyloric stenosis were present at surgery

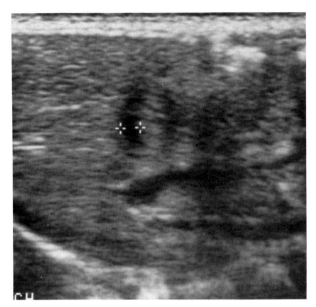

FIG 26–14.
Transverse scan in a proven case of hypertrophic pyloric stenosis. Note that the echogenicity in the near field and far field is greater than that seen in the lateral aspects of the thickened pyloric muscle.

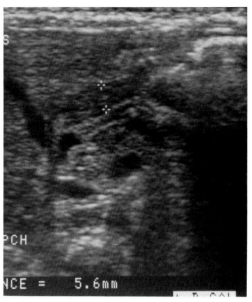

FIG 26–15.
Longitudinal scan of hypertrophic pyloric stenosis demonstrates the muscle thickness to be 5.6 mm, well beyond the normal range and characteristic of hypertrophic pyloric stenosis.

of the transducer, depending upon the anatomy of the specific case.

An experienced examiner can frequently make the diagnosis just by qualitative assessment of the thickness of the pyloric wall, but great interest has been paid to trying to determine accurate measurements of the pyloric wall thickness, length, and luminal channel length. In order to perform the measurements accurately, great care must be taken to image the pylorus properly. On the transverse scans, the pylorus should look like a doughnut with the echolucent hypertrophied muscle surrounding the echogenic gastric mucosa (Fig 26–13). Although asymmetry in the "doughnut" can sometimes be seen, most often careful positioning will show a high degree of symmetry. The echolucent ring of hypertrophied muscle may sometimes appear nonuniform on the transverse scan. Typically, the near and far fields appear more echogenic than the sides (Fig 26–14). Spevak and her colleagues have shown this to be a technical artifact secondary to the anisotropic effect of the sound passing obliquely through the circular muscle. On longitudinal scans, the hypertrophied muscle should be of equal thickness on both sides of the echogenic central mucosa (Fig 26–15).

Swischuk and his colleagues have described a number of pitfalls in the sonographic diagnosis of pyloric stenosis. The most important of these is mistaking the antrum for the pylorus, but careful examination usually separates out these two anatomical areas. Other diseases which can mimic pyloric stenosis on sonographic examination are antropyloric gastritis, with or without ulcer disease, and chronic granulomatous disease of childhood. Swischuk also points out the need for careful technical examination, as inaccurate placement of the transducer or an overfilled stomach with a posteriorly directed an-

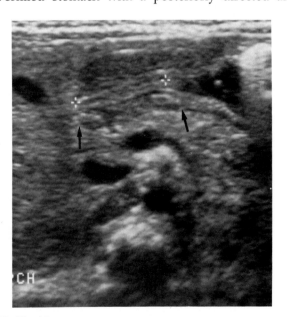

FIG 26–16.
Longitudinal scan demonstrates the length of the pyloric canal as demonstrated by the cursor marks. The length of the hypertrophied pyloric muscle *(arrows)* can also be demonstrated.

trum may simulate a thickened pylorus or lead to a false-negative diagnosis.

The pyloric muscle thickness should be measured on both transverse and longitudinal scans, and these measurements should be in close agreement. The boundary between the antrum and pyloric muscle can usually be identified, with an appearance not unlike that seen on barium studies. The length of the pyloric muscle can be measured, then, in longitudinal position (Fig 26–16). In the same position, the length of the pyloric channel (see Fig 26–16), as demonstrated by the echogenic gastric mucosa, can also be measured. Cohen et al. have demonstrated a US double track sign which they believe is reliable.

In the original descriptions of the technique by Teele and Smith and by Blumhagen, a measurement of pyloric wall thickness of 4 mm was judged to be the upper limit of normal. In later reports, measurements of pyloric muscle length suggested a normal upper limit of 17 mm, while the pyloric channel length was felt to be up to 13 mm in normal patients.

Subsequent to the initial reports, a number of studies have been performed suggesting that, in fact, the measurements separating normal from ab-

TABLE 26–1.

Pyloric Measurements in the Diagnosis of HPS*

	Stunden et al.	Blumhagen et al.
Pyloric muscle thickness (mm)		
With HPS	3–5	3.5–6.0
Without HPS	1–3	1.0–3.1
Pyloric canal length (mm)		
With HPS	18–28	11–25
Without HPS	5–14	5–22
Pyloric muscle length (mm)		
With HPS	NA	14–29
Without HPS	NA	5.0–26.5
Pyloric diameter (mm)		
With HPS	9–19	NA
Without HPS	7–13	NA

*HPS = hypertrophic pyloric stenosis; NA = not available.

normal were somewhat smaller than originally anticipated. Stunden et al. studied 200 consecutive infants with persistent vomiting. The authors demonstrated measurements shown in Table 26–1 for overall diameter of the pylorus, thickness of the pyloric muscle, and length of the pyloric canal. Although there was a statistically significant difference in all

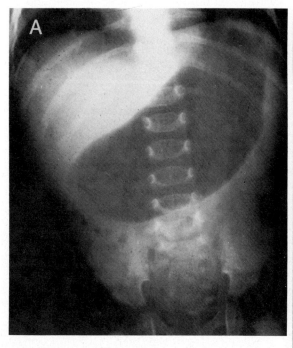
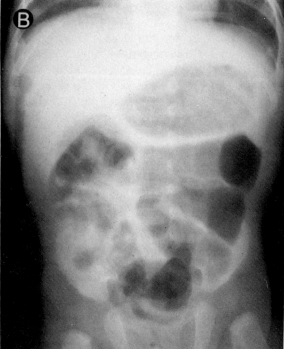

FIG 26–17.
Plain films in pyloric stenosis. **A,** kidney-ureter-bladder study (KUB) demonstrating marked dilatation of the stomach with little gas in the distal bowel in a patient with documented pyloric stenosis. **B,** KUB in a child with surgically documented pyloric stenosis, demonstrating a relatively normal-sized gastric air bubble for a crying baby and gas throughout the rest of the gastrointestinal tract, including the colon.

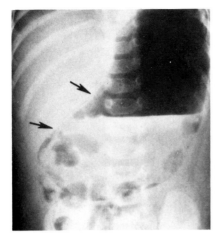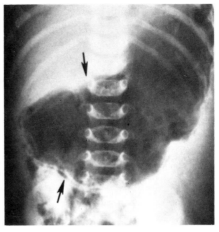

FIG 26–18.
Gastric pneumatosis. Upright and supine views of the abdomen in a 6-week-old girl with pyloric stenosis. The stomach is distended with gas and liquid. Intramural gas can be identified *(arrows)*. The pneumatosis disappeared within 24 hours after decompression with gastric intubation. (Courtesy of Dr. J. Leonidas, New Hyde Park, Long Island.)

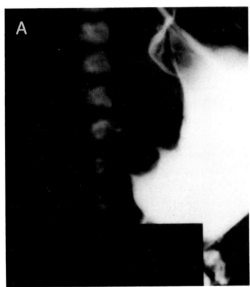

FIG 26–19.
A, typical upper GI series in a patient with pyloric stenosis. The markedly narrowed pylorus curves upward and posteriorly to the duodenal bulb which shows an impression of the hypertrophied muscle in the base. The hypertrophied muscle can also be seen impressing itself on the lesser curvature of the stomach, causing the "pyloric tit" to appear slightly above it. The barium column narrows sharply as it enters the pylorus causing the "beak sign." **B,** a *portion* of an upper GI series in a patient with pyloric stenosis demonstrates a linear filling defect in the barium column, suggesting an antral web. **C,** a little later in the study, the characteristic string sign of pyloric stenosis is seen. Both the pyloric stenosis and antral web were corrected at surgery.

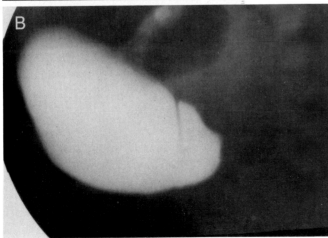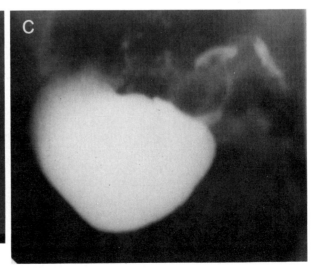

measurements between the normal group and the group with pyloric stenosis, there was a very small overlap between normals and abnormals based on diameter and muscle wall thickness. However, there was complete separation of the two groups based on canal length.

Blumhagen et al. did a similar study on 319 infants in whom they measured the thickness of the pyloric muscle, the length of the pyloric muscle, and the length of the pyloric channel. In their study, there was significant overlap between normals and abnormals in measurement of channel length, less overlap in measurement of muscle length, and no overlap in measurement of muscle thickness. The actual values from both studies are given in Table 26–1.

O'Keeffe et al. studied antropyloric muscle wall thickness in 145 babies with vomiting or regurgitation. All babies with measurements of 3 mm or more had pyloric stenosis while none of the babies with measurements less than 2 mm had HPS. Of the six infants with measurements of 2.0 to 2.9 mm, two had HPS; two, pylorospasm; and one each had milk allergy and gastritis.

Westra et al., on the other hand, found that none of the three measurements was satisfactory for absolutely differentiating abnormal from normal patients and devised a formula for pyloric volume which, in their experience, was more reliable than any of the other indicators. Finkelstein and colleagues suggest that the volume of retained fluid in the stomach can be a guide to the likelihood of pyloric stenosis being present. They recommend measuring gastric contents before deciding which imaging study to perform, using the volume as a predictor of the likelihood of pyloric stenosis being

present. Like Cohen and Haller, we have not found this a useful technique.

Although the value of measurements of the pylorus varies from one study to another, most experienced sonographers have become very comfortable with the technique. In our experience, the criteria of Blumhagen et al. have proved 100% accurate.

Keller et al. compared US measurements of the thickened pylorus with measurements at surgery, finding excellent correlation in each of 17 cases. The sonographic measurement was actually smaller than the anatomical measurement in all cases.

The major argument against using US as the primary imaging modality for pyloric stenosis has been made by Foley et al. They point out that US may be quite accurate in the diagnosis of HPS, but will not be diagnostic in infants with vomiting from other causes. In the latter case, the barium upper GI series is more valuable. In a cost-benefit analysis of vomiting infants, they suggest that the use of US for the initial evaluation of vomiting in infants increases the cost of diagnosis without significant decrease in either morbidity or mortality. Nevertheless, most pediatric radiologists use US as the initial diagnostic imaging study when there is a high index of suspicion based on history and physical examination.

Prior to the advent of real-time US imaging, contrast upper GI series was used for diagnosis and may still be more widely utilized than US by radiologists with limited pediatric sonographic experience. The upper GI series is also utilized when US is normal or equivocal. Riggs and Long described eight plain film findings which are suggestive of the diagnosis when present, but we have never found an instance when an abnormal plain film has precluded the need for US or barium study. Indeed, the plain

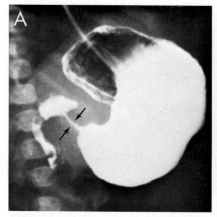
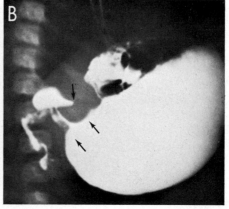

FIG 26–20.
Characteristic findings of hypertrophic pyloric stenosis in a 7-week-old boy with a 4-week history of vomiting. **A,** the pyloric canal is narrowed and elongated *(arrows)* and the base of the duodenal bulb is stretched by the pyloric mass. **B,** the pyloric canal is narrow, demonstrating a double string sign. Indentation of the hypertrophied muscle on the lesser curvature is identified by the *double arrows.*

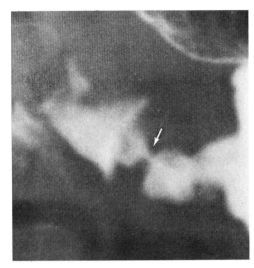

FIG 26–21.
Incomplete pyloromyotomy. This 9-month-old infant had been treated surgically for pyloric stenosis 7½ months earlier. He continued to vomit and did not gain weight adequately. The distal portion of the pyloric channel *(arrow)* at the base of the duodenal bulb did not widen under lengthy fluoroscopic observation. The site of incomplete pyloromyotomy was identified and corrected at surgery.

film may be quite normal even when HPS is present (Fig 26–17). In rare instances, pyloric stenosis is associated with isolated gastric pneumatosis which disappears after the stomach is decompressed (Fig 26–18).

In order to obtain a technically satisfactory barium study, a nasogastric tube should be passed and the stomach emptied. We try to place the tube in the antrum with the patient in the prone oblique position so as not to require large amounts of contrast

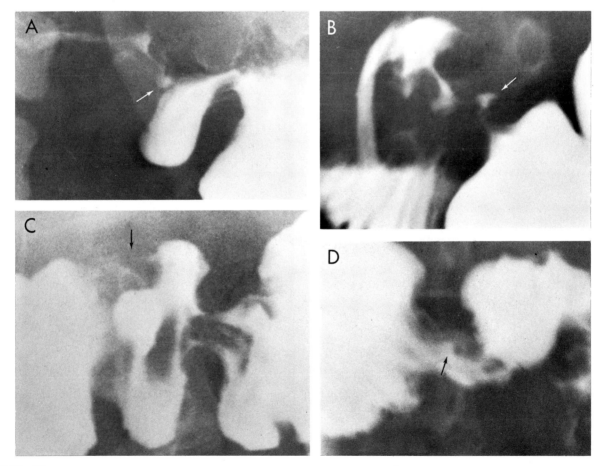

FIG 26–22.
Peptic ulcers. **A,** postbulbar ulcer *(arrow)* in a 9-year-old girl with a long history of vomiting and weight loss. **B,** pyloric channel ulcer *(arrow)* in a 6-year-old boy. **C,** large duodenal ulcer *(arrow)* in the bulb of a boy 9 years of age. Note the marked deformity of the duodenal bulb and the edematous folds. **D,** small channel ulcer *(arrow)* in an 11-year-old boy with abdominal pain and melena.

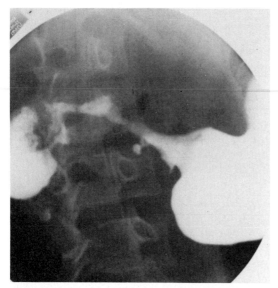

FIG 26–23.
A polypoid "button" gastric ulcer in the pyloric channel with marked narrowing and fibrosis of the chronically inflamed pylorus.

material. Barium is injected via the tube under fluoroscopic control and spot films are taken as needed.

Most of the infants, those with and without HPS, will show some degree of pylorospasm. Generally, barium will finally pass the antropyloric region within 1 to 10 minutes, but may be delayed as long as 20 to 25 minutes. Spasm is not a definitive

sign of HPS but may mimic it on both US and barium study. When spasm is severe, Currarino suggests putting the infant supine and pressing into the abdomen from right to left. With HPS, the pyloric muscle mass pushes into the distal body of the barium-filled stomach, permitting a diagnosis to be made. We prefer using an anticholingeric, although this is rarely necessary. If the barium does not pass the pylorus because of severe HPS, the US scan will be markedly abnormal even to the less experienced sonographer.

The radiographic signs of HPS are remarkably constant from one patient to another (Fig 26–19). The pyloric channel is narrowed (the "string sign") and almost always curved upward posteriorly. Barium may be caught between folds overlying the hypertrophied muscle, and parallel lines (the "double string sign") may be seen (Fig 26–20). The enlarged muscle mass looks much like an "apple-core lesion" with undercutting of the distal antrum and proximal duodenal bulb, although the latter may be seen in normal patients. The "shoulder sign" and the "pyloric tit" are at the juncture of the stomach wall and hypertrophied pyloric muscle. The "beak sign" is noted as the thick muscle narrows the barium column as it enters the pyloric channel. Virtually all of the above signs can be seen transiently in infants, especially those with some degree of spasm. The study should be continued sufficiently long to docu-

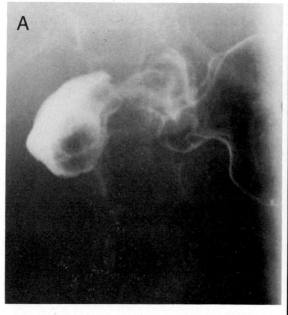

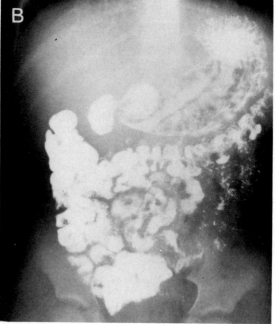

FIG 26–24.
Giant duodenal ulcer, confirmed at endoscopy, in a 7-year-old boy with vomiting and hematemesis **(A)**. Persistent barium in the ulcer at 2 hours after ingestion **(B)** is a useful diagnostic sign.

ment the persistence of the findings in order to assure the diagnosis of pyloric stenosis. On occasion, an associated antral web or diaphragm may be identified (see Fig 26–19).

Following pyloromyotomy, both the US and the barium gastrointestinal study may remain abnormal for several months, even in asymptomatic patients. Thus, the diagnosis of incomplete surgical repair requires a history of persistent vomiting as well as a positive imaging study (Fig 26–21).

Several attempts have been made to treat HPS by peroral balloon dilatation. Hayashi et al. performed this procedure on six patients. In five patients, the muscular ring was incompletely disrupted, and pyloromyotomy was necessary. In the sixth patient, the ring was disrupted, but the mucosa was torn, requiring surgical repair.

The most common antropyloric abnormality mimicking HPS on upper GI series is spasm. As noted, pharmacologic agents may be necessary to make a definitive differentiation. Although spasm may also make the pyloric muscle appear thicker on US, this is a transient phenomenon usually distinguishable from HPS. Gastric and duodenal ulcers and gastritis (see below) can mimic the findings of HPS, especially on US.

PEPTIC ULCER DISEASE

Gastric and duodenal ulcers occur in both neonates and older children but with some differences. Gastric ulcers are much more common than duodenal ulcers in the newborn and most typically present with free intraperitoneal air from perforation or with

hematemesis. Neonatal ulcer disease is discussed more thoroughly in Chapter 52.

Peptic ulcer disease in children beyond the newborn period is much like that in adults. In the study of Drumm et al., the ages ranged from 3 months to 17 years. Duodenal ulcers are three times as commonly diagnosed as gastric ulcers in infants and children. Drumm et al. reported that ulcers in children under age 10 years were more likely to be associated with other diseases, whereas those in adolescents and teenagers were likely to be primary. Most of the diseases reported to be associated with peptic ulcers are treated with ulcerogenic drugs which may be the immediate cause of the ulcers. Patients with cystic fibrosis may have a deficient defense mechanism because of abnormal intestinal mucus, but they are often treated with ulcerogenic drugs and are subject to intense emotional stress and the etiology of ulcers in them is probably multifactorial. Patients with Zollinger-Ellison syndrome have severe abdominal pain, intractable peptic ulcers, and gastric hypersecretion. Non-beta islet cell tumors of the pancreas are implicated as the cause. Rarely seen in children, the syndrome has been described in patients as young as 7 years old.

The radiologic appearance of ulcers in children is much like that in adults (Fig 26–22). Barium is the contrast material of choice unless perforation is suspected in which case a low osmolar nonionic contrast agent should be used. Gastric ulcers are more likely to be in the antrum. Ulcers in both stomach and duodenum will demonstrate a barium-filled niche with radiating folds representing surrounding mucosal inflammation. In the gastric antrum, "button ulcers" may be seen (Fig 26–23). Giant duodenal

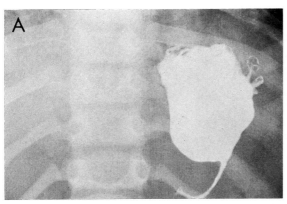
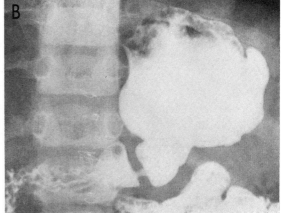

FIG 26–25.
Severe necrotizing gastritis due to zinc chloride. **A,** 8 weeks after ingestion of soldering solution, the distal third of the stomach is constricted to a lumen a few millimeters in diameter with almost complete obstruction of the pylorus. **B,** 13 months after surgery, function of the deformed, remaining portion of the stomach is normal.

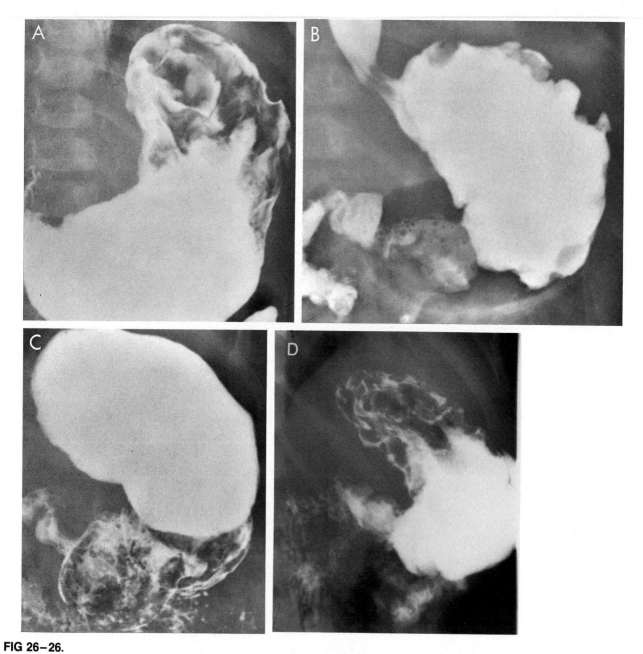

FIG 26–26.
Ménétrier disease. **A,** prone and **B,** supine projections of the stomach show rugal hypertrophy in a 3½-year-old girl with periorbital edema. Hypoproteinemia was found on laboratory studies. **C,** 3 months later, serum protein values were normal as were the gastric rugae. **D,** giant rugal hypertrophy in a 2-year-old boy with hyperproteinemia, diffuse edema, and pleural effusions. Note the body and antrum of the stomach are normal.

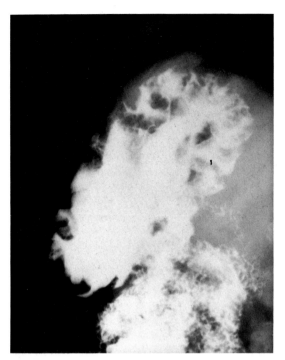

FIG 26–27.
Lymphangiectasia of the stomach demonstrates giant rugal hypertrophy involving all parts of the stomach.

ulcers are even more rare in children than in adults (Fig 26–24). They usually require surgical therapy.

The study of Drumm et al. confirms the high false-negative rate of single contrast barium studies for ulcer disease when compared with endoscopy that has been demonstrated previously in adults. Double contrast studies of the stomach and duodenum may have a higher sensitivity but are difficult

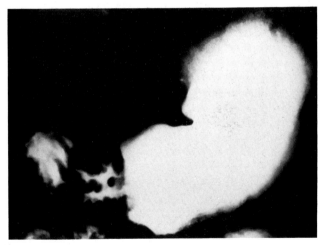

FIG 26–28.
Eosinophilic gastritis. The gastric antrum is narrowed with polypoid filling defects in this adolescent girl with peripheral eosinophilia. Diagnosis was documented by biopsy. Note the proximal portion of the stomach is entirely normal.

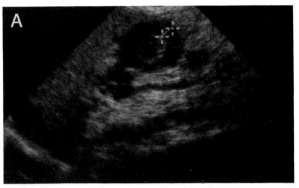

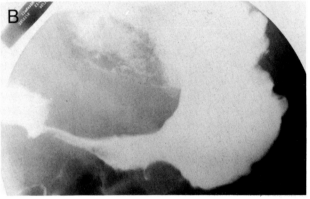

FIG 26–29.
Chronic granulomatous disease of childhood in a 2-year-old boy. **A,** US demonstrates persistently marked enlargement of the antropyloric wall. **B,** upper GI series demonstrates a long narrowed antrum and pylorus which were fixed on fluoroscopic examination.

to perform in young children and usually result in a higher radiation dose at any age. As with antral gastritis, duodenal ulcers may be associated with *Campylobacter pyloris.* Endoscopy appears to be the most sensitive diagnostic procedure.

Although US is not used routinely in evaluation for ulcer disease, Hayden et al. found 7 children of 600 being investigated for vomiting who had US abnormalities with gastric ulcers demonstrated by other means. The US abnormalities included thickening of the antropyloric mucosa, elongation of the antropyloric canal, persistent spasm, and delayed gastric emptying.

GASTRITIS

Gastritis is a nonspecific term for inflammation of the mucosa of the stomach. A number of etiologies have been implicated in childhood gastritis, and the common ones are discussed below.

Chemical gastritis is secondary to the ingestion of a variety of substances and can be of extreme severity and even lead to death. Although alkali ingestion more commonly causes esophagitis (see Chapter 25),

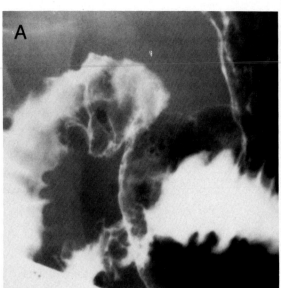

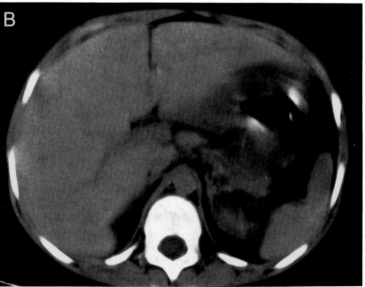

FIG 26–30.
A and **B,** Crohn disease. Marked mucosal fold hypertrophy of the duodenal bulb and postbulbar portion of the duodenum was shown at endoscopy and biopsy to be secondary to previously undetected Crohn disease.

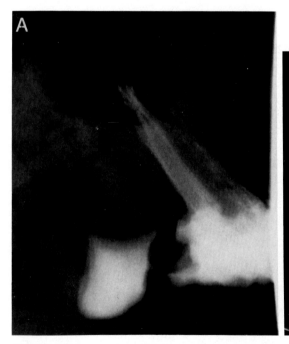

FIG 26–31.
Graft-vs-host disease. **A,** upper GI series demonstrates the body of the stomach to be rigid with effacement of the mucosa secondary to submucosal infiltration. **B,** CT scan demonstrates marked edema of the gastric wall in this 14-year-old girl who had had bone marrow transplant for acute lymphocytic leukemia. Similar findings have been described elsewhere in the gastrointestinal tract.

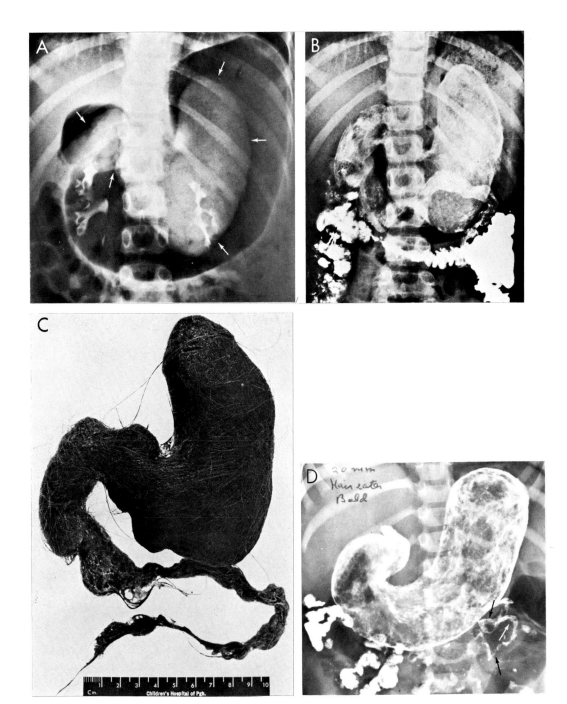

FIG 26–32.
Trichobezoar in a 10-year-old girl with anemia and left upper quadrant mass. **A,** a large soft-tissue mass is seen in the dilated, air-filled stomach *(arrows).* **B,** barium is trapped in the trichobezoar, demonstrating the mass extending through the duodenum and into the proximal jejunum. **C,** surgical specimen. **D,** trichobezoar in a 20-month-old girl. The mass of hair fills the gastric lumen. The *arrows* demonstrate pieces of the trichobezoar in the duodenum and jejunum.

about 20% of patients who ingest these substances will also develop mild to moderate degrees of antral gastritis. More common agents implicated in the direct production of gastritis are calcium chloride, zinc chloride, iron sulfate tablets, and acids (Fig 26–25).

Following the ingestion of corrosive agents, plain films, including horizontal-beam radiographs, should be obtained to exclude free air prior to any contrast studies being performed. If there is no evidence of perforation, double contrast studies of the stomach are most useful if they can be performed. The most common of the corrosive agents used is calcium chloride. It is likely that some free hydrochloric acid is formed in the stomach by hydrolysis of calcium chloride and it is this acid which is the direct cause of the severe gastritis. Most commonly, by the time contrast studies are performed, there has already been severe edema, spasm, and narrowing of the distal stomach. Secondary calcification in the gastric wall, with cicatricial constrictions, has been found several weeks after the original ingestion. Extensive necrosis of the stomach, with almost complete obstruction, has been reported from the ingestion of zinc chloride also. Again, typically, the distal body and antrum of the stomach are primarily involved. Ingested ferrous sulfate tablets can lead to complete gastric outlet obstruction with scarring of the antrum. Vomiting and hematemesis generally occur almost immediately after ingestion, and death has been reported.

Intramural air in the stomach has been reported in cases of gastritis, although it is more common in adults than in children. More commonly, gastric pneumatosis will be secondary to gastric outlet obstruction, small intestinal obstruction, or necrotizing enterocolitis in the newborn.

Campylobacter pyloris has been described in association with gastritis and peptic ulcer disease since 1982. Antral gastritis is present in virtually every patient, adult, or child from whom the organism is cultured, and gastric or duodenal ulcers have been described in many. Morrison et al. described a pattern of enlarged gastric folds in the body and antropyloric regions of the stomach in half of their patients with biopsy-proven *Campylobacter* infection.

Markedly enlarged gastric folds, so-called giant rugal hypertrophy, are more typically associated with *Ménétrier disease*. This is an uncommon, self-limited disease in children which may not be the same as the adult disease. The cause in children is unknown. Hypersensitivity response, autoimmune disease, and cytomegalovirus (CMV) infection have all been implicated but not proved. The children usually present with abdominal pain or with nausea

and vomiting. Because of an associated protein-losing enteropathy, peripheral edema, ascites, and pleural effusions are frequently found. Gastric hemorrhage is rare. On barium study, there is marked enlargement of the fundal rugae, especially along the greater curvature, with sparing of the antropyloric region (Fig 26–26). US demonstrates thickened mucosa and rugal hypertrophy when the stomach is empty or partially filled, according to Gassner et al. When the stomach is completely filled with fluid, the hypertrophied rugae characteristically collapse. Markedly enlarged gastric rugae may also be seen in gastrointestinal lymphangiectasia (Fig 26–27).

Infectious gastritis has been described in adults with acquired immunodeficiency syndrome (AIDS). Falcone et al. described 11 patients with AIDS who

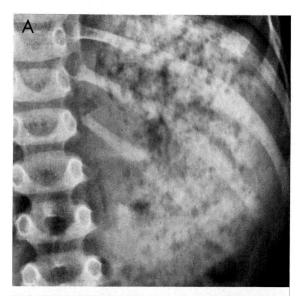

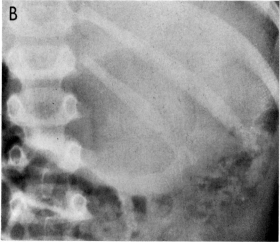

FIG 26–33.
Food simulating a gastric bezoar in a 3-year-old girl. **A,** shortly after a breakfast of four bowls of dry cereal was consumed. **B,** 24 hours later, the stomach appears normal.

had gastric abnormalities. Five of these had infections with CMV, *Toxoplasma gondii*, or *Cryptosporidium*; the other six had Kaposi sarcoma or lymphoma.

Eosinophilic gastritis has been reported, occurring both alone and, more commonly, as part of a more diffuse gastroenteritis involving particularly the small intestine. It is typically of an allergic or hypersensitivity etiology and generally responds well to steroids. The disease usually causes a strikingly nodular pattern in the gastric antrum with relative sparing of the body and fundus (Fig 26–28).

Chronic granulomatous disease of childhood (CGD) is a syndrome of recurrent infection, usually bacterial or fungal, whose underlying pathophysiology is one of disordered phagocytosis. The most common gastrointestinal manifestation is chronic antral gastritis (Fig 26–29). US examination demonstrates an abnormally thick (>4 mm) antropyloric wall. This finding simulates HPS but occurs in patients beyond infancy. Upper GI series reveals narrowing of the

antropyloric lumen secondary to chronic inflammation and fibrosis. Surgical intervention is generally not required.

Crohn disease is more common in the upper gastrointestinal tract than has been thought. Lenaerts et al. reported involvement of the esophagus, stomach, and duodenum in 69 of 230 children. In 13 of the patients, radiologic studies were negative. However, these studies were not performed using double contrast technique which is imperative to find the aphthous ulcers which characterize the early stages of the disease. These will be found most typically in the antrum, pylorus, and duodenum (Fig 26–30), but can be seen in the more proximal stomach as well as the distal esophagus.

Graft-vs.-host disease (GVHD) most typically affects the distal small intestine and the colon, but can affect the stomach. The findings are nonspecific, but suggestive when other clinical signs of GVHD are present. Mucosal inflammation and irregularity may

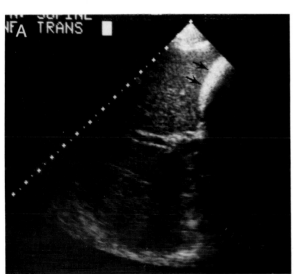

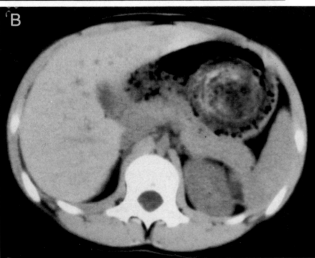

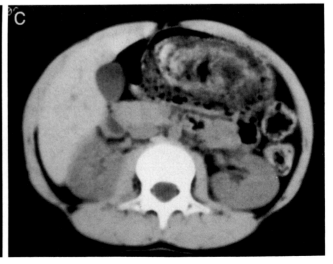

FIG 26–34.
Gastric bezoar. **A,** transverse US scan in the epigastrium demonstrates a broad band of increased echogenicity in the region of the stomach *(arrows),* with clear shadowing posteriorly. This appearance persists irrespective of the angle or plane of imaging. CT cuts through the fundus **(B)** and antrum **(C)** of the stomach demonstrate an intragastric mass consisting of compressed concentric rings with entrapped air, debris, and barium (from an upper GI series 10 days previously). (From Newman B, Girdany BR: *Pediatr Radiol* 1990; 20:526. Used by permission.)

be identified on barium studies, while CT or US, as well as barium studies, may demonstrate thickening of the gastric wall (Fig 26–31). In the acute phase, this is related to edema. In the chronic phase, fibrosis is a more likely diagnosis. Patients with GVHD may also acquire CMV gastroenteritis, and the imaging findings are indistinguishable from GVHD itself.

Duodenitis has been a historically contentious subject for radiologists. It is an uncommon finding in children who are more likely to have antral gastritis than duodenditis. Large mucosal folds in the duodenal bulb are best seen on double contrast upper gastrointestinal examination. However, Levine et al., in a series of 50 adults having upper GI series and endoscopy, found the radiographs to have 50% false-positive and 50% false-negative results.

BEZOARS

Occasionally, ingested materials accumulate in the stomach and form nonopaque foreign bodies called bezoars. *Trichobezoars,* or hairballs, result usually from the swallowing of hair plucked from the head or fibers from fur rugs, garments, or woolen clothing and blankets. Over a period of time, an intralu-

minal mass develops, representing matted hair and trapped food particles, taking the shape of the stomach (Fig 26–32). Young girls are the most commonly affected. Alternatively, certain foods may simulate bezoars on plain film examination, but the findings disappear with time (Fig 26–33). *Phytobezoars,* or foodballs, are composed of mucilaginous masses; they develop most frequently following the ingestion of high-fiber vegetables and fruits. Swallowed shellac or tar may also form gastric foreign bodies.

Plain film examination of patients with bezoars may show an appearance like that of the stomach shortly after the ingestion of a meal. Horizontal-beam plain films typically demonstrate a rim of air surrounding the intragastric mass. Bezoars of all types produce filling defects in the stomach after the ingestion of barium. After the free barium has been expelled from the stomach, the barium that has adhered to the surface of the bezoar, and has been absorbed by it, casts a persistent, mottled shadow of increased density. Small bezoars are frequently movable, may be of almost any shape, and are found in any position.

Newman and Girdany have demonstrated the US and CT characteristics of trichobezoars (Fig 26–34). US demonstrates a broad band of increased echogenicity in the stomach with prominent acoustic shadowing. CT demonstrates an intragastric mass with entrapped air and debris. Large milk curds may remain in the stomach long after the organ has emptied itself of liquid and simulate hairballs and fiber balls. This is most typically seen in the newborn and may reflect states of hydration and types of formula

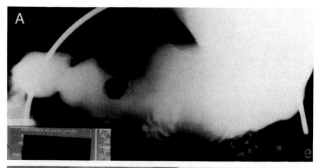

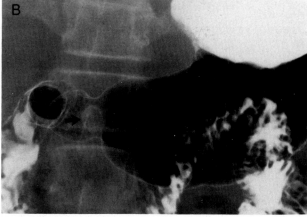

FIG 26–35.
Solitary benign gastric polyp in a 14-year-old boy seen on single **(A)** and double **(B)** contrast examinations. No evidence of polyposis syndromes was found on extensive evaluation.

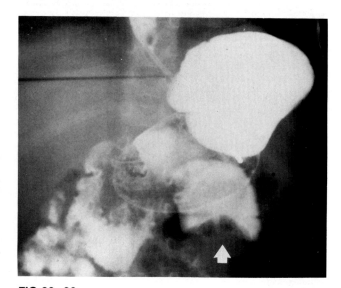

FIG 26–36.
Inflammatory fibroid polyp of the jejunum presenting with symptoms of gastric outlet obstruction. (Same patient as in Fig 26–4.)

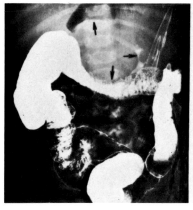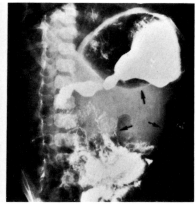

FIG 26–37.
Gastric teratoma. Frontal and oblique views of a barium enema and upper GI series demonstrate a large mass impinging on the stomach and transverse colon. At surgery, the mass was found to arise directly from the stomach and teratoma was documented histologically.

used. Grosfeld et al. have noted the changing pattern of bezoar formation, particularly in prematurely born infants. In 35 of 40 infants and children studied by them, alimentary tract bezoars were related to medical therapy.

TUMORS AND TUMORLIKE CONDITIONS

True neoplasms of the stomach are relatively uncommon in childhood. Polyps have been described in several of the polyposis syndromes, including Peutz-Jeghers syndrome and Gardner syndrome, as well as familial polyposis. Double contrast studies of the stomach are most useful for evaluation of these polyps (Fig 26–35).

Inflammatory fibroid polyps are more typically seen in the small intestine (Fig 26–36), but can appear anywhere in the upper gastrointestinal tract, including the stomach and duodenum. In fact, reports of these lesions in the stomach and duodenum have been appearing with increasing frequency. Their cause is unclear and they have gone by a variety of names in the past. The histologic appearance varies slightly between areas and the gastric lesions frequently contain elements histologically characterized as neurilemmomas. They are always benign, can be either polypoid or sessile, originate in the submucosa, and are best seen on double contrast

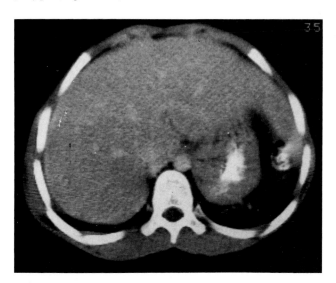

FIG 26–38.
Non-Hodgkin lymphoma of the stomach in a 14-year-old boy. The wall of the entire stomach is uniformly thickened on CT scan. Findings were confirmed at laparotomy.

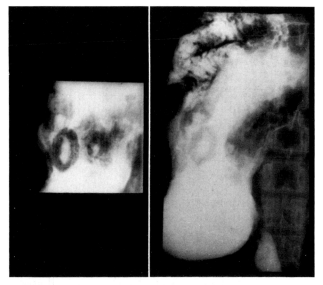

FIG 26–39.
Upper GI series in a 16-year-old boy with diffuse non-Hodgkin lymphoma demonstrates "bull's-eye" lesions throughout the stomach which were confirmed at endoscopy and microscopy to be lymphoma.

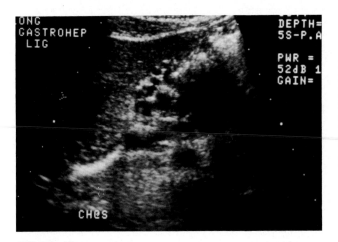

FIG 26–40.
US of the gastrohepatic ligament demonstrates multiple dilated vessels within the ligament virtually diagnostic of varices.

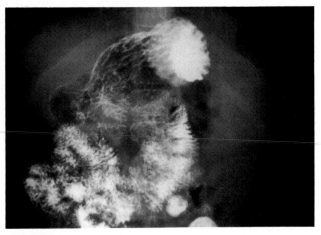

FIG 26–41.
Gastric varices in an 8-year-old boy with cavernous transformation of the portal vein and massive splenomegaly. Note the serpiginous filling defects throughout the fundus and lesser curvature of the stomach. Varices were confirmed by endoscopy.

studies of the stomach or duodenum. They are also easily identified on CT.

Gastric teratomas have been described in neonates and young infants, predominantly affecting boys. They most commonly present with evidence of proximal gastrointestinal obstruction or gastrointestinal hemorrhage (Fig 26–37).

Malignant lesions of the stomach are extremely rare. Carcinomas have been described in teenagers. The most common malignancy involving the stomach in children is lymphoma, usually of the non-Hodgkin variety. These lesions present with markedly enlarged gastric folds, usually in the body or pyloric region. CT typically shows marked thickening of the gastric wall due to diffusely infiltrative tumor (Fig 26–38). Rarely, they may present as "bull's-eye" lesions simulating melanomatous lesions in adults (Fig 26–39).

Both benign and malignant tumors of smooth muscle have been described in the stomach. Leiomyoma, leiomyoblastoma, and leiomyosarcoma have all been seen, although quite rarely in children. Since they are typically submucosal, the diagnosis can be made by barium study, but thickening of the submucosal region on US or CT is usually more suggestive of the correct diagnosis. CT is particularly useful to demonstrate the extragastric component of the tumor which may occur with the malignant varieties.

Other than the inflammatory polyps, primary neoplasms of the duodenum are extraordinarily rare. Both the stomach and the duodenum may be affected by tumors arising elsewhere in the abdomen which invade or displace them.

VARICES

Patients with portal hypertension may develop gastric and duodenal varices in addition to those in the esophagus. On US or CT, varices may be found in the gastrohepatic ligament (Fig 26–40) and the gastric wall. On barium studies, gastric varices are most commonly found in the fundus and along the lesser curvature, appearing as serpiginous filling defects (Fig 26–41). A similar appearance may less commonly be seen in the antrum or the proximal duodenum.

REFERENCES

Hypertrophic Pyloric Stenosis

Blumhagen JD: The role of ultrasonography in the evaluation of vomiting in infants. *Pediatr Radiol* 1986; 16:267–270.

Blumhagen JD, Maclin L, Krauter D, et al: Sonographic diagnosis of hypertrophic pyloric stenosis. *Am J Roentgenol* 1988; 150:1367.

Blumhagen JD, Noble HGS: Muscle thickness in hypertrophic pyloric stenosis: Sonographic determination. *Am J Roentgenol* 1983; 140:221–223.

Breaux CW Jr, Georgeson KE, Royal SA, et al: Changing patterns in the diagnosis of hypertrophic pyloric stenosis. *Pediatrics* 1988; 81:213.

Cohen HL, Haller JO: Hypertrophic pyloric stenosis: Volumetric measurement of nasogastric aspirate to determine imaging modality (letter). *Radiology* 1991; 179:877.

Cohen HL, Schechter S, Mastel AL, et al: Ultrasonic "double track" sign in hypertrophic pyloric stenosis. *J Ultrasound Med* 1987; 6:136.

Currarino G: The value of double contrast examination of the stomach with pressure "spots" in the diagnosis of infantile hypertrophic pyloric stenosis. *Radiology* 1964; 83:873–878.

Finkelstein MS, Mandell GA, Tarbell KV: Hypertrophic pyloric stenosis: volumetric measurement of nasogastric aspirate to determine the imaging modality. *Radiology* 1990; 177:759.

Foley LC, Slovis TL, Campbell JB, et al: Evaluation of the vomiting infant. *Am J Dis Child* 1989; 143:660.

Forman HP, Leonidas JC, Kronfeld CD: A rational approach to the diagnosis of hypertrophic pyloric stenosis: Do the results match the claims? *J Pediatr Surg* 1990; 25:202.

Geer LL, Gaisie G, Mandell VS, et al: Evolution of pyloric stenosis in the first week of life. *Pediatr Radiol* 1985; 15:205–206.

Haller JO, Cohen HL: Hypertrophic pyloric stenosis: diagnosis using US. *Radiology* 1986; 161:335.

Hayashi AH, Giacomantonio JM, Lau HYC, et al: Balloon catheter dilatation for hypertrophic pyloric stenosis. *J Pediatr Surg* 1990; 25:1119.

Jamroz GA, Blocker SH, McAlister WH: Radiographic findings after incomplete pyloromyotomy. *Gastrointest Radiol* 1986; 11:139–141.

Keller H, Waldmann D, Greiner P: Comparison of preoperative sonography with intraoperative findings in congenital hypertrophic pyloric stenosis. *J Pediatr Surg* 1987; 22:950.

Konvolinka CW, Wernuth CR: Hypertrophic pyloric stenosis in older infants. *Am J Dis Child* 1971; 122:76–79.

Latchaw LA, Jacir NN, Harris BH: The development of pyloric stenosis during transpyloric feedings. *J Pediatr Surg* 1989; 24:823.

Mandell GA: Association of antral diaphragms and hypertrophic pyloric stenosis. *Am J Roentgenol* 1978; 131:203–206.

O'Keeffe FN, Stansberry SD, Swischuk LE, Hayden CK: Antropyloric muscle thickness at US in infants: What is normal? *Radiology* 1991; 178:827.

Okorie NM, Dickson JA, Carver RA, et al: What happens to the pylorus after pyloromyotomy? *Arch Dis Child* 1988; 63:1339.

Riggs W Jr., Long L: The value of the plain film roentgenogram in pyloric stenosis. *Am J Roentgenol* 1971; 112:77–82.

Sauerbrei EE, Paloschi GGB: The ultrasonic features of hypertrophic pyloric stenosis, with emphasis on the postoperative appearance. *Radiology* 1983; 147:503–506.

Shuman FI, Darling DB, Fisher JH: The radiographic diagnosis of congenital hypertrophic pyloric stenosis. *J Pediatr* 1967; 71:70–74.

Spevak MR, Ahmadjian JM, Kleinman PK, et al: Sonography of hypertrophic pyloric stenosis: Frequency and cause of nonuniform echogenicity of the thickened pyloric muscle. *Am J Roentgenol* 1992; 158:129.

Steinicke O, Roelsgaard M: Radiographic follow-up in hypertrophic pyloric stenosis. *Acta Paediatr Scand* 1960; 49:4–16.

Stunden RJ, LeQuesne GW, Little KET: The improved ultrasound diagnosis of hypertrophic pyloric stenosis. *Pediatr Radiol* 1986; 16:200.

Swischuk LE, Hayden CK Jr, Stansberry SD: Sonographic pitfalls in imaging of the antropyloric region in infants. *Radiographics* 1989; 9:437.

Teele RL, Smith EH: Ultrasound in the diagnosis of idiopathic hypertrophic pyloric stenosis. *N Engl J Med* 1977; 296:1149–1150.

Weiskittel DA, Leary DL, Blane CE: Ultrasound diagnosis of evolving pyloric stenosis. *Gastrointest Radiol* 1989; 14:22.

Westra SJ, de Groot CJ, Smits NJ, et al: Hypertrophic pyloric stenosis: use of the pyloric volume measurement in early US diagnosis. *Radiology* 1989; 172:615.

Peptic Ulcer Disease

Block WM: Chronic gastric ulcer in childhood: A critical analysis of the literature with report of a case in an eleven year old boy. *Am J Dis Child* 1963; 85:566–574.

Drumm B, Rhoads JM, Stringer DA, et al: Peptic ulcer disease in children: Etiology, clinical findings and clinical course. *Pediatrics* 1988; 82:410–414.

Dunn S, Weber TR, Grosfeld JL, et al: Acute peptic ulcer in childhood. *Arch Surg* 1983; 118:656–660.

Hayden CK Jr, Swischuk LE, Rytting JE: Gastric ulcer disease in infants: US findings. *Radiology* 1987; 164:131–134.

Kumar D, Spitz L: Peptic ulceration in children. *Surg Gynecol Obstet* 1984; 159:63–66.

Purelekar SG, Lubert M: Ultrasound demonstration of giant duodenal ulcer. *Gastrointest Radiol* 1983; 8:29–31.

Rosenquist CJ: Clinical and radiographic features of giant duodenal ulcer. *Clin Radiol* 1969; 20:324.

Gastritis

Baker A, Volberg F, Sumner T, et al: Childhood Ménétrier's disease: Four new cases and discussion of the literature. *Gastrointest Radiol* 1986; 11:131.

Bar-Ziv J, Barki Y, Weizman Z, Urkin J: Transient protein-losing gastropathy (Ménétrier's disease) in childhood. *Pediatr Radiol* 1988; 18:82–84.

Bowen A III, Gibson MD: Chronic granulomatous disease with gastric antral narrowing. *Pediatr Radiol* 1980; 10:119–120.

Burns B, Gay BB: Ménétrier's disease of the stomach in children. *Am J Roentgenol* 1968; 103:300–306.

Chalouplea JC, Gay BB, Caplan D: *Campylobacter* gastritis simulating Ménétrier's disease by upper gastrointestinal radiography. *Pediatr Radiol* 1990; 20:200–201.

Coad NAG, Shah KJ: Ménétrier's disease in childhood associated with cytomegalovirus infection: A case report and review of the literature. *Br J Radiol* 1986; 59:615–620.

Derchi LE, Biggi GARE, Cicio GR, et al: Sonographic findings of Ménétrier's disease: A case report. *Gastrointest Radiol* 1982; 7:323–325.

Dohmen K, Harada M, Ishibashi M, et al: Ultrasonographic studies on abdominal complications in patients receiving marrow-ablative chemotherapy and bone marrow or blood stem cell transplantation. *JCU* 1991; 19:321.

Drumm B, O'Brien A, Cutz E, Sherman P: *Campylobacter pylori*–associated primary gastritis in children. *Pediatrics* 1987; 80:192–195.

Falcone S, Murphy BJ, Weinfeld A: Gastric manifestations of AIDS: Radiographic findings on upper gastrointestinal examination. *Gastrointest Radiol* 1991; 16:95.

Franken EA Jr: Caustic damage of the gastrointestinal tract: Roentgen features. *Am J Roentgenol Radium Ther Nucl Med* 1973; 118:77–85.

Gassner I, Strasser K, Bart G, et al: Sonographic appearance of Ménétrier's disease in a child. *J Ultrasound Med* 1990; 9:537.

Gelfand DW, Dale WJ, Ott DJ, et al: Duodenitis: Endoscopic-radiologic correlation in 272 patients. *Radiology* 1985; 157:577–581.

Griscom NT, Kirkpatrick JA, Girdany BR, et al: Gastric antral narrowing in chronic granulomatous disease of childhood. *Pediatrics* 1974; 54:456–460.

Kopen PA, McAlister WH: Upper gastrointestinal and ultrasound examinations of gastric antral involvement in chronic granulomatous disease. *Pediatr Radiol* 1984; 14:91–93.

Lenaerts C, Roy CC, Vaillancourt M, et al: High incidence of upper gastrointestinal tract involvement in children with Crohn disease. *Pediatrics* 1989; 83:777.

Leonidas JC, Beatty EC, Wenner HA: Ménétrier disease and cytomegalovirus infection in childhood. *Am J Dis Child* 1973; 126:806–808.

Levine MS, Turner D, Ekberg O, et al: Duodenitis: A reliable radiologic diagnosis? *Gastrointest Radiol* 1991; 16:99.

Manson DE, Stringer DA, Durie PR, et al: The radiologic and endoscopic investigation and etiologic classification of gastritis in children. *J Can Assoc Radiol* 1990; 41:201.

Marks MP, Lanza MV, Kahlstrom EJ, et al: Pediatric hypertrophic gastropathy. *Am J Roentgenol* 1986; 147:1031–1034.

Mashako MNL, Cezard JP, Navarro J, et al: Crohn's disease lesions in the upper gastrointestinal tract: Correlation between clinical, radiological, endoscopic, and histologic features in adolescents and children. *J Pediatr Gastroenterol* 1989; 8:442.

McDonald GB, Shulman HM, Sullivan KM, et al: Intestinal and hepatic complications of human bone marrow transplantation. Part I. *Gastroenterology* 1986; 90:460.

Morrison S, Dahms BB, Hoffenberg E, et al: Enlarged gastric folds in association with *Campylobacter pylori* gastritis. *Radiology* 1989; 171:819–821.

Ott DG, Gelfand DW, Wu WC, et al: Sensitivity of single- vs. double-contrast radiology in erosive gastritis. *Am J Roentgenol* 1982; 138:263–266.

Pugh TF, Fitch SJ: Invasive gastric candidiasis. *Pediatr Radiol* 1986; 16:67–68.

Scharschmidt BF: The natural history of hypertrophic gastropathy (Ménétrier's disease). Report of a case with 16-year follow-up and review of 120 cases from the literature. *Am J Med* 1977; 63:644–652.

Teele RL, Katz AJ, Goldman H, et al: Radiographic features of eosinophilic gastroenteritis (allergic gastroenteropathy) of childhood. *Am J Roentgenol* 1979; 132:575–580.

Theoni RF, Goldberg HI, Ominsky S, et al: Detection of gastritis by single and double contrast radiography. *Radiology* 1983; 148:621–626.

Tootla F, Lucas RJ, Bernacki EG, et al: Gastroduodenal Crohn's disease. *Arch Surg* 1976; 3:855–857.

Turner CJ, Lipitz LR, Pastore RA: Antral gastritis. *Radiology* 1974; 113:305–312.

Bezoars

Grosfeld JL, Schreiner RL, Franken EA: The changing pattern of gastrointestinal bezoars in infants and children. *Surgery* 1980; 16:301.

McCracken S, Jongeward R, Silver TM, et al: Gastric trichobezoar: Sonographic findings. *Radiology* 1986; 161:123–124.

Naik DR, Bolia A, Boon AW: Demonstration of a lactobezoar by ultrasound. *Br J Radiol* 1987; 60:506–508.

Newman B, Girdany BR: Gastric trichobezoars—sonographic and computed tomographic appearance. *Pediatr Radiol* 1990; 20:526.

Tumors and Tumorlike Conditions

Bahk YW, Ahn JS, Choi HJ: Lymphoid hyperplasia of the stomach presenting as umbilicated polypoid lesions. *Radiology* 1971; 100:277–280.

Bowen B, Ros PR, McCarthy MJ, et al: Gastrointestinal teratomas: CT and US appearance with pathologic correlation. *Radiology* 1987; 162:431–433.

Denzler TB, Harned RK, Pergam CJ: Gastric polyps in familial polyposis coli. *Radiology* 1979; 130:63–66.

Dixon WL, Fazzari PJ: Carcinoma of the stomach in a child. *JAMA* 1976; 235: 2414–2415.

Dunnick NR, Harell GS, Parker BR: Multiple "bull's-eye" lesions in gastric lymphoma. *Am J Roentgenol* 1976; 126:965.

Lichtman S, Hayes G, Stringer DA, et al: Chronic intussusception due to antral myoepithelioma. *J Pediatr Surg* 1986; 21:955–956.

Megibow AJ, Balthazar EJ, Hulnick DH, et al: CT evaluation of gastrointestinal leiomyomas and leiomyosarcomas. *Am J Roentgenol* 1985; 144:727–731.

Odes HS, Krawiec J, Yanai-Inbar I, et al: Benign lymphoid hyperplasia of the stomach. *Pediatr Radiol* 1981; 10:244–246.

Schneider K, Dickerhoff R, Bertele RM: Malignant gastric sarcoma—diagnosis by ultrasound. *Pediatr Radiol* 1986; 16:69–70.

Shimer GR, Helwig EB: Inflammatory fibroid polyps of the intestine. *Am J Clin Pathol* 1984; 81:708.

Siegel MJ, Shackelford GD: Gastric teratomas in infants: Report of 2 cases. *Pediatr Radiol* 1978; 7:197–200.

Wurlitzer FP, Mares AJ, Isaacs H Jr, et al: Smooth muscle tumors of the stomach in childhood and adolescence. *J Pediatr Surg* 1973; 8:421–427.

27

The Small Intestine

Imaging studies
Hereditary and developmental disorders
Functional and infiltrative diseases
Infectious diseases

Crohn disease
Acquired small-intestinal obstruction
Intussusception
Tumors

The small intestine is a long, convoluted, musculo-membranous tube that begins at the pylorus and ends at the ileocecal valve. Its length and pattern are variable; its three major divisions are the duodenum, jejunum, and ileum. The jejunum accounts for approximately three fifths of the small bowel; the remaining two fifths is ileum. The proximal third of the small intestine commonly fills the left upper abdominal quadrant, the middle third occupies the midportion of the abdomen and the right upper quadrant, and the terminal third lies on the right side of the abdomen and pelvis. The caliber of the lumen gradually diminishes from proximal to distal, the diameter of the terminal ileum being about one third smaller than the first portion of the jejunum. The external surface of the tube is smooth and devoid of permanent folds or creases. The internal surface is thrown into transverse and spiral folds, the plicae circulares of the submucosa, which are covered by the villous folds of mucous membrane. These folds greatly increase the secreting and absorbing surface and facilitate digestion by retarding the passage of the intestinal content. The embryologic development of the small intestine is described in Chapter 22.

IMAGING STUDIES

Plain radiographs are often nonspecific in patients with small-intestinal disease but are extremely useful in identifying adynamic ileus, intestinal obstruction, free air secondary to intestinal perforation, pathologic calcification, and masses large enough to displace normal structures. The *contrast small-intestinal series* remains the mainstay of small-bowel imaging. Barium is still the most frequently used contrast agent with the more expensive water-soluble non-ionic agents reserved for specific indications such as potential perforations. Although *ultrasound* (US) is limited by the intraluminal air of the intestine, it can often identify thickened bowel wall, intestinal and mesenteric masses, including abscesses and intussusceptions, and has increasing utility in a variety of disease entities as discussed throughout this chapter. *Computed tomography* (CT) has ever-increasing utility in the intestinal tract. Good opacification of the bowel lumen is critical for adequate CT evaluation of the intestine and mesentery. CT is useful in a wide variety of disorders including, but not limited to, inflammatory bowel disease and its complications, intra-abdominal abscesses, and mass lesions. *Scintigraphy* plays a limited role in small-bowel disease but may be useful in cases of abdominal pain or intestinal bleeding, especially when ectopic gastric mucosa is suspected. The value of scintigraphy in inflammatory disease of the intestinal tract is still debated. *Magnetic resonance* (MR) imaging of intestinal disease has been little studied in children. Intestinal motion and the lack of a satisfactory intestinal contrast agent severely limits the usefulness of MR except in evaluation of mass lesions.

HEREDITARY AND DEVELOPMENTAL DISORDERS

Most abnormalities of the small intestine of genetic or developmental origin present in the newborn period and are discussed in Chapter 52. Patients with *midgut malrotation* who do not develop volvulus at birth may remain asymptomatic throughout life (Fig 27–1). Midgut volvulus can present beyond infancy, but most patients with malrotation who present with intestinal obstruction later in life do so because of crossing peritoneal (Ladd) bands. As described in

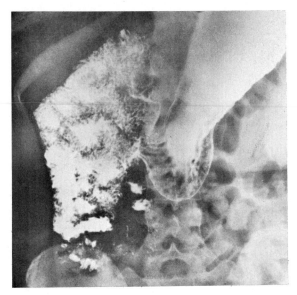

FIG 27–1.
Nonobstructive malrotation of the midgut of a 15½-year-old girl. The jejunum is on the right side of the abdomen and there is no evidence of duodenal obstruction.

Chapter 22, failure of normal rotation of the midgut as it returns from the extraembryonic coelom results in malfixation of the mesentery. Hence, bands of peritoneum may cross anterior to loops of bowel which are caught between the bands and the posterior wall of the peritoneal cavity. The most common site of obstruction is at the third portion of the duodenum (Fig 27–2), but the bands may obstruct anywhere in the upper abdomen, including the colon. Malrotation presenting beyond infancy may have unusual manifestations. Jackson et al. de-

scribed a 16-month-old boy with malrotation and intermittent midgut volvulus who presented with failure to thrive and intestinal malabsorption. The normal alignment of the superior mesenteric artery and vein as seen on US, MR, and CT is sometimes inverted in patients with malrotation, with the vein being found to the left of the artery. This may be a helpful clue in patients with unexplained abdominal pain, according to Shatzkes et al. Zerin and Di Pietro, however, point out that complete inversion of the vessels can be secondary to adjacent masses and that partial inversion of the vessels can be found in normal persons. The same authors used sonography to study nine patients with proven malrotation. Six of them had inversion and three did not.

Duodenal obstruction secondary to *annular pancreas* and associated duodenal stenosis also presents most commonly in the newborn (see Chapters 23 and 52), but may present later in infancy (Fig 27–3) or childhood and even in adults. Affected patients present with intermittent vomiting. Upper gastrointestinal (GI) series in older patients reveals partial obstruction of the descending limb of the duodenum. The prominent gastric and proximal duodenal dilatation seen on plain radiographs of the abdomen in infants is usually not found in older patients. Other congenital obstructive lesions of the duodenum such as webs and diaphragms may also present beyond infancy.

Several different types of developmental cysts may present in infancy or later in childhood, depending largely on the size of the cyst. The most frequent location for a *duplication cyst* of the intestinal

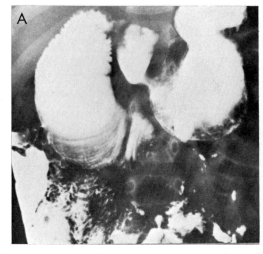
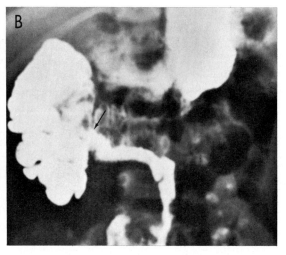

FIG 27–2.
Incomplete obstruction of the third portion of the duodenum secondary to duodenal bands in a boy 5 years of age. **A,** the first and second portions of the duodenum are markedly dilated. The small intestine distal to the usual site of the ligament of Treitz lies below the duodenum and to the right. **B,** delayed film demonstrates the terminal ileum and cecum to be on the right although the cecum is higher than its usual position.

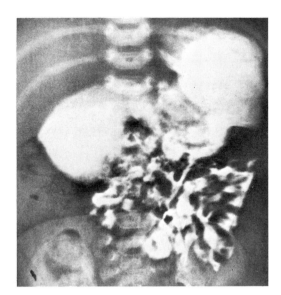

FIG 27–3.
Incomplete obstruction of the second portion of the duodenum secondary to an annular pancreas in a 1-year-old infant.

tract is the region of the terminal ileum and ileocecal valve. The next most common areas are the esophagus, stomach, and duodenum, but they can be located anywhere in the GI tract. Multiple duplications have been reported. Duplication cysts, by definition, contain mucosal and muscular layers. The majority are localized, somewhat spherical, and noncommunicating. Some duplication cysts are tubular, paralleling significant lengths of bowel, and may communicate with the normal intestinal lumen.

Presenting symptoms depend on the location and size of the duplication. Obstruction can occur anywhere there is a duplication cyst and is the most frequent cause of symptoms. Many are large enough to be palpable. Abdominal pain may be related to distention of the cyst or peptic disease if the cyst contains gastric mucosa. Distal ileal duplication may cause intussusception, and volvulus may occur at any site in the small intestine where a duplication is present. GI bleeding may occur from a communicating duplication containing gastric mucosa.

Plain radiographic examination is usually unrewarding unless the duplication is large enough to cause a mass effect on adjacent structures, intestinal obstruction is present, or calcification in the wall is identified (Fig 27–4). Sonography identifies the duplication as anechoic (Fig 27–4,*B*). Sometimes a specific sonographic diagnosis can be suggested if the echogenic mucosa surrounded by a thin hypoechoic halo representing the muscular layer is identified. Occasionally, the cysts will be multilocular. Echogenic debris may be seen, probably secondary to hemorrhage or mucosal secretions. Caspi et al. described an infected duplication with mixed echogenicity that mimicked a pelvic abscess. Those duplications containing gastric mucosa may be identified by technetium 99m pertechnetate scintigraphy. CT is not indicated once sonography demonstrates the cystic nature of the duplication but will show low attenuation surrounded by an enhancing wall. Contrast studies of the intestinal tract may demon-

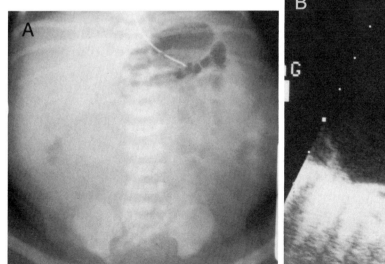

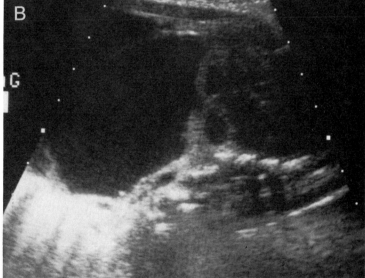

FIG 27–4.
Ileal duplication cyst. **A,** plain film of the abdomen in a newborn infant demonstrates a paucity of bowel gas and marked abdominal distention. **B,** abdominal US demonstrates a large hypoechoic structure with acoustic enhancement adjacent to thickened loops of small intestine. At surgery, multiple noncommunicating ileal duplication cysts were found.

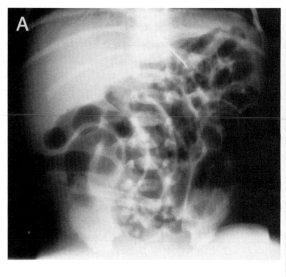

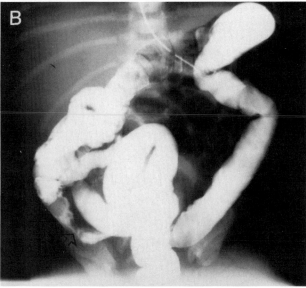

FIG 27–5.
Ileal duplication cyst. **A,** plain radiograph of the abdomen demonstrates multiple dilated loops of small intestine. **B,** barium enema with reflux through the ileocecal valve demonstrates an intramural pressure defect on the terminal ileum *(arrow)*. At surgery, an ileal duplication cyst was identified and removed.

strate the lumen of communicating duplications, but are more likely to demonstrate just the mass effect (Fig 27–5).

Other intraperitoneal cysts arise within the mesentery or omentum. Ros et al. point out that the terms "mesenteric cyst" and "omental cyst" are synonymous and include a group of lesions which have differing histologic and radiographic features. They include enteric duplication cysts with their enteric lining, double muscle layer, and neural elements, as discussed above. *Lymphangiomas* (Fig 27–6) have only an endothelial lining, are usually multiloculated, and may contain chyle. They typically present as painless abdominal distention with a palpable mass. The cyst may be adherent to small intestine, causing partial obstruction and vomiting and requiring surgical resection of involved bowel loops. Plain films show a large mass displacing intestinal loops. Dilated loops may be seen in patients with partial obstruction. GI contrast studies show displacement

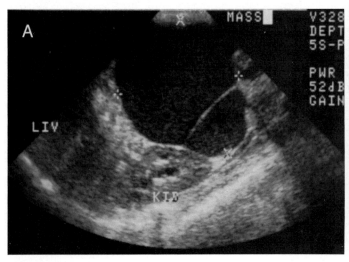

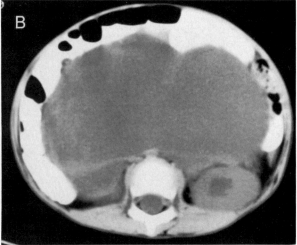

FIG 27–6.
Mesenteric lymphangioma. **A,** longitudinal sonogram through the upper abdomen demonstrates a septated, hypoechoic mass abutting the liver *(LIV)* and right kidney *(KID)*. **B,** CT scan confirms the massive fluid-filled structure displacing contrast-filled loops of bowel. The right-sided septation is again seen, even in an unenhanced scan.

of bowel with no communication. Sonography demonstrates the multilocular nature of the mass with fine septations. Most of the mass is anechoic, but some of the loculated spaces may be hypoechoic or even echogenic, depending on the chyle or blood content. Echogenic debris is commonly seen. CT also demonstrates the septa and loculation. The attenuation values of the fluid range from near-fat to near-water, depending on the content of the fluid. The septa may enhance with intravenous contrast injection. MR studies of patients with lymphangioma show characteristics of the cyst ranging from fluid with low-intensity signal on T1 weighted images to fat with high-intensity signal.

Nonpancreatic pseudocysts can arise in the mesentery. They have a fibrous wall without a lining. They are frequently hemorrhagic or infected with increased echogenicity on sonography and increased attenuation values on CT compared with water. *Enteric cysts* are much like duplication cysts but have an enteric lining without a muscle layer and with no ganglion cells. Mesothelial cysts have a mesothelial lining, are unilocular, and are anechoic on US. *Intraperitoneal teratomas* are typically cystic (Fig 27–7). Identification of multitissue origin, especially when fat and calcium are seen, can lead to the correct diagnosis. Since there is sufficient overlap of imaging findings among the different types of cysts, histologic examination is the only sure diagnostic study, but the characteristics of lymphangioma, a more difficult surgical problem than the other types, may lead in some cases to the correct preoperative diagnosis.

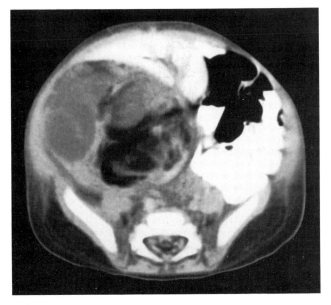

FIG 27–7.
Intraperitoneal teratoma. CT scan demonstrates a large intraperitoneal mass with multiple components of different attenuation values equal to those of water and of fat displacing bowel loops. A benign teratoma was removed at surgery.

FUNCTIONAL AND INFILTRATIVE DISEASES

There are a large number of diseases of disparate etiologies which affect the small intestine in similar, thus nonspecific, ways. Abnormalities of intestinal motility are frequently associated with abnormalities of mucosal folds identified on contrast examinations of the small bowel and with intestinal dilatation, either generalized or focal. *Celiac disease* is the most common cause of intestinal malabsorption in childhood. The disease is also known as nontropical sprue or gluten enteropathy because the cause is gluten intolerance. Gluten is a protein present in the food grains most commonly used by humans. Most affected children present with failure to thrive, abdominal distention, and diarrhea. Diarrhea is considered one of the hallmarks of the disease but is not present in 10% of patients with celiac disease. Affected adolescents have delayed puberty, anorexia, and clinical findings related to the hypocalcemia and hypoproteinemia of malabsorption. Imaging studies are only adjunctive at best, and diagnosis relies on a combination of clinical findings and small-bowel biopsy. Plain films in patients with celiac disease may show nonspecific small-bowel dilatation. The classic findings on barium small-bowel series are dilatation, thickened mucosal folds, flocculation, and segmentation. The last two findings, however, are uncommonly seen with modern-day barium preparations. The mucosal folds may be abnormal with thinning or thickening and reversal of the mucosal patterns of jejunum and ileum. The duodenum may show mucosal erosions or thickened nodular folds. CT is not indicated for evaluation, but, if performed, may demonstrate mesenteric lymphadenopathy which resolves with the institution of a gluten-free diet.

Intestinal lymphangiectasia is a severe protein-losing enteropathy characterized by dilatation of intestinal lymphatics resulting in protein loss as lymph leaks into the lumen of the intestine. The disease can be secondary to developmental abnormalities of the intestinal lymphatics which may be associated with abnormal lymphatics elsewhere in the body. Intestinal lymphangiectasia has been found in patients with Noonan syndrome. Lymphangiectasia can also be secondary to diseases which cause obstruction of the intestinal lymphatics or increase in the intralymphatic pressure. Patients typically have diarrhea and hypoproteinemia. Symptoms related to malabsorption may also be present. Barium studies are nonspecific with mild dilatation and thickened folds (Fig 27–8). A substantial number of affected children may have normal barium examinations. Sonographic findings have been described, but are nonspecific and related to the edema with thickening of the walls of the intestine and gallbladder, ascites, and a thickened mesentery.

Patients with *immunodeficiency syndromes* may have a clinical and radiographic picture similar to that in patients with celiac disease. Some affected patients will have radiographic findings of lymphoid hyperplasia, especially prominent in the distal ileum. Small, relatively uniform polypoid mucosal filling defects are seen, characteristically with a central barium-filled umbilication. The latter is not seen uniformly, however, but its presence in a number of the polypoid defects suggests the correct nature of the lesions. Reactive lymphoid hyperplasia can also be seen in patients with gastroenteritis, both infectious and allergic, and in some otherwise normal persons. Lymphoid hyperplasia of the terminal ileum may act as a lead point for ileocolic intussusception.

Other causes of *protein-losing enteropathy* include allergic gastroenteropathy, Whipple disease (Fig 27–9), inflammatory bowel disease, infectious mononucleosis, and polyarteritis nodosa; Menetrier disease is discussed in Chapter 26. The radiologic

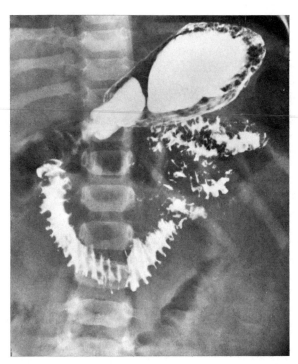

FIG 27–9.
Whipple disease in a 2½-year-old boy. Upper GI series demonstrates marked thickening of the duodenal and jejunal folds.

findings in the GI tract may be nonspecific or related to underlying intestinal disease such as regional enteritis.

Cystic fibrosis (CF) may present in the newborn period with meconium ileus (see Chapter 52). Older children show duodenal abnormalities such as dilatation, thickened folds, and filling defects which may represent abnormal collections of mucus adherent to the mucosa. Patients with CF have a surprisingly high rate of duodenal ulcer disease which has suggested the lack of a protective mechanism in the duodenum because of the abnormal secretions. As patients live longer, the most prominent intestinal abnormality is the distal intestinal obstruction syndrome (DIOS), formerly known as meconium ileus equivalent. Patients present with colicky abdominal pain and a palpable right lower quadrant mass, representing impacted fecal material in the ileocolic region. Since mild to severe constipation is a common concomitant of CF, the term DIOS is reserved for those patients who also have signs and symptoms of small-bowel obstruction. Plain films show small-bowel dilatation with air-fluid levels and bubbly fecal material in the right lower quadrant (Figs 27–10 and 27–11). Although most patients respond to enemas using mucolytic agents, we still occasionally perform contrast enemas under fluoroscopic control. Gastrografin (diatrizoate meglumine) is the most

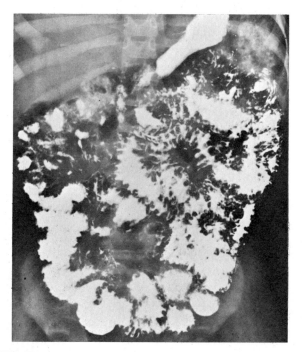

FIG 27–8.
Small-bowel series in a 3½-year-old girl with intestinal lymphangiectasia demonstrates mucosal folds which are markedly coarsened and thickened.

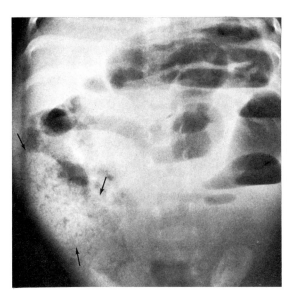

FIG 27–10.
Distal intestinal obstructive syndrome in a 2-month-old infant with cystic fibrosis. Upright radiograph of the abdomen demonstrates bubbly stool in the right lower quadrant *(arrows)* with multiple air-fluid levels suggestive of distal small-intestinal obstruction.

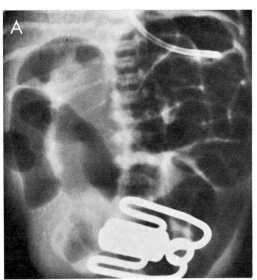

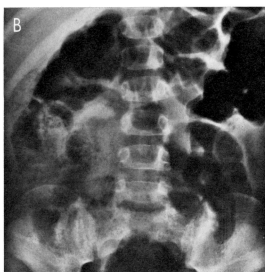

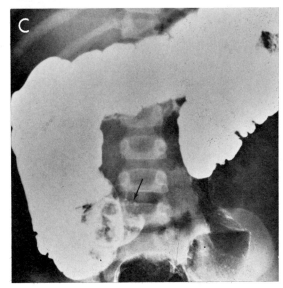

FIG 27–11.
Distal intestinal obstructive syndrome in a patient with cystic fibrosis. **A,** plain film of the abdomen in a newborn infant demonstrates multiple dilated loops of small intestine in this patient with meconium ileus. Six years later, the patient presented with clinical signs of obstruction and a palpable right lower quadrant mass. **B,** plain film of the abdomen demonstrates inspissated fecal material in the right lower quadrant and multiple dilated loops of small intestine. **C,** barium enema demonstrates inspissated fecal material in the cecum and terminal ileum *(arrow).*

widely used agent but is very expensive in the volumes needed for teen-agers and adults who are the most likely affected CF patients. We have had good success using a hypertonic solution of powdered sodium diatrizoate in warm water. For best results, reflux into the terminal ileum is necessary. Patients with CF may also have malabsorption with dilated intestinal loops showing thickened folds. Patients with *Schwachman syndrome* may have malabsorption with nonspecific findings on barium studies.

Graft-versus-host disease (GVHD) is a reaction of donor lymphocytes against host cells. Although GVHD can be seen in patients undergoing solid organ transplantation, it is more common in patients undergoing bone marrow transplantation. Furthermore, bone marrow transplantation is more commonly performed in children than is solid organ transplantation because of its utility in hematologic and immunodeficiency states as well as leukemia, lymphoma, and widespread malignancies such as metastatic neuroblastoma. Acute GVHD occurs within the first 3 months following transplantation. Patients with GI manifestations have severe diarrhea and crampy abdominal pain. Frequent accompaniments are skin rash, liver dysfunction, and hematologic complications. Plain films show a pattern of adynamic ileus with separation of bowel loops, thickening of the bowel wall, and air-fluid levels. Less commonly seen are pneumatosis intestinalis and ascites. On occasion, the abdomen may be completely gasless. Contrast studies are usually not necessary but will show severe edema of the bowel

wall, poor coating of the mucosa, luminal narrowing, and rapid transit time. Chronic fibrosis, not unlike that seen in chronic radiation enteritis, may occur. Sonography reveals thickening of the bowel wall, sometimes with a sonolucent ring in the submucosal layer (Fig 27–12,*A*). The bowel lumina are filled with fluid, and ascites can be identified. Concomitant findings can be seen on CT which can also demonstrate mesenteric thickening (Fig 27–12,*B*).

Henloch-Schönlein purpura is an idiopathic anaphylactoid reaction characterized by a diffuse angiitis. In the small intestine, the disease manifests itself with bleeding into the bowel wall, causing submucosal filling defects (Fig 27–13). Findings related to the angiitis on contrast studies include segmental dilatation and stenosis, bowel wall thickening with separation of bowel loops, and coarsening and loss of the normal mucosal fold pattern. The submucosal hematomas may act as a lead point for intussusception. The characteristic skin rash is usually diagnostic but the GI manifestations may precede its appearance.

INFECTIOUS DISEASES

The most common intestinal infection in children in North America and Europe is viral gastroenteritis. Parasites and bacteria as well as viruses are worldwide causative agents of acute gastroenteritis in children. The resultant severe diarrhea and vomiting with subsequent dehydration is, tragically, still a leading cause of childhood morbidity and mortality

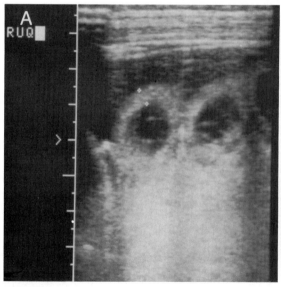
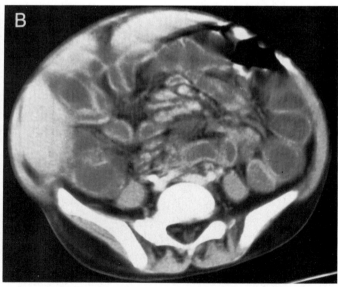

FIG 27–12.
Graft-versus-host disease. **A,** sonogram of the right upper quadrant demonstrates markedly thickened bowel wall surrounded by ascitic fluid. **B,** CT scan demonstrates edematous bowel wall throughout the small intestine.

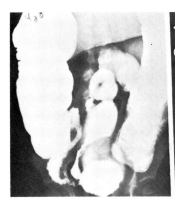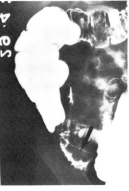

FIG 27–13.
Henoch-Schönlein purpura. Barium enema performed in a 4-year-old boy with a 7-day history of vomiting, bloody diarrhea, and abdominal pain. Filling *(left)* and postevacuation *(right)* films from a barium enema demonstrate marginal filling defects in the distal ileum *(arrow)*. The diagnosis of Henoch-Schönlein purpura was made when the characteristic rash developed during hospitalization.

throughout the underdeveloped countries of the world.

Viral gastroenteritis in the United States is most commonly secondary to rotavirus infection. Associated upper respiratory symptoms are common and may precede the GI presentation which usually begins with vomiting, followed by severe watery diarrhea. Imaging studies are not generally indicated, but plain films are occasionally requested to rule out other causes for the patient's symptoms. The most common finding is fluid-filled loops of nondilated

bowel with multiple air-fluid levels on horizontal-beam radiographs. Depending on the time course and degree of motility disturbance, nonobstructive dilatation of bowel loops may occur (Fig 27–14). The fluid-filled loops may give the false impression of separation of loops by ascites (see Fig 22–25). Barium studies are not indicated but, if performed for other reasons, will show dilution of barium from fluid retention, minimal thickening of mucosal folds, and either rapid or delayed transit time, depending on the chronicity of the disease. Disordered peristalsis is commonly seen. Capitanio and Greenberg described pneumatosis intestinalis in two infants with rotavirus enteritis.

Bacterial enterocolitis is much less common than the viral form. *Shigella, Salmonella, Escherichia coli, Yersinia enterocolitica,* and *Campylobacter fetus* are the most commonly identified bacterial agents in the United States. *Vibrio cholerae* is the most common infectious bacterial agent in Asia. The symptoms are similar to those of viral gastroenteritis, but frequently are accompanied by high fever and systemic toxicity. Typhoid fever and tuberculosis are less commonly seen than in prior years and are less common in children than in adults. The plain film findings in bacterial gastroenterocolitis are similar to those described above for viral disease. Contrast studies in those cases caused by the common bacteria are also nonspecific. *Yersinia,* typhoid, and tuberculosis all have a predilection for the terminal ileum (Fig 27–15) and *Yersinia* may simulate Crohn disease

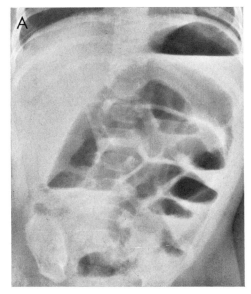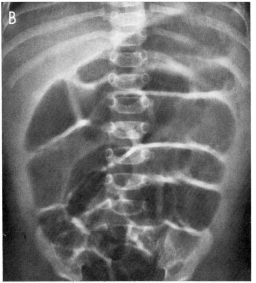

FIG 27–14.
Gastroenteritis. **A,** upright view of the abdomen demonstrates multiple dilated loops of bowel with air-fluid levels approximately at the same level within each individual loop. Gas is seen within the rectosigmoid region. **B,** supine view of the abdomen demonstrates multiple dilated loops of bowel.

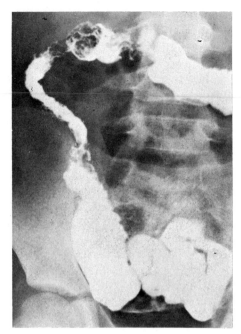

FIG 27–15.
Ileocecal tuberculosis. Persistent spasm and stenosis of the terminal ileum, cecum, and ascending colon are identified.

(Fig 27–16). A cobblestone pattern may be seen. Typhoid may cause prominent lymphoid hyperplasia. Puylaert et al. diagnosed typhoid fever in a 12-year-old girl with the sonographic findings of enlarged mesenteric lymph nodes and mural thickening of the terminal ileum and cecum accompanied by hepatic portal lymphadenopathy and splenomegaly.

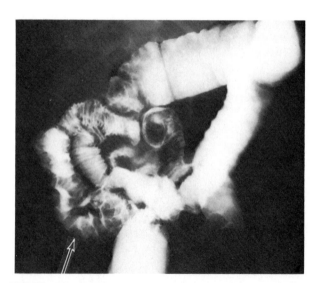

FIG 27–16.
Yersinia enterocolitis. Barium enema demonstrates "thumbprinting" in the cecum and ascending colon in a 1-year-old girl. The ileum is dilated with thickened folds. Yersinia enterocolitica was cultured from mesenteric nodes removed at the time of exploratory laparotomy.

Yersinia can cause mesenteric adenitis with associated abdominal pain sometimes mimicking appendicitis. Matsumoto et al. performed sonography on eight children and young adults with Yersinia terminal ileitis. Thickening of the ileal wall was present in all eight patients and mesenteric lymphadenopathy in six. Tuberculous involvement of the terminal ileum may cause small-bowel obstruction, presumably from adherent bowel loops. Ascites may be present. Pulmonary tuberculosis is probably the source of the GI infection and chest radiographs should always be obtained in suspected cases.

Parasitic enterocolitis is most frequently caused by *Giardia lamblia* in the Western Hemisphere and usually results from drinking contaminated water. In the western United States, virtually all of the natural mountain streams have become infested with *Giardia*. Although the protozoan easily infects otherwise normal people, it is an especially common etiologic agent in patients with acquired immunodeficiency syndrome (AIDS) who develop enteritis. On barium studies, giardiasis produces thickened mucosal folds in the duodenum and jejunum associated with rapid transit time and dilution of the contrast material (Fig 27–17).

Helminthic enteritis can be caused by a variety of worms of which *Ascaris lumbricoides* causes the

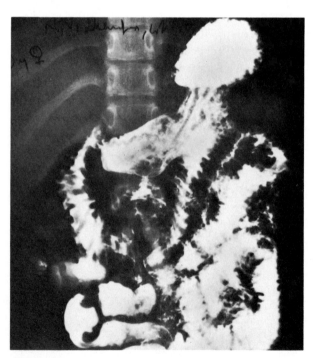

FIG 27–17.
Giardiasis. Small intestinal examination in a 10-year-old girl with a history of nausea, vomiting, diarrhea, and weight loss. The mucosal folds of the duodenum and proximal jejunum are markedly thickened. Giardia was identified in the stool.

most striking and diagnostic radiographic abnormalities. The disease results from swallowed larvae which grow into adult worms in the intestinal tract. Barium studies outline the characteristic vermiform organisms which may appear singly or in clumps. The live worms may ingest barium, permitting visualization of their intestinal tracts. Infections with *Strongyloides stercoralis,* tapeworms, roundworms, and hookworms may all occur.

AIDS is substantially less common in children than in adults, but the number of infected children is growing. Most early cases in children were secondary to transmission of the human immunodeficiency virus (HIV) through contaminated blood products. Patients treated for hemophilia are at particular risk. Presently, according to Haney et al., 80% or more of affected children have acquired the virus from their mothers via transplacental passage. The presenting symptoms and signs are nonspecific and related to the affected organ systems. Enteritis is most frequently caused by the common pathogens described above, but may follow infection with opportunistic organisms such as cytomegalovirus (CMV), *Mycobacterium avium-intracellulare,* and the ubiquitous fungi, especially *Candida albicans.* Extrapulmonic *Pneumocystis carinii* infection is being reported with increasing frequency. Candidiasis most commonly affects the esophagus, but any of the organisms can infect any part of the GI tract. Nonspecific edema of the affected intestine is the most frequently found abnormality on barium studies. Effacement of the mucosal pattern is common, especially with *Cryptosporidium* infection. Sivit et al. described an 8-month-old girl who developed small-bowel obstruction secondary to adhesions formed by serosal plaques of CMV infection. *Pneumatosis intestinalis* has been reported although the cause is unclear. Sonography and CT demonstrate thickening of the bowel wall with intra-abdominal and retroperitoneal lymphadenopathy being the most frequent finding. Both Kaposi sarcoma and lymphoma have been reported in the intestine, mesentery, and pancreas of affected children, but less frequently than in adults.

CROHN DISEASE

Crohn disease is also commonly known as regional enteritis, with the terms segmental enteritis and terminal ileitis less frequently used. The peak incidence is in young adulthood, but 25% of patients present in childhood, adolescence, or the teen-age years. The disease has been reported in infants less than 1 year of age. Crohn disease is characterized by seg-

mental transmural granulomatous inflammation of the intestine. It may be localized to one segment or involve several segments with normal bowel between them. The terminal ileum is the most frequently involved segment, but the disease has been described everywhere in the GI tract from the mouth to the rectum. The intestinal lumen is narrowed by edematous and fibrotic thickening of the wall and by spasm. The mucosal layer is extensively destroyed, and ulcers are usually present.

Most children with Crohn disease present with the insidious onset of GI symptoms, including diarrhea, abdominal pain, anorexia, abdominal mass, or fistula in ano. Extraintestinal manifestations of the disease may accompany or precede the GI symptoms and include failure to thrive with delayed puberty, fever, aphthous stomatitis, arthralgias, arthritis, sacroiliitis, and erythema nodosum. Digital clubbing is found in 25% to 33% of affected children. A smaller number of patients present acutely with right lower quadrant pain and fever mimicking appendicitis.

Plain film evaluation of the abdomen in patients with inflammatory bowel disease may be normal. During an acute exacerbation of the disease, plain films are more likely to show nonspecific abnormalities such as adynamic ileus and bowel wall thickening. Occasionally, a focally abnormal loop with edematous wall can be identified, strongly suggesting acute inflammation.

Barium contrast small-intestinal series continues to be the most frequently utilized diagnostic imaging examination in the evaluation of the jejunoileal manifestations of regional enteritis. The terminal ileum is the most frequently involved area (Fig 27–18), but more proximal disease with sparing of the terminal ileum has been reported. The earliest change is granularity, probably reflecting mucosal edema. More prominent mural edema and increased mucosal secretion result in the thickening of mucosal folds and effacement of the mucosal pattern. More typical early findings include nodular irregularity with linear and transverse ulceration. The characteristic "rose-thorn ulcer" is less commonly seen and is not pathognomonic, as once believed. Extensive ulceration can lead to a spiculated appearance. The intersection of multiple linear and transverse ulcers leads to a cobblestone appearance (Fig 27–19). This pattern has also been described as pseudopolypoid but this is inaccurate because these "pseudopolyps" are really areas of maintained mucosa adjacent to denuded areas and ulcers filled with barium. Spasm of involved segments is frequently seen.

Edema, fibrosis, and spasm lead to narrowing of

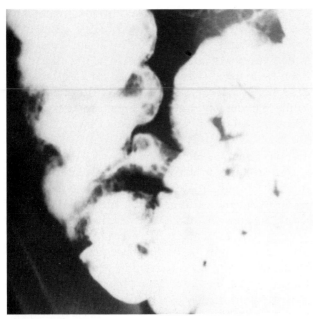

FIG 27–18.
Crohn disease. Coned-down view of the ileocecal valve demonstrates the typical "bird-beak" deformity of the terminal ileum and thickening of the wall, causing separation from the ileocecal valve.

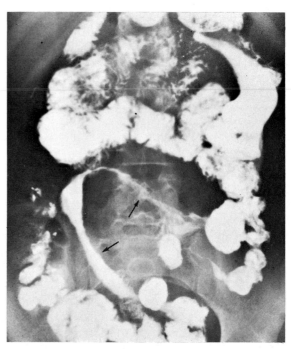

FIG 27–20.
Crohn disease in a 14-year-old girl. Small-bowel series demonstrates markedly narrowed and rigid loop of jejunum. The *upper arrow* points to an extreme narrowing, the so-called string sign.

the intestinal lumen which may be so profound as to be labeled the "string sign" (Fig 27–20). The narrowing is accompanied by persistent ulcers. The mesentery becomes inflamed, thickened, and fibrotic, causing separation and retraction of bowel loops. Enlarged mesenteric lymph nodes may cause mass

effect on adjacent loops of bowel (Fig 27–21). Postinflammatory polyps may be seen. These are filiform projections of submucosa covered by mucosa on all sides, as described by Buck et al. They represent healing of undermined mucosal and submucosal remnants and ulcers and are almost always multiple.

The diagnostic accuracy of barium studies is quite good. Lipson et al. compared barium small-bowel series with ileoscopy and biopsy results in 46

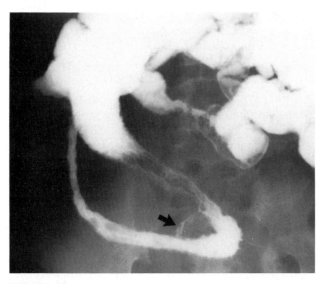

FIG 27–19.
Coned-down view of the distal ileum in a patient with documented Crohn disease demonstrates marked separation of bowel loops secondary to mesenteric thickening, a cobblestone pattern in the bowel mucosa, and multiple "rose-thorn ulcers" throughout the affected loop. A walled-off fistulous tract *(arrow)* was identified.

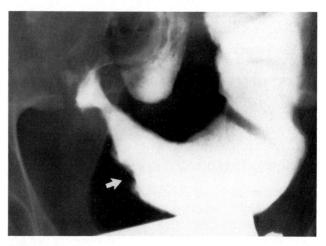

FIG 27–21.
Coned-down view of the proximal ileum in a patient with Crohn disease. Extrinsic filling defects secondary to mesenteric adenopathy are identified *(arrow)*.

children with suspected regional enteritis of the terminal ileum. Although ileoscopy agreed with the biopsy results in all 20 positive cases, the small-bowel series had a sensitivity of 90% and a specificity of 96%. The major source of misdiagnosis was pronounced lymphoid hyperplasia on the barium study which led to diagnostic errors in 2 cases.

Imaging studies other than small-bowel series are being used with increasing frequency in the evaluation of patients with regional enteritis, although this is more the case in adults than in children. Nuclear scintigraphy using a variety of radiopharmaceuticals can be used to identify areas of active inflammation, although with questionable success in some studies, and have been successful in differentiating primary bowel disease from adjacent abscesses. As pointed out by Stringer, these studies are not often performed in children because of concern over the long-range effects of the isotopes used, particularly indium-111.

US is not used for primary diagnosis in Crohn disease but is more apt to be requested for evaluation of complications such as abscesses. Sonography can, however, demonstrate thickening of the bowel wall and separation of bowel loops. The bowel wall appears stiff as well as thickened and no peristalsis in the affected loop can be demonstrated. A halo of submucosal edema may give a targetlike appearance to the bowel wall when seen transversely and a "double-track" appearance when imaged longitudinally. Large abscesses can be identified but small abscesses are difficult to distinguish from matted loops of inflamed bowel.

CT is becoming more widely used in adults with regional enteritis, but in children is reserved for the evaluation of complications. CT readily identifies bowel wall thickening, luminal narrowing and stricture formation, and mesenteric changes such as lymphadenopathy, fibrofatty proliferation, and phlegmon formation.

The major intra-abdominal complications of regional enteritis are enteroenteric fistulas, sinus tracts, and abscesses (Fig 27–22). CT is the most sensitive imaging study for elucidation of these complications. Barium studies can identify fistulas if the examination is carefully monitored so that premature filling of a bowel loop can be seen. Sinus tracts to the skin can be injected. We use water-soluble contrast for such injections in the event of an unanticipated intraperitoneal leak. Abscesses are among the most common complications of regional enteritis. CT will identify over 90% of abscesses and is the best modality for their guided percutaneous drainage.

Findings similar to those of Crohn disease can be seen in other inflammatory diseases. *Behçet syndrome* is a multiorgan process with inflammatory changes and ulceration anywhere in the GI tract. The esophagus, terminal ileum (Fig 27–23), and right colon are most commonly affected.

ACQUIRED SMALL-INTESTINAL OBSTRUCTION

Many of the lesions which cause small intestinal obstruction are congenital or developmental and are discussed in Chapter 52. The more common congenital lesions which present after infancy are discussed above. Acquired intestinal obstruction in older children may be due to either intrinsic or extrinsic abnormalities affecting the small intestine. The plain film findings may help identify the level of obstruction but in many cases may show nonspecific changes of incomplete obstruction or adynamic ileus.

Although adynamic (paralytic) ileus can simulate mechanical obstruction on plain films, certain signs, if present, are useful in distinguishing the two entities. Supine radiographs of the abdomen show dilated loops of bowel in both entities. The lack of rectal gas is not a useful sign, especially in young children, because air rises out of the dependent rectum on supine films. Generalized adynamic ileus causes both small intestine and colon to dilate while obstruction usually causes proximal dilatation with reduced caliber of the distal bowel. Air-fluid levels on horizontal-beam films can be seen with both mechanical and adynamic ileus. In the former, they are relatively short and are at different levels in the same loop of bowel (Fig 27–24), while in the latter, they are longer and at the same level within a loop (see Fig 27–14). Decubitus views are frequently more successful in demonstrating the long levels of adynamic ileus than are upright films. Unfortunately, there are a significant number of children in whom differentiation is not possible. This is especially true of children with a focal ileus affecting the small intestine but not the colon. There are other children in whom partial small-intestinal obstruction mimics adynamic ileus. CT has been used in adults to identify obstruction, particularly of the closed-loop variety, but this is rarely, if ever, a necessary procedure in children.

Incarcerated hernias are a less frequent cause of small-intestinal obstruction than previously, possibly owing to the increased performance of elective outpatient herniorrhaphy. Most incarcerated hernias are inguinal and, occasionally, umbilical. The diagnosis is made on clinical grounds, but plain films

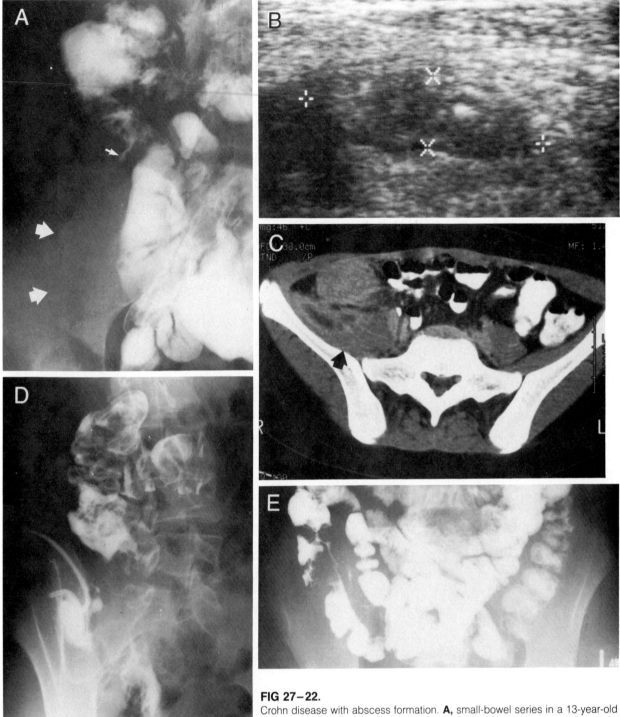

FIG 27–22.
Crohn disease with abscess formation. **A,** small-bowel series in a 13-year-old girl with known Crohn disease who presented with fevers and right lower quadrant tenderness. A walled-off fistulous tract *(arrow)* leads to a right lower quadrant mass *(large arrows)*, causing separation of bowel loops and extrinsic compression defect on the barium-filled small intestine. **B,** sonographic examination of the right lower quadrant demonstrates an area of hypoechogenicity with a bright echo within it. **C,** CT scan through the right lower quadrant demonstrates a large abscess *(arrow)* deep to the markedly thickened and edematous cecum. Under CT guidance, a drainage tube was placed. **D,** 8 days later, injection of contrast material through the drainage tube demonstrates communication with the small bowel. **E,** 6 weeks later, small-bowel series demonstrates leak of contrast material from the markedly narrowed terminal ileum into a small residual mass. The patient was asymptomatic at the time of this examination.

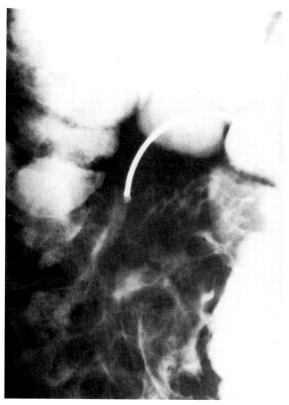

FIG 27–23.
Behçet syndrome. Coned-down pressure spot film of the terminal ileum in a patient with known Behçet syndrome demonstrates a cobblestone pattern similar to that seen in Crohn disease. (Courtesy of Dr. P.S. Moskowitz, Los Gatos, Calif.)

may be used to confirm the diagnosis and to rule out bowel perforation (Fig 27–25).

Adhesions are a common cause of obstruction in patients who have undergone prior abdominal surgery. Adhesive bands can obstruct the small intestine even at a site distant from the original surgical site. Plain films are useful in corroborating the clinical suspicion and in ruling out intestinal perforation (Fig 27–26). Adhesions can also occur in children who have had peritonitis, usually from appendicitis or inflammatory bowel disease.

Duodenal hematomas are generally secondary to blunt abdominal trauma and are discussed in Chapter 30. Occasionally, they may occur in patients with a bleeding disorder who have a diagnostic or therapeutic procedure involving the duodenum. We have seen one child who was severely thrombocytopenic following bone marrow transplantation for leukemia. Endoscopic biopsy of the duodenum was performed to confirm the suspected diagnosis of GVHD. Several days later, the patient developed jaundice. US and CT examination revealed a massive duodenal hematoma with partial obstruction of the common bile duct (Fig 27–27).

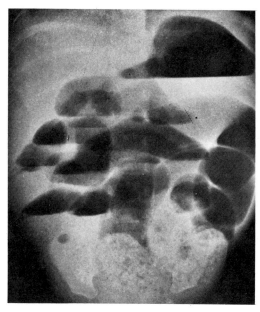

FIG 27–24.
Small-intestinal obstruction secondary to postoperative adhesions. Upright film of the abdomen demonstrates multiple air-fluid levels at different levels throughout the abdomen.

The superior mesenteric artery syndrome is a condition in which the third portion of the duodenum is trapped between the superior mesenteric artery (SMA) and the root of the mesentery. Originally described in young adult women, the syndrome usually occurs in asthenic persons who develop vomiting following sudden weight loss secondary to ei-

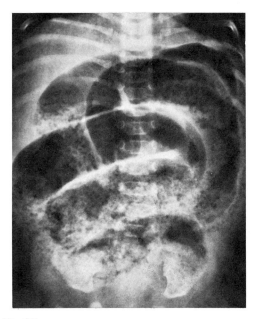

FIG 27–25.
Intestinal obstruction secondary to incarcerated inguinal hernia. Supine film of the abdomen demonstrates multiple dilated loops of small intestine.

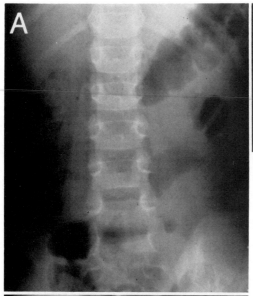

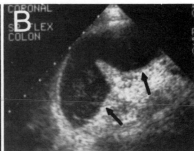

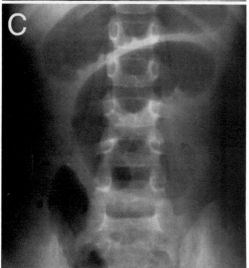

FIG 27–26.
Postoperative adhesions causing intestinal obstruction. **A,** focally dilated loops of bowel in a 4-year-old girl 3 weeks following surgery for a ruptured appendix. **B,** coronal sonogram demonstrates dilated fluid-filled loops of bowel *(arrows)*. **C,** plain film 2 days later shows a markedly dilated air-fluid loop of bowel in the midportion of the abdomen. Adhesions were lysed at exploratory laparotomy.

ther illness or voluntary dieting. Subsequently, the syndrome was described in adolescents, but its existence as a real entity has been doubted by many. Marchant et al. reviewed their experience with 13 patients ranging in age from 4 to 18 years in whom the SMA syndrome was treated surgically in 9 children with resolution of symptoms. Plain films may show gastric dilatation but the stomach may be decompressed by the vomiting. Barium study shows a high-grade partial obstruction of the third portion of the duodenum (Fig 27–28). Fluoroscopy demonstrates to-and-fro motion of the barium in the dilated proximal portions of the duodenum. The findings are not specific and may be seen with Ladd bands and focal ileus or functional obstruction of the proximal jejunum, as may be seen with inflammatory bowel disease. Ortiz et al. described SMA syndrome

in five members of a family of eight, raising the question of genetic disposition.

An acute form of SMA syndrome following scoliosis treatment has been called the *cast syndrome* since it was initially identified in children being casted for scoliosis. We have also seen the syndrome following the placement of spinal rods even without a cast. Presumably, the abrupt straightening of the spine changes the angle at which the SMA leaves the aorta, causing duodenal compression. Massive gastric dilatation is the rule and gastric perforation has been described (Fig 27–29). Decompression by nasogastric tube is usually effective.

Duodenal dilatation is a common manifestation of *intestinal pseudo-obstruction*. This entity is discussed in Chapter 28. Another congenital abnormality which can mimic obstruction is segmental dilata-

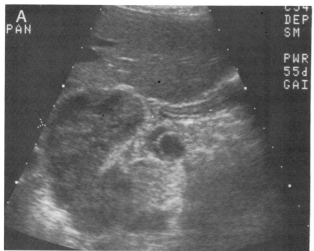

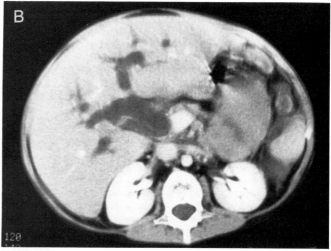

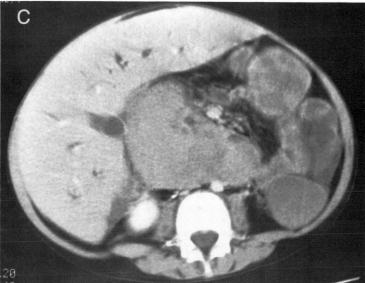

FIG 27–27.
Duodenal hematoma secondary to endoscopic biopsy in a thrombocytopenic patient. **A,** sonogram demonstrates a hypoechoic lesion in the region of the pancreatic head and duodenum. **B,** CT scan through the upper abdomen demonstrates marked dilatation of the common bile duct and intrahepatic ducts. **C,** CT scan slightly more inferiorly demonstrates a large intramural hematoma of the duodenum. The hematoma resolved gradually over a prolonged course.

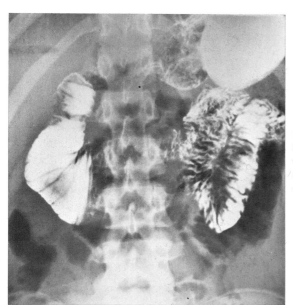

FIG 27–28.
Superior mesenteric artery syndrome in a 15-year-old boy with 4 weeks of vomiting and a 32-lb weight loss. The second and third portions of the duodenum are markedly dilated secondary to a partial obstruction. The distal bowel was normal.

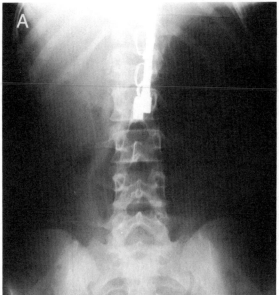

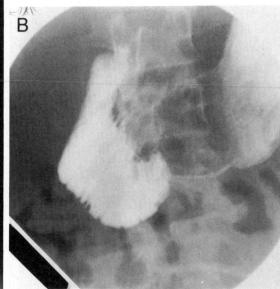

FIG 27–29.
Cast syndrome. **A,** supine film of the abdomen 1 day after insertion of corrective rods for scoliosis demonstrates massive dilatation of the stomach. **B,** spot film from an upper GI series demonstrates characteristic obstruction of the duodenum at the level of the third portion. The symptoms resolved over the course of 1 week with nasogastric tube drainage.

tion of the small bowel. This rare disorder is characterized by segmental dilatation which may appear as a single dilated loop with an air-fluid level on plain film and a focally dilated loop of bowel, usually ileum, on barium study (Fig 27–30). Transit time is normal and surgery is curative.

INTUSSUSCEPTION

Intussusception is the invagination or telescoping of one portion of intestine into the contiguous distal segment (Fig 27–31). The proximal segment is known as the intussusceptum while the distal portion is the intussuscipiens. Idiopathic intussusception is the most common cause of small-intestinal obstruction in the infant-toddler age group, with the peak incidence between 2 months and 3 years of life. About 50% of the affected patients present during the first year of life with another 24% during the second year. Idiopathic intussusception has been described in newborns and in adults, but its appearance outside the peak age group should always alert one to the possibility of a pathologic lead point, as discussed at the end of this section. Approximately two thirds of patients are boys. Over 90% of intussusceptions are ileocolic, enteroenteric and colocolic being uncommon. Some investigators believe, however, that undiagnosed ileoileal intussusception may be the lead point for ileocolic intussusception. Other

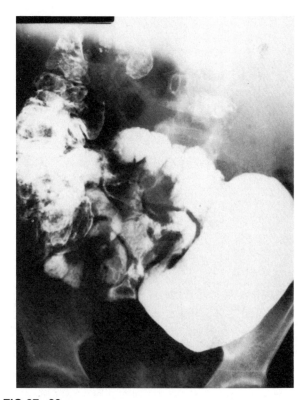

FIG 27–30.
Segmental dilatation of the small bowel. Small bowel series demonstrates dilatation of a focal loop of ileum in the left lower quadrant. The patient's symptoms were relieved following removal of the abnormal portion of small intestine. **(Courtesy of Dr. John Ratcliffe, Brisbane.)**

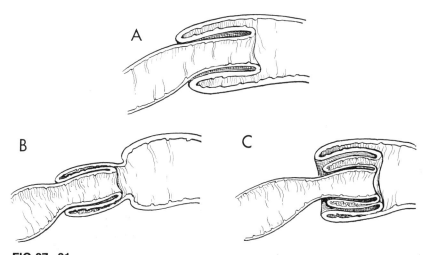

FIG 27–31.
The common types of infantile intussusception, in longitudinal section. **A,** ileocecal; **B,** ileoileal, a type not visualized by barium enema; **C,** ileoileocecal (double intussusception).

authors have postulated hypertrophied Peyer patches or reactive lymphoid hyperplasia of the terminal ileum as lead points.

The affected child usually has a history of abrupt onset of intermittent abdominal pain, sometimes following a prodromal period with symptoms of upper respiratory infection or, rarely, gastroenteritis. The bouts of pain quickly come closer together and vomiting or diarrhea may ensue. Lethargy is a frequent occurrence, often quite profound. In some cases, lethargy may be the presenting complaint in a patient with only minimal GI symptoms. Vomiting or diarrhea may lead to dehydration, which exaggerates the lethargy. Blood may appear in the stool. The mixture of stool, blood, and blood clots has been described as having a currant jelly appearance which, when present, is highly suggestive of intussusception. Patients who delay in seeking medical attention may become toxic with fever, leukocytosis, and peritoneal signs on physical examination. Otherwise, physical examination is either unremarkable or discloses a palpable abdominal mass most commonly located in the right upper quadrant but which can be found anywhere in the course of the colon. On rare occasions, the intussusception may be seen or palpated at the anus.

Plain abdominal radiographs are indicated regardless of how high the clinical index of suspicion is for the diagnosis of intussusception. Eklöf and Hartelius compared plain film findings in patients with proven intussusception to those with suspected intussusception who were later found not to have the disease (Table 27–1). The combination of diminished colonic stool and gas, especially when accom-

panied by a visible soft-tissue mass, makes the likelihood of intussusception very high (Fig 27–32). In some patients, the plain film will be normal. A horizontal-beam film is useful to rule out bowel perforation and to evaluate the degree of obstruction. White and Blane recommend a cross-table lateral horizontal-beam film as more likely to demonstrate the soft-tissue mass than the supine film. Johnson and Woisard point out on the cross-table lateral film an inappropriate craniocaudal separation of gas-filled bowel loops in the upper abdomen, representing the gasless telescoped bowel interposed between the site of

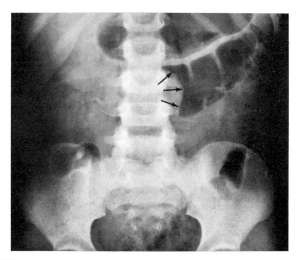

FIG 27–32.
Ileocolic intussusception in a 4½-year-old patient. The leading edge of the intussusceptum is seen within the air column of the transverse colon *(arrows).* No gas can be seen in the cecum or ascending colon. The intussusception was successfully reduced with hydrostatic pressure.

TABLE 27–1.

Plain Film Analysis in Patients With Suspected Intussusception*

Findings	Confirmed Intussusception (100 Patients) No. of Cases	Suspected Intussusception Normal on Follow-up (100 Patients) No. of Cases
Sparse intestinal gas	89	45
Sparse fecal content	82	19
Discernible liver tip	66	58
Discernible mass	61	5
Small bowel in right upper quadrant	58	28
Air-fluid levels–nondilated bowel	56	75
Normal fecal content	18	81
Normal gas pattern	11	55
Air-fluid levels–dilated bowel	8	3
Ascites	0	0

*Modified from Eklöf O, Hartelius H: *Pediatr Radiol* 1980; 9:199.

initiation of the intussusception and the leading edge of the intussusceptum. This sign was present in 4 of 12 patients, a mass was seen in 5 patients, and no specific sign was present in 3, all of whom had documented intussusception.

Sonography is being used with increasing frequency in patients in whom intussusception is suspected but whose clinical presentation and plain film findings are nondiagnostic. In other circumstances, when sonography is performed for evaluation of acute abdominal discomfort, an unsuspected intussusception may be found. Sonography is not indicated when there is a high clinicoradiologic suspicion of intussusception. The sonographic findings are very suggestive, if not pathognomonic. On transverse scan, a "doughnut" configuration may be seen. There is a central echogenic area representing the mucosa of the intussusceptum and a larger sonolucent rim representing the edematous wall of the intussusceptum, according to Swischuk et al. In other cases, a "target" will be seen with concentric rings of alternating sonolucency and echogenicity. If there is fluid in the lumen of the intussusceptum, the central core may appear sonolucent, with the next layer being the echogenic mucosa (Fig 27–33). Depending on the degree of edema and compression of the bowel wall, the layers of the intussuscipiens may also be seen, producing the appearance of multiple concentric rings. On longitudinal scan, the appearance of the doughnut has been likened to a kidney with the sonolucent wall being reniform and surrounding the echogenic mucosa which simulates the kidney's peripelvic fat. These characteristic signs will be found along the course of the intussuscep-

tion, but are most easily recognized near the leading edge of the intussusceptum. Swischuk and Stansberry reported the sonographic detection of small amounts of free intraperitoneal fluid in two patients with uncomplicated intussusception. A lead point is rarely seen with sonography, even in patients ultimately shown to have one at barium enema or surgery. Pracros et al. reported the sonographic findings in a series of 145 patients with intussusception, all of whom had a positive sonogram. Of 8 patients who had lead points, identified at surgery or by other means, only 2 were identified at sonography. Adamsbaum et al. described the sonographic appearance of an enterogenous cyst acting as a lead point in which the cyst was just distal to the "pseudokidney." Kenney, however, described a similar appearance in a patient in whom fluid was trapped in intussuscepted mesentery.

CT is not part of the evaluation of suspected intussusception, but may demonstrate intussusception when performed for other reasons. Knowles et al. used CT to diagnose transient intussusception in two adults with regional enteritis and severe abdominal pain.

Hydrostatic reduction of ileocolic intussusception under fluoroscopic control is probably the earliest therapeutic procedure introduced into pediatric radiology. Although there are significant procedural variations among experienced radiologists, certain principles are generally accepted. Absolute contraindications to radiologic reduction are intestinal perforation, frank peritonitis, and hypovolemic shock. Even patients with prolonged symptoms before diagnosis and small-intestinal obstruction on plain

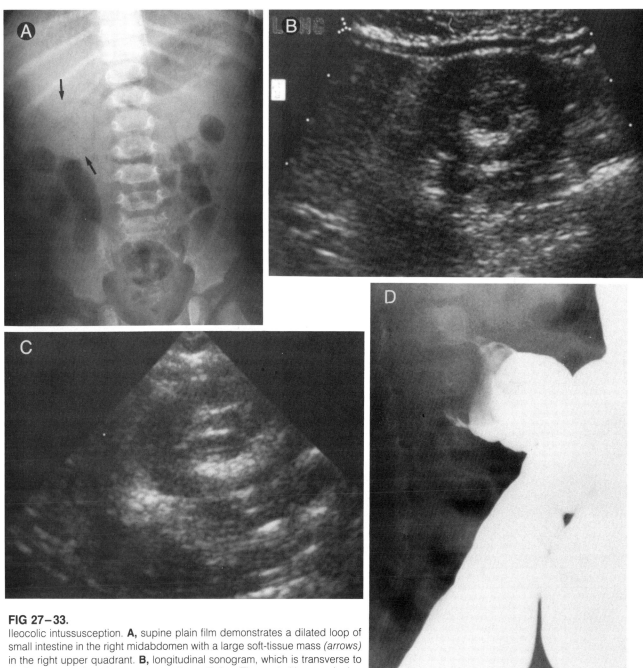

FIG 27–33.
Ileocolic intussusception. **A,** supine plain film demonstrates a dilated loop of small intestine in the right midabdomen with a large soft-tissue mass *(arrows)* in the right upper quadrant. **B,** longitudinal sonogram, which is transverse to the intussusception, demonstrates a "target" sign. The central lucency is due to fluid within the lumen which is surrounded by an echogenic layer surrounded by another lucent layer representing edema in the wall of the intussusceptum. **C,** longitudinal scan of the intussusception demonstrates a pseudokidney sign with the edematous wall surrounding the echogenic mucosa. **D,** barium enema demonstrates the characteristic "coiled-spring" appearance of intussusception in the hepatic flexure.

films may have their intussusceptions reduced, but with a lower success rate than in uncomplicated cases. Stephenson et al. report a higher success rate with proximal intussusception than with more distal ones. Fever, leukocytosis, and abdominal tenderness may be signs of early peritonitis, but are nonspecific abnormalities. An abdominal physical examination by an experienced surgeon is a useful pre-caution before undertaking fluoroscopically monitored reduction.

The likelihood of success seems to be enhanced if the patient is well hydrated and sedated for the procedure. Some experienced pediatric radiologists use a balloon catheter to help maintain a high pressure head, but many others are concerned about the development thereby of a closed-loop obstruction

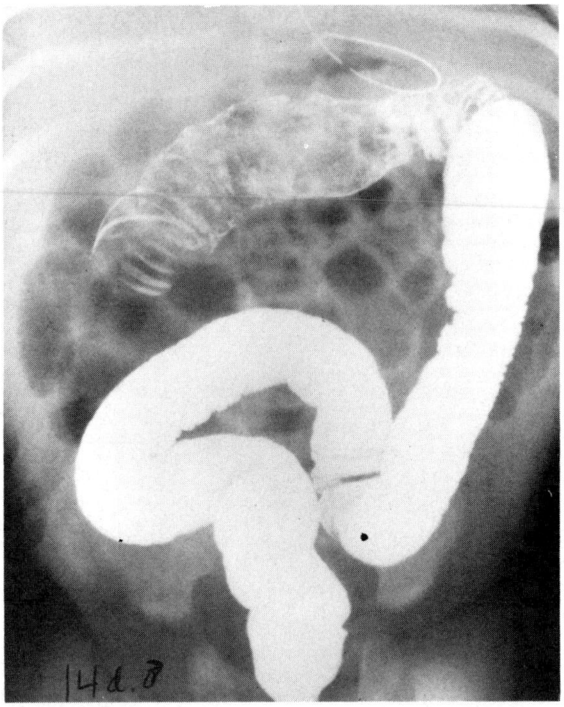

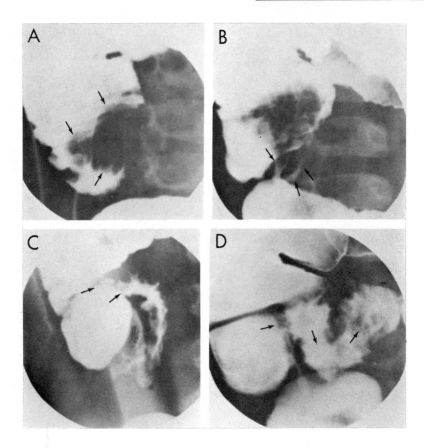

FIG 27–34.
Intussusception. Barium enema demonstrates a coiled-spring appearance in a 14-day-old infant. Note the lack of fecal material in the descending colon, the sigmoid colon, and the rectum.

FIG 27–35.
Serial changes at the ileocecal valve during hydrostatic reduction of an intussusception in an 18-month-old infant. **A,** the intussusceptum has been moved proximally from the transverse colon into the cecum where it causes a filling defect. **B,** the appendix is beginning to fill, and the cecal filling defect is smaller. **C,** the terminal ileum is beginning to fill, and cecal filling defect has disappeared. **D,** the terminal ileum is normally dilated with normal mucosal relief.

with a possibly increased hazard of perforation. A large rubber catheter with tight taping together of the buttocks usually produces a sufficient seal if reduction is possible and has a "safety valve" function if reduction cannot be performed. A commonly used technique is the "rule of threes." The hydrostatic pressure is kept at 3 ft and three attempts at reduction are made for 3 minutes each. Many experienced pediatric radiologists, however, will use higher pressures and perform more frequent attempts for longer periods of time. Palpation of the abdomen increases the intra-abdominal pressure in an uncontrolled fashion and should not be performed.

When the barium column meets the head of the intussusceptum, a concave filling defect appears.

This frequently presents a curvilinear spiral pattern that resembles the coil of a bedspring (Fig 27–34). The appearance is produced by a steady puddling of the barium in the compressed lumen between the head and the sleeve of the invagination and is not present until the barium mixture has worked itself into the folds between the intussusceptum and the intussuscipiens. The concavity flattens, and the head of the barium column moves unevenly toward the ileocecal valve.

When barium flows freely through the valve, reduction of the colonic portion of the intussusception is usually complete (Fig 27–35). A relatively dilute barium mixture produces better visualization of the individual loops of bowel near the ileocecal valve,

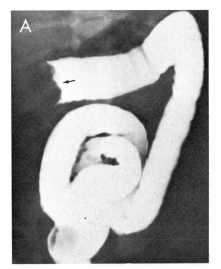

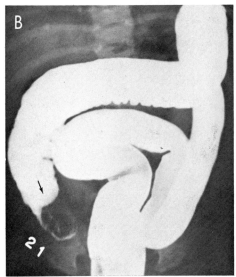
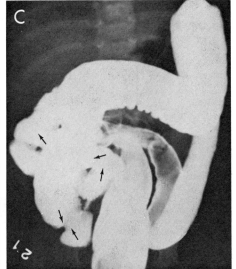

FIG 27–36.
Progressive changes during hydrostatic reduction of an ileocecal intussusception in a 3-month-old infant. **A,** the intussusceptum is identified in the proximal transverse colon. **B,** following initiation of hydrostatic reduction, the intussusceptum is moved retrograde into the cecum where it presents as a large filling defect. **C,** complete reduction of the intussusception with reflux into multiple loops of small intestine *(arrows)*. There continues to be some edematous swelling of the ileocecal valve *(lower arrows)*.

which may be swollen, particularly in long-standing intussusception. The edematous valve, which can simulate an incomplete reduction of the intussusception or lead point, may remain swollen for several days. US can confirm that the filling defect is caused by the edematous margins of the ileocecal valve. In ileoileocolic intussusception, the ileocolic component may be reduced completely, with persistence of the ileoileal lesions in the small bowel.

The end point of a successful reduction is flooding of the small bowel with contrast material to prove the ileocolic intussusception has been reduced and to reduce an ileoileal intussusception which may have acted as a lead point (Figs 27–36 and 27–37). Reported rates of successful hydrostatic reduction are about 85%. Approximately 5% of these patients will have recurrence, half within 48 hours. A successful second reduction can frequently be accomplished. When hydrostatic reduction fails, patients are brought to surgery. A phenomenon well known to surgeons is easy manual reduction after induction of anesthesia. Collins et al. were able to reduce 21 of 31 intussusceptions by contrast enemas in the operating room after the children were anesthetized. Each patient had had a failed previous attempt at reduction in the radiology department.

Although barium is the traditional contrast material used for hydrostatic reduction, some centers advocate using water-soluble contrast agents because of presumed decreased hazard in the event of perforation. Campbell's survey of 40 children's hospitals published in 1989 revealed that 34 institutions used barium all the time and 3 others used it most of the time. Schmitz-Rode et al., based on results of an experimental study, suggest that lower-viscosity contrast agents such as water-soluble media, especially when used with a large-bore tube, are theoretically more successful than barium, although not as successful as air (see below).

Pneumatic reduction of intussusception under fluoroscopic control has been practiced in China for several decades and is gaining wider acceptance in the rest of the world. Specific devices for control of pressure are required with most studies being performed at 80 to 120 mm Hg (Fig 27–38). Success rates and complication rates are similar to those in hydrostatic reduction. Advocates of pneumatic reduction point out its ease, the reduced likelihood of peritonitis in the event of perforation, and the reduced expense, at least when compared with the use of water-soluble contrast materials. The pneumatic reductions are usually faster, reducing radiation exposure. As with hydrostatic reduction, the filling of large portions of small bowel is necessary for assurance of adequate reduction. Hedlund et al., however, described three patients in whom extensive reflux of air occurred without successful reduction. They point out the importance of examining the cecum for a persistent filling defect even after air refluxes into the small intestine.

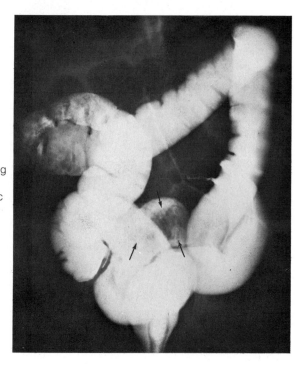

FIG 27–37.
Residual ileoileal intussusception *(arrows)* in the terminal ileum following hydrostatic reduction of the colic component of an ileoileocolic intussusception, the leading edge of which was originally in the splenic flexure.

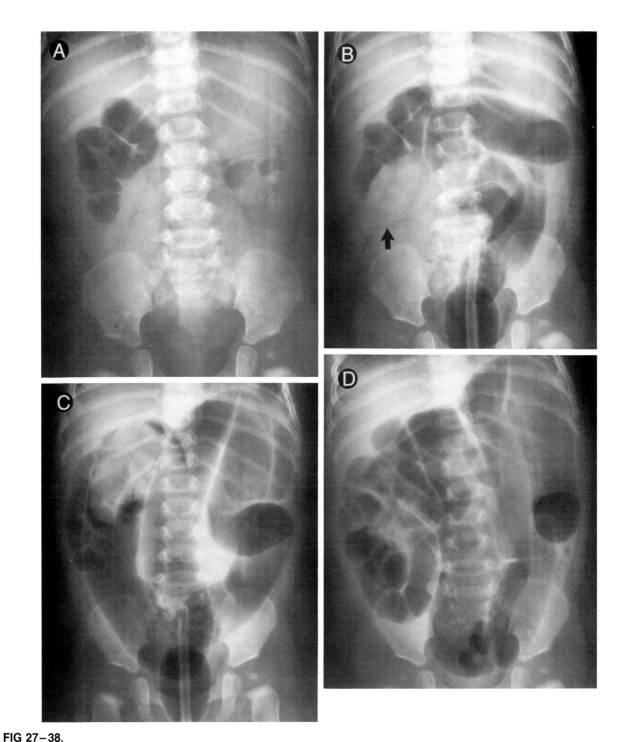

FIG 27–38.
Pneumatic reduction of intussusception. **A,** plain film demonstrates a dilated loop of small intestine in the right upper quadrant. A mass was palpated in this region. **B,** initial injection of air into the colon demonstrates a right upper quadrant mass *(arrow).* **C,** further distention of the colon with air reveals the mass to better ad-vantage. At this point, the pressure was changed from 60 to 80 mm Hg. **D,** following complete reduction of the intussusception, numerous air-filled loops of small intestine are seen and a soft-tissue mass is no longer present. **(Courtesy of Dr. Liu Ai-Qin, Macao.)**

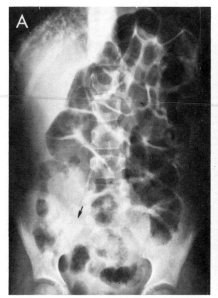
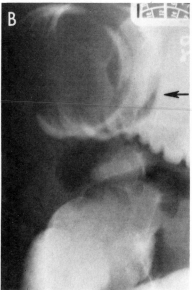

FIG 27–39.
Ileocolic intussusception in an 8½-year-old child with cystic fibrosis. **A,** plain film demonstrates a soft-tissue mass *(arrow)* in the right lower quadrant. Dilated small bowel loops are seen. **B,** spot film in the transverse colon demonstrates characteristic findings of intussusception. Successful hydrostatic reduction was accomplished.

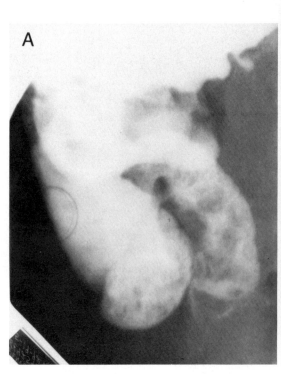
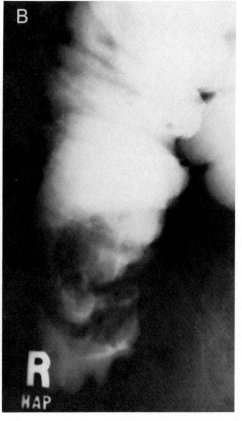

FIG 27–40.
Intussusception in a 42-year-old man with cystic fibrosis. **A,** filled film of the colon and terminal ileum during water-soluble contrast enema in an attempt to relieve symptoms of distal intestinal obstruction syndrome. Several fecal masses cause filling defects. **B,** postevacuation film demonstrates multiple loops of small intestine within the cecum. The patient experienced no pain.

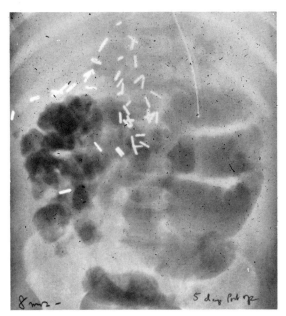

FIG 27–41.
Intestinal obstruction is seen on the plain film of an 8-month-old patient 5 days following removal of a right-sided Wilms tumor. Small intestinal intussusception was relieved surgically.

The most worrisome complication of hydrostatic or pneumatic reduction is intestinal perforation which occurs at sites of bowel necrosis, usually in the colon. Campbell's study of hydrostatic reduction reported 55 perforations in over 14,000 cases (0.4%) with one death. Stein et al. reported 7 perforations in 199 cases (2.8%) and no deaths with pneumatic reduction. Shiels et al. reported no perforations in 75 patients who underwent pneumatic reduction.

Approximately 5% of intussusceptions in child-hood are secondary to lead points. In the older child, adolescent, and teen-ager, lymphoma of the small bowel, usually Burkitt, is the lead point. Duplication cysts, polyps, and other congenital lesions act as lead points. Patients with CF with chronic constipation have a higher-than-normal incidence of intussusception (Figs 27–39 and 27–40). Postoperative intussusception is being recognized with increasing frequency. Plain film findings are those of small intestinal obstruction (Fig 27–41). Contrast studies are usually not rewarding since the majority are enteroenteric. West et al. reported 36 patients with postoperative intussusception of which 5 were ileocolic and 31 involved only small bowel. Hydrostatic reduction was successful in 2 cases of ileocolic intussusception and 1 case of distal ileoileal intussusception.

TUMORS

Tumors of the small intestine, benign or malignant, are rare in children. Polyposis of the small bowel usually occurs in children with the polyposis syndromes, which are described in Chapter 28. Patients usually present with blood in the stools and crampy abdominal pain secondary to recurrent enteroenteric intussusceptions. Distal ileal polyps may produce ileocolic intussusception. Barium studies reveal polypoid filling defects. The polyps can also be identified on sonography and CT. In children with blue rubber bleb nevus syndrome, hemangiomas can cause polypoid defects in the stomach, colon, and small bowel. Tyrrel et al. reported the CT diagnosis of intussusception in a young woman with the blue

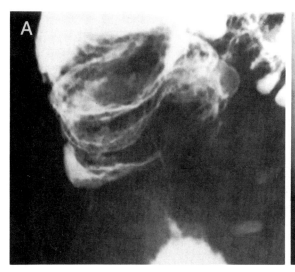

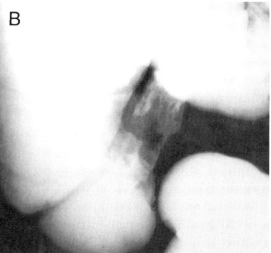

FIG 27–42.
Burkitt lymphoma presenting as intussusception. **A,** spot film from a barium enema demonstrates an intussusceptum within the cecum. **B,** reflux into the small intestine reveals an ileocecal mass which proved to be Burkitt lymphoma.

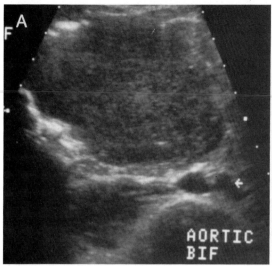
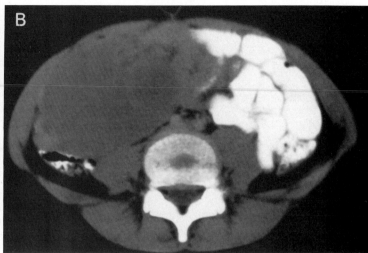

FIG 27–43.
Burkitt lymphoma in a 14-year-old boy who presented with a large abdominal mass. **A,** sonogram demonstrates a hypoechoic mass anterior to the aortic bifurcation which on multiple scans extended both superiorly and inferiorly. **B,** CT scan demonstrates the mass extending from just in front of the psoas muscle to the anterior abdominal wall. Percutaneous needle biopsy under US control demonstrated Burkitt lymphoma.

rubber bleb nevus syndrome. Unusual tumors in childhood include lipomas, fibromas, neurofibromas, and leiomyomas.

Malignant tumors of the small intestine in children, other than lymphoma, are exceedingly rare. The benign tumors mentioned above have their malignant counterparts. Patients with several of the polyposis syndromes can develop GI malignancies. Malignant carcinoid has been reported in children.

Burkitt lymphoma is a B cell lymphoma with a predilection for abdominal organs, particularly the distal ileum. It is the most common lead point in children over the age of 4 years with ileocolic intussusception (Fig 27–42). Patients present with variable symptoms, including nausea, vomiting, change in bowel habits, GI bleeding, or a right lower quadrant mass. Half of all patients with the sporadic form of Burkitt lymphoma (formerly called American Burkitt) have involvement of the terminal ileum, and in 25% of patients the disease is limited to this site. Mesenteric lymph nodes are usually involved. Plain film findings may be normal, show evidence of obstruction secondary to intussusception, or show a noncalcified mass. If a mass is obvious, either clinically or radiographically, sonography is the appropriate imaging study. Lymphoma is often hypoechoic or anechoic, so sonography may enable a specific diagnosis to be suggested (Fig 27–43). The small-bowel lesion is usually eccentric and the lumen is frequently dilated. The involved lymph nodes may be focal or may infiltrate the mesentery and encase the mesenteric vessels. The nodal masses are also of decreased echogenicity. CT also shows the mesenteric masses and infiltration of bowel wall with dilatation of bowel lumen. Both sonography and CT may demonstrate ascites. Barium studies may show polypoid involvement of the mucosa, infiltration of the wall, dilatation and ulceration of the bowel wall, or effacement of the mucosa mimicking inflammatory bowel disease. The effect of the adjacent mesenteric masses can be seen. The tumor may also involve other abdominal sites, and careful evaluation of the retroperitoneal organs, the liver, and the spleen is mandatory during sonography and CT.

REFERENCES

Hereditary and Developmental Disorders

Adamsbaum C, Sellier N, Helardot P: Ileocolic intussusception with enterogenous cyst: Ultrasonic diagnosis. *Pediatr Radiol* 1989; 19:325.

Barr LL, Hayden CK Jr, Stansberry SD, et al: Enteric duplication cysts in children: Are their ultrasonographic wall characteristics diagnostic? *Pediatr Radiol* 1990; 20:326.

Bender TM, Ledesma-Medina J, Oh KS: Radiographic manifestations of anomalies of the gastrointestinal tract. *Radiol Clin North Am* 1991; 29:335.

Bowen B, Ros PR, McCarthy MJ, et al: Gastrointestinal teratomas: CT and US appearance with pathologic correlation. *Radiology* 1987; 162:431.

Bower RJ, Sieber WKN, Kiesewetter WB: Alimentary tract duplications in children. *Ann Surg* 1978; 188:669.

Caspi B, Schachter M, Lancet M: Infected duplication cyst of ileum masquerading as an adnexal abscess-ultrasonographic feature *JCU* 1989; 17:431.

Egelhoff JC, Bisset GS III, Strife JL: Multiple enteric duplications in an infant. *Pediatr Radiol* 1986; 16:160.

Geer LL, Mittelstaedt CA, Staab EV, et al: Mesenteric cyst: sonographic appearance with CT correlation. *Pediatr Radiol* 1984; 14:102.

Gilchrist AM, Sloan JM, Logan CJH, et al: Case report: gastrointestinal bleeding due to multiple ileal duplications diagnosed by scintigraphy and barium studies. *Clin Radiol* 1990; 41:134.

Haller JO, Schneider M, Kassner EG, et al: Sonographic evaluation of mesenteric and omental masses in children. *AJR* 1978; 130:269.

Harvey PJ, Whitley NO: CT of benign cystic abdominal masses in children. *AJR* 1984; 142:1279.

Ilstad ST, Tollerud DJ, Weiss RG, et al: Duplications of the alimentary tract. *Ann Surg* 1988; 208:184.

Jackson A, Bisset R, Dickson AP: Malrotation and midgut volvulus presenting as malabsorption. *Clin Radiol* 1989; 40:536.

Lamont AC, Starinsky R, Cremin BJ: Ultrasonic diagnosis of duplication cysts in children. *Br J Radiol* 1984; 57:463.

McAlister WH, Siegel MJ: Pediatric radiology case of the day. *AJR* 1989; 152:1328.

Nicolet V, Grignon A, Filiatrault D, et al: Sonographic appearance of an abdominal cystic lymphangioma. *J Ultrasound Med* 1984; 3:85.

Rifkin MD, Kurtz AB, Pasto ME: Mesenteric chylous (lymph-containing) cyst. *Gastrointest Radiol* 1983; 8:267.

Ros PR, Olmsted WW, Moser RP Jr, et al: Mesenteric and omental cysts: Histologic classification with imaging correlation. *Radiology* 1987; 164:327.

Shatzkes D, Gordon DH, Haller JO, et al: Malrotation of the bowel: malalignment of the superior mesenteric artery-vein complex shown by CT and MR. *J Comput Assist Tomogr* 1990; 14:93.

Teele RL, Henschke CT, Tapper D: The radiographic and ultrasonographic evaluation of enteric duplication cysts. *Pediatr Radiol* 1980; 10:9.

Vasquez R, Oates E, Sarno RC, et al: Incidental discovery of a large duplication cyst during Meckel's scintigraphy. *Clin Nucl Med* 1989; 14:537.

Zerin JM, Di Pietro MA: Mesenteric vascular anatomy at CT: Normal and abnormal appearances. *Radiology* 1991; 179:739.

Zerin JM, Di Pietro MA: Superior mesenteric vascular anatomy at US in patients with surgically proved malrotation of the midgut. *Radiology* 1992; 183:693.

Functional and Infiltrative Diseases

Bartram CI, Small E: The intestinal radiological changes in older people with pancreatic cystic fibrosis. *Br J Radiol* 1971; 44:195.

Berk RN, Lee FA: The late gastrointestinal manifestations of cystic fibrosis of the pancreas. *Radiology* 1973; 106:337.

Bova JG, Friedman AC, Weser E, et al: Adaptation of the ileum in nontropical sprue: Reversal of the jejunoileal fold pattern. *AJR* 1985; 144:299.

Djurhuus MJ, Lykkegaard E, Pock-Steen OC: Gastrointestinal radiological findings in cystic fibrosis. *Pediatr Radiol* 1973; 1:113.

Dorne HL, Jequier S: Sonography of intestinal lymphangiectasia. *J Ultrasound Med* 1986; 5:13.

Fisk JD, Shulman HM, Greening RR, et al: Gastrointestinal radiographic features of human graft-vs-host disease. *AJR* 1981; 136:329.

Glasier CM, Siegel MJ, McAlister WH, et al: Henoch-Schönlein syndrome in children: Gastrointestinal manifestations. *AJR* 1981; 136:1081.

Gorske K, Winchester P, Grossman H: Unusual protein-losing enteropathies in children. *AJR* 1969; 92:739.

Haworth EM, Hodson CJ, Pringle EM, et al: The value of radiological investigations of the alimentary tract in children with the celiac syndrome. *Clin Radiol* 1968; 107:158.

Herzog DB, Logan R, Looistra JB: The Noonan syndrome with intestinal lymphangiectasia. *J Pediatr* 1976; 88:270.

Jones B, Bayless TM, Fishman EK, et al: Lymphadenopathy in celiac disease: Computed tomographic observations. *AJR* 1984; 142:1127.

Jones B, Bayless TM, Hamilton SR, et al: "Bubbly" duodenal bulb in celiac disease: Radiologic-pathologic correlation. *AJR* 1984; 142:119.

Jones B, Fishman EK, Kramer SS, et al: Computed tomography of gastrointestinal inflammation after bone marrow transplantation. *AJR* 1986; 146:691.

Koletzko S, Stringer DA, Cleghorn GJ, et al: Lavage treatment of distal intestinal obstruction syndrome in children with cystic fibrosis. *Pediatrics* 1989; 83:727.

Lanning P, Simila S, Sioramo I, et al: Lymphatic abnormalities in Noonan's syndrome. *Pediatr Radiol* 1978; 7:106.

Maile CW, Frick MP, Crass JR, et al: The plain abdominal radiograph in acute gastrointestinal graft-vs-host disease. *AJR* 1985; 145:289.

Marn CS, Gore RM, Chahremani GG: Duodenal manifestations of nontropical sprue. *Gastrointest Radiol* 1986; 11:30.

Martinez-Frontanilla LA, Silverman L, Meagher DP Jr: Intussusception in Henoch-Schönlein purpura: Diagnosis with ultrasound. *J Pediatr Surg* 1988; 23:375.

Miyamoto K, Fukuda Y, Urushibara K, et al: Ultrasonographic findings in duodenum caused by Schönlein-Henoch purpura. *JCU* 1989; 17:299.

Rubinstein S, Moss RB, Lewiston NJ: Constipation and meconium ileus equivalent in patients with cystic fibrosis. *Pediatrics* 1986; 78:473.

Schimmelpenninck M, Zwaan F: Radiographic features of

small intestinal injury in graft-versus-host disease. *Gastrointest Radiol* 1982; 7:29.

Taussig LM, Saldino RM, di Sant'Agnese PA: Radiographic abnormalities of the duodenum and small bowel in cystic fibrosis of the pancreas (mucoviscidosis). *Radiology* 1973; 106:369.

Weizman Z, Stringer DA, Durie PR: Radiologic manifestations of malabsorption: A nonspecific finding. *Pediatrics* 1984; 74:530.

Infectious Diseases

Bohrer SP: Typhoid perforation of the ileum. *Br J Radiol* 1966; 39:37.

Bradford BF, Abdenour GE Jr, Frank JL, et al: Usual and unusual radiologic manifestations of acquired immunodeficiency syndrome (AIDS) and human immunodeficiency virus (HIV) infection in children. *Radiol Clin North Am* 1988; 26:341.

Brandon J, Glick SN, Teplick SK: Intestinal giardiasis: The importance of serial filming. AJR 1985; 144:581.

Brody PA, Fertig S, Aron JM: *Campylobacter* enterocolitis: Radiographic features. AJR 1982; 139:1199.

Capitanio MA, Greenberg SB: Pneumatosis intestinalis in two infants with rotavirus gastroenteritis. *Pediatr Radiol* 1991; 21:361.

Eckberg O, Sjostrum B, Brahme F: Radiological findings in *Yersinia* ileitis. *Radiology* 1977; 123:15.

Haney PJ, Yale-Loehr AJ, Nussbaum AR, et al: Imaging of infants and children with AIDS. AJR 1989; 152:1033.

Hodes HL: Gastroenteritis with special reference to rotavirus. *Adv Pediatr* 1980; 27:195.

Jones B, Fishman EK: CT of the gut in the immunocompromised host. *Radiol Clin North Am* 1989; 27:763.

Katz M: Parasitic infections. *J Pediatr* 1975; 87:165.

Matsumoto T, Iida M, Sakai T, et al: *Yersinia* terminal ileitis: Sonographic findings in eight patients. AJR 1991; 156:965.

Nagi B, Duggal R, Gupta R, et al: Tuberculous peritonitis in children. *Pediatr Radiol* 1987; 17:282.

Puylaert JBCM, Kristjánsdóttir S, Golterman KL, et al: Typhoid fever: Diagnosis by using sonography. *Am J Roentgenol* 1989; 153:745.

Sivit CJ, Josephs SH, Taylor GA, et al: Pneumatosis intestinalis in children with AIDS. AJR 1990; 155:133.

Sivit CJ, Taylor GA, Patterson K, et al: Bowel obstruction in an infant with AIDS. AJR 1990; 154:803.

Crohn Disease

Balthazar EJ: CT of the gastrointestinal tract: Principles and interpretation. *AJR* 1991; 156:23.

Berlinger L, Redmond P, Purow EK, et al: Computed tomography in Crohn's disease. *Am J Gastroenterol* 1982; 77:533.

Buck JL, Dachman AH, Sobin LH: Polypoid and pseudopolypoid manifestations of inflammatory bowel disease. *Radiographics* 1991; 11:293.

Desai RK, Tagliabue JR, Wegryn SA, et al: CT evaluation of wall thickening in the alimentary tract. *Radiographics* 1991; 1:771.

Dinker E, Dittrich M, Peters H, et al: Real-time ultrasound in Crohn's disease: Characteristic features and clinical implications. *Pediatr Radiol* 1986; 16:8.

Dubois RS, Rothschild J, Silverman A, et al: The varied manifestations of Crohn's disease in children and adolescents. *Am J Gastroenterol* 1978; 69:203.

Gore RM: CT of inflammatory bowel disease. *Radiol Clin North Am* 1989; 27:717.

Jabra AA, Fishman EK, Taylor GA: Crohn disease in the pediatric patient: CT evaluation. *Radiology* 1991; 179:495.

Jones B, Fishman EK, Hamilton SR, et al: Submucosal accumulation of fat in inflammatory bowel disease: CT/pathologic correlation. *J Comput Assist Tomogr* 1986; 10:759.

Kirks DR, Currarino G: Regional enteritis in children: Small bowel disease with normal terminal ileum. *Pediatr Radiol* 1978; 7:10.

Lindquist BL, Jarnerot G, Wickbom G: Clinical and epidemiological aspects of Crohn's disease in children and adolescents. *Scand J Gastroenterol* 1984; 19:502.

Lipson A, Bartram CI, Williams CB, et al: Barium studies and ileoscopy compared in children with suspected Crohn's disease. *Clin Radiol* 1990; 41:5.

Park RHR, McKillop JH, Duncan A, et al: Can [111]indium autologous mixed leucocyte scanning accurately assess disease extent and activity in Crohn's disease? *Gut* 1988; 29:821.

Riddlesberger MM Jr: CT of complicated inflammatory bowel disease in children. *Pediatr Radiol* 1985; 15:384.

Scott WW Jr, Fishman EK, Kuhlman JE, et al: Computed tomography evaluation of the sacroiliac joints in Crohn disease: Radiologic/clinical correlation. *Skeletal Radiol* 1990; 19:207.

Shirkhoda A: Diagnostic pitfalls in abdominal CT. *Radiographics* 1991; 11:969.

Stringer DA: Imaging inflammatory bowel disease in the pediatric patient. *Radiol Clin North Am* 1987; 25:93.

Stringer DA, Cleghorn GJ, Durie PR, et al: Behçet's syndrome involving the gastrointestinal tract—a diagnostic dilemma in childhood. *Pediatr Radiol* 1986; 16:131.

Tolia V, Kuhns LR, Chang CH, et al: Comparison of indium-111 scintigraphy and colonoscopy with histologic study in children for evaluation of colonic chronic inflammatory bowel disease. *J Pediatr Gastroenterol Nutr* 1991; 12:336.

Vlymen WJ, Moskowitz PS: Roentgenographic manifestations of esophageal and intestinal involvement in Behçet's disease in children. *Pediatr Radiol* 1981; 10:193.

Yeh H-C, Rabinowitz JG: Granulomatous enterocolitis: Findings by ultrasonography and computed tomography. *Radiology* 1983: 149:253.

Acquired Small-Intestinal Obstruction

Akin JT Jr: The anatomic basis of vascular compression of the duodenum. *Surg Clin North Am* 1974; 64:1361.

Marchant EA, Alvear DT, Fagelman KM: True clinical entity of vascular compression of the duodenum in adolescence. *Surg Gynecol Obstet* 1989; 168:381.

Munns SW: Hyperalimentation for superior mesenteric artery (cast) syndrome following correction of spinal deformity. *J Bone Joint Surg [Am]* 1984; 66:1175.

Ortiz C, Cleveland RH, Blickman JG, et al: Familial superior mesenteric artery syndrome. *Pediatr Radiol* 1990; 20:588.

Pentlow BD, Dent RG: Acute vascular compression of the duodenum in anorexia nervosa. *Br J Surg* 1981; 68:665.

Ratcliffe J, Tait J, Lisle D, et al: Segmental dilatation of the small bowel: Report of three cases and literature review. *Radiology* 1989; 171:827.

Intussusception

Adamsbaum C, Sellier N, Helardot P: Ileocolic intussusception with enterogenous cyst: Ultrasonic diagnosis. *Pediatr Radiol* 1989; 325.

Alzen G, Funke G, Truong S: Pitfalls in the diagnosis of intussusception. *JCU* 1989; 17:481.

Bisset GS III, Kirks DR: Intussusception in infants and children: diagnosis and therapy. *Radiology* 1988; 168:141.

Campbell JB: Contrast media in intussusception. *Pediatr Radiol* 1989; 19:293.

Collins DL, Pinckney LE, Miller KE: Hydrostatic reduction of ileocolic intussusception: A second attempt in the operating room with general anesthesia. *J Pediatr* 1989; 115:204.

Ein SH, Stephen CA: Intussusception: 354 cases in 10 years. *J Pediatr Surg* 1971; 6:16.

Eklöf O, Hartelius H: Reliability of the abdominal plain film diagnosis in pediatric patients with suspected intussusception. *Pediatr Radiol* 1980; 9:199.

Hedlund GL, Johnson JF, Strife JL: Ileocolic intussusception: extensive reflux of air preceding pneumatic reduction. *Radiology* 1990; 174:187.

Johnson JF, Woisard KK: Ileocolic intussusception: New sign on the supine cross-table lateral radiograph. *Radiology* 1989; 170:483.

Kenney IJ: Ultrasound in intussusception: A false cystic lead point. *Pediatr Radiol* 1990; 20:348.

Knowles MC, Fishman EK, Kuhlman JE, et al: Transient intussusception in Crohn disease: CT evaluation. *Radiology* 1989; 170:814.

Markowitz RI, Meyer JJ: Pneumatic versus hydrostatic reduction of intussusception (editorial). *Radiology* 1992; 183:623.

Pracros JP, Tran-Minh VA, Morin De Finfe CH, et al: Acute intestinal intussusception in children. Contribution of ultrasonography (145 cases). *Ann Radiol (Paris)* 1987; 30:525.

Schmitz-Rode T, Müller-Leisse C, Alzen G: Comparative examination of various rectal tubes and contrast media for the reduction of intussusceptions. *Pediatr Radiol* 1991; 21:341.

Shiels WE II, Bisset GS III, Kirks DR: Simple device for air reduction of intussusception. *Pediatr Radiol* 1990; 20:472.

Shiels WE II, Maves CK, Hedlund GL, et al: Air enema for diagnosis and reduction of intussusception: Clinical experience and pressure correlates. *Radiology* 1991; 181:169.

Stein M, Alton DJ, Daneman A: Pneumatic reduction of intussusception: five-year experience. *Radiology* 1992; 183:681.

Stephenson CA, Seibert JJ, Strain JDO, et al. Intussusception: Clinical and radiographic factors influencing reducibility. *Pediatr Radiol* 1989; 20:57.

Stringer DA, Ein EH: Pneumatic reduction: Advantages, risks, and indications (invited commentary). *Pediatr Radiol* 1990; 20:475.

Swischuk LE, Hayden CK, Boulden T: Intussusception: Indications for ultrasonography and an explanation of the doughnut and pseudokidney signs. *Pediatr Radiol* 1985; 15:388.

Swischuk LE, Stansberry SD: Ultrasonographic detection of free peritoneal fluid in uncomplicated intussusception. *Pediatr Radiol* 1991; 21:350.

West KW, Stephens B, Rescorla FJ, et al: Postoperative intussusception: experience with 36 cases in children. *Surgery* 1988; 104:781.

White SJ, Blane CE: Intussusception: Additional observations on the plain radiograph. AJR 1983; 139:511.

Tumors

Alford B, Coccia P, L'Heureux P: Roentgenographic features of American Burkitt's lymphoma. *Radiology* 1977; 124:763.

Dunnick NR, Reaman GH, Head GL, et al: Radiographic manifestations of Burkitt's lymphoma in American patients. AJR 1979; 132:1.

Jenkin RD, Sonley MJ, Stephens CA, et al: Primary gastrointestinal tract lymphoma in childhood. *Radiology* 1969; 92:763.

Magrath IT: Malignant non-Hodgkin's lymphomas, in Pizzo PA, Poplack DG (eds): *Principles and Practice of Pediatric Oncology,* Philadelphia, JB Lippincott, 1989, pp 433–434.

Miller JH, Hindman BW, Lam AH: Ultrasound in the evaluation of small bowel lymphoma in children. *Radiology* 1980; 135:409.

Tyrrel RT, Baumgartner BR, Montemayor KA: Blue rubber bleb nevus syndrome: CT diagnosis of intussusception. AJR 1990; 154:105.

Vade A, Blane CE: Imaging of Burkitt lymphoma in pediatric patients. *Pediatr Radiol* 1985; 15:123.

28

The Colon

ANATOMY AND DEVELOPMENT

The colon, or large intestine, extends from the cecum in the right lower quadrant to the anus. The cecum and ascending colon are usually fixed by peritoneal attachments, although the cecum can be on a mesentery which makes it mobile during imaging examinations. The ascending colon extends to the hepatic flexure which is subjacent to the underside of the liver. The transverse colon extends across the upper abdomen and is on a mesentery, allowing it substantial positional mobility. The highest visualized point in the left upper quadrant on barium enema, the radiographic splenic flexure, is actually the distal end of the transverse colon. The anatomical splenic flexure is the most proximal fixed point of the descending colon. The fixed colon descends into the left lower quadrant where the mobile sigmoid colon on a mesentery runs between the descending colon and rectum. The colon in children, especially the sigmoid and transverse components, is often more redundant than in adults. The cecum in young children may be relatively more cephalad than it is in older children or adults.

The proximal colon, from cecum to mid- or distal-transverse colon, is derived from the embryonic midgut and receives its blood supply from the superior mesenteric artery. It participates in the extracoelomic migration of the midgut described in Chapter 22. The portion of colon from the transverse colon through the rectum is derived from the hindgut and receives its blood supply from the inferior mesenteric artery. In the early embryo, it empties into the cloaca along with portions of the genitourinary tract, but is separated by a developing septum from these structures.

The anal canal is formed by the joining of the distalmost portion of the hindgut to an invagination of the ectoderm of the embryonic rump.

IMAGING STUDIES

Plain films are useful in the evaluation of colonic disease. The air-filled colon is usually easily distinguished from small bowel in children beyond 1 year of age. This differentiation is not always easy in infants. The supine film shows the anatomy well and is satisfactory for the evaluation of stool content, intramural air, and pathologic calcifications. A horizontal-beam film is valuable when anatomical or functional obstruction or free air is a concern.

The standard examination of the colon continues to be the *contrast enema*. Barium is still the most commonly used contrast medium with water-soluble agents being reserved for patients with potential perforations or for therapeutic interventions. Double contrast barium enemas, as described in adults, can easily be performed in children, even in infants, and are especially useful in patients with suspected mucosal lesions such as inflammatory bowel disease or in the evaluation of children with lower intestinal bleeding or suspected of having polyps.

Sonography is useful in specific diseases such as appendicitis, neutropenic colitis, and tumors. It is also very useful in the search for complications of colonic disease such as abscesses. *Computed tomography* (CT) is also useful in the evaluation of tumors, abscesses, and other intra-abdominal, extracolonic manifestations of colonic disease. *Magnetic resonance* (MR) imaging has yet to achieve a defined role in the evaluation of colonic diseases.

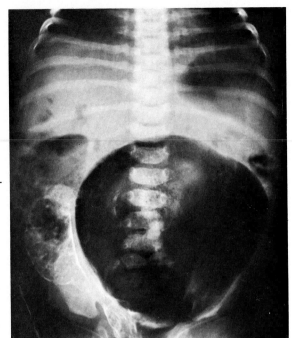

FIG 28–1.
Congenital duplication of the colon in a 7-week-old infant. At surgery, the gas-filled cyst was seen to communicate with the lumen of the colon. (Courtesy of Dr. H. Thompson, Tucson.)

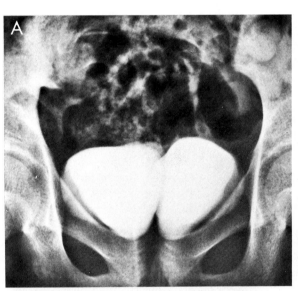

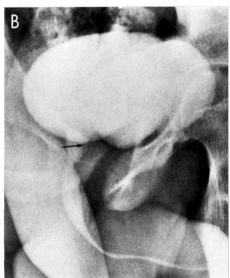

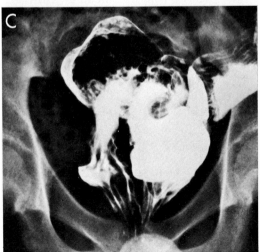

FIG 28–2.
Duplication of the bladder and entire colon in a 15-year-old boy who had been treated in the newborn period for anal atresia. **A,** frontal film of the pelvis after excretory urography shows two bladders. Each upper urinary tract emptied into the bladder on its side. **B,** voiding urethrogram. A single urethra *(arrow)* originated from the right side. **C,** barium enema demonstrates two rectums. Surgical exploration revealed duplication of the colon from appendix to rectum.

CONGENITAL AND DEVELOPMENTAL ABNORMALITIES

The majority of congenital and developmental abnormalities of the colon present in the newborn period and are discussed in Chapter 52. *Duplication cysts* are much less frequently found in the colon than in the small bowel and are usually localized. Noncommunicating cysts may be palpable or lead to symptoms of obstruction, if large. Sonography demonstrates an anechoic mass. Contrast enemas show an extraluminal mass effect. Localized duplications occasionally communicate with the lumen and can fill with air or contrast material (Fig 28–1). A rare entity is complete duplication of the colon which is associated with duplication of the urinary bladder (Fig 28–2).

In patients with *midgut malrotation,* the cecum is usually in the midpelvis and the ascending colon is midline, running cephalad to join with a shortened distal transverse colon and left colon, which are in normal position (Fig 28–3). In rare circumstances, peritoneal bands cross anterior to the transverse colon, causing partial obstruction (Fig 28–4). When the

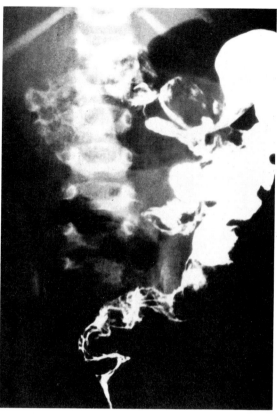

FIG 28–4.
Peritoneal bands. AP view of the abdomen following barium enema demonstrates partial obstruction of the transverse colon by peritoneal bands crossing anterior to it. The cecum is malpositioned. (Courtesy of Dr. William Schey, Chicago.)

left kidney is ectopic or absent, the splenic flexure may be positioned more medially and inferiorly than is the normal situation (Fig 28–5).

COLONIC AGANGLIONOSIS

Functional disorders of the colon produce clinical and radiologic findings of constipation, obstruction, or both, without a mechanical defect being identified. They can be developmental, as with colonic aganglionosis, or acquired, as with some forms of intestinal pseudo-obstruction.

Colonic aganglionosis, or Hirschsprung disease, occurs in about 1 in 5,000 live births. It presents in the newborn period in 80% of cases and its manifestations in neonates are discussed in Chapter 52. Beyond the neonatal period, aganglionosis can present at any age, even in adults, although it is more frequently identified in younger children. The disease results from absence of the myenteric plexus secondary to failure of migration of neural crest cells throughout the total length of the gastrointestinal

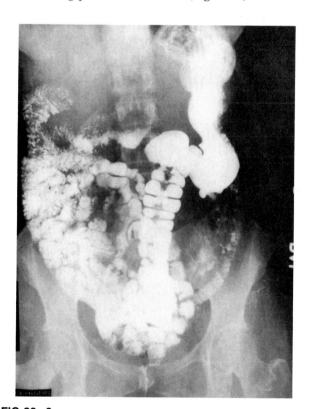

FIG 28–3.
AP view of the abdomen in a young woman with symptoms of duodenal ulcer disease shows complete malrotation of the midgut. The cecum and ascending colon are in the midline while the portions of the colon derived from the embryonic hindgut are in normal position.

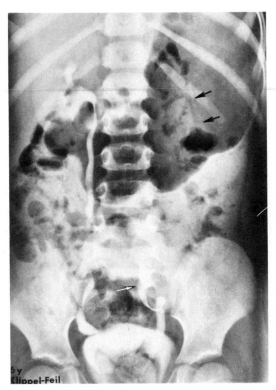

FIG 28–5.
Excretory urogram in a 6-year-old boy with Klippel-Feil syndrome demonstrates a pelvic kidney *(lowest arrow)* on the *left.* The *upper arrows* show the medial position of the splenic flexure.

(GI) tract. Since the normal migration is continuous from proximal to distal, that portion of the GI tract distal to the site of arrest is aganglionic. Skip areas are not seen (Fig 28–6). So-called zonal aganglionosis has been described, but the focal lack of ganglion cells is probably secondary to a different cause. It is extremely rare. The transition from innervated to aganglionic bowel is found in the anorectosigmoid region in 73% of patients, the descending colon in 14%, and the more proximal colon in 10%, according to Swenson et al. Total colonic aganglionosis occurs in 3% of patients. Nearly all patients who present beyond infancy have short-segment disease involving only the distal colon. Since the normal myenteric plexus cells are necessary for relaxation of the colon, the pathophysiology is persistent irregular contraction of the aganglionic segment causing functional obstruction.

Males are more frequently affected than females in short-segment aganglionosis while the sex incidence is equal with long-segment disease. A familial incidence has been identified in some patients with total aganglionosis and long-segment involvement. The disease is associated with trisomy 21 in about 3% of cases and with a variety of other congenital abnormalities in sporadic instances.

Patients beyond infancy present with a history of constipation usually dating to the first weeks of life, although the onset of symptoms is sometimes delayed. Fecal soiling is very rare and its presence is

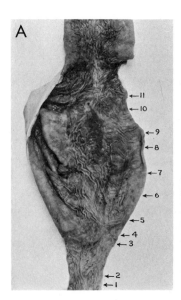

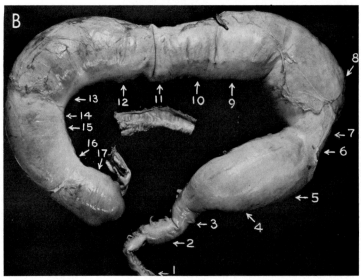

FIG 28–6.
Absence of the myenteric plexus in the rectum and terminal segment of the sigmoid colon in congenital megacolon. **A,** photograph of an enlarged colon that shows the small rectum distal to the dilated sigmoid. In blocks of tissue taken from sites marked by *arrows,* there were no ganglion cells in levels *1–7;* a few at level *8;* and normal numbers at levels *9–11.* **B,** photograph of an entire megacolon that shows the small rectum. There were no ganglion cells at levels *1–4;* scanty ganglion cells at levels *5–7;* and normal numbers at levels *8–17.* **(From Whitehouse FR, Kernohan JW:** *Arch Intern Med* **1948; 82:75. Used by permission.)**

suggestive of psychogenic constipation rather than aganglionosis. The classic presentation of the wan, lethargic patient with protuberant abdomen, but otherwise wasted-appearing and with failure to thrive, is very uncommon other than in areas of the world that are medically underserved. Definitive diagnosis is made by distal colonic biopsy, but radio-

graphic evaluation is useful in differentiating aganglionosis from other causes of megacolon and for evaluating the length of the involved colon segment.

Plain film examination reveals extensive amounts of stool throughout a dilated colon. Depending on the level of transition, a small distal colon empty of stool may be identified (Fig 28–7). Di-

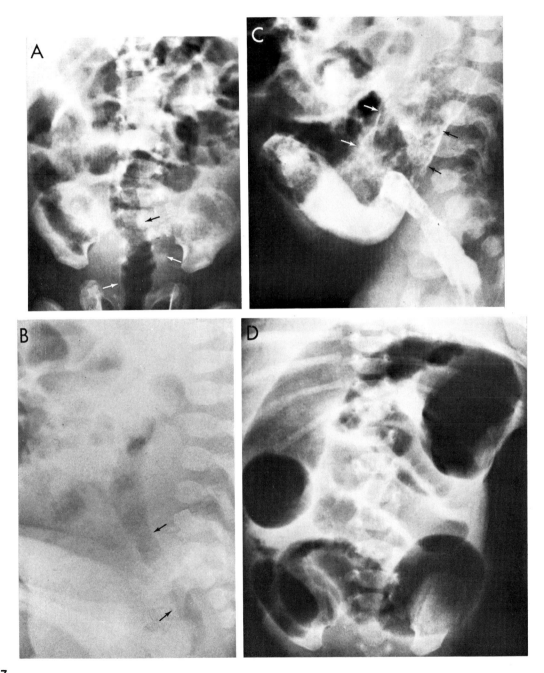

FIG 28–7.
Aganglionic megacolon in a 6-week-old infant with a history of abdominal distention and constipation. **A,** frontal and **B,** lateral films of the abdomen demonstrate the small caliber of the air-filled rectum *(arrows).* **C,** lateral view of a barium enema demonstrates a transition zone between the narrowed rectosigmoid colon and the dilated descending colon. **D,** frontal film 3 days after the barium enema demonstrates the abdomen to be distended with markedly dilated loops of colon. Some dilatation of small bowel is also seen. The baby required emergency transverse colostomy for necrotizing enterocolitis of Hirschsprung disease.

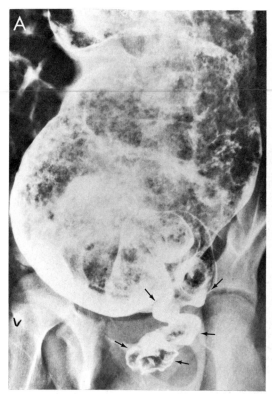 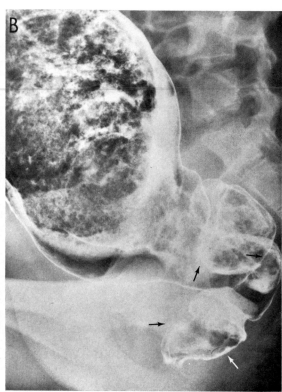

FIG 28–8.
Megacolon secondary to aganglionosis of the rectum and distal sigmoid colon. **A,** oblique and **B,** lateral projections of barium enema demonstrate an abrupt transition from the narrow caliber of the rectosigmoid to the large caliber of the more proximal sigmoid colon. This 14-year-old girl had been obstipated since birth.

lated, air-filled loops of small intestine may be seen but the signs of intestinal obstruction frequently present in newborns are uncommon in older children.

Although water-soluble contrast enemas are often recommended in newborns with intestinal obstruction, barium enema is the examination of choice to evaluate the constipated child for aganglionosis. Historically, patients do not receive a bowel preparation before barium enema because the presence of stool in the dilated portion of the bowel makes the identification of a transition zone easier. The older the patient, however, the less likely cleaning enemas are to cause confusion. Rosenfield et al. have shown that digital rectal examination preceding barium enema does not interfere with making the diagnosis. A large-bore straight rubber catheter cut to have only a single end-hole is inserted no more than a centimeter into the anal canal and taped in place. The buttocks of young children can be taped tightly. Initial filling takes place with the patient recumbent, left side down, and spot films of the rectum in lateral projection are obtained, following which the patient is turned supine and anteroposterior (AP) films obtained. The examination is terminated if the charac-

teristic findings of aganglionosis are present. If not, the examination is continued until a transition zone is identified or until the colon is filled.

The most frequently identified sign of aganglionosis on barium enema is the presence of a transition zone between a variably narrowed, stool-free aganglionic distal segment and a dilated, stool-filled proximal segment (Figs 28–8 and 28–9). The transition zone cannot always be identified, but it is more reliably present in older children than in neonates. Although the radiographic transition zone does not correspond exactly to the histologic transition zone, it is close enough to be a guide to the surgeon. The final decision as to the true level of transition is made in the operating room with serial biopsies and frozen sections until normal ganglion cells are found. In general, the normal rectum is more capacious than the sigmoid colon. This relationship may be reversed with anorectal aganglionosis and has led to the derivation of a "rectosigmoid index." There are so many factors that affect colonic caliber in this disease, however, that a quantitative assessment of the rectosigmoid relationship may be misleading.

Since the aganglionic segment has disordered motor function, irregular contraction waves will be

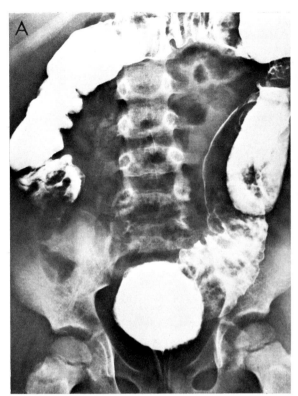

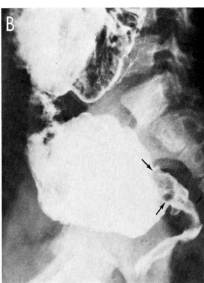

FIG 28–9.
Aganglionosis of the rectum in a 5-year-old boy. **A,** frontal and **B,** lateral projections of the barium enema demonstrate the transition zone between the small caliber of the rectum and the large sigmoid *(arrows).*

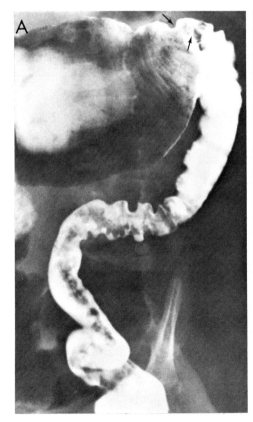

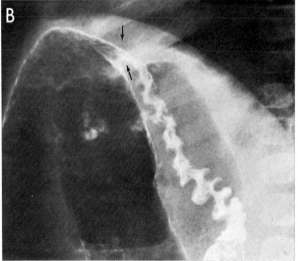

FIG 28–10.
Long-segment aganglionosis with the transition zone near the splenic flexure *(arrows)* in an 8-month-old boy. **A,** oblique and **B,** lateral views of the area of the descending colon demonstrate irregular hypertonic contraction waves throughout the aganglionic segment.

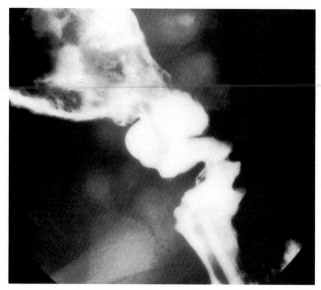

FIG 28–11.
Rectal aganglionosis. Lateral view of a barium enema demonstrates spiky irregular contractions of the aganglionic segment of the rectum.

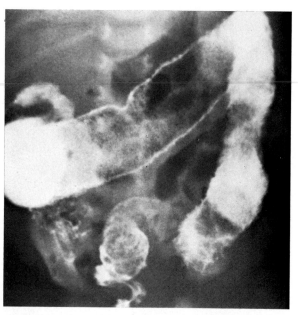

FIG 28–12.
Enterocolitis in a 3-week-old boy with aganglionic megacolon. Contrast enema demonstrates a granular appearance to the mucosa with small ulcerations.

seen in about 40% of patients. These can be either smooth (Fig 28–10) or spiky (Fig 28–11) and are a very reliable diagnostic indicator when present. When the diagnosis cannot be made at the time of the enema, delayed films may be helpful. By 24 hours after an enema which completely filled the colon, the barium should have moved to the left side of the colon, and by 48 hours, it should be gone except for minor rectal residual. Retention at 48 hours is suspect for aganglionosis but certainly not diagnostic. Rosenfield et al. found a pattern of mixed stool and barium on delayed films a useful sign, but it is seen uncommonly.

The major complication of colonic aganglionosis is enterocolitis (Fig 28–12). This is a potentially fatal entity seen in the first month of life and is discussed in Chapter 52. In rare instances, older children who have had surgical therapy for aganglionosis develop acute distention which usually responds to conservative treatment (Fig 28–13). The distention may be secondary to a very short segment of aganglionic bowel which is left in place to permit the anus to remain in its normal anatomical position.

MISCELLANEOUS FUNCTIONAL DISORDERS

Neuronal intestinal dysplasia is a much rarer form of myenteric plexus abnormality in which most children present with constipation, although rectal bleeding has been described. Clinically, colonic involvement may mimic aganglionosis, but histologic examination reveals hyperplastic submucosal and myenteric plexuses, giant neurons, and ganglia within the lamina propria. The abnormal neuromuscular activity leads to intestinal pseudo-obstruction. Barium enema demonstrates a flaccid megacolon. Small-bowel series shows poor motor activity of the involved portions of the intestine with focal areas of dilatation and delayed passage of barium. Neuronal dysplasia has been found in the proximal intestine of patients with colonic aganglionosis and can be associated with neurofibromatosis and multiple endocrine neoplasia (MEN) syndrome type IIB. MEN syndrome type IIA can also mimic the presentation of colonic aganglionosis, but rectal biopsy shows giant ganglia.

Intestinal pseudo-obstruction has been associated with non-neurogenic causes, including scleroderma; amyloidosis; endocrinopathies, especially hypothyroidism (Fig 28–14); drugs; and electrolyte disturbances. These entities affect the intestinal smooth muscle leading to disordered motility. An idiopathic form of myopathic intestinal pseudo-obstruction is being described with increasing frequency. These children present with periodic vomiting, abdominal distention, constipation, urinary retention, and weight loss. Plain films demonstrate dilated loops of bowel with air-fluid levels suggestive of obstruction but which really represent severe adynamic ileus (Fig 28–15). Barium studies are nonspecific, showing poor motor activity in affected parts of

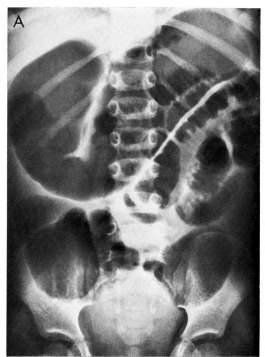
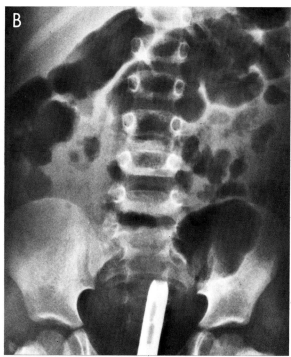

FIG 28–13.
Postoperative distal obstruction. **A,** supine view of the abdomen demonstrates marked gaseous distention of the colon and distal small intestine in a 3-year-old boy who had had surgery for agan- glionic megacolon 2 years previously. He had been well until the current episode of acute abdominal distress. **B,** decompression was obtained by placement of a rectal tube.

the bowel. Megacolon is typically found with con- trast enema. Associated myogenic abnormalities of the urinary tract may be found.

Psychogenic constipation is a pejorative term used for children who develop severe constipation with- out gross or microscopic pathologic abnormalities. In many instances, no definite emotional disturbance is recognized, and a better, although ambiguous, term is *functional constipation*. Patients typically stool nor- mally during the first year or two of life, but the dis- ease has been reported in infants. The affected chil- dren suffer severe constipation, which may lead to

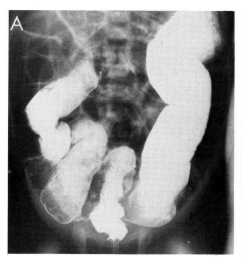
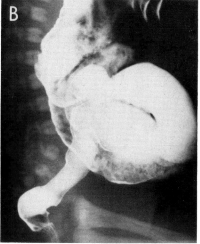

FIG 28–14.
A, frontal and **B,** lateral views of the abdomen following barium en- ema in a patient with congenital hypothyroidism. Obstipation was present before the other signs of hypothyroidism became manifest. An apparent transition from small-caliber rectum to dilated sigmoid mimics aganglionosis. (Courtesy of Dr. F.A. Lee, Pasadena, Calif.)

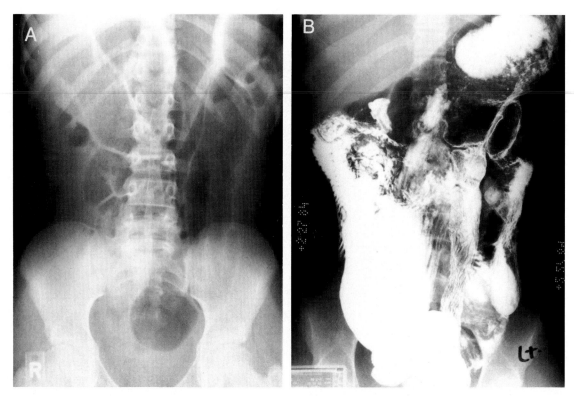

FIG 28–15.
Intestinal pseudo-obstruction. **A,** plain film of the abdomen demonstrates diffuse gaseous dilatation of the small bowel. **B,** small-intestinal series reveals diffuse dilatation of the bowel with no focal obstructive lesion identified. At surgery, no mechanical obstruction was identified. Ganglion cells were present in the myenteric plexus, but were abnormal.

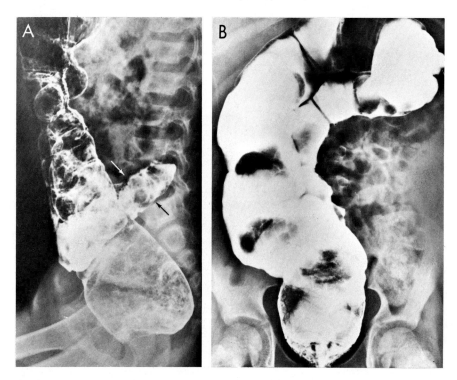

FIG 28–16.
Functional (psychogenic)megacolon. **A,** lateral projection following barium enema demonstrates markedly enlarged rectum which is filled with stool. The normal rectal shelf is well seen. **B,** frontal projection during barium enema demonstrates scybalous material throughout the distal colon down to and including the low rectum. A rectal biopsy demonstrated normal ganglion cells.

anal fissures and painful defecation. Encopresis is very common in this disease as opposed to colonic aganglionosis in which it virtually never occurs. Plain films demonstrate a capacious rectum filled with scybalous material. Stool may back up all the way to the cecum, and secondary small-bowel dilatation may be seen. Contrast studies are usually not necessary but, if performed, will show a colon dilated to the anus and filled with fecal material (Fig 28–16). Anal aganglionosis may give a similar appearance.

INFLAMMATORY AND INFECTIOUS DISEASES

Nonspecific chronic ulcerative colitis is an idiopathic inflammatory disease of the colon affecting older children and young adults. An infantile form has been described which is devastating and often fatal (Fig 28–17). The disease is characterized by mucosal inflammation, edema, and ulceration. It is accompanied by submucosal edema in the early stages and fibrosis in the later stages. Transmural disease is uncommon. The disease may be localized in the distal colon or spread to involve the entire colon and the terminal ileum. Fatal outcomes are less common recently than in years past but still occur. Colonic carcinoma is a frequent complication, especially in patients who present with total colonic involvement or who respond poorly to therapy. Although the cancers do not arise in childhood, prophylactic total colectomy is often offered to patients in the high-risk group.

Bloody diarrhea may appear explosively in as many as one third of affected patients, but the majority present with progressive chronic diarrhea. Many children present with non-GI symptoms of which severe growth retardation is the most common and clinically striking. Arthritis may precede the colon symptoms. Typically, it is monarticular or pauciarticular, affecting large joints. Seronegative spondyloarthropathy is seen in some affected males. Skin rashes, uveitis, digital clubbing, stomal ulcers, and hepatic dysfunction may occur in variable numbers of children but less frequently than in adults.

Plain films are most frequently nonspecific but may show evidence of mucosal edema (Fig 28–18,A). Occasional patients present with toxic megacolon in which marked dilatation of the large bowel, primarily the transverse colon, is seen. These patients should not undergo contrast enemas because of the high risk of perforation.

Double contrast barium enema is the imaging procedure of choice. Stringer et al. have demonstrated its efficacy in children in whom it is almost comparable to endoscopy for diagnosis. The disease always affects the rectum with contiguous proximal involvement. Skip areas do not occur although different parts of the colon may not be equally affected. The earliest change seen with air-contrast enema is a fine granularity of the colonic mucosa. This may be accompanied by haustral thickening secondary to edema of the submucosa. The mucosa becomes progressively more irregular as the disease progresses, and ulcers can be seen (Fig 28–18,B). In the early

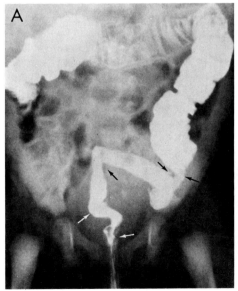
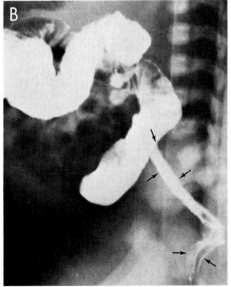

FIG 28–17.
Infantile ulcerative colitis in a 3-week-old girl with rectal bleeding. **A,** frontal and **B,** lateral projections during barium enema demonstrate tubular narrowing of the rectum and sigmoid colon with an abrupt transition zone. The findings were suggestive of aganglionosis, but biopsy revealed ulcerative colitis.

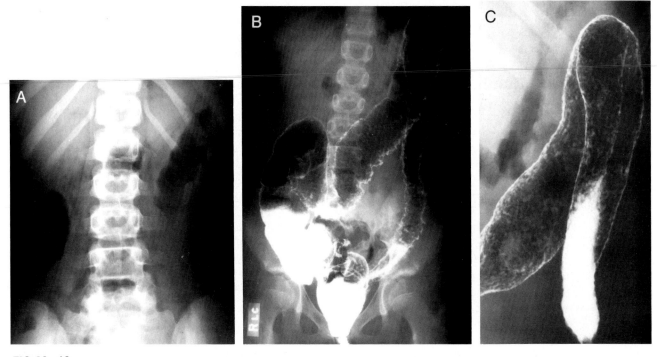

FIG 28–18.
Ulcerative colitis in a 14-year-old girl. **A,** plain film demonstrates thumbprinting of the distal transverse colon, suggesting mucosal and submucosal edema. **B,** double contrast enema demonstrates granularity and irregularity of the colonic mucosa. Small ulcer- ations are seen throughout the transverse colon and the descending colon. The entire colon was involved. **C,** coned-down view of the splenic flexure demonstrates multiple areas of pseudopolyps.

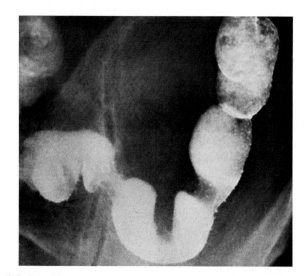

FIG 28–19.
Innominate grooves. Coned-down view of the distal descending and proximal sigmoid colon demonstrates regular, small spicula- tions which should not be confused with the ulceration of inflam- matory bowel disease. The innominate grooves are less commonly seen in children than in adults.

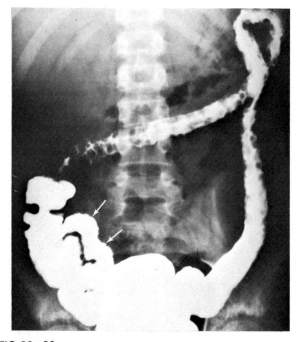

FIG 28–20.
Ulcerative colitis with pseudopolyposis and backwash ileitis in a 15-year-old boy. There are multiple round marginal filling defects in the transverse and descending portions of the colon, reflecting retained islands of normal mucosa between areas of denuded mu- cosa. The terminal ileum is rigid and lacks a normal mucosal pat- tern.

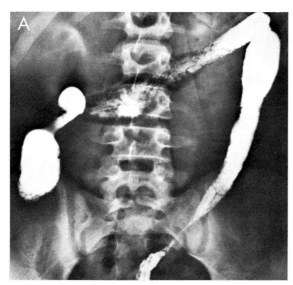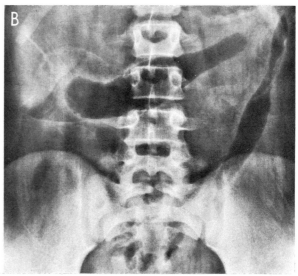

FIG 28–21.
Advanced ulcerative colitis. **A,** following barium enema, the shortened, narrow, stiff, smooth, tubular appearance is evident. **B,** the air-filled colon on plain film demonstrates strikingly similar findings.

stages, they may be small enough to be confused with normal innominate grooves (Fig 28–19), but the associated mucosal irregularity and edema should lead to the correct interpretation. The ulcers may become large, so-called collar-button ulcers. Pseudopolyposis may occur when islands of residual mucosa are surrounded by areas of denuded mucosa (Figs 28–18,C and 28–20). The colonic wall becomes stiff, shortened, and tubular, the "lead-pipe" colon, secondary to fibrosis of the submucosa (Fig 28–21). With total colonic involvement, the terminal ileum

may also be involved, so-called backwash ileitis (Fig 28–22). Late-stage disease produces presacral thickening, and retroperitoneal fibrosis is a rare complication (Fig 28–23).

Crohn disease is discussed in Chapter 27. The disease can affect the colon as well as the small intestine. An important differentiating feature from ulcerative colitis is the frequent sparing of the rectum and the presence of skip areas with involved portions of colon separated from one another by uninvolved portions. Ulceration and edema are noted on air-

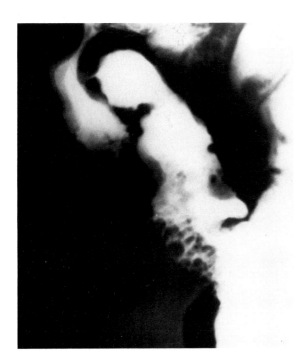

FIG 28–22.
Backwash ileitis in a teen-age boy with ulcerative colitis. Although the terminal ileum is distensible, it is irregular with marginal filling defects and mucosal inflammation. The cecum is markedly fibrotic and contracted.

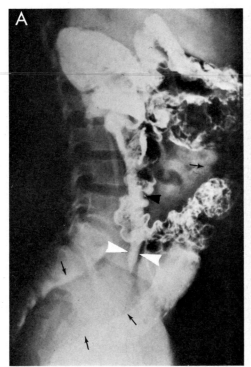 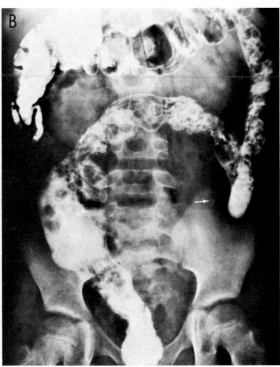

FIG 28–23.
Ulcerative colitis with pseudopolyposis and retroperitoneal fibrosis.
A, lateral view following excretory urography and barium enema demonstrates marked thickening of the presacral soft tissues *(arrows)*. The anterior margin of the sacrum is sclerotic. The ureters are dilated *(arrowheads)*. **B,** frontal projection demonstrates the rectum and sigmoid to be fixed by the retroperitoneal fibrosis *(arrow)*, the presence of which was confirmed at surgery.

contrast barium enemas. The ulcers are initially small and superficial (aphthous) but eventually develop the characteristic rose-thorn configuration. A cobblestone pattern like that in the small intestine may be seen (Fig 28–24,*A* and *B*). As in the small intestine, fistulas, sinus tracts, and abscesses can develop (Fig 28–24,*C*). Crohn disease is more likely to lead to colonic strictures than is ulcerative colitis.

Pseudomembranous colitis is characterized by fever, diarrhea, and colonic mucositis. The condition most commonly follows antibiotic therapy, often in debilitated or postoperative patients (Fig 28–25). The toxin produced by *Clostridium difficile* is the most important cause of antibiotic-associated pseudomembranous colitis, but it may also be responsible for enterocolitis in infants and children who have not received antibiotics. The radiographic findings are similar to those of the other colidites, and the diagnosis is a clinical one.

The *hemolytic-uremic syndrome* (HUS) usually has a GI prodrome preceding clinical evidence of renal involvement. Evidence implicates a bacterial toxin. Colitis is common and barium enema is frequently requested before the correct diagnosis has been made. The findings are nonspecific, but thumbprint-

ing is a frequent manifestation (Fig 28–26). Tochen and Campbell reported toxic megacolon in HUS. Liebhaber et al. reported a case of HUS with colonic perforation (Fig 28–27).

Behçet syndrome can affect virtually any part of the GI tract. Severe ulceration in the colon can occur although the radiographic findings are not specific (Fig 28–28).

Patients with *radiation colitis* do not usually undergo imaging examinations during the acute phase when diarrhea is the prominent clinical feature. Eventually, fibrosis may occur, leading to the affected portions of the colon being stiff with fibrotic walls and loss of the normal mucosal pattern (Fig 28–29). The normally mobile portions of the colon are fixed.

Neutropenic colitis is a specific entity in patients with hematopoietic disorders. In children, acute lymphocytic leukemia is the most common underlying disease with acute myelogenous leukemia also being associated with the colitis. Although the colitis may be due to bacterial overgrowth in immunocompromised patients, the leukemic children are almost invariably in relapse rather than remission. The prognosis is grave with most affected leukemic chil-

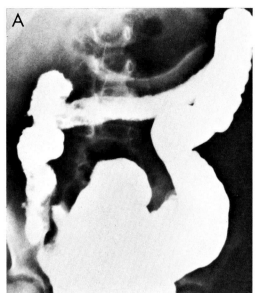

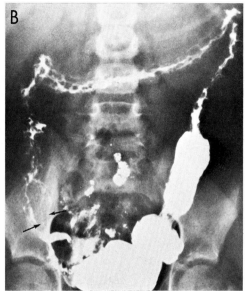

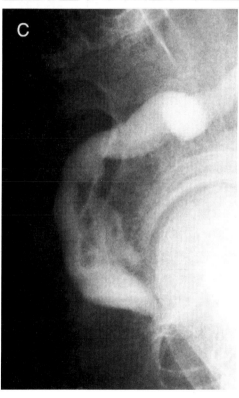

FIG 28–24.
Crohn disease of the terminal ileum and colon in a 10-year-old girl with failure to thrive and vague abdominal complaints. **A,** barium enema demonstrates the mucosal margins of the cecum and ascending and transverse portions of the colon to be irregular with small rounded filling defects. **B,** film of the abdomen taken at the completion of a small-intestinal series demonstrates the characteristic cobblestone pattern of granulomatous colitis. The *arrows* demonstrate the irregular narrowed terminal ileum. **C,** water soluble-contrast enema in another patient with longstanding Crohn disease reveals perforation of the anterior rectal wall with leakage into an extrarectal cavity.

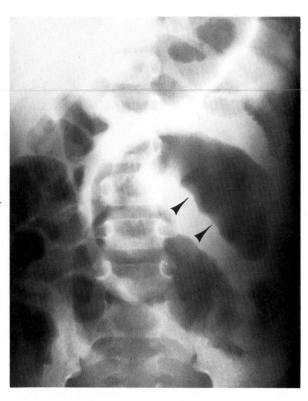

FIG 28–25.
Pseudomembranous colitis secondary to *Clostridium* toxin. AP view of the abdomen in a 7-year-old boy who received 1 week of antibiotic therapy for otitis media demonstrates dilatation of a dilated loop of sigmoid colon with typical thumbprinting *(arrowheads).*

dren dying. The disease most often affects the cecum, hence the other commonly used name, typhlitis. Abdominal pain, diarrhea, and distended abdomen are the most common presenting symptoms. The patients are often too ill to come to the radiology department and portable radiography and sonography are the most commonly performed stud-

ies. The radiographs show focal ileus in the right lower quadrant. Often a sentinel loop of dilated terminal ileum may be seen. We have had two patients who developed pneumatosis coli as a preterminal event (Fig 28–30). Sonography demonstrates a markedly thickened cecal wall which may be either hyperechoic or hypoechoic. Intraluminal fluid may

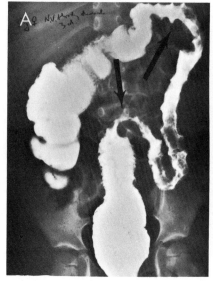

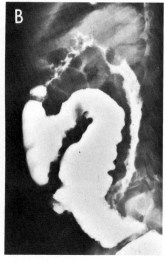

FIG 28–26.
Hemolytic-uremic syndrome. **A,** frontal and **B,** lateral films following barium enema demonstrate irregular, narrow, spiculated areas from the distal transverse colon to the distal sigmoid colon *(ar-*
rows). The clinical and radiographic gastrointestinal abnormalities preceded the abnormalities of the kidneys and blood.

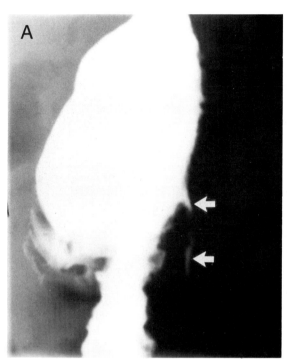

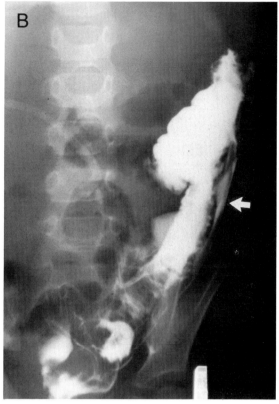

FIG 28–27.
Hemolytic-uremic syndrome. **A,** coned-down view of the hepatic flexure during barium enema demonstrates a fistulous tract *(arrows).* **B,** delayed film demonstrates extravasated contrast material *(arrow)* tracking along the lateral paracolic gutter. **(From Liebhaber MI, Parker BR, Morton JA, et al: *Am J Dis Child* 1977; 131:1168. Used by permission.)**

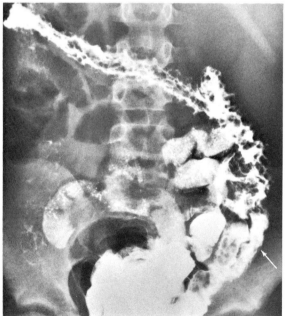

FIG 28–28.
Behçet syndrome. Barium enema demonstrates a cobblestone pattern in the colon with coarse ulceration. The patient also had ulcerative esophagitis. **(Courtesy of Dr. W. Berdon, New York City.)**

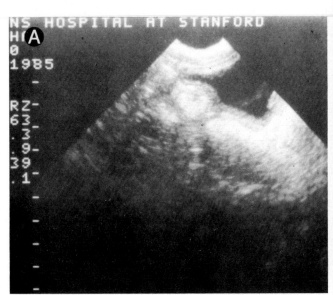

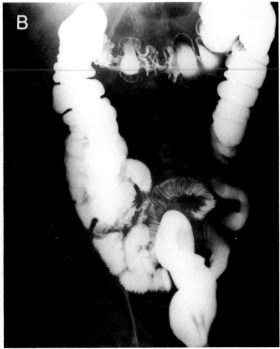

FIG 28–29.
Radiation colitis. **A,** pelvic ultrasound in an 8-year-old boy who had received radiation therapy for a pelvic tumor 3 years prior to the study. The echogenic area adjacent to the bladder is fixed bowel with no peristalsis. **B,** barium enema demonstrates narrowing, rigidity, and loss of haustration in the distal descending and sigmoid portions of the colon.

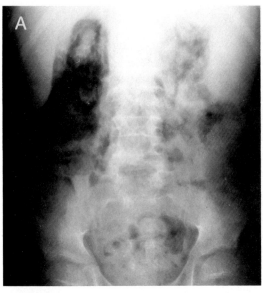

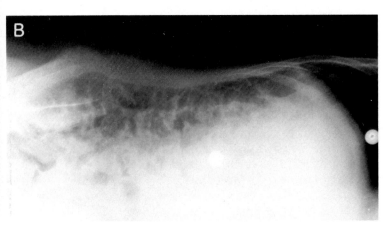

FIG 28–30.
Neutropenic colitis. **A,** AP and **B,** decubitus views of the abdomen of a 9-year-old boy with leukemia and chemotherapy-induced neutropenia demonstrate air diffusely throughout the colonic wall. This film was obtained 10 days following an episode of acute neutropenic colitis.

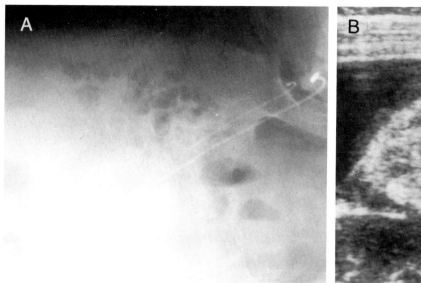

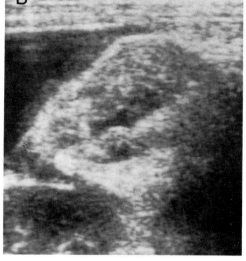

FIG 28–31.
Neutropenic colitis. **A,** right-side-up decubitus view of the abdomen in an 11-year-old girl with leukemia and severe abdominal pain demonstrates a mottled appearance in the right lower quadrant. **B,** sonogram of the right lower quadrant demonstrates the cecal wall to be markedly thickened. Fluid is seen within the cecal lumen and ascites is present.

be identified (Fig 28–31). Sonography can also identify associated ascites. If the cecum has perforated, an abscess may be seen.

The infectious colidites are usually caused by the same agents discussed in Chapter 27 in the section on infectious diseases. Imaging studies are rarely needed and usually show a nonspecific colitis when performed.

APPENDICITIS

The vermiform appendix serves no significant physiologic function in humans, but inflammation of this atavistic organ is the most common reason for abdominal surgery in children. Early diagnosis is important since morbidity increases after the appendix perforates. Death from appendicitis, even in the most complicated cases, is much rarer in children than in adults but certainly occurs. On the other hand, since the history and physical findings in children with suspected appendicitis are often atypical, patients without appendicitis are often sent to surgery. According to Kottmeier, 11% to 32% of children undergoing appendectomy have a normal appendix. Therefore, imaging examinations can play a useful adjunctive role when the clinical findings are ambiguous.

According to Shandling and Fallis, the actual incidence of appendicitis in children is unknown, but the annual rate of appendectomy in the United States is about four in 1,000 children under age 14

years. Appendicitis occurs most frequently in children over 2 years of age, but can occur in infancy and even in the neonate. The disease occurs secondary to obstruction of the appendix. Transmural inflammation occurs rapidly. Young children are par-

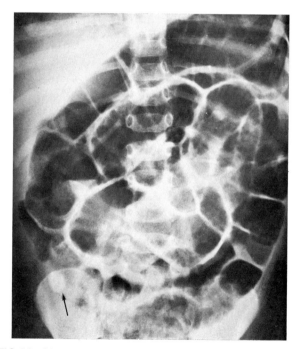

FIG 28–32.
Acute appendicitis with abscess formation. AP view of the abdomen demonstrates marked distention of the small intestine and colon with a right lower quadrant appendicolith *(arrow)* in a 14-month-old boy with peritonitis and periappendiceal abscess.

ticularly susceptible to perforation because delayed diagnosis is more frequent than in older children and adults. Perforation can lead to generalized peritonitis, but a local abscess adjacent to the appendix is more likely because the perforation is usually contained by the omentum. Pain, vomiting, and anorexia are common symptoms, but younger children often do not localize the pain to the right lower quadrant. Abdominal tenderness, fever, and leukocytosis are common accompaniments. Surgery is performed without imaging studies when the diagnosis is clinically obvious.

Patients with appendicitis and an atypical clinical presentation often undergo plain film radiography. Pain usually leads to abdominal splinting with subsequent scoliosis of the lumbar spine, concave toward the side of pain. Dilated loops of bowel are seen, sometimes focally in the right lower quadrant, more often throughout the abdomen when perforation has occurred (Fig 28–32). When an abscess has formed, a mass effect on the air-filled cecum may be seen. On horizontal-beam films, a right lower quadrant air-fluid level that has no discernible mucosal pattern is presumptive evidence of an abscess (Fig 28–33). Abscesses most commonly have a mottled appearance on supine films, but a featureless air collection may be seen as well. The radiographic appearance of distal small-intestinal obstruction may be found in patients with appendiceal abscesses.

Appendicoliths are calcific concretions in the appendix that are considered compelling evidence of appendicitis in symptomatic patients. Most surgeons will operate on these children without further imaging studies. According to Shimkin, they occur in up to 50% of children with appendicitis. They may be round or oval, uniformly calcified or, more frequently, lamellated. Appendicoliths are multiple 30% of the time (Fig 28–34).

Before the introduction of sonographic evaluation of appendicitis, barium enemas were requested in patients in whom the diagnosis was not clinically evident. Nonfilling of the appendix was considered a positive sign for appendicitis, but this finding is also present in 5% to 10% of normal persons. Cecal spasm is seen and a mass effect on the cecum may be present if an abscess has formed. All of these signs are nonspecific and can be found in other conditions. Barium enemas are rarely performed any longer in patients suspected of having appendicitis.

The role of sonography in the evaluation of possible appendicitis was described by Puylaert in 1986. Numerous studies demonstrating its efficacy in adults have appeared as well as several recent series

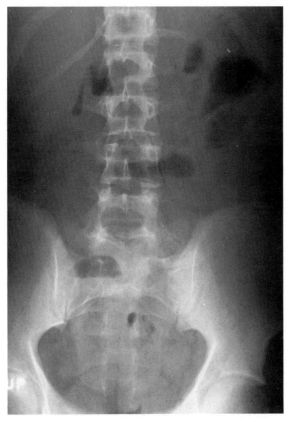

FIG 28–33.
Upright view of the abdomen in a 15-year-old boy with signs and symptoms of appendicitis. A featureless air-fluid level is noted in the right lower quadrant. CT scan confirmed the presence of the abscess which was drained under CT control.

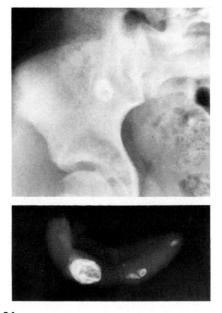

FIG 28–34.
Calcified appendicoliths are seen in a coned-down AP view of the right lower quadrant and in the resected appendix of a 10-year-old girl with acute appendicitis.

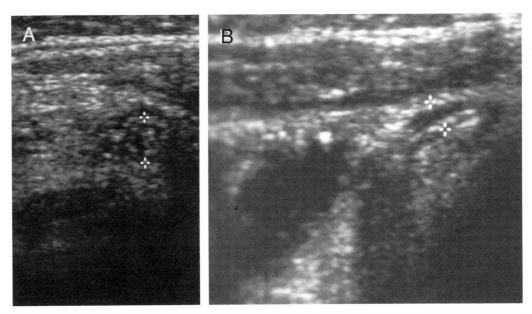

FIG 28–35.
Left lower quadrant appendicitis. **A,** transverse and **B,** longitudinal sonograms of the left lower quadrant in an 11-year-old boy who complained of left lower quadrant pain. The cecum was identified in the right lower quadrant, but a typical "target lesion" was noted

in the left lower quadrant. At surgery, a very long appendix, extended from the tip of the cecum in the right lower quadrant, crossed the midline to the left lower quadrant and a small, walled-off perforation was identified.

in children. A 5.0- or 7.5-MHz linear array transducer is used, depending on the size of the patient and the depth of the appendix from the skin. Transverse and longitudinal scans are performed over the point of maximal tenderness. Graded compression displaces other loops of bowel, permits higher-resolution imaging, and differentiates compressible normal bowel from the inflamed noncompressible appendix. If the appendix is not identified, a complete scan of the lower abdomen and pelvis should be performed because of the variability of appendiceal position (Fig 28–35). The normal sonographic anat-

omy of the right lower quadrant was well described by Abu-Yousef and Franken.

The inflamed appendix almost always measures more than 6 mm in diameter in children as well as adults and is noncompressible (Fig 28–36). A target sign has been described with the order of hypoechoic and hyperechoic layers, depending on the acuity of the process. In most instances of obstructive appendicitis, as typically found in children, the center of the target is hypoechoic because of fluid or pus in the lumen of the appendix (Fig 28–37,A). This is surrounded by a circle of echogenic mucosa

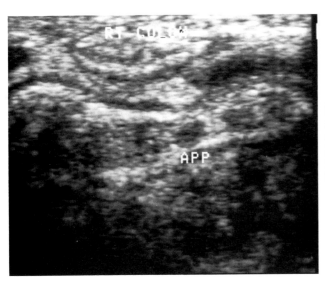

FIG 28–36.
Appendicitis. Longitudinal view of the appendix using the graded compression technique demonstrates the failure of the appendiceal lumen to narrow significantly with compression performed using a linear array transducer. The noncompressed appendix measured 9 mm in transverse diameter.

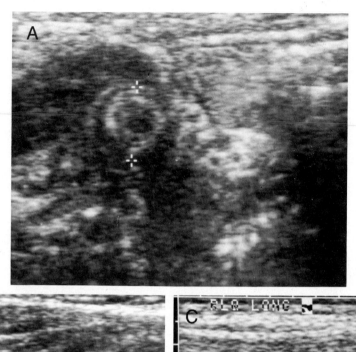

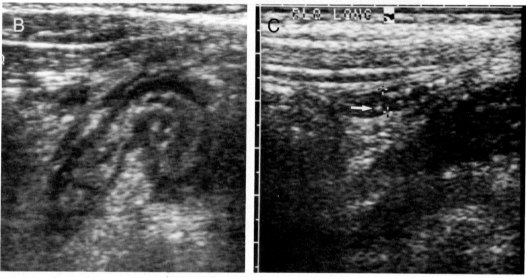

FIG 28–37.
Sonograms of patients with appendicitis. **A,** transverse sonogram of the appendix demonstrates the characteristic "target sign." In this case, the innermost portion is sonolucent, compatible with fluid or pus. **B,** longitudinal view of another patient demonstrates the alternating hyperechoic and hypoechoic layers with an outermost hypoechoic layer, suggesting periappendiceal fluid. **C,** longitudinal sonogram of the right lower quadrant demonstrates a dilated, noncompressible appendix. The bright echo within the appendix represents an appendicolith with acoustic shadowing *(arrow).*

which is, in turn, surrounded by a hypoechoic edematous appendiceal wall. When the appendix is not markedly inflamed, and the lumen is collapsed, multiple concentric rings corresponding to the layers of the appendiceal wall may be identified. Longitudinal images will be comparable in nature but ovoid rather than circular (Fig 28–37,B). Appendicoliths will be seen more commonly than on plain films since not all of them calcify (Fig 28–37,C). Perforation and abscess formation can be identified at sonography by the presence of periappendiceal fluid, intraperitoneal fluid, and a mass of mixed echoge-

nicity (Fig 28–38). Perforation without abscess may lead to a false-negative examination since the decompressed appendix may be difficult to find. The presence of unexplained fluid, however, should alert the examiner to the possibility, and further studies such as CT or scintigraphy should be undertaken.

The role of CT in appendicitis in children is limited. CT is more sensitive than ultrasound (US) for the detection of an abscess. CT may be useful in patients with perforation who have false-negative sonograms if signs of inflammation in the right

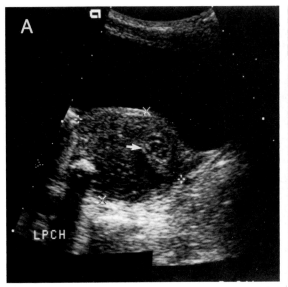 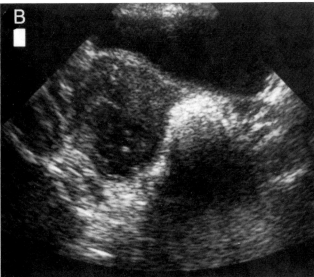

FIG 28–38.
Periappendiceal abscesses. **A,** transverse sonogram of the pelvis demonstrates a large mass of mixed echogenicity behind the bladder. Within the mass is the appendix *(arrow)* showing a typical target sign. **B,** longitudinal sonogram in another patient demonstates a mass of mixed echogenicity behind the bladder. In this case, the appendix itself was not seen because of decompression secondary to perforation.

lower quadrant are identified. CT is particularly well suited for percutaneous drainage guidance (Fig 28–39).

Scintigraphic studies may also be useful in the diagnosis of appendicitis. Navarro and Weber used indium 111–labeled white blood cells and found them particularly useful when perforation has led to a false-negative sonogram. Menneman et al. used technetium 99m–labeled white blood cells in the evaluation of acute appendicitis in children. They found the scan useful to rule out appendicitis in that they had no false-negatives. However, 24% of their cases had abnormal but nondiagnostic studies.

Although most abscesses will be adjacent to the appendix, distant spread can occur. Diffuse peritonitis is less common in children over age 2 than in infants. Slovis et al. described three patients with hepatic abscesses and two patients with portal pylephlebitis following complicated appendicitis. Zerin described an intrathoracic appendiceal abscess in a 10-year-old girl with a previously undetected Bochdalek hernia.

NEOPLASMS

Colonic neoplasms are rare in children. The majority are benign juvenile polyps. The hereditary polyposis syndromes are less common, and primary malignancies of great rarity. The double contrast enema is the examination of choice in children who present with rectal bleeding or who are suspected, for any reason, of having a benign or malignant colonic neoplasm. Scattered reports have suggested that sonography may be helpful in determining the depth of wall involvement in colorectal tumors, and CT is useful for staging colorectal carcinomas. These cancers are so rare in children that they can reasonably be evaluated, as are those in adults when they occur.

Juvenile polyps have been considered either postinflammatory in nature or hamartomatous. They may be single or multiple, sessile or pedunculated, and are benign with no reported tendency to become malignant (Fig 28–40). The majority are diagnosed in children under age 10 years who present with painless rectal bleeding. Most juvenile polyps occur in the rectosigmoid region and are less frequently found in the transverse, ascending, and cecal portions of the colon, in that order. They are typically under 2 cm in diameter and may be as small as 2 to 3 mm. *Juvenile polyposis coli* is an uncommon syndrome consisting of multiple juvenile polyps found in children who have a family history of colorectal malignancy. Associated abnormalities include midgut malrotation, amyotonia congenita, hypertelorism, and hydrocephalus. Juvenile polyps are found in the *Cronkhite-Canada syndrome* which does not occur in children.

Adenomatous polyps are found in several of the inherited polyposis syndromes (Table 28–1) and

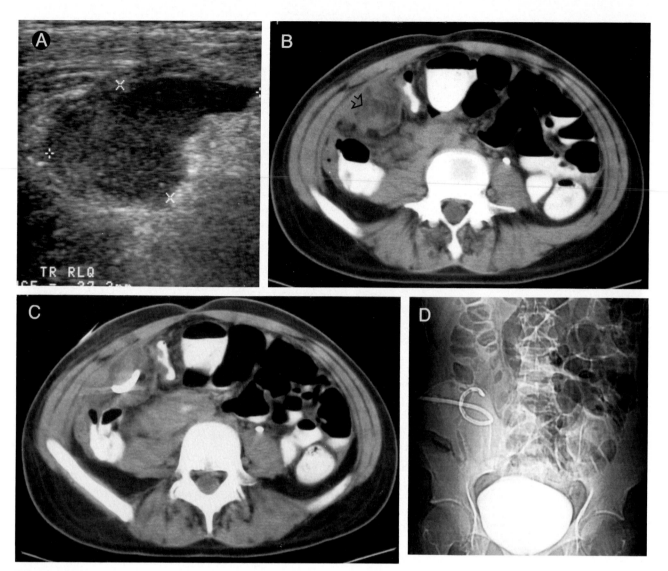

FIG 28–39.
Percutaneous drainage of an appendiceal abscess. **A,** transverse sonogram through the right lower quadrant demonstrates a large mass of mixed echogenicity. The appendix itself was not identified. **B,** CT scan demonstrates a mass in the right lower quadrant *(arrow)* of mixed attenuation characteristic of an abscess. **C,** a percutaneous drainage catheter was placed under CT control. The tip of the catheter can be seen within the center of the abscess cavity. **D,** CT scanogram following placement of the catheter demonstrates its course and positioning in the right lower quadrant.

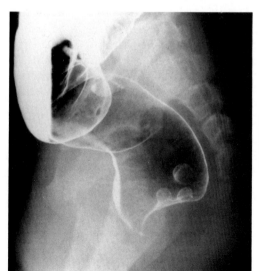

FIG 28–40.
Prone view of the rectum following double contrast barium enema demonstrates multiple sessile and pedunculated juvenile polyps, all of which measured less than 2 cm in diameter. No polyps were identified in the remainder of the colon.

TABLE 28–1.
The Inherited Gastrointestinal Polyposis Syndromes*

Syndrome	Gastrointestinal Lesions	Pathologic Nature of Polyps	Extraintestinal Lesions	Predisposition to Cancer	Inheritance
Familial adenomatous colonic polyposis	Polyposis limited to colon and rectum	Adenomatous	None	Marked (colonic adenocarcinoma develops in most untreated patients)	Autosomal dominant
Peutz-Jeghers syndrome	Generalized polyposis, but polyps of small intestine are consistent	Hamartomatous	Melanin spots of lips, buccal mucosa, and digits	About 2%–3% risk of GI cancer, often involving duodenal region	Autosomal dominant
Gardner syndrome	Polyps of colon and rectum (rarely small intestine)	Adenomatous	Osseous and soft-tissue tumors, usually multiple (globoid osteomas of the mandible with overlying fibromas are characteristic); also seen are osteomas of the calvaria with overlying fibromas, epidermoid cysts, lipomas, and especially after an operation, desmoid tumors and wound fibromatosis	Marked, as in familial adenomatous colonic polyposis but with additional risk of carcinoma of pancreaticoduodenal region	Autosomal dominant
Generalized juvenile polyposis	Usually colon and rectum but may involve small intestine and stomach	Hamartomatous	None	Probable, but magnitude of risk uncertain	Autosomal dominant
Turcot syndrome	Colonic polyps	Adenomatous	Tumors of brain	In brain (not reported in GI tract)	Autosomal recessive

*From Erbe RW: *N Engl J Med* 1976; 294:1101. Used by permission.

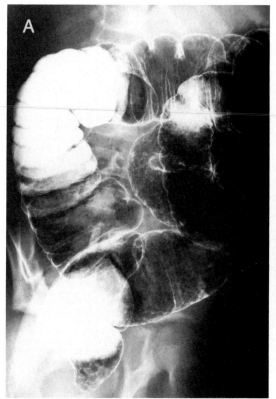
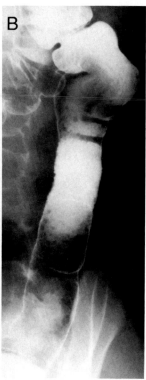

FIG 28–41.

Familial adenomatous polyposis. **A,** double contrast barium enema in an 11-year-old boy whose father had had a total colectomy for familial polyposis. Numerous mucosal filling defects of varying sizes are seen throughout the entire colon. None of the lesions appears umbilicated. The patient underwent total colectomy at the age of 15. **B,** coned-down view of the descending colon during air-contrast barium enema in the patient's sister aged 9 years. Multiple filling defects seen en face are similar to those seen in lymphoid hyperplasia (compare with Fig 28–42). Note the marginal filling defects, however, which suggest the presence of polyps. Colonoscopy confirmed the diagnosis of familial adenomatous polyposis.

have significant malignant potential. Familial polyposis is an autosomal dominant disorder characterized by numerous tiny adenomatous polyps scattered throughout the colon. The majority of patients have a family history of colonic polyps or cancers. Others may develop their disease as a result of a new genetic mutation. All immediate family members, even if asymptomatic, should be studied for polyposis. The malignant potential approaches 100%, and total colectomy is usually performed. Rectal bleeding, diarrhea, and crampy abdominal pain are the common presenting symptoms. Double contrast barium enema demonstrates a myriad of tiny polyps which have been likened to a shag carpet (Fig 28–41). The appearance is reminiscent of lymphoid hyperplasia (Fig 28–42), but the polyps are of variable size, do not have central umbilication, and affect the whole colon. Lymphoid hyperplasia shows filling defects of uniform size, many of which have central umbilication, and is predominantly found in the left colon with progressively diminished involvement in the more proximal portions of the colon (see below).

Gardner syndrome is an autosomal dominant disorder in which adenomatous polyps of the colon are associated with multiple osseous and soft-tissue tumors, the more common of which are cranial and facial osteomas. The potential for cancers of the colon and of the pancreas is high. *Turcot syndrome* is an autosomal recessive disease which presents more commonly in adults than in children. Although adenomatous polyps are found in the colon, they usually do not become malignant. Malignant brain tumors do develop, however. The polyps in *Peutz-Jeghers syndrome* are more likely to be found in the proximal portions of the GI tract than in the colon (Fig 28–43). These polyps are hamartomatous and the malignant potential is low. If colonic polyps are present, however, they may be adenomatous with malignant potential. The characteristic clinical appearance is melanosis of the lips, buccal mucosa, and digits.

Colorectal carcinoma is quite rare in children. It is

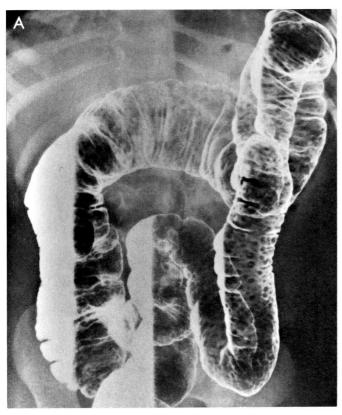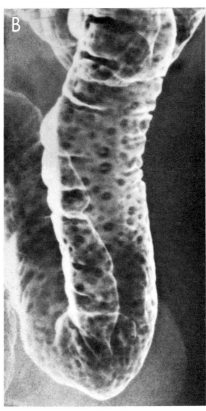

FIG 28–42.
Lymphoid hyperplasia demonstrating multiple umbilicated polypoid filling defects throughout the colon, although more prominently seen in the left colon than in the right. **A,** right lateral decubitus view and **B,** sigmoid and descending portions of the colon demonstrate the filling defects to be of relatively uniform size, many of them having a central umbilication. (Courtesy of Dr. Marie Capitanio, Philadelphia.)

usually found in teen-age boys but has been reported even in infancy and in patients of both sexes. Although there is an increased incidence of carcinoma in patients with polyposis syndromes, these cancers usually do not appear until adulthood. Mu-

cinous adenocarcinoma is the most common histologic variety in children. There is some evidence that environmental factors or diet may be involved in childhood colonic cancers. Chromosomal abnormalities have been discovered in patients with predis-

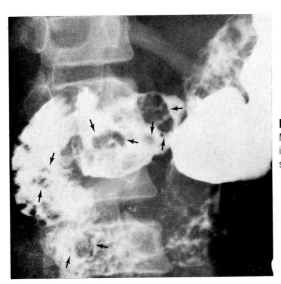

FIG 28–43.
Multiple polyposis of the duodenum in a 12-year-old boy who also had polyps in the stomach, small intestine, and colon. Examination of his mouth demonstrated the typical melanin patches of Peutz-Jeghers syndrome.

posing polyposis syndromes and with the sporadic variety of colon cancer. The most common symptoms are pain, change in bowel habits, weight loss and anorexia, anemia, rectal bleeding, and an abdominal mass. Plain film findings may be normal, show irregularity in the bowel gas pattern, or demonstrate partial obstruction. The mucinous tumors may have punctate calcification in the primary area (Fig 28–44,A) and in metastatic deposits. Air-contrast barium enema demonstrates findings like those described in adults. Because diagnosis is often delayed due to a low index of suspicion on the part of physicians, the tumors tend to be larger at presentation than is frequently true in adults (Figs 28–44,B and 28–45). Cures have not been reported other than following complete surgical resection. Initial metastases are to liver, lymph nodes, and other intra-abdominal sites. Generalized carcinomatosis may occur.

The colon is a less frequent primary site for the development of *lymphoma* than is the small intestine. The characteristics are similar with a large hypoechoic mass usually extending well beyond the bowel itself (Fig 28–46). CT characteristics are similar to those discussed in Chapter 27.

Benign lymphoid hyperplasia is not a neoplasm but may be mistaken for polyposis (see Fig 28–42). The filling defects seen on air-contrast barium enema represent patches of lymphoid tissue in the mucosa and submucosa with an increased size and number of lymph follicles. They are uniform, frequently umbilicated, and found predominantly in the left side of the colon. They are typically 2 to 3 mm in diameter. Larger hyperplastic lymphoid patches may be seen in patients with inflammatory bowel disease and hypogammaglobulinemia. Rectal bleeding has been described with benign lymphoid hyperplasia, but the association is probably fortuitous.

MISCELLANEOUS DISORDERS

Volvulus of the colon is quite rare in childhood. *Cecal volvulus* may occur in children with a malpositioned cecum secondary to partial midgut malrotation. Plain films show the dilated cecum displaced to the midabdomen (Fig 28–47) and the diagnosis can be confirmed by contrast enema. *Sigmoid volvulus* is equally rare in children and may be related to a congenital defect in the sigmoid mesentery. The sigmoid can rotate 180 degrees causing ischemia, infarction, perforation, and peritonitis. Plain films demonstrate a dilated loop of bowel extending from the left lower quadrant to the right upper quadrant (Fig 28–48). Contrast enema will demonstrate the spiral torsion and may actually cause the sigmoid to untwist. Reinarz et al. described splenic flexure volvulus as a complication of intestinal pseudo-obstruction in infancy.

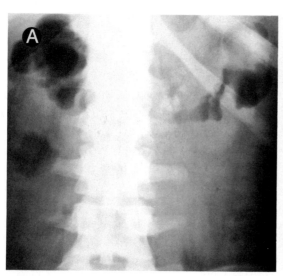

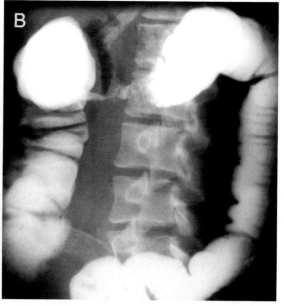

FIG 28–44.
Carcinoma of the colon in a 16-year-old boy. **A,** plain film of the abdomen demonstrates focal narrowing in the midportion of the transverse colon with associated stippled calcifications. **B,** oblique view during barium enema demonstrates a circumferential mass in the same area. Histologic examination confirmed the diagnosis of mucinous adenocarcinoma of the colon.

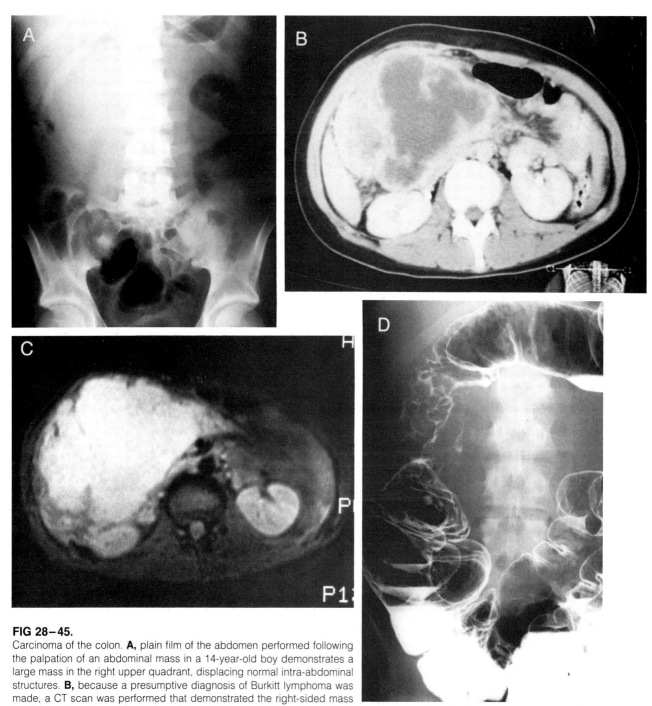

FIG 28–45.
Carcinoma of the colon. **A,** plain film of the abdomen performed following the palpation of an abdominal mass in a 14-year-old boy demonstrates a large mass in the right upper quadrant, displacing normal intra-abdominal structures. **B,** because a presumptive diagnosis of Burkitt lymphoma was made, a CT scan was performed that demonstrated the right-sided mass to have central areas of nonenhancement which were initially thought to be areas of necrosis within a lymphomatous tumor. **C,** T2-weighted spin-echo MR image of the right upper quadrant demonstrated the marked irregularity of the mass and the high signal intensity suggestive of malignant tumor. **D,** following a needle biopsy, which revealed signet cells, a barium enema was performed, demonstrating a large infiltrating carcinoma of the right side of the colon. Histologic examination confirmed the diagnosis of mucinous adenocarcinoma of the colon.

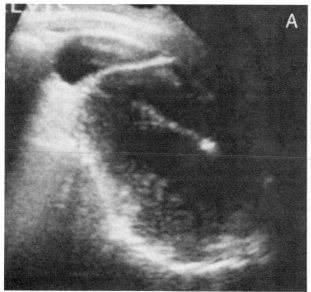
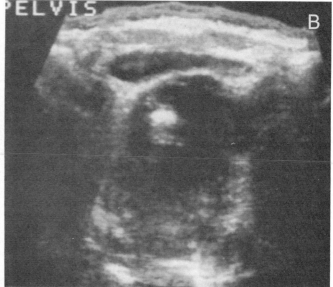
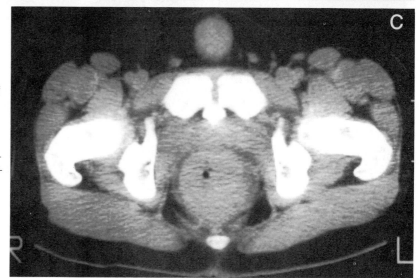

FIG 28–46.
Perirectal lymphoma in a 14-year-old boy.
A, longitudinal and **B,** transverse sonograms of
the pelvis demonstrate a large hypoechoic
mass completely surrounding the rectum. The
bright shadow contained within the mass is residual rectal gas. Displacement of the bladder
is noted. **C,** CT scan through the pelvis demonstrates the markedly narrowed rectal lumen surrounded by the mass of lymphomatous tissue.
Histologic examination revealed lymphocytic
lymphoma.

FIG 28–47.
Cecal volvulus. AP view of the abdomen in a 20-year-old man with abdominal distention and vomiting demonstrates a markedly distended
cecum in the low portion of the abdomen *(arrows)*. Note the typical "cof-
fee-bean" configuration. **(Courtesy of Dr. Donald Darling, Boston.)**

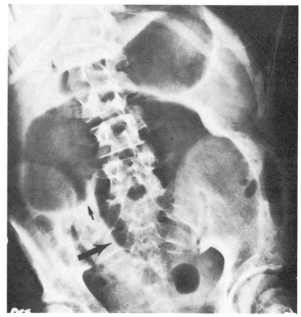

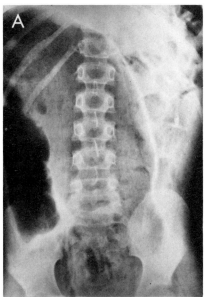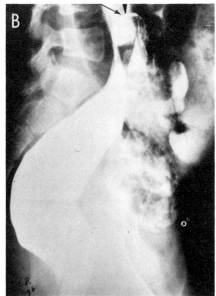

FIG 28–48.
Sigmoid volvulus in a 10-year-old boy with acute crampy abdominal pain. **A,** AP view of the abdomen demonstrates a markedly dilated loop of colon extending from the left lower quadrant to the right upper quadrant. **B,** lateral view of barium enema demonstrates a spiral twist at the level of the sigmoid torsion *(arrow).* (Courtesy of Dr. Eugene Blank, Portland, Ore.)

Pneumatosis coli is itself a benign disorder but is often a sign of grave underlying disease. It is most commonly seen in adults with chronic partial obstruction. In children, it has been seen in patients with cystic fibrosis, leukemia, collagen-vascular disorders, acquired immunodeficiency syndrome (AIDS), neutropenic colitis (see Fig 28–30), and following organ transplantation (Fig 28–49), presumably secondary to drug therapy. It is a rare complication of steroid therapy. Patients may have asymptomatic pneumatosis coli for months. Pneumoperitoneum rarely, if ever, occurs. Pneumatosis coli may be seen in newborns with necrotizing enterocolitis in whom it is a more ominous finding (see Chapter 52).

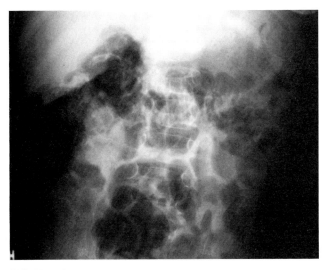

FIG 28–49.
Pneumatosis coli in a 4-year-old boy 5 months following cardiac transplantation. Note the air in the wall of the transverse colon outlining the mucosa, which appears as a thin white line.

REFERENCES

Congenital and Developmental Disorders

Kangarloo H, Sample WF, Hansen G, et al: Ultrasonic evaluation of abdominal gastrointestinal tract duplication in children. *Radiology* 1979; 131:191.

Kottra JJ, Dodds WJ: Duplication of the large bowel. AJR 1971; 113:310.

Sonada N, Matsuzaki S, Ono A, et al: Duplication of the caecum in a neonate simulating intussusception. *Pediatr Radiol* 1985; 15:427.

Yucesan S, Zorludemir V, Olcay I: Complete duplication of the colon. *J Pediatr Surg* 1986; 21:962.

Colonic Aganglionosis

Cremin BJ: The early diagnosis of Hirschsprung's disease. *Pediatr Radiol* 1974; 2:23.

Haney PJ, Hill JL, Chen-Chik JS: Zonal colonic aganglionosis. *Pediatr Radiol* 1982; 12:258.

Johnson JF, Cronk RL: The pseudotransition zone in long segment Hirschsprung's disease. *Pediatr Radiol* 1980; 10:87.

Kilcoyne RF, Taybi HT: Conditions associated with congenital megacolon. *Am J Roentgenol Radium Ther Nucl Med* 1970; 108:615.

Krishnamurthy S, Schuffler MD: Pathology of neuromuscular disorders of the small intestine and colon. *Gastroenterology* 1987; 93:610.

Pochaczevsky R, Leonidas JC: The "rectosigmoid index": A measurement for the early diagnosis of Hirschsprung's disease. AJR 1975; 123:770.

Rosenfield NS, Ablow RC, Markowitz RI, et al: Hirschsprung disease: Accuracy of the barium enema examination. *Radiology* 1984; 150:393.

Schey WL, White H: Hirschsprung's disease. Problems in the roentgen interpretation. AJR 1971; 112:105.

Schiller M, Levy P, Shawa RA, et al: Familial Hirschsprung's disease—report of 22 affected siblings in four families. *J Pediatr Surg* 1990; 25:322.

Siegel MJ, Shackelford GD, McAlister WH: The rectosigmoid index. *Radiology* 1981; 139:497.

Swenson O, Sherman JO, Fisher JH: Diagnosis of congenital megacolon: an analysis of 501 patients. *J Pediatr Surg* 1973; 8:587.

Whitehouse FR, Kernohan JW: Myenteric plexus in congenital megacolon. *Arch Intern Med* 1948; 82:75.

Yunis E, Sieber WK, Akers DR: Does zonal aganglionosis really exist? *Pediatr Pathol* 1983; 1:33.

Other Functional Disorders

Case Records of the Massachusetts General Hospital: Intestinal neuronal dysplasia associated with long-segment Hirschsprung's disease. *N Engl J Med* 1991; 325:1865.

Glassman M, Spivak W, Mininberg D, et al: Chronic idiopathic intestinal pseudo-obstruction: A commonly misdiagnosed disease in infants and children. *Pediatrics* 1989; 83:603.

Khan AH, Desjardins JG, Youssef S, et al: Gastrointestinal manifestations of Sipple syndrome in children. *J Pediatr Surg* 1987; 22:719.

Puri P, Lake BD, Nixon HH, et al: Neuronal colonic dysplasia: An unusual association of Hirschsprung's disease. *J Pediatr Surg* 1977; 12:681.

Schärli AF, Meier-Ruge W: Localized and disseminated forms of neuronal intestinal dysplasia mimicking Hirschsprung's disease. *J Pediatr Surg* 1981; 16:164.

Shuffler MD: Chronic intestinal pseudo-obstruction syndromes. *Med Clin North Am* 1981; 1331–1357.

Staple TW, McAlister WH, Anderson MS: Plexiform neurofibromatosis of the colon simulating Hirschsprung's disease. AJR 1964; 91:840.

Inflammatory and Infectious Diseases

Abramson SJ, Berdon WE, Baker DH: Childhood typhlitis: Its increasing association with acute myelogenous leukemia. *Radiology* 1983; 146:61.

Archibald RB, Nelson JA: Necrotizing enterocolitis in acute leukemia: Radiographic findings. *Gastrointest Radiol* 1978; 3:63.

Atkinson GO Jr, Gay BB, Ball TI Jr, et al: *Yersinia enterocolitica* colitis in infants: Radiographic changes. *Radiology* 1983; 146:113.

Balachandran S, Hayden CK Jr, Swischuk LE: Filiform polyposis in a child with Crohn disease. *Pediatr Radiol* 1984; 14:171.

Bartlett JG: Antimicrobial agents implicated in *Clostridium difficile* toxin–associated diarrhea or colitis. *Johns Hopkins Med J* 1981; 149:6.

Bolandi L, Ferrentino M, Trevisani F, et al: Sonographic appearance of pseudomembranous colitis. *J Ultrasound Med* 1985; 4:489.

Brunner D, Feifarek C, McNeely D, et al: CT of pseudomembranous colitis. *Gastrointest Radiol* 1984; 9:73.

Cammerer RC, et al: Clinical spectrum of pseudomembranous colitis. *JAMA* 1976; 235:2502.

Chamovitz BN, Hartstein AI, Alexander SR, et al: *Campylobacter jejuni*–associated hemolytic-uremic syndrome in a mother and daughter. *Pediatrics* 1983; 71:253.

Davidson M, Bloom AA, Kugler MK: Chronic ulcerative colitis of childhood: An evaluative review. *J Pediatr* 1965; 67:471.

Devroede GJ, Taylor WF, Sauer WG, et al: Cancer risk and life expectancy of children with ulcerative colitis. *N Engl J Med* 1971; 285:17.

Diner WC, Barnard HJ: Toxic megacolon. *Semin Roentgenol* 1973; 8:433.

Eklöf O, Gierup J: The retrorectal soft tissue space in children: normal variations and appearances in granulomatous colitis. AJR 1970; 108:624.

Frick MP, Maile CW, Crass JR, et al: Computed tomography of neutropenic colitis. AJR 1984; 143:763.

Goldstein SJ, Crooks DJM: Colitis in Behçet's syndrome: Two new cases. *Radiology* 1978; 128:321.

Gore RM, Marn CS, Kirby DF, et al: CT findings in ulcerative, granulomatous and indeterminate colitis. AJR 1984; 143:279.

Grand RJ, Homer DR: Approaches to inflammatory bowel disease in childhood and adolescence. *Pediatr Clin North Am* 1975; 22:835.

Hamilton JR, Bruce GA, Abdourhaman M, et al: Inflammatory bowel disease in children and adolescents. *Adv Pediatr* 1979; 26:311.

Hunter TB, Bjelland JC: Gastrointestinal complications of leukemia and its treatment. AJR 1984; 142:513.

Hymans JS, Berman MM, Helgason H: Nonantibiotic-associated enterocolitis caused by *Clostridium difficile* in an infant. *J Pediatr* 1981; 99:750.

Joffe N: Diffuse mucosal granularity in double-contrast studies of Crohn's disease of the colon. *Clin Radiol* 1981; 32:85.

Karjoo M, McCarthy B: Toxic megacolon of ulcerative colitis in infancy. *Pediatrics* 1976; 57:962.

Karmali MA, Steele BT, Petric M, et al: Sporadic cases of

haemolytic-uraemic syndrome associated with faecal cytotoxin and cytotoxin-producing *Escherichia coli* in stools. *Lancet* 1983; 1:619.

Kawanami T, Bowen A, Girdany BR: Enterocolitis: Prodrome of the hemolytic-uremic syndrome. *Radiology* 1984; 151:91.

Kelvin FM, Oddson TA, Rice RP, et al: Double contrast barium enema in Crohn disease and ulcerative colitis. *AJR* 1978; 131:207.

Kirks DR: The radiology of enteritis due to hemolytic-uremic syndrome. *Pediatr Radiol* 1982; 12:179.

Liebhaber MI, Parker BR, Morton JA, et al: Abdominal mass and colonic perforation in a case of the hemolytic-uremic syndrome. *Am J Dis Child* 1977; 131:1168.

Loughran CR, Tappin JA, Whitehouse GH: The plain abdominal radiograph in pseudomembranous colitis due to *Clostridium difficile*. *Clin Radiol* 1982; 33:277.

McNamara MJ, Chalmers AG, Morgan M, et al: Typhlitis in acute childhood leukemia: radiological features. *Clin Radiol* 1986; 37:83.

Stringer DA, Cleghorn GJ, Daneman A, et al: Behçet's syndrome involving the gastrointestinal tract: A diagnostic dilemma in childhood. *Pediatr Radiol* 1986; 16:131.

Stringer DA, Sherman PM, Jakowenko N: Correlation of double-contrast high-density barium enema, colonoscopy, and histology in children with special attention to disparities. *Pediatr Radiol* 1986; 16:298.

Tochen ML, Campbell JR: Colitis in children with the hemolytic-uremic syndrome. *J Pediatr Surg* 1977; 12:213.

Vlymen WJ, Moskowitz PS: Roentgenographic manifestations of esophageal and intestinal involvement in Behçet's disease in children. *Pediatr Radiol* 1981; 10:193.

Wagner ML, Rosenberg HS, Fernbach JJ, et al: Typhlitis: A complication of leukemia in childhood. *AJR* 1971; 109:341.

Winthrop JD, Balfe DM, Shackelford GD, et al: Ulcerative and granulomatous colitis in children. *Radiology* 1985; 154:657.

Appendicitis

Abu-Yousef MM, Franken EA Jr: An overview of graded compression sonography in the diagnosis of acute appendicitis. *Semin US CT MR* 1989; 10:352.

Borushok KF, Jeffrey RB Jr, Laing FC, et al: Sonographic diagnosis of perforation in patients with acute appendicitis. *AJR* 1990; 154:275.

Fedyshin P, Kelvin FM, Rice RP: Nonspecificity of barium enema findings in acute appendicitis. *AJR* 1984; 143:99.

Garcia CJ, Rosenfield NS: The barium enema in the diagnosis of acute appendicitis. *Semin US CT MR* 1989; 10:314.

Jeffrey RB Jr, Laing FC, Townsend RR: Acute appendicitis: Sonographic criteria based on 250 cases. *Radiology* 1988; 167:327.

Johnson JF, Coughlin WF: Plain film diagnosis of appen-

diceal perforation in children. *Semin US CT MR* 1989; 10:306.

Kao SCS, Smith WL, Abu-Yousef MM, et al: Acute appendicitis in children: Sonographic findings. *AJR* 1989; 153:375.

Kottmeier PK: Appendicitis, in Welch KJ, Randolph JG, Ravitch MM, et al (eds): *Pediatric Surgery*. St Louis, Mosby–Year Book, 1986, pp 989–994.

Menneman PL, Marcus CS, Inkelis SH, et al: Evaluation of children with possible appendicitis using technetium 99m leukocyte scan. *Pediatrics* 1990; 85:838.

Navarro DA, Weber PM: Indium-111 imaging in appendicitis. *Semin US CT MR* 1989; 10:321.

Nunez D Jr, Yrizarry JM, Casillas VJ, et al: Percutaneous management of appendiceal abscesses. *Semin US CT MR* 1989; 10:348.

Puylaert JB: Acute appendicitis: US evaluation using graded compression. *Radiology* 1986; 158:355.

Rice RP, Thompson WM, Fedyshin PJ, et al: The barium enema in appendicitis: spectrum of appearances and pitfalls. *Radiographics* 1984; 4:393.

Shandling B, Fallis JC: Acute appendicitis, in Behrman RE, Vaughn VC III (eds): *Nelson Textbook of Pediatrics*. Philadelphia, WB Saunders, 1987, pp 810–813.

Shimkin PM: Radiology of acute appendicitis. *AJR* 1978; 130:1001.

Slovis TL, Haller JO, Cohen HL, et al: Complicated appendiceal inflammatory disease in children: Pylephlebitis and liver abscess. *Radiology* 1989; 171:823.

Van Sonnenberg E, Wittich GR, Gasola G, et al: Periappendiceal abscesses: Percutaneous drainage. *Radiology* 1987; 163:23.

Vignault F, Filiatrault D, Brandt ML, et al: Acute appendicitis in children: evaluation with US. *Radiology* 1990; 176:501.

Zerin JM: Intrathoracic appendicitis in a ten-year-old girl. *Invest Radiol* 1990; 25:1162.

Neoplasms

Bartram CI, Thornton A: Colonic polyp patterns in familial polyposis. *AJR* 1984; 142:305.

Berk RN: Polypoid lesions of the colon. *Postgrad Radiol* 1981; 1:29.

Bryne WJ, Jimenez JF, Euler AR, et al: Lymphoid polyps (focal lymphoid hyperplasia) of the colon in children. *Pediatrics* 1982; 69:598.

Capitanio MA, Kirkpatrick JA: Lymphoid hyperplasia of the colon in children: Roentgen observations. *Radiology* 1970; 94:323.

Cremin BJ, Louw JH: Polyps in the large bowel in children. *Clin Radiol* 1970; 21:195.

Dodds WJ: Clinical and roentgen features of the intestinal polyposis syndromes. *Gastrointest Radiol* 1976; 1:127.

Erbe RW: Inherited gastrointestinal-polyposis syndromes. *N Engl J Med* 1976; 295:1101.

Franken EA, Bixler D, Fitzgerald JF, et al: Juvenile polyposis of the colon. *Ann Radiol (Paris)* 1975; 18:499.

Howell J, Pringle K, Kirschner B, et al: Peutz-Jeghers polyps causing colocolic intussusception in infancy. *J Pediatr Surg* 1981; 16:82.

Lamego CM, Torloni H: Colorectal adenocarcinoma in childhood and adolescence. Report of 11 cases and review of the literature. *Pediatr Radiol* 1989; 19:504.

Laufer I, deSa D: Lymphoid follicular pattern: A normal feature of the pediatric colon. AJR 1978; 130:51.

Lewis CT, Riley WE, Georgeson K, et al: Carcinoma of the colon and rectum in patients less than 20 years of age. *South Med J* 1990; 83:383.

Pratt CB, George SL: Epidemic colon cancer in children and adolescents, in Correa P, Haenszel W (eds): *Epidemiology of Cancer of the Digestive Tract.* Boston, Martinus Nijhoff, 1982, pp 127–145.

Radin DR, Fortgang KC, Zee CS, et al: Turcot syndrome: A case with spinal cord and colonic neoplasms. AJR 1984; 142:475.

Rao BN, Pratt CB, Fleming ID, et al: Colon carcinoma in children and adolescents. *Cancer* 1985; 55:1322.

Schatello CR, Pickren WJ, Grace JT Jr: Generalized juvenile gastrointestinal polyposis. A hereditary syndrome. *Gastroenterology* 1970; 58:699.

Miscellaneous Disorders

Andersen JF, Eklöf O, Thomasson B: Large bowel volvulus in children. *Pediatr Radiol* 1981; 11:129.

Berger RB, Hillmeier AC, Stahl RS, et al: Volvulus of the ascending colon: An unusual complication of nonrotation of the midgut. *Pediatr Radiol* 1982; 12:298.

Campbell JR, Blank E: Sigmoid volvulus in children. *Pediatrics* 1974; 53:702.

Hernanz-Schulman M, Kirkpatrick J Jr, Schwachman H, et al: Pneumatosis intestinalis in cystic fibrosis. *Radiology* 1986; 160:497.

Kirks DR, Swischuk LE, Merten DF, et al: Cecal volvulus in children. AJR 1981; 136:419.

Knight PJ, Morse TS: Splenic flexure volvulus. *J Pediatr Surg* 1981; 16:744.

Reinarz S, Smith WL, Franken EA, et al: Splenic flexure volvulus: A complication of pseudoobstruction in infancy. AJR 1985; 145:1303.

Sivit CJ, Josephs SH, Taylor GA, et al: Pneumatosis intestinalis in children with AIDS. AJR 1990; 155:133.

Wood RE, Herman CJ, Johnson KW, et al: Pneumatosis coli in cystic fibrosis. *Am J Dis Child* 1985; 129:246.

Yeager AM, Kanof ME, Kramer SS, et al: Pneumatosis intestinalis in children after allogeneic bone marrow transplantation. *Pediatr Radiol* 1987; 17:18.

29

Abdominal Masses

The explosive expansion of the diagnostic imaging armamentarium during the past several decades has greatly changed the formerly conventional approach to the evaluation of abdominal masses in infants and children. Along with this increased capability, however, has come increased financial cost and increased confusion on the part of physicians as to the selection of the proper imaging studies in a particular clinical situation. The purpose of this brief chapter is to summarize an imaging approach to abdominal masses that is widely advocated by pediatric radiologists. Specific information and relevant illustrative material is found in the appropriate sections of this book.

Regardless of the anatomical site of origin and ultimate diagnosis, the first imaging examination in a child of any age with an abdominal mass should be plain film radiography. The plain film can identify dilated loops of bowel which may be mistaken for a mass by the clinician; may contain pathologic calcification, the presence of which may aid in diagnosis; and can identify associated bony abnormalities such as congenital defects, metastases, or invasion by tumor, which may direct the further workup. Of major importance, the plain film often can suggest the correct nature of a gastrointestinal problem, such as obstruction or intussusception, and lead directly to a diagnostic contrast examination.

If a mass is not clearly of gastrointestinal origin, sonography is the next appropriate imaging examination. Since the majority of palpable masses in children are cystic, fluid-filled, and benign, sonography allows that differentiation and usually discriminates between intraperitoneal and retroperitoneal masses.

Further imaging evaluation is directed by the combined results of plain film and sonographic studies.

In the oft-quoted study by Melicow and Uson, 57% of abdominal masses in infants and children are enlarged organs. Hepatomegaly, splenomegaly, and renomegaly usually can be differentiated from other types of masses by the examining pediatrician. Patients with organomegaly may require imaging evaluation, but the thrust of studies of childhood masses has been directed to pathologic conditions causing a variably discrete mass rather than generalized enlargement of the affected organ. As a generalization, 90% of abdominal masses in infants and children are retroperitoneal or pelvic and half of these are related to the urinary tract.

ABDOMINAL MASSES IN THE NEWBORN

According to studies by Melicow and Uson, Griscom, and Kirks et al., 55% of all palpable abdominal masses not representing organomegaly or gastrointestinal tract lesions are renal in origin. Sonography usually identifies these abnormalities as being genitourinary. Hydronephrosis accounts for 45% of the renal masses and renal cystic dysplasia (multicystic dysplastic kidney) accounts for 27%, although some studies suggest an equal incidence. The more common causes of hydronephrosis include ureteropelvic junction obstruction; reflux nephropathy, especially in boys with posterior urethral valves; ectopic ureterocele, usually associated with duplication and obstruction of the ipsilateral collecting system; prune-belly syndrome; and ureterovesical junction obstruction. Further evaluation of those lesions usually requires cystourethrography, either scintigraphic or radiographic, and, sometimes, excretory urography. Radioisotopic renal studies can give useful information about renal function.

Renal cystic dysplasia has several characteristic sonographic appearances which permit the correct diagnosis. These are described in detail in Chapter 32. Further imaging studies are rarely, if ever, indicated except for the 15% of patients in whom the lesions are bilateral. These patients require tests of renal function, often including a radioisotopic renogram, in order to plan the proper therapeutic approach.

Renal masses that are solid by sonography are most likely to be mesoblastic nephroma in the newborn. True Wilms tumors are seen uncommonly in the newborn but certainly are in the differential diagnosis. Mesoblastic nephroma and Wilms tumor have similar imaging characteristics and cannot be distinguished as long as the Wilms tumor is contained by the renal capsule. Computed tomography (CT) is useful to identify extrarenal spread, which occurs with Wilms tumor but not with mesoblastic nephroma. Since mesoblastic nephroma is so much more common than Wilms tumor in the neonate, some experienced pediatric surgeons are willing to operate on these babies with plain films and sonography as the only imaging studies.

Polycystic renal disease and renal vein thrombosis present as nephromegaly rather than discrete masses. Nephroblastomatosis also presents with nephromegaly and is less common than polycystic disease and renal vein thrombosis.

Adrenal masses account for 15% of retroperitoneal masses in the neonate. The major differential considerations are adrenal hemorrhage, neuroblastoma, and teratoma. Plain films may demonstrate the upper quadrant mass if it is large enough, but the lack of retroperitoneal fat and overlying bowel gas may make detection of small lesions difficult. Calcifications in neuroblastoma and teratoma are less common in neonates than in older children.

Adrenal hemorrhage often appears hyperechoic in its early stage but eventually liquefies and becomes progressively smaller with time. Although liquefaction of the hemorrhage usually occurs within 2 to 3 days, we have had several patients in whom the sonographic appearance did not change for several weeks. Nevertheless, serial sonography is the appropriate imaging evaluation. The major differential diagnosis of a hyperechoic adrenal mass is neuroblastoma. Since the prognosis for neonatal neuroblastoma is excellent, there is no harm in following an adrenal mass for up to 3 to 4 weeks. If by the end

of that time, the mass remains unchanged, the presumptive diagnosis changes to neuroblastoma, and the workup continues as discussed below. Neonatal adrenal teratomas may be calcified on plain films, but this occurs less commonly than in older children. Sonography is usually diagnostic because of its ability to demonstrate the multitissue origin of the mass. If sonography is not definitive, magnetic resonance (MR) is useful because of its sensitivity to the presence of fat, a typical component of teratomas.

Pelvic masses in girls account for 15% of masses in neonates. The most common is an ovarian cyst. Plain films may be misleading as the cysts may be so large as to simulate a mass of abdominal rather than pelvic origin. These cysts are characteristically anechoic. Sonography can identify the pelvic origin of even the largest cysts although there can be some confusion between a massive ovarian cyst extending into the abdomen and a massive mesenteric cyst extending into the pelvis. The latter are often lymphangiomas, however, and may be hypoechoic rather than anechoic. We have had one case of an ectopic ureter draining into the vagina with a focal ureterocele simulating an ovarian mass on ultrasound (US).

Hydrocolpos is not common in the newborn, and the diagnosis is often missed because it is not considered in the differential diagnosis. Careful pelvic sonography usually enables the correct diagnosis to be made. Hydrometrocolpos is even less common than hydrocolpos, but the presence of a fluid-filled endometrial cavity associated with an inferior midline cystic structure should lead to the correct diagnosis. Rare, tragic instances of inadvertent hysterectomy have occurred when hydrocolpos or hydrometrocolpos have been mistaken for an ovarian cyst. MR is useful if there is a question and the presence of unilateral renal agenesis or hypoplasia strongly supports the diagnosis of hydrocolpos secondary to congenital vaginal stenosis. The most common presacral tumors are teratoma, neuroblastoma, and endodermal sinus tumor. MR is a useful adjunct to sonography in these cases because of its greater sensitivity to invasion of local structures.

Gastrointestinal lesions account for 15% of masses in the neonate. Most of them will have plain film findings leading to appropriate contrast studies. Meconium cysts associated with intestinal atresia are often calcified, and the obstructive bowel pattern is seen. Patients with meconium ileus may have a palpable mass in the right lower quadrant. Plain films will demonstrate the characteristic bubbly pattern of meconium, and dilated proximal loops of intestine may be seen. Intestinal duplication cysts large enough to be palpated are usually anechoic. If the echogenic mucosal layer is seen, sonography may be diagnostic, but, more commonly, the differential diagnosis is between duplication and mesenteric cysts. These lesions are anechoic or hypoechoic, benign in appearance, and usually do not require further imaging studies unless the surgeon requires additional information on the impact of the cyst on neighboring structures. CT is helpful in those uncommon instances.

Hepatobiliary masses account for only 5% of neonatal abdominal masses. Plain films may show a right upper quadrant mass. Calcification is not necessarily helpful because hepatoblastomas and infantile hemangioendotheliomas can calcify, as can Wilms tumor, neuroblastoma, and adrenal teratomas. Sonography can identify the hepatic origin of the mass, however. A solid hepatic mass should be evaluated with Doppler US and MR. Hydrops of the gallbladder and hepatic cysts are well demonstrated sonographically. Sonography usually suggests the correct diagnosis in patients with choledochal cysts and further evaluation with biliary scintigraphy and cholangiography gives appropriate preoperative information.

ABDOMINAL MASSES IN OLDER INFANTS AND CHILDREN

Renal masses account for over half of all abdominal masses in older infants and children just as they do in neonates. In these patients, however, about half of the renal masses are solid on sonographic examination, nearly all of them Wilms tumors. Sonography is useful for evaluation of the inferior vena cava and right atrium in Wilms tumor patients but CT or MR is also indicated. Both CT and MR can evaluate extrarenal extension, vascular invasion, body wall involvement, and liver metastases. Contrast-enhanced CT is the cross-sectional examination of choice in most centers. MR is more sensitive to respiratory artifact than is CT and is a longer examination. Its multiplanar and "angiographic" abilities, however, make it likely that MR will supersede CT in the evaluation of Wilms tumor as more rapidly performed scanning sequences become available. An advantage for CT at present is the outmoded requirement of the National Wilms' Tumor Study for excretory urography. A kidney-ureter-bladder (KUB) examination obtained following contrast-enhanced CT suffices to meet this requirement for patients enrolled in the study.

Sonographically demonstrable hydronephrosis accounts for most of the other palpable renal masses in this age group. The causes are largely the same as those listed for the neonate. Diseases causing nephromegaly, such as nephroblastomatosis and polycystic renal disease, are more likely to be discovered for reasons other than a palpable abdominal mass.

Fully a quarter of palpable abdominal masses in this age group will be identified by sonography as being retroperitoneal and extrarenal. About 90% of these lesions will be solid by sonographic criteria and represent neuroblastoma, ganglioneuroblastoma, and ganglioneuroma. Further cross-sectional imaging studies are invariably obtained, and both CT and MR have their adherents. Unenhanced CT will demonstrate intratumoral calcification in 90% of neuroblastomas, but the additional information gleaned from CT and MR makes this finding of less importance than was true in earlier times. MR has the advantage of demonstrating invasion of the neural foramina and the spinal canal to much better advantage than does CT. They can both demonstrate regional lymphadenopathy and hepatic metastases. With the advent of faster MR scanning techniques, the increased use of intravenous MR contrast agents, and the development of satisfactory oral MR contrast agents, it is likely that MR will become the definitive imaging examination in patients with retroperitoneal neurogenic tumors.

About 5% of extrarenal retroperitoneal tumors are teratomas, most of them adrenal in origin. Sonography is usually able to identify the multitissue origin of the tumor. CT and MR are more sensitive to extracapsular spread, denoting malignancy, than is sonography. They are both capable of demonstrating the fatty component of the tumor with CT more likely to demonstrate calcification.

An additional 5% of tumors in this region are those which can arise from any of the retroperitoneal tissues. They are invariably solid on sonography and CT or MR will be useful in evaluation since even the benign lesions such as neurofibromatosis and juvenile fibromatosis may involve vital structures and cause significant morbidity and even death. Retroperitoneal lymphoma rarely presents as a clinically palpable mass.

Pelvic masses account for about 25% of palpable masses in this age group and may be found in boys or girls. In boys, they are most likely to be abscesses secondary to appendiceal perforation with their characteristic sonographic appearance. Further imaging evaluation is not necessary if the patient is going to surgery, but CT is an excellent guide for percutaneous drainage. Solid pelvic masses in boys without symptoms of infection represent tumors, almost all malignant, of which rhabdomyosarcoma is the most common. MR is extremely valuable in the evaluation of these tumors, especially in terms of local extension.

Pelvic masses in girls may also be abscesses, appendiceal in the younger girls and both appendiceal and tubo-ovarian in sexually active adolescents and teen-agers. Sonography is usually sufficiently diagnostic to preclude the need for additional imaging studies. Hydrocolpos and hydrometrocolpos both are found in adolescents, usually near the time of menarche. Sonography is usually diagnostic. If there is any doubt, MR is useful because of its sensitivity to intrauterine blood and the lack of gonadal radiation which accompanies CT. Ovarian masses are usually benign if completely anechoic but a substantial percentage of the malignant ovarian tumors have both cystic and solid components. Any pelvic mass that is sonographically solid, in whole or in part, should be considered malignant until proved otherwise, and further evaluation by MR is warranted. The exception is teratoma which may have solid components. As with teratomas elsewhere, sonography is usually sufficient unless malignancy is suspected. A number of other tumors, most of them malignant, can arise in the female pelvis, the most common being rhabdomyosarcoma. Endodermal sinus tumors may arise as solid pelvic masses or as the solid components of a teratoma.

Intraperitoneal masses, other than abscesses, are most likely to be mesenteric cysts if anechoic or hypoechoic. These will generally be found in the infant-toddler age group. Cystic duplications of the gastrointestinal tract are usually discovered early if large enough to be palpable. Choledochal cysts may be found in older children but rarely as a palpable mass. Intraperitoneal masses in older children are frequently hyperechoic although lymphoma arising from the bowel or mesentery may appear hypoechoic. The majority of hyperechoic intraperitoneal lesions are hepatic in origin. Hemangioendothelioma, cavernous hemangioma, hepatoblastoma, and hepatocellular carcinoma are all differential possibilities, depending on the age of the patient, and MR is the most useful imaging examination for evaluation, especially when MR angiography is performed.

Although one can never predict future changes in the rapidly advancing field of diagnostic imaging, the evaluation of the newborn or child with a palpable abdominal mass should always begin with plain abdominal radiography to be followed either by a gastrointestinal contrast study or sonography depending on the findings. For those patients requiring further evaluation, MR is becoming increasingly useful because of its sensitivity to tissue characteristics and its multiplanar and angiographic capabilities. CT is clearly useful for nonhepatic intraperitoneal masses and as a guide for interventional procedures.

REFERENCES

Donaldson JS, Shkolnik A: Pediatric renal masses. *Semin Roentgenol* 1988; 23:194.

Griscom NT: The roentgenology of neonatal abdominal masses. AJR 1965; 93:447.

Kirks DR, Merten DF, Grossman H, et al: Diagnostic imaging of pediatric abdominal masses: An overview. *Radiol Clin North Am* 1981; 19:527.

Kirks DR, Rosenberg ER, Johnson DG, et al: Integrated imaging of neonatal renal masses. *Pediatr Radiol* 1985; 15:147.

Mahaffey SM, Ryckman FC, Martin LW: Clinical aspects of abdominal masses in children. *Semin Roentgenol* 1988; 23:161.

Melicow MD, Uson AC: Palpable abdominal masses in infants and children: A report based on a review of 653 cases. *J Urol* 1959; 81:705.

Parker BR, Moore SG: Imaging studies in the diagnosis of pediatric malignancies, in Pizzo PA, Poplack DG (eds): *Principles and Practice of Pediatric Oncology*, ed 2. Philadelphia, JB Lippincott, 1992.

Teele RL, Share JC: The abdominal mass in the neonate. *Semin Roentgenol* 1988; 23:175.

30

Abdominal Trauma

Blunt abdominal trauma, most often due to vehicular accidents, frequently causes multiple intra-abdominal injuries; in the past, many children have been subjected to exploratory surgery to evaluate the extent of possible hidden injury. Since the advent of noninvasive radiologic imaging techniques, including scintigraphy, ultrasonography (US), and especially computed tomography (CT), the radiologist has been better able to accurately assess the extent of abdominal injury and thus allow conservative, nonoperative therapy in many cases.

Penetrating abdominal trauma occurs following gunshot wounds, stabbing, and other similar injury. If there is any question that a wound has extended intraperitoneally, a sinogram with water-soluble contrast medium allows quick, accurate diagnosis. The presence of large amounts of free intraperitoneal gas suggests penetrating injury to the colon or other gas-containing viscus and is generally considered an indication for surgery.

SECTION 1

Imaging Evaluation

Radiologic assessment of the child with suspected abdominal injury begins with communication with the clinician. The nature of the suspected injury and the condition of the child determine the urgency, appropriateness, and extent of the radiologic investigation. The other important factor is the availability of CT, which is usually the examination of choice following plain radiography. If CT scanning is not available, a combination of radionuclide and US procedures with conventional examinations such as intravenous urography and occasionally arteriography may yield much useful information.

PLAIN FILM

Plain film examination is indicated in virtually every case unless the child is so severely injured that immediate lifesaving maneuvers are needed. A frontal chest film and a complete abdominal series, modified according to the patient's age and condition, are usually indicated if abdominal injury is suspected. Skeletal survey is often indicated. The imaging procedures used next depend on the plain film findings, on whether or not CT is available, and on the condition of the child.

CONVENTIONAL CONTRAST STUDIES

Conventional contrast studies, including excretory urography, upper gastrointestinal (GI) series, and barium enema may be useful. Renal injury often occurs in blunt abdominal trauma; this topic is discussed in greater detail in Chapter 37. When serious renal injury is evaluated with an intravenous urogram, our experience is that the extent of renal injury is significantly underestimated by urography when compared with CT scanning; therefore we reserve excretory urography either for suspected minimal injury or as an emergency procedure to make certain that there are two functioning kidneys before emergency abdominal surgery is performed.

The presence of gross or microscopic hematuria suggests renal injury but does not correlate well with the severity of injury. A positive physical examination appears to be a much better predictor of the presence of significant renal injury. Multiple organ injuries are associated with renal injury in children involved in motor vehicle accidents, whereas the kidney tends to be the only organ injured if there is a history of a direct blow to the kidney. Therefore, in a patient with a history of a direct blow to the kidney and who has hematuria but normal findings on physical examination, either US or intravenous urography may be performed; if physical findings are positive, CT is suggested for more complete evaluation.

Contrast examinations of the gastrointestinal tract are useful for localization of a suspected perforation or if a duodenal or mesenteric hematoma is suspected. Pancreatic injury is best evaluated by US or CT.

SCINTIGRAPHY

Scintigraphy has been used successfully to diagnose hepatic, splenic, and renal injury. The anatomical detail visualized is less than with CT. Moreover, radionuclide techniques cannot reveal intraperitoneal bleeding or bowel, mesenteric, and pancreatic injury. In addition, scintigraphy is relatively organ-specific.

ULTRASOUND

Ultrasonography is also useful in the diagnosis of acute abdominal injury, particularly if CT is not available. Hematomas are seen as sonolucent areas in or around organs, but complete visualization of the entire abdomen is often difficult. In our practice, US is used primarily to follow the size of a known hepatic or perirenal hematoma rather than in initial patient evaluation. US is sensitive for the detection of intraperitoneal fluid. Doppler US is useful to evaluate flow in major intra-abdominal vessels.

COMPUTED TOMOGRAPHY

Technique

Computed tomography is the most useful imaging tool in the evaluation of the acutely injured child. Careful attention to technique is required for high-quality examinations. Patient motion can prevent a successful examination, so some degree of patient cooperation is required. If the patient cannot hold still or if sedation is clinically contraindicated, then CT probably should not be attempted.

For optimal pediatric abdominal CT, both oral and intravenous contrast enhancement should be used. Some centers have been reluctant to use oral contrast media in children who may need to go to surgery or who will need to have contrast media injected intravenously. We have used oral contrast media, usually dilute Gastrografin (meglumine diatrizoate) for 15 years in most of our patients who have had CT for evaluation of abdominal trauma and have had no instances of aspiration in that period of time. The children who are injured rarely have empty stomachs when they are injured, and adding a contrast agent to their existing gastric contents has had no deleterious effect. Many times oral contrast material is not necessary, but it does allow better visualization of the duodenum and its use increases the likelihood that a bowel perforation or intraluminal hematoma will be detected.

Intravenous contrast material, preferably nonionic, should be injected as a bolus of 3 mL/kg. It is possible to use 1 to 2 mL/kg and obtain good vascular and organ opacification if ultrafast CT or conventional CT with spiral or helical scanning is available.

In suspected abdominal injury, our protocol is to obtain images following contrast enhancement from the umbilicus to the lung bases using 6-mm slices at

8-mm increments. If an abnormality is noted at the lung bases, additional images may be obtained through the thorax. Additional images are also obtained through the pelvis to exclude intrapelvic accumulations of large amounts of peritoneal fluid.

Selection of Patients for CT

Not every child with abdominal trauma is a suitable candidate for CT scanning; some children require immediate surgery; others need nothing more than careful clinical evaluation. The protocol followed at the Children's Hospital of Buffalo for patients with abdominal trauma is shown in Figure 30–1. Table 30–1 lists the indications for CT as practiced at the Children's Hospital of Buffalo and elsewhere. In general, the patients in the high-yield category tend to have a 50% or greater chance of significant intra-abdominal injury. In the low-yield category, positive findings are usually found in less than 10% of patients. Despite the fact that the incidence of positive findings is low in these children, other factors may justify proceeding with abdominal CT depending on the circumstances of the individual case.

TABLE 30–1.

Indications for Computed Tomography

High Yield	Low Yield
Severe trauma	"Unevaluable abdomen"
Motor vehicle accident	Serious neurologic injury
Child abuse	Injury requiring general
Direct blow to the abdomen	anesthesia
Positive laboratory findings	Microscopic hematuria with
Gross hematuria	normal physical examination
Elevated liver enzymes	
Progressive signs of blood	
loss	
Positive physical findings	
Bruise	
Focal abdominal tenderness	
Lap-belt sign	

Angiography is now rarely used to evaluate acute abdominal injury because of the availability of CT. If CT scans show the vascular integrity of the kidney to be violated (Fig 30–2), emergency surgery rather than arteriography is needed. Angiography is most useful in cases of suspected posttraumatic arteriovenous malformations and of posttraumatic renovascular hypertension.

ABDOMINAL TRAUMA

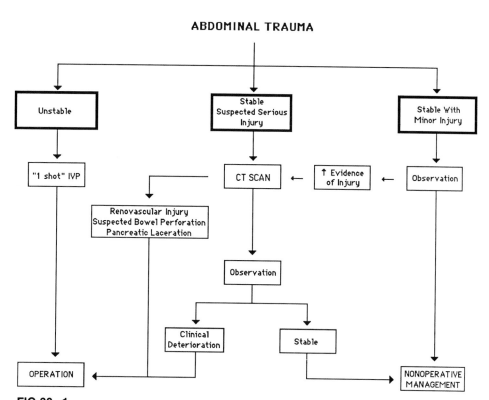

FIG 30–1.
Protocol currently followed at the Children's Hospital of Buffalo for evaluation of the child with abdominal trauma. IVP, intravenous pyelography.

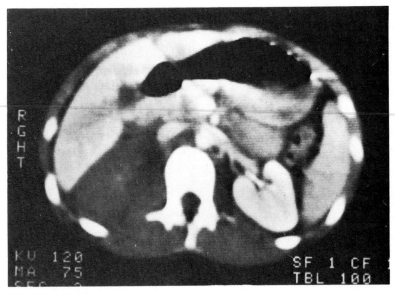

FIG 30–2.
Renovascular injury in a 12-year-old girl struck by an automobile. CT reveals opacification of the aorta, inferior vena cava, and left kidney. The right kidney is nonperfused. Avulsion of the right renal artery was found at surgery.

SECTION 2

Radiographic and CT Findings

GENERAL RADIOGRAPHIC FINDINGS

The plain film evaluation for abdominal injury should include a frontal chest radiograph, and supine, left lateral decubitus, and cross-table lateral views of the abdomen. The findings of abdominal trauma on plain films are nonspecific; nonetheless, they should be carefully searched for because they may provide the first clue to a serious injury.

A *hematoma* can be suspected if normal gas shadows are displaced or effaced. A mass associated with partial or complete small bowel obstruction suggests duodenal or jejunal hematoma. *Pancreatic pseudocysts* usually are diagnosed only after CT or US examinations. *Pneumoperitoneum* suggests a ruptured viscus and is best appreciated on a left lateral decubitus film. *Intraperitoneal fluid,* which suggests hemorrhage, is harder to recognize on radiographs than is free gas. Classic findings include central displacement of the bowel loops and bulging flanks. This de-

gree of fluid, however, is usually obvious clinically. Of more importance is the radiologist's ability to detect smaller amounts of fluid. Jorulf suggests that, with careful technique, it is possible to detect as little as 25 mL of free intraperitoneal fluid. The signs of intraperitoneal and extraperitoneal fluid collections have been described by Whalen. Those that seem useful in children include the "dog-ear" sign in the pelvis, loss of visualization of the inferior angle of the liver, and displacement of the colon medially away from the flank stripe (Fig 30–3,*A*). If the findings of the plain film study are equivocal for the presence of fluid, either US or CT can be used to establish a firm diagnosis.

GENERAL CT FINDINGS

The presence of fluid in the peritoneal cavity suggests strongly that there is visceral injury. The distri-

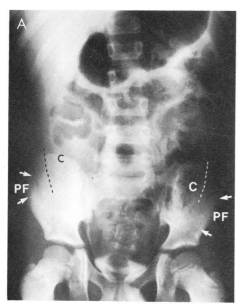

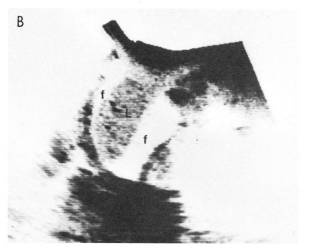

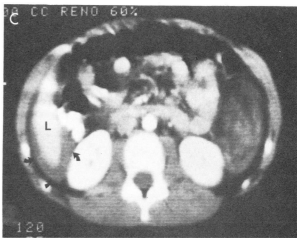

FIG 30–3.
Free intraperitoneal blood. **A,** excretory urogram in a 7-year-old boy with a ruptured liver. Note the displacement of the colonic wall *(C, dotted line)* away from the properitoneal fat line *(PF, arrows)* bilaterally, which indicates fluid in the flanks. **B,** a US study through the Morison pouch in a patient with free intraperitoneal blood clearly shows the sonolucent fluid *(f)* surrounding the liver *(L).* **C,** a CT study through the Morison pouch in the same patient shows the free intraperitoneal blood as relatively low-density material surrounding the tip of the liver *(L)* and lying medial to the kidney *(arrow).*

bution of fluid depends on its site of origin, the amount, and the position of the patient. Fluid tends to accumulate first in the retrovesical area and the lateral paravesical spaces. Large amounts of fluid will extend up the lateral paracolic gutters. Small amounts of blood in the right upper quadrant can first be recognized around the tip of the liver and anterior to the kidney in the Morison pouch (Fig 30–3,*B* and *C*). Blood originating in the left upper quadrant from splenic lacerations accumulates first in a perisplenic location, but is often visible also in the paracolic gutters and the Morison pouch.

The attenuation of the fluid on CT depends on its age and nature. Urine is of water density; infected peritoneal fluid ranges from 0 to 30 Hounsfield units (HU), and fresh blood from 30 to 40 HU. Intraperitoneal fluid, including blood, is of lower attenuation than most abdominal viscera; therefore fluid usually appears relatively hypodense com-

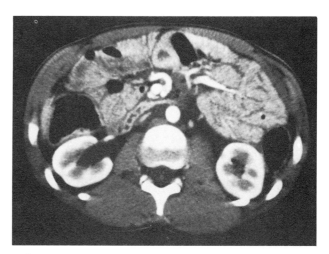

FIG 30–4.
Hypoperfusion syndrome. There is free intraperitoneal fluid, a small inferior vena cava, ascites, and marked enhancement of the viscera. The patient died of head injuries.

pared with the surrounding organs. Clotted blood is often of slightly greater attenuation and may appear denser than the surrounding organ. Injected contrast media can enhance the rim of a resolving hematoma; its center has low attenuation. Differentiating an abscess from an infected hematoma by CT may be impossible.

CT findings suggesting hypovolemic shock in children have been described, and include diffuse dilatation of the intestine with fluid; abnormally intense contrast enhancement of the organs, including the bowel wall and mesentery; decreased caliber of the abdominal aorta and inferior vena cava; and moderate to large peritoneal fluid collections. These findings may vary depending on therapy and the timing of the examination but in general are associated with severe injury and a poor outcome (Fig 30–4).

SECTION 3

Specific Injuries

GASTROINTESTINAL INJURIES

Perforation of the stomach or other hollow viscus occurs most commonly following a violent injury such as an automobile accident but can also be due to child abuse. The most common gastrointestinal injury following blunt abdominal trauma is to the duodenum, which may be injured either singly or in combination with trauma to the pancreas. Many such injuries occur in older children when they are thrown against the handlebar of a bicycle; if seen in a child younger than 3 years of age, the presence of this injury should suggest child abuse.

Plain radiographic findings may be those of partial or complete obstruction of the duodenum, usually in the second or third portion. Occasionally the hematoma is large enough to appear as a mass, especially if it involves the jejunum or mesentery. An upper GI series provides a definite diagnosis, showing the classic coiled-spring appearance.

Plain films and GI series are, however, relatively insensitive in the diagnosis of retroperitoneal duodenal rupture. Toxopus et al. were able to diagnose retroperitoneal rupture correctly in only one third of cases, and Kelly et al. found that none of six patients with retroperitoneal duodenal rupture was correctly diagnosed by plain film studies. It is possible to diagnose duodenal rupture by CT if conventional studies fail to establish the diagnosis (Fig 30–5,*A* and *B*).

US can be used to monitor the size of a hematoma. The ultrasonic appearance of a hematoma depends on the age of the injury. Fresh unclotted or homogeneously clotted blood is usually hypoechoic. Once lysis and fragmentation of the clot occur, the mass becomes more complex and fluid-fluid levels and septa may be observed. US, however, is insensitive to detection of free air.

The CT appearance of duodenal and mesenteric hematomas depends on the age of the injury and the attenuation of the surrounding structures. Fresh blood may appear as either relatively increased or decreased attenuation, depending on the attenuation of the adjacent viscera (Fig 30–6). As the hematoma ages, its relative attenuation diminishes.

CT is very accurate in the diagnosis of solid organ injury; its accuracy in injury to the mesentery and bowel is less well established but in our experience appears to be about 75%. Since most children with intra-abdominal injury are now managed nonoperatively, it is important that bowel injury, which may require surgery, be diagnosed accurately by CT. A careful search must be made for free intraperitoneal air; the findings can be quite subtle (see Fig 30–5,*A* and *B*) and require the radiologist to carefully window and level the images at the console to differentiate free air from intraperitoneal fat. There can be confusion as to whether air is intraluminal or extraluminal; often this can be resolved by obtaining additional images with the patient in a decubitus position. Other signs suggesting bowel or mesenteric injury are a focal hematoma, localized thickening of the bowel, bowel wall enhancement, which is often best appreciated on an unenhanced scan, and findings of fluid in the peritoneal cavity with no evidence of solid organ injury. Such children need care-

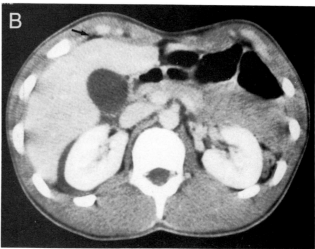

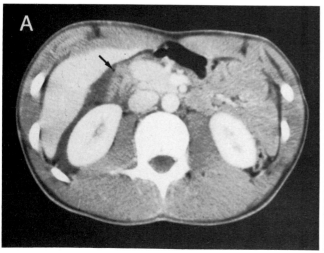

FIG 30–5.

Subtle bowel perforation with a tiny amount of free air. The patient was a 15-year-old boy who was beaten by a gang. **A,** contrast-enhanced CT (CECT) reveals fluid in the subhepatic space. A tiny air bubble *(arrow)* is present, and the duodenum is collapsed. No oral contrast medium was given to this patient. **B,** CT scan section more superior to **A** reveals a slightly larger collection of air *(arrow)* anterior to the liver. At surgery a duodenal perforation was discovered.

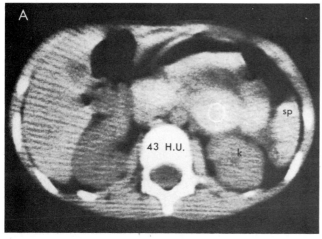

FIG 30–6.

Duodenal hematoma due to child abuse. Unenhanced, intravenous (IV) contrast-enhanced, and IV and oral contrast-enhanced sections from a CT examination in this patient. **A,** unenhanced CT scan shows a hematoma *(white circle)* anterior to the kidney *(K)* and medial to the spleen *(sp)* as a relatively high-attenuation lesion (43 HU). This study was made approximately 24 hours following injury. **B,** after a bolus of contrast enhancement, the hematoma, because of its avascular nature, appears of relatively lower attenuation *(a, aorta; c, vena cava; p, pancreas; k, kidney; sp, spleen).* **C,** following oral ingestion of Gastrografin, the hematoma *(arrows)* has a coiled-spring appearance in the proximal jejunum *(j).* The duodenum *(d)* is dilated but not completely obstructed.

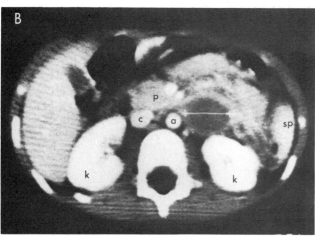

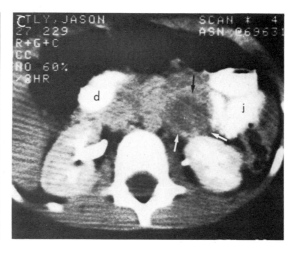

ful clinical observation and may benefit from peritoneal lavage after the CT scan, contrast-enhanced studies of the gastrointestinal tract, or follow-up CT scans.

The history can also be very helpful in assessment of bowel injuries. Child abuse and handlebar injury are well known to be associated with duodenal, jejunal, pancreatic, and mesenteric injury. A lap-belt injury also is likely to be associated with bowel injury. Vertebral fracture due to lap-belt injury can be difficult to appreciate on transaxial CT images. It should be suspected if a large soft-tissue hematoma is noted—this is nearly always present (Fig 30–7, *A*). The fracture is more apparent on a lateral radiograph of the spine, even a "scout view" prior to CT scanning (Fig 30-7, *B*). If a vertebral fracture is suspected, magnetic resonance (MR) provides definitive evaluation (Fig 30–7,*C*).

PANCREATIC INJURIES

Pancreatic injuries often escape early detection in children. Abdominal pain, bilious vomiting, signs of inflammation, and increased serum amylase levels are usually present. In early childhood, trauma is the most common cause of pancreatitis which may be complicated by sepsis, shock, and late development of pseudocysts. Pancreatic injury accounts for between 5 % and 10% of solid intra-abdominal organ injury in children. Plain film examination can lead the radiologist to suspect either pancreatitis or pseudocyst formation. Twenty percent of patients have pleural effusion. Localized ileus, in the form of a dilated duodenum or the "colon cutoff sign," is highly suggestive of pancreatitis. Free intraperitoneal fluid may be present and the gastrocolic space may be increased.

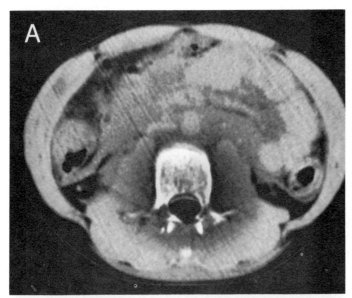

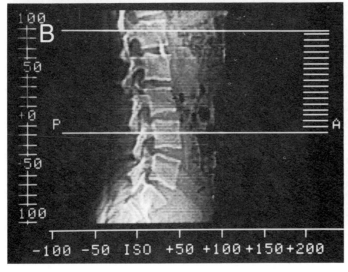

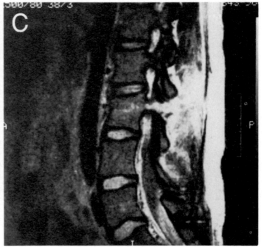

FIG 30–7.
Lap belt fracture with soft tissue hematoma and bowel perforation. Twelve-year-old female injured in a motor vehicle accident. Patient was riding in the back seat and restrained by a lap belt. **A,** nonenhanced CT image reveals a large subcutaneous hematoma posterior to the erector spinae muscles. Also noted is a small fragment of bone avulsed from the fractured vertebral body. The jejunum is markedly thickened and a subsequent diagnosis of bowel perforation was established. **B,** lateral scout radiograph obtained prior to the CT scan revealed mild anterior wedging of the L-3 vertebral body. **C,** mildly T-2 weighted parasagittal MR image reveals a transverse fracture extending through the vertebral pedicle. Also noted is a large area of edema and hemorrhage in the subcutaneous tissues posteriorly and traumatic herniation of the L2-3 disk.

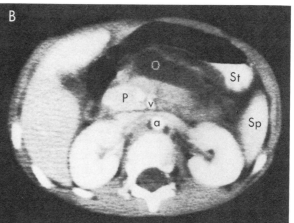

FIG 30–8.
Fracture of the body of the pancreas. CECT in an 8-year-old boy hit by an automobile. There is a massive transverse fracture in the body of the pancreas with peripancreatic and subhepatic fluid collections. This patient died of head injuries.

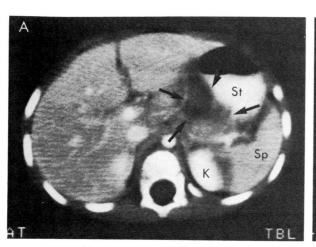

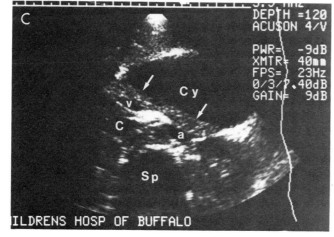

FIG 30–9.
Pancreatic pseudocyst. **A,** CT scan demonstrates an oblique fracture of the liver along the falciform ligament and a fluid collection *(arrows)* medial and posterior to the stomach (*K*, kidney; *Sp*, spleen; *St*, stomach). **B,** a lower CT cut reveals the fluid collection anterior to the pancreas. (*St*, stomach; *Sp*, spleen; *a*, aorta; *v*, superior vena cava; *P*, pancreas **C,** US examination clearly demonstrates this pancreatic pseudocyst (*Sp*, spine; *C*, vena cava; *v*, portal vein; *Cy*, pseudocyst; *arrows*, pancreas), **D,** a follow-up US scan reveals a marked decrease in the size of the cyst, which was then punctured under US guidance and did not recur (*c*, vena cava; *Sp*, spine; *a*, aorta; *Cy*, pseudocyst).

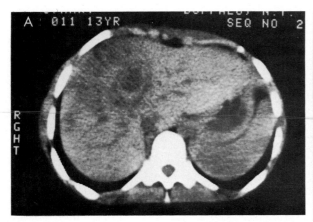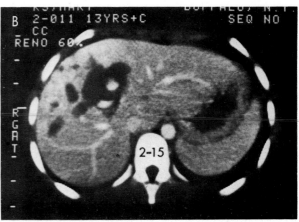

FIG 30–10.
Large intrahepatic hematoma. **A,** unenhanced CT scan of a 13-year-old girl kicked by a horse. A large hematoma is seen in the right lobe of the liver as an ill-defined, low-density area. **B,** the he-matoma is now seen much more clearly following contrast enhancement. The vascular radicles of the liver are well demonstrated.

US and CT are the primary modalities used to visualize the pancreas. Despite the superb US studies usually obtained, a localized ileus may prevent complete examination in the injured patient. If a complete evaluation by US is not possible, CT is then performed and usually results in good anatomical delineation of the pancreas and surrounding organs. Parapancreatic fluid collections are easily recognized, and the presence of fluid in either the lesser sac or the anterior pararenal space should suggest possible pancreatic injury. Fractures which involve the body of the pancreas can be demonstrated on good-quality CT images (Fig 30–8). In our experience, and also that of Sikuit, pancreatic trauma is correctly recognized by CT only about 70% of the time. Formation and evolution of pseudocysts can be assessed. Pseudocysts occur 1 to 2 weeks following injury (Fig 30–9). They may be drained percutaneously and their size monitored by US.

HEPATIC INJURIES

Hepatic injury can be strongly suspected if the liver transaminase levels are elevated (aspartate aminotransferase >450 IU/L, and alanine aminotransferase >250 IU/L). Plain radiographic examination is limited to the detection of gross alterations in the size or shape of the liver. Radiographic detection of fluid in the peritoneal cavity should raise the possibility of liver injury. Liver scintigraphy, a good screening method for detecting severe intrahepatic injury, is somewhat limited by its relative organ specificity, relatively poor definition of anatomy, and inability to show intraperitoneal bleeding.

A complete evaluation of the liver by US can be difficult, particularly near the dome. US may be better suited for monitoring the progress of a known liver injury than for establishing the initial diagnosis.

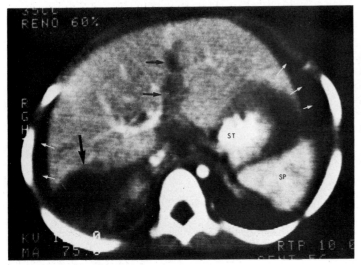

FIG 30–11.
Deep hepatic laceration in the left lower lobe and massive injury to the posterior right lobe of the liver in a 3-year-old boy who was run over by a bus. The liver was crushed against the spine and extensively lacerated anteriorly *(small black arrows)*. A large hematoma is noted posterior to the liver *(large black arrow)*, and blood is seen in the peritoneal cavity bilaterally *(white arrows)*. Despite the massive injury, this patient was treated conservatively, and the lesions healed completely with only a small area of calcification remaining in the posterior aspect of the right lobe of the liver *(ST, stomach; SP, spleen)*.

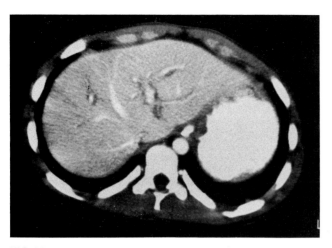

FIG 30–12.
Periportal tracking as a sign of hepatic injury. Note the low attenuation surrounding the portal venous branches but not the branches of the hepatic veins. On a lower CT scan section (not shown), a small periportal hepatic laceration was present but was appreciated only in retrospect after visualization of the extensive periportal tracking.

On CT, liver injury can be classified as: (1) contusions—ill-defined areas of decreased attenuation after contrast enhancement; (2) hematomas—focal, well-defined areas which may be isointense on unenhanced studies but which are seen to be avascular following contrast enhancement (Fig 30–10); (3) lacerations, which may be either linear or stellate; (4) fractures are lacerations extending from one hepatic surface to an opposing one; and (5) large segmental areas of devascularization (Fig 30–11). A common associated finding in hepatic injury is the presence of areas of hypoattenuation surrounding portal venous branches (periportal tracking) (Fig 30–12). While usually associated with obvious hepatic, abnormality, occasionally this finding is seen with only a small or barely perceptible hepatic injury. Its presence in an injured child should prompt a careful search of the CT scan for a subtle intrahepatic injury. Free blood in the peritoneal cavity implies a capsular tear. Subcapsular hematoma is classically lenticular-shaped (Fig 30–13).

The posterior segment of the right lobe of the liver is most frequently injured. Right-sided injuries tend to involve the peripheral portions of the liver, and the less common left-sided injuries tend to be deeper and complex. Right-sided injuries are associated with injury to the right kidney and adrenal as well as the right lower lobe of the lung (Fig 30–14). Left lobe injuries (Fig 30–15) are associated with injury to the pancreas, spleen, and, less often, the left kidney.

Usually, conservative therapy is feasible even when free intraperitoneal blood is detected. Serial follow-up scans may be performed to exclude potential complications, such as bile leakage. On follow-up scans, the injured area initially coalesces into a larger defect of lower attenuation. This area then gradually diminishes in size and increases in attenuation until it becomes isodense with adjacent normal tissue, and consequently invisible. Occasionally, calcifications develop in the injured areas.

BILIARY INJURIES

Biliary damage can occur with any liver injury. Blood in the gallbladder is seen as fluid of greater attenuation than bile. If bile leakage is suspected, the diagnosis can be confirmed with a technetium 99m iminodiacetic acid (IDA) scan. On CT, bilomas in the liver are circumscribed, low-attenuation, avascular areas. Communication with the biliary tree can be demonstrated by percutaneous transhepatic cholangiography.

SPLENIC INJURIES

The plain film diagnosis is neither specific nor sensitive but rib fractures, pneumothorax, elevation of the left hemidiaphragm, enlargement of the spleen shadow, and signs of free intraperitoneal blood should be sought. US and radionuclide scanning are both accurate noninvasive methods of diagnosing splenic hematoma, but CT is now the preferred technique for imaging splenic injury. Fractures and lacerations are best appreciated after enhancement with contrast medium and are seen as irregular, in-

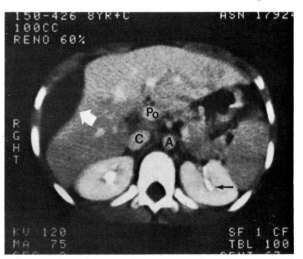

FIG 30–13.
Lenticular subcapsular hematoma *(white arrow)* of the right lobe of the liver *(A,* aorta; *C,* vena cava; *P_o,* portal vein; *small black arrow,* normal-appearing kidney).

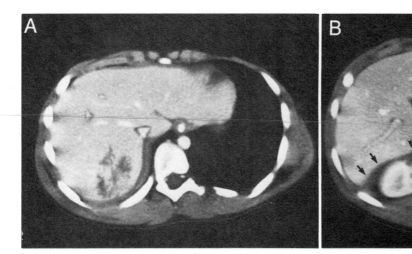

FIG 30–14.

Injury to the posterior right lobe of the liver associated with multiple organ injury. The patient was a 10-year-old boy. **A,** CECT scan reveals a stellate laceration in the posterior segment of the right lobe of the liver. Periportal tracking and a halo of blood are noted around the inferior vena cava and the portal venous radicles. Pleural effusion and a right lung contusion were noted on a higher scan level (not shown). **B,** lower section reveals a small amount of blood in the hepatorenal space *(arrows)* and there is a fracture of the anterior medial aspect of the right kidney *(arrowheads).*

trasplenic, low-attenuation defects. On CT scans, splenic injuries range from single, wedge-shaped, low-attenuation areas to complex shattering fractures (Fig 30–16). They may be accompanied by either subcapsular hematoma or intraperitoneal bleeding. Subcapsular hematomas appear as crescentic, low-attenuation fluid collections that flatten or indent the lateral margins of the spleen.

In a series at Children's Hospital of Buffalo, 79% of patients diagnosed as having splenic injury were managed conservatively without development of the long-term complications of splenic rupture, cyst, or splenosis. Delayed rupture of the spleen is now

thought to represent delayed bleeding from an occult subcapsular hematoma. Initial CT scanning should define this defect and facilitate the management of these patients. In our series, treatment usually consisted of 2 weeks of bed rest followed by limited activity at home until healing of the parenchymal defect and resolution of the hematoma were apparent on CT (Fig 30–17). Commonly, the CT scan showed no sequelae in the spleen. Some patients showed a residual scar, and a few showed a 1- to 2-cm focal area of low density.

Of all the abdominal viscera, the spleen is the most difficult to image consistently well on CT.

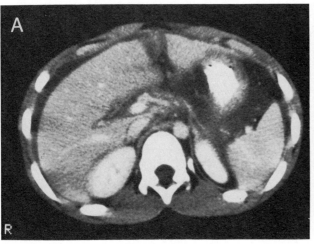
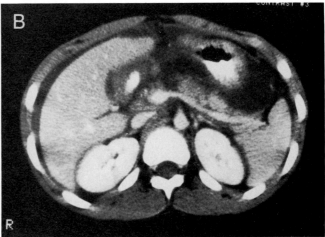

FIG 30–15.

Injury to the left lobe of the liver associated with pancreatic fracture, **A,** there is hemoperitoneum and a complete fracture through the lateral segment of the left lobe of the liver. **B,** more inferior section reveals a transverse section through the body of the pancreas. The splenic vein, however, is intact.

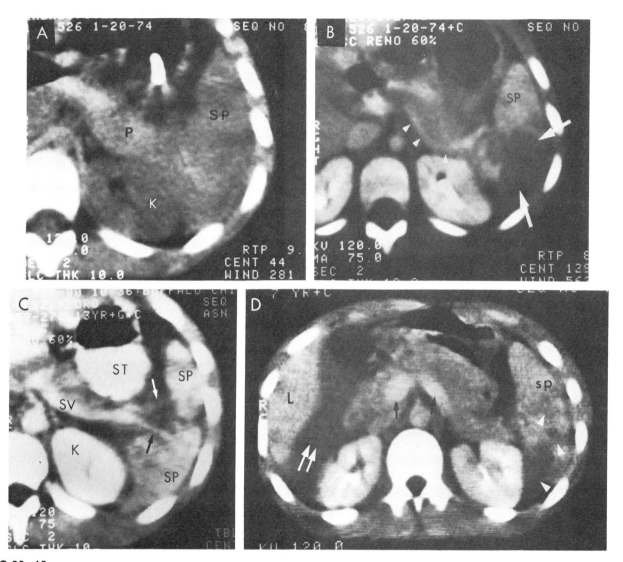

FIG 30–16.
Splenic fractures **A,** unenhanced CT scan of the spleen. Artifacts are caused by the tip of the nasogastric tube in the stomach. Splenic margins are ill defined, but a hematoma cannot be seen clearly (K, kidney; SP, spleen; P, pancreas). **B,** same patient. The nasogastric tube has been removed from the stomach, thereby decreasing the artifacts. After IV enhancement, shattering of the posterior aspect of the spleen (SP) is noted (arrows) and integrity of the splenic vein (arrowheads) is demonstrated. **C,** transverse fracture through the midspleen (SP). A branch of the splenic vein (SV) drains each half of the shattered spleen. This injury was treated conservatively and healed without complication (K, kidney; ST, stomach). **D,** 17-year-old hemophilia patient who, following a disagreement with his brother, suffered extensive abdominal injury. Note the shattered spleen (white arrowheads) and massive free intraperitoneal blood (double white arrows). The splenic and portal veins are partially opacified (black arrows). Because of uncontrollable bleeding, this patient underwent a splenectomy (L, liver; sp, spleen).

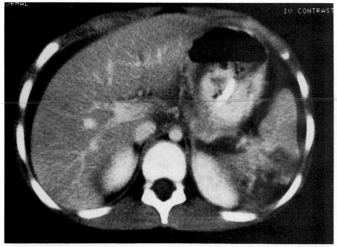

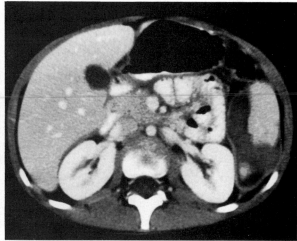

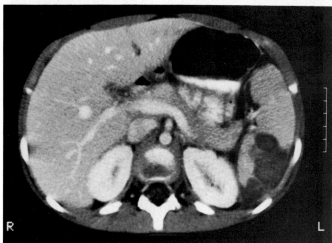

FIG 30–17.
Massive splenic hematoma with CT evidence of healing. **A,** contrast-enhanced CT scan image of a 10-year-old girl who suffered massive splenic hematoma as the result of a motor vehicle accident. Also noted is perisplemic and free intraperitoneal blood. **B,** follow-up CECT scan two weeks later reveals an encapsulated hematoma surrounding the inferior aspect of the spleen. **C,** CECT scan image, more superior to **B,** revealed considerable healing with the remaining intrasplenic hematoma now much better defined and showing beginning encapsulation, A follow-up scan two months later (not shown) revealed only a small scar in this region.

Slight respiratory motion can cause artifacts from the ribs. Furthermore, following bolus enhancement, the normal spleen does not show enhancement as homogeneously as the liver. Nonetheless, if a technically satisfactory examination can be obtained, splenic injury can be confidently diagnosed or excluded by CT. In questionable cases, a radionuclide or US scan may be obtained, or the CT study may be repeated.

REFERENCES

Balthazar EJ, Hulnick D, Megibow AJ, et al.: Computed tomography of intramural intestinal hemorrhage and bowel ischemia. *J Comput Assist Tomogr* 1987; 11:67.

Berger PE, Kuhn JP: Computed tomography of blunt abdominal trauma in childhood. *Am J Roentgenol* 1981; 136:105.

Berger PE, Kuhn JP, Brusehaber J: Techniques for computed tomography in infants and children. *Radiol Clin North Am* 1981; 19:399.

Brick SH, Taylor GA, Potter BM, et al.: Hepatic and splenic injury in children: Role of CT in the decision for laparotomy. *Radiology* 1987; 164:643.

Brody AS, Seidel FG, Kuhn JP: CT evaluation of blunt abdominal trauma in children: Comparison of ultrafast and conventional CT. *Am J Roentgenol* 1989; 153:803.

Bulas DI, Taylor GA, Eichelberger MR: The value of CT in detecting bowel perforation in children after blunt abdominal trauma. *Am J Roentgenol* 1989; 153:561.

Cobb LM, Vinocur CD, Wagner CW, et al.: Intestinal perforation due to blunt trauma in children in an era of increased nonoperative treatment. *J Trauma* 1986; 26:461.

Dodds WJ, Taylor AJ, Erickson SJ, et al.: Traumatic fracture of the pancreas: CT characteristics. *J Comput Assist Tomogr* 1990; 14:375.

Federle MP, Brant-Zawadzki M: *Computed Tomography in Evaluation of Trauma.* Baltimore, Williams & Wilkins, 1986.

Filiatrault D, Longpre D, Patriquin H, et al: Investigation of childhood blunt abdominal trauma: A practical approach using ultrasound as the initial diagnostic modality. *Pediatr Radiol* 1987; 17:373.

Gay SB, Sistrom CL: Computed tomographic evaluation of blunt abdominal trauma, *Radiol Clin North Am* 1992; 30:367.

Glaser GM, Buy JN, Moss AA, et al: CT detection of duodenal perforation. *Am J Roentgenol* 1981; 173:333.

Goodman LR, Aprahamian C: Changes in splenic size after abdominal trauma. *Radiology* 1990; 176:629.

Hara H, Babyn PS, Bourgeois D: Significance of bowel wall enhancement on CT following blunt trauma in childhood. *J Comput Assist Tomogr* 1992; 16(1):94–98.

Hayashi K, Futagawa S, Kozaki S, et al: Ultrasound and CT diagnosis of intramural duodenal hematoma. *Pediatr Radiol* 1988; 18:167.

Hayes CW, Conway WF, Walsh JW, et al: Seat belt injuries: Radiologic findings and clinical correlation. *Radiographics* 1991:11:23.

Hennes HM, Smith DS, Schneider K, et al.: Elevated liver transaminase levels in children with blunt abdominal trauma: A predictor of liver injury. *Pediatrics* 1990; 86:87.

Hofer GA, Cohen AJ: CT signs of duodenal perforation secondary to blunt abdominal trauma. *J Comput Assist Tomogr* 1989; 13:430.

Jorulf H: Roentgen diagnosis of intraperitoneal fluid. *Acta Radiol Suppl (Stockh)* 1975; 343-85.

Kane NM, Cronan JJ, Dorfman GS, et al: Pediatric abdominal trauma: Evaluation by computed tomography. *Pediatrics* 1988; 82:11.

Karnaze GC, Sheedy PF, Stevens DH, et al: Computed tomography in duodenal rupture due to blunt abdominal trauma. *J Comput Assist Tomogr* 1981; 5:267.

Karp M, Cooney D, Berger PE, et al: The role of CT in the evaluation of blunt abdominal trauma in childhood. *J Pediatr Surg* 1981; 16:316.

Karp MP, Cooney DR, Pros GA, et al: The non-operative management of pediatric hepatic trauma. *J Pediatr Surg* 1983; 18:512–518.

Karp MP, Jewett TC Jr, Kuhn JP, et al: Impact of CT and non-operative therapy on the child with renal trauma. *J Pediatr Surg* 1986; 21:617.

Kaufman RA, Babcock DS: An approach to imaging the upper abdomen in the injured child. *Semin Roentgenol* 1984; 19:308.

Kaufman RA, Towbin R, Babcock DS, et al: Upper abdominal trauma in children: Imaging evaluation. *Am J Roentgenol* 1984; 142:449.

Kelly G, Norton L, Moore G, et al: The continual challenge of duodenal injuries. *J Trauma* 1978; 18:160.

Kirks DR, Caron KH, Bisset GS: CT of blunt Abdominal Trauma in children: An anatomic "snapshot in time." *Radiology* 1992; 182:631–632.

Kuhn JP, Berger PE: Computed tomography of blunt abdominal trauma in children. *Radiol Clin North Am* 1981; 19:503.

Kuhn JP: Diagnostic imaging for the evaluation of abdominal trauma in children. *Pediatr Clin North Am* 1985; 32:1427.

Lieu TA, Fleisher GR, Mahboubi S, et al: Hematuria and clinical findings as indications for intravenous pyelography in pediatric blunt renal trauma. *Pediatrics* 1988; 82:216.

Macrander SJ, Lawson TL, Foley WD, et al: Periportal tracking in hepatic trauma: CT features. *J Comput Assist Tomogr* 1989; 13:952.

Mercer S, Legrand L, Stringel G, et al: Delay in diagnosing gastrointestinal injury after blunt abdominal trauma in children. *Can J Surg* 1985; 28:138.

Meyer DM, Thal ER, Weigelt JA, et al: Evaluation of computed tomography and diagnostic peritoneal lavage in blunt abdominal trauma. *J Trauma* 1989; 29:1168.

Orwig D, Federle MP: Localized clotted blood as evidence of visceral trauma on CT: The sentinel clot sign. *Am J Roentgenol* 1989; 153:747

Rizzo MJ, Federle MP, Griffiths BG: Bowel and mesenteric injury following blunt abdominal trauma: Evaluation with CT. *Radiology* 1989; 173:143.

Schiffman MA: Nonoperative management of blunt abdominal trauma in pediatrics. *Emerg Med Clin North Am* 1989; 7:519.

Sivit CJ, Eichelberger MR, Taylor GA, et al: Blunt pancreatic trauma in children: CT diagnosis. *Am J Roentgenol* 1992; 158:1097–1100.

Sivit CJ, Peclet M, Taylor GA: CT demonstration of life-threatening intraperitoneal bleeding. *Radiology* 1989; 171:430.

Sivit CJ, Taylor GA, Bulas DI, et al: Significance of peritoneal fluid in children following blunt trauma. *Radiology* 1991; 178:185.

Sivit CJ, Taylor GA, Eichelberger MR: Visceral injury in battered children: A changing perspective. *Radiology* 1989; 173:659.

Stalker HP, Kaufman RA, Stedje K: The significance of hematuria in children after blunt abdominal trauma. *Am J Roentgenol* 1990; 154:569.

Stalker HP, Kaufman RA, Towbin R: Patterns of liver injury in childhood: CT analysis. *Am J Roentgenol* 1986; 147:1199.

Taylor GA, Eichelberger MR: Abdominal CT in children with neurologic impairment following blunt trauma. *Ann Surg* 1989; 210:229.

Taylor GA, Eichelberger MR, Potter BM: Hematuria: A marker of abdominal injury in children after blunt trauma. *Ann Surg* 1988; 208:688.

Taylor GA, Fallat ME, Eichelberger MR: Hypovolemic shock in children: Abdominal CT manifestation. *Radiology* 1987; 164:479.

Taylor GA, Fallat ME, Potter BM, et al: The role of computed tomography in blunt abdominal trauma in children. *J Trauma* 1988; 28:1660.

Taylor GA, Guion CJ, Potter BM, et al: CT of blunt abdominal trauma in children. *Am J Roentgenol* 1989; 153:555.

Toxopus MD, Lucas LE, Krabbenhoft AL: Roentgen features in blunt retroperitoneal rupture. *Radiology* 1972; 115:281.

Whalen JP: *Radiology of the Abdomen: Anatomic Basis.* Philadelphia, Lea & Febiger, 1976.

Wolfman NT, Bechtold RE, Scharling ES, et al: Blunt upper abdominal trauma: Evaluation by CT. *Am J Roentgenol* 1992; 158:493–501.